SAUNDERS

Q&A Review for the NCLEX-RN® EXAMINATION

SAUNDERS

EDITION 4

Q&A Review *for the* NCLEX-RN® EXAMINATION

LINDA ANNE SILVESTRI, MSN, RN

Instructor of Nursing
Salve Regina University
Newport, Rhode Island

President
Nursing Reviews, Inc.
and
Professional Nursing Seminars, Inc.
Charlestown, Rhode Island

Instructor
NCLEX-RN® and NCLEX-PN® Review Courses

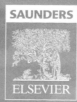

SAUNDERS

ELSEVIER

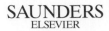

SAUNDERS
ELSEVIER

11830 Westline Industrial Drive
St. Louis, Missouri 63146

SAUNDERS Q&A REVIEW FOR THE NCLEX-RN® EXAMINATION   ISBN: 978-1-4160-4850-3
Copyright © 2009 by Saunders, an imprint of Elsevier Inc.

Notice

Knowledge and best practice in this field are constantly changing. As new research and experience broaden our knowledge, changes in practice, treatment and drug therapy may become necessary or appropriate. Readers are advised to check the most current information provided (i) on procedures featured or (ii) by the manufacturer of each product to be administered, to verify the recommended dose or formula, the method and duration of administration, and contraindications. It is the responsibility of the practitioner, relying on their own experience and knowledge of the patient, to make diagnoses, to determine dosages and the best treatment for each individual patient, and to take all appropriate safety precautions. To the fullest extent of the law, neither the Publisher nor the Author assumes any liability for any injury and/or damage to persons or property arising out or related to any use of the material contained in this book.

The Publisher

NCLEX® and NCLEX-RN® are registered trademarks and service marks of the National Council of State Boards of Nursing, Inc.

Library of Congress Cataloging-in-Publication Data
Silvestri, Linda Anne.
    Saunders Q&A review for the NCLEX-RN examination / Linda Anne Silvestri. -- Ed. 4.
        p. ; cm.
    Includes bibliographical references.
    ISBN 978-1-4160-4850-3 (pbk. : alk. paper)
    1. Nursing--Examinations, questions, etc. I. Title. II. Title: Q&A review for the
NCLEX-RN examination. III. Title: Saunders Q and A review for the NCLEX-RN examination.
    [DNLM: 1. Nursing Care--Examination Questions. WY 18.2 S587sq 2009]
    RT55.S4875 2009
    610.73076--dc22

                                                                2008043082

Managing Editor: Nancy O'Brien
Developmental Editor: Todd McKenzie
Publishing Services Manager: Anne Altepeter
Senior Project Manager: Doug Turner
Multimedia Producer: David Rushing
Designer: Amy Buxton

Printed in the United States of America
Last digit is the print number: 9 8 7 6 5 4 3 2

To my father,
ARNOLD LAWRENCE
My memories of his love, support, and words of encouragement
will remain in my heart forever!
and
To my many nursing students, past, present, and future:
their inspiration has brought many professional rewards to my life!

About the Author

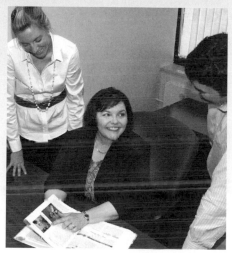

Linda Anne Silvestri

As a child, I dreamed of becoming a nurse or a teacher. Initially I chose to become a nurse because I really wanted to help others, especially those who were ill. Then I realized that both of my dreams could come true: I could be a nurse and a teacher. So I pursued my dreams.

I received my diploma in nursing at Cooley Dickinson Hospital School of Nursing in Northampton, Massachusetts. Afterward I worked at Baystate Medical Center in Springfield, Massachusetts. At Baystate Medical Center, I cared for clients in acute medical-surgical units, the intensive care unit, the emergency department, pediatric units, and other acute care units. Later I received an associate degree from Holyoke Community College in Holyoke, Massachusetts, my BSN from American International College in Springfield, Massachusetts, and my MSN from Anna Maria College in Paxton, Massachusetts, with a dual major in Nursing Management and Patient Education. I am now a PhD in Nursing candidate at the University of Nevada, Las Vegas, and I am planning to do research related to predictors of NCLEX outcomes using Artificial Neural Networking. I am also a member of the Honor Society of Nursing, Sigma Theta Tau International, Phi Kappa Phi, the Western Institute of Nursing, and the Eastern Nursing Research Society.

As a native of Springfield, Massachusetts, I began my teaching career as an instructor of medical-surgical nursing and leadership-management nursing at Baystate Medical Center School of Nursing in 1981. In 1989, I relocated to Rhode Island and began teaching advanced medical-surgical nursing and psychiatric nursing to RN and LPN students at the Community College of Rhode Island. While teaching there, a group of students approached me for assistance in preparing for the NCLEX. I have always had a very special interest in test success for nursing students because of my own personal experiences with testing. Success with testing was never easy for me, and as a student I needed to find methods and strategies that would bring success. My own difficult experiences and my desire and dedication to assist nursing students to overcome the obstacles associated with testing inspired me to write the many products that would foster success with testing.

My experiences as a student, nursing educator, and item writer for the NCLEX aided me as I developed a comprehensive review course to prepare nursing graduates for the NCLEX. In 1994, I began teaching medical-surgical nursing at Salve Regina University in Newport, Rhode Island, and remain there as an adjunct faculty member. I also prepare nursing students at Salve Regina University for the NCLEX-RN.

I established Professional Nursing Seminars, Inc., in 1991 and Nursing Reviews, Inc., in 2000. Both companies are dedicated to conducting review courses for the NCLEX-RN and the NCLEX-PN and helping nursing graduates to achieve their goals of becoming Registered Nurses and/or Licensed Practical/Vocational Nurses.

Today, I conduct review courses for the NCLEX throughout New England and am the successful author of numerous review products. I am so pleased that you have decided to join with me in your journey to success in testing for nursing examinations and for the NCLEX-RN!

Contributors

Cara M. Chenette, RN, BSN
Graduate, Department of Nursing
Salve Regina University
Newport, Rhode Island;
Staff Nurse, Concord Hospital
Concord, New Hampshire

Laurent W. Valliere, BS
Vice President
Professional Nursing Seminars, Inc.
Charlestown, Rhode Island

ITEM WRITERS

Katherine Dimmock, JD, EdD, MSN, RN
Dean and CEO
Columbia College of Nursing, Inc.
Milwaukee, Wisconsin

Mary Dowell, PhD, RNC
Associate Dean, Professor
College of Nursing
University of Mary Hardin Baylor
Belton, Texas

Marilyn Johnessee Greer, MS, RN
Associate Professor of Nursing
Rockford College
Rockford, Illinois

Donna Russo, RN, MSN, CCRN
Nursing Instructor
Frankford Hospital School of Nursing
Philadelphia, Pennsylvania

Sharon Souter, RN, PhD
Director of the Bachelor of Nursing Program
Patty Hanks Shelton School of Nursing
Abilene, Texas

Linda Turchin, RN, BSN, MSN
Assistant Professor of Nursing
Fairmont State University
Fairmont, West Virginia

Cheryle I. Whitney, RN, MSN, BC
President
ciwhitney & associates, L.L.C.
The Woodlands, Texas

The author and publisher would also like to acknowledge the following individuals for contributions to the previous editions of this book:

Marianne P. Barba, MS, RN
Coventry, Rhode Island

Nancy Blasdell, MSN, RN
Kingston, Rhode Island

Rebecca S. Blaszczak, RN
Newport, Rhode Island

Barbara Bono-Snell, MS, RN, CS
Liverpool, New York

Netta Moncur Bowen, MSN, RN
Sanford, Florida

Carolyn Pierce Buckelew, RNCS, NC, CHyp
Perth Amboy, New Jersey

Janis M. Byers, MSN, RNC
Sewickley, Pennsylvania

Penny S. Cass, PhD, RN
Kokomo, Indiana

Deborah H. Chatham, RN, MS, CS
Gulfport, Mississippi

Tom Christenbery, MSN, RN
Nashville, Tennessee

Anita M. Creamer, RN, MS, CS
Warwick, Rhode Island

Barbara A. Dagastine, EdMSN, RN
Troy, New York

Jean DeCoffe, MSN, RN
Milton, Massachusetts

DeAnna Jan Emory, MS, RN
Muskogee, Oklahoma

Mary E. Farrell, MS, RN, CCRN
Salem, Massachusetts

Patsy H. Fasnacht, MSN, RN, CCRN
Lancaster, Pennsylvania

Dona Ferguson, MSN, RN, C
Mays Landing, New Jersey

Thomas E. Folcarelli, MSN, RN
Newport, Rhode Island

Florence Hayes Gibson, MSN, CNS
Monroe, Louisiana

Alma V. Harkey, RNC, MSN, ACCE
Cape Girardeau, Missouri

Joyce Ellen Heil, BSN, CCRN
Pittsburgh, Pennsylvania

Barbara Hicks, DSN, RN
Sylacauga, Alabama

Mary Ann Hogan, RN, CS, MSN
Amherst, Massachusetts

Noreen M. Houck, MS, RN
Syracuse, New York

Amy Lawyer Hudson, RN, MSN
Helene, Arkansas

Frances E. Johnson, MS, RNC
Berrien Springs, Michigan

Deborah Klaas, RN, PhD
Flagstaff, Arizona

June Peterson Larson, RN, MS
Vermillion, South Dakota

Suzanne K. Marnocha, RN, MSN, CCRN
Oshkosh, Wisconsin

Ellen Frances McCarty, PhD, RN, CS
Newport, Rhode Island

Connie M. Metzler, MSN, RN
Lancaster, Pennsylvania

Patricia A. Miller, MSN, RN
Springfield, Massachusetts

Jo Ann Barnes Mullaney, PhD, RN, CS
Newport, Rhode Island

Kathleen Ann Ohman, RN, MS, EdD
St. Joseph, Minnesota

Lynda C. Opdyke, RN, MSN
Charlotte, North Carolina

MaeDella Perry, RN, MSN
Augusta, Georgia

Lisa A. Ruth-Sahd, MSN, RN, CEN, CCRN
York, Pennsylvania

Jeanine T. Seguin, MS, RN, CS
Keuka Park, New York

Alberta Elaine Severs, MSN, MA, RN
Lincoln, Rhode Island

Kimberly Sharpe, MS, RN
Syracuse, New York

Susan Sienkiewicz, MA, RN, CS
Lincoln, Rhode Island

Yvonne Marie Smith, MSN, RN, CCRN
Canton, Ohio

Judith Stamp, MS, RN
Troy, New York

Yvonne Nazareth Stringfield, EdD, RN
Nashville, Tennessee

Mattie Tolley, RN, MS
Weatherford, Oklahoma

Johanna M. Tracy, MSN, RN, CS
Trenton, New Jersey

Joyce I. Turnbull, RN, MN
San Jose, California

Paula A. Viau, PhD, RN
Kingston, Rhode Island

Carol Warner, RN, CPN, MSN
Bethlehem, Pennsylvania

Deborah Williams, EdD, RN
Bowling Green, Kentucky

CONSULTANT

Nicole Marie Vallerie, BSN, RN
Professional Nurse I—Pediatrics
Hasbro Children's Hospital
Providence, Rhode Island

Preface

"Success is climbing a mountain, facing the challenge of obstacles, and reaching the top of the mountain."
Linda Anne Silvestri, MSN, RN

Welcome to *Saunders Pyramid to Success!*

AN ESSENTIAL RESOURCE FOR TEST SUCCESS

Saunders Q&A Review for the NCLEX-RN® Examination is one in a series of products designed to assist you in achieving your goal of becoming a registered nurse. This text and CD package provides you with more than 5200 practice NCLEX-RN test questions based on the 2007 NCLEX-RN test plan.

The 2007 test plan for the NCLEX-RN identifies a framework based on *Client Needs*. The Client Needs categories include Physiological Integrity, Safe and Effective Care Environment, Health Promotion and Maintenance, and Psychosocial Integrity. *Integrated Processes* are also identified as a component of the test plan. These include Caring, Communication and Documentation, Nursing Process, and Teaching and Learning. This book has been uniquely designed and includes chapters that describe each specific component of the 2007 NCLEX-RN test plan framework and chapters that contain practice questions specific to each component.

NCLEX-RN® TEST PREPARATION

This book begins with information regarding NCLEX-RN preparation. Chapter 1 addresses all of the information related to the 2007 NCLEX-RN test plan and the testing procedures related to the examination. This chapter answers all of the questions that you may have regarding the testing procedures.

Chapter 2 provides information to the foreign-educated nurse about the process of obtaining a license to practice as a registered nurse in the United States.

Chapter 3 discusses the NCLEX-RN from a nonacademic viewpoint and emphasizes a holistic approach for your individual test preparation. This chapter identifies the components of a structured study plan, anxiety-reducing techniques, and personal focus issues. Nursing students also want to hear what other students have to say about their experiences with the NCLEX-RN and what it is really like to take this examination. Chapter 4 is a story of success written by a nursing graduate who recently took the NCLEX-RN and addresses the issue of what the examination is all about.

Chapter 5, "Test-Taking Strategies," includes all of the important strategies that will assist in teaching you how to read a question, how not to read into a question, and how to use the process of elimination and various other strategies to select the correct response from the options presented.

CLIENT NEEDS

Chapters 6 through 10 address the 2007 NCLEX-RN test plan component, Client Needs. Chapter 6 describes each category of Client Needs as identified by the test plan and lists any subcategories, the percentage of test questions for each category, and some of the content included on the NCLEX-RN. Chapters 7 through 10 contain practice test questions related specifically to each category of Client Needs. Chapter 7 comprises questions related to Physiological Integrity; Chapter 8 contains questions dealing with Safe and Effective Care Environment; Chapter 9 is made up of questions concerned with Health Promotion and Maintenance; and Chapter 10 contains Psychosocial Integrity questions.

INTEGRATED PROCESSES

Chapters 11 and 12 address the Integrated Processes as identified in the NCLEX-RN test plan. Chapter 11 describes each Integrated Process. Chapter 12 contains practice test questions related specifically to each Integrated Process, including Caring, Communication and Documentation, Nursing Process, and Teaching and Learning.

COMPREHENSIVE TEST

A comprehensive test is included at the end of this book. It consists of 300 practice questions representative of the components of the 2007 test plan framework for NCLEX-RN.

SPECIAL FEATURES OF THE BOOK

Book Design

The book is designed with a unique two-column format. The left column presents the practice questions, answer options, and coding areas while the right column provides the corresponding answers, rationales, test-taking strategies, and references. The two-column format makes the review easier so that you do not have to flip through pages in search of answers and rationales.

Practice Questions

While preparing for the NCLEX-RN, students have a strong need to review practice test questions. Each chapter contains practice test questions in the NCLEX-RN format. This book contains more than 1800 practice questions that are in the multiple-choice format or in one of the alternate item test question formats used in the NCLEX-RN examination. The accompanying software includes all of the questions from the book, including the alternate item test question formats, plus an additional 3400 questions and heart and lung sound questions for a total of more than 5200 test questions.

Multiple-Choice Questions

This book contains more than 1800 practice questions in NCLEX format, most of which are multiple-choice questions reflective of what you will encounter on the NCLEX-RN examination. The accompanying software includes all of the multiple-choice questions from the book, plus additional multiple-choice, alternate item format, and heart and lung sound questions for a total of more 5,200 questions.

Alternate Item Format Questions

Chapters 7, 8, 9, 10, and 12 and the Comprehensive Test contain alternate item format questions. These questions may be presented as a fill-in-the-blank question, a multiple-response question, a prioritizing (ordered response) question, a figure/illustration question (hot spot), or a chart/exhibit question. These types of questions provide you practice in prioritizing, decision-making, and critical thinking skills. The accompanying software includes all of the alternate item format questions from the book, plus an abundance of additional questions in the alternate item format.

Heart and Lung Sound Questions

Also found on the accompanying CD are heart and lung sound questions representative of content addressed in the 2007 test plan for the NCLEX-RN exam. Each of these questions is in the NCLEX-style format and presents an audio sound as a component of the question.

Answer Sections for Practice Questions

Each practice question is accompanied by the correct answer, rationale, test-taking strategy, question categories, and a reference source. The structure of the answer section is unique and provides the following information for every question:

- **Rationale:** The rationale provides you significant information regarding both correct and incorrect options.
- **Test-Taking Strategy:** The test-taking strategy describes the logic for selecting the correct option and assists you in selecting an answer to a question on which you must guess. Specific suggestions for review are identified in the test-taking strategy.
- **Question Categories:** Each question is identified based on the categories used by the NCLEX-RN test plan. Additional content area categories are provided with each question to assist you in identifying areas in need of review. The categories identified with each question include Level of Cognitive Ability, Client Needs, Integrated Process, and the specific nursing Content Area. All categories are identified by their full names so that you do not need to memorize codes or abbreviations.
- **Reference:** The reference source and page number are listed for you so that you can easily find the information you need to review in your undergraduate nursing textbooks.

NCLEX-RN® REVIEW SOFTWARE

Packaged in this book you will find an NCLEX-RN review CD. This software contains more than 5200 questions: all 1810 from the book, plus more than 3400 additional questions. It contains multiple-choice questions and the alternate item formats, including fill-in-the-blank questions, multiple-response questions, prioritizing (ordered response) questions, figure/illustration (hot spot) questions, and chart/exhibit questions. This Windows- and Macintosh-compatible program offers three testing modes for review of the questions.

- **Quiz:** Ten randomly chosen questions on Client Needs, Integrated Process, or a specific Content Area. After you answer all 10 questions, the results are given and a review of the answer, rationale, and test-taking strategy, as well as a reference source, are provided.

- **Study:** All questions in a selected Client Needs, Integrated Process, or Content Area. The answer, rationale, test-taking strategy, question categories, and reference source appear after answering each question.
- **Examination:** One hundred questions randomly chosen from selected content areas from the entire pool of more than 5200 questions. The answer, rationale, test-taking strategy, question categories, reference source, and results appear after you answer all 100 questions.

The CD allows you to customize your review and determine your areas of strength and weakness. It also provides you with a wealth of practice test questions while simulating the NCLEX-RN experience on computer.

HOW TO USE THIS BOOK

Saunders Q&A Review for the NCLEX-RN® Examination is especially designed to help you with your successful journey to the peak of the Pyramid to Success: becoming a registered nurse. As you begin your journey through this book, you will be introduced to all of the important points regarding the NCLEX-RN examination, the process of testing, and the unique and special tips regarding how to prepare yourself both academically and nonacademically for this important examination. Read the chapter from the nursing graduate who recently passed the NCLEX-RN and consider what the graduate had to say about the examination. The test-taking strategy chapter will provide you with important strategies that will guide you in selecting the correct option or assist you in guessing the answer. Read this chapter and practice these strategies as you proceed through your journey with this book.

Once you have read the introductory components of this book, it is time to begin the practice questions. As you read through each question and select an answer, be sure to read the rationale and the test-taking strategy. The rationale provides you with significant information regarding both the correct and incorrect options, and the test-taking strategy provides you with the logic for selecting the correct option. The strategy also identifies the content area that you need to review if you had difficulty with the question. Use the reference source provided so that you can easily find the information you need to review.

As you work your way through *Saunders Q&A Review for the NCLEX-RN® Examination* and identify your areas of strength and weakness, you can return to the companion book, *Saunders Comprehensive Review for the NCLEX-RN® Examination*, to focus your study on these areas. The companion book and its accompanying CD provide you with a comprehensive review of all areas of the nursing content reflected in the 2007 NCLEX-RN test plan.

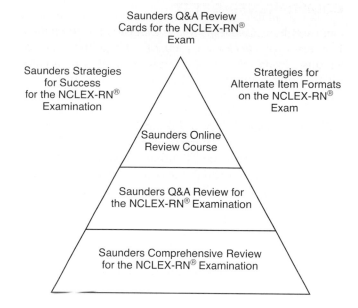

Other extremely valuable resources that will ensure your success in testing are *Saunders Strategies for Success for the NCLEX-RN® Examination, Strategies for Alternate Item Formats on the NCLEX-RN® Examination,* and *Saunders Q&A Review Cards for the NCLEX-RN® Exam. Saunders Strategies for Success for the NCLEX-RN® Examination* and its accompanying CD provide all of the test-taking strategies that will help you pass your nursing examinations and the NCLEX-RN examination. The chapters describe specific test-taking strategies, include several sample questions that illustrate how to use the strategy, and provide an additional total of 500 practice questions, including multiple choice and alternate item format questions.

Strategies for Alternate Item Formats on the NCLEX-RN® Examination focuses specifically on the alternate item format questions that will appear on your nursing examinations and on the NCLEX-RN examination. This resource is organized by the Client Needs component of the test plan, provides an accompanying CD, and includes over 275 alternate item format questions including fill-in-the blank, multiple response, prioritizing (ordered response), figure/illustration (hot spot), and chart/exhibit questions. A total of 15 heart and lung sound questions are also included on the accompanying CD.

Saunders Q&A Review Cards for the NCLEX-RN® Exam provides you with 1000 NCLEX-RN review questions, including all types of alternate item questions, in a convenient flashcard format. This is the perfect portable study resource that you can use anytime and anywhere. Review questions are on the front of each card and are organized by Client Needs, consistent with the current NCLEX-RN test plan. Answers are included on the back of the card, along with rationales, test-taking strategies, and Integrated Process categories.

Also available to ensure your success is *Saunders Online Review Course for the NCLEX-RN® Examination.* This resource contains a total of 10 modules and 47 lessons. Every lesson contains content for review, illustrations, animations, practice questions, and a case study followed by questions related to the case study. Each module is followed by a 100-question exam that contains questions representative of the content in the module lessons. There is also a diagnostic Pretest Exam that generates an individualized study calendar to guide your review through the course, a Comprehensive (Cumulative) Exam, and a CAT (computerized adaptive testing) Exam. The course provides you with a systematic and individualized method for preparing to take the NCLEX examination.

To obtain any of these resources that will prepare you for your nursing exams and the NCLEX-RN exam, visit the Elsevier Health Sciences Web site at www.elsevierhealth.com.

Good Luck with your journey through the *Saunders Pyramid to Success.* I wish you continued success throughout your new career as a Registered Nurse!

Linda Anne Silvestri, MSN, RN

Acknowledgments

There are many individuals who in their own ways have contributed to my success in making my professional dreams become a reality. My sincere appreciation and warmest thanks is extended to all of them.

First, I want to acknowledge my parents, who opened my door of opportunity in education. I thank my mother, Frances Mary, for all of her love, support, and assistance as I continuously worked to achieve my professional goals. I thank my father, Arnold Lawrence, who always provided insightful words of encouragement. My memories of his love and support will always remain in my heart. I also thank my best friend and love of my life, Larry; my sister, Dianne Elodia; my brother, Lawrence Peter; and my niece, Gina Marie, who were continuously supportive, giving, and helpful during my research and preparation of this publication.

I want to thank my nursing students at the Community College of Rhode Island who approached me in 1991 and persuaded me to assist them in preparing to take the NCLEX-RN examination. Their enthusiasm and inspiration led to the commencement of my professional endeavors in conducting review courses for the NCLEX-RN exam for nursing students. I also thank the numerous nursing students who have attended my review courses for their willingness to share their needs and ideas. Their input has certainly added a special uniqueness to this publication.

I wish to acknowledge all of the nursing faculty who taught in my review courses for the NCLEX-RN exam. Their commitment, dedication, and expertise have certainly assisted nursing students in achieving success with the NCLEX-RN exam. Additionally, I want to acknowledge Laurent W. Valliere for his contribution to this publication, for teaching in my review courses for the NCLEX-RN exam, and for his commitment and dedication in assisting my nursing students to prepare for the NCLEX-RN exam from a non-academic point of view. A special thank you also goes to Cara M. Chenette, RN, BSN, for writing a chapter for this book about her experiences with preparing for and taking the NCLEX-RN examination!

I sincerely acknowledge and thank three very important individuals from Elsevier. I thank Nancy O'Brien, managing editor, for all of her assistance throughout the preparation of this edition and for her continuous enthusiasm, support, and expert professional guidance. Thank you also to Lauren Harms, editorial assistant, who assisted in organizing the work submitted by contributors. And, a very special thank you extends to my new developmental editor, Todd McKenzie, who provided me with a tremendous amount of support throughout this publication. Todd did outstanding work in maintaining order for the enormous amount of work that I submitted for manuscript production. Thank you Nancy, Lauren, and Todd!

A special thank you and acknowledgment goes to three important individuals, Nicole Valliere, Dianne E. Ventrice, and Lawrence Fiorentino. Nicole, thank you for all of your expert input and revisions. To Dianne and Lawrence, I thank you both for your continuous support and dedication to my work in both the NCLEX exam review courses and in reference support and other secretarial responsibilities for the fourth edition of this book.

I want to acknowledge all of the staff at Elsevier for their tremendous help throughout the preparation and production of this publication. A special thank you to all of them. I thank all of the special people in the production department, Doug Turner, project manager; Anne Altepeter, publishing services manager; David Rushing, multimedia producer; and Amy Buxton, designer, who all played such significant roles in finalizing this publication. I sincerely thank those in the marketing department who helped with the promotion of this book, including Bob Boehringer, senior segment marketing director; Kathy Mantz, group segment manager; Dan Hughes, marketing manager; and Shelle Goggins, marketing coordinator.

I would also like to acknowledge Patricia Mieg, former educational sales representative, who encouraged me to submit my ideas and initial work for the first edition of this book to the W.B. Saunders Company.

I want to acknowledge all of the item writers who updated and provided many of the practice questions and all of the previous contributors who provided contributions to this book. A very special thank you to all of you!

I also need to thank Salve Regina University for the opportunity to educate nursing students in the baccalaureate nursing program and for its support as I researched and wrote this publication. I would like to especially acknowledge my colleagues, Dr. Peggy Matteson, Dr. Ellen McCarty, Dr. JoAnn Mullaney, and Dr. Bethany Sykes for all of their support and encouragement.

I wish to acknowledge the Community College of Rhode Island, which provided me the opportunity to educate nursing students in the Associate Degree of Nursing Program, and a special thank you to Patricia Miller, MSN, RN, and Michelina McClellan, MS, RN, from Baystate Medical Center School of Nursing in Springfield, Massachusetts, who were my first mentors in nursing education.

Lastly, a very special thank you to all my nursing students, past, present, and future. All of you light up my life! Your love and dedication to the profession of nursing and your commitment to provide health care will bring never ending rewards!

Linda Anne Silvestri, MSN, RN

Contents

NCLEX-RN® Preparation

The NCLEX-RN® Examination

PYRAMID TO SUCCESS

Welcome to *Saunders Q&A Review for the NCLEX-RN® Examination*, the second component of the Pyramid to Success! At this time, you have completed your first path toward the peak of the pyramid with *Saunders Comprehensive Review for the NCLEX-RN® Examination*. Now it is time to continue that journey to become a registered nurse with *Saunders Q&A Review for the NCLEX-RN® Examination*.

As you begin your journey through this book, you will be introduced to all of the important points regarding the NCLEX-RN examination, the process of testing, and the unique and special tips regarding how to prepare yourself academically and nonacademically for this very important examination. You will read what a nursing graduate who passed the NCLEX-RN examination has to say about the examination. All of those important test-taking strategies are detailed. These details will guide you in selecting the correct option or in selecting an answer when you need to guess.

Saunders Q&A Review for the NCLEX-RN® Examination contains more than 5200 NCLEX-RN–style practice questions. The chapters have been developed to provide a description of the components of the NCLEX-RN test plan, including the Client Needs and the Integrated Processes. In addition, chapters have been prepared to contain practice questions specific to each category of Client Needs and the Integrated Processes.

In each chapter that contains practice questions, a rationale, test-taking strategy, and reference source containing a page number are provided with each question. Each question is coded on the basis of the Level of Cognitive Ability, Client Needs category, Integrated Process, and the content area being tested. The rationale contains significant information regarding both the correct and incorrect options. The test-taking strategy maps out a logical path for selecting the correct option and identifies the content area to review, if necessary. The reference source and page number provide easy access to the information that you need to review. After you complete the *Saunders Comprehensive Review for the NCLEX-RN® Examination* and the *Saunders Q&A Review for the NCLEX-RN® Examination*, you will be ready for the *Saunders Online Review Course for the NCLEX-RN® Examination*. Additional products in the Saunders Pyramid to Success include *Saunders Strategies for Success for the NCLEX-RN® Examination, Saunders Strategies for Alternate Item Formats on the NCLEX-RN® Examination*, and the *Saunders Q&A Review Cards for the NCLEX-RN® Exam*. These products are described below.

The *Saunders Online Review Course for the NCLEX-RN® Examination* addresses all areas of the test plan identified by the National Council of State Boards of Nursing (NCSBN). The course contains a pretest that provides feedback regarding your strengths and weaknesses and that generates an individualized study schedule in a calendar format. Content review includes practice questions and case studies, figures and illustrations, a glossary, and animations and videos. A cumulative examination and a computer adaptive test (CAT) are also key components of the online review course. The types of practice questions in this course include multiple choice, fill-in-the-blank, multiple response, ordered response (those that require you to prioritize), and questions containing figures that may require you to use the computer mouse to answer.

The *Saunders Strategies for Success for the NCLEX-RN® Examination* focuses on the test-taking strategies that will help you pass your nursing examinations while in nursing school and will prepare you for the NCLEX-RN examination. The chapters describe all of the test-taking strategies and include several sample questions that illustrate how to use the test-taking strategy. Five hundred practice questions accompany this book, and all of the practice questions, including multiple-choice and alternate item–format questions, reflect the framework and content identified in the current NCLEX-RN test plan.

The *Saunders Strategies for Alternate Item Formats on the NCLEX-RN® Examination* differs from the other products in the Saunders Pyramid to Success in that it contains only alternate item–format questions. It provides all the information you need about all types of alternate item–format questions that may appear on your nursing examinations and on the NCLEX-RN examination. It contains 265 practice alternate item–format questions and 15 heart and lung sounds questions to prepare you for your nursing examinations and that most important examination, the NCLEX-RN.

The *Saunders Q&A Review Cards for the NCLEX-RN® Exam* is organized specifically by the test plan framework of the current NCLEX-RN test plan. This product provides 1000 practice test questions on portable, easy-to-use cards. The question is on the front of the card and the answer, rationale, test-taking strategy, and Integrated Process code are on the back of the card. This product includes both multiple-choice questions and alternate item–format questions, including fill-in-the-blank, multiple-response, ordered-response (prioritizing), image ("hot spot" questions), and chart/exhibit questions. All of the products in the Saunders Pyramid to Success can be obtained online by visiting www.elsevierhealth.com or by calling (800) 545-2522.

Let's continue our journey up the Pyramid to Success.

THE EXAMINATION PROCESS

An important step in the Pyramid to Success is to become as familiar as possible with the examination process. A significant amount of anxiety can occur in candidates facing the challenge of this examination. Knowing what the examination is all about and knowing what you will encounter during the process of testing will assist in alleviating fear and anxiety. The information contained in this chapter addresses the procedures related to the development of the NCLEX-RN examination test plan, the components of the test plan, and the answers to the questions most commonly asked by nursing students and graduates preparing to take the NCLEX-RN examination. The information contained in this chapter related to the test plan is from the NCSBN Web site at www.ncsbn.org and from the *2007 NCLEX-RN® Detailed Test Plan*, National Council of State Boards of Nursing, Inc., Chicago, 2006. You can obtain additional information regarding the test and its development by accessing the NCSBN Web site or by writing to the National Council of State Boards of Nursing, 111 E. Wacker Drive, Suite 2900, Chicago, Illinois 60601.

COMPUTER ADAPTIVE TEST

The acronym *CAT* stands for *computer adaptive test*, which means that the examination is created as the test-taker answers each question. All of the test questions are categorized based on the test plan structure and the level of difficulty of the question. As you answer a question, the computer determines your competency based on the answer that you selected. If you selected a correct answer to a question, the computer scans the question bank and selects a more difficult question. If you selected an incorrect answer, the computer scans the question bank and selects an easier question. This process continues until the test plan requirements are met and a reliable pass or fail decision is made.

When a test question is presented on the computer screen, you must answer it or the test will not move on. This means that you will not be able to skip questions, go back and review questions, or go back and change answers. Remember, in a CAT examination, once an answer is recorded, all subsequent questions administered depend, to an extent, on the answer selected for that question. Skipping and returning to earlier questions is not compatible with the logical methodology of a CAT. The inability to skip questions or go back to change previous answers is not a disadvantage; you cannot fall into the "trap" of changing correct answers to incorrect ones with the CAT system.

When faced with a question that contains unfamiliar content, you may need to guess at the answer. There is no penalty for guessing on this examination. Remember, in the majority of the questions, the answer is right there in front of you. If you need to guess, use your nursing knowledge to its fullest extent and use the test-taking strategies that you practice in this review program.

You do not need any computer experience to take this examination. A keyboard tutorial is provided and administered to all test-takers at the start of the examination. The tutorial instructs you on the use of the on-screen optional calculator, the use of the mouse, and how to record an answer. In addition to the traditional four-option multiple-choice questions, the tutorial also provides instructions on how to respond to alternate item–format questions. A proctor is present to explain the use of the computer to ensure your full understanding of how to proceed.

DEVELOPMENT OF THE TEST PLAN AND ITEM WRITERS

The test plan for the NCLEX-RN examination is developed by the NCSBN. As an initial step in the test's development, the NCSBN considers the legal scope of nursing practice as governed by state laws and regulations, including the nurse practice act, and uses these laws to define the areas on the examination that will assess the competence of a candidate (test-taker) for licensure.

The NCSBN also conducts a practice analysis study to determine the framework for the test plan for the examination. The participants in this study include newly licensed registered nurses from all types of basic education programs. The NCSBN provides participants with a list of nursing activities and asks them about the frequency of performing these specific activities, their impact on maintaining client safety, and the setting where the activities were performed. A panel of experts at the NCSBN analyzes the results of the study and makes decisions regarding the test plan framework. Because nursing practice continues to change, the NCSBN conducts this study every 3 years. The results of this study (conducted in 2005) provided the structure for the test plan that was implemented in April 2007.

The NCSBN selects question (item) writers after an extensive application process. The writers are registered nurses who hold a master's level or higher degree. Many of the writers are nursing educators, although a nurse currently employed in clinical nursing practice who meets specific eligibility criteria may be selected to participate in this process. Question writers voluntarily submit an application to become a writer and must meet specific criteria established by the council to be accepted as participants in the process.

THE TEST PLAN

The content of the NCLEX-RN examination reflects the activities that a newly licensed, entry-level registered nurse must be able to perform to provide clients with safe and effective nursing care. The questions are written to address Level of Cognitive Ability, Client Needs, and Integrated Process as identified in the test plan developed by the NCSBN (Box 1-1).

Levels of Cognitive Ability

The examination for licensure as a registered nurse may include questions at the cognitive levels of knowledge, comprehension, application, and analysis. However, the majority of the questions are written at the application or higher levels of cognitive ability, such as the analysis level, because the practice of nursing requires critical thinking in decision making. This means that the test-taker will be required to analyze and apply the information provided in the test question. Box 1-2 presents an example of a question that requires you to analyze data to determine the nursing intervention.

Client Needs

In the test plan implemented in April 2007, the NCSBN identified a test plan framework based on Client Needs. The NCSBN identifies four major categories of Client Needs. Some of these categories are further divided into subcategories. The Client Needs categories include Physiological Integrity, Safe and Effective Care Environment, Health Promotion and Maintenance,

---

Box 1-1 ▲ EXAMINATION QUESTIONS

Each Examination Question Addresses:
A Level of Cognitive Ability
A Client Needs category
An Integrated Process

Box 1-2 ▲ LEVEL OF COGNITIVE ABILITY

Question
A nurse is caring for a client diagnosed with tuberculosis. The client is receiving rifampin (Rifadin) 600 mg orally daily. Which laboratory finding would indicate to the nurse that the client is experiencing an adverse reaction?
1 A total bilirubin of 0.5 mg/dL
2 A white blood cell count of 6000/μL
3 A sedimentation rate of 15 mm/hr
4 An alkaline phosphatase of 25 units/dL

Answer: 4
Rationale: This question requires you to determine the adverse reactions associated with this medication and to analyze each of the laboratory values identified in the options. Adverse reactions or toxic effects of rifampin include hepatotoxicity, hepatitis, blood dyscrasias, Stevens-Johnson syndrome, and antibiotic-related colitis. The nurse monitors for increased liver function, bilirubin, blood urea nitrogen, and uric acid levels because elevations indicate an adverse reaction. The normal alkaline phosphatase is 4.5 to 13 King-Armstrong units/dL. The normal total bilirubin level is less than 1.5 mg/dL. A normal white blood cell count is 4500 to 11,000/μL. The normal sedimentation rate is 0 to 30 mm/hr.
Level of Cognitive Ability: Analysis

Reference:
McKenry, L., Tressier, E., & Hogan, M. (2006). *Mosby's pharmacology in nursing* (22nd ed., p. 1059). St. Louis: Mosby.

---

and Psychosocial Integrity (Table 1-1). Refer to Chapter 6 for a detailed description of the categories of Client Needs and the NCLEX-RN examination.

Integrated Processes

The NCSBN identifies four processes that are fundamental to the practice of nursing. These processes are a component of the test plan and are incorporated throughout the major categories of Client Needs. Box 1-3 identifies these processes. Refer to Chapter 11 for a detailed description of the Integrated Processes and the NCLEX-RN examination.

Table 1-1 ▲ CLIENT NEEDS CATEGORIES AND PERCENTAGE OF QUESTIONS

PHYSIOLOGICAL INTEGRITY	
Basic Care and Comfort	6%-12%
Pharmacological and Parenteral Therapies	13%-19%
Reduction of Risk Potential	13%-19%
Physiological Adaptation	11%-17%
SAFE AND EFFECTIVE CARE ENVIRONMENT	
Management of Care	13%-19%
Safety and Infection Control	8%-14%
HEALTH PROMOTION AND MAINTENANCE	6%-12%
PSYCHOSOCIAL INTEGRITY	6%-12%

From National Council of State Boards of Nursing. (2007). *2007 NCLEX-RN® Detailed Test Plan.* Chicago: Author.

Box 1-3 ▲ INTEGRATED PROCESSES

Caring
Communication and documentation
Teaching and learning
Nursing process
    Assessment
    Analysis
    Planning
    Implementation
    Evaluation

TYPES OF QUESTIONS ON THE EXAM

The types of questions that may be administer on the examination include multiple choice, fill-in-the-blank, multiple response, prioritizing (ordered response), chart/exhibit, and questions that contain a figure or illustration (hot spot). Some questions may require you to use the mouse component of the computer system. For example, you may be presented with a visual that displays the arterial vessels of an adult client. In this visual, you may be asked to "point and click" (using the mouse) on the area where the dorsalis pedis pulse can be felt. The NCSBN provides specific directions to guide you in your process of testing. Be sure to read these directions as they appear on the computer screen.

Multiple Choice

Most of the questions that you will be asked to answer will be in the multiple-choice format. These questions provide you with data about a particular client situation and four answers or options.

Fill-in-the-Blank

Fill-in-the-blank questions may ask you to perform a medication calculation, determine an intravenous flow rate, or calculate an intake or output record. You will need to type in your answer. (See Box 1-4 for an example.)

Box 1-4 ▲ FILL-IN-THE-BLANK

Question
A physician's order reads: acetaminophen (Tylenol Extra Strength) liquid, 650 mg orally every 4 hours prn for pain. The medication label reads: 500 mg/15 mL. The nurse prepares how many milliliters to administer one dose?
Answer: _____ mL

Answer: 19.5

Formula:

$$\frac{Desired}{Available} \times Volume = mL$$

$$\frac{650\ mg}{500\ mg} \times 15\ mL = 19.5\ mL$$

Rationale: In this question you need to use the formula for calculating a medication dose. Once the dose is determined, you will need to type in your answer. Always follow the specific directions noted on the computer screen when answering the question. Also, remember that there will be an on-screen calculator on the computer for your use if needed.

Reference:
Kee, J., & Marshall, S. (2009). *Clinical calculations: With applications to general and specialty areas* (6th ed., p. 86). Philadelphia. Saunders.

Multiple Response

For a multiple-response question, you will be asked to select or check all of the options, such as nursing interventions, that relate to the information in the question. No partial credit is given if some correct options are selected. You need to do exactly as the question asks, which is to select all that apply. (See Box 1-5 for an example.)

Prioritizing (Ordered Response)

In this type of question, you will be asked to use the computer mouse to drag and drop your nursing actions in order of priority. Information will be presented in a question and, based on the data, you need to determine what you will do first, second, third, and so forth. (See Box 1-6 for an example.)

Figure or Illustration

A question with a figure or illustration will ask you to answer the question based on the figure or illustration. The question could contain a chart, table, or a figure

Box 1-5 ▲ MULTIPLE RESPONSE

Question
A nurse is preparing to remove a nasogastric tube from a client. Which of the following actions would the nurse take to perform this procedure? Select all that apply.
- ☐ 1. Place the client in a supine position.
- ☒ 2. Assess for the presence of bowel sounds.
- ☒ 3. Untape the nasogastric tube from the client's nose.
- ☒ 4. Ask the client to hold his breath during removal of the tube.
- ☐ 5. Keep the tube attached to the prescribed amount of suction during removal.
- ☒ 6. Instill 20 mL of air into the nasogastric tube to displace secretions back into the client's stomach.

Rationale: In a multiple-response question, you will be asked to select or check all of the options, such as nursing actions, that relate to the information in the question. To answer this question, visualize the procedure and think about airway patency, preventing aspiration, and preventing mucosal irritation to identify the correct interventions. After explaining the procedure for tube removal to the client, the nurse would assess for the presence of bowel sounds. The tube would not be removed if bowel sounds are absent. The nurse would don clean gloves, place the client in an upright position, and place a towel across the client's chest. The suction is turned off and the nasogastric tube is disconnected from the suction tube. The nurse instills 20 mL of air into the nasogastric tube to displace secretions back into the client's stomach and decrease the client's risk of aspiration. The nasogastric tube is untaped from the client's nose. The client is instructed to hold his or her breath during removal of the tube, and the tube is pulled out in one quick, steady motion.

Reference:
Harkreader, H., Hogan, M.A., & Thobaben, M. (2007). *Fundamentals of nursing: Caring and clinical judgment* (3rd ed., pp. 631-632). Philadelphia: Saunders.

Box 1-6 ▲ PRIORITIZING (ORDERED RESPONSE)

Question
The nurse cares for a client upon arrival in the post-anesthesia care unit following a colectomy. List in order of priority the actions that the nurse takes. (Number 1 is the first action and number 6 is the last performed.)
___ Checks for airway patency
___ Checks abdominal dressing
___ Measures the respiratory rate
___ Evaluates heart rate and rhythm
___ Asks the client about any concerns
___ Documents postoperative findings

Answer: 1, 4, 2, 3, 5, 6
Rationale: This question asks you to prioritize nursing actions. Postoperative care begins by evaluating the client's ABCs—airway, breathing, and circulation; thus the nurse assesses airway patency first to ensure adequate oxygenation to body organs and tissues. Next, the rate and quality of the client's respirations are determined, and breath sounds are auscultated throughout all lung fields to ensure adequate ventilation. The client's heart rate and rhythm are determined and the client's blood pressure is checked following respiratory assessment and according to the hierarchy of the ABCs. After the ABCs are complete, the nurse assesses the neurological status, the remaining organ systems, and other assessments including dressings, drains, tubes, and pain as part of a comprehensive assessment. Finally, a psychosocial assessment is done, and the nurse documents assessment findings.

References:
Lewis, S., Heitkemper, M., Dirksen, S., O'Brien, P., & Bucher, L. (2007). *Medical-surgical nursing: Assessment and management of clinical problems* (7th ed., pp. 377-378). St. Louis: Mosby.
Potter, P., & Perry, A. (2005). *Fundamentals of nursing* (6th ed., pp. 1628-1630). St. Louis: Mosby.

or illustration. You also may be asked to use the computer mouse to "point and click" on a specific area in the visual. A visual or image may appear in any type of question, including a multiple-choice question. (See Box 1-7 for an example.)

Chart/Exhibit Questions

In this type of question, you will be presented with a problem and a chart/exhibit. You will need to refer to the information in the chart/exhibit in order to answer the question. (See Box 1-8 for an example.)

REGISTERING TO TAKE THE EXAMINATION

The initial step in the registration process is to submit an application to the state board of nursing in the state in which you intend to obtain licensure. You need to obtain information from the board of nursing regarding the specific registration process because the process may vary from state to state. In most states, you may register for the examination through the Internet, by mail, or by telephone. The NCLEX candidate Web site is www.vue.com/nclex. Following the registration instructions and completing the registration forms precisely and accurately is important. Registration forms not properly completed or not accompanied by the proper fees in the required method of payment will be returned to you

Box 1-7 ▲ VISUAL OR ILLUSTRATION

Question

The nurse notes this rhythm displayed on a client's cardiac monitor. Based on this rhythm, the nurse should take which appropriate action?
1 Contact the physician.
2 Prepare to administer atropine sulfate.
3 Ask the client to perform the Valsalva maneuver.
4 Document the rhythm in the client's medical record.

Answer: 4
Rationale: In this question you are provided with a figure of a rhythm strip and asked something about it. Focus on the characteristics of the rhythm. Noting that the rhythm identifies normal sinus rhythm will direct you to the correct option. Also note that all of the incorrect options identify nursing actions that indicate that the rhythm is an abnormal one.

Reference:
Ignatavicius, D., & Workman, M. (2006). *Medical-surgical nursing: Critical thinking for collaborative care* (5th ed., p. 716). Philadelphia: Saunders.

Box 1-8 ▲ CHART/EXHIBIT

Question
The nurse reviews the history and physical examination documented in the medical record of a client requesting a prescription for oral contraceptives. The nurse determines that oral contraceptives are contraindicated because of which documented item?

Client's Medical Record		
History and Physical	Medications	Laboratory Results
Item 1. Has renal calculi		
Item 2. Blood pressure: 128/72 mmHg		
Item 3. Had thrombotic stroke at age 35		
Item 4. Apical heart rate: 72 beats per minute		

Answer: 3
Rationale: This chart/exhibit question provides data from the client's medical record and asks you to identify the item that is a contraindication to the use of oral contraceptives. Oral contraceptives are contraindicated in women with a history of any of the following: thrombophlebitis and thromboembolic disorders; cardiovascular or cerebrovascular diseases (including stroke); any estrogen-dependent cancer or breast cancer, or benign or malignant liver tumors; impaired liver function; hypertension; and diabetes mellitus with vascular involvement. Adverse effects of oral contraceptives include increased risk of superficial and deep venous thrombosis, pulmonary embolism, thrombotic stroke (or other types of strokes), myocardial infarction, and accelerations of preexisting breast tumors.

References:
Kee, J., & Hayes, E. (2006). *Pharmacology: A nursing process approach* (5th ed., p. 846). St. Louis: Mosby.
Murray, S., & McKinney, E. (2006). *Foundations of maternal-newborn nursing* (4th ed., p. 843). Philadelphia: Saunders.

and will delay testing. You must pay a fee for taking the examination, and you also may have to pay additional fees to the board of nursing in the state in which you are applying. You will be sent a confirmation indicating that your registration was received. If you do not receive a confirmation within 4 weeks of submitting your registration, you should contact the candidate services. Information regarding this contact can be obtained at the NCLEX candidate Web site at www.vue.com/nclex.

AUTHORIZATION TO TEST

Once your eligibility to test has been determined by the board of nursing for the state in which you are seeking licensure, your registration form is processed and an Authorization to Test (ATT) form will be sent to you. You cannot make an appointment until the board of nursing declares eligibility and you receive an ATT form. The examination takes place at a Pearson Professional Center, and you can make an appointment through the Internet (www.vue.com/nclex) or by telephone. You can schedule an appointment at any Pearson Professional Center. You do not have to take the examination in the same state in which you are seeking licensure. A confirmation of your appointment will be sent to you.

The ATT form contains important information, including your test authorization number, candidate identification number, and an expiration date. Note the expiration date on the form because you must test by that date. You also need to take your ATT form to the test center on the day of your examination. You will not be admitted to the examination if you do not have it.

If for any reason you need to cancel or reschedule your appointment to test, you can make the change on the candidate Web site (www.vue.com/nclex) or by calling candidate services. The change needs to be made 1 full business day (24 hours) before your scheduled appointment. If you fail to arrive for the examination or fail to cancel your appointment to test without providing appropriate notice, you will forfeit your examination fee and your ATT will be invalidated. This information will be reported to the board of nursing in the state in which you have applied for licensure, and you will be required to register and pay the testing fees again.

It is important that you arrive at the testing center at least 30 minutes before the test is scheduled. If you arrive late for the scheduled testing appointment, you may be required to forfeit your examination appointment. If it is necessary to forfeit your appointment, you will need to reregister for the examination and pay an additional fee. The board of nursing will be notified that you did not test. A few days before your scheduled date of testing, take the time to drive to the testing center to determine its exact location, the length of time required to arrive to that destination, and any potential obstacles that might delay you, such as road construction, traffic, or parking sites.

SPECIAL TESTING CIRCUMSTANCES

If you require special testing accommodations, you should contact the board of nursing before submitting a registration form. The board of nursing will provide the procedures for the request. The board of nursing must authorize special testing accommodations. Following board of nursing approval, the NCSBN reviews the requested accommodations and also must approve the request. If the request is approved, the testing appointment must be made by the NCLEX program coordinator, whom you can contact by calling NCLEX candidate services. If it is necessary, you must cancel or reschedule an appointment through the NCLEX program coordinator.

THE TESTING CENTER

The test center is designed to ensure complete security of the testing process. Strict candidate identification requirements have been established. To be admitted to the testing center, you must bring the ATT form, along with two forms of identification. Both forms of identification must be signed and current or nonexpired, and one must contain a recent photograph of you. The name on the photograph identification must be the same as the name on the ATT form. A digital fingerprint, signature, and photograph will be taken at the test center and will accompany the NCLEX examination results to confirm your identity. Additionally, if you leave the testing room for any reason, you may be required to

have your fingerprint taken again to be readmitted to the room.

Personal belongings are not allowed in the testing room. Secure storage will be provided for you; however, storage space is limited, so you must plan accordingly. In addition, the testing center will not assume responsibility for your personal belongings. The testing waiting areas are generally small, so friends or family members who accompany you are not permitted to wait in the testing center while you are taking the examination.

Once you have completed the admission process and a brief orientation, the proctor will escort you to the assigned computer. You will be seated at an individual work space area that includes computer equipment, appropriate lighting, an erasable note board, and a marker. No items, including unauthorized scratch paper, are allowed into the testing room. Electronic devices such as watches, beepers, or cell phones are not allowed in the testing room. Eating, drinking, and the use of tobacco are not allowed in the testing room. You will be observed at all times by the test proctor during the examination. Additionally, video and audio recording of all test sessions occurs. Pearson Professional Centers has no control over the sounds made by typing on the computer by others. If these sounds are distracting, raise your hand to summon the proctor. Earplugs are available on request.

You must follow the directions given by the test center staff and must remain seated during the test, except when authorized to leave. If you feel that you have a problem with the computer, need an additional note board, need to take a break, or need the test proctor for any reason, you must raise your hand.

TESTING TIME

The maximum testing time is 6 hours, and this period includes the tutorial, the sample items, all breaks, and the examination. All breaks are optional, and if you decide to take a break, you must leave the testing room. When you return, you may be required to provide a fingerprint to be readmitted to the testing room.

LENGTH OF THE EXAMINATION

The minimum number of questions that you will need to answer is 75. Of these 75 questions, 60 will be operational (scored) questions and 15 will be pretest (unscored) questions. The maximum number of questions in the test is 265.

The pretest questions are questions that may be presented as scored questions on future examinations. These pretest questions are not identified as such. In other words, you do not know which questions are the pretest questions.

PASS OR FAIL DECISIONS

All of the examination questions are categorized by test plan area and level of difficulty. This is an important point to keep in mind when you consider how the computer makes a pass or fail decision because a pass or fail decision is not based on a percentage of correctly answered questions.

After the minimum number of questions have been answered (75 questions), the computer compares the test-taker's ability level to the standard required for passing. The standard required for passing is set based on the expert judgment of several individuals appointed by the NCSBN. If the test-taker is clearly above the passing standard, then the test-taker passes the examination. If the test-taker is clearly below the passing standard, then the test-taker fails the examination. If the computer is not able to determine clearly whether the test-taker has passed or failed because the test-taker's ability is close to the passing standard, then the computer continues asking questions. After each question, the computer determines the test-taker's ability, and when it becomes clear on which side of the passing standard the test-taker falls (above the standard or below the standard), the examination ends. If the test-taker is administered the maximum number of questions (265 questions), the computer will make a pass or fail decision by recomputing the test-taker's final ability level, based on every question answered, and comparing it with the passing standard. If the ability level is above the passing standard, the test-taker passes. If the ability level is not above the passing standard, the test-taker fails.

If the examination ends because the test-taker has run out of time, the computer may not have enough information to make a clear pass-or-fail decision. If this is the situation, the computer will review the test-taker's performance during testing. If the test-taker's ability was consistently above the passing standard specifically on the last 60 questions, the test-taker passes. If the test-taker's ability falls below the passing standard, even once, the test-taker fails.

COMPLETING THE EXAMINATION

Once the examination has ended, you will complete a brief computer-delivered questionnaire about your testing experience. After you complete this questionnaire, you need to raise your hand to summon the test proctor. The test proctor will collect and inventory all note boards and then permit you to leave.

PROCESSING RESULTS

Every computerized examination is scored twice—once by the computer at the testing center and again after the examination is transmitted to Pearson Professional Centers.

No results are released at the test center. The board of nursing will mail your results to you about 1 month after you take the examination. You should not call Pearson Professional Centers, the NCSBN, candidate services, or the state board of nursing for results. In some states, results can be obtained via the state Web site or via an NCSBN telephone results service. Information about obtaining NCLEX results by this method can be obtained on the NCSBN Web site under candidate services.

CANDIDATE PERFORMANCE REPORT

A candidate performance report is provided to a test-taker who failed the examination. This report provides test-takers with information about their strengths and weaknesses in relation to the test plan and provides a guide for studying and retaking the examination. The test-taker should refer to the state board of nursing in the state in which licensure is sought for procedures regarding the time period for retaking the examination.

INTERSTATE ENDORSEMENT

Because the NCLEX-RN examination is a national examination, you can apply to take the examination in any state. Once licensure is received, you can apply for Interstate Endorsement, which is obtaining another license in another state to practice nursing in that state. The procedures and requirements for Interstate Endorsement may vary from state to state, and these procedures can be obtained from the state board of nursing in the state in which endorsement is sought. You may also be allowed to practice nursing in another state if the state has enacted the Nurse Licensure Compact. The state boards of nursing can be accessed via the NCSBN Web site at www.ncsbn.org.

NURSE LICENSURE COMPACT

It may be possible to hold one license from the state of residency and practice nursing in another state under the mutual recognition model of nursing licensure, if the state has enacted the Nurse Licensure Compact. To obtain information about the Nurse Licensure Compact and the states that have entered this interstate compact, access the NCSBN Web site at www.ncsbn.org.

ADDITIONAL INFORMATION ABOUT THE EXAMINATION

Additional information regarding the NCLEX-RN examination can be obtained from the National Council of State Boards of Nursing, Inc., 111 East Wacker Drive, Suite 2900, Chicago, Illinois 60601. The telephone number for the testing service is (866) 293-9600. The Web site is www.ncsbn.org.

REFERENCES

Harkreader, H., Hogan, M.A., & Thobaben, M. (2007). *Fundamentals of nursing: Caring and clinical judgment* (3rd ed.). Philadelphia: Saunders.

Ignatavicius, D., & Workman, M. (2006). *Medical-surgical nursing: Critical thinking for collaborative care* (5th ed.). Philadelphia: Saunders.

Kee, J., & Hayes, E. (2006). *Pharmacology: A nursing process approach* (5th ed.). St. Louis: Mosby.

Kee, J., & Marshall, S. (2009). *Clinical calculations: With applications to general and specialty areas* (6th ed.). Philadelphia: Saunders.

Lewis, S., Heitkemper, M., Dirksen, S., O'Brien, P., & Bucher, L. (2007). *Medical-surgical nursing: Assessment and management of clinical problems* (7th ed.). St. Louis: Mosby.

McKenry, L., Tressier, E., & Hogan, M. (2006). *Mosby's pharmacology in nursing* (22nd ed.). St. Louis: Mosby.

Murray, S., & McKinney, E. (2006). *Foundations of maternal-newborn nursing* (4th ed.). Philadelphia: Saunders.

National Council of State Boards of Nursing. (2007). *2007 NCLEX-RN® detailed test plan*. Chicago: Author.

National Council of State Boards of Nursing Web site: www.ncsbn.org.

Potter, P., & Perry, A. (2005). *Fundamentals of nursing* (6th ed.). St. Louis: Mosby.

Preparation for the NCLEX-RN® Examination: Transitional Issues for the Foreign-Educated Nurse

This chapter provides information regarding the certification processes that must be pursued to become a registered nurse in the United States. An important factor to consider as you pursue this process is that some of the requirements may vary from state to state. Therefore, as a first step in the process, you need to contact the board of nursing in the state in which you are planning to obtain licensure. You can obtain contact information for each state board of nursing through the National Council of State Boards of Nursing (NCSBN) Web site at www.ncsbn.org. Once you have accessed the NCSBN Web site, select the link titled "Boards of Nursing." Additionally, you can write to the NCSBN regarding the NCLEX exam. The address is National Council of State Boards of Nursing, Inc., 111 East Wacker Drive, Suite 2900, Chicago, Illinois 60601. The telephone number for the NCSBN is (312) 525-3600; the fax number is (312) 279-1032.

An additional step in the process of obtaining information about becoming a registered nurse in the United States is to access the NCSBN Web site at www.ncsbn.org and obtain information provided for international nurses in the NCLEX Web site link. The NCSBN provides information about some of the data that you will need to obtain as an international nurse seeking licensure as a registered nurse in the United States and the credentialing agencies.

This chapter provides information about The Commission on Graduates of Foreign Nursing Schools (CGFNS) credentialing program. The NCSBN Web site (www.ncsbn.org) can provide information about additional credentialing agencies. The credentialing agency needs to follow the standards identified by the professional credentialing associations such as the National Association of Credential Evaluation

Services (NACES) (www.naces.org). Therefore it is important to obtain contact information about credentialing agencies from the NCSBN. Additionally, because criteria can change, it is recommended that you access the NCSBN Web site to obtain the most up-to-date information about the credentialing process and obtaining a license to practice as a registered nurse in the United States.

VISASCREEN

U.S. immigration law requires certain health care professionals to successfully complete a screening program before receiving an occupational visa (Section 343 of the Illegal Immigration Reform and Immigration Responsibility Act of 1996). Therefore you are required to obtain a VisaScreen certificate.

The CGFNS is an organization that offers this federal screening program. The International Commission on Health Care Professions, a division of the CGFNS, administers the VisaScreen. The VisaScreen components include an educational analysis, license verification, assessment of proficiency in the English language, and an examination that tests nursing knowledge. This chapter describes each of these components. Once the applicant successfully achieves each of the components, the applicant is presented with a VisaScreen certificate. You can obtain information related to the VisaScreen through the CGFNS Web site at www.cgfns.org.

Educational Analysis

The educational analysis component requires the following:
1. Applicant must present proof of completion of senior secondary school education, separate from any professional certification.

2. Applicant must present proof of completion from a government-approved professional health care program of at least 2 years in length.
3. Applicant must provide documentation that he or she has completed a minimum number of clock and/or credit hours in specific theoretical and clinical areas while in nursing school.

Licensure Verification

The applicant must present all current and past licensure for review.

Proficiency in the English Language

The applicant must submit proof of a passing score on an approved U.S. Department of Education and Health and Human Services English language proficiency examination. Box 2-1 lists English proficiency examinations and testing organizations. The credentialing agency will also provide information about English language proficiency examinations.

Testing Nursing Knowledge

An examination to test nursing knowledge includes the following:
1. The 1-day qualifying examination that is administered as part of the process for obtaining a CGFNS Certificate tests nursing knowledge; therefore a CGFNS Certificate provides proof of adequate nursing knowledge.

Box 2-1 ▲ ENGLISH LANGUAGE PROFICIENCY EXAM AND TESTING ORGANIZATIONS

> **TESTS ADMINISTERED BY THE EDUCATIONAL TESTING SERVICE (ETS) WORLDWIDE**
> Test of English as a Foreign Language (TOEFL)
> The Test of English for International Communication (TOEIC)
> *Contact Information:*
>   Educational Testing Service (ETS)
>   P.O. Box 6151
>   Princeton, NJ 08541-6151
>   Telephone: (609) 771-7100
>   Email: toefl@ets.org
>
> **INTERNATIONAL ENGLISH LANGUAGE TESTING SYSTEM (IELTS)**
> *Contact Information:*
>   International English Language Testing System (IELTS)
>   IELTS Administrator
>   Cambridge Examinations and IELTS International
>   100 East Corson Street, Suite 200
>   Pasadena, CA 91103
>   Telephone: (626) 564-2954
>   Web site: www.ielts.org

This qualifying examination is described in Components of the CGFNS Certification Program.
2. A foreign-educated nurse who is licensed and practicing nursing in the United States also is required to obtain a VisaScreen; if the nurse does not have a CGFNS Certificate, the nurse may be granted eligibility to take the NCLEX exam to provide proof of nursing knowledge.

STATE REQUIREMENTS

Most states in the United States require that you receive certification from the CGFNS or another credentialing agency before you can be eligible to take the NCLEX exam. If the state in which you intend to obtain licensure does not require certification, it may require submission of some of the same documents that the CGFNS or other credentialing agency requires. Therefore, in addition to what the CGFNS or other credentialing agency requires, a state may require the following:
1. Proof of citizenship or lawful alien status.
2. Official transcripts of educational credentials sent directly to the agency and board of nursing from the school of nursing.
3. Validation of theoretical instruction and clinical practice in a variety of nursing areas, including but not limited to medical nursing, surgical nursing, pediatric nursing, maternity and newborn nursing, community and public health nursing, and mental health nursing. Validation of professional nursing course work may also be required.
4. Copy of nursing license and/or diploma.
5. Proof of proficiency in the English language.
6. Photographs of the applicant.
7. Application fees.

THE COMMISSION ON GRADUATES OF FOREIGN NURSING SCHOOLS

The CGFNS provides a certification program for nurses educated and licensed outside of the United States.

The certificate program offered by the CGFNS is a requirement of most state boards of nursing, and the certificate may be required before you can take the NCLEX exam. The certificate program ensures that you are eligible and qualified to meet licensure and other practice requirements in the United States, and it predicts your success on the NCLEX exam. This program also assists you in obtaining your VisaScreen certificate. You can obtain additional information relating to the CGFNS and its certification program through the CGFNS Web site at www.cgfns.org.

Eligibility for the CGFNS Certification Program

The CGFNS Certification Program is designed for nurses educated outside of the United States who hold an initial and current registration/licensure as a first-level general registered nurse. According to the CGFNS, a first-level nurse is called a *registered nurse* or *professional nurse* in most countries. As a general nurse, the foreign-educated nurse must have obtained theoretical instruction and clinical practice in a variety of nursing areas. These nursing areas include but are not limited to medical nursing, surgical nursing, pediatric nursing, maternity and newborn nursing, community public health nursing, and mental health nursing. If the nurse educated outside of the United States does not meet these requirements, the nurse is not eligible for the certification program.

Components of the CGFNS Certification Program

The CGFNS Certification Program contains three parts, and you must complete all parts successfully to be awarded a CGFNS Certificate. The three parts include a credentials review, a 1-day qualifying examination that tests nursing knowledge, and an English language proficiency examination. You can take the qualifying and English language proficiency examinations at various locations throughout the world. This provides the applicant the opportunity to obtain the CGFNS Certificate before coming to the United States. These three parts of the certificate program are described next.

Credentials Review

The CGFNS requires validation of education and a licensing history of the applicant to ensure that the applicant has the appropriate credentials to seek certification. The CGFNS must receive transcripts and validation documents from the nursing program and licensing agency. The CGFNS does not accept transcripts and validation documents from the applicant. The specific credentialing requirements are similar to those needed for the VisaScreen certificate and include the following:
1. Completion of a senior secondary school education
2. Graduation from a government-approved nursing program of at least 2 years in length
3. Acquisition of theoretical instruction and clinical practice in the areas of medical nursing, surgical nursing, pediatric nursing, maternity and newborn nursing, community public health nursing, and mental health nursing
4. Possession of a full and unrestricted license or registration to practice as a first-level general nurse in the country where he or she completed their general nursing education
5. Possession of a current license or registration as a first-level general nurse

Qualifying Examination

The qualifying examination tests the applicant's knowledge in nursing in the areas of adult health, pediatrics, maternity and newborn, mental health, and community

public health. The examination is designed to ensure that the applicant has the knowledge to provide nursing care to various client groups at the same level as recent U.S. nursing graduates.

English Language Proficiency Examination

The applicant must take and pass an English language proficiency examination. You can take the examination before or after the qualifying examination. The English language proficiency examination needs to be taken from a testing organization that is approved by the CGFNS, and the applicant must apply directly with the testing organization to take the examination. The scores must be sent directly to the CGFNS from the testing organization. The CGFNS will not accept test scores from the applicant. Box 2-1 lists the types of English proficiency examinations, approved testing organizations, and their contact information. The CGFNS or other credentialing agency will provide you with current information about these approved testing organizations.

The CGFNS or other credentialing agency may identify certain applicants as exempt from the English language proficiency requirement. For an applicant to be exempt, the applicant must meet all of the following criteria: native language is English; country of nursing education was Australia, Canada (except Quebec), New Zealand, United Kingdom, or Trinidad and Tobago, and language of instruction and language of textbooks was English. Because these criteria may change, it is recommended that you obtain current information from the credentialing agency.

Once you successfully have met each of the three required components of the CGFNS Certification Program, the CGFNS will issue a certificate of completion. Unless the state in which you intend to obtain licensure indicates additional requirements and if you have received your VisaScreen certificate, you will be eligible to take the NCLEX exam.

REGISTERING TO TAKE THE NCLEX® EXAM

If you are planning to take the examination in the United States, the initial step in the registration process is to submit an application to the state board of nursing in the state in which you intend to obtain licensure. You need to obtain information from the board of nursing regarding the specific registration process because the process may vary from state to state. In most states, you may register for the examination through the Web, by mail, or by telephone. The NCLEX candidate Web site is www.vue.com/nclex. You must follow the registration instructions and complete the registration forms precisely and accurately. Registration forms not properly completed or not accompanied by the proper fees in the required method of payment will be returned to you and will delay testing. You must pay a fee for taking the examination, and you also may have to pay additional fees to the board of nursing in the state in which you are applying. You will be sent a confirmation indicating that your registration was received. If you do not receive a confirmation within 4 weeks of submitting your registration, you should contact the candidate services. You can obtain information regarding candidate services at the candidate Web site at www.vue.com/nclex.

Once the board of nursing in the state in which you request licensure has verified your eligibility to take the examination, the board will process your registration form and send you an Authorization to Test (ATT) form. You cannot make an appointment until the board of nursing declares eligibility and you receive an ATT form. The examination will take place at a Pearson Professional Center, and you can make an appointment through the Web or by telephone. You can schedule an appointment at any Pearson Professional Center. You do not have to take the examination in the same state in which you are seeking licensure. A confirmation of your appointment will be sent to you. For additional information regarding the NCLEX exam and testing procedures, refer to Chapter 1. You can also obtain information about the registration process and testing procedures from the NCSBN Web site at www.ncsbn.org.

NCLEX examination testing abroad is also available in some countries. Some international sites that provide this testing are Australia, Canada, England, Germany, Hong Kong, India, Japan, Mexico, Puerto Rico, South Korea, and Taiwan. Additional international sites may also be available and it is recommended that you visit the NCLEX Web site for current information about international testing sites. These testing sites provide the nurse who is interested in becoming a licensed nurse in the United States an opportunity to pass the NCLEX examination before traveling to the United States.

PREPARING TO TAKE THE NCLEX® EXAM

The challenge that is presented to you is one that requires patience and endurance. The positive result of your endeavor certainly will reward you professionally and give you the personal satisfaction of knowing you have become part of a family of highly skilled professionals, the registered nurse. You have successfully completed the requirements to become eligible to take the NCLEX exam, and now you have one more important goal to achieve: to pass the exam.

I highly recommend adequate preparation for the NCLEX examination because the examination is difficult. An important step that you have taken in preparing is that you are using this book, *Saunders Q&A Review for the NCLEX-RN® Examination*, which provides you with more than 5200 practice questions based on the NCLEX-RN examination test plan framework. The companion book, *Saunders Comprehensive Review for the NCLEX-RN® Examination*, provides both a thorough content review

and more than 4200 additional practice questions based on the NCLEX-RN test plan. Additional resources to prepare you for this examination are the *Saunders Strategies for Success for the NCLEX-RN® Examination, Saunders Strategies for Alternate Item Formats on the NCLEX-RN® Examination, Saunders Q&A Review Cards for the NCLEX-RN® Exam,* and the *Saunders Online Review Course for the NCLEX-RN® Examination*. These products are described below. All of these products can be obtained online by visiting www.elsevierhealth.com or by calling (800) 545-2522 in the United States or (800) 460-3110 outside the United States.

The *Saunders Strategies for Success for the NCLEX-RN®* Examination focuses on the test-taking strategies that will help you prepare for the NCLEX-RN examination. The chapters describe all of the test-taking strategies and include several sample questions that illustrate how to use the test-taking strategy. There are a total of 500 practice questions that accompany this book and all of the practice questions are reflective of the framework and the content identified in the current NCLEX-RN test plan and include multiple-choice and alternate item format questions.

The *Saunders Strategies for Alternate Item Formats on the NCLEX-RN® Examination* differs from all of the other products in that it contains only alternate item format questions. It provides you with all of the information that you need about all types of alternate item format questions that may appear on the NCLEX-RN examination. It contains 265 practice alternate item format questions and 15 heart and lung sounds questions.

The *Saunders Q&A Review Cards for the NCLEX-RN® Exam* is organized specifically by the test plan framework of the current NCLEX-RN test plan. This product provides 1000 practice test questions on portable, easy-to-use cards. The question is on the front of the card and the answer, rationale, test-taking strategy, and Integrated Process code are on the back of the card. This product includes both multiple-choice questions and alternate item format questions including fill-in-the-blank, multiple response, prioritizing (ordered response), image (hot spot questions), and chart/exhibit questions.

The *Saunders Online Review Course for the NCLEX-RN® Examination* addresses all areas of the test plan identified by the NCSBN. The course contains a pretest that provides feedback regarding your strengths and weaknesses and generates an individualized study schedule in a calendar format. Content review includes practice questions and case studies, figures and illustrations, a glossary, and animations and videos. A cumulative examination and a computer adaptive test are also key components of the online review course. The types of practice questions in this course include multiple choice, fill-in-the-blank, multiple response, prioritizing (ordered response), and questions containing figures that may require you to use the computer mouse to answer.

Lastly, never lose sight of your goal. Patience and dedication will contribute significantly to your achieving the status of registered nurse. Remember, success is climbing a mountain, facing the challenge of obstacles, and reaching the top of the mountain. I wish you the best success in your journey and beginning your career as a registered nurse in the United States of America.

REFERENCES

Commission on Graduates of Foreign Nursing Schools. Web site http://www.cgfns.org.

Educational Testing Service, Princeton, New Jersey. Email toefl@ets.org.

International English Language Testing System. Web site http://www.ielts.org.

National Council of State Boards of Nursing. Web site http://www.ncsbn.org.

Profiles to Success

LAURENT W. VALLIERE

Preparing to take the National Council Licensure Examination (NCLEX-RN®) can produce a great deal of anxiety in the nursing graduate. You may be thinking that the NCLEX-RN is the most important examination that you will ever have to take and that it reflects the culmination of everything that you have worked so hard for. The NCLEX-RN is an important examination because achieving that nursing license defines the beginning of your career as a registered nurse. A vital ingredient to your success on the NCLEX involves avoiding negative thoughts that allow this examination to seem overwhelming and intimidating. Such thoughts will take full control over your destiny (Box 3-1).

Box 3-1 ▲ PROFILES TO SUCCESS

- Avoid negative thoughts that allow the examination to seem overwhelming and intimidating.
- Develop a comprehensive plan to prepare for the examination.
- Examine the study methods and strategies that you used in preparing for examinations during nursing school.
- Develop realistic time goals.
- Select a study time period and study place that will be most conducive to your success.
- Commit to your own special study methods and strategies.
- Incorporate a balance of exercise with adequate rest and relaxation time in your preparation schedule.
- Maintain healthy eating habits.
- Learn to control anxiety.
- Remember that discipline and perseverance will automatically bring control.
- Remember that this examination is all about you.
- Remember that your self-confidence and the belief in yourself will lead you to success!

Nursing graduates preparing for the NCLEX must develop a comprehensive plan to prepare for this examination. The most important component in developing a plan is identifying the study patterns that guided you to your nursing degree. It is important to begin your planning by reflecting on all of the personal and academic challenges you experienced during your nursing education. Take time to focus on the thoughts, feelings, and emotions that you experienced before taking an examination while in your nursing program. Examine the methods that you used in preparing for that examination both academically and from the standpoint of how you dealt with the anxiety that parallels the experience of facing an examination.

These factors are very important considerations in preparing for the NCLEX. The reason that these factors are so important is because they identify the patterns that worked for you. Think about this for a moment. Your own methods of study must have worked, or you would not be at the point of preparing for the NCLEX-RN.

Each individual requires his or her own methods of preparing for an examination. Graduate nurses who have taken the NCLEX-RN will probably share their experiences and methods of preparing for this challenge with you. It is very helpful to listen to what they tell you. These graduates can provide you with important strategies that they have used. Listen closely to what they have to say, but remember that this examination is all about you. Your identity and what you require in terms of preparation are most important.

Reflect on the methods and strategies that worked for you throughout your nursing program. Do not think that you need to develop new methods and strategies to prepare for the NCLEX. Use what has worked for you. Take some time to reflect on these strategies, write them down on a large blank card, sign your name, and write "RN" after your name. Post this card in a place where you will see it every morning. Commit to your own special strategies. These strategies reflect your profile and identity, and will lead you to success!

A frequent concern of graduates preparing for the NCLEX relates to deciding whether they should study alone or become a part of a study group. Examining your profile will easily direct you in making this decision. Again, reflect on what has worked for you throughout your nursing program as you prepared for examinations. Remember, your needs are most important. Address your own needs and do not become pressured by peers who are encouraging you to join a study group, if this is not your normal pattern for study. Additional pressure is not what you need at this important time of your life.

Nursing graduates preparing for the NCLEX frequently inquire about the best method of preparing. First, remember that you are prepared. In fact, you began preparing for this examination on the first day that you entered your nursing program.

The task that you are faced with is to review, in a comprehensive manner, all of the nursing content that you learned in your nursing program. It can become totally overwhelming to look at your bookshelf, which is overflowing with the nursing books that you used during nursing school, and your challenge becomes monumental when you look at the boxes of nursing lecture notes that you have accumulated. It is unrealistic to even think that you could read all of those nursing books and lecture notes in preparation for the NCLEX. These books and lecture notes should be used as a reference source, if needed, during your preparation for the NCLEX.

Saunders Comprehensive Review for the NCLEX-RN® Examination has identified for you all of the important nursing content areas relevant to the examination. During the comprehensive review, you should have noted the areas that are unfamiliar or unclear to you. Be sure that you have taken the time to become familiar with these areas. Now, progress through the Pyramid to Success and test your knowledge in this book, *Saunders Q&A Review for the NCLEX-RN® Examination.* You may identify nursing content areas that require further review. Take the time to review, as you are guided to do in this book.

Your profile to success requires that you develop realistic time goals to prepare for the NCLEX. It is necessary to take the time to examine your life and all of the commitments that you may have. These commitments may include family, work, and friends. As you develop your goals, remember to plan time for fun and exercise. To achieve success, you require a balance of both work time and enjoyment time. If you do not plan for some leisure time, you will become frustrated and perhaps even angry.

These sorts of feelings will block your ability to focus and concentrate. Remember that you need time for yourself.

Goal development may be a relatively easy process because you have probably been juggling your life commitments ever since you entered nursing school. Remember that your goal is to identify a daily time frame and time period for you to use in reviewing and preparing for the NCLEX. Open your calendar and identify days on which life commitments will not allow you to spend this time preparing. Block those days off and do not consider them as a part of your review time. Identify the time that is best for you in terms of your ability to concentrate and focus, so that you can accomplish the most in your identified time frame. Be sure that you consider a time that is quiet and free of distractions. Many individuals find that the morning hours provide the most productive hours, whereas others may find the afternoon and evening hours most productive. Remember that this examination is all about you, so select the time period that will be most conducive to your success.

The place of study is also very important. Select a place that is quiet and comfortable for study—where you normally do your studying and preparing. If studying at home in your own environment is your normal pattern, be sure to free yourself of distractions during your scheduled preparation time. If you are not able to free yourself of distractions, you may consider spending your preparation time in a library. When selecting your place of study, reflect on what worked best for you during your nursing program.

Selecting the amount of daily preparation time can be a dilemma for many graduates preparing for the NCLEX. It is very important to set a realistic time period that can be adhered to on a daily basis. Set a time frame that will provide you with quality time and a time frame that can be achieved. If you set a time frame that is not realistic and cannot be achieved every day, you will become frustrated. This frustration will block your journey toward the peak of the Pyramid to Success.

The best suggestion is to spend at least 2 hours daily for NCLEX preparation. Two hours is a realistic time period, both in terms of spending quality time and of adhering to a time frame. You may find that after 2 hours your ability to focus and concentrate will diminish. You may, however, find that on some days you are able to spend more than the scheduled 2 hours; if you can and feel as though your ability to concentrate and focus is still present, then do so.

Discipline and perseverance will automatically bring control. Control will provide you with the momentum that will sweep you to the peak in the Pyramid to Success.

Discipline yourself to spend time preparing for the NCLEX every day. Daily preparation is very important because it maintains a consistent pattern and keeps you in synchrony with the mind flow needed on the day you are scheduled to take the NCLEX examination. Some days you may think about skipping your scheduled preparation time because you are not in the mood for study or because you just do not feel like studying. On these days, practice discipline and persevere. Stand yourself up, shake off those thoughts of skipping a day of preparation, take a deep breath, and get the oxygen flowing throughout your body. Look in the mirror, smile, and say to yourself "This time is for me and I can do this!" Look at your card that displays your name with "R.N." after it, and get yourself to that special study place. Remember that discipline and perseverance will bring control!

In the profile to success, academic preparation directs the path to the peak of the Pyramid to Success. There are, however, additional factors that will influence successful achievement to the peak. These factors include your ability to control anxiety, physical stamina, the amount of rest and relaxation you get, your self-confidence, and the belief in yourself that you will achieve success on the NCLEX. You need to take time to think about these important factors and incorporate these factors into your daily preparation schedule.

Anxiety is a common concern among students preparing to take the NCLEX. Feeling some anxiety is normal and will keep your senses sharp and alert. A great deal of anxiety, however, can block your process of thinking and hamper your ability to focus and concentrate. You have already practiced the task of controlling anxiety when you took examinations in nursing school. Now you need to continue with this practice and incorporate this control on a daily basis. Each day, before beginning your scheduled preparation time, sit in your quiet special study place, close your eyes, and take a slow deep breath. Fill your body with oxygen, hold your breath to a count of four, then exhale slowly through your mouth. Continue with this exercise and repeat it four to six times. This exercise helps relieve your mind of any unnecessary chatter and delivers oxygen to all of your body tissues and to your brain. On your scheduled day for taking the NCLEX, after the necessary pretesting procedures, you will be escorted to your test computer. Practice this breathing exercise before beginning the examination. Use this exercise during the examination if you feel yourself becoming anxious and distracted and if you are having difficulty focusing or concentrating. Remember that breathing will move that oxygen to your brain!

Physical stamina is a necessary component of readiness for the NCLEX. Plan to incorporate a balance of exercise with adequate rest and relaxation time in your preparation schedule. It is also important that you maintain healthy eating habits. Begin to practice these healthy habits now, if you have not already done so. There are a few points to keep in mind each day as you plan your daily meals. Three balanced meals are important, with snacks, such as fruits, included between meals. Remember that food items that contain fat will slow you down and food items that contain caffeine will cause nervousness and sometimes shakiness.

These items need to be avoided. Healthy foods that are high in carbohydrates work best to supply you with your energy needs. Remember that your brain can work like a muscle. It requires those carbohydrates. In addition, be sure that you include those needed fruits and vegetables in your diet (Box 3-2).

If you are the type of individual who is not a breakfast eater, work on changing that habit. Practice the habit of eating breakfast now, as you are preparing for the NCLEX. Attempt to provide your brain with energy in the morning with some form of complex carbohydrate food. It will make a difference. On your scheduled day for the NCLEX, feed your brain and eat a healthy breakfast. In addition, on this very important day, bring some form of snack such as a fruit or bagel for break time, and feed your brain again so that you will have the energy to concentrate, focus, and complete your examination.

Adequate rest, relaxation, and exercise are important in your preparation process. Many graduates preparing for the NCLEX have difficulty sleeping, particularly the night before the examination. Begin now to develop methods that will assist in relaxing your body and mind and allow you to obtain a restful sleep. You may already have a particular method developed to help you sleep. If not, it may be helpful to try the breathing exercise while you lie in bed to assist in eliminating any "mind chatter" that is present. It is also helpful to visualize your favorite and most peaceful place while you do these breathing exercises. Graduates have also stated that listening to quiet music and relaxation tapes has assisted in helping them relax and sleep. Begin to practice some of these helpful methods now, while you are preparing for the NCLEX. Identify those that work best for you. The night before your scheduled examination is an important one. Spend time having some fun, get to bed early, and incorporate the relaxation method that you have been using to help you sleep.

Confidence and belief that you have the ability to achieve success will bring your goals to fruition. Reflect on your profile maintained during your nursing education. Your confidence and belief in yourself, along with

Box 3-2 ▲ HEALTHY EATING HABITS

Eat three balanced meals each day.
Include snacks, such as fruits and vegetables, between meals.
Avoid food items that contain fat.
Avoid food items that contain caffeine.
Consume healthy foods that are high in complex carbohydrates.

your academic achievements, have brought you to the status of graduate nurse. Now you are facing one more important challenge (Box 3-3).

Can you meet this challenge successfully? Yes, you can! There is no reason to think otherwise, if you have taken all of the necessary steps to ensure that profile to success. Each morning, place your feet on the floor, stand tall, take a deep breath, and smile. Take both hands and imagine yourself brushing off any negative feelings. Look at your card that bears your name with the letters "RN" after it, and tell yourself "Yes, I can do this successfully!"

Believe in yourself, and you will reach the peak of the Pyramid to Success!

Congratulations, and I wish you continued success in your career as a Registered Nurse!

Box 3-3 ▲ CRITICAL WORDS

BELIEVE
In your success every day.

PLAN
The study strategies that work for you.

CONTROL
Always maintain command of your emotions, and breathe.

PRACTICE
Review, review, review: Practice questions, practice questions, and more practice questions!

SUCCEED
Believe, plan, control, and practice: "Yes I can!"

The NCLEX-RN® Examination: From a New Graduate's Perspective

CARA CHENETTE, BSN, RN

Congratulations! What an accomplishment it is to have made it this far. As someone who has just been through the experience of a nursing degree and sitting for the NCLEX-RN examination, I can honestly say that I know what you are going through and you WILL be okay! I am so glad that I can take this opportunity to share my experience with you, as well as offer some feedback to you; some things that I wish someone would have shared with me to make the experience a little less stressful (and as I know, this time in your life needs no added stress!).

I earned my nursing degree at a 4-year BSN program. I had always wanted to have a bachelor's degree and nursing was something I had considered as far back as I can remember. I am not a "book smart" person and knew that if I wanted to be a nurse, I would have to work hard and not lose focus. My driver's education instructor in high school always said that "driving is a privilege, not a right," and I applied that philosophy to nursing. I often made the decision to spend a little more time studying than to do what was popular at the moment among my peers. I did find time to have fun with my friends, and I often found creative ways to study with my four roommates (all nursing majors) rather than be out at a party. Doing little things like going to the gym before class so I wouldn't lose time when I could be studying in the afternoon, or going to the library in the 2-hour break I had in the middle of the day instead of going home to take a nap were things that I believe not only helped me make it through nursing school, but also prepared me for the task of self-study for the NCLEX-RN examination.

I was also a person who had to be employed throughout college and was very worried that my job would interfere with my ability to maintain the GPA I needed to graduate as a nurse. I tried a few different things to start with, but found that an on-campus job was most beneficial. While it didn't pay as much as other jobs, it did allow me the flexibility to bring my books with me and work hours that were most practical for my schedule. I never worked before a test or paper was due and often studied with friends at their campus jobs. I did work during the summer and school breaks at a doctor's office. This allowed me to get my foot in the door in the nursing profession. While it was not the best decision to work there during the school year, as it was out of state and demanding of my time, it did introduce me to what would be expected of me as a nurse, and eventually it became the field of nursing that I went into.

Graduation came quickly and I found myself faced with the reality that my preparation for the NCLEX-RN was no longer at the suggestion of my professors, but was now completely my responsibility. I prepared for the NCLEX using the Elsevier Pyramid to Success products. I stopped "reading" nursing material as a method of studying, as I was used to doing in school, and I started practicing NCLEX questions on the computer using the Elsevier products. Because the NCLEX-RN examination is on the computer, it is most beneficial to use the computer to do practice questions. I found my habits of studying in a book very hard to break, but am extremely glad that I did. I got used to doing 100 to 200 questions on the computer every day and found that it made me less intimidated when I had to do the same number of questions when sitting for the NCLEX-RN.

In college, I had been a part of a very successful "study group." Two other nursing student friends and I found that we had complementary styles of studying and improved our grades once we started studying together. This was great for college, but I found that after college when I moved back home several states away from my study buddies, I was lost as to how to study alone. I had studied for so long with these two girls, I had forgotten how to successfully study by myself. It took me a few weeks to find an effective method of studying without my group. Looking back on it, I wish that I had started studying this way long before I graduated from college. That way my grades would have indicated whether I was successful in my method and it would have alleviated some of the stress right before the NCLEX.

I also found that my best time to study was in the afternoon, between two and six o'clock. I wish someone had suggested that I schedule the NCLEX-RN examination at that time. Because I am generally a morning person, I decided to schedule it for the first appointment of the day at the testing center. After a few days, I realized that I had to modify my studying so that I was used to answering questions at that time in the morning. This was something I wish I had thought of because it did add a degree of stress that was unnecessary.

It is important to find a place to study that is quiet and comfortable for you. I found that the best place for me to study was on the porch of my house. My porch had no clocks or phones. I am a horrible clock watcher and there were times I was more interested in seeing how long I had been studying than actually focusing on studying. It was easy to ignore my house phone ringing, but it was even easier to study when I couldn't hear it ring. Taking those seemingly little distractions away from study time made a huge difference for me.

My style of study was simple. I did questions on the computer, reviewed the answers after, and used the text that went along with the questions to explain the answer to questions I answered incorrectly. I did multiple sets of 10 questions at a time for the first few weeks, so that I would get used to doing questions on the computer. I would do a different content area a day, sometimes a few content areas if I had done very well, until all the content areas were covered. Then I started doing 100 to 200 questions at a time. I found that this was not hard because I was so used to doing questions. I also did small things that were helpful, like writing lab values that I had a hard time remembering and putting them on Post-it notes throughout my house where they could be easily seen ("sodium" on the salt shaker, etc.). I also made charts for things like standard and transmission-based precautions, med-math, heart rhythms, and other lab values, and took them everywhere I went. You would be surprised at the amount of time you have to look at them. I remember one particular time when I was waiting in line at the bank and I was able to completely memorize the precautions.

For me, it was the best decision not to take the NCLEX-RN examination right after graduation. I knew that I still had a lot to prepare for and that it would be premature for me to take it right away. I graduated in May and scheduled the NCLEX-RN in August. Looking back on it, I would have done this a little differently. I still would have waited as I did, but I would not have scheduled my test on a Friday, especially the Friday of a holiday weekend (Labor Day). I tend to be a somewhat nervous person and waiting the whole weekend, plus the holiday, to find out about the test was nothing short of torture.

I should have taken it at a time when I could have found out my results at the soonest possible time.

After I had scheduled the examination, I did not tell anyone when I was taking it. I did not feel as though I needed the additional pressure that would come with multiple people knowing. I did not want to think that I would somehow be letting them down if I failed. Only my mother knew, as she was the one who drove me to the exam (I did not want to drive myself . . . something that sounds silly to me now). When I was hired at my job, I let the director of my nursing unit know when my exam was and asked for the week of the exam off. I did this upon being hired, so it was no problem. I had the entire week off to devote to NCLEX preparation. I would suggest to anyone to take the time off and I really felt as though the last week of my studying was the biggest factor in my passing the exam. I was focused and knew that I could pass the NCLEX-RN.

For some reason that I will never understand, I had a great night's sleep the night before the examination. At this point, I had mentally prepared myself for the test, to the point where I was walking around my house, saying out loud, "I got this." I went to bed early, looked over some last-minute material, and fell asleep. I woke the next morning in plenty of time to get ready without rushing. I still had the confidence I had the night before, and got ready without second-guessing my ability to take the test to the best of my capacity. I layered my clothes, because I wanted to make sure that being too hot or cold was not an issue that would cause me to be distracted. I did eat breakfast in the car on the way and it goes without saying that eating something was a good idea.

I got to the testing center in plenty of time. I checked in, provided my fingerprint as requested, showed them my driver's license, and signed a few things. The check-in process took much less time than I had anticipated and I was glad that it didn't act as much of a distraction before the test. Right after I was done checking in, they brought me to the computer room, gave me some last-minute instructions, and I was left to do my test. I sat at the computer, looked at the screen, and said again, "I got this." I started with the tutorial at the beginning that explained how the process worked. The test began promptly after the tutorial. Something that I hadn't planned on was that my computer screen was somewhat old and had a consistent "wavy" line. This threw me off a little, but it was presumptuous of me to think that they would have brand new, mint-condition computers.

I took the test question by question. I didn't allow myself to think about questions that I had already answered. I wanted to focus on the one in front of me and get everything else out of my head. Any time I got thrown off, I just reminded myself, "I got this" and continued. I also never allowed myself to think, "what if?" If I looked at a question and thought, "well, if the patient something" or "this would be right if," I stopped and read the question over again as if it was the first time

I was seeing it. Usually, after reading it the second time, the answer was apparent to me.

I was given a tip by a family member that I took to heart and used during the NCLEX-RN examination. She told me that if I am there long enough to take a break, which is offered at various points throughout the test, to take the break. She explained that you need to get up and move around and stop looking at the computer for a minute to clear your head. I was offered a break and walked to the bathroom of the testing center. There, thinking about endorphins and adrenalin, I jumped up and down for a minute. I didn't think about anything I had just done and wanted to refresh my mind before sitting back down. It really helped to just move for a minute.

When I sat back down, I looked at the test as if I was starting at question number one. To me, I was going to do the best I could regardless of how many questions I answered incorrectly in the previous hour. There were many questions I knew, some I could reason through, and some I just didn't know. I didn't allow myself to get frustrated with those questions. I kept thinking of myself in the situation and what would be safe and effective for the patient. Trying to make the questions as simple and matter-of fact as possible seemed to help me through the ones I had little to no clue about.

Contrary to popular belief, those who have to answer the entire 265 questions do survive the test and can pass. I am proof. I had to answer every last question that test could offer. I remember that, because I was faced with all the questions, knowing which question I had last was somewhat stressful. I took twice as long on that question as I did on most and made extra sure that I was clicking on the right button.

The screen does temporarily shut off after you finish. Like someone had told me, you think that there is something wrong with the computer because the screen spontaneously turns black. A posttest questionnaire does eventually pop up, and I completed it (it does not take very long). The experience was then over, and I gathered my belongings and left the center.

A friend of mine, who took the test before me, told me that one goes through a gauntlet of emotions after the test, and I agree. At times I was sure I passed and there were times that I knew I had failed miserably. After a day or two, I was mentally prepared for whether I had passed or failed. I had thought about it enough to be okay with either, knowing that if I failed I just needed some more test preparation and my ability to be a nurse would not be affected by the results of the test. I did, however, keep studying every day just in case.

I was at work when I found out the results. Being afraid that I would push medications with a null and void temporary license, I checked my state's board of nursing Web site close to what seemed like a million times. In the afternoon, I saw that there were now numbers next to my name, and under the word "License" it said the word "Valid." I jumped out of my seat, ran down the hallway (which was less than professional), grabbed my nursing preceptor, ran her to the computer, and pointed at it, speechless. For some time at work, I was known as "the girl who runs when she is excited."

It is hard to explain the feeling you have when you pass and you WILL pass. You have an immense sense of accomplishment because you know you succeeded based on all of your hard work. No one was telling you to do it and you made the decision to put in the time, study, and practice questions. I can honestly say it was one of the few times in my life that I was truly proud of myself and I still can't believe that I did it!

I wish you good luck. You can do it. You have the ability to pass the NCLEX-RN examination. You have the knowledge, whether you believe it or not. Make a plan, practice, don't watch the clock, and trust in yourself. You've got this!

Test-Taking Strategies

I. Pyramid to Success (Box 5-1)

II. How to Avoid Reading Into the Question (Box 5-2)

A. Pyramid Points
1. Avoid asking yourself, "Well, what if . . .?" because this will lead you right into the "forbidden," that is, reading into the question.
2. Focus only on the information in the question, read every word, and make a decision regarding what the question is asking.
3. Look for the strategic words in the question, such as *immediate, initial, first, priority, side effect,* or *toxic effect.* Strategic words make a difference with regard to what the question is asking.
4. In multiple-choice questions, multiple-response questions, or questions that require you to number in order of priority, read every choice or option before selecting answers.
5. Always use the process of elimination when choices or options are presented. Once you have eliminated options, reread the question before selecting your final choice or choices.
6. With questions that require you to fill in the blank, focus on the information in the question and determine what the question is asking. If the question requires you to calculate a medication dose, an intravenous flow rate, or intake and output amounts, recheck your work in calculating and always use the on-screen calculator to verify the answer.
7. Avoid asking yourself the "forbidden" words "Well, what if . . .?" when deciding on an answer to a question.

B. The Ingredients of a Question (Box 5-3)
1. The ingredients of a question include the event (which is a client or clinical situation), the event query, and the options or answers. A fill-in-the-blank question does not contain options, and some figure or illustration ("hot spot") questions may or may not contain options.

2. The event provides you with the content about the client or clinical situation that you need to think about in answering the question.
3. The event query asks something specific about the content of the event.
4. The options are all of the answers provided with the question.
5. In a multiple-choice question, there are four options and you must select one. Read every option carefully and think about the event and the event query as you use the process of elimination.
6. In a multiple-response question, there are several options and you must select all options that apply to the event in the question. Visualize the event, and use your nursing knowledge and your clinical experiences to answer the question.
7. In a prioritizing (ordered response) question, you will be required to list in order of priority certain nursing interventions or other data. Visualize the event, and use your nursing knowledge and clinical experiences to answer the question.

Box 5-1 ▲ PYRAMID TO SUCCESS

Avoid asking yourself, "Well, what if . . .?" because this will lead you right into reading into the question!

Focus only on the information in the question, read every word, and make a decision regarding what the question is asking!

Look for the strategic words in the question. Strategic words make a difference with regard to what the question is asking!

Always use the process of elimination when choices or options are presented. Once you have eliminated options, reread the question before selecting your final choice or choices!

Determine whether the question is a positive or negative event query!

Use all of your nursing knowledge, your clinical experiences, and your test-taking skills and strategies to answer the question!

8. A chart/exhibit question usually contains options. Read the question carefully and all of the information in the chart/exhibit before selecting an answer.

III. The Strategic Words (Boxes 5-4 and 5-5)

A. Strategic words focus your attention on a critical point to consider when answering the question and will assist you in eliminating the incorrect options.

B. Some strategic words may indicate that all of the options are correct and that it will be necessary to prioritize in order to select the correct option (see Box 5-9).

C. As you read the question, look for the strategic words. Strategic words make a difference with regard to what the question is asking.

Box 5-2 ▲ PRACTICE QUESTION: AVOIDING THE "WHAT IF . . .?" SYNDROME AND READING INTO THE QUESTION

A nurse is changing the tapes on a tracheostomy tube. The client coughs and the tube is dislodged. The initial nursing action is to:

1 Call the physician to reinsert the tube.
2 Ventilate the client using a manual resuscitation bag and face mask.
3 Cover the tracheostomy site with a sterile dressing to prevent infection.
4 Call the respiratory therapy department to reinsert the tracheostomy tube.

Answer: 2
Test-Taking Strategy: Now you may immediately think, "The tube is dislodged and I need a physician!" Read the question carefully and note the strategic word "initial." Focus on the subject: the tube is dislodged. The question is asking you for a nursing action so that is what you need to look for as you eliminate the incorrect options. Eliminate options 1 and 4 because they are comparable or alike and delay the initial intervention needed. Eliminate option 3 because this action will block the airway. If the tube is dislodged, the initial nursing action is to ventilate the client using a manual resuscitation bag and face mask. Additionally, use of the ABCs—airway, breathing, and circulation—will direct you to the correct option. Remember, avoid reading into the question!

Reference:
Ignatavicius, D., & Workman, M. (2006). *Medical-surgical nursing: Critical thinking for collaborative care* (5th ed., p. 553). Philadelphia: Saunders.

Box 5-4 ▲ COMMON STRATEGIC WORDS

Best	Initial
Early or late	Most appropriate or
First	least appropriate
Immediate	Most likely or least likely

Box 5-3 ▲ MULTIPLE-CHOICE QUESTION: EVENT, EVENT QUERY, AND OPTIONS

Event: A client has two chest tubes inserted into the right pleural space following thoracic surgery. The two chest tubes are attached to chest drainage systems.
Event Query: To promote optimal respiratory functioning, the nurse plans to implement which of the following?
Options:
1 Milk and strip the chest tubes once a shift.
2 Position the client only on the back and on the right side.
3 Encourage the client to cough and deep breathe every hour.
4 Maintain the client on bedrest until the chest tubes are removed.

Answer: 3
Test-Taking Strategy: Focus on the subject, to promote optimal respiratory functioning. Option 1 is eliminated first because milking and stripping a chest tube is done only with a physician's order or when allowed by agency policy. Bedrest (option 4) does not promote respiratory function and is eliminated next. From the remaining options, recalling that positioning is done according to surgeon preference directs you to option 3.

References:
Black, J., & Hawks, J. (2005). *Medical-surgical nursing: Clinical management for positive outcomes* (7th ed., pp. 1857-1859). Philadelphia: Saunders.
Monahan, F., Sands, J., Neighbors, M., Marek, J., & Green, C. (2007). *Phipps medical-surgical nursing: Health and illness perspectives* (8th ed., p. 652). St. Louis: Mosby.

Box 5-5 ▲ PRACTICE QUESTION: STRATEGIC WORDS

A client with a diagnosis of heart failure reports the occurrence of sudden shortness of breath and dyspnea. The nurse takes which immediate action?
1 Calls the physician
2 Administers oxygen
3 Elevates the head of the bed
4 Prepares to administer furosemide (Lasix)

Answer: 3
Test-Taking Strategy: Note the strategic word "immediate." Focusing on this strategic word and the client's symptoms (shortness of breath and dyspnea) will direct you to the correct option. Note that the question is asking for an immediate nursing action, so look for that as you eliminate each incorrect option. Remember to look for strategic words!

Reference:
Ignatavicius, D., & Workman, M. (2006). *Medical-surgical nursing: Critical thinking for collaborative care* (5th ed., p. 756). Philadelphia: Saunders.

IV. The Subject of the Question (Box 5-6)

A. The subject of the question is the specific topic about which the question is asking.
B. Identifying the subject of the question helps eliminate incorrect options and directs you to the correct option.

V. Positive and Negative Event Queries (Boxes 5-7 and 5-8)

A. A positive event query uses strategic words that ask you to select the correct option; for example, the event query may read: "Which statement by a client indicates an understanding of the side effects of the prescribed medication?"
B. A negative event query uses strategic words that ask you to select an incorrect option; for example, the event query may read: "Which statement by a client indicates a need for further teaching about the side effects of the prescribed medication?"

Box 5-7 ▲ PRACTICE QUESTION: POSITIVE EVENT QUERY

The nurse has provided discharge instructions regarding nitroglycerin therapy to the client with angina. Which statement by the client indicates an understanding of home use of the nitroglycerin?
1 "If I use a nitroglycerin and the pain does not subside in 15 minutes, I should go to the hospital."
2 "When I have pain, I should lie down and place a tablet under my tongue. If unrelieved in 5 minutes, I should take another tablet."
3 "When I have chest pain, I should put a tablet under my tongue. If I have a burning sensation, I should call my doctor immediately."
4 "When I experience chest pain, I can continue what I'm doing. If it doesn't go away in 10 minutes, I should use a nitroglycerin tablet."

Answer: 2
Test-Taking Strategy: This question identifies an example of a positive event query. Note the strategic words "indicates an understanding." The client taking sublingual nitroglycerin should lie down upon taking the medication because lightheadedness and dizziness may occur as a result of postural hypotension. The client should use up to three tablets at 5-minute intervals before seeking medical attention. A burning sensation is a common side effect of nitroglycerin. Nitroglycerin should be taken with the onset of anginal pain. The client should repeat nitroglycerin if relief is not obtained with the first or second dose. Remember that positive event queries ask you to select an option that is a *correct* item or statement!

References:
Hodgson, B., & Kizior, R. (2008). *Saunders nursing drug handbook 2008* (p. 847). St. Louis: Saunders.
Lehne, R. (2007). *Pharmacology for nursing care* (6th ed., p. 583). St. Louis: Saunders.

Box 5-6 ▲ THE SUBJECT OF THE QUESTION

The nurse is planning to teach a client in skeletal leg traction about measures to increase bed mobility. Which item would be most helpful for this client?
1 Television
2 Fracture bedpan
3 Overhead trapeze
4 Reading materials

Answer: 3
Test-Taking Strategy: Focus on the subject, to increase bed mobility. Also note the strategic words "most helpful." The use of an overhead trapeze is extremely helpful in assisting a client to move about in bed and to get on and off the bedpan. Television and reading materials are helpful in reducing boredom and providing distraction. A fracture bedpan is useful in reducing discomfort with elimination. Remember, focus on the subject!

References:
Black, J., & Hawks, J. (2005). *Medical-surgical nursing: Clinical management for positive outcomes* (7th ed., p. 636). Philadelphia: Saunders.
Monahan, F., Sands, J., Neighbors, M., Marek, J., & Green, C. (2007). *Phipps' medical-surgical nursing: Health and illness perspectives* (8th ed., pp. 1528-1529, 1535). St. Louis: Mosby.

Box 5-8 ▲ PRACTICE QUESTION: NEGATIVE EVENT QUERY

A nurse has provided medication instructions to a client who will be taking warfarin sodium (Coumadin) indefinitely. Which statement by the client indicates a need for further teaching?
1 "I need to use a soft toothbrush."
2 "I need to use a straight razor for shaving."
3 "I need to avoid drinking alcohol while taking this medication."
4 "I need to carry identification about the medication being taken."

Answer: 2
Test-Taking Strategy: This question identifies an example of a negative event query question. Note the strategic words "need for further teaching." These strategic words indicate that you need to select an option that identifies an incorrect client statement. Recalling that warfarin sodium is an anticoagulant and that the client is at risk for bleeding will direct you to the correct option. Remember that negative event queries ask you to select an option that is an *incorrect* item or statement!

Reference:
Skidmore-Roth, L. (2008). *Mosby's nursing drug reference* (21st ed., p. 1069). St. Louis: Mosby.

VI. Questions That Require Prioritizing

A. Questions in the examination may require you to use the skill of prioritizing nursing actions.
B. Look for the strategic words in the question that indicate the need to prioritize (Box 5-9).
C. Remember, when a question requires prioritization, all options may be correct and you need to determine the correct order of action.

Box 5-9 ▲ COMMON STRATEGIC WORDS THAT INDICATE THE NEED TO PRIORITIZE

Best
Essential
First
Highest priority
Immediate
Initial
Most appropriate or least appropriate
Most important
Most likely or least likely
Next
Primary
Vital

Box 5-10 ▲ PRACTICE QUESTION: USE OF THE ABCs

A client with a compound (open) fracture of the radius has a cast applied in the emergency department. The nurse provides home care instructions and tells the client to seek medical attention if which of the following occurs?
1 Numbness and tingling are felt in the fingers.
2 The cast feels heavy and damp after 24 hours of application.
3 The entire cast feels warm in the first 24 hours after application.
4 Bloody drainage is noted on the cast during the first 6 hours after application.

Answer: 1
Test-Taking Strategy: Use the ABCs—airway, breathing, and circulation—as a guide to direct you to the correct option. A limb encased in a cast is at risk for nerve damage and diminished circulation from increased pressure caused by edema. Signs of increased pressure and diminished circulation from the cast include numbness, tingling, and increased pain. Remember to use the ABCs—airway, breathing, and circulation—to prioritize.

Reference:
Monahan, F., Sands, J., Neighbors, M., Marek, J., & Green, C. (2007). *Phipps' medical-surgical nursing: Health and illness perspectives* (8th ed., p. 1536). St. Louis: Mosby.

D. Strategies to use for prioritizing include the ABCs (airway, breathing, and circulation); Maslow's Hierarchy of Needs theory; and the steps of the nursing process.
E. The ABCs (Box 5-10)
   1. Use the ABCs—airway, breathing, and circulation—when selecting an answer or determining the order of priority.
   2. Remember the order of priority: (1) airway, (2) breathing, and (3) circulation.
   3. Airway is always the first priority!
F. Maslow's Hierarchy of Needs Theory (Box 5-11 and Figure 5-1)
   1. According to Maslow's Hierarchy of Needs theory, physiological needs are the priority, followed by safety and security needs, love and belonging needs, self-esteem needs, and finally self-actualization needs; therefore, select the option or determine the order of priority by addressing physiological needs first
   2. When a physiological need is not addressed in the question or noted in one of the options, continue to use Maslow's Hierarchy of Needs theory as a guide and look for the option that addresses safety
G. Steps of the Nursing Process
   1. Use the steps of the nursing process to prioritize.
   2. The steps include assessment, analysis, planning, implementation, and evaluation and are followed in this order.

Box 5-11 ▲ PRACTICE QUESTION: MASLOW'S HIERARCHY OF NEEDS THEORY

A community health nurse is caring for a group of homeless people. In planning for the potential needs of this group, what is the priority concern?
1 Finding affordable housing for the group
2 Setting up a 24-hour crisis center and hotline
3 Ensuring the availability of peer support through structured groups
4 Meeting the basic needs to ensure that adequate food, shelter, and clothing are available

Answer: 4
Test-Taking Strategy: Use Maslow's Hierarchy of Needs theory to answer the question. Option 4 addresses basic physiological needs. Although options 1, 2, and 3 are also appropriate actions, option 4 is the priority concern. Remember to use Maslow's Hierarchy of Needs theory to prioritize.

Reference:
Potter, P., & Perry, A. (2005). *Fundamentals of nursing* (6th ed., pp. 51-52, 143). St. Louis: Mosby.

a. Assessment
   (1) Assessment questions address the process of gathering subjective and objective data relative to the client, confirming those data, and communicating and documenting the data.
   (2) Remember that assessment is the first step in the nursing process.
   (3) When you are asked to select your first, immediate, or initial nursing action, follow the steps of the nursing process to prioritize when selecting the correct option.
   (4) Look for strategic words in the options that reflect assessment (Box 5-12).
   (5) If an option contains the concept of assessment or the collection of client data, the best choice is to select that option (Box 5-13).
   (6) If an assessment action is not one of the options, follow the steps of the nursing process as your guide to select your first, immediate, or initial action.
   (7) Possible exception to the guideline: If the question presents an emergency situation, read carefully; in an emergency situation, an intervention may be the priority!

b. Analysis (Box 5-14)
   (1) Analysis questions are the most difficult questions because they require understanding of the principles of physiological responses and require interpretation of the data based on assessment.
   (2) Analysis questions require critical thinking and determining the rationale for therapeutic interventions that may be addressed in the question.

Box 5-12 ▲ ASSESSMENT: STRATEGIC WORDS

Ascertain
Assess
Check
Collect
Determine
Find out
Gather
Identify
Monitor
Observe
Obtain information
Recognize

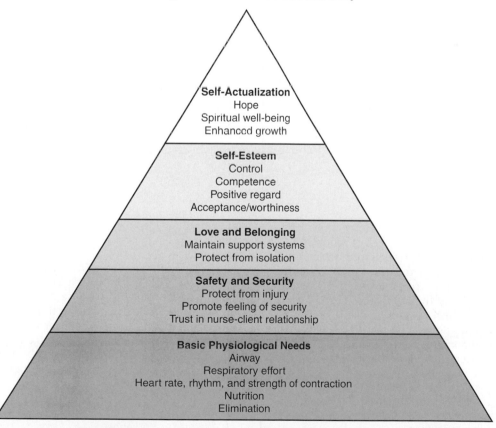

Nursing Priorities From Maslow's Hierarchy

Self-Actualization
Hope
Spiritual well-being
Enhanced growth

Self-Esteem
Control
Competence
Positive regard
Acceptance/worthiness

Love and Belonging
Maintain support systems
Protect from isolation

Safety and Security
Protect from injury
Promote feeling of security
Trust in nurse-client relationship

Basic Physiological Needs
Airway
Respiratory effort
Heart rate, rhythm, and strength of contraction
Nutrition
Elimination

Figure 5-1 Using Maslow's Hierarchy to establish priorities. (From Harkreader, H., Hogan, M.A., & Thobaben, M. (2007). *Fundamentals of nursing: Caring and clinical judgment* (3rd ed., p. 209). Philadelphia: Saunders.)

Box 5-13 ▲ PRACTICE QUESTION: THE NURSING PROCESS—ASSESSMENT

The nurse develops a plan of care for an older client with diabetes mellitus. The nurse plans to first:
1 Structure menus for adherence to diet.
2 Teach with videotapes showing insulin administration to ensure competence.
3 Encourage dependence on others to prepare the client for the chronicity of the disease.
4 Determine the client's ability to read label markings on syringes and blood glucose monitoring equipment

Answer: 4

Test-Taking Strategy: Note the strategic word "first." Use the steps of the nursing process to answer the question, remembering that assessment is the first step. The only option that addresses assessment is option 4. Options 1, 2, and 3 address the implementation step of the nursing process. Remember that assessment is the first step in the nursing process.

References:
Black, J., & Hawks, J. (2005). *Medical-surgical nursing: Clinical management for positive outcomes* (7th ed., pp. 154, 1265-1266). Philadelphia: Saunders.
Meiner, S., & Leuckenotte, A. (2006). *Gerontologic nursing* (3rd ed., pp. 544-545). St. Louis: Mosby.

Box 5-14 ▲ PRACTICE QUESTION: THE NURSING PROCESS—ANALYSIS

A client had arterial blood gases drawn, and the results are: pH 7.34, $Paco_2$ of 37 mm Hg, Pao_2 of 79, HCO_3^- of 19 mEq/L. The nurse interprets that the client is experiencing:
1 Metabolic acidosis
2 Metabolic alkalosis
3 Respiratory acidosis
4 Respiratory alkalosis

Answer: 1

Test-Taking Strategy: Metabolic acidosis occurs when the pH falls below 7.35 and the bicarbonate level falls below 22 mEq/L. With respiratory acidosis, the pH drops below 7.35 and the carbon dioxide level rises above 45 mm Hg. With respiratory alkalosis, the pH rises above 7.45 and the carbon dioxide level falls below 35 mm Hg. With metabolic alkalosis, the pH rises above 7.45 and the bicarbonate level rises above 26 mEq/L. Remember that analysis is the second step of the nursing process.

References:
Ignatavicius, D., & Workman, M. (2006). *Medical-surgical nursing: Critical thinking for collaborative care* (5th ed., p. 282). Philadelphia: Saunders.
Pagana, K., & Pagana, T. (2005). *Mosby's diagnostic and laboratory test reference* (7th ed., p. 119). St. Louis: Mosby.

(3) Analysis questions may address the formulation of a nursing diagnosis and the communication and documentation of the results of the process of analysis.
c. Planning (Box 5-15)
   (1) Planning questions require prioritizing nursing diagnoses, determining goals and outcome criteria for goals of care, developing the plan of care, and communicating and documenting the plan of care.
   (2) Regarding nursing diagnoses, remember that actual client problems rather than potential or at-risk client problems will most likely be the priority.
d. Implementation (Box 5-16)
   (1) Implementation questions address the process of organizing and managing care, counseling and teaching, providing care to achieve established goals, supervising and coordinating care, and communicating and documenting nursing interventions.
   (2) Focus on a nursing action rather than on a medical action when you are answering a question, unless the question is asking you what prescribed medical action is anticipated.
   (3) On the NCLEX-RN exam, the only client that you need to be concerned about is the client described in the question that you are answering. Avoid the "what if . . .?

Box 5-15 ▲ PRACTICE QUESTION: THE NURSING PROCESS—PLANNING

A nurse is assigned to care for a child with juvenile rheumatoid arthritis. The nurse reviews the plan of care, knowing that which of the following is a priority nursing diagnosis?
1 Acute pain, related to inflammatory process
2 Risk for self-care deficit related to immobility
3 Risk for injury related to impaired physical mobility
4 Disturbed body image related to activity intolerance

Answer: 1

Test-Taking Strategy: This question relates to planning nursing care and asks you to identify the priority nursing diagnosis. Use Maslow's Hierarchy of Needs theory, remembering that physiological needs (option 1) receive highest priority. Option 2 identifies a risk for a problem, not an actual problem. Option 4 addresses self-esteem needs. Option 3 addresses safety and security needs. Remember, planning is the third step of the nursing process.

Reference:
Wong, D., Hockenberry, M., Perry, S., Lowdermilk, D., & Wilson, D. (2006). *Maternal-child nursing care* (3rd ed., p. 1834). St. Louis: Mosby.

syndrome" and remember that the client in the question on the computer screen is your only assigned client.

    (4) Answer the question from a textbook and ideal perspective, and remember that the nurse has all the time and resources needed and readily available at the client's bedside. Avoid the "what if…? syndrome" and remember that you do not need to run to the treatment room to obtain supplies, such as sterile gloves because the sterile gloves will be at the client's bedside.

  e. Evaluation (Box 5-17)

    (1) Evaluation questions focus on comparing the actual outcomes of care with the expected outcomes, and communicating and documenting findings.

    (2) These questions focus on assisting in determining the client's response to care and in identifying factors that may interfere with achieving expected outcomes.

    (3) In an evaluation question, watch for negative event queries because they are frequently used in evaluation type questions.

VII. Client Needs

A. Physiological Integrity

  1. These questions test the concepts that the nurse provides comfort and assistance in the performance of activities of daily living, and provides care related to the administration of medications and parenteral therapies.

  2. These questions also address the nurse's ability to reduce the client's potential for developing complications or health problems related to treatments, procedures, or existing conditions, and providing care to clients with acute, chronic, or life-threatening physical health conditions

  3. Focus on Maslow's Hierarchy of Needs theory in these types of questions and remember that physiological needs are a priority and are addressed first.

  4. Use the ABCs (airway, breathing, and circulation) and the steps of the nursing process when selecting an option addressing physiological integrity.

B. Safe and Effective Care Environment

  1. These questions test the concepts that the nurse provides nursing care, collaborates with other health care team members to facilitate effective client care, and protects clients, significant others, and health care personnel from environmental hazards.

  2. Focus on safety in these types of questions, and remember the importance of handwashing, call bells, bed positioning, the appropriate use of side rails, and the use of standard and other precautions.

C. Health Promotion and Maintenance

  1. These questions test the concepts that the nurse provides and assists in directing nursing care to promote and maintain health.

  2. Content addressed in these questions relates to assisting the client and significant other(s) during the normal expected stages of growth and development from conception through advanced old age, and providing client care related to the prevention and early detection of health problems.

Box 5-16 ▲ PRACTICE QUESTION: THE NURSING PROCESS—IMPLEMENTATION

A nurse is checking the fundus in a postpartum woman and notes that the uterus is soft and spongy. Which nursing action is appropriate initially?

1 Notify the physician.
2 Encourage the mother to ambulate.
3 Massage the fundus gently until firm.
4 Document fundal position, consistency, and height.

Answer: 3
Test-Taking Strategy: Implementation questions address the process of organizing and managing care. Note the strategic word "initially." If the fundus is boggy (soft), it should be massaged gently until firm, observing for increased bleeding or clots. Remember that implementation is the fourth step of the nursing process.

Reference:
Murray, S., & McKinney, E. (2006). *Foundations of maternal-newborn nursing* (4th ed., p. 409). Philadelphia: Saunders.

Box 5-17 ▲ PRACTICE QUESTION: THE NURSING PROCESS—EVALUATION

A client has just taken a dose of trimethobenzamide (Tigan). The nurse evaluates that the medication has been effective if the client states relief of:

1 Heartburn
2 Constipation
3 Abdominal pain
4 Nausea and vomiting

Answer: 4
Test-Taking Strategy: Note the strategic words "medication has been effective." These words indicate that this is an evaluation-type question. Recalling that this medication is an antiemetic will direct you to option 4. Remember that evaluation is the fifth step of the nursing process.

Reference:
Skidmore-Roth, L. (2008). *Mosby's nursing drug reference* (21st ed., p. 1034). St. Louis: Mosby.

3. Use teaching and learning concepts if the question addresses client teaching, remembering that client willingness, desire, and readiness to learn are the first priorities.
4. Watch for negative event queries because they are frequently used in questions that address health promotion and maintenance and client education.

D. Psychosocial Integrity
1. These questions test the concepts that the nurse provides nursing care that promotes and supports the emotional, mental, and social well-being of the client and significant others.
2. Content addressed in these questions relates to supporting and promoting the client or significant others' ability to cope, adapt, or problem-solve in situations such as illnesses, disabilities, or stressful events such as abuse, neglect, or violence.
3. In this Client Needs category, you may be asked communication-type questions that relate to how you would respond to a client, a client's family member or significant other, or other health care team members.
4. Use therapeutic communication techniques to answer communication questions because of their effectiveness in the communication process.
5. Remember to select the option that focuses on the thoughts, feelings, concerns, anxieties, or fears of the client, client's family member, or significant others' (Box 5-18).

VIII. Eliminating Comparable or Alike Options (Box 5-19)

A. When reading the options, look for options that are comparable or alike; these options will include a similar concept or nursing action.
B. Comparable or alike options can be eliminated as possible answers.

IX. Eliminate Options That Contain Close-ended Words (Box 5-20)

A. Eliminate options that contain close-ended words because these words infer a fixed or extreme meaning; these types of options are usually incorrect.
B. Close-ended words include *all*, *always*, *every*, *must*, *none*, *never*, and *only*.
C. Options that contain words that are open-ended, such as *may*, *usually*, *normally*, *commonly*, or *generally*, should be considered as a possible correct option.

X. Look for the Umbrella Option (Box 5-21)

A. When answering a question, look for the umbrella option.
B. The umbrella option is one that is a broad or universal statement and usually contains the concepts of the other options within it.
C. The umbrella option will be the correct answer.

Box 5-18 ▲ PRACTICE QUESTION: COMMUNICATION

A client with a diagnosis of major depression says to the nurse, "I should have died. I've always been a failure." The nurse should make which therapeutic response to the client?
1 "I see a lot of positive things in you."
2 "You still have a great deal to live for."
3 "Feeling like a failure is part of your illness."
4 "You've been feeling like a failure for some time now?"

Answer: 4
Test-Taking Strategy: Use the techniques that facilitate therapeutic communication to answer this question. Remember to address the client's feelings and concerns. Option 4 is the only option that is stated in the form of a question and is open-ended, thus encouraging the verbalization of feelings. Remember, use therapeutic communication techniques and focus on the client.

Reference:
Stuart, G., & Laraia, M. (2005). *Principles and practice of psychiatric nursing* (8th ed., pp. 30-34). St. Louis: Mosby.

Box 5-19 ▲ PRACTICE QUESTION: ELIMINATE COMPARABLE OR ALIKE OPTIONS

A clinic nurse instructs an adolescent with iron-deficiency anemia about the administration of oral iron preparations. The nurse tells the adolescent that it is best to take the iron with:
1 Cola
2 Soda
3 Ginger ale
4 Tomato juice

Answer: 4
Test-Taking Strategy: Note that options 1, 2, and 3 are comparable or alike options in that they are carbonated beverages. Iron should be administered with vitamin C–rich fluids because vitamin C enhances the absorption of the iron preparation. Tomato juice contains a high content of ascorbic acid (vitamin C). Cola, soda, and ginger ale do not contain vitamin C. Remember, eliminate comparable or alike options!

References:
Hockenberry, M., Wilson, D., & Winkelstein, M. (2005). *Wong's Essentials of pediatric nursing* (7th ed., p. 1519). St. Louis: Mosby.
McKinney, E., James, S., Murray, S., & Ashwill, J. (2005). *Maternal-child nursing* (2nd ed., p. 657). St. Louis: Saunders.

XI. Use the Guidelines for Delegating and Assignment-Making (Box 5-22)

A. You may be asked a question that will require you to decide how you will delegate a task or assign clients to other health care providers.

B. Focus on the information in the question and what task or assignment is to be delegated.

C. Once you have determined what task or assignment is to be delegated, consider the client's needs and match the client's needs with the scope of practice of the health care providers identified in the question.

D. The nurse practice act and any practice limitations define which aspects of care can be delegated and which must be performed by the registered nurse.

E. Generally, noninvasive interventions such as skin care, range of motion exercises, ambulation, grooming, and hygiene measures can be assigned to a nursing assistant.

F. A licensed practical nurse can perform the tasks that a nursing assistant can perform and additionally can generally perform certain invasive tasks such as applying dressings, suctioning, urinary catheterization, and administering medications orally or by subcutaneous or intramuscular injections.

G. The registered nurse can perform the tasks that a licensed practical nurse can perform and is responsible for assessment and planning care, analyzing client data, implementing and evaluating client care, supervising care, initiating teaching, and administering medications intravenously.

XII. Answering Pharmacology Questions (Box 5-23)

A. If you are familiar with the medication, use nursing knowledge to answer the question.

B. Remember that the question will identify both the generic name and the trade name of the medication.

C. If the question identifies a medical diagnosis, then try to make a relationship between the medication and the diagnosis; for example, you can determine that cyclophosphamide (Cytoxan) is an antineoplastic medication if the question refers to a client with breast cancer who is taking this medication.

D. Try to determine the classification of the medication being addressed to assist in answering the question; identifying the classification will assist in determining a medication action and/or side effects; for example diltiazem (Cardizem) is a cardiac medication.

Box 5-20 ▲ PRACTICE QUESTION: ELIMINATE OPTIONS THAT CONTAIN CLOSE-ENDED WORDS

A client will undergo a barium swallow, and the nurse provides preprocedure instructions to the client. The nurse instructs the client to:

1 Avoid eating or drinking after midnight before the test.
2 Limit self to only two cigarettes on the morning of the test.
3 Have a clear liquid breakfast only on the morning of the test.
4 Take all routine medications with a glass of water on the morning of the test.

Answer: 1
Test-Taking Strategy: Note the close-ended word "only" in options 2 and 3, and "all" in option 4. Remember to eliminate options that contain close-ended words because these options are usually incorrect. Also note that options 2, 3, and 4 are comparable or alike options in that they all involve taking in something on the morning of the examination. Remember to eliminate options that contain close-ended words!

Reference:
Ignatavicius, D., & Workman, M. (2006). *Medical-surgical nursing: Critical thinking for collaborative care* (5th ed., p. 1243). Philadelphia: Saunders.

Box 5-21 ▲ PRACTICE QUESTION: LOOK FOR THE UMBRELLA OPTION

A nurse is teaching health education classes to a group of expectant parents and the topic is preventing mental retardation caused by congenital hypothyroidism. The nurse tells the parents that the most effective means of preventing this disorder is:

1 Vitamin intake
2 Neonatal screening
3 Adequate protein intake
4 Limiting alcohol consumption

Answer: 2
Test-Taking Strategy: Focus on the subject, preventing mental retardation caused by congenital hypothyroidism. Congenital hypothyroidism is the most common preventable cause of mental retardation. Neonatal screening is the only means of early diagnosis and subsequent prevention of mental retardation. Options 1, 3, and 4 are measures to prevent all birth defects. Also note that neonatal screening is the umbrella option and is a broad statement or intervention. Remember to look for the umbrella option!

References:
Murray, S., & McKinney, E. (2006). *Foundations of maternal-newborn nursing* (4th ed., p. 533). Philadelphia: Saunders.
Wong, D., Hockenberry, M., Perry, S., Lowdermilk, D., & Wilson, D. (2006). *Maternal-child nursing care* (3rd ed., p. 742). St. Louis: Mosby.

Box 5-22 ▲ PRACTICE QUESTION: USE THE GUIDELINES FOR DELEGATING AND ASSIGNMENT-MAKING

A nurse is planning the client assignments for the day and has a licensed practical nurse (LPN) and a nursing assistant on the nursing team. Which client would the nurse most appropriately assign to the LPN?
1 A client who is scheduled for an electrocardiogram and a chest radiograph
2 A client with stable congestive heart failure who has early stage Alzheimer's disease
3 A client who was treated for dehydration and is weak and needs assistance with bathing
4 A client with emphysema who is receiving oxygen at 2 L by nasal cannula and becomes dyspneic on exertion

Answer: 4
Test-Taking Strategy: The nurse would most appropriately assign the client with emphysema to the LPN. This client has an airway problem and has the highest priority needs of the clients presented in the options. The clients described in options 1, 2, and 3 can be cared for appropriately by the nursing assistant. Remember to match the client's needs with the scope of practice of the health care provider.

Reference:
Huber, D. (2006). *Leadership and nursing care management* (3rd ed., pp. 546-550). Philadelphia: Saunders.

Box 5-23 ▲ PRACTICE QUESTION: ANSWERING PHARMACOLOGY QUESTIONS

The nurse is preparing to administer atenolol (Tenormin) to a client. The nurse checks which of the following before administering the medication?
1 Temperature
2 Blood pressure
3 Potassium level
4 Blood glucose level

Answer: 2
Test-Taking Strategy: Focus on the name of the medication. Recall that most beta-blocker medication names end with the letters "lol" and that these medications are used to treat hypertension. This will direct you to option 2. Remember to focus on the medication name when answering pharmacology questions!

Reference:
Hodgson, B., & Kizior, R. (2007). *Saunders nursing drug handbook 2007* (p. 97). Philadelphia: Saunders.

E. Recognize the common side effects associated with each medication classification and then relate the appropriate nursing interventions to each side effect; for example, if a side effect is hypertension, then the associated nursing intervention would be to monitor the blood pressure.

F. Learn medications that belong to a classification by commonalities in their medication names; for example, medications that are xanthine bronchodilators end with the letters "line," for example, theophylline.

G. Look at the medication name and use medical terminology to assist in determining the medication action; for example, Lopressor lowers (lo) the blood pressure (pressor).

H. If the question requires a medication calculation, remember that a calculator is available on the computer. Talk yourself through each step to be sure the answer makes sense, and recheck the calculation before answering the question, particularly if the answer seems like an unusual dosage.

I. Pharmacology: Pyramid Points to Remember
1. Generally, the client should not take an antacid with medication because the antacid will affect the absorption of the medication.
2. Enteric-coated and sustained-release tablets should not be crushed; additionally, capsules should not be opened.
3. The client should never adjust or change a medication dose or abruptly stop taking a medication.
4. The nurse never adjusts or changes the client's medication dosage and never discontinues a medication.
5. The client needs to avoid taking any over-the-counter medications or any other medications such as herbal preparations unless they are approved for use by the health care provider.
6. The client needs to avoid consuming alcohol.
7. Medications are never administered if the order is difficult to read, is unclear, or identifies a medication dose that is not a normal one.

REFERENCES

Black, J., & Hawks, J. (2005). *Medical-surgical nursing: Clinical management for positive outcomes* (7th ed.). Philadelphia: Saunders.

Harkreader, H., Hogan, M.A., & Thobaben, M. (2007). *Fundamentals of nursing: Caring and clinical judgment* (3rd ed.). Philadelphia: Saunders.

Hockenberry, M., & Wilson, D. (2007). *Wong's nursing care of infants and children* (8th ed.). St. Louis: Mosby.

Hockenberry, M., Wilson, D., & Winkelstein, M. (2005). *Wong's Essentials of pediatric nursing* (7th ed.). St. Louis: Mosby.

Hodgson, B., & Kizior, R. (2008). *Saunders nursing drug handbook 2008.* Philadelphia: Saunders.

Huber, D. (2006). *Leadership and nursing care management* (3rd ed.). Philadelphia: Saunders.

Ignatavicius, D., & Workman, M. (2006). *Medical-surgical nursing: Critical thinking for collaborative care* (5th ed.). Philadelphia: Saunders.

Lehne, R. (2007). *Pharmacology for nursing care* (6th ed.). St. Louis: Saunders.

Lowdermilk, D., & Perry, S. (2006). *Maternity nursing* (7th ed.). St. Louis: Mosby.

McKinney, E., James, S., Murray, S., & Ashwill, J. (2005). *Maternal-child nursing* (2nd ed.). St. Louis: Saunders.

Meiner, S., & Leuckenotte, A. (2006). *Gerontologic nursing* (3rd ed.). St. Louis: Mosby.

Monahan, F., Sands, J., Neighbors, M., Marek, J., & Green, C. (2007). *Phipps' medical-surgical nursing: Health and illness perspectives* (8th ed.). St. Louis: Mosby.

Murray, S., & McKinney, E. (2006). *Foundations of maternal-newborn nursing* (4th ed.). Philadelphia: Saunders.

National Council of State Boards of Nursing. Web site http://www.ncsbn.org/.

National Council of State Boards of Nursing. (2007). *2007 NCLEX-RN® detailed test plan.* Chicago: Author.

Pagana, K., & Pagana, T. (2005). *Mosby's diagnostic and laboratory test reference* (7th ed.). St. Louis: Mosby.

Potter, P., & Perry, A. (2005). *Fundamentals of nursing* (6th ed.). St. Louis: Mosby.

Skidmore-Roth, L. (2008). *Mosby's nursing drug reference* (21st ed.). St. Louis: Mosby.

Stuart, G., & Laraia, M. (2005). *Principles and practice of psychiatric nursing* (8th ed.). St. Louis: Mosby.

Wong, D., Hockenberry, M., Perry, S., Lowdermilk, D., & Wilson, D. (2006). *Maternal-child nursing care* (3rd ed.). St. Louis: Mosby.

Client Needs

Client Needs and the NCLEX-RN® Test Plan

In the new test plan, which was implemented in April 2007, the National Council of State Boards of Nursing (NCSBN) identified a test plan framework that was based on Client Needs. This framework was selected on the basis of the findings in a practice analysis study of newly licensed registered nurses in the United States. This study identified the nursing activities performed by entry-level nurses. Also, according to the NCSBN, the Client Needs categories provide a structure for defining nursing actions and competencies across all settings for all clients. The NCSBN identifies four major categories of Client Needs. Some of these categories are further divided into subcategories, and the percentage of test questions in each subcategory is identified (Table 6-1).

The information contained in this chapter related to the test plan was obtained from the NCSBN Web site www.ncsbn.org and from the NCSBN *2007 NCLEX-RN® Detailed Test Plan*. Additional information regarding the test and its development can be obtained by accessing the NCSBN Web site at www.ncsbn.org or by writing to the National Council of State Boards of Nursing, 111 E. Wacker Drive, Suite 2900, Chicago, Illinois 60601.

PHYSIOLOGICAL INTEGRITY

The Physiological Integrity category includes four subcategories: Basic Care and Comfort, Pharmacological and Parenteral Therapies, Reduction of Risk Potential, and Physiological Adaptation. The NCSBN describes the content tested in each subcategory. Basic Care and Comfort (6% to 12%) addresses content that tests the knowledge, skills, and ability required to provide comfort and assistance to the client in the performance of activities of daily living. Pharmacological and Parenteral Therapies (13% to 19%) addresses content that tests the knowledge, skills, and ability required to administer medications and parenteral therapies. Reduction of Risk Potential (13% to 19%) addresses content that tests the knowledge, skills, and ability required to prevent complications or health problems related to the client's condition, or any prescribed treatments or procedures. Physiological Adaptation (11% to 17%) addresses content that tests the knowledge, skills, and ability required to provide care to clients with acute, chronic, or life-threatening conditions.

The NCSBN identifies nursing content related to the subcategories of this Client Needs category (Box 6-1). See Box 6-2 for examples of questions in this Client Needs category, and refer to Chapter 7 for practice questions reflective of this Client Needs category.

Table 6-1 ▲ CLIENT NEEDS CATEGORIES AND PERCENTAGE OF QUESTIONS ON NCLEX-RN®

CLIENT NEEDS CATEGORY	PERCENTAGE OF QUESTIONS
PHYSIOLOGICAL INTEGRITY	
Basic Care and Comfort	6-12
Pharmacological and Parenteral Therapies	13-19
Reduction of Risk Potential	13-19
Physiological Adaptation	11-17
SAFE AND EFFECTIVE CARE ENVIRONMENT	
Management of Care	13-19
Safety and Infection Control	8-14
HEALTH PROMOTION AND MAINTENANCE	6-12
PSYCHOSOCIAL INTEGRITY	6-12

Portions copyright by the National Council of State Boards of Nursing, Inc. All rights reserved.

Box 6-1 ▲ NCLEX-RN® CONTENT: PHYSIOLOGICAL INTEGRITY

BASIC CARE AND COMFORT
Alternative therapies
Assistive devices, such as canes, walkers, and crutches
Comfort and palliative care including nonpharmacological comfort interventions
Complementary therapies
Elimination
Hydration
Hygiene
Immobility
Mobility
Nutrition
Oral hygiene
Rest and sleep

PHARMACOLOGICAL AND PARENTERAL THERAPIES
Administration and monitoring of blood and blood products
Administration of intravenous therapy
Adverse effects of medications and parenteral therapies
Care of central venous access devices
Contraindications to medications and parenteral therapies
Expected effects of medications and parenteral therapies
Medication and intravenous administration and dosage calculation

Pain management
Parenteral nutrition
Pharmacological agents, actions, interactions, side effects, adverse effects, and toxic effects
Types of parenteral fluids

REDUCTION OF RISK POTENTIAL
Assessment of body systems
Diagnostic tests: preprocedure and postprocedure care
Monitoring laboratory values
Potential for alterations in body systems
Potential for complications of diagnostic tests, procedures, treatments, and surgery
Therapeutic treatments and procedures
Vital signs assessment

PHYSIOLOGICAL ADAPTATION
Care to the client receiving radiation therapy
Fluid and electrolyte imbalances
Managing illnesses
Infectious diseases
Managing medical emergencies
Pathophysiology related to diseases and conditions
Providing respiratory care
Unexpected responses to therapies, treatments, and procedures

From National Council of State Boards of Nursing. (2007). *2007 NCLEX-RN® detailed test plan.* Chicago: Author. Portions copyright by the National Council of State Boards of Nursing, Inc. All rights reserved.

Box 6-2 ▲ PHYSIOLOGICAL INTEGRITY QUESTIONS

BASIC CARE AND COMFORT
A client with right-sided weakness needs to learn how to use a cane for home maintenance of mobility. The nurse plans to teach the client to position the cane by holding it with the:
1 Left hand and 6 inches lateral to the left foot
2 Right hand and 6 inches lateral to the right foot
3 Left hand and placing the cane in front of the left foot
4 Right hand and placing the cane in front of the right foot

Answer: 1
Rationale: This question addresses content related to the use of an assistive device in the subcategory Basic Care and Comfort in the Client Needs category of Physiological Integrity. The client is taught to hold the cane on the opposite side of the weakness because, with normal walking, the opposite arm and leg move together (called *reciprocal motion*). The cane is placed 6 inches lateral to the fifth toe.

References:
Ignatavicius, D., & Workman, M. (2006). *Medical-surgical nursing: Critical thinking for collaborative care* (5th ed., pp. 125-126). Philadelphia: Saunders.
Potter, P., & Perry, A. (2005). *Fundamentals of nursing* (6th ed., pp. 948-949). St. Louis: Mosby.

PHARMACOLOGICAL AND PARENTERAL THERAPIES
A nurse is caring for a client with hypertension who is receiving torsemide (Demadex) 5 mg orally daily. Which of the following would indicate to the nurse that the client might be experiencing an adverse reaction related to the medication?
1 A chloride level of 98 mEq/L
2 A sodium level of 135 mEq/L
3 A potassium level of 3.1 mEq/L
4 A blood urea nitrogen (BUN) of 15 mg/dL

Answer: 3
Rationale: This question addresses content related to the adverse effect of a medication in the subcategory Pharmacological and Parenteral Therapies in the Client Needs category of Physiological Integrity. Torsemide is a loop diuretic. The medication can produce acute, profound water loss; volume and electrolyte depletion; dehydration; decreased blood volume; and circulatory collapse. Option 3 is the only option that indicates an electrolyte depletion because the normal potassium level is 3.5 to 5.1 mEq/L. The normal sodium level is 135 to 145 mEq/L. The normal chloride level is 98 to 107 mEq/L. The normal BUN is 5 to 20 mg/dL.

Reference:
Lehne, R. (2007). *Pharmacology for nursing care* (6th ed., p. 447). St. Louis: Saunders.

Continued

Box 6-2 ▲ PHYSIOLOGICAL INTEGRITY QUESTIONS—cont'd

REDUCTION OF RISK POTENTIAL

The nurse is caring for a client scheduled to undergo a renal biopsy. To minimize the risk of postprocedure complications, the nurse reports which of the following laboratory results to the physician before the procedure?

1 Potassium: 3.8 mEq/L
2 Serum creatinine: 1.2 mg/dL
3 Prothrombin time: 15 seconds
4 Blood urea nitrogen (BUN): 18 mg/dL

Answer: 3

Rationale: This question addresses a potential postprocedure complication of a diagnostic test in the subcategory Reduction of Risk Potential in the Client Needs category of Physiological Integrity. Postprocedure hemorrhage is a complication after renal biopsy. Because of this, prothrombin time is assessed before the procedure. The normal prothrombin time range is 11 to 12.5 seconds. The nurse ensures that these results are available and reports abnormalities promptly. The normal BUN is 5 to 20 mg/dL, the normal serum creatinine is 0.6 to 1.3 mg/dL, and the normal potassium is 3.5 to 5.1 mEq/L.

Reference:

Ignatavicius, D., & Workman, M. (2006). *Medical-surgical nursing: Critical thinking for collaborative care* (5th ed., p. 883, 1672-1673). St. Louis: Saunders.

PHYSIOLOGICAL ADAPTATION

A pregnant client tells a nurse that she felt wetness on her peri-pad and that she found some clear fluid. The nurse immediately inspects the perineum and notes the presence of the umbilical cord. The nurse's initial action is to:

1 Notify the physician.
2 Monitor the fetal heart rate.
3 Transfer the client to the delivery room.
4 Place the client in Trendelenburg position.

Answer: 4

Rationale: This question addresses an acute and life-threatening physical health condition in the subcategory Physiological Adaptation in the Client Needs category of Physiological Integrity. On inspection of the perineum, if the umbilical cord is noted, the nurse immediately places the client into Trendelenburg position while pushing the presenting part upward to relieve the cord compression. This position is maintained, the physician is notified, and the nurse monitors the fetal heart rate. The client is transferred to the delivery room when prescribed by the physician.

Reference:

Lowdermilk, D., & Perry, S. (2006). *Maternity nursing* (7th ed., p. 811). St. Louis: Mosby.

Box 6-3 ▲ NCLEX-RN® CONTENT: SAFE AND EFFECTIVE CARE ENVIRONMENT

MANAGEMENT OF CARE

Advance directives
Case management
Client advocacy and client rights, including confidentiality, information security, and informed consent
Concepts of management
Consultation with members of the health care team
Continuity of care
Delegation and supervision
Education
Establishing priorities
Ethical practice and legal responsibilities
Information technology
Performance improvement

Referrals
Resource management

SAFETY AND INFECTION CONTROL

Accident and error prevention
Disaster planning, security plans, and emergency response planning
Ergonomic principles
Handling hazardous and infectious materials
Injury prevention, including home safety
Medical and surgical asepsis
Reporting unusual occurrences
Safe use of equipment, restraints, and safety devices
Standard and other precautions

From National Council of State Boards of Nursing (2007). *2007 NCLEX-RN® detailed test plan.* Chicago: Author. Portions copyright by the National Council of State Boards of Nursing, Inc. All rights reserved.

SAFE AND EFFECTIVE CARE ENVIRONMENT

The Safe and Effective Care Environment category includes two subcategories: (1) Management of Care and (2) Safety and Infection Control. The NCSBN describes the content tested in each subcategory. Management of Care (13% to 19%) addresses content that tests the knowledge, skills, and ability required to enhance the care delivery setting to protect clients, families, significant others, visitors, and health care personnel. Safety and Infection Control (8% to 14%) addresses content that tests the knowledge, skills, and ability required to protect clients, families, significant others, visitors, and health care personnel from health and environmental hazards.

Box 6-4 ▲ SAFE AND EFFECTIVE CARE ENVIRONMENT QUESTIONS

MANAGEMENT OF CARE

A registered nurse is planning the client assignments for the day. Which of the following is the most appropriate assignment for the nursing assistant?

1 A client requiring colostomy irrigation
2 A client receiving continuous tube feedings
3 A client who requires stool specimen collections
4 A client who has difficulty swallowing food and fluids

Answer: 3

Rationale: This question addresses content related to delegation in the subcategory Management of Care in the Client Needs category of Safe and Effective Care Environment. Work that is delegated to others must be done consistent with the individual's level of expertise and licensure or lack of licensure. In this situation, the most appropriate assignment for the nursing assistant is to care for the client who requires stool specimen collections. The client with difficulty swallowing food and fluids is at risk for aspiration. Colostomy irrigations and tube feedings are not performed by unlicensed personnel. Remember, the health care provider needs to be competent and skilled to perform the assigned task or activity.

Reference:

Huber, D. (2006). *Leadership and nursing care management* (3rd ed., pp. 546-550). Philadelphia: Saunders.

SAFETY AND INFECTION CONTROL

A client diagnosed with tuberculosis (TB) is scheduled to go to the radiology department for a chest radiograph. Which nursing intervention would be appropriate when preparing to transport the client?

1 Apply a mask to the client.
2 Apply a mask and gown to the client.
3 Apply a mask, gown, and gloves to the client.
4 Notify the radiology department so that the personnel can be sure to wear a mask when the client arrives.

Answer: 1

Rationale: This question addresses content related to airborne precautions in the subcategory Safety and Infection Control in the Client Needs category of Safe and Effective Care Environment. Clients known or suspected of having TB should wear a mask when out of the hospital room to prevent the spread of the infection to others. Gown and gloves are not necessary.

References:

Ignatavicius, D., & Workman, M. (2006). *Medical-surgical nursing: Critical thinking for collaborative care* (5th ed., pp. 644-645). Philadelphia: Saunders.

Potter, P., & Perry, A. (2005). *Fundamentals of nursing* (6th ed., pp. 788, 797). St. Louis: Mosby.

The NCSBN identifies nursing content related to the subcategories of this Client Needs category (Box 6-3). See Box 6-4 for examples of questions in this Client Needs category, and refer to Chapter 8 for practice questions reflective of this Client Needs category.

HEALTH PROMOTION AND MAINTENANCE

The Health Promotion and Maintenance category (6% to 12%) addresses the principles related to growth and development. According to the NCSBN, this Client Needs category also addresses content that tests the knowledge, skills, and ability required to assist the client, family members, and/or significant others to prevent health problems, to recognize alterations in health, and to develop health practices that promote and support wellness.

The NCSBN identifies nursing content related to this Client Needs category (Box 6-5). See Box 6-6 for examples of questions in this Client Needs category, and refer to Chapter 9 for practice questions reflective of this Client Needs category.

Box 6-5 ▲ NCLEX-RN® CONTENT: HEALTH PROMOTION AND MAINTENANCE

Antepartum, intrapartum, and postpartum periods
Care to the newborn
Developmental stages and transitions
Expected body image changes
Family planning and family systems
Growth and development and the aging process
Health and wellness and preventing disease
Health screening and promotion programs
High-risk behaviors
Human sexuality
Immunizations
Lifestyle choices
Physical assessment techniques
Self-care principles
Teaching and learning

From National Council of State Boards of Nursing (2007). *2007 NCLEX-RN® detailed test plan.* Chicago: Author. Portions copyright by the National Council of State Boards of Nursing, Inc. All rights reserved.

Box 6-6 ▲ HEALTH PROMOTION AND MAINTENANCE QUESTIONS

A postpartum nurse has instructed a new mother on how to bathe her newborn infant. The nurse demonstrates the procedure to the mother and on the following day asks the mother to perform the procedure. Which observation by the nurse indicates that the mother is performing the procedure correctly?
1 The mother cleans the ears and then moves to the eyes and the face.
2 The mother begins to wash the newborn infant by starting with the eyes and face.
3 The mother washes the arms, chest, and back followed by the neck, arms, and face.
4 The mother washes the entire newborn infant's body and then washes the eyes, face, and scalp.

Answer: 2
Rationale: This question addresses the postpartum period in the Client Needs category of Health Promotion and Maintenance. Bathing should start at the eyes and face and with the cleanest area first. Next, the external ears and behind the ears are cleaned. The newborn infant's neck should be washed because formula, lint, or breast milk often accumulates in the folds of the neck. Hands and arms are then washed. The newborn infant's legs are washed next, with the diaper area washed last. Remember to always start with the cleanest area of the body first and proceed to the dirtiest area.

Reference:
Wong, D., Hockenberry, M., Perry, S., Lowdermilk, D., & Wilson, D. (2006). *Maternal-child nursing care* (3rd ed., p. 763). St. Louis: Mosby.

A client with atherosclerosis asks a nurse about dietary modifications to lower the risk of heart disease. The nurse encourages the client to eat which of the following foods that will lower this risk?
1 Fresh cantaloupe
2 Broiled cheeseburger
3 Baked chicken with skin
4 Mashed potato with gravy

Answer: 1
Rationale: This question addresses health and wellness in the Client Needs category of Health Promotion and Maintenance. To lower the risk of heart disease, the diet should be low in saturated fat, with the appropriate number of total calories. The diet should include fewer red meats and more white meat, with the skin removed. Dairy products used should be low in fat, and foods with large amounts of empty calories should be avoided. Fresh fruits and vegetables are naturally low in fat.

Reference:
Grodner, M., Long, S., & DeYoung, S. (2004). *Foundations and clinical applications of nutrition: A nursing approach* (3rd ed., p. 587). St. Louis: Mosby

PSYCHOSOCIAL INTEGRITY

The Psychosocial Integrity category (6% to 12%) addresses content that tests the knowledge, skills, and ability required to promote and support the client, family, and/or significant others' ability to cope, adapt, and/or solve problems during stressful events. According to the NCSBN, this Client Needs category also addresses the emotional, mental, and social well-being of the client, family, or significant other, and the knowledge, skills, and ability required to care for the client with an acute or chronic mental illness.

The NCSBN identifies nursing content related to this Client Needs category (Box 6-7). See Box 6-8 for examples of questions in this Client Needs category, and refer to Chapter 10 for practice questions reflective of this Client Needs category.

Box 6-7 ▲ NCLEX-RN® CONTENT: PSYCHOSOCIAL INTEGRITY

Abuse and neglect
Behavioral interventions
Chemical dependency
Coping mechanisms
Crisis interventions
Cultural diversity
Domestic violence
Grief and loss and end-of-life issues
Mental health concepts
Religious and spiritual issues
Sensory/perceptual alterations
Sexual abuse
Situational role changes
Stress management
Support systems
Therapeutic interactions
Unexpected body image changes

From National Council of State Boards of Nursing (2007). *2007 NCLEX-RN® detailed test plan.* Chicago: Author. Portions copyright by the National Council of State Boards of Nursing, Inc. All rights reserved.

Box 6-8 ▲ PSYCHOSOCIAL INTEGRITY QUESTIONS

The nurse is planning care for a client who is experiencing anxiety following a myocardial infarction. Which priority nursing intervention should be included in the plan of care?
1 Answer questions with factual information.
2 Limit family involvement during the acute phase.
3 Provide detailed explanations of all procedures.
4 Administer an antianxiety medication to promote relaxation.

Answer: 1
Rationale: This question addresses content related to fear and anxiety in the Client Needs category of Psychosocial Integrity. Accurate information reduces fear, strengthens the nurse–client relationship, and assists the client in dealing realistically with the situation. Providing detailed information may increase the client's anxiety. Information should be provided simply and clearly. The client's family may be a source of support for the client. Limiting family involvement may or may not be helpful. Medication should not be used unless necessary.

Reference:
Black, J., & Hawks, J. (2005). *Medical-surgical nursing: Clinical management for positive outcomes* (7th ed., p. 1723). Philadelphia: Saunders.

A nurse in the mental health clinic is performing an initial assessment of a family with a diagnosis of domestic violence. Which of the following factors would the nurse initially want to include in the assessment?
1 The coping style of each family member
2 The family's ability to use community resources
3 The family's anger toward the intrusiveness of the nurse
4 The family's denial of the violent nature of their behavior

Answer: 1
Rationale: This question addresses domestic violence in the Client Needs category of Psychosocial Integrity. Note the strategic word "initially." The initial family assessment includes a careful history of each family member. Options 2, 3, and 4 address the family. Option 1 addresses each family member.

Reference:
Stanhope, M., & Lancaster, J. (2008). *Public health nursing: Population-centered health care in the community* (7th ed., pp. 845-848). St. Louis: Mosby.

REFERENCES

Black, J., & Hawks, J. (2005). *Medical-surgical nursing: Clinical management for positive outcomes* (7th ed.). Philadelphia: Saunders.

Grodner, M., Long, S., & DeYoung, S. (2004). *Foundations and clinical applications of nutrition: A nursing approach.* (3rd ed.). St. Louis: Mosby.

Huber, D. (2006). *Leadership and nursing care management* (3rd ed.). Philadelphia: Saunders.

Ignatavicius, D., & Workman, M. (2006). *Medical-surgical nursing: Critical thinking for collaborative care* (5th ed.). Philadelphia: Saunders.

Lehne, R. (2007). *Pharmacology for nursing care* (6th ed.). St. Louis: Saunders.

Lowdermilk, D., & Perry, S. (2006). *Maternity nursing* (7th ed.). St. Louis: Mosby.

National Council of State Boards of Nursing (NCSBN). Web site: www.ncsbn.org.

National Council of State Boards of Nursing (2007). *2007 NCLEX-RN® detailed test plan.* Chicago: Author.

Potter, P., & Perry, A. (2005). *Fundamentals of nursing* (6th ed.). St. Louis: Mosby.

Stanhope, M., & Lancaster, J. (2008). *Public health nursing: Population-centered health care in the community* (7th ed.). St. Louis: Mosby.

Wong, D., Hockenberry, M., Perry, S., Lowdermilk, D., & Wilson, D. (2006). *Maternal-child nursing care* (3rd ed.). St. Louis: Mosby.

Physiological Integrity

1. A client has an arteriovenous (AV) fistula in place in the right upper extremity for hemodialysis treatments. When planning care for this client, which of the following measures should the nurse implement to promote client safety?

1 Use the fistula for all venipunctures and intravenous infusions.

2 Ensure that small clamps are attached to the AV fistula dressing.

3 Take blood pressures only on the right arm to ensure accuracy.

4 Assess the fistula for the presence of a bruit and thrill every 4 hours.

Level of Cognitive Ability: Application
Client Needs: Physiological Integrity
Integrated Process: Nursing Process/Planning
Content Area: Adult Health/Renal

Answer: 4

Rationale: Arteriovenous fistulas are created by anastomosis of an artery and a vein within the subcutaneous tissues to create access for hemodialysis. Fistulas should be evaluated for presence of thrills (palpate over the area) and bruits (auscultate with a stethoscope) as an assessment of patency.

Test-Taking Strategy: Use the process of elimination and knowledge of arteriovenous fistulas to answer this question. Immediately eliminate option 2 because this refers to care of an AV shunt in which there is an external cannula that can become disconnected. If accidental disconnection occurs, the small clamps can be used to occlude the ends of the cannula. Blood pressure measurement, insertion of intravenous access, and venipuncture should never be performed on the affected extremity because of the potential for infection and clotting of the fistula, thus eliminating options 1 and 3. The only option that relates to this subject is option 4. Review care of the client with an AV fistula if you had difficulty with this question.

Reference
Ignatavicius, D., & Workman, M. (2006). *Medical-surgical nursing: Critical thinking for collaborative care* (5th ed., p. 1755). Philadelphia: Saunders.

2. A client is due in hydrotherapy for a burn dressing change. To ensure that the procedure is most tolerable for the client, the nurse takes which of the following actions?

1 Ensures that the client has a robe and slippers

2 Administers an analgesic 20 minutes before therapy

3 Sends dressing supplies with the client to hydrotherapy

4 Administers the intravenous antibiotic 30 minutes before therapy

Answer: 2

Rationale: The client should receive pain medication approximately 20 minutes before a burn dressing change. This will help the client tolerate an otherwise painful procedure. Antibiotics are timed evenly around the clock and not necessarily in relation to timing of burn dressing changes. Dressing supplies are generally available in the hydrotherapy area and do not need to be sent with the client. A robe and slippers are beneficial for the client's comfort if traveling by wheelchair, but pain medication is more essential.

Test-Taking Strategy: Use Maslow's Hierarchy of Needs theory and focus on the strategic words "most tolerable." This will direct you to option 2. Review care of the burn client if you had difficulty with this question.

Level of Cognitive Ability: Application
Client Needs: Physiological Integrity
Integrated Process: Nursing Process/
   Implementation
Content Area: Adult Health/Integumentary

References

Black, J., & Hawks, J. (2005). *Medical-surgical nursing: Clinical management for positive outcomes* (7th ed., p. 1451). Philadelphia: Saunders.
Monahan, F., Sands, J., Neighbors, M., Marek, J., & Green, C. (2007). *Phipps medical-surgical nursing: Health and illness perspectives* (8th ed., p. 1932). St. Louis: Mosby.

---

3. The nurse is caring for a client with heart failure who has a magnesium level of 1.4 mg/dL. The nurse should:
   1 Monitor the client for irregular heart rhythms.
   2 Encourage the intake of antacids with phosphate.
   3 Teach the client to avoid foods high in magnesium.
   4 Provide a diet of ground beef, eggs, and chicken breast.

Level of Cognitive Ability: Application
Client Needs: Physiological Integrity
Integrated Process: Nursing Process/Planning
Content Area: Fundamental Skills

Answer: 1

Rationale: The normal magnesium level ranges from 1.8 to 3.0 mg/dL. The nurse avoids administering phosphate in the presence of hypomagnesemia because it aggravates the condition. The client should be monitored for dysrhythmias because magnesium plays an important role in myocardial nerve cell impulse conduction; thus, hypomagnesemia increases the client's risk of ventricular dysrhythmias. The nurse instructs the client to consume foods rich in magnesium; ground beef, eggs, and chicken breast are low in magnesium.

Test-Taking Strategy: Recalling the normal magnesium level and noting that the client is experiencing hypomagnesemia will direct you to option 1. Also, use of the ABCs—airway, breathing, and circulation—will direct you to the correct option. Review this electrolyte disorder and its treatment if you had difficulty with this question.

References

Black, J., & Hawks, J. (2005). *Medical-surgical nursing: Clinical management for positive outcomes* (7th ed., p. 1582). Philadelphia. Saunders.
Chernecky, C., & Berger, B. (2008). *Laboratory tests and diagnostic procedures* (5th ed., p. 744). Philadelphia: Saunders.

---

4. A nurse is preparing to care for a client following parathyroidectomy. The nurse plans care anticipating which postoperative order?
   1 Maintain the endotracheal tube for 36 hours.
   2 Take a rectal temperature only until discharge.
   3 Ensure that intravenous calcium preparations are available.
   4 Place the client in a flat position with the head and neck immobilized.

Level of Cognitive Ability: Application
Client Needs: Physiological Integrity
Integrated Process: Nursing Process/Planning
Content Area: Adult Health/Endocrine

Answer: 3

Rationale: Hypocalcemia is a potentially life-threatening complication following parathyroidectomy, and the nurse should ensure that intravenous calcium preparations are readily available. Semi-Fowler's position is the position of choice to assist in lung expansion and prevent edema. Rectal temperatures are not required. Tympanic temperatures can be taken. The client will not necessarily have an endotracheal tube.

Test-Taking Strategy: Eliminate option 2 first because of the close-ended word "only." Next, focusing on the anatomical location of the surgical procedure will assist in eliminating option 4. From the remaining options, recalling that the client will not necessarily have an endotracheal tube and noting the words "36 hours" in option 1 will assist in eliminating this option. Review care of the client following parathyroidectomy if you had difficulty with this question.

Reference
Lewis, S., Heitkemper, M., Dirksen, S., O'Brien, P., & Bucher, L. (2007). *Medical-surgical nursing: Assessment and management of clinical problems* (7th ed., p. 1311). St. Louis: Mosby.

---

5. A client with a wound infection and osteo-myelitis is to receive hyperbaric oxygen therapy. During the therapy, the nurse implements which priority intervention?

1 Maintains an intravenous access
2 Ensures that oxygen is being delivered
3 Provides emotional support to the client's family
4 Administers sedation to prevent claustrophobia

Level of Cognitive Ability: Application
Client Needs: Physiological Integrity
Integrated Process: Nursing Process/ Implementation
Content Area: Delegating/Prioritizing

Answer: 2
Rationale: Hyperbaric oxygen therapy is a process by which oxygen is administered at greater than atmospheric pressure. When oxygen is inhaled under pressure, the level of tissue oxygen is greatly increased. The high levels of oxygen promote the action of phago-cytes and promote healing of the wound. Because the client is placed in a closed chamber, the administration of oxygen is of primary importance. Although options 1, 3, and 4 may be appropriate interventions, option 2 is the priority.

Test-Taking Strategy: Note the strategic word "priority." Use the ABCs—airway, breathing, and circulation—to direct you to option 2. Review nursing care related to this therapy if you had difficulty with this question.

References
Black, J., & Hawks, J. (2005). *Medical-surgical nursing: Clinical management for positive outcomes* (7th ed., p. 414). Philadelphia: Saunders.
Lewis, S., Heitkemper, M., Dirksen, S., O'Brien, P., & Bucher, L. (2007). *Medical-surgical nursing: Assessment and management of clinical problems* (7th ed., p. 1670). St. Louis: Mosby.

---

6. The nurse is caring for a client with a herniated lumbar intervertebral disk. The nurse plans to place the client in which position to minimize the pain?

1 Flat with the knees raised
2 High Fowler's posit1ion with the foot of the bed flat
3 Semi-Fowler's position with the foot of the bed flat
4 Semi-Fowler's position with the knees slightly raised

Level of Cognitive Ability: Application
Client Needs: Physiological Integrity
Integrated Process: Nursing Process/Planning
Content Area: Adult Health/Neurological

Answer: 4
Rationale: Clients with low back pain are often more comfortable in the semi-Fowler's position with the knees raised sufficiently to flex the knees (William's position). This relaxes the muscles of the lower back and relieves pressure on the spinal nerve root. Keeping the foot of the bed flat will enhance extension of the spine. Keeping the bed flat with the knees raised would excessively stretch the lower back and put the client at risk for thrombophlebitis.

Test-Taking Strategy: Use the process of elimination. Focus on the client's diagnosis and the subject, the position that will minimize pain. Visualize each of the positions, noting that option 4 places the least amount of pressure on the spine. Review care of the client with a herniated lumbar intervertebral disk if you had difficulty with this question.

References
Ignatavicius, D., & Workman, M. (2006). *Medical-surgical nursing: Critical thinking for collaborative care* (5th ed., p. 979). Philadelphia: Saunders.
Lewis, S., Heitkemper, M., Dirksen, S., O'Brien, P., & Bucher, L. (2007). *Medical-surgical nursing: Assessment and management of clinical problems* (7th ed., p. 1684). St. Louis: Mosby

7. A mother arrives at the emergency department with her child, stating that she just found the child sitting on the floor next to an empty bottle of aspirin. On assessment, the nurse notes that the child is drowsy but conscious. The nurse anticipates that the physician will prescribe which of the following?
1 Ipecac syrup
2 Activated charcoal
3 Magnesium citrate
4 Magnesium sulfate

Level of Cognitive Ability: Application
Client Needs: Physiological Integrity
Integrated Process: Nursing Process/Planning
Content Area: Child Health

Answer: 2
Rationale: Whereas ipecac is administered to induce vomiting in certain poisoning situations, it is not recommended as the initial treatment in the hospital setting for ingestion of salicylates. This is because ipecac does not totally remove the poison from the child's system. In this situation, the child is conscious and the ingested substance (aspirin) would not damage the esophagus or lungs from vomiting. However, activated charcoal would be prescribed as an antidote in this poisoning situation, because its action is to absorb ingested toxic substances and thus decrease absorption. Options 3 and 4 are unrelated to treatment for this occurrence.

Test-Taking Strategy: Use the process of elimination. Eliminate options 3 and 4 first because they are unrelated to the subject of poisoning. From the remaining options, note that the child is conscious. It is also important to remember that ipecac is not recommended for use in the home setting and that, of the two antidotes remaining, activated charcoal will remove the poisoning from the child's system. This will direct you to option 2. Review measures to treat aspirin poisoning if you had difficulty with this question.

Reference
Hockenberry, M., Wilson, D., & Winkelstein, M. (2005). *Wong's essentials of pediatric nursing* (7th ed., pp. 452-454). St. Louis: Mosby

---

8. A client with myasthenia gravis is admitted to the hospital, and the nursing history reveals that the client is taking pyridostigmine (Mestinon). The nurse assesses the client for side effects of the medication and asks the client about the presence of:
1 Mouth ulcers
2 Muscle cramps
3 Feelings of depression
4 Unexplained weight gain

Level of Cognitive Ability: Application
Client Needs: Physiological Integrity
Integrated Process: Nursing Process/Assessment
Content Area: Pharmacology

Answer: 2
Rationale: Mestinon is an acetylcholinesterase inhibitor. Muscle cramps and small muscle contractions are side effects and occur as a result of overstimulation of neuromuscular receptors. Options 1, 3, and 4 are not associated with this medication.

Test-Taking Strategy: Recall that myasthenia gravis is a neuromuscular disorder. Select the option that is most closely associated with this disorder. This will direct you to option 2. Review the side effects associated with this medication if you had difficulty with this question.

Reference
Skidmore-Roth, L. (2008). *Mosby's nursing drug reference* (21st ed., p. 871). St. Louis: Mosby.

9. A client with a fractured right ankle has a short leg cast applied in the emergency department. During discharge teaching, the nurse provides which information to the client to prevent complications?

1 Trim the rough edges of the cast after it is dry.
2 Weight-bearing on the right leg is allowed once the cast feels dry.
3 Expect burning and tingling sensations under the cast for 3 to 4 days.
4 Keep the right ankle elevated above the heart level with pillows for 24 hours.

Level of Cognitive Ability: Application
Client Needs: Physiological Integrity
Integrated Process: Teaching and Learning
Content Area: Adult Health/Musculoskeletal

Answer: 4

Rationale: Leg elevation is important to increase venous return and decrease edema, which can cause compartment syndrome, a major complication of fractures and casting. Weight-bearing on a fractured extremity is prescribed by the physician during follow-up examination, after radiographs are obtained. Additionally, a walking heel or cast shoe may be added to the cast if the client is allowed to bear weight and walk on the affected leg. Although the client may feel heat after the cast is applied, burning and/or tingling sensations indicate nerve damage or ischemia and are not expected. These complaints should be reported immediately. Option 1 is incorrect. The client and/or family may be taught how to "petal" the cast to prevent skin irritation and breakdown, but rough edges, if trimmed, can fall into the cast and cause a break in skin integrity.

Test-Taking Strategy: Focus on the subject, to prevent complications. Use the process of elimination and the ABCs—airway, breathing, and circulation. Option 4 is associated with maintenance of circulation. Review client teaching points related to cast care if you had difficulty with this question.

References

Ignatavicius, D., & Workman, M. (2006). *Medical-surgical nursing: Critical thinking for collaborative care* (5th ed., p. 1198). Philadelphia: Saunders.
Lewis, S., Heitkemper, M., Dirksen, S., O'Brien, P., & Bucher, L. (2007). *Medical-surgical nursing: Assessment and management of clinical problems* (7th ed., pp. 1646-1647). St. Louis: Mosby.

10. An older adult female client with a fractured left tibia has a long leg cast and is using crutches to ambulate. In caring for the client, the nurse assesses for which sign or symptom that indicates a complication associated with crutch walking?

1 Left leg discomfort
2 Weak biceps brachii
3 Triceps muscle spasms
4 Forearm muscle weakness

Level of Cognitive Ability: Analysis
Client Needs: Physiological Integrity
Integrated Process: Nursing Process/Assessment
Content Area: Adult Health/Musculoskeletal

Answer: 4

Rationale: Forearm muscle weakness is a sign of radial nerve injury caused by crutch pressure on the axillae. When a client lacks upper body strength, especially in the flexor and extensor muscles of the arms, he or she frequently allows weight to rest on the axillae and on the crutch pads instead of using the arms for support while ambulating with crutches. Leg discomfort is expected as a result of the injury. Triceps muscle spasms may occur as a result of increased muscle use but is not a complication of crutch walking. Weak biceps brachii is a common physical assessment finding in older adults and is not a complication of crutch walking.

Test-Taking Strategy: Focus on the subject, a complication of crutch walking. When asked about a complication of the use of crutches, think about nerve injury caused by crutch pressure on the axillae. This will direct you to option 4. Review this complication if you had difficulty with this question.

References

Meiner, S., & Leuckenotte, A. (2006). *Gerontologic nursing* (3rd ed., pp. 604-605). St. Louis: Mosby.
Potter, P., & Perry, A. (2005). *Fundamentals of nursing* (6th ed., pp. 948-949). St. Louis: Mosby.

11. A client with myasthenia gravis is experiencing prolonged periods of weakness, and the physician orders an edrophonium (Tensilon) test. A test dose is administered and the client becomes weaker. The nurse interprets this test result as:
    1 Normal
    2 Positive
    3 Myasthenic crisis
    4 Cholinergic crisis

Level of Cognitive Ability: Analysis
Client Needs: Physiological Integrity
Integrated Process: Nursing Process/Analysis
Content Area: Adult Health/Neurological

Answer: 4
Rationale: A Tensilon test may be performed to determine whether increasing weakness in a previously diagnosed myasthenic client is a result of cholinergic crisis (overmedication with anticholinesterase drugs) or myasthenic crisis (undermedication with cholinesterase inhibitors). Worsening of the symptoms after the test dose of medication is administered indicates a cholinergic crisis.

Test-Taking Strategy: Focus on the subject; the client becomes weaker after edrophonium is administered. Recalling that edrophonium is a short-acting anticholinesterase and that the treatment for myasthenia gravis includes administration of an anticholinesterase will assist in answering the question. If the client's symptoms worsen after administration of edrophonium, then the client is likely experiencing overmedication. Review this test and the interpretation of results if you had difficulty with this question.

References
Chernecky, C., & Berger, B. (2008). *Laboratory tests and diagnostic procedures* (5th ed., pp. 1053-1054). Philadelphia: Saunders.
Ignatavicius, D., & Workman, M. (2006). *Medical-surgical nursing: Critical thinking for collaborative care* (5th ed., p. 1014). Philadelphia: Saunders.

12. The nurse notes an isolated premature ventricular contraction (PVC) on the cardiac monitor. The appropriate nursing action is to:
    1 Prepare for defibrillation.
    2 Continue to monitor the rhythm.
    3 Notify the physician immediately.
    4 Prepare to administer lidocaine hydrochloride (Xylocaine).

Level of Cognitive Ability: Application
Client Needs: Physiological Integrity
Integrated Process: Nursing Process/Implementation
Content Area: Adult Health/Cardiovascular

Answer: 2
Rationale: As an isolated occurrence, the PVC is not life-threatening. In this situation, the nurse should continue to monitor the client. Frequent PVCs, however, may be precursors of more life-threatening rhythms, such as ventricular tachycardia and ventricular fibrillation. If this occurs, the physician needs to be notified.

Test-Taking Strategy: Focus on the information in the question and note the strategic word "isolated." This should direct you to the option that addresses continued monitoring. Also, use of the ABCs—airway, breathing, and circulation—will direct you to option 2. Review the implications of PVCs and the associated interventions if you had difficulty with this question.

References
Black, J., & Hawks, J. (2005). *Medical-surgical nursing: Clinical management for positive outcomes* (7th ed., pp. 1682-1683). Philadelphia: Saunders.
Lewis, S., Heitkemper, M., Dirksen, S., O'Brien, P., & Bucher, L. (2007). *Medical-surgical nursing: Assessment and management of clinical problems* (7th ed., p. 854). St. Louis: Mosby.

13. The nurse is caring for a client admitted to the hospital with the diagnosis of active tuberculosis. The nurse determines that the diagnosis was confirmed by a:
1 Tine test
2 Chest x-ray
3 Mantoux test
4 Sputum culture

Level of Cognitive Ability: Analysis
Client Needs: Physiological Integrity
Integrated Process: Nursing Process/Assessment
Content Area: Adult Health/Respiratory

Answer: 4
Rationale: A sputum culture showing *Mycobacterium tuberculosis* confirms the diagnosis of tuberculosis. Usually three sputum samples are obtained for the acid-fast smear. After the initiation of medication therapy, sputum samples are obtained again to determine the effectiveness of therapy. A positive tine or Mantoux test indicates exposure to tuberculosis but does not confirm the presence of *Mycobacterium tuberculosis*. A positive chest radiograph may indicate the presence of tuberculosis lesions, but again does not confirm active disease.

Test-Taking Strategy: Note the strategic words "active" and "confirmed" in the query of the question. Active tuberculosis can only be confirmed by the presence of the bacilli. The sputum culture is the only method of determining the presence of this organism. Review tests associated with diagnosing tuberculosis if you had difficulty with this question.

Reference
Ignatavicius, D., & Workman, M. (2006). *Medical-surgical nursing: Critical thinking for collaborative care* (5th ed., p. 641). Philadelphia: Saunders.

---

14. A clinic nurse prepares to assess the fundal height on a client who is in the second trimester of pregnancy. When measuring the fundal height, the nurse will most likely expect the measurement to:
1 Be less than gestational age.
2 Correlate with gestational age.
3 Be greater than gestational age.
4 Have no correlation to gestational age.

Level of Cognitive Ability: Analysis
Client Needs: Physiological Integrity
Integrated Process: Nursing Process/Assessment
Content Area: Maternity/Antepartum

Answer: 2
Rationale: Until the third trimester, the measurement of fundal height will, on average, correlate with the gestational age. Options 1, 3, and 4 are incorrect.

Test-Taking Strategy: Note the strategic words "most likely." Focus on the subject, second trimester and fundal height. Recall the correlation of fundal height and gestational age to direct you to option 2. Review this prenatal assessment if you had difficulty with this question.

Reference
Wong, D., Hockenberry, M., Perry, S., Lowdermilk, D., & Wilson, D. (2006). *Maternal-child nursing care.* (3rd ed., p. 273). St. Louis: Mosby.

---

15. A pregnant client tells a nurse that she felt wetness on her peri-pad and found some clear fluid. The nurse immediately inspects the perineum and notes the presence of the umbilical cord. The nurse's initial action is to:
1 Notify the physician.
2 Monitor the fetal heart rate.
3 Transfer the client to the delivery room.
4 Place the client in the Trendelenburg position.

Answer: 4
Rationale: On inspection of the perineum, if the umbilical cord is noted, the nurse immediately places the client in the Trendelenburg position while gently pushing the presenting part upward to relieve the cord compression. This position is maintained and the physician is notified. The nurse monitors the fetal heart rate. The client is transferred to the delivery room when prescribed by the physician.

Test-Taking Strategy: Note the strategic words "presence of the umbilical cord," which indicates the need for an immediate action on the nurse's part to prevent or relieve cord compression. The only action that will achieve this is option 4. The physician is notified after the client is positioned. Review nursing actions for this complication if you had difficulty with this question.

Level of Cognitive Ability: Application
Client Needs: Physiological Integrity
Integrated Process: Nursing Process/
Implementation
Content Area: Maternity/Intrapartum

References
McKinney, E., James, S., Murray, S., & Ashwill, J. (2005). *Maternal-child nursing* (2nd ed., pp. 695-696). St. Louis: Saunders.
Murray, S., & McKinney, E. (2006). *Foundations of maternal-newborn nursing* (4th ed., p. 325). Philadelphia: Saunders.
Wong, D., Hockenberry, M., Perry, S., Lowdermilk, D., & Wilson, D. (2006). *Maternal-child nursing care.* (3rd ed., p. 479). St. Louis: Mosby.

---

16. A nurse admits a newborn infant to the nursery. On assessment of the infant, the nurse palpates the anterior fontanel and notes that it feels soft. The nurse determines that this finding indicates:
    1 Dehydration
    2 A normal finding
    3 Increased intracranial pressure
    4 Decreased intracranial pressure

Level of Cognitive Ability: Analysis
Client Needs: Physiological Integrity
Integrated Process: Nursing Process/Assessment
Content Area: Maternity/Postpartum

Answer: 2
Rationale: The anterior fontanel is normally 2 to 3 cm in width, 3 to 4 cm in length, and diamond-like in shape. It can be described as soft, which is normal, or full and bulging, which could indicate increased intracranial pressure. Conversely, a depressed fontanel could mean that the infant is dehydrated.

Test-Taking Strategy: Use the process of elimination. Focusing on the strategic word "soft" will direct you to option 2. Review the normal findings related to the fontanels if you had difficulty with this question.

References
McKinney, E., James, S., Murray, S., & Ashwill, J. (2005). *Maternal-child nursing* (2nd ed., p. 521). St. Louis: Saunders.
Murray, S., & McKinney, E. (2006). *Foundations of maternal-newborn nursing* (4th ed., p. 479). Philadelphia: Saunders.

---

17. A client with acquired immunodeficiency syndrome (AIDS) is admitted to the hospital for chills, fever, nonproductive cough, and pleuritic chest pain. A diagnosis of *Pneumocystis jiroveci* pneumonia is made and the client is started on intravenous (IV) pentamidine (Pentam-300). Which of the following should the nurse plan to carry out to safely administer the medication?
    1 Infuse over 1 hour and allow the client to ambulate.
    2 Infuse over 1 hour with the client in a supine position.
    3 Administer over 30 minutes with the client in a reclining position.
    4 Administer an IV push over 15 minutes with the client in a supine position.

Level of Cognitive Ability: Application
Client Needs: Physiological Integrity
Integrated Process: Nursing Process/Planning
Content Area: Adult Health/Immune

Answer: 2
Rationale: IV pentamidine is infused over 1 hour with the client supine to minimize severe hypotension and dysrhythmias. Options 1, 3, and 4 are inaccurate in either the length of time that pentamidine is administered or the client's position.

Test-Taking Strategy: Use the process of elimination. Eliminate options 3 and 4 first because these timeframes are very short for an IV medication. From the remaining options, recalling that the medication causes hypotension will direct you to option 2, which addresses both the supine position and the longest time of administration. Review this medication if you had difficulty with this question.

References
Gahart, B., & Nazareno, A. (2006). *2006 Intravenous medications* (22nd ed., p. 969). St. Louis: Mosby.
Hodgson, B., & Kizior, R. (2007). (p. 915). *Saunders nursing drug handbook 2007.* Philadelphia: Saunders.

18. The nurse is caring for a client who has been transferred to the surgical unit after a pelvic exenteration. During the postoperative period, the client complains of pain in the calf area. What action should the nurse take?
   1 Ask the client to walk and observe the gait.
   2 Lightly massage the calf area to relieve the pain.
   3 Check the calf area for temperature, color, and size.
   4 Administer prn morphine as prescribed for postoperative pain.

Level of Cognitive Ability: Application
Client Needs: Physiological Integrity
Integrated Process: Nursing Process/ Implementation
Content Area: Adult Health/Cardiovascular

Answer: 3
Rationale: The nurse monitors for postoperative complications such as deep vein thrombosis, pulmonary emboli, and wound infection. Pain in the calf area could indicate a deep vein thrombosis. Change in color, temperature, or size of the client's calf could also indicate this complication. Options 1 and 2 could result in an embolus if in fact the client had a deep vein thrombosis. Administering pain medication for this client complaint is not the appropriate nursing action. Further assessment needs to take place.

Test-Taking Strategy: Focus on the information in the question and use the steps of the nursing process. Assessment is the first step. Option 3 is the only option that addresses assessment. Review postoperative complications and appropriate interventions if you had difficulty with this question.

Reference
Ignatavicius, D., & Workman, M. (2006). *Medical-surgical nursing: Critical thinking for collaborative care* (5th ed., p. 1848). Philadelphia: Saunders.

---

19. A prenatal client with a history of rheumatic heart disease is experiencing unusual episodes of a nonproductive cough on minimal exertion. The nurse interprets that this assessment finding may be an early manifestation of which potential complication?
   1 Chronic hypertension
   2 Right-sided heart failure
   3 Eisenmenger's syndrome
   4 Cardiac decompensation

Level of Cognitive Ability: Analysis
Client Needs: Physiological Integrity
Integrated Process: Nursing Process/Assessment
Content Area: Maternity/Antepartum

Answer: 4
Rationale: A cough that occurs with minimal exertion is a sign of pulmonary edema, which leads to cardiac decompensation in a pregnant client who has a history of rheumatic heart disease. Elevated blood pressure would be the assessment finding for a client with chronic hypertension. Eisenmenger's syndrome is a right-to-left or bidirectional shunting with elevated pulmonary vascular resistance, thus a nonproductive cough would be a late manifestation of this complication. A nonproductive cough is also a late manifestation of right-sided heart failure.

Test-Taking Strategy: Note the strategic words "early manifestation." An early subjective symptom and objective sign of cardiac decompensation for a pregnant client with a cardiac disorder is a frequent cough that worsens with exertion. Review the signs of cardiac decompensation for a pregnant client with an underlying cardiac disorder if you had difficulty with this question.

References
Lowdermilk, D., & Perry, A. (2006). *Maternity nursing* (7th ed., p. 695). St. Louis: Mosby.
Murray, S., & McKinney, E. (2006). *Foundations of maternal-newborn nursing* (4th ed., pp. 672, 676). Philadelphia: Saunders.

---

20. A nurse is performing an assessment on a client with a diagnosis of chronic angina pectoris who is receiving sotalol (Betapace) 80 mg orally daily. Which assessment finding indicates that the client is experiencing a side effect of the medication?
   1 Dry mouth
   2 Palpitations
   3 Diaphoresis
   4 Difficulty swallowing

Answer: 2
Rationale: Sotalol is a beta-adrenergic blocking agent. Side effects include bradycardia, palpitations, an irregular heartbeat, difficulty breathing, signs of congestive heart failure, and cold hands and feet. Gastrointestinal disturbances, anxiety and nervousness, and unusual tiredness and weakness can also occur. Options 1, 3, and 4 are not side effects of this medication.

Level of Cognitive Ability: Analysis
Client Needs: Physiological Integrity
Integrated Process: Nursing Process/Assessment
Content Area: Pharmacology

Test-Taking Strategy: Note that the question presents a client with chronic angina pectoris, a cardiac disorder. Remember that medication names ending with "lol" (sotalol) are beta-blockers, which are commonly used for cardiac disorders. Note that option 2 is the only option that is directly cardiac related. Review the side effects of sotalol if you had difficulty with this question.

References
Hodgson, B., & Kizior, R. (2007). *Saunders nursing drug handbook 2007.* (p. 1073). Philadelphia: Saunders.
Skidmore-Roth, L. (2008). *Mosby's nursing drug reference* (21st ed., p. 939). St. Louis: Mosby.

---

21. Before performing a venipuncture to initiate continuous intravenous (IV) therapy, a nurse should:
   1 Inspect the IV solution and expiration date.
   2 Apply a cool compress to the affected area.
   3 Secure a padded armboard above the IV site.
   4 Apply a tourniquet below the venipuncture site.

Level of Cognitive Ability: Application
Client Needs: Physiological Integrity
Integrated Process: Nursing Process/ Implementation
Content Area: Fundamental Skills

Answer: 1
Rationale: IV solutions should be free of particles or precipitates to prevent trauma to veins or a thromboembolic event; in addition, the nurse avoids administering IV solutions whose expiration date has passed to prevent infection. A tourniquet is applied above the chosen vein site to halt venous return and engorge the vein; this makes the vein easier to puncture. Cool compresses cause vasoconstriction, making the vein less visible, smaller, and more difficult to puncture. Arm boards are applied after the IV is started and are used only if necessary.

Test-Taking Strategy: Note the strategic word "before" and use the steps of the nursing process. Option 1 is the only option that reflects assessment, the first step of the nursing process. Review nursing interventions related to initiating an IV if you had difficulty with this question.

Reference
Potter, P., & Perry, A. (2005). *Fundamentals of nursing* (6th ed., pp. 1162, 1164). St. Louis: Mosby.

---

22. A nurse is caring for a client who had an allogenic liver transplant and is receiving tacrolimus (Prograf) daily. Which finding indicates to the nurse that the client is experiencing an adverse reaction to the medication?
   1 Hypotension
   2 Photophobia
   3 Profuse sweating
   4 Decrease in urine output

Level of Cognitive Ability: Analysis
Client Needs: Physiological Integrity
Integrated Process: Nursing Process/Assessment
Content Area: Pharmacology

Answer: 4
Rationale: Tacrolimus is an immunosuppressant medication used in the prophylaxis of organ rejection in clients receiving allogenic liver transplants. Frequent side effects include headache, tremor, insomnia, paresthesia, diarrhea, nausea, constipation, vomiting, abdominal pain, and hypertension. Adverse reactions and toxic effects include nephrotoxicity and pleural effusion. Nephrotoxicity is characterized by an increasing serum creatinine level and a decrease in urine output.

Test-Taking Strategy: First, determine the medication classification. Note the client's diagnosis and look at the medication name Prograf, "Pro" meaning "for" and "graf" meaning "graft," to identify the action of the medication: to prevent transplant rejection. This will assist in identifying the medication classification as immunosuppressant. Next, recalling that nephrotoxicity is an adverse effect of the medication will direct you to option 4. Review the adverse effects of this medication if you had difficulty with this question.

References
Hodgson, B., & Kizior, R. (2007). *Saunders nursing drug handbook 2007.* (p. 1093). Philadelphia: Saunders.
Lehne, R. (2007). *Pharmacology for nursing care.* (6th ed., p. 800). St. Louis: Saunders.

---

23. A client was admitted to the hospital 24 hours ago after sustaining blunt chest trauma. The nurse monitors for which earliest clinical manifestation of acute respiratory distress syndrome (ARDS)?
  1 Cyanosis and pallor
  2 Diffuse crackles and rhonchi on chest auscultation
  3 Increase in respiratory rate from 18 to 30 breaths per minute
  4 Haziness or "white-out" appearance of lungs on chest radiograph

Level of Cognitive Ability: Analysis
Client Needs: Physiological Integrity
Integrated Process: Nursing Process/Assessment
Content Area: Adult Health/Respiratory

Answer: 3
Rationale: Acute respiratory distress syndrome usually develops within 24 to 48 hours after an initiating event, such as chest trauma. In most cases, tachypnea and dyspnea are the earliest clinical manifestations as the body compensates for mild hypoxemia through hyperventilation. Cyanosis and pallor are late findings and are the result of severe hypoxemia. Breath sounds in the early stages of ARDS are usually clear but then progress to diffuse crackles and rhonchi as pulmonary edema occurs. Chest radiographic findings may be normal during the early stages but will show diffuse haziness or "white-out" appearance in the later stages.

Test-Taking Strategy: Note the strategic words "earliest clinical manifestation." Remember that with ARDS initial presenting symptoms are tachypnea, dyspnea, and restlessness as hypoxia develops. Knowing the definition of tachypnea and possible etiologies will direct you to option 3. Review the early clinical manifestations of ARDS if you had difficulty with this question.

References
Ignatavicius, D., & Workman, M. (2006). *Medical-surgical nursing: Critical thinking for collaborative care* (5th ed., pp. 658-659). Philadelphia: Saunders.
Lewis, S., Heitkemper, M., Dirksen, S., O'Brien, P., & Bucher, L. (2007). *Medical-surgical nursing: Assessment and management of clinical problems* (7th ed., pp. 524, 1813, 1815). St. Louis: Mosby.

---

24. A nurse is caring for a client with Buck's traction and is monitoring the client for complications of the traction. Which assessment finding indicates a complication?
  1 Weak pedal pulses
  2 Drainage at the pin sites
  3 Complaints of discomfort
  4 Warm toes with brisk capillary refill

Level of Cognitive Ability: Analysis
Client Needs: Physiological Integrity
Integrated Process: Nursing Process/Analysis
Content Area: Adult Health/Musculoskeletal

Answer: 1
Rationale: Weak pedal pulses are a sign of vascular compromise, which can be caused by pressure on the tissues of the leg by the elastic bandage or prefabricated boot used to secure this type of traction.

Test-Taking Strategy: Use the process of elimination and prioritization of care to answer this question. Eliminate option 2 because Buck's traction does not use pins. Discomfort is an expected finding, so option 3 can be eliminated. Eliminate option 4 because warm toes with brisk capillary refill are normal findings. Focus on the ABCs—airway, breathing, and circulation—to direct you to option 1, indicative of vascular compromise. Review care of the client with Buck's traction if you had difficulty with this question.

References
Ignatavicius, D., & Workman, M. (2006). *Medical-surgical nursing: Critical thinking for collaborative care* (5th ed., p. 1201). Philadelphia: Saunders.
Monahan, F., Sands, J., Neighbors, M., Marek, J., & Green, C. (2007). *Phipps' medical-surgical nursing: Health and illness perspectives* (8th ed., p. 1535). St. Louis: Mosby.

25. A prenatal client has been diagnosed with a vaginal infection from the organism *Candida albicans*. Which finding(s) should the nurse expect to note on assessment of the client?
1 Costovertebral angle pain
2 Pain, itching, and vaginal discharge
3 Absence of any signs and symptoms
4 Proteinuria, hematuria, edema, and hypertension

Level of Cognitive Ability: Analysis
Client Needs: Physiological Integrity
Integrated Process: Nursing Process/Assessment
Content Area: Maternity/Antepartum

Answer: 2
Rationale: Clinical manifestations of a *Candida* infection include pain, itching, and a thick, white vaginal discharge. Proteinuria, edema, and hypertension are signs of gestational hypertension. Hematuria, proteinuria, and costovertebral angle pain are clinical manifestations associated with urinary tract infections.

Test-Taking Strategy: Use the process of elimination, focusing on the subject: vaginal infection. Note the relationship between the subject and option 2. Review the signs of a vaginal *Candida* infection if you had difficulty with this question.

Reference
Murray, S., & McKinney, E. (2006). *Foundations of maternal-newborn nursing* (4th ed., pp. 910-911). Philadelphia: Saunders.

---

26. A prenatal client is suspected of having iron deficiency anemia. Which finding should the nurse expect to note regarding the client's status?
1 Excess fluid volume
2 Deficient fluid volume
3 A low hemoglobin and hematocrit level
4 A high hemoglobin and hematocrit level

Level of Cognitive Ability: Analysis
Client Needs: Physiological Integrity
Integrated Process: Nursing Process/Assessment
Content Area: Maternity/Antepartum

Answer: 3
Rationale: When the hemoglobin level is below 11 mg/dL, iron deficiency is suspected. An indirect index of the oxygen-carrying capacity is the packed red blood cell volume or hematocrit level. Pathological anemia of pregnancy is primarily caused by iron deficiency. Options 1 and 2 are nursing diagnoses that are not noted in iron deficiency anemia.

Test-Taking Strategy: Use the process of elimination. Note the words "deficiency" in the question and "low" in option 3. Review the manifestations of iron deficiency anemia if you had difficulty with this question.

Reference
Murray, S., & McKinney, E. (2006). *Foundations of maternal-newborn nursing* (4th ed., p. 677). Philadelphia: Saunders.

---

27. A nurse is caring for a postpartum client. Which finding would make the nurse suspect endometritis in this client?
1 Breast engorgement
2 Elevated white blood cell count
3 Lochia rubra on the second day postpartum
4 Fever over 38° C, beginning 2 days postpartum

Level of Cognitive Ability: Analysis
Client Needs: Physiological Integrity
Integrated Process: Nursing Process/ Assessment
Content Area: Maternity/Postpartum

Answer: 4
Rationale: The presence of fever of 38° C or more on 2 successive days of the first 10 postpartum days (not counting the first 24 hours after birth) is indicative of a postpartum infection. Endometritis is the most common cause of postpartum infection until proven otherwise. Lochia rubra on the second day postpartum is a normal finding. The white blood cell count of a postpartum woman is normally elevated. Thus, this method of detecting infection is not of great value in the puerperium. Breast engorgement is also a normal response in the postpartum period and is not associated with endometritis.

Test-Taking Strategy: Use the process of elimination, focusing on the subject: endometritis. Recalling the normal findings in the postpartum period will assist in eliminating options 1, 2, and 3. Review the signs of endometritis if you had difficulty with this question.

References

Murray, S., & McKinney, E. (2006). *Foundations of maternal-newborn nursing* (4th ed., pp. 747-748). Philadelphia: Saunders.

Wong, D., Hockenberry, M., Perry, S., Lowdermilk, D., & Wilson, D. (2006). *Maternal-child nursing care* (3rd ed., p. 668). St. Louis: Mosby.

---

28. A nurse is performing an assessment on a postterm infant. Which physical characteristic should the nurse expect to observe?

1 Peeling of the skin
2 Smooth soles without creases
3 Lanugo covering the entire body
4 Vernix that covers the body in a thick layer

Level of Cognitive Ability: Analysis
Client Needs: Physiological Integrity
Integrated Process: Nursing Process/Assessment
Content Area: Maternity/Postpartum

Answer: 1

Rationale: The postterm infant (born after the 42nd week of gestation) exhibits dry, peeling, cracked, almost leather-like skin over the body, which is called *desquamation.* The preterm infant (born between 24 and 37 weeks of gestation) exhibits thick vernix covering the body, smooth soles without creases, and lanugo covering the entire body.

Test-Taking Strategy: Use the process of elimination, focusing on the subject—the postterm infant. Recalling that the postterm infant is born after the 42nd week of gestation will direct you to option 1. Review the characteristics of preterm and postterm infants if you had difficulty with this question.

References

McKinney, E., James, S., Murray, S., & Ashwill, J. (2005). *Maternal-child nursing* (2nd ed., p. 741). St. Louis: Saunders.

Murray, S., & McKinney, E. (2006). *Foundations of maternal-newborn nursing* (4th ed., pp. 499-500). Philadelphia: Saunders.

---

29. A postterm infant, delivered vaginally, is exhibiting tachypnea, grunting, retractions, and nasal flaring. The nurse interprets that these assessment findings are indicative of:

1 Hypoglycemia
2 Respiratory distress syndrome
3 Meconium aspiration syndrome
4 Transient tachypnea of the newborn

Level of Cognitive Ability: Analysis
Client Needs: Physiological Integrity
Integrated Process: Nursing Process/Analysis
Content Area: Maternity/Postpartum

Answer: 3

Rationale: Tachypnea, grunting, retractions, and nasal flaring are symptoms of respiratory distress related to meconium aspiration syndrome (MAS). MAS occurs often in postterm infants and develops when meconium in the amniotic fluid enters the lungs during fetal life or at birth. Transient tachypnea of the newborn is primarily found in infants delivered via cesarean section. Respiratory distress syndrome is a complication of preterm infants. The symptoms noted in the question are unrelated to hypoglycemia.

Test-Taking Strategy: Use the process of elimination, focusing on the symptoms identified in the question. Option 1 is eliminated first because hypoglycemia is not a respiratory condition. From the remaining options, recalling the complications that can occur in a postterm infant will direct you to option 3. Review these complications if you had difficulty with this question.

References

McKinney, E., James, S., Murray, S., & Ashwill, J. (2005). *Maternal-child nursing* (2nd ed., pp. 741, 746-748). St. Louis: Saunders.

Murray, S., & McKinney, E. (2006). *Foundations of maternal-newborn nursing* (4th ed., pp. 804-805). Philadelphia: Saunders.

30. A nurse is caring for a client who had an orthopedic injury of the leg requiring surgery and application of a cast. Postoperatively, which nursing assessment is of highest priority?
1 Monitoring for heel breakdown
2 Monitoring for bladder distention
3 Monitoring for extremity shortening
4 Monitoring for loss of blanching ability of toe nailbeds

Level of Cognitive Ability: Analysis
Client Needs: Physiological Integrity
Integrated Process: Nursing Process/Assessment
Content Area: Delegating/Prioritizing

Answer: 4
Rationale: With cast application, concern for compartment syndrome development is of the highest priority. If postsurgical edema compromises circulation, the client will demonstrate numbness, tingling, loss of blanching of toenail beds, and pain that will not be relieved by opioids. Although bladder distention, extremity lengthening or shortening, or heel breakdown can occur, these complications are not potentially life-threatening complications.

Test-Taking Strategy: Use the ABCs—airway, breathing, and circulation—to answer the question. Assessment for circulation to the foot, including observations for numbness and tingling as well as ability of the nailbeds to blanch, will direct you to option 4. Review postoperative assessment following orthopedic surgery if you had difficulty with this question.

References
Black, J., & Hawks, J. (2005). *Medical-surgical nursing: Clinical management for positive outcomes* (7th ed., pp. 1483, 1537). Philadelphia: Saunders.
Ignatavicius, D., & Workman, M. (2006). *Medical-surgical nursing: Critical thinking for collaborative care* (5th ed., p. 343). Philadelphia: Saunders.

31. A nurse is caring for a client who is receiving cyclosporine (Gengraf). Which of the following indicates to the nurse that the client is experiencing an adverse reaction to the medication?
1 Acne
2 Sweating
3 Joint pain
4 Hyperkalemia

Level of Cognitive Ability: Analysis
Client Needs: Physiological Integrity
Integrated Process: Nursing Process/Analysis
Content Area: Pharmacology

Answer: 4
Rationale: Cyclosporine is an immunosuppressant medication used in the prophylaxis of organ rejection. Adverse effects include nephrotoxicity, infection, hypertension, tremor, and hirsutism. Additionally, neurotoxicity, gastrointestinal effects, hyperkalemia, and hyperglycemia can occur. Options 1, 2, and 3 are not associate with this medication.

Test-Taking Strategy: Focus on the name of the medication to recall that it is an immunosuppressant used to prevent organ rejection. Next, use the process of elimination and remember that this medication causes hyperkalemia. Review the adverse effects of this medication if you had difficulty with the question.

Reference
Hodgson, B., & Kizior, R. (2007). *Saunders nursing drug handbook 2007* (p. 302). Philadelphia: Saunders.

32. A nurse is caring for a client with hypertension receiving torsemide (Demadex) 5 mg orally daily. Which of the following would indicate to the nurse that the client might be experiencing an adverse reaction related to the medication?
1 A chloride level of 98 mEq/L
2 A sodium level of 135 mEq/L
3 A potassium level of 3.1 mEq/L
4 A blood urea nitrogen (BUN) of 15 mg/dL

Level of Cognitive Ability: Analysis
Client Needs: Physiological Integrity
Integrated Process: Nursing Process/Analysis
Content Area: Pharmacology

Answer: 3
Rationale: Torsemide (Demadex) is a loop diuretic. The medication can produce acute, profound water loss, volume and electrolyte depletion, dehydration, decreased blood volume, and circulatory collapse. Option 3 is the only option that indicates an electrolyte depletion because the normal potassium level is 3.5 to 5.1 mEq/L. The normal sodium level is 135 to 145 mEq/L. The normal chloride level is 98 to 107 mEq/L. The normal blood BUN is 5 to 20 mg/dL.

Test-Taking Strategy: Use the process of elimination and knowledge of normal laboratory values to assist in selecting option 3, because this is the only abnormal laboratory value presented. Review this content if you are unfamiliar with this medication or these normal laboratory values.

Reference
Hodgson, B., & Kizior, R. (2007). *Saunders nursing drug handbook 2007* (p. 1156). Philadelphia: Saunders.

33. During history taking of a client admitted with newly diagnosed Hodgkin's disease, which of the following would the nurse expect the client to report?
1 Weight gain
2 Night sweats
3 Severe lymph node pain
4 Headache with minor visual changes

Level of Cognitive Ability: Analysis
Client Needs: Physiological Integrity
Integrated Process: Nursing Process/Assessment
Content Area: Adult Health/Oncology

Answer: 2
Rationale: Assessment of a client with Hodgkin's disease most often reveals enlarged, painless lymph nodes, fever, malaise, and night sweats. Weight loss may be present if metastatic disease occurs. Headache and visual changes may occur if brain metastasis is present.

Test-Taking Strategy: Use the process of elimination. Eliminate options 3 and 4 first because they are comparable or alike in that they relate to discomfort. Weight gain is rarely the symptom of a cancer diagnosis, so eliminate option 1. Review content related to Hodgkin's disease if you had difficulty with this question.

References
Black, J., & Hawks, J. (2005). *Medical-surgical nursing: Clinical management for positive outcomes* (7th ed., p. 2412). Philadelphia: Saunders.
Lewis, S., Heitkemper, M., Dirksen, S., O'Brien, P., & Bucher, L. (2007). *Medical-surgical nursing: Assessment and management of clinical problems* (7th ed., p. 723). St. Louis: Mosby.

34. A nurse is assessing a 3-day-old preterm neonate with a diagnosis of respiratory distress syndrome (RDS). Which assessment finding indicates that the neonate's respiratory status is improving?
1 Edema of the hands and feet
2 Presence of a systolic murmur
3 Urine output of 1 to 3 mL/kg/hour
4 Respiratory rate between 60 and 70 breaths per minute

Level of Cognitive Ability: Analysis
Client Needs: Physiological Integrity
Integrated Process: Nursing Process/Evaluation
Content Area: Maternity/Postpartum

Answer: 3
Rationale: Increased urination is an early sign that the neonate's respiratory condition is improving. Lung fluid, which occurs in RDS, moves from the lungs into the bloodstream as the condition improves and the alveoli open. This extra fluid circulates to the kidneys, which results in increased voiding. Systolic murmurs usually indicate the presence of a patent ductus arteriosus, which is a common complication of RDS. Respiratory rates above 60 are indicative of tachypnea, which is a sign of respiratory distress. Edema of the hands and feet occurs within the first 24 hours as a result of low protein concentrations, a decrease in colloidal osmotic pressure, and transudation of fluid from the vascular system to the tissues.

Test-Taking Strategy: Use the process of elimination. Note the subject: respiratory status is improving. Option 3 is the only normal finding and indicates a normal urine output, which would indicate resolution of excess lung fluid. Review content related to RDS if you had difficulty answering the question.

References
McKinney, E., James, S., Murray, S., & Ashwill, J. (2005). *Maternal-child nursing* (2nd ed., p. 726). St. Louis: Saunders.
Murray, S., & McKinney, E. (2006). *Foundations of maternal-newborn nursing* (4th ed., p. 770). Philadelphia: Saunders.

35. A nurse is caring for a term newborn. Which assessment finding would predispose the newborn to the occurrence of jaundice?
1 Presence of a cephalhematoma
2 Infant blood type of O negative
3 Birth weight of 8 pounds 6 ounces
4 A negative direct Coombs' test result

Level of Cognitive Ability: Analysis
Client Needs: Physiological Integrity
Integrated Process: Nursing Process/Assessment
Content Area: Maternity/Postpartum

Answer: 1
Rationale: Enclosed hemorrhage, such as with cephalhematoma, predisposes the newborn to jaundice by producing an increased bilirubin load as the cephalhematoma resolves and is absorbed into the circulatory system. A negative direct Coombs' test result indicates that there are no maternal antibodies on fetal erythrocytes. The birth weight in option 3 is within the acceptable range for a term newborn and therefore does not contribute to an increased bilirubin level. The classic Rh incompatibility situation involves an Rh-negative mother with an Rh-positive fetus/newborn.

Test-Taking Strategy: Use the process of elimination. Recalling the risk factors associated with jaundice and the association between hemorrhage and jaundice will direct you to option 1. Review the risk factors associated with jaundice if you had difficulty with this question.

References
McKinney, E., James, S., Murray, S., & Ashwill, J. (2005). *Maternal-child nursing* (2nd ed., p. 529). St. Louis: Saunders.
Murray, S., & McKinney, E. (2006). *Foundations of maternal-newborn nursing* (4th ed., p. 480). Philadelphia: Saunders.

---

36. Which assessment is most important for the nurse to make before advancing a client from liquid to solid food?
1 Bowel sounds
2 Chewing ability
3 Current appetite
4 Food preferences

Level of Cognitive Ability: Analysis
Client Needs: Physiological Integrity
Integrated Process: Nursing Process/Assessment
Content Area: Fundamental Skills

Answer: 2
Rationale: It may be necessary to modify a client's diet to a soft or mechanical chopped diet if the client has difficulty chewing because of the risk of aspiration. Food preferences should be ascertained on admission assessment. Appetite will affect the amount of food eaten, but not the type of diet ordered. Bowel sounds should be present before introducing any diet, including liquids.

Test-Taking Strategy: Use the process of elimination. Focusing on the subject, advancing a diet from liquid to solid, will direct you to option 2 because the primary difference between a liquid and a solid diet is that the food needs mechanical processing before it can be safely swallowed. Review nursing considerations related to dietary measures if you had difficulty with this question.

References
Grodner, M., Long, S., & DeYoung, S. (2004). *Foundations and clinical applications of nutrition: A nursing approach* (3rd ed., pp. 416-417). St. Louis: Mosby.
Lewis, S., Heitkemper, M., Dirksen, S., O'Brien, P., & Bucher, L. (2007). *Medical-surgical nursing: Assessment and management of clinical problems* (7th ed., p. 1544). St. Louis: Mosby.

37. A nurse is assessing a client who is diagnosed with cystitis. Which assessment finding is inconsistent with the typical clinical manifestations noted in this disorder?
1 Hematuria
2 Low back pain
3 Urinary retention
4 Burning on urination

Level of Cognitive Ability: Analysis
Client Needs: Physiological Integrity
Integrated Process: Nursing Process/Assessment
Content Area: Adult Health/Renal

Answer: 3
Rationale: Clinical manifestations of cystitis usually include urinary frequency, urgency, dysuria, inability to void, or voiding only small amounts. The urine may be cloudy, with hematuria and bacteriuria. The client may complain of pain that is suprapubic or in the lower back. Nonspecific signs include fever, chills, malaise, and nausea and vomiting. Some clients may be asymptomatic, particularly the older client.

Test-Taking Strategy: Use the process of elimination. Noting the strategic word "inconsistent" guides you to look for an incorrect option. First, eliminate options 1 and 4, because they are commonly associated with cystitis. From the remaining options, recalling that urgency and frequency, not urinary retention, are signs of cystitis directs you to select option 3. Review the clinical manifestations of cystitis if you had difficulty with this question.

Reference
Ignatavicius, D., & Workman, M. (2006). *Medical-surgical nursing: Critical thinking for collaborative care* (5th ed., p. 1681). Philadelphia: Saunders.

---

38. The nurse is caring for an obese client on a weight loss program. Which method should the nurse use to most accurately assess the program's effectiveness?
1 Monitor intake and output.
2 Check serum protein levels.
3 Calculate daily caloric intake.
4 Weigh the client after toileting.

Level of Cognitive Ability: Analysis
Client Needs: Physiological Integrity
Integrated Process: Nursing Process/Assessment
Content Area: Fundamental Skills

Answer: 4
Rationale: The most accurate measurement of weight loss is weighing of the client at the same time of the day, in the same clothes, and using the same scale. Options 1, 2, and 3 measure nutrition and hydration status.

Test-Taking Strategy: Use the process of elimination. Focus on the subject, weight loss, and note the strategic words "most accurately assess." Assessing weight will most accurately identify weight changes. Review care of the client on a weight loss program if you had difficulty with this question.

Reference
Lewis, S., Heitkemper, M., Dirksen, S., O'Brien, P., & Bucher, L. (2007). *Medical-surgical nursing: Assessment and management of clinical problems* (7th ed., p. 979). St. Louis: Mosby.

---

39. A client has fallen and sustained a leg injury. Which question would the nurse ask the client to help determine if the injury caused a fracture?
1 "Is the pain a dull ache?"
2 "Is the pain sharp and continuous?"
3 "Does the discomfort feel like a cramp?"
4 "Does the pain feel like the muscle was stretched?"

Answer: 2
Rationale: Fracture pain is generally described as sharp, continuous, and increasing in frequency. Bone pain is often described as a dull, deep ache. Strains result from trauma to a muscle body or to the attachment of a tendon from overstretching or overextension. Muscle injury is often described as an aching or cramping pain, or soreness.

Test-Taking Strategy: Use the process of elimination, focusing on the subject—a fracture. Recalling that a new injury such as a fracture is more likely to be described as sharp will direct you to option 2. Review the clinical manifestations of a fracture if you had difficulty with this question.

Level of Cognitive Ability: Application
Client Needs: Physiological Integrity
Integrated Process: Nursing Process/Assessment
Content Area: Adult Health/Musculoskeletal

References
Black, J., & Hawks, J. (2005). *Medical-surgical nursing: Clinical management for positive outcomes* (7th ed., pp. 622, 652). Philadelphia: Saunders.
Monahan, F., Sands, J., Neighbors, M., Marek, J., & Green, C. (2007). *Phipps' Medical-surgical nursing: Health and illness perspectives* (8th ed., pp. 1524-1525). St. Louis: Mosby.

---

40. Which of the following arterial blood gases (ABGs) should the nurse anticipate in the client with a nasogastric tube attached to continuous suction?
  1 pH 7.25 P_{CO_2} 55, HCO_3 24
  2 pH 7.30 P_{CO_2} 38, HCO_3 20
  3 pH 7.48 P_{CO_2} 30, HCO_3 23
  4 pH 7.49 P_{CO_2} 38, HCO_3 30

Level of Cognitive Ability: Analysis
Client Needs: Physiological Integrity
Integrated Process: Nursing Process/Analysis
Content Area: Fundamental Skills

Answer: 4
Rationale: The anticipated arterial blood gas in the client with a nasogastric tube to continuous suction is metabolic alkalosis due to loss of acid. In uncompensated metabolic alkalosis the pH will be elevated (greater than 7.45), bicarbonate will be elevated (greater than 27 mEq/mL), and the P_{CO_2} will be within normal limits (35 to 45 mm Hg).

Test-Taking Strategy: Focus on the data in the question and note that the question addresses a gastrointestinal situation. Eliminate options 1 and 2 because they both identify a respiratory imbalance. From the remaining options, remember that acid will be removed with nasogastric suctioning, so an alkalotic condition will result. This will direct you to option 4. Review ABG analysis and causes of acid base disturbances if you had difficulty with this question.

Reference
Lewis, S., Heitkemper, M., Dirksen, S., O'Brien, P., & Bucher, L. (2007). *Medical-surgical nursing: Assessment and management of clinical problems* (7th ed., pp. 335, 337). St. Louis: Mosby.

---

41. A nurse obtains a fingerstick glucose reading of 425 mg/dL on a client who was recently started on parenteral nutrition (PN). What nursing action is appropriate at this time?
  1 Stop the PN.
  2 Administer insulin.
  3 Notify the physician.
  4 Decrease the flow rate of the PN.

Level of Cognitive Ability: Application
Client Needs: Physiological Integrity
Integrated Process: Nursing Process/Implementation
Content Area: Fundamental Skills

Answer: 3
Rationale: Hyperglycemia is a complication of PN, and the nurse reports abnormalities to the physician. Options 1, 2, and 4 are not done without a physician's order.

Test-Taking Strategy: Use the process of elimination. Note that options 1, 2, and 4 are not within the scope of nursing practice and require a physician's order. A blood glucose greater than 400 mg/dL requires notification of the physician. Review the complications associated with PN if you had difficulty with this question.

Reference
Ignatavicius, D., & Workman, M. (2006). *Medical-surgical nursing: Critical thinking for collaborative care* (5th ed., p. 1433). Philadelphia: Saunders.

42. A client with urolithiasis is scheduled for extracorporeal shock wave lithotripsy (ESWL). The nurse assesses to ensure that which of the following items are in place or maintained before sending the client for the procedure?
1 IV line and a Foley catheter
2 NPO status and a Foley catheter
3 Signed informed consent, NPO status, and an IV line
4 Signed informed consent and clear liquid restriction preprocedure

Level of Cognitive Ability: Analysis
Client Needs: Physiological Integrity
Integrated Process: Nursing Process/Assessment
Content Area: Adult Health/Renal

Answer: 3
Rationale: ESWL is done with conscious sedation or general anesthesia. The client must sign an informed consent form for the procedure and must be NPO for the procedure. The client needs an IV line for the procedure as well. A Foley catheter is not needed.

Test-Taking Strategy: Use the process of elimination. Begin to answer by eliminating options 1 and 2, because a Foley catheter is not needed for this procedure. From the remaining options, recalling that the procedure is invasive and that the client is premedicated before the procedure will direct you to option 3. Review the preprocedure preparation for ESWL if you had difficulty with this question.

Reference
Ignatavicius, D., & Workman, M. (2006). *Medical-surgical nursing: Critical thinking for collaborative care* (5th ed., pp. 304, 1699). Philadelphia: Saunders.

---

43. A client has developed atrial fibrillation and has a ventricular rate of 150 beats per minute. The nurse assesses the client for:
1 Flat neck veins
2 Nausea and vomiting
3 Hypotension and dizziness
4 Hypertension and headache

Level of Cognitive Ability: Analysis
Client Needs: Physiological Integrity
Integrated Process: Nursing Process/Assessment
Content Area: Adult Health/Cardiovascular

Answer: 3
Rationale: The client with uncontrolled atrial fibrillation with a ventricular rate over 100 beats per minute is at risk for low cardiac output caused by loss of atrial kick. The nurse assesses the client for palpitations, chest pain or discomfort, hypotension, pulse deficit, fatigue, weakness, dizziness, syncope, shortness of breath, and distended neck veins.

Test-Taking Strategy: Use the process of elimination. Recalling that flat neck veins are normal or indicate hypovolemia will assist in eliminating option 1. Remembering that nausea and vomiting are associated with vagus nerve activity, not a tachycardic state, will assist you in eliminating option 2. From the remaining options, thinking of the effects of a falling cardiac output will direct you to option 3. Review the symptoms related to atrial fibrillation if you had difficulty with this question.

Reference
Ignatavicius, D., & Workman, M. (2006). *Medical-surgical nursing: Critical thinking for collaborative care* (5th ed., p. 728). Philadelphia: Saunders.

---

44. A preschooler with a history of cleft palate repair comes to the clinic for a routine well-child checkup. To determine whether this child is experiencing a long-term effect of cleft palate, the nurse asks the parent which question?
1 "Does the child play with an imaginary friend?"
2 "Was the child recently treated for pneumonia?"
3 "Is the child unresponsive when given directions?"
4 "Has the child had any difficulty swallowing food?"

Answer: 3
Rationale: Unresponsiveness may be an indication that the child is experiencing hearing loss. A child who has a history of cleft palate should be routinely checked for hearing loss. Options 2 and 4 are unrelated to cleft palate after repair. Option 1 is normal behavior for a preschool child. Many preschoolers with vivid imaginations have imaginary friends.

Test-Taking Strategy: Use the process of elimination, focusing on the subject—a long-term effect. Recalling that hearing loss can occur in a child with cleft palate will direct you to option 3. Review the long-term effects of cleft palate if you had difficulty with this question.

Level of Cognitive Ability: Analysis
Client Needs: Physiological Integrity
Integrated Process: Nursing Process/Assessment
Content Area: Child Health

References
Hockenberry, M., & Wilson, D. (2007). *Nursing care of infants and children* (8th ed., p. 465). St. Louis: Mosby.
McKinney, E., James, S., Murray, S., & Ashwill, J. (2005). *Maternal-child nursing* (2nd ed., p. 1111). St. Louis: Saunders.

---

45. A nurse is performing a respiratory assessment on a client being treated for an asthma attack. The nurse determines that the client's respiratory status is worsening if which of the following occurs?
1 Loud wheezing
2 Wheezing on expiration
3 Noticeably diminished breath sounds
4 Wheezing during inspiration and expiration

Level of Cognitive Ability: Analysis
Client Needs: Physiological Integrity
Integrated Process: Nursing Process/Analysis
Content Area: Adult Health/Respiratory

Answer: 3
Rationale: Noticeably diminished breath sounds are an indication of severe obstruction and impending respiratory failure. Wheezing is not a reliable manifestation to determine the severity of an asthma attack. Clients with minor attacks may experience loud wheezes, whereas others with severe attacks may not wheeze. The client with severe asthma attacks may have no audible wheezing because of the decrease of airflow. For wheezing to occur, the client must be able to move sufficient air to produce breath sounds. Wheezing usually occurs first on expiration. As the asthma attack progresses, the client may wheeze during both inspiration and expiration.

Test-Taking Strategy: Use the ABCs—airway, breathing, and circulation. Note the strategic words "client's respiratory status is worsening." Remember that diminished breath sounds indicate obstruction and impending respiratory failure; this will direct you to select option 3. Review care of the client experiencing an asthma attack if you had difficulty with this question.

References
Ignatavicius, D., & Workman, M. (2006). *Medical-surgical nursing: Critical thinking for collaborative care* (5th ed., p. 587). Philadelphia: Saunders.
Lewis, S., Heitkemper, M., Dirksen, S., O'Brien, P., & Bucher, L. (2007). *Medical-surgical nursing: Assessment and management of clinical problems* (7th ed., p. 612). St. Louis: Mosby.

---

46. The nurse is assessing the casted extremity of a client for signs of infection. Which of the following findings is indicative of infection?
1 Dependent edema
2 Diminished distal pulse
3 Coolness and pallor of the skin
4 Presence of a "hot spot" on the cast

Level of Cognitive Ability: Application
Client Needs: Physiological Integrity
Integrated Process: Nursing Process/Assessment
Content Area: Adult Health/Musculoskeletal

Answer: 4
Rationale: Signs and symptoms of infection under a casted area include a musty odor or purulent drainage from the cast or the presence of "hot spots," which are areas on the cast that are warmer than others. The physician should be notified if any of these occur.

Test-Taking Strategy: Use the process of elimination. Eliminate options 1, 2, and 3 because coolness and pallor of the skin, diminished arterial pulse, and edema all signify impaired circulation in the distal extremity. Focus on the subject—infection. Thinking about the signs of infection (i.e., redness, swelling, heat, and drainage) will direct you to option 4. The "hot spot" on the cast could signify infection underneath that area. Review the signs and symptoms of infection if you had difficulty with this question.

References
Black, J., & Hawks, J. (2005). *Medical-surgical nursing: Clinical management for positive outcomes* (7th ed., pp. 633-634). Philadelphia: Saunders.
Monahan, F., Sands, J., Neighbors, M., Marek, J., & Green, C. (2007). *Phipps' medical-surgical nursing: Health and illness perspectives* (8th ed., p. 1536). St. Louis: Mosby.

47. A home care nurse assesses a client with chronic obstructive pulmonary disease (COPD) who is complaining of increased dyspnea. The client is on home oxygen via a concentrator at 2 L per minute, and the client's respiratory rate is 22 breaths per minute. The appropriate nursing action is to:

1 Determine the need to increase the oxygen.

2 Reassure the client that there is no need to worry.

3 Conduct further assessment of the client's respiratory status.

4 Call emergency services to take the client to the emergency department.

Level of Cognitive Ability: Application
Client Needs: Physiological Integrity
Integrated Process: Nursing Process/ Implementation
Content Area: Adult Health/Respiratory

Answer: 3

Rationale: Obtaining further assessment data is the appropriate nursing action. Reassuring the client that there is "no need to worry" is inappropriate. Calling emergency services is a premature action. Oxygen is not increased without the approval of the physician, especially because the client with COPD can retain carbon dioxide.

Test-Taking Strategy: Use the process of elimination. Eliminate option 2 first because it is an inappropriate communication technique and dismisses the client's complaint of dyspnea. Option 4 can be eliminated because calling emergency services is a premature action and no data supports the notion that an emergency exists. Remember that oxygen is not increased without physician approval, and there is no evidence to support that the client is exhibiting tissue hypoxia. Recalling the steps of the nursing process will direct you to option 3. Review care of the client with COPD if you had difficulty with this question.

Reference
Black, J., & Hawks, J. (2005). *Medical-surgical nursing: Clinical management for positive outcomes* (7th ed., p. 1822). Philadelphia: Saunders.

---

48. A client with schizophrenia tells the nurse, "I stopped taking my chlorpromazine (Thorazine) because of the way it made me feel." Which side effect is the nurse likely to note during further assessment of the client's complaint?

1 Drowsiness

2 Nervousness

3 Hand tremors

4 Increased urination

Level of Cognitive Ability: Analysis
Client Needs: Physiological Integrity
Integrated Process: Nursing Process/Assessment
Content Area: Pharmacology

Answer: 1

Rationale: Side effects of chlorpromazine can include hypotension, dizziness and fainting especially with parenteral use, drowsiness, blurred vision, dry mouth, lethargy, constipation or diarrhea, nasal congestion, peripheral edema, and urinary retention. Options 2, 3, and 4 are not side effects of chlorpromazine.

Test-Taking Strategy: Use the process of elimination. Eliminate options 2 and 3 first because they are comparable or alike. Next, focus on the name of the medication. Recall that most phenothiazine medication names end with "zine" and that a side effect of these medications is drowsiness. Review this information if you are unfamiliar with the side effects of this medication.

Reference
Hodgson, B., & Kizior, R. (2007). *Saunders nursing drug handbook 2007* (p. 242). Philadelphia: Saunders.

---

49. The home care nurse is making follow-up visits to a client following renal transplant. The nurse assesses the client for which signs of acute graft rejection?

1 Hypotension, graft tenderness, and anemia

2 Hypertension, oliguria, thirst, and hypothermia

3 Fever, hypertension, graft tenderness, and malaise

4 Fever, vomiting, hypotension, and copious amounts of dilute urine

Answer: 3

Rationale: Acute rejection usually occurs within the first 3 months after transplant, although it can occur for up to 2 years post-transplant. The client exhibits fever, hypertension, malaise, and graft tenderness. Treatment is immediately begun with corticosteroids and possibly also with monoclonal antibodies and antilymphocyte agents.

Level of Cognitive Ability: Analysis
Client Needs: Physiological Integrity
Integrated Process: Nursing Process/Assessment
Content Area: Adult Health/Renal

Test-Taking Strategy: Use the process of elimination. Begin to answer this question by eliminating options 1 and 4, because hypotension is not part of the clinical picture with graft rejection. Additionally, option 4 can be eliminated because the client rejecting a transplanted kidney would experience oliguria versus copious amounts of urine output. From the remaining options, recalling that fever rather than hypothermia accompanies this complication will direct you to option 3. Review the signs of acute graft rejection if you had difficulty with this question.

References

Black, J., & Hawks, J. (2005). *Medical-surgical nursing: Clinical management for positive outcomes* (7th ed., p. 969). Philadelphia: Saunders.

Ignatavicius, D., & Workman, M. (2006). *Medical-surgical nursing: Critical thinking for collaborative care* (5th ed., p. 1762). Philadelphia: Saunders.

50. A nurse is caring for a client diagnosed with a skin infection who is receiving tobramycin sulfate (Nebcin) intravenously every 8 hours. Which of the following would indicate to the nurse that the client is experiencing an adverse reaction related to the medication?
1 A total bilirubin of 0.5 mg/dL
2 A sedimentation rate of 15 mm/hour
3 A blood urea nitrogen (BUN) of 30 mg/dL
4 A white blood cell count (WBC) of 6000 cells/mm³

Level of Cognitive Ability: Analysis
Client Needs: Physiological Integrity
Integrated Process: Nursing Process/Analysis
Content Area: Pharmacology

Answer: 3
Rationale: Adverse reactions or toxic effects of tobramycin sulfate include nephrotoxicity as evidenced by an increased BUN and serum creatinine; irreversible ototoxicity as evidenced by tinnitus, dizziness, ringing or roaring in the ears, and reduced hearing; and neurotoxicity as evidenced by headaches, dizziness, lethargy, tremors, and visual disturbances. A normal WBC is 4500 to 11,000 cells/mm³. The normal sedimentation rate is 0 to 30 mm/hour. The normal total bilirubin level is less than 1.5 mg/dL. The normal BUN is 5 to 20 mg/dL.

Test-Taking Strategy: Use the process of elimination and knowledge of normal laboratory values to assist in directing you to option 3, because this is the only abnormal laboratory value presented in the options. Review this content if you are unfamiliar with this medication or these laboratory values.

References

Gahart, B., & Nazareno, A. (2006). *2006 Intravenous medications* (22nd ed., p. 1174). St. Louis: Mosby.

Lehne, R. (2007). *Pharmacology for nursing care* (6th ed., p. 1000). St. Louis: Saunders.

51. A nurse hears the alarm sound on the telemetry monitor, looks at the monitor, and notes that a client is in ventricular tachycardia. The nurse rushes to the client's room. Upon reaching the client's bedside, the nurse would take which action first?
1 Call a code.
2 Prepare for cardioversion.
3 Prepare to defibrillate the client.
4 Check the client's level of consciousness.

Answer: 4
Rationale: Determining unresponsiveness is the first assessment action to take. When a client is in ventricular tachycardia, there is a significant decrease in cardiac output. However, assessing for unresponsiveness helps to determine whether the client is affected by the decreased cardiac output. If the client is unconscious, then the ABCDs—airway, breathing, circulation, defibrillation—of cardiopulmonary resuscitation or basic life support are initiated.

Level of Cognitive Ability: Application
Client Needs: Physiological Integrity
Integrated Process: Nursing Process/
  Implementation
Content Area: Delegating/Prioritizing

Test-Taking Strategy: Note the strategic word "first." Use the steps of cardiopulmonary resuscitation or basic life support to answer the question. Remember that determining unresponsiveness is the first action. Review the nursing actions that you should take if a client experiences ventricular tachycardia, if you had difficulty with this question.

References
Black, J., & Hawks, J. (2005). *Medical-surgical nursing: Clinical management for positive outcomes* (7th ed., pp. 1682-1685). Philadelphia: Saunders.
Ignatavicius, D., & Workman, M. (2006). *Medical-surgical nursing: Critical thinking for collaborative care* (5th ed., pp. 729, 731). Philadelphia: Saunders.

---

52. The nurse assesses a preoperative client. Which question should the nurse ask the client, to help determine the client's risk for developing malignant hyperthermia in the perioperative period?

1 "Have you ever had heat exhaustion or heat stroke?"

2 "What is the normal range for your body temperature?"

3 "Do you or any of your family members have frequent infections?"

4 "Do any of your family members have problems with general anesthesia?"

Level of Cognitive Ability: Application
Client Needs: Physiological Integrity
Integrated Process: Nursing Process/Assessment
Content Area: Fundamental Skills

Answer: 4
Rationale: Malignant hyperthermia is a genetic disorder in which a combination of anesthetic agents (the muscle relaxant succinylcholine and inhalation agents such as halothanes) trigger uncontrolled skeletal muscle contractions that can quickly lead to a potentially fatal hyperthermia. Questioning the client about the family history of general anesthesia problems may reveal this as a risk for the client. Options 1, 2, and 3 are unrelated to this surgical complication.

Test-Taking Strategy: Use the process of elimination. Recalling that this disorder is genetic will direct you to option 4. Review the characteristics of malignant hyperthermia if you had difficulty with this question.

References
Black, J., & Hawks, J. (2005). *Medical-surgical nursing: Clinical management for positive outcomes* (7th ed., p. 298). Philadelphia: Saunders.
Monahan, F., Sands, J., Neighbors, M., Marek, J., & Green, C. (2007). *Phipps' medical-surgical nursing: Health and illness perspectives* (8th ed., p. 287). St. Louis: Mosby.

---

53. A client has developed oral mucositis as a result of radiation to the head and neck. The nurse should teach the client to incorporate which of the following measures in his or her daily home care routine?

1 Oral hygiene should be performed in the morning and evening.

2 High-protein foods such as peanut butter should be incorporated in the diet.

3 A glass of wine per day will not pose any further harm to the oral cavity.

4 A combination of a weak saline and water solution should be used to rinse the mouth before and after each meal.

Answer: 4
Rationale: Oral mucositis (irritation, inflammation, and/or ulceration of the mucosa) commonly occurs in clients receiving radiation to the head and neck. Measures need to be taken to soothe the mucosa as well as provide effective cleansing of the oral cavity. A combination of a weak saline and water solution is an effective cleansing agent.

Test-Taking Strategy: Knowing the definition of mucositis will help you to eliminate incorrect options. First, eliminate option 3, knowing that alcohol will have a further drying and irritating effect on the mucosa. Next, eliminate option 2, knowing that although high-protein foods are necessary, peanut butter would not be a good choice because of its consistency. From the remaining options, choose option 4 over option 1 because of the frequency. Review the care of the client experiencing mucositis if you had difficulty with this question.

Level of Cognitive Ability: Application
Client Needs: Physiological Integrity
Integrated Process: Teaching and Learning
Content Area: Adult Health/Oncology

References
Ignatavicius, D., & Workman, M. (2006). *Medical-surgical nursing: Critical thinking for collaborative care* (5th ed., p. 496). Philadelphia: Saunders.
Lewis, S., Heitkemper, M., Dirksen, S., O'Brien, P., & Bucher, L. (2007). *Medical-surgical nursing: Assessment and management of clinical problems* (7th ed., p. 298). St. Louis: Mosby.

---

54. A nursing instructor has taught a student about the protective structures of the brain and asks the student to identify the membranes that surround the brain and spinal cord. The student responds correctly by stating that these are the:

1 Meninges
2 Basal ganglia
3 Gray matter areas
4 Corticospinal tract

Level of Cognitive Ability: Comprehension
Client Needs: Physiological Integrity
Integrated Process: Teaching and Learning
Content Area: Adult Health/Neurological

Answer: 1

Rationale: The meninges, three membranes that surround the brain and spinal cord, are predominantly for protection. Each layer (pia mater, arachnoid, and dura mater) is a separate membrane. The basal ganglia consist of subcortical gray matter buried deep in the cerebral hemispheres. The basal ganglia, along with the corticospinal tract, is important in controlling complex motor activity.

Test-Taking Strategy: Focus on the subject, the membranes that surround the brain and spinal cord. Eliminate options 2, 3, and 4 because they have a similar function and are important in controlling complex motor activity. Review the anatomy and physiology of the brain if you had difficulty with this question.

Reference
Black, J., & Hawks, J. (2005). *Medical-surgical nursing: Clinical management for positive outcomes* (7th ed., pp. 2002-2004). Philadelphia: Saunders.

---

55. A client has been taking an antihypertensive for approximately 2 months. A home care nurse monitoring the effects of therapy determines that drug tolerance has developed if which of the following are noted in the client?

1 Decrease in weight
2 Output greater than intake
3 Decrease in blood pressure
4 Gradual rise in blood pressure

Level of Cognitive Ability: Analysis
Client Needs: Physiological Integrity
Integrated Process: Nursing Process/Assessment
Content Area: Pharmacology

Answer: 4

Rationale: Drug tolerance can develop in a client taking an antihypertensive, which is evident by rising blood pressure levels. The physician should be notified, who may then increase the medication dosage or add a diuretic to the medication regimen. The client is also at risk of developing fluid retention, which would be manifested as dependent edema, intake greater than output, and an increase in weight. This would also warrant adding a diuretic to the course of therapy.

Test-Taking Strategy: Use the process of elimination. Recall the definition of drug tolerance; that is, as one adjusts to a medication, the therapeutic effect diminishes. These concepts will direct you to option 4. Review the definition of drug tolerance if you had difficulty with this question.

References
Hodgson, B., & Kizior, R. (2007). *Saunders nursing drug handbook 2007* (pp. 753-754). Philadelphia: Saunders.
McKenry, L., Tressier, E., & Hogan, M. (2006). *Mosby's pharmacology in nursing* (22nd ed., p. 565). St. Louis: Mosby.

56. A client with a known history of panic disorder comes to the emergency department and states to the nurse, "Please help me. I think I'm having a heart attack." What is the priority nursing action?
1 Check the client's vital signs.
2 Encourage the client to use relaxation techniques.
3 Identify the manifestations related to the panic disorder.
4 Determine what the client's activity involved when the pain started.

Level of Cognitive Ability: Application
Client Needs: Physiological Integrity
Integrated Process: Nursing Process/
   Implementation
Content Area: Mental Health

Answer: 1
Rationale: Clients with panic disorders can experience acute physical symptoms, such as chest pain and palpitations. The priority is to assess the client's physical condition to rule out a physiological disorder. Although options 2, 3, and 4 may be appropriate at some point in the care of the client, they are not the priority.

Test-Taking Strategy: Use Maslow's Hierarchy of Needs theory, recalling that physiological needs are the priority. Also, use of the ABCs—airway, breathing, and circulation—will direct you to option 1. Review care of the client with a panic disorder who develops physiological manifestations if you had difficulty with this question.

References
Ignatavicius, D., & Workman, M. (2006). *Medical-surgical nursing: Critical thinking for collaborative care* (5th ed., pp. 755-756). Philadelphia: Saunders.
Varcarolis, E., Carson, V., & Shoemaker, N. (2006). *Foundations of psychiatric mental health nursing* (5th ed., p. 233). Philadelphia: Saunders.

---

57. A client with trigeminal neuralgia (tic douloureux) asks the nurse for a snack and something to drink. Which of the following selections should the nurse provide for the client?
1 Hot cocoa with honey and toast
2 Vanilla wafers and lukewarm milk
3 Hot herbal tea with graham crackers
4 Iced coffee and peanut butter and crackers

Level of Cognitive Ability: Application
Client Needs: Physiological Integrity
Integrated Process: Nursing Process/
   Implementation
Content Area: Adult Health/Neurological

Answer: 2
Rationale: Because mild tactile stimulation of the face of clients with trigeminal neuralgia can trigger pain, the client needs to eat or drink lukewarm, nutritious foods that are soft and easy to chew. Extremes of temperature will cause trigeminal pain.

Test-Taking Strategy: Use the process of elimination. Note the similarity between options 1, 3, and 4. These options contain hot or iced items and foods that are mechanically difficult to chew and swallow. Review care of the client with trigeminal neuralgia if you had difficulty with this question.

References
Black, J., & Hawks, J. (2005). *Medical-surgical nursing: Clinical management for positive outcomes* (7th ed., pp. 2153-2154). Philadelphia: Saunders.
Lewis, S., Heitkemper, M., Dirksen, S., O'Brien, P., & Bucher, L. (2007). *Medical-surgical nursing: Assessment and management of clinical problems* (7th ed., p. 1583). St. Louis: Mosby.

---

58. A child is admitted to the orthopedic nursing unit after spinal rod insertion for the treatment of scoliosis. Which assessment is most important in the immediate postoperative period?
1 Pain level
2 Ability to flex and extend the feet
3 Ability to turn using the logroll technique
4 Capillary refill, sensation, and motion in all extremities

Answer: 4
Rationale: When the spinal column is manipulated during surgery, altered neurovascular status is a possible complication; therefore, neurovascular checks including circulation, sensation, and motion should be done at least every 2 hours. Level of pain is an important postoperative assessment, but circulatory status is more important. Assessment of flexion and extension of the lower extremities is a component of option 4, which includes checking motion. Logrolling is performed by nurses.

Level of Cognitive Ability: Analysis
Client Needs: Physiological Integrity
Integrated Process: Nursing Process/Assessment
Content Area: Child Health

Test-Taking Strategy: Use the ABCs—airway, breathing, and circulation—and the process of elimination. Option 4 addresses circulatory status. Review priority nursing assessments following spinal rod insertion if you had difficulty with this question.

References

Hockenberry, M., Wilson, D., & Winkelstein, M. (2005). *Wong's essentials of pediatric nursing* (7th ed., p. 1176). St. Louis: Mosby.
McKinney, E., James, S., Murray, S., & Ashwill, J. (2005). *Maternal-child nursing* (2nd ed., p. 1444). St. Louis: Saunders.

---

59. A nurse has just finished assisting the physician in placing a central intravenous (IV) line. Which of the following is a priority nursing intervention after central line insertion?

 1 Prepare the client for a chest radiograph.
 2 Assess the client's temperature to monitor for infection.
 3 Label the dressing with the date and time of catheter insertion.
 4 Monitor the blood pressure (BP) to assess for fluid volume overload.

Level of Cognitive Ability: Application
Client Needs: Physiological Integrity
Integrated Process: Nursing Process/ Implementation
Content Area: Delegating/Prioritizing

Answer: 1

Rationale: A major risk associated with central line placement is the possibility of a pneumothorax developing from an accidental puncture of the lung. Assessing the results of a chest radiograph is one of the best methods to determine if this complication has occurred and to verify catheter tip placement before initiating intravenous (IV) therapy. A temperature elevation related to central line insertion would not likely occur immediately after placement. Labeling the dressing site is important but is not the priority. Although BP assessment is always important in assessing a client's status after an invasive procedure, fluid volume overload is not a concern until IV fluids are started.

Test-Taking Strategy: Use the process of elimination and note the strategic words "has just finished" and "priority nursing intervention." Recall that assessment of accurate placement is essential before initiating IV therapy. Review care of the client following central line placement if you had difficulty with this question.

Reference

Ignatavicius, D., & Workman, M. (2006). *Medical-surgical nursing: Critical thinking for collaborative care* (5th ed., p. 255). Philadelphia: Saunders.

---

60. A nurse is admitting a client suspected of having tuberculosis (TB) to the hospital. The nurse understands that the most accurate method for confirming the diagnosis is:

 1 A chest radiograph positive for lung lesions
 2 A positive purified protein derivative test (PPD)
 3 A sputum culture positive for *Mycobacterium tuberculosis*
 4 Obtaining data about the client's long history of hemoptysis

Level of Cognitive Ability: Analysis
Client Needs: Physiological Integrity
Integrated Process: Nursing Process/Assessment
Content Area: Adult Health/Respiratory

Answer: 3

Rationale: The most accurate means of confirming the diagnosis of TB is by sputum culture. Establishing the presence of *Mycobacterium tuberculosis* is essential for a definitive diagnosis. Hemoptysis is not a common finding and is usually associated with more advanced cases of TB. A positive PPD indicates exposure to TB. A chest radiograph does not confirm the diagnosis of TB. Lung lesions may be indicative of diseases other than TB.

Test-Taking Strategy: Note the strategic words "confirming the diagnosis." Consider which test or data would be most definitive. The actual presence of *Mycobacterium tuberculosis* in the sputum culture is the most accurate method, directing you to option 3. Review the diagnostic tests related to TB if you had difficulty with this question.

Reference

Ignatavicius, D., & Workman, M. (2006). *Medical-surgical nursing: Critical thinking for collaborative care* (5th ed., p. 641). Philadelphia: Saunders.

61. A child has just returned from surgery and has a hip spica cast. A priority nursing action at this time is to:
1 Elevate the head of the bed.
2 Abduct the hips, using pillows.
3 Turn the child on the right side.
4 Assess the child's circulatory status.

Level of Cognitive Ability: Application
Client Needs: Physiological Integrity
Integrated Process: Nursing Process/ Implementation
Content Area: Child Health

Answer: 4
Rationale: During the first few hours after a cast is applied, the chief concern is swelling that may cause the cast to act as a tourniquet and obstruct circulation, resulting in compartment syndrome. Therefore, circulatory assessment is the priority. Elevating the head of the bed of a child in a hip spica cast would cause discomfort. Using pillows to abduct the hips is not necessary because a hip spica cast immobilizes the hip and knee. Turning the child side to side at least every 2 hours is important because it allows the body cast to dry evenly and prevents complications related to immobility; however, it is not a higher priority than checking circulation.

Test-Taking Strategy: Use the process of elimination and the ABCs—airway, breathing, and circulation—to answer this question. Also, use the nursing process to answer this question. Because assessment is the first step in the nursing process, it is likely that the priority is to assess. Review nursing care following application of a spica cast if you had difficulty with this question.

Reference
Hockenberry, M., Wilson, D., & Winkelstein, M. (2005). *Wong's essentials of pediatric nursing* (7th ed., pp. 1157-1158). St. Louis: Mosby.

62. A nurse is assessing a client with a brainstem injury. In addition to performing the Glasgow Coma Scale, the nurse plans to:
1 Perform arterial blood gases.
2 Assist with a lumbar puncture.
3 Perform a pulmonary wedge pressure.
4 Check cranial nerve functioning and respiratory rate and rhythm.

Level of Cognitive Ability: Application
Client Needs: Physiological Integrity
Integrated Process: Nursing Process/Planning
Content Area: Adult Health/Neurological

Answer: 4
Rationale: Assessment should be specific to the area of the brain involved. Assessing the respiratory status and cranial nerve function is a critical component of the assessment process in a client with a brainstem injury. Options 1, 2, and 3 are not necessary, based on the data in the question.

Test-Taking Strategy: Use the process of elimination. Recall the anatomical location of the respiratory center to direct you to option 4. Remember that the respiratory center is located in the brainstem. Review content and nursing care related to brainstem injuries if you had difficulty with this question.

References
Ignatavicius, D., & Workman, M. (2006). *Medical-surgical nursing: Critical thinking for collaborative care* (5th ed., pp. 1044, 1049). Philadelphia: Saunders.
Monahan, F., Sands, J., Neighbors, M., Marek, J., & Green, C. (2007). *Phipp's medical-surgical nursing: Health and illness perspectives* (8th ed., p. 1383). St. Louis: Mosby.

63. A client has had a Miller-Abbott tube in place for 24 hours. Which assessment finding indicates that the tube is located in the intestine?
1 The client is nauseous.
2 Bowel sounds are absent.
3 Aspirate from the tube has a pH of 7.
4 The abdominal radiograph report indicates that the end of the tube is above the pylorus.

Answer: 3
Rationale: The Miller-Abbott tube is a nasoenteric tube that is used to decompress the intestine and to correct a bowel obstruction. The end of the tube should be located in the intestine. The pH of the gastric fluid is acidic, and the pH of the intestinal fluid is alkaline (7 or higher). Location of the tube can also be determined by radiographs.

Level of Cognitive Ability: Analysis
Client Needs: Physiological Integrity
Integrated Process: Nursing Process/Analysis
Content Area: Adult Health/Gastrointestinal

Test-Taking Strategy: Use the process of elimination. Focus on the subject—a Miller-Abbott tube and its intestinal location. Recalling that intestinal fluid is alkaline will direct you to option 3. Review the purpose and nursing care of a client with a Miller-Abbott tube if you had difficulty with this question.

References
Black, J., & Hawks, J. (2005). *Medical-surgical nursing: Clinical management for positive outcomes* (7th ed., p. 745). Philadelphia: Saunders.
Ignatavicius, D., & Workman, M. (2006). *Medical-surgical nursing: Critical thinking for collaborative care* (5th ed., p. 1329). Philadelphia: Saunders.

---

64. While a client with myxedema is being admitted to the hospital, the client reports having experienced a lack of energy, cold intolerance, and puffiness around the eyes and face. The nurse knows that these symptoms are caused by a lack of production of which hormone(s)?

1 Luteinizing hormone (LH)
2 Adrenocorticotropic hormone (ACTH)
3 Triiodothyronine (T_3) and thyroxine (T_4)
4 Prolactin (PRL) and growth hormone (GH)

Level of Cognitive Ability: Comprehension
Client Needs: Physiological Integrity
Integrated Process: Nursing Process/Analysis
Content Area: Adult Health/Endocrine

Answer: 3
Rationale: Although all of these hormones originate from the anterior pituitary, only T_3 and T_4 are associated with the client's symptoms. Myxedema results from inadequate thyroid hormone levels (T_3 and T_4). Low levels of thyroid hormone result in an overall decrease in the basal metabolic rate, affecting virtually every body system and leading to weakness, fatigue, and a decrease in heat production. A decrease in LH results in the loss of secondary sex characteristics. A decrease in ACTH is seen in Addison's disease. PRL stimulates breast milk production by the mammary glands, and GH affects bone and soft tissue by promoting growth through protein anabolism and lipolysis.

Test-Taking Strategy: Use the process of elimination. Recalling that myxedema is associated with the thyroid gland will assist in making a relationship between what the question is asking about and option 3. Review content and laboratory values related to myxedema if you had difficulty with this question.

Reference
Lewis, S., Heitkemper, M., Dirksen, S., O'Brien, P., & Bucher, L. (2007). *Medical-surgical nursing: Assessment and management of clinical problems* (7th ed., p. 1306). St. Louis: Mosby.

---

65. A 33-year old female is admitted to the hospital with a suspected diagnosis of Graves' disease. Which symptom related to the client's menstrual cycle would the client likely report?

1 Amenorrhea
2 Metrorrhagia
3 Menorrhagia
4 Dysmenorrhea

Level of Cognitive Ability: Analysis
Client Needs: Physiological Integrity
Integrated Process: Nursing Process/Assessment
Content Area: Adult Health/Endocrine

Answer: 1
Rationale: Amenorrhea or a decreased menstrual flow is common in the client with Graves' disease. Dysmenorrhea, metrorrhagia, and menorrhagia are also disorders related to the female reproductive system; however, they do not manifest in the presence of Graves' disease.

Test-Taking Strategy: Focus on the client's suspected diagnosis. Thinking about the pathophysiology associated with Graves' disease will direct you to option 1. Review the clinical manifestations of Graves' disease if you had difficulty with this question.

References
Ignatavicius, D., & Workman, M. (2006). *Medical-surgical nursing: Critical thinking for collaborative care* (5th ed., p. 1488). Philadelphia: Saunders.
Lewis, S., Heitkemper, M., Dirksen, S., O'Brien, P., & Bucher, L. (2007). *Medical-surgical nursing: Assessment and management of clinical problems* (7th ed., p. 1300). St. Louis: Mosby.

66. A client with gestational hypertension (GH) is in active labor. The nurse most likely expects to note which assessment finding?
1 Negative proteinuria
2 Increased urine output
3 Increased blood pressure
4 Decreased brachial reflexes

Level of Cognitive Ability: Analysis
Client Needs: Physiological Integrity
Integrated Process: Nursing Process/Assessment
Content Area: Maternity/Intrapartum

Answer: 3
Rationale: The major symptom of GH is increased blood pressure. As the disease progresses, it is possible that increased brachial reflexes, decreased fetal heart rate and variability, and decreased urine output will occur, particularly during labor.

Test-Taking Strategy: Use the process of elimination. Noting the name of the disorder will easily direct you to option 3. Review the manifestations associated with GH if you had difficulty with this question.

References
McKinney, E., James, S., Murray, S., & Ashwill, J. (2005). *Maternal-child nursing* (2nd ed., p. 631). St. Louis: Saunders.
Wong, D., Hockenberry, M., Perry, S., Lowdermilk, D., & Wilson, D. (2006). *Maternal-child nursing care.* (3rd ed., pp. 371-372). St. Louis: Mosby.

---

67. A nurse has just administered a purified protein derivative (PPD) skin test to a client who is at low risk for developing tuberculosis. The nurse determines that the test is positive if which of the following occurs?
1 An induration of 15 mm
2 The presence of a wheal
3 A large area of erythema
4 Client complains of constant itching

Level of Cognitive Ability: Analysis
Client Needs: Physiological Integrity
Integrated Process: Nursing Process/Assessment
Content Area: Adult Health/Respiratory

Answer: 1
Rationale: An induration of 15 mm or more is considered positive for clients in low-risk groups. Erythema is not a positive reaction. The presence of a wheal would indicate that the skin test was administered appropriately. Itching is not an indication of a positive PPD.

Test-Taking Strategy: Focus on the subject—a positive test—and note that the client is at low risk for developing tuberculosis. This will direct you to option 1. Review the interpretation of PPD results if you had difficulty with this question.

References
Black, J., & Hawks, J. (2005). *Medical-surgical nursing: Clinical management for positive outcomes* (7th ed., p. 1846). Philadelphia: Saunders.
Chernecky, C., & Berger, B. (2008). *Laboratory tests and diagnostic procedures* (5th ed., pp. 758-759). Philadelphia: Saunders.

---

68. A nurse is performing an otoscopic examination on a client with a suspected diagnosis of mastoiditis. The nurse would expect to note which of the following if this disorder was present?
1 A mobile tympanic membrane
2 A transparent tympanic membrane
3 A pearly colored tympanic membrane
4 A thick and immobile tympanic membrane

Level of Cognitive Ability: Analysis
Client Needs: Physiological Integrity
Integrated Process: Nursing Process/Assessment
Content Area: Adult Health/Ear

Answer: 4
Rationale: Otoscopic examination in a client with mastoiditis reveals a red, dull, thick, and immobile tympanic membrane with or without perforation. Options 1, 2, and 3 indicate normal findings in an otoscopic examination.

Test-Taking Strategy: Use the process of elimination and knowledge of normal assessment findings on an ear examination to direct you to option 4, the only abnormal finding. Review the assessment findings associated with this disorder if you had difficulty with this question.

References
Black, J., & Hawks, J. (2005). *Medical-surgical nursing: Clinical management for positive outcomes* (7th ed., p. 1983). Philadelphia: Saunders.
Ignatavicius, D., & Workman, M. (2006). *Medical-surgical nursing: Critical thinking for collaborative care* (5th ed., p. 1130). Philadelphia: Saunders.

69. A nurse is reviewing the record of a client with a disorder involving the inner ear. Which of the following would the nurse most likely expect to note documented as an assessment finding in this client?
1 Complaints of tinnitus
2 Complaints of burning in the ear
3 Complaints of itching in the affected ear
4 Complaints of severe pain in the affected ear

Level of Cognitive Ability: Analysis
Client Needs: Physiological Integrity
Integrated Process: Nursing Process/Assessment
Content Area: Adult Health/Ear

Answer: 1
Rationale: Tinnitus is the most common complaint of clients with ear disorders, especially disorders involving the inner ear. Symptoms of tinnitus can range from mild ringing in the ear that can go unnoticed during the day to a loud roaring in the ear that can interfere with the client's thinking process and attention span. The assessment findings noted in options 2, 3, and 4 are not specifically noted in the client with an inner ear disorder.

Test-Taking Strategy: Focus on the subject—inner ear disorder. Recalling the function of the inner ear will direct you to option 1. Review this content if you had difficulty with this question or are unfamiliar with the signs and symptoms associated with an inner ear disorder.

Reference
Ignatavicius, D., & Workman, M. (2006). *Medical-surgical nursing: Critical thinking for collaborative care* (5th ed., p. 1131). Philadelphia: Saunders.

---

70. A nurse has an order to administer hydroxyzine (Vistaril) to a client by the intramuscular route. Before administering the medication, the nurse tells the client that:
1 Excessive salivation is a side effect.
2 There will be some pain at the injection site.
3 There will be relief from nausea within 5 minutes
4 The client will have increased alertness for about 2 hours.

Level of Cognitive Ability: Application
Client Needs: Physiological Integrity
Integrated Process: Nursing Process/ Implementation
Content Area: Pharmacology

Answer: 2
Rationale: Hydroxyzine is an antiemetic and sedative/hypnotic that may be used in conjunction with opioid analgesics for added effect. The injection can be extremely painful. Medications administered by the intramuscular route generally take 20 to 30 minutes to become effective. Hydroxyzine causes dry mouth and drowsiness as side effects.

Test-Taking Strategy: Use the process of elimination, and read each option carefully. Eliminate options 1 and 4 first because they are the least likely effects. From the remaining options, noting that the medication is administered by the intramuscular route will direct you to option 2. Review the side effects of this medication if you had difficulty with this question.

Reference
Skidmore-Roth, L. (2008). *Mosby's nursing drug reference* (21st ed., p. 543). St Louis: Mosby.

---

71. A client with diabetes mellitus has a blood glucose level of 644 mg/dL. The nurse interprets that this client is most at risk of developing which type of acid-base imbalance?
1 Metabolic acidosis
2 Metabolic alkalosis
3 Respiratory acidosis
4 Respiratory alkalosis

Level of Cognitive Ability: Analysis
Client Needs: Physiological Integrity
Integrated Process: Nursing Process/Analysis
Content Area: Adult Health/Endocrine

Answer: 1
Rationale: Diabetes mellitus can lead to metabolic acidosis. When the body does not have sufficient circulating insulin, the blood glucose level rises. At the same time, the cells of the body use all available glucose. The body then breaks down glycogen and fat for fuel. The by-products of fat metabolism are acidotic and can lead to the condition known as *diabetic ketoacidosis*. Options 2, 3, and 4 are incorrect.

Test-Taking Strategy: Use the process of elimination. Noting the client's diagnosis will assist in eliminating options 3 and 4. From the remaining options, remember that the client with diabetes mellitus is at risk for developing metabolic acidosis. Review the causes of metabolic acidosis if you had difficulty with this question.

Reference
Ignatavicius, D., & Workman, M. (2006). *Medical-surgical nursing: Critical thinking for collaborative care* (5th ed., pp. 283, 1501). Philadelphia: Saunders.

72. The nurse reviews the client's most recent blood gas results that include a pH of 7.43, P_{CO_2} of 31 mm Hg, and HCO_3 of 21 mEq/L. Which acid-base imbalance does the nurse use to interpret these results?

1 Compensated metabolic acidosis
2 Compensated respiratory alkalosis
3 Uncompensated respiratory acidosis
4 Uncompensated metabolic alkalosis

Level of Cognitive Ability: Analysis
Client Needs: Physiological Integrity
Integrated Process: Nursing Process/Analysis
Content Area: Fundamental Skills

Answer: 2
Rationale: The normal pH is 7.35 to 7.45, the normal P_{CO_2} is 35 to 45 mm Hg, and the normal HCO_3 is 22 to 27 mEq/L. The pH is elevated in alkalosis and low in acidosis. In a respiratory condition, the pH and the P_{CO_2} move in opposite directions—that is, the pH rises and the P_{CO_2} drops (alkalosis) or vice versa (acidosis). In a metabolic condition, the pH and the bicarbonate move in the same direction; if the pH is low, the bicarbonate level will be low, also. In this client, the pH is at the high end of normal, indicating compensation and alkalosis. The P_{CO_2} is low, indicating a respiratory condition (opposite direction of the pH).

Test-Taking Strategy: Remember that in a respiratory imbalance you will find that the pH and P_{CO_2} move in opposite directions. Therefore, options 1 and 4 are eliminated first. Next, remember that the pH is elevated with alkalosis, but compensation has occurred, as evidenced by a normal pH. Option 2 reflects a respiratory alkalotic condition and compensation because the P_{CO_2} is below normal but the pH is at the high end of normal. Review the steps related to reading blood gas values if you had difficulty with this question.

References
Black, J., & Hawks, J. (2005). *Medical-surgical nursing: Clinical management for positive outcomes* (7th ed., p. 252). Philadelphia: Saunders.
Ignatavicius, D., & Workman, M. (2006). *Medical-surgical nursing: Critical thinking for collaborative care* (5th ed., pp. 278-279). Philadelphia: Saunders.

73. The nurse is caring for a client with a nasogastric tube that is attached to low suction. Which acid-base disorder is most likely to occur in this client?

1 Metabolic acidosis
2 Metabolic alkalosis
3 Respiratory acidosis
4 Respiratory alkalosis

Level of Cognitive Ability: Analysis
Client Needs: Physiological Integrity
Integrated Process: Nursing Process/Assessment
Content Area: Fundamental Skills

Answer: 2
Rationale: Loss of gastric fluid via nasogastric suction or vomiting causes metabolic alkalosis because of the loss of hydrochloric acid (HCl), an acid secreted in the stomach. Thus, the loss of hydrogen ions in the HCl results in alkalosis. Because the respiratory system is not involved, the alkalosis must be metabolic.

Test-Taking Strategy: Eliminate options 1 and 3 first, because the loss of HCl would cause an alkalotic condition. Because the question addresses a situation other than a respiratory one, the acid-base disorder would be metabolic alkalosis. Review the causes of metabolic alkalosis if you had difficulty with this question.

References
Black, J., & Hawks, J. (2005). *Medical-surgical nursing: Clinical management for positive outcomes* (7th ed., p. 255). Philadelphia: Saunders.
Lewis, S., Heitkemper, M., Dirksen, S., O'Brien, P., & Bucher, L. (2007). *Medical-surgical nursing: Assessment and management of clinical problems* (7th ed., p. 1081). St. Louis: Mosby.

74. The nurse reviews the results of a blood chemistry profile for a client who has late-stage salicylate poisoning and metabolic acidosis. Which serum study does the nurse review for data about the client's acid-base balance?

1 Sodium
2 Potassium
3 Magnesium
4 Phosphorus

Level of Cognitive Ability: Analysis
Client Needs: Physiological Integrity
Integrated Process: Nursing Process/Analysis
Content Area: Fundamental Skills

Answer: 2
Rationale: A client with late-stage salicylate poisoning is at risk for metabolic acidosis because acetylsalicylic acid increases the client's hydrogen ion (H^+) concentration, decreases the pH, and creates a bicarbonate deficit. Hyperkalemia develops as the body attempts to compensate for the influx of H^+ by moving H^+ into the cell and potassium out of the cell; thus, potassium accumulates in the body. Clinical manifestations of metabolic acidosis include the clinical indicators of hyperkalemia, including hyperpnea, central nervous system depression, twitching, and seizures. Options 1, 3, and 4 are not a primary concern.

Test-Taking Strategy: Knowledge about the effect of an influx of H^+ in an acid-base disorder and the potassium shifts that occur will direct you to option 2. Review the pathophysiology associated with acid-base imbalances if you had difficulty with this question.

References
Black, J., & Hawks, J. (2005). *Medical-surgical nursing: Clinical management for positive outcomes* (7th ed., p. 256). Philadelphia: Saunders.
Lewis, S., Heitkemper, M., Dirksen, S., O'Brien, P., & Bucher, L. (2007). *Medical-surgical nursing: Assessment and management of clinical problems* (7th ed., p. 335). St. Louis: Mosby.

75. An emergency department nurse prepares to treat a child with acetaminophen (Tylenol) overdose. The nurse reviews the physician's orders, expecting that which of the following will be prescribed?

1 Protamine sulfate
2 Succimer (Chemet)
3 Acetylcysteine (Mucomyst)
4 Vitamin K (AquaMEPHYTON)

Level of Cognitive Ability: Analysis
Client Needs: Physiological Integrity
Integrated Process: Nursing Process/Analysis
Content Area: Child Health

Answer: 3
Rationale: Acetylcysteine (Mucomyst) is the antidote for acetaminophen overdose. It is administered orally or via nasogastric tube in a diluted form with water, juice, or soda. It can also be administered intravenously. Vitamin K is the antidote for warfarin (Coumadin). Protamine sulfate is the antidote for heparin. Succimer (Chemet) is used in the treatment of lead poisoning.

Test-Taking Strategy: Knowledge regarding the antidote for acetaminophen overdose is required to answer this question. Remember that acetylcysteine (Mucomyst) is the antidote for acetaminophen overdose. Learn the major antidotes for medication overdose if you are unfamiliar with them.

References
Hockenberry, M., & Wilson, D. (2007). *Nursing care of infants and children* (8th ed., p. 683). St. Louis: Mosby.
Hodgson, B., & Kizior, R. (2007). *Saunders nursing drug handbook 2007* (p. 13). Philadelphia: Saunders.

76. A client receives a prescription for 1000 mL of intravenous (IV) 0.9% normal saline solution. Which statement guides the nurse during the administration of this solution? The solution:

1 Affects the plasma osmolarity
2 Is the same solution as sodium chloride 0.45%
3 Is isotonic with the plasma and other body fluids
4 Is hypertonic with the plasma and other body fluids

Level of Cognitive Ability: Application
Client Needs: Physiological Integrity
Integrated Process: Nursing Process/ Implementation
Content Area: Fundamental Skills

Answer: 3
Rationale: Sodium chloride 0.9% (not sodium chloride 0.45%) is the same solution as normal saline 0.9%. This solution is isotonic (not hypertonic), and isotonic solutions are frequently used for IV infusion because they do not affect the plasma osmolarity.

Test-Taking Strategy: Focus on the percentage of the solution: 0.9%. This will assist in eliminating option 2. From the remaining options, note the relationship between the name of the solution, normal saline, and the word "isotonic." Remember that "normal saline" is isotonic and would not affect plasma osmolarity. Review the tonicity of IV fluids if you had difficulty with this question.

References
Black, J., & Hawks, J. (2005). *Medical-surgical nursing: Clinical management for positive outcomes* (7th ed., p. 210). Philadelphia: Saunders.
Gahart, B., & Nazareno, A. (2006). *2006 Intravenous medications* (22nd ed., pp. 1114-1115). St. Louis: Mosby.

---

77. A client who has fallen from a ladder and fractured three ribs has arterial blood gas (ABG) results of pH 7.38, P_{CO_2} 38 mm Hg, P_{O_2} 86 mm Hg, and HCO_3 23 mEq/L. The nurse interprets that the client's ABGs indicate which of the following?

1 Normal results
2 Metabolic acidosis
3 Metabolic alkalosis
4 Respiratory acidosis

Level of Cognitive Ability: Analysis
Client Needs: Physiological Integrity
Integrated Process: Nursing Process/Analysis
Content Area: Adult Health/Respiratory

Answer: 1
Rationale: Normal ABG results include a pH of 7.35 to 7.45, a P_{CO_2} of 35 to 45 mm Hg, a P_{O_2} of 80 to 100, and an HCO_3 of 22 to 27 mm Hg. The client's results fall in the normal range.

Test-Taking Strategy: Specific knowledge of the normal ABG levels is needed to answer this question. Recalling these normal levels will direct you to option 1. Review these normal levels if you had difficulty with this question.

References
Black, J., & Hawks, J. (2005). *Medical-surgical nursing: Clinical management for positive outcomes* (7th ed., p. 252). Philadelphia: Saunders.
Chernecky, C., & Berger, B. (2008). *Laboratory tests and diagnostic procedures* (5th ed., pp. 210-214). Philadelphia: Saunders.

---

78. An adult client has undergone a lumbar puncture to obtain cerebrospinal fluid (CSF) for analysis. The nurse assesses for which of the following values that should be negative if the CSF is normal?

1 Protein
2 Glucose
3 Red blood cells
4 White blood cells

Level of Cognitive Ability: Analysis
Client Needs: Physiological Integrity
Integrated Process: Nursing Process/Assessment
Content Area: Adult Health/Neurological

Answer: 3
Rationale: The adult with normal CSF has no red blood cells in the CSF. The client may have small levels of white blood cells (0 to 8 cells/mm^3). Protein (15 to 45 mg/dL) and glucose (45 to 74 mg/dL) are normally present in CSF.

Test-Taking Strategy: Use the process of elimination and note the strategic word "normal" in the question. Recalling that the presence of red blood cells would indicate blood vessel rupture or meningeal irritation will direct you to option 3. Review normal CSF values if you had difficulty with this question.

References
Ignatavicius, D., & Workman, M. (2006). *Medical-surgical nursing: Critical thinking for collaborative care* (5th ed., p. 943). Philadelphia: Saunders.
Lewis, S., Heitkemper, M., Dirksen, S., O'Brien, P., & Bucher, L. (2007). *Medical-surgical nursing: Assessment and management of clinical problems* (7th ed., pp. 1461, 1464). St. Louis: Mosby.

79. A client with a burn injury receives a prescription for a regular diet. Which is the best meal for the nurse to provide to the client to promote wound healing?
  1 Peanut butter and jelly sandwich, apple, tea
  2 Chicken breast, broccoli, strawberries, milk
  3 Veal chop, boiled potatoes, Jell-O, orange juice
  4 Pasta with tomato sauce, garlic bread, ginger ale

Level of Cognitive Ability: Analysis
Client Needs: Physiological Integrity
Integrated Process: Nursing Process/ Implementation
Content Area: Fundamental Skills

Answer: 2
Rationale: The meal with the best potential to promote wound healing includes nutrient-rich food choices including protein, such as chicken and milk, and vitamin C, such as broccoli and strawberries. The remaining options include one or more items with a low nutritional value, especially the tea, jelly, Jell-O, and ginger ale.

Test-Taking Strategy: Knowledge that protein and vitamin C are necessary for wound healing assists in selecting the option that contains those nutrients, and the option with the most nutrients is the best choice. Eliminate options 1 and 3 first because jelly and Jell-O have no nutrient value related to healing. From the remaining options, select option 2 over option 4 because option 2 contains foods with greater nutritional value. Review foods high in protein and vitamin C if you had difficulty with this question.

Reference
Nix, S. (2005). *Williams' basic nutrition & diet therapy* (12th ed., pp. 427-428). St. Louis: Mosby.

---

80. A nurse caring for a client with a neurological disorder is planning care to maintain nutritional status. The nurse is concerned about the client's swallowing ability. Which of the following food items would the nurse plan to avoid in this client's diet?
  1 Spinach
  2 Custard
  3 Scrambled eggs
  4 Mashed potatoes

Level of Cognitive Ability: Application
Client Needs: Physiological Integrity
Integrated Process: Nursing Process/Planning
Content Area: Adult Health/Neurological

Answer: 1
Rationale: In general, flavorful, warm, or well-chilled foods with texture stimulate the swallowing reflex. Soft and semisoft foods such as custards or puddings, egg dishes, and potatoes are usually effective. Raw vegetables, chunky vegetables such as diced beets, and stringy vegetables such as spinach, corn, and peas are foods commonly excluded from the diet of a client with a poor swallowing reflex.

Test-Taking Strategy: Note the strategic words "swallowing ability" and "avoid." Use the process of elimination to select option 1 as the food that is stringy and with the least amount of substance or consistency. Review feeding measures for a client with altered swallowing ability if you had difficulty with this question.

References
Grodner, M., Long, S., & DeYoung, S. (2004). *Foundations and clinical applications of nutrition: A nursing approach* (3rd ed., pp. 501-504). St. Louis: Mosby.
Nix, S. (2005). *Williams' basic nutrition & diet therapy* (12th ed., pp. 325-326). St. Louis: Mosby.

---

81. A nurse reviews the assessment data of a client admitted to the hospital with a diagnosis of anxiety. The nurse assigns priority to which assessment finding?
  1 Temperature 99.4° F, flat affect
  2 Fist clenched and pounding table
  3 Tearful, withdrawn, and isolated
  4 Blood pressure 160/100 mm Hg; pulse 120 beats per minute; respirations 18 breaths per minute

Answer: 2
Rationale: Anxiety can lead to behavior that is harmful to the client and others. If safety is threatened, this is the priority. Tearfulness, withdrawal, isolation, and elevated vital signs are abnormal findings. However, these findings are not life-threatening, although they should be monitored. After the client's mental status is addressed and the client's safety is ensured, the nurse should attend to the elevated vital signs.

Level of Cognitive Ability: Analysis
Client Needs: Physiological Integrity
Integrated Process: Nursing Process/Analysis
Content Area: Delegating/Prioritizing

Test-Taking Strategy: Note the strategic word "priority," and focus on the client's diagnosis. Remembering that client safety and safety of others is the priority will direct you to option 2. Review the priority interventions for anxiety if you had difficulty with this question.

Reference

Varcarolis, E., Carson, V., & Shoemaker, N. (2006). *Foundations of psychiatric mental health nursing* (5th ed., pp. 232-233, 243). Philadelphia: Saunders.

---

82. A client is resuming a diet after a Billroth II procedure. To minimize complications from eating, the nurse teaches the client to avoid doing which of the following?
1 Lying down after eating
2 Eating a diet high in protein
3 Drinking liquids with meals
4 Eating six small meals per day

Level of Cognitive Ability: Application
Client Needs: Physiological Integrity
Integrated Process: Nursing Process/
  Implementation
Content Area: Adult Health/Gastrointestinal

Answer: 3
Rationale: The client who has had a Billroth II procedure is at risk for dumping syndrome. The client should avoid drinking liquids with meals to prevent this syndrome. The client should be placed on a dry diet that is high in protein, moderate in fat, and low in carbohydrates. Frequent small meals are encouraged, and the client should avoid concentrated sweets.

Test-Taking Strategy: Note the strategic word "avoid." Focusing on the diagnosis (surgical procedure) and recalling that dumping syndrome is a complication of this surgical procedure will direct you to option 3. Review the complications of gastric surgery and the prevention and management of the complications if you had difficulty with this question.

Reference

Monahan, F., Sands, J., Neighbors, M., Marek, J., & Green, C. (2007). *Phipps' medical-surgical nursing: Health and illness perspectives* (8th ed., p. 1226). St. Louis: Mosby.

---

83. A nurse is preparing to administer diazepam (Valium) by the intravenous (IV) route to a client who is having a seizure. The nurse plans to:
1 Administer the prescribed dose over at least 60 minutes.
2 Administer the prescribed dose by IV push directly into the vein.
3 Dilute the prescribed dose in 50 mL of 5% dextrose in water.
4 Mix the prescribed dose into the existing IV of 5% dextrose in normal saline.

Level of Cognitive Ability: Application
Client Needs: Physiological Integrity
Integrated Process: Nursing Process/Planning
Content Area: Pharmacology

Answer: 2
Rationale: Intravenous diazepam is given by IV push directly into a large vein (reduces the risk of thrombophlebitis), at a rate no greater than 1 mg per minute. It should not be mixed with other medications or solutions and can be diluted only with normal saline.

Test-Taking Strategy: Use the process of elimination. Eliminate options 3 and 4 first because they are comparable or alike. From the remaining options, focusing on the client situation will direct you to option 2. Review the procedure for the administration of IV diazepam if you had difficulty with this question.

Reference

Skidmore-Roth, L. (2008). *Mosby's nursing drug reference* (21st ed., p. 354). St. Louis: Mosby.

84. A nurse is closely monitoring a child with increased intracranial pressure who has been exhibiting decorticate posturing. The nurse notes that the child suddenly exhibits decerebrate posturing and interprets that this change in the child's condition indicates which of the following?
1 An insignificant finding
2 An improvement in condition
3 Decreasing intracranial pressure
4 Deteriorating neurological function

Level of Cognitive Ability: Analysis
Client Needs: Physiological Integrity
Integrated Process: Nursing Process/Analysis
Content Area: Child Health

Answer: 4
Rationale: The progression from decorticate to decerebrate posturing usually indicates deteriorating neurological function and warrants physician notification. Options 1, 2, and 3 are inaccurate interpretations.

Test-Taking Strategy: Use the process of elimination. Eliminate options 2 and 3 first because they are comparable or alike. From the remaining options, recalling the significance of decerebrate posturing will assist in eliminating option 1. Review the significance of decorticate and decerebrate posturing if you had difficulty with this question.

Reference
Hockenberry, M., Wilson, D., & Winkelstein, M. (2005). *Wong's essentials of pediatric nursing* (7th ed., pp. 1015-1016). St. Louis: Mosby.

85. A nurse caring for a hospitalized infant is monitoring for increased intracranial pressure (ICP) and notes that the anterior fontanel bulges when the infant cries. Based on this assessment finding, which action would the nurse take?
1 Document the findings
2 Lower the head of the bed
3 Place the infant on NPO status
4 Notify the physician immediately

Level of Cognitive Ability: Application
Client Needs: Physiological Integrity
Integrated Process: Nursing Process/
  Implementation
Content Area: Child Health

Answer: 1
Rationale: The anterior fontanel is diamond-shaped and located on the top of the head. It should be soft and flat in a normal infant, and it normally closes by 12 to 18 months of age. The posterior fontanel closes by 2 to 3 months of age. A bulging or tense fontanel may result from crying or increased ICP. Noting a bulging fontanel when the infant cries is a normal finding that should be documented and monitored. It is not necessary to notify the physician. Options 2 and 3 are inappropriate actions.

Test-Taking Strategy: Use the process of elimination, and focus on the information in the question. Note the strategic words "bulges when the infant cries." This should provide you with the clue that this is a normal finding. Remember that a bulging or tense fontanel may result from crying. Review normal assessment findings in an infant if you had difficulty with this question.

References
Hockenberry, M., & Wilson, D. (2007). *Nursing care of infants and children* (8th ed., p. 1617). St. Louis: Mosby.
McKinney, E., James, S., Murray, S., & Ashwill, J. (2005). *Maternal-child nursing* (2nd ed., p. 1497). St. Louis: Saunders.

86. A nurse is assessing the vital signs of a 3-year-old child hospitalized with a diagnosis of croup and notes that the respiratory rate is 28 breaths per minute. Based on this finding, which nursing action is appropriate?
1 Administer oxygen.
2 Notify the physician.
3 Document the findings.
4 Reassess the respiratory rate in 15 minutes.

Answer: 3
Rationale: The normal respiratory rate for a 3-year-old child is approximately 20 to 30 breaths per minute. Because the respiratory rate is normal, options 1, 2, and 4 are unnecessary actions. The nurse would document the findings.

Test-Taking Strategy: Recalling that the normal respiratory rate for a 3-year-old child is approximately 20 to 30 breaths per minute will direct you to option 3. Review the normal vital signs in a 3-year-old child if you had difficulty with this question.

Level of Cognitive Ability: Application
Client Needs: Physiological Integrity
Integrated Process: Nursing Process/
  Implementation
Content Area: Child Health

References
Hockenberry, M., Wilson, D., & Winkelstein, M. (2005). *Wong's essentials of pediatric nursing* (7th ed., pp. 800-801). St. Louis: Mosby.
Wong, D., Hockenberry, M., Perry, S., Lowdermilk, D., & Wilson, D. (2006). *Maternal-child nursing care.* (3rd ed., p. 1913). St. Louis: Mosby.

---

87. A nurse is performing an assessment on a female client who is suspected of having mittelschmerz. Which does the nurse expect to note on assessment of the client?
1 Experiences pain during intercourse
2 Has pain at the onset of menstruation
3 Experiences profuse vaginal bleeding
4 Has sharp pelvic pain during ovulation

Level of Cognitive Ability: Comprehension
Client Needs: Physiological Integrity
Integrated Process: Nursing Process/Assessment
Content Area: Fundamental Skills

Answer: 4
Rationale: Mittelschmerz (middle pain) refers to pelvic pain that occurs midway between menstrual periods or at the time of ovulation. The pain is caused by growth follicle within the ovary, or rupture of the follicle and subsequent spillage of follicular fluid and blood into the peritoneal space. The pain is fairly sharp and is felt on the right or left side of the pelvis. It generally lasts 1 to 3 days, and slight vaginal bleeding may accompany the discomfort.

Test-Taking Strategy: Use the process of elimination. Recalling that mittelschmerz is "middle pain" will direct you to option 4. Review this disorder if you are unfamiliar with it.

References
McKinney, E., James, S., Murray, S., & Ashwill, J. (2005). *Maternal-child nursing* (2nd ed., p. 776). St. Louis: Saunders.
Murray, S., & McKinney, E. (2006). *Foundations of maternal-newborn nursing* (4th ed., p. 895). Philadelphia: Saunders.

---

88. A client is diagnosed with endometriosis and asks the nurse to describe this condition. The nurse tells the client that endometriosis is:
1 Extrauterine endometrial tissue
2 Known as primary dysmenorrhea
3 A process that halts menstruation
4 A pain that occurs during ovulation

Level of Cognitive Ability: Comprehension
Client Needs: Physiological Integrity
Integrated Process: Nursing Process/
  Implementation
Content Area: Fundamental Skills

Answer: 1
Rationale: Endometriosis is defined as the presence of tissue outside the uterus that resembles the endometrium in structure, function, and response to estrogen and progesterone during the menstrual cycle. Primary dysmenorrhea refers to menstrual pain without identified pathology. Amenorrhea, the cessation of menstruation for a period of at least three cycles or 6 months in a woman who has established a pattern of menstruation, can result from a variety of causes. Mittelschmerz refers to pelvic pain that occurs midway between menstrual periods coinciding with ovulation.

Test-Taking Strategy: Use the process of elimination. Note the relationship between "endometriosis" in the question and "endometrium" in the correct option. Review this disorder if you had difficulty with this question.

References
McKinney, E., James, S., Murray, S., & Ashwill, J. (2005). *Maternal-child nursing* (2nd ed., pp. 777-778). St. Louis: Saunders.
Murray, S., & McKinney, E. (2006). *Foundations of maternal-newborn nursing* (4th ed., pp. 896-897). Philadelphia: Saunders.

89. A client calls the physician's office to schedule an appointment because a home pregnancy test was performed and the results are positive. The nurse determines that the home pregnancy test identified the presence of which of the following in the urine?

1 Estrogen
2 Progesterone
3 Follicle-stimulating hormone (FSH)
4 Human chorionic gonadotropin (hCG)

Level of Cognitive Ability: Comprehension
Client Needs: Physiological Integrity
Integrated Process: Nursing Process/Assessment
Content Area: Maternity/Antepartum

Answer: 4
Rationale: In early pregnancy, hCG is produced by trophoblastic cells that surround the developing embryo. This hormone is responsible for positive pregnancy tests. Options 1, 2, and 3 are incorrect.

Test-Taking Strategy: Knowledge regarding the changes caused by placental hormones in early pregnancy is required to answer this question. Remember that hCG is responsible for positive pregnancy tests. Review this pregnancy test if you are unfamiliar with it.

References
Chernecky, C., & Berger, B. (2008). *Laboratory tests and diagnostic procedures* (5th ed., pp. 896-897). Philadelphia: Saunders.
Murray, S., & McKinney, E. (2006). *Foundations of maternal-newborn nursing* (4th ed., pp. 126-127). Philadelphia: Saunders.

---

90. A hepatitis B screen is performed on a pregnant client and the results indicate the presence of antigens in the maternal blood. Which of the following should the nurse anticipate to be prescribed?

1 Obtain serum liver enzymes.
2 Repeat hepatitis B screen in 1 week.
3 Administer antibiotics during pregnancy.
4 Administer hepatitis vaccine and hepatitis B immune globulin to the neonate within 12 hours after birth.

Level of Cognitive Ability: Analysis
Client Needs: Physiological Integrity
Integrated Process: Nursing Process/Analysis
Content Area: Maternity/Antepartum

Answer: 4
Rationale: A hepatitis B screen is performed to detect the presence of antigens in maternal blood. If antigens are present, the neonate should receive the hepatitis vaccine and hepatitis B immune globulin within 12 hours after birth. Obtaining serum liver enzymes, retesting the maternal blood in a week, and administering antibiotics are inappropriate actions and would not decrease the chance of the neonate contracting the hepatitis B virus.

Test-Taking Strategy: Use the process of elimination. Eliminate options 1, 2, and 3 because they are actions that would not decrease a chance of the neonate contracting the hepatitis B virus. Recall that the concern is the effect on the fetus and neonate, which will lead you to option 4. Review the purpose and the significance of the hepatitis B screen if you had difficulty with this question.

References
McKinney, E., James, S., Murray, S., & Ashwill, J. (2005). *Maternal-child nursing* (2nd ed., p. 664). St. Louis: Saunders.
Murray, S., & McKinney, E. (2006). *Foundations of maternal-newborn nursing* (4th ed., pp. 687-688). Philadelphia: Saunders.

---

91. A prenatal client is experiencing pain in the calf when she walks. Which action is appropriate for the nurse to implement?

1 Instruct the client to restrict walking.
2 Assess for the presence of Homans' sign.
3 Tell the client that this is normal during pregnancy.
4 Instruct the client to elevate the legs consistently throughout the day.

Answer: 2
Rationale: If a woman complains of calf pain during walking, it could be an indication of venous thrombosis of the lower extremities. The appropriate nursing action should be to assess for Homans' sign, which would assist in determining the presence of venous thrombosis. It is not appropriate to tell the mother that this is normal during pregnancy. Ambulation is an important exercise, and the woman should be encouraged to ambulate during pregnancy. Although it is important to elevate the legs during pregnancy, elevating the legs consistently is not an appropriate nursing action.

Level of Cognitive Ability: Application
Client Needs: Physiological Integrity
Integrated Process: Nursing Process/
Implementation
Content Area: Maternity/Antepartum

Test-Taking Strategy: Note the strategic word "appropriate." Use the steps of the nursing process to assist in answering the question. Option 2 is the only option that addresses assessment. Review normal and abnormal expectations in the prenatal period if you had difficulty with this question.

Reference

McKinney, E., James, S., Murray, S., & Ashwill, J. (2005). *Maternal-child nursing* (2nd ed., p. 482). St. Louis: Saunders.

---

92. A nurse is performing an assessment on a client seen in the health care clinic for a first prenatal visit. The nurse asks the client when the first day of the last menstrual period (LMP) was, and the client reports February 9, 2010 . Using Nägele's rule, the nurse determines that the estimated date of confinement is:

    1 October 7, 2010
    2 October 16, 2010
    3 November 7, 2010
    4 November 16, 2010

Level of Cognitive Ability: Comprehension
Client Needs: Physiological Integrity
Integrated Process: Nursing Process/Assessment
Content Area: Maternity/Antepartum

Answer: 4

Rationale: Accurate use of Nägele's rule requires that the woman have a regular 28-day menstrual cycle. To calculate the estimated date of confinement, the nurse would add 7 days to the first day of the LMP, subtract 3 months, and then add 1 year. First day of last menstrual period: February 9, 2010; add 7 days: February 16, 2010; subtract 3 months: November 16, 2009; and add 1 year, November 16, 2010.

Test-Taking Strategy: Use Nägele's rule to answer this question. Be careful when following the steps to determine the estimated date of confinement using this rule. Read all of the options carefully, noting the dates and years before selecting an option. Review Nägele's rule if you had difficulty with this question.

Reference

Murray, S., & McKinney, E. (2006). *Foundations of maternal-newborn nursing* (4th ed., p. 131). Philadelphia: Saunders.

---

93. The nurse prepares to access an implanted vascular port. Which should the nurse implement first?

    1 Apply a cool compress.
    2 Palpate the vascular port.
    3 Anchor the vascular port.
    4 Cleanse the site with alcohol.

Level of Cognitive Ability: Application
Client Needs: Physiological Integrity
Integrated Process: Nursing Process/
Implementation
Content Area: Fundamental Skills

Answer: 2

Rationale: Before accessing an implanted vascular port, the nurse must palpate the port to locate the center of the septum because the nurse needs to know where to insert the needle to avoid more than one needle stick for the client. The nurse then applies the cool compress to the insertion site to provide mild pain relief for the needle stick, cleanses the site with alcohol, anchors the port with the nondominant hand, and avoids contamination of the septum.

Test-Taking Strategy: Use the steps of the nursing process, remembering that assessment is the first step. Palpation is an assessment technique. Review the concepts related to implanted vascular ports if you had difficulty answering this question.

References

Ignatavicius, D., & Workman, M. (2006). *Medical-surgical nursing: Critical thinking for collaborative care* (5th ed., p. 251). Philadelphia: Saunders.

Potter, P., & Perry, A. (2005). *Fundamentals of nursing* (6th ed., pp. 1159-1160). St. Louis: Mosby.

94. A nurse is preparing to measure the fundal height of a client whose fetus is 28 weeks' gestation. To perform the procedure, the nurse should place the client:

1 In a standing position
2 In the Trendelenburg position
3 Supine with the head of the bed elevated to 45 degrees
4 Supine with her head on a pillow and knees slightly flexed

Level of Cognitive Ability: Application
Client Needs: Physiological Integrity
Integrated Process: Nursing Process/Assessment
Content Area: Maternity/Antepartum

Answer: 4
Rationale: When measuring fundal height, the client lies in a supine (back) position with her head on a pillow and knees slightly flexed. The standing position, Trendelenburg (head lowered), or supine with the head elevated to 45 degrees would not give an accurate measurement.

Test-Taking Strategy: Visualize this assessment technique to direct you to option 4. Options 1, 2, or 3 would not give an accurate measurement. Review the procedure for measuring fundal height if you had difficulty with this question.

Reference
Wong, D., Hockenberry, M., Perry, S., Lowdermilk, D., & Wilson, D. (2006). *Maternal-child nursing care* (3rd ed., pp. 272-273). St. Louis: Mosby.

---

95. A nurse is measuring the fundal height on a client who is 36 weeks' gestation when the client complains of feeling lightheaded. The nurse determines that the client's complaint is most likely caused by:

1 Fear
2 Anemia
3 A full bladder
4 Compression of the vena cava

Level of Cognitive Ability: Analysis
Client Needs: Physiological Integrity
Integrated Process: Nursing Process/Analysis
Content Area: Maternity/Antepartum

Answer: 4
Rationale: Compression of the inferior vena cava and aorta by the uterus may cause supine hypotension syndrome (vena cava syndrome) late in pregnancy. Having the client turn onto her left side or elevating the left buttock during fundal height measurement will correct or prevent the problem. Options 1, 2, and 3 are unrelated to this syndrome.

Test-Taking Strategy: Focus on the information in the question. Recalling that compression of the inferior vena cava and aorta by the uterus may cause supine hypotension syndrome will direct you to option 4. Review vena cava syndrome and its causes if you had difficulty with this question.

Reference
Wong, D., Hockenberry, M., Perry, S., Lowdermilk, D., & Wilson, D. (2006). *Maternal-child nursing care* (3rd ed., p. 286). St. Louis: Mosby.

---

96. A nurse in the prenatal clinic is monitoring a client who is pregnant with twins. The nurse monitors the client closely for which priority complication that is associated with a twin pregnancy?

1 Hemorrhoids
2 Postterm labor
3 Maternal anemia
4 Gestational diabetes

Level of Cognitive Ability: Application
Client Needs: Physiological Integrity
Integrated Process: Nursing Process/Assessment
Content Area: Maternity/Antepartum

Answer: 3
Rationale: Maternal anemia often occurs in twin pregnancies because of a greater demand for iron by the fetuses. Option 2 is incorrect because twin pregnancies often end in prematurity. Hemorrhoids occur in twin pregnancy but would not be as high a priority as anemia. Option 4 is not a complication of a twin pregnancy.

Test-Taking Strategy: Focus on the subject—twin pregnancy—and note the strategic words "priority." Thinking about the physiological occurrences of a twin pregnancy will direct you to option 3. Review the risks associated with a twin pregnancy if you had difficulty with this question.

Reference
Wong, D., Hockenberry, M., Perry, S., Lowdermilk, D., & Wilson, D. (2006). *Maternal-child nursing care* (3rd ed., p. 295). St. Louis: Mosby.

97. A clinic nurse is assessing a prenatal client with heart disease. The nurse carefully assesses the client's vital signs, weight, and fluid and nutritional status to detect for complications caused by:
1 Rh incompatibility
2 Fetal cardiomegaly
3 The increase in circulating blood volume
4 Hypertrophy and increased contractility of the heart

Level of Cognitive Ability: Application
Client Needs: Physiological Integrity
Integrated Process: Nursing Process/Assessment
Content Area: Maternity/Antepartum

Answer: 3
Rationale: Pregnancy taxes the circulating system of every woman because both the blood volume and cardiac output increase. Options 1, 2, and 4 are not directly associated with pregnancy in a client with a cardiac condition.

Test-Taking Strategy: Use the process of elimination and focus on the client of the question. Eliminate options 1 and 2 first because they address the fetus, not the prenatal client. From the remaining options, recalling the changes that take place in the woman during pregnancy will direct you to option 3. Also, remember that hypertrophy of the heart may occur in cardiac disease, but the outcome would be a decrease in contractility, not an increase. Review the pathophysiology in relation to cardiac disease in the pregnant client if you had difficulty with this question.

Reference
McKinney, E., James, S., Murray, S., & Ashwill, J. (2005). *Maternal-child nursing* (2nd ed., pp. 654-655). St. Louis: Saunders.

---

98. The nurse assists the provider with a liver biopsy performed at the bedside. Which position does the nurse place the client in after the biopsy?
1 Supine with the head elevated on one pillow
2 Semi-Fowler's with two pillows under the legs
3 Left side-lying with a small pillow under the puncture site
4 Right side-lying with a folded towel under the puncture site

Level of Cognitive Ability: Application
Client Needs: Physiological Integrity
Integrated Process: Nursing Process/ Implementation
Content Area: Fundamental Skills

Answer: 4
Rationale: Following a liver biopsy, the nurse positions the client on the right side with a small pillow or folded towel under the puncture site for 2 hours. This position compresses the liver against the chest wall at the biopsy site.

Test-Taking Strategy: Use knowledge regarding the anatomy of the body and principles of hemostasis to answer this question. Remember that the liver is on the right side of the body, and, by applying pressure at the puncture site, the nurse helps prevent the escape of blood or bile. Review care of the client following a liver biopsy if you had difficulty with this question.

Reference
Pagana, K., & Pagana, T. (2005). *Mosby's diagnostic and laboratory test reference* (7th ed., p. 597). St. Louis: Mosby.

---

99. A client has a prescription for "enemas until clear" before bowel surgery, so the nurse prepares the equipment and solution. The nurse assists the client into which position to administer the enema?
1 Prone
2 Right side-lying
3 Left-lateral Sims'
4 Right-lateral Sims'

Answer: 3
Rationale: When administering an enema, the nurse places the client in a left Sims' position exposing the rectal area and allowing the enema solution to flow by gravity in the natural direction of the colon. Lying on the right side prevents administration of an effective enema because the solution will not flow against gravity to reach the colon. In the prone position, the client is lying on the stomach.

Level of Cognitive Ability: Comprehension
Client Needs: Physiological Integrity
Integrated Process: Nursing Process/
  Implementation
Content Area: Fundamental Skills

Test-Taking Strategy: Use knowledge regarding the anatomy of the bowel to answer the question. This will assist in eliminating options 2 and 4. From the remaining options, visualize the procedure for administering an enema and eliminate option 1 because in the prone position, the client is lying on the stomach. Review the procedure for administering an enema if you had difficulty with this question.

Reference
Potter, P., & Perry, A. (2005). *Fundamentals of nursing* (6th ed., pp. 1399). St. Louis: Mosby.

---

100. A provider has just inserted a Cantor (nasointestinal) tube in a client with a bowel obstruction. When the procedure is complete, the nurse assists the client into which of the following positions initially to maximize the effect of the tube?
  1 Left side
  2 Right Sims'
  3 Semi-Fowler's
  4 High Fowler's

Level of Cognitive Ability: Comprehension
Client Needs: Physiological Integrity
Integrated Process: Nursing Process/
  Implementation
Content Area: Fundamental Skills

Answer: 3
Rationale: The Cantor tube is a single-lumen, weighted tube. The weight of the tube carries the tube by gravity. The nurse positions the client to protect the airway and facilitate breathing. Although high Fowler's is frequently used to facilitate breathing, it is more likely to increase intraabdominal pressure and, therefore, is contraindicated for a bowel obstruction.

Test-Taking Strategy: Note the type of tube being inserted. Understanding the effect of peristalsis will guide you to option 3 because this position involves effective, smooth muscle action to propel contents of the gastrointestinal tract through the gastrointestinal system. Review nursing care related to the client with a Cantor tube if you had difficulty with this question.

Reference
Ignatavicius, D., & Workman, M. (2006). *Medical-surgical nursing: Critical thinking for collaborative care* (5th ed., p. 1329). Philadelphia: Saunders.

---

101. A nurse is caring for a client following a supratentorial craniotomy. The nurse places a sign above the client's bed stating that the client should be maintained in which of the following positions?
  1 Prone
  2 Supine
  3 Semi-Fowler's
  4 Dorsal recumbent

Level of Cognitive Ability: Application
Client Needs: Physiological Integrity
Integrated Process: Nursing Process/
  Implementation
Content Area: Adult Health/Neurological

Answer: 3
Rationale: Following supratentorial surgery (surgery above the brain's tentorium), the client's head is usually elevated 30 degrees to promote venous outflow through the jugular veins and modulate intracranial pressure (ICP). Options 1, 2, and 4 are incorrect positions following this surgery because they are likely to increase ICP.

Test-Taking Strategy: Use the process of elimination. A helpful strategy is to remember: supra, above the brain's tentorium, head up. Also note that options 1 and 2 are comparable or alike in that they are flat positions; option 4 is eliminated because the increased intraabdominal pressure from this position is more likely to inhibit venous return from the brain. Review positioning following craniotomy surgery if you had difficulty with this question.

Reference
Ignatavicius, D., & Workman, M. (2006). *Medical-surgical nursing: Critical thinking for collaborative care* (5th ed., p. 1058). Philadelphia: Saunders.

102. A nurse is reviewing the records of recently admitted clients to the postpartum unit. The nurse determines that which new client would be at least risk for developing a puerperal infection?
1 A client with a history of previous infections
2 A client who had an excessive number of vaginal exams
3 A client who underwent a vaginal delivery of the newborn
4 A client who experienced prolonged rupture of the membranes

Level of Cognitive Ability: Analysis
Client Needs: Physiological Integrity
Integrated Process: Nursing Process/Assessment
Content Area: Maternity/Antepartum

Answer: 3
Rationale: Risk factors associated with puerperal infection include a history of previous infections, cesarean births, trauma, prolonged rupture of the membranes, prolonged labor, excessive number of vaginal examinations, and retained placental fragments.

Test-Taking Strategy: Note the strategic words "at least risk" and focus on the subject—developing a puerperal infection. Eliminate option 1 first because of its relationship to infection. Next, eliminate option 4 because of the word "prolonged" and option 2 because of the word "excessive." Review the risk factors associated with puerperal infection if you had difficulty with this question.

References
McKinney, E., James, S., Murray, S., & Ashwill, J. (2005). *Maternal-child nursing* (2nd ed., p. 712). St. Louis: Saunders.
Murray, S., & McKinney, E. (2006). *Foundations of maternal-newborn nursing* (4th ed., pp. 746-747). Philadelphia: Saunders.

---

103. A nurse in the delivery room assists with the delivery of a newborn infant. Following delivery, the nurse prevents heat loss in the newborn infant resulting from conduction by:
1 Wrapping the newborn in a blanket
2 Closing the doors to the delivery room
3 Drying the newborn with a warm blanket
4 Placing a warm pad on the crib before placing the newborn in the crib

Level of Cognitive Ability: Application
Client Needs: Physiological Integrity
Integrated Process: Nursing Process/ Implementation
Content Area: Maternity/Postpartum

Answer: 4
Rationale: Hypothermia caused by conduction occurs when the newborn infant is on a cold surface, such as a cold pad or mattress. Warming the crib pad will assist in preventing hypothermia by conduction. Evaporation of moisture from a wet body dissipates heat along with the moisture. Keeping the newborn infant dry by drying the wet newborn infant at birth will prevent hypothermia via evaporation. Convection occurs as air moves across the newborn infant's skin from an open door and heat is transferred to the air. Radiation occurs when heat from the newborn infant radiates to a colder surface.

Test-Taking Strategy: Note the strategic word "conduction" in the question to assist in selecting the correct option. Recalling that conduction occurs when a baby is on a cold surface will assist in directing you to option 4. Review these heat loss concepts if you had difficulty with this question.

References
McKinney, E., James, S., Murray, S., & Ashwill, J. (2005). *Maternal-child nursing* (2nd ed., p. 510). St. Louis: Saunders.
Murray, S., & McKinney, E. (2006). *Foundations of maternal-newborn nursing* (4th ed., p. 299). Philadelphia: Saunders.

104. A nurse provides a class to new mothers on newborn care. When teaching cord care, the nurse tells the new mothers:

1 If antibiotic ointment has been applied to the cord, it is not necessary to do anything else to it.
2 All that is necessary is to wash the cord with antibacterial soap and allow it to air dry once a day.
3 Apply alcohol to the cord, ensuring that all areas around the cord are cleaned two to three times a day.
4 Apply alcohol thoroughly to the cord, being careful not to move the cord because it will cause the newborn infant pain.

Level of Cognitive Ability: Application
Client Needs: Physiological Integrity
Integrated Process: Teaching and Learning
Content Area: Maternity/Postpartum

Answer: 3
Rationale: The cord and base needs to be cleansed with alcohol (or another substance as prescribed) thoroughly, two to three times per day. The steps are (1) lift the cord, (2) wipe around the cord starting at the top, (3) clean the base of the cord, and (4) fold the diaper below the umbilical cord to allow the cord to air dry and to prevent contamination from urine. Continuation of cord care is necessary until the cord falls off within 7 to 14 days. The infant does not feel pain in this area. Water and soap are not necessary; in fact, the cord should be kept from getting wet. Antibiotic ointment is not normally prescribed.

Test-Taking Strategy: Use the process of elimination. Simply recalling that the cord should be cleansed two to three times a day will direct you to the correct option. Review the principles related to cord care if you had difficulty with this question.

Reference
Lowdermilk, D., & Perry, A. (2004). *Maternity & women's health care* (8th ed., p. 728). St. Louis: Mosby.

---

105. A nurse is monitoring a preterm newborn infant for signs of respiratory distress syndrome (RDS). The nurse monitors the infant for:

1 Acrocyanosis, emphysema, and interstitial edema.
2 Acrocyanosis, apnea, pneumothorax, and grunting.
3 Barrel-shaped chest, hypotension, and bradycardia.
4 Cyanosis, tachypnea, retractions, grunting respirations, and nasal flaring.

Level of Cognitive Ability: Application
Client Needs: Physiological Integrity
Integrated Process: Nursing Process/Assessment
Content Area: Maternity/Postpartum

Answer: 4
Rationale: The newborn infant with RDS may present with clinical signs of cyanosis, tachypnea or apnea, nasal flaring, chest wall retractions, or audible grunts. Acrocyanosis, the bluish discoloration of the hands and feet, is associated with immature peripheral circulation and is not uncommon in the first few hours of life. Options 1, 2, and 3 do not indicate clinical signs of RDS.

Test-Taking Strategy: Use the process of elimination. Recalling that acrocyanosis may be a normal sign in a newborn infant will assist in eliminating options 1 and 2. From the remaining options, it is necessary to be familiar with the signs of RDS. Also, note the relationship between the diagnosis and the signs noted in option 4. Review the signs of RDS if you had difficulty with this question.

References
Hockenberry, M., Wilson, D., & Winkelstein, M. (2005). *Wong's essentials of pediatric nursing* (7th ed., p. 273). St. Louis: Mosby.
McKinney, E., James, S., Murray, S., & Ashwill, J. (2005). *Maternal-child nursing* (2nd ed., p. 526). St. Louis: Saunders.

---

106. A nurse is preparing to assess the apical heart rate of a newborn infant. The nurse performs the procedure and notes that the heart rate is normal if which of the following is noted?

1 A heart rate of 90 beats per minute
2 A heart rate of 140 beats per minute
3 A heart rate of 180 beats per minute
4 A heart rate of 190 beats per minute

Answer: 2
Rationale: The normal heart rate in a newborn infant is 100 to 170 beats per minute. Options 1, 3, and 4 are incorrect. Option 1 indicates bradycardia, and options 3 and 4 indicate tachycardia.

Test-Taking Strategy: Focus on the subject—a newborn infant. Recalling the normal heart rate for a newborn infant will direct you to the correct option. Review this content if you are unfamiliar with this normal finding.

Level of Cognitive Ability: Analysis
Client Needs: Physiological Integrity
Integrated Process: Nursing Process/Assessment
Content Area: Maternity/Postpartum

Reference
McKinney, E., James, S., Murray, S., & Ashwill, J. (2005). *Maternal-child nursing* (2nd ed., p. 526). St. Louis: Saunders.

---

107. A nurse reviews the electrolyte values of a client with congestive heart failure, notes that the potassium level is low, and notifies the physician. The physician prescribes a dose of intravenous (IV) potassium chloride. When administering the IV potassium chloride, the nurse plans to:

1 Inject it as a bolus.
2 Use a filter in the IV line.
3 Dilute it per medication instructions.
4 Apply cool compresses to the IV site during administration.

Level of Cognitive Ability: Application
Client Needs: Physiological Integrity
Integrated Process: Nursing Process/Planning
Content Area: Pharmacology

Answer: 3
Rationale: Potassium chloride is very irritating to the vein and needs to be diluted to prevent phlebitis. Potassium chloride is never administered as a bolus injection. A filter is not necessary for potassium solutions. Cool compresses would constrict the blood vessel, which could possibly be more irritating to the vein.

Test-Taking Strategy: Use the process of elimination. Recalling that potassium chloride is always diluted before administration will eliminate option 1. From the remaining options, noting the words "per medication instructions" in option 3 will direct you to this option. Review the procedure for administering IV potassium chloride if you had difficulty with this question.

References
Gahart, B., & Nazareno, A. (2006). *2006 Intravenous medications* (22nd ed., p. 1021). St. Louis: Mosby.
Hodgson, B., & Kizior, R. (2007). *Saunders nursing drug handbook 2007* (p. 947). Philadelphia: Saunders.

---

108. A childbirth educator tells a class of expectant parents that it is standard routine to instill a medication into the eyes of a newborn infant as a preventive measure against ophthalmia neonatorum. The educator tells the class that the medication currently used for the prophylaxis of ophthalmia neonatorum is:

1 Vitamin K injection
2 Penicillin ophthalmic eye ointment
3 Neomycin ophthalmic eye ointment
4 Erythromycin ophthalmic eye ointment

Level of Cognitive Ability: Application
Client Needs: Physiological Integrity
Integrated Process: Teaching and Learning
Content Area: Maternity/Postpartum

Answer: 4
Rationale: Ophthalmic erythromycin 0.5% ointment is a broad-spectrum antibiotic and is used prophylactically to prevent ophthalmia neonatorum, an eye infection acquired from the newborn infant's passage through the birth canal. Infection from these organisms can cause blindness or serious eye damage. Erythromycin is effective against *Neisseria gonorrhoeae* and *Chlamydia trachomatis*. Vitamin K is administered to the newborn infant to prevent abnormal bleeding, and it promotes liver formation of the clotting factors II, VII, IX, and X. Options 2 and 3 are incorrect.

Test-Taking Strategy: Focusing on the subject—eye medication—will assist in eliminating option 1. From the remaining options, recalling that erythromycin is a broad-spectrum antibiotic will direct you to option 4. Review initial care of the newborn infant if you had difficulty with this question.

References
McKinney, E., James, S., Murray, S., & Ashwill, J. (2005). *Maternal-child nursing* (2nd ed., p. 555). St. Louis: Saunders.
Murray, S., & McKinney, E. (2006). *Foundations of maternal-newborn nursing* (4th ed., p. 513). Philadelphia: Saunders.

109. An infant has been found to be human immunodeficiency virus (HIV) positive. When teaching the infant's mother, the nurse should instruct the mother to:

1 Check the anterior fontanel for bulging and the sutures for widening each day.
2 Provide meticulous skin care to the infant and change the infant's diaper after each voiding or stool.
3 Feed the infant in an upright position with the head and chest tilted slightly back to avoid aspiration.
4 Feed the infant with a special nipple and burp the infant frequently to decrease the tendency to swallow air.

Level of Cognitive Ability: Application
Client Needs: Physiological Integrity
Integrated Process: Teaching and Learning
Content Area: Maternity/Postpartum

Answer: 2
Rationale: Meticulous skin care helps protect the HIV-infected infant from secondary infections. Feeding the infant in an upright position, using a special nipple, and bulging fontanels are unrelated to the pathology associated with HIV.

Test-Taking Strategy: Read the question carefully and use the process of elimination. The question specifically asks for instructions to be given to the mother regarding HIV. Although options 1, 3, and 4 may be correct or partially correct, the content does not specifically relate to care of the infant infected with HIV. Review care of an infant infected with HIV if you had difficulty with this question.

References
McKinney, E., James, S., Murray, S., & Ashwill, J. (2005). *Maternal-child nursing* (2nd ed., p. 666). St. Louis: Saunders.
Murray, S., & McKinney, E. (2006). *Foundations of maternal-newborn nursing* (4th ed., p. 813). Philadelphia: Saunders.

---

110. Following assessment and diagnostic evaluation, it has been determined that the client has Lyme disease, stage II. The nurse assesses the client for which of the following that is most indicative of this stage?

1 Lethargy
2 Headache
3 Erythematous rash
4 Neurological deficits

Level of Cognitive Ability: Analysis
Client Needs: Physiological Integrity
Integrated Process: Nursing Process/Assessment
Content Area: Adult Health/Integumentary

Answer: 4
Rationale: Stage II of Lyme disease develops within 1 to 6 months in most untreated individuals. The most serious problems in this stage include cardiac conduction defects and neurological disorders such as Bell's palsy and paralysis. These problems are not usually permanent. Flulike symptoms (headache and lethargy) and a rash appear in stage I.

Test-Taking Strategy: Use the process of elimination. Recalling that a rash and flulike symptoms occur in stage I will assist you in eliminating options 1, 2, and 3 and direct you to the correct option. Review the clinical manifestations associated with each stage of Lyme disease if you had difficulty with this question.

References
Ignatavicius, D., & Workman, M. (2006). *Medical surgical nursing. Critical thinking for collaborative care* (5th ed., p. 418). Philadelphia: Saunders
Lewis, S., Heitkemper, M., Dirksen, S., O'Brien, P., & Bucher, L. (2007). *Medical-surgical nursing: Assessment and management of clinical problems* (7th ed., p. 1714). St. Louis: Mosby.

---

111. A nurse is caring for a client with a diagnosis of pemphigus. On assessment of the client, the nurse looks for which hallmark sign characteristic of this condition?

1 Homans' sign
2 Chvostek's sign
3 Nikolsky's sign
4 Trousseau's sign

Answer: 3
Rationale: A hallmark sign of pemphigus is Nikolsky's sign, which is when the epidermis can be rubbed off by slight friction or injury. Other characteristics include flaccid bullae that rupture easily and emit a foul-smelling drainage, leaving crusted, denuded skin. The lesions are common on the face, back, chest, and umbilicus. Even slight pressure on an intact blister may cause spread to adjacent skin. Homans' sign, a sign of thrombosis in the leg, is discomfort in the calf on forced dorsiflexion of the foot. Chvostek's sign, seen in tetany, is a spasm of the facial muscles elicited by tapping the facial nerve in the region of the parotid gland. Trousseau's sign is a sign for tetany, in which carpal spasm can be elicited by compressing the upper arm with a blood pressure cuff inflated above the systolic pressure and causing ischemia to the nerves distally.

Level of Cognitive Ability: Analysis
Client Needs: Physiological Integrity
Integrated Process: Nursing Process/Assessment
Content Area: Adult Health/Integumentary

Test-Taking Strategy: Use the process of elimination. Eliminate options 2 and 4 first because they are comparable or alike and both relate to tetany. From the remaining options, recalling that Homans' sign is related to thrombophlebitis will direct you to option 3. Review these various signs if you had difficulty with this question.

References

Black, J., & Hawks, J. (2005). *Medical-surgical nursing: Clinical management for positive outcomes* (7th ed., p. 1418). Philadelphia: Saunders.

Monahan, F., Sands, J., Neighbors, M., Marek, J., & Green, C. (2007). *Phipp's medical-surgical nursing: Health and illness perspectives* (8th ed., p. 1890). St. Louis: Mosby.

---

112. Following tonsillectomy, which of the following fluid or food items is appropriate to offer to the child?
  1 Jell-O
  2 Cold ginger ale
  3 Vanilla pudding
  4 Cool Cherry Kool-Aid

Level of Cognitive Ability: Application
Client Needs: Physiological Integrity
Integrated Process: Nursing Process/Implementation
Content Area: Child Health

Answer: 1
Rationale: Following tonsillectomy, clear, cool liquids should be administered. Citrus, carbonated, and extremely hot or cold liquids need to be avoided because they may irritate the throat. Red liquids need to be avoided because they give the appearance of blood if the child vomits. Milk and milk products (pudding) are avoided because they coat the throat and cause the child to clear the throat, thus increasing the risk of bleeding.

Test-Taking Strategy: Note the strategic word "appropriate." Avoiding foods and fluids that may irritate or cause bleeding is the concern. This will assist in eliminating options 2 and 3. The word "cherry" in option 4 should be the clue that this is not an appropriate food item. Review dietary measures following tonsillectomy if you had difficulty with this question.

Reference

Hockenberry, M., Wilson, D., & Winkelstein, M. (2005). *Wong's essentials of pediatric nursing* (7th ed., pp. 796-797). St. Louis: Mosby.

---

113. A nurse is checking postoperative orders and planning care for a 110-pound child after spinal fusion. Morphine sulfate, 8 mg subcutaneously every 4 hours prn for pain, is prescribed. The pediatric drug reference states that the safe dose is 0.1 to 0.2 mg/kg/dose every 2 to 4 hours. From this information, the nurse determines that:
  1 The dose is too low.
  2 The dose is too high.
  3 The dose is within the safe dosage range.
  4 There is not enough information to determine the safe dose.

Answer: 3
Rationale: Use the formula to determine the dosage parameters. Convert pounds to kilograms by dividing weight by 2.2: 110 lb. divided by 2.2 = 50 kg.

Dosage parameters:
0.1 mg/kg/dose × 50 kg = 5 mg
0.2 mg/kg/dose × 50 kg = 10 mg

Dosage is within the safe dosage range.

Test-Taking Strategy: Identify the strategic components of the question and what the question is asking. In this case, the question asks for the safe dosage range for medication. Change pounds to kilograms. Calculate the dosage parameters using the safe dose range identified in the question and the child's weight in kg. Use a calculator to verify the answer. Review medication calculations if you had difficulty with this question.

Level of Cognitive Ability: Analysis
Client Needs: Physiological Integrity
Integrated Process: Nursing Process/Analysis
Content Area: Child Health

Reference
Kee, J., & Marshall, S. (2004). *Clinical calculations: With applications to general and specialty areas* (4th ed., pp. 235-236). Philadelphia: Saunders.

---

114. A nurse is performing a physical assessment on a client and is testing the client's reflexes. What action would the nurse take to assess the pharyngeal reflex?
 1 Ask the client to swallow.
 2 Pull down on the lower eyelid.
 3 Shine a light toward the bridge of the nose.
 4 Stimulate the back of the throat with a tongue depressor.

Level of Cognitive Ability: Application
Client Needs: Health Promotion and Maintenance
Integrated Process: Nursing Process/Assessment
Content Area: Adult Health/Neurological

Answer: 4
Rationale: The pharyngeal (gag) reflex is tested by touching the back of the throat with an object, such as a tongue depressor. A positive response to this reflex is considered normal. The corneal light reflex is tested by shining a penlight toward the bridge of the nose at a distance of 12 to 15 inches (light reflection should be symmetrical in both corneas). Asking the client to swallow assesses the swallowing reflex. To assess the palpebral conjunctiva, the nurse would pull down and evert the lower eyelid.

Test-Taking Strategy: Focus on the type of reflex addressed in the question. Recalling that "pharyngeal" refers to the pharynx, or back of the throat, will assist in determining how this reflex is tested and direct you to option 4. Review assessment of reflexes if you had difficulty with this question.

References
Black, J., & Hawks, J. (2005). *Medical-surgical nursing: Clinical management for positive outcomes* (7th ed., p. 2035). Philadelphia: Saunders.
Lewis, S., Heitkemper, M., Dirksen, S., O'Brien, P., & Bucher, L. (2007). *Medical-surgical nursing: Assessment and management of clinical problems* (7th ed., p. 521). St. Louis: Mosby.
Wilson, S., & Giddens, J. (2005). *Health assessment for nursing practice* (3rd ed., pp. 306, 309, 624). St. Louis: Mosby.

---

115. A pediatric nurse specialist provides an educational session to the nursing students about childhood communicable diseases. A nursing student asks the pediatric nurse specialist to describe the signs and symptoms associated with the most common complication of mumps. The pediatric nurse specialist responds, knowing that which of the following signs or symptoms is indicative of the most common complication of this communicable disease?
 1 Pain
 2 Deafness
 3 Nuchal rigidity
 4 A red swollen testicle

Level of Cognitive Ability: Analysis
Client Needs: Physiological Integrity
Integrated Process: Teaching and Learning
Content Area: Child Health

Answer: 3
Rationale: The most common complication of mumps is aseptic meningitis, with the virus being identified in the cerebrospinal fluid. Common signs include nuchal rigidity, lethargy, and vomiting. A red swollen testicle may be indicative of orchitis. Although this complication appears to cause most concern among parents, it is not the most common complication. Although mumps is one of the leading causes of unilateral nerve deafness, it does not occur frequently. Muscular pain, parotid pain, or testicular pain may occur, but pain does not indicate a sign of a common complication.

Test-Taking Strategy: Use the process of elimination. Recalling that aseptic meningitis is the most common complication of mumps will direct you to option 3. Review the complications associated with mumps if you had difficulty with this question.

References
Hockenberry, M., Wilson, D., & Winkelstein, M. (2005). *Wong's essentials of pediatric nursing* (7th ed., pp. 440-441). St. Louis: Mosby.
McKinney, E., James, S., Murray, S., & Ashwill, J. (2005). *Maternal-child nursing* (2nd ed., pp. 1026-1027). St. Louis: Saunders.

116. A 5-year-old child is hospitalized with Rocky Mountain spotted fever (RMSF). The nursing assessment reveals that the child was bitten by a tick 2 weeks ago. The child presents with complaints of headache, fever, and anorexia, and the nurse notes a rash on the palms of the hands and soles of the feet. The nurse reviews the physician's orders and anticipates that which of the following medications will be prescribed?

1 Ganciclovir (Cytovene)
2 Amantadine (Symmetrel)
3 Doxycycline (Vibramycin)
4 Amphotericin B (Fungizone)

Level of Cognitive Ability: Analysis
Client Needs: Physiological Integrity
Integrated Process: Nursing Process/Analysis
Content Area: Child Health

Answer: 3
Rationale: The nursing care of a child with RMSF will include the administration of doxycycline. An alternative medication is chloramphenicol. Amphotericin B is used for fungal infections. Ganciclovir is used to treat cytomegalovirus. Amantadine is used to treat Parkinson's disease.

Test-Taking Strategy: Knowledge regarding the treatment plan associated with RMSF is required to answer this question. Remember that RMSF is treated with doxycycline. Review this content if you are unfamiliar with this treatment plan or with the medications identified in the options.

Reference
Hockenberry, M., Wilson, D., & Winkelstein, M. (2005). *Wong's essentials of pediatric nursing* (7th ed., p. 1119). St. Louis: Mosby.

---

117. A nursing instructor assigns a student nurse to present a clinical conference to the student group about brain tumors in children younger than 3 years of age. The nursing student prepares for the conference and includes which of the following information in the presentation?

1 Radiation is the treatment of choice.
2 The most significant symptoms are headaches and vomiting.
3 Head shaving is not required before removal of the brain tumor.
4 Surgery is not normally performed because of the risk of functional deficits occurring as a result of the surgery.

Level of Cognitive Ability: Application
Client Needs: Physiological Integrity
Integrated Process: Teaching and Learning
Content Area: Child Health

Answer: 2
Rationale: The hallmark symptoms of children with brain tumors are headaches and vomiting. The treatment of choice is total surgical removal of the tumor without residual neurological damage. Before surgery, the child's head will be shaved, although every effort is made to shave only as much hair as is necessary. Radiation therapy is avoided in children younger than 3 years of age due to the toxic side effects on the developing brain, particularly in very young children.

Test-Taking Strategy: Use the process of elimination. Eliminate options 3 and 4 first because of the close-ended word "not." From the remaining options, recalling that the treatment of choice is total surgical removal of the tumor will direct you to option 2. Review this content if you are unfamiliar with the clinical manifestations and interventions associated with a brain tumor.

Reference
Hockenberry, M., Wilson, D., & Winkelstein, M. (2005). *Wong's essentials of pediatric nursing* (7th ed., p. 1035). St. Louis: Mosby.

---

118. A magnetic resonance imaging (MRI) scan is prescribed for a client with a suspected brain tumor. Which prescription does the nurse prepare to administer to the client before the procedure?

1 An opioid
2 A sedative
3 A corticosteroid
4 An antihistamine

Answer: 2
Rationale: An MRI scan is a noninvasive diagnostic test that visualizes the body's tissues, structure, and blood flow. The client is positioned on a padded table and moved into a cylinder-shaped scanner. Relaxation techniques, an eye mask, and sedation are used before the procedure to reduce claustrophobic effects; however, because the client must remain very still during the scan, the nurse avoids oversedating the client to ensure client cooperation. There is no useful purpose for administering an, opioid, corticosteroid, or antihistamine.

Level of Cognitive Ability: Analysis
Client Needs: Physiological Integrity
Integrated Process: Nursing Process/Analysis
Content Area: Fundamental Skills

Test-Taking Strategy: Focus on the diagnostic test. Recalling that claustrophobia is a concern will direct you to option 2. Review this diagnostic test if you are unfamiliar with it.

Reference
Chernecky, C., & Berger, B. (2008). *Laboratory tests and diagnostic procedures* (5th ed., pp. 750-751). Philadelphia: Saunders.

---

119. Tretinoin (Retin-A) gel is prescribed for a client with acne. The client calls the clinic nurse and tells the nurse that her skin has become very red and is beginning to peel. The nurse makes which statement to the client?
1 "Notify the physician."
2 "Discontinue the medication."
3 "Come to the clinic immediately."
4 "This is a normal occurrence with the use of this medication."

Level of Cognitive Ability: Application
Client Needs: Physiological Integrity
Integrated Process: Nursing Process/
   Implementation
Content Area: Pharmacology

Answer: 4
Rationale: Tretinoin decreases cohesiveness of the epithelial cells, increasing cell mitosis and turnover. It is potentially irritating, particularly when used correctly. Within 48 hours of use, the skin generally becomes red and begins to peel. Options 1, 2, and 3 are incorrect statements to the client.

Test-Taking Strategy: Use the process of elimination. Options 1 and 3 can be eliminated first because they are comparable or alike. Eliminate option 2 next because it is not within the scope of nursing practice to advise a client to discontinue a medication. Review the effects of this medication if you had difficulty with this question.

Reference
Skidmore-Roth, L. (2008). *Mosby's nursing drug reference* (21st ed., p. 1025). St. Louis: Mosby.

---

120. A child is hospitalized with a diagnosis of lead poisoning, and chelation therapy is prescribed. The nurse caring for the child would prepare to administer which of the following medications?
1 Ipecac syrup
2 Activated charcoal
3 Sodium bicarbonate
4 Calcium disodium edetate (EDTA)

Level of Cognitive Ability: Application
Client Needs: Physiological Integrity
Integrated Process: Nursing Process/Planning
Content Area: Child Health

Answer: 4
Rationale: EDTA is a chelating agent that is used to treat lead poisoning. Sodium bicarbonate may be used in salicylate poisoning. Ipecac syrup may be prescribed for use in the hospital setting but would not be used to treat lead poisoning. Activated charcoal is used to decrease absorption in certain poisoning situations.

Test-Taking Strategy: Focus on the subject—treatment related to lead poisoning. Think about the classifications of the medications in the options. Recalling that EDTA is a chelating agent will direct you to option 4. Review this treatment if you are unfamiliar with it.

References
Mosby. (2007). *Mosby's nursing drug reference* (20th ed., p. 978). St. Louis: Mosby.
Hockenberry, M., Wilson, D., & Winkelstein, M. (2005). *Wong's essentials of pediatric nursing* (7th ed., p. 458). St. Louis: Mosby.

121. A nurse is performing pin site care on a client in skeletal traction. Which finding would the nurse expect to note when assessing the pin sites?
1 Loose pin sites
2 Clear drainage from the pin sites
3 Purulent drainage from the pin sites
4 Redness and swelling around the pin sites

Level of Cognitive Ability: Analysis
Client Needs: Physiological Integrity
Integrated Process: Nursing Process/Assessment
Content Area: Adult Health/Musculoskeletal

Answer: 2
Rationale: A small amount of clear drainage ("weeping") may be expected after cleaning and removing crusting around the pin sites. Redness and swelling around the pin sites and purulent drainage may be indicative of an infection. Pins should not be loose, and, if this is noted, the physician should be notified.

Test-Taking Strategy: Use the process of elimination. Option 1 is not an expected finding and can be eliminated first because loose pins would not provide a secure hold with the traction. Eliminate options 3 and 4 next because they are comparable or alike and indicate signs of infection. Review assessment of pin sites in the client with skeletal traction if you had difficulty with this question.

Reference
Ignatavicius, D., & Workman, M. (2006). *Medical-surgical nursing: Critical thinking for collaborative care* (5th ed., pp. 1201-1202). Philadelphia: Saunders.

---

122. A nurse is caring for a client who has been placed in Buck's extension traction while awaiting surgical repair of a fractured femur. The nurse prepares to perform a complete neurovascular assessment of the affected extremity and plans to assess:
1 Vital signs and bilateral lung sounds.
2 Pain level and for the presence of edema in the affected extremity.
3 Warmth of the skin and the temperature in the affected extremity.
4 Color, sensation, movement, capillary refill, and pulse of the affected extremity.

Level of Cognitive Ability: Application
Client Needs: Physiological Integrity
Integrated Process: Nursing Process/Assessment
Content Area: Adult Health/Musculoskeletal

Answer: 4
Rationale: A complete neurovascular assessment of an extremity includes color, sensation, movement, capillary refill, and pulse of the affected extremity.

Test-Taking Strategy: Focus on the strategic words "complete neurovascular assessment of the affected extremity." Options 2 and 3 identify only some of the components of a neurovascular assessment while option 1 does not identify any. Use the ABCs—airway, breathing, and circulation—to direct you to option 4. Review the components of a neurovascular assessment if you had difficulty with this question.

References
Black, J., & Hawks, J. (2005). *Medical-surgical nursing: Clinical management for positive outcomes* (7th ed., pp. 628, 644). Philadelphia: Saunders.
Monahan, F., Sands, J., Neighbors, M., Marek, J., & Green, C. (2007). *Phipp's medical-surgical nursing: Health and illness perspectives* (8th ed., pp. 1527-1528). St. Louis: Mosby.

---

123. A client in the emergency department has a cast applied. The client arrives at the nursing unit, and the nurse prepares to transfer the client into the bed by:
1 Placing ice on top of the cast.
2 Supporting the cast with the fingertips only.
3 Asking the client to support the cast during transfer.
4 Using the palms of the hands and soft pillows to support the cast.

Level of Cognitive Ability: Application
Client Needs: Physiological Integrity
Integrated Process: Nursing Process/Planning
Content Area: Adult Health/Musculoskeletal

Answer: 4
Rationale: The palms or the flat surface of the extended fingers should be used when moving a wet cast to prevent indentations. Pillows are used to support the curves of the cast to prevent cracking or flattening of the cast from the weight of the body. Half-full bags of ice may be placed next to the cast to prevent swelling, but this would be done after the client is placed in bed. Asking the client to support the cast during transfer is inappropriate.

Test-Taking Strategy: Focusing on the strategic words "transfer the client into the bed" will assist in eliminating option 1. Eliminate option 3 next because it is inappropriate to ask the client to support the cast. From the remaining options, eliminate option 2 because of the close-ended word "only" in this option. Review care of the client in a newly applied plaster cast if you had difficulty with this question.

References
Ignatavicius, D., & Workman, M. (2006). *Medical-surgical nursing: Critical thinking for collaborative care* (5th ed., p. 1198). Philadelphia: Saunders.
Monahan, F., Sands, J., Neighbors, M., Marek, J., & Green, C. (2007). *Phipps' medical-surgical nursing: Health and illness perspectives* (8th ed., p. 1536). St. Louis: Mosby.

---

124. A physician orders the deflation of the esophageal balloon of a Sengstaken-Blakemore tube in a client. The nurse prepares for the procedure, knowing that the deflation of the esophageal balloon places the client at risk for:

1 Gastritis
2 Increased ascites
3 Esophageal necrosis
4 Recurrent hemorrhage from the esophageal varices

Level of Cognitive Ability: Analysis
Client Needs: Physiological Integrity
Integrated Process: Nursing Process/Planning
Content Area: Adult Health/Gastrointestinal

Answer: 4
Rationale: A Sengstaken-Blakemore tube is inserted in clients with cirrhosis who have ruptured esophageal varices. It has esophageal and gastric balloons. The esophageal balloon exerts pressure on the ruptured esophageal varices and stops the bleeding. The pressure of the esophageal balloon is released at intervals to decrease the risk of trauma to the esophageal tissues, including esophageal rupture or necrosis. When the balloon is deflated, the client may begin to bleed again from the esophageal varices.

Test-Taking Strategy: Focus on the subject and recall the purpose of the esophageal balloon of the Sengstaken-Blakemore tube. Remembering that the esophageal balloon exerts pressure on ruptured esophageal varices and stops the bleeding will assist in directing you to option 4. Review the complications associated with this type of tube if you are unfamiliar with it.

References
Black, J., & Hawks, J. (2005). *Medical-surgical nursing: Clinical management for positive outcomes* (7th ed., pp. 1345-1346). Philadelphia: Saunders.
Ignatavicius, D., & Workman, M. (2006). *Medical-surgical nursing: Critical thinking for collaborative care* (5th ed., pp. 1378-1379). Philadelphia: Saunders.

---

125. A physician tells a nurse that a client can be given droperidol (Inapsine) for relief of postoperative nausea. The nurse anticipates that the physician will order the medication by which of the following routes?

1 Oral
2 Intranasal
3 Intravenous
4 Subcutaneous

Level of Cognitive Ability: Analysis
Client Needs: Physiological Integrity
Integrated Process: Nursing Process/Analysis
Content Area: Pharmacology

Answer: 3
Rationale: Droperidol may be administered by the intramuscular (IM) or intravenous (IV) routes. The IV route is the route used when relief of nausea is needed. The IM route may be used when the medication is used as an adjunct to anesthesia. Options 1, 2, and 4 are not routes of administration of this medication.

Test-Taking Strategy: Focus on the data in the question. Noting that this is a postoperative client will direct you to option 3. Review this medication if you had difficulty with this question.

Reference
Skidmore-Roth, L. (2008). *Mosby's nursing drug reference* (21st ed., p. 397). St. Louis: Mosby.

---

126. A nurse is teaching the parents of a child with celiac disease about dietary measures. In the teaching plan, the nurse will instruct the parents to:

1 Restrict corn and rice in the diet.
2 Restrict fresh vegetables in the diet.
3 Substitute grain cereals with pasta products.
4 Read all label ingredients carefully to avoid hidden sources of gluten.

Answer: 4
Rationale: Gluten is found primarily in the grains of wheat and rye. Corn and rice become substitute foods. Gluten is added to many foods as hydrolyzed vegetable protein that is derived from cereal grains, therefore labels need to be read. Corn and rice as well as vegetables are acceptable in a gluten-free diet. Many pasta products contain gluten. Grains are frequently added to processed foods for thickness or fillers.

Level of Cognitive Ability: Application
Client Needs: Physiological Integrity
Integrated Process: Teaching and Learning
Content Area: Child Health

Test-Taking Strategy: Use the process of elimination, recalling that a gluten-free diet is required in celiac disease. Select option 4 because it is the umbrella option. Review the dietary mea sures in celiac disease if you had difficulty with this question.

Reference
Hockenberry, M., Wilson, D., & Winkelstein, M. (2005). *Wong's essentials of pediatric nursing* (7th ed., p. 886). St. Louis: Mosby.

---

127. A 45-year-old client is admitted to the hospital for evaluation of recurrent runs of ventricular tachycardia noted on Holter monitoring. The client is scheduled for electrophysiology studies (EPS) the following morning. Which statement should the nurse include in a teaching plan for this client?
  1 "You will continue to take your medications until the morning of the test."
  2 "You will be sedated during the procedure and will not remember what has happened."
  3 "This test is a noninvasive method of determining the effectiveness of your medication regimen."
  4 "During the procedure, a special wire is used to increase the heart rate and produce the irregular beats that caused your signs and symptoms."

Level of Cognitive Ability: Application
Client Needs: Physiological Integrity
Integrated Process: Nursing Process/
  Implementation
Content Area: Adult Health/Cardiovascular

Answer: 4
Rationale: The purpose of EPS is to study the heart's electrical system. During this invasive procedure, a special wire is introduced into the heart to produce dysrhythmias. To prepare for this procedure, the client should be NPO for 6 to 8 hours before the test, and all antidysrhythmics are held for at least 24 hours before the test in order to study the dysrhythmias without the influence of medications. Because the client's verbal responses to the rhythm changes are extremely important, sedation is avoided if possible.

Test-Taking Strategy: Note the relationship between the words "recurrent runs of ventricular tachycardia" in the question and "produce the irregular beats" in option 4. Review this procedure if you had difficulty with this question.

Reference
Chernecky, C., & Berger, B. (2008). *Laboratory tests and diagnostic procedures* (5th ed., pp. 470-471). Philadelphia: Saunders.

---

128. A nurse is providing diet teaching to a client with congestive heart failure (CHF). The nurse tells the client to avoid which of the following?
  1 Sherbet
  2 Steak sauce
  3 Apple juice
  4 Leafy green vegetables

Level of Cognitive Ability: Application
Client Needs: Physiological Integrity
Integrated Process: Teaching and Learning
Content Area: Adult Health/Cardiovascular

Answer: 2
Rationale: Steak sauce is high in sodium. Leafy green vegetables, any juice (except tomato or V8 brand vegetable), and sherbet are all low in sodium. Clients with CHF should monitor sodium intake.

Test-Taking Strategy: Note the strategic word "avoid." Use the process of elimination, noting that options 1, 3, and 4 are comparable or alike in that they are low-sodium foods. Recalling that the client with CHF should limit sodium intake will direct you to option 2. Review dietary measures for the client with CHF if you had difficulty with this question.

Reference
Ignatavicius, D., & Workman, M. (2006). *Medical-surgical nursing: Critical thinking for collaborative care* (5th ed., p. 763). Philadelphia: Saunders.

129. The home care nurse is developing a plan of care for an older client with diabetes mellitus who has gastroenteritis. In order to maintain food and fluid intake to prevent dehydration, the nurse plans to:

1 Offer water only until the client is able to tolerate solid foods.
2 Withhold all fluids until vomiting has ceased for at least 4 hours.
3 Encourage the client to take 8 to 12 ounces of fluid every hour while awake.
4 Maintain a clear liquid diet for at least 5 days before advancing to solids to allow inflammation of the bowel to dissipate.

Level of Cognitive Ability: Application
Client Needs: Physiological Integrity
Integrated Process: Nursing Process/Planning
Content Area: Adult Health/Endocrine

Answer: 3

Rationale: The client should be offered liquids containing both glucose and electrolytes. Small amounts of fluid may be tolerated, even when vomiting is present. The diet should be advanced as tolerated and include a minimum of 100 to 150 grams of carbohydrates daily. Offering water only and maintaining liquids for 5 days will not prevent dehydration but may promote it in this client.

Test-Taking Strategy: Eliminate options 1 and 2 because of the words "only" and "all" in these options, respectively. From the remaining options, note the words "for at least 5 days" in option 4. Thinking about the subject—a client with diabetes mellitus and preventing dehydration—will assist in eliminating this option. Review sick day rules for a client with diabetes mellitus if you had difficulty with this question.

References
Ignatavicius, D., & Workman, M. (2006). *Medical-surgical nursing: Critical thinking for collaborative care* (5th ed., p. 1545). Philadelphia: Saunders.
Monahan, F., Sands, J., Neighbors, M., Marek, J., & Green, C. (2007). *Phipps' medical-surgical nursing: Health and illness perspectives* (8th ed., p. 1154). St. Louis: Mosby.

---

130. A client is unable to expectorate sputum for a sputum sample, and the nurse is preparing to obtain the sample via saline inhalation. The nurse instructs the client to inhale the warm saline vapor via nebulizer by:

1 Holding the nebulizer under the nose
2 Keeping the lips closed lightly over the mouthpiece
3 Keeping the lips closely tightly over the mouthpiece
4 Alternating one vapor breath with one breath from room air

Level of Cognitive Ability: Comprehension
Client Needs: Physiological Integrity
Integrated Process: Nursing Process/ Implementation
Content Area: Fundamental Skills

Answer: 2

Rationale: The inhalation of warm saline vapor helps the client to cough productively because the vapor condenses on the tracheobronchial mucosa and stimulates the production of secretions leading to a cough. The client is told to lightly cover the mouthpiece with the lips and avoid forming a tight seal. The client inhales the vaporized saline until coughing results. Options 1, 3, and 4 are incorrect.

Test-Taking Strategy: Note that options 2 and 3 are opposite actions in that one option says to keep the lips closed tightly over the mouthpiece whereas the other says to keep the lips closed lightly over the mouthpiece. Visualizing this procedure will direct you to option 2. Review this variation of procedure for obtaining a sputum sample if you had difficulty with the question.

References
Chernecky, C., & Berger, B. (2008). *Laboratory tests and diagnostic procedures* (5th ed., pp. 1034-1035). Philadelphia: Saunders.
Potter, P., & Perry, A. (2005). *Fundamentals of nursing* (6th ed., pp. 1435-1438). St. Louis: Mosby.

131. The nurse has completed tracheostomy care for a client whose tracheostomy tube has a nondisposable inner cannula. Immediately before reinserting the inner cannula, which is the best nursing action for the nurse to complete?
1 Rinsing it in sterile water
2 Suctioning the client's airway
3 Tapping it against a sterile basin
4 Drying it with loosely woven gauze

Level of Cognitive Ability: Application
Client Needs: Physiological Integrity
Integrated Process: Nursing Process/
  Implementation
Content Area: Fundamental Skills

Answer: 3
Rationale: After washing and rinsing the inner cannula, the nurse taps it dry to remove large water droplets; then, the nurse inserts the cannula into the tracheostomy and turns it clockwise to lock it into place. The nurse avoids shaking the inner cannula to prevent contamination. A wet cannula should not be inserted into a tracheostomy because water is a lung irritant. Suctioning is not performed without an inner cannula in place. Fine-mesh sterile gauze may be used to dry the inner cannula because it is less likely than loosely woven gauze to deposit debris on the cannula.

Test-Taking Strategy: Use the process of elimination and focus on the subject—reinserting the inner cannula. Note the strategic word "nondisposable" and visualize the procedure. Eliminate option 1 because a wet cannula should not be inserted and option 2 because you would not suction a client without the inner cannula in place. Eliminate option 4 because loosely woven gauze would deposit debris. Review the procedure for tracheotomy care if you had difficulty with this question.

References
Ignatavicius, D., & Workman, M. (2006). *Medical-surgical nursing: Critical thinking for collaborative care* (5th ed., p. 558). Philadelphia: Saunders.
Lewis, S., Heitkemper, M., Dirksen, S., O'Brien, P., & Bucher, L. (2007). *Medical-surgical nursing: Assessment and management of clinical problems* (7th ed., p. 546). St. Louis: Mosby.

132. A nurse suspects that an air embolism has occurred when the client's central venous catheter disconnects from the IV tubing. The nurse immediately places the client in which position?
1 Trendelenburg's on the left side
2 Trendelenburg's on the right side
3 Reverse Trendelenburg's on the left side
4 Reverse Trendelenburg's on the right side

Level of Cognitive Ability: Application
Client Needs: Physiological Integrity
Integrated Process: Nursing Process/
  Implementation
Content Area: Fundamental Skills

Answer: 1
Rationale: If the client develops an air embolism, the immediate action is to place the client in Trendelenburg's position on the left side. This position raises the client's feet higher than the head and traps any air in the right atrium. If necessary, the air can then be directly removed by intracardiac aspiration. Options 2, 3, and 4 are incorrect positions because reverse Trendelenburg's elevates the head, puts the air in a dependent position, and increases the risk of a cerebral embolism; lying on the right side places the air in a dependent position, rendering it more likely to migrate.

Test-Taking Strategy: Visualize each position in the options. Recalling that the goal of action is to trap air in the right atrium will direct you to option 1. Review immediate care of a client with an air embolism if you had difficulty with this question.

Reference
Black, J., & Hawks, J. (2005). *Medical-surgical nursing: Clinical management for positive outcomes* (7th ed., p. 1833). Philadelphia: Saunders.

133. An anxious client enters the emergency department seeking treatment for a laceration of the finger. The client's vital signs are pulse 106 beats per minute, blood pressure (BP) 158/88 mm Hg, and respirations 28 breaths per minute. After cleansing the injury and reassuring the client, the nurse rechecks the vital signs and notes a pulse of 82 beats per minute, BP 130/80 mm Hg, and respirations 20 breaths per minute. The nurse determines that the change in vital signs is caused by:

1 Cooling effects of the cleansing agent
2 Early clinical indicators of cardiogenic shock •
3 Client's adaptation to the air conditioning
4 Fall in sympathetic nervous system discharge

Level of Cognitive Ability: Comprehension
Client Needs: Physiological Integrity
Integrated Process: Nursing Process/Analysis
Content Area: Fundamental Skills

Answer: 4
Rationale: Physical or emotional stress triggers a sympathetic nervous system stimulation. Increased epinephrine and norepinephrine cause tachycardia, high blood pressure, and tachypnea. Stress reduction, then, returns these parameters to baseline as the sympathetic discharge falls. Options 1 and 3 are unrelated to the changes in vital signs. Because the client's vital signs remain within normal limits, the client exhibits no indication of cardiogenic shock.

Test-Taking Strategy: Eliminate options 1 and 3 first because they are comparable or alike. Next note that the client is anxious and has an injury. These two pieces of information guide you to think about the body's response to stress. Recalling the relationship of stress to the sympathetic nervous system will direct you to option 4. Review the effects of physical stress on the vital signs if you had difficulty with this question.

Reference
Lewis, S., Heitkemper, M., Dirksen, S., O'Brien, P., & Bucher, L. (2007). *Medical-surgical nursing: Assessment and management of clinical problems* (7th ed., pp. 747-748, 766). St. Louis: Mosby.

---

134. The nurse schedules multiple diagnostic procedures for the client with heart failure who has activity intolerance. The procedures ordered include an echocardiogram, a chest radiograph (CXR), and a computed axial tomography (CAT) scan. Which is the best schedule for the nurse to plan to meet the needs of this client safely and effectively?

1 CAT scan and CXR in the morning, and echocardiogram on the following morning
2 CXR and echocardiogram together in the morning, and CAT scan in the afternoon of the same day
3 Echocardiogram in the morning, and CXR and CAT scans together in the afternoon of the same day
4 CXR in the morning, echocardiogram in the afternoon, and CAT scan in the morning of the following day

Level of Cognitive Ability: Analysis
Client Needs: Physiological Integrity
Integrated Process: Nursing Process/Planning
Content Area: Fundamental Skills

Answer: 4
Rationale: CAT scans are always performed in radiology and CXR and echocardiograms can be done at the bedside; however, the best results usually occur when the test is performed in the related department. As long as the client is stable and transportation is provided, the nurse can schedule each procedure in its department with two procedures on 1 day separated by a rest period, and the remaining procedure the next day. The nurse should plan the CXR or echocardiogram for the afternoon because, if the client's condition deteriorates after the first procedure, the nurse can order a portable CXR or echocardiogram.

Test-Taking Strategy: Focus on the subject—activity intolerance. Recalling that the client will do best if activities are spaced will direct you to option 4. Review interventions for the client with activity intolerance if you had difficulty with this question.

References
Black, J., & Hawks, J. (2005). *Medical-surgical nursing: Clinical management for positive outcomes* (7th ed., p. 1667). Philadelphia: Saunders.
Monahan, F., Sands, J., Neighbors, M., Marek, J., & Green, C. (2007). *Phipps' medical-surgical nursing: Health and illness perspectives* (8th ed., pp. 814, 827-828). St. Louis: Mosby.

135. The nurse is preparing to initiate an intravenous nitroglycerin drip on a client with acute myocardial infarction. In the absence of an invasive (arterial) monitoring line, the nurse prepares to have which piece of equipment for use at the bedside?

1 Defibrillator
2 Pulse oximeter
3 Central venous pressure (CVP) tray
4 Noninvasive blood pressure monitor

Level of Cognitive Ability: Application
Client Needs: Physiological Integrity
Integrated Process: Nursing Process/Planning
Content Area: Adult Health/Cardiovascular

Answer: 4
Rationale: Nitroglycerin dilates both arteries and veins, causing peripheral blood pooling, thus reducing preload, afterload, and myocardial workload. This action accounts for the primary side effect of nitroglycerin, which is hypotension. In the absence of an arterial monitoring line, the nurse should have a noninvasive blood pressure monitor for use at the bedside.

Test-Taking Strategy: Use the process of elimination, noting the strategic words "absence of an invasive (arterial) monitoring line." Recalling the purpose of this type of monitoring device and the action of nitroglycerin will direct you to option 4. Review nursing responsibilities when administering a nitroglycerin drip if you had difficulty with this question.

References
Gahart, B., & Nazareno, A. (2006). *2006 Intravenous medications* (22nd ed., p. 900). St. Louis: Mosby.
Ignatavicius, D., & Workman, M. (2006). *Medical-surgical nursing: Critical thinking for collaborative care* (5th ed., p. 855). Philadelphia: Saunders.

---

136. A client in labor has a concurrent diagnosis of sickle cell anemia. Which action has priority to assist in preventing a sickling crisis from occurring during labor?

1 Reassure the client.
2 Prevent bearing down.
3 Maintain strict asepsis.
4 Administer oxygen throughout labor.

Level of Cognitive Ability: Application
Client Needs: Physiological Integrity
Integrated Process: Nursing Process/ Implementation
Content Area: Maternity/Intrapartum

Answer: 4
Rationale: During the labor process, the client with sickle cell anemia is at high risk for being unable to meet the oxygen demands of labor. Administering oxygen will prevent sickle cell crisis during labor. Options 1 and 3 are appropriate actions but are unrelated to sickle cell crisis. Option 2 is inappropriate.

Test-Taking Strategy: Note the strategic word "priority." Focus on the client's diagnosis and use the ABCs—airway, breathing, and circulation—to direct you to option 4. Review care of the client with sickle cell anemia in labor if you had difficulty with this question.

References
McKinney, E., James, S., Murray, S., & Ashwill, J. (2005). *Maternal-child nursing* (2nd ed., p. 659). St. Louis: Saunders.
Murray, S., & McKinney, E. (2006). *Foundations of maternal-newborn nursing* (4th ed., p. 679). Philadelphia: Saunders.

---

137. A client is scheduled for computed tomography (CT) of the kidneys to rule out renal disease. As an essential preprocedure component of the nursing assessment, the nurse plans to ask the client about a history of:

1 Familial renal disease
2 Frequent antibiotic use
3 Long-term diuretic therapy
4 Allergy to shellfish or iodine

Answer: 4
Rationale: The client undergoing any type of diagnostic testing involving possible dye administration should be questioned about allergy to shellfish or iodine. This is essential to identify the risk for potential allergic reaction to contrast dye, which may be used. The other items are also useful as part of the assessment but are not as critical as the allergy determination in the preprocedure period.

Level of Cognitive Ability: Application
Client Needs: Physiological Integrity
Integrated Process: Nursing Process/Assessment
Content Area: Adult Health/Renal

Test-Taking Strategy: Note the strategic words "essential" and "preprocedure component." Because the question indicates that CT of the kidneys is planned, the items in the options are evaluated against their potential connection to this aspect of care. Recalling that contrast dye may be used during CT to enhance visualization of the kidneys will direct you to option 4. Review client assessment related to diagnostic testing if you had difficulty with this question.

References
Black, J., & Hawks, J. (2005). *Medical-surgical nursing: Clinical management for positive outcomes* (7th ed., pp. 93, 101). Philadelphia: Saunders.
Potter, P., & Perry, A. (2005). *Fundamentals of nursing* (6th ed., pp. 1480-1481). St. Louis: Mosby.

---

138. The nurse assists a client who has a renal disorder collect a 24-hour urine specimen. Which does the nurse implement to ensure proper collection of the 24-hour specimen?
1 Strain the specimen before pouring the urine into the container.
2 Save all urine, beginning with the urine voided at the start time.
3 Have the client void at the start time and discard the specimen.
4 Once completed, refrigerate the urine collection until picked up by the laboratory.

Level of Cognitive Ability: Application
Client Needs: Physiological Integrity
Integrated Process: Nursing Process/ Implementation
Content Area: Fundamental Skills

Answer: 3
Rationale: The nurse asks the client to void at the beginning of the collection period and discards this urine sample because this urine has been stored in the bladder for an undetermined length of time. All urine thereafter is saved in an iced or refrigerated container. The client is asked to void at the finish time, and this sample is the last specimen added to the collection. Straining the urine is contraindicated for timed urine collections. The container is labeled, placed on fresh ice, and sent to the laboratory immediately.

Test-Taking Strategy: Focusing on the subject—a 24-hour urine collection—will assist in eliminating options 1 and 2. For the remaining options, think about the procedure. The container is sent to the laboratory immediately to prevent an alteration in the results. Review this procedure if you had difficulty with this question.

Reference
Ignatavicius, D., & Workman, M. (2006). *Medical-surgical nursing: Critical thinking for collaborative care* (5th ed., p. 1666). Philadelphia: Saunders.

---

139. A nurse is caring for a client in active labor. Which priority action should the nurse perform to prevent fetal heart rate decelerations?
1 Prepare the client for a cesarean delivery.
2 Monitor the fetal heart rate every 30 minutes.
3 Encourage upright or side-lying maternal positions.
4 Increase the rate of the oxytocin (Pitocin) infusion.

Answer: 3
Rationale: Side-lying and upright positions such as walking, standing, and squatting can improve venous return and encourage effective uterine activity. The nurse should discontinue an oxytocin infusion in the presence of fetal heart rate decelerations, thereby reducing uterine activity and increasing uteroplacental perfusion. Monitoring the fetal heart rate every 30 minutes will not prevent fetal heart rate decelerations. There are many nursing actions to prevent fetal heart rate decelerations, without necessitating surgical intervention.

Level of Cognitive Ability: Application
Client Needs: Physiological Integrity
Integrated Process: Nursing Process/
   Implementation
Content Area: Maternity/Intrapartum

Test-Taking Strategy: Use the process of elimination and focus on the subject—"to prevent fetal heart rate decelerations." Options 1, 2, and 4 will not prevent fetal heart rate decelerations. Side-lying and upright positions will improve venous return and encourage effective uterine activity. Review nursing interventions for the client in labor if you had difficulty with this question.

References
McKinney, E., James, S., Murray, S., & Ashwill, J. (2005). *Maternal-child nursing* (2nd ed., p. 406). St. Louis: Saunders.
Murray, S., & McKinney, E. (2006). *Foundations of maternal-newborn nursing* (4th ed., p. 325). Philadelphia: Saunders.

---

140. A client with diabetes mellitus is at 36 weeks' gestation. The client has had weekly nonstress tests for the last 3 weeks, and the results have been reactive. This week, the nonstress test was nonreactive after 40 minutes. Based on these results, the nurse should anticipate the client will be prepared for:
   1 A contraction stress test
   2 Immediate induction of labor
   3 Hospitalization with continuous fetal monitoring
   4 A return appointment in 2 to 7 days to repeat the nonstress test

Level of Cognitive Ability: Analysis
Client Needs: Physiological Integrity
Integrated Process: Nursing Process/Planning
Content Area: Maternity/Antepartum

Answer: 1
Rationale: A nonreactive nonstress test needs further assessment. There are not enough data in the question to indicate that the procedures in options 2 and 3 are necessary at this time. To send the client home for 2 to 7 days may place the fetus in jeopardy. A contraction stress test is the next test needed to further assess the fetal status.

Test-Taking Strategy: Use the process of elimination, focusing on the subject—a change in test results from reactive to nonreactive. Options 2 and 3 can be eliminated first because they are unnecessary at this time. Option 4 can be eliminated next because repeating the test at a later time is not a safe intervention, especially considering the fact that previous test results were reactive. Review the meanings of the test results related to a nonstress test if you had difficulty with this question.

Reference
Wong, D., Hockenberry, M., Perry, S., Lowdermilk, D., & Wilson, D. (2006). *Maternal-child nursing care* (3rd ed., p. 230). St. Louis: Mosby.

---

141. A nurse is administering magnesium sulfate to a client for severe preeclampsia. During the administration of the medication, the nurse:
   1 Schedules a daily ultrasound to assess fetal movement
   2 Schedules a nonstress test every 4 hours to assess fetal well-being
   3 Assesses the client's temperature every 2 hours because the client is at high risk for infection
   4 Assesses for signs and symptoms of labor because the client's level of consciousness may be altered

Answer: 4
Rationale: Because of the sedative effect of the magnesium sulfate, the client may not perceive labor. This client is not at high risk for infection. A nonstress test may be done, but not every 4 hours. Daily ultrasounds are not necessary for this client.

Test-Taking Strategy: Use the nursing process to answer the question. Assessment is the first step; therefore, eliminate options 1 and 2. From the remaining options, knowledge that the client is not at high risk for infection will assist in directing you to option 4. Review nursing responsibilities when administering magnesium sulfate if you had difficulty with this question.

Level of Cognitive Ability: Application
Client Needs: Physiological Integrity
Integrated Process: Nursing Process/
  Implementation
Content Area: Maternity/Antepartum

Reference
Wong, D., Hockenberry, M., Perry, S., Lowdermilk, D., & Wilson, D. (2006). *Maternal-child nursing care* (3rd ed., p. 383). St. Louis: Mosby.

---

142. A client's nasogastric (NG) tube stops draining. Which should the nurse implement first to maintain client safety?
 1 Instill 30 to 60 mL of air.
 2 Verify the tube placement.
 3 Clamp the tube for 2 hours.
 4 Retract the tube by 2 inches.

Level of Cognitive Ability: Application
Client Needs: Physiological Integrity
Integrated Process: Nursing Process/
  Implementation
Content Area: Fundamental Skills

Answer: 2
Rationale: If a client's nasogastric tube stops draining, the nurse verifies placement first to ensure that the tube remains in the stomach. After checking the equipment and verifying a prescription for tube irrigation, the nurse irrigates the tube with 30 to 60 mL of the fluid per agency procedure. Clamping the tube increases the risk of aspiration and is contraindicated; besides, this intervention cannot unclog a tube. Pulling out the tube can displace the tube and place the client at risk for aspiration. Replacement of the tube is the last step if other actions are unsuccessful.

Test-Taking Strategy: Focus on the subject—the tube stopped draining. Eliminate options 1, 3, and 4 because these interventions increase client risk of aspiration. Also use the steps of the nursing process; option 2 is the only assessment action. Review care of the client with an NG tube if you had difficulty with this question.

Reference
Ignatavicius, D., & Workman, M. (2006). *Medical-surgical nursing: Critical thinking for collaborative care* (5th ed., p. 1666). Philadelphia: Saunders.

---

143. A nurse is planning to give a tepid tub bath to a child who has hyperthermia. The nurse plans to:
 1 Obtain isopropyl alcohol to add to the bath water.
 2 Allow 5 minutes for the child to soak in the bath water.
 3 Have cool water available to add to the warm bath water.
 4 Warm the water to the same body temperature of the child.

Level of Cognitive Ability: Application
Client Needs: Physiological Integrity
Integrated Process: Nursing Process/Planning
Content Area: Child Health

Answer: 3
Rationale: Adding cool water to an already warm bath allows the water temperature to slowly drop. The child is able to gradually adjust to the changing water temperature and will not experience chilling. Alcohol is toxic and contraindicated for tepid sponge or tub baths. To achieve the best cooling results, the water temperature should be at least 2 degrees lower than the child's body temperature. The child should be in a tepid tub bath for 20 to 30 minutes to achieve maximum results.

Test-Taking Strategy: Use the process of elimination. Eliminate option 1, recalling that alcohol is toxic as well as irritating to the skin. Eliminate option 4 because water that is the same as body temperature will not reduce hyperthermia. Eliminate option 2 because of the 5-minute timeframe. Review measures for hyperthermia and the procedure for giving a tepid bath to a child if you had difficulty with this question.

Reference
Hockenberry, M., Wilson, D., & Winkelstein, M. (2005). *Wong's essentials of pediatric nursing* (7th ed., pp. 732-733). St. Louis: Mosby.

144. A nurse is assigned to care for a child who is 1 day postoperative following a surgical repair of a cleft lip. Which nursing intervention is appropriate when caring for this child's surgical incision?
1 Rinse the incision with sterile water after feeding.
2 Clean the incision only when serous exudate forms.
3 Rub the incision gently with a sterile cotton-tipped swab.
4 Replace the Logan bar carefully after cleaning the incision.

Level of Cognitive Ability: Application
Client Needs: Physiological Integrity
Integrated Process: Nursing Process/ Implementation
Content Area: Child Health

Answer: 1
Rationale: The incision should be rinsed with sterile water after every feeding. Rubbing alters the integrity of the suture line. Rather, the incision should be patted or dabbed. The purpose of the Logan bar is to maintain the integrity of the suture line. Removing the Logan bar on the first postoperative day would increase tension on the surgical incision.

Test-Taking Strategy: Use the process of elimination. Eliminate options 2 and 3 first because of the word "only" in option 2 and "rub" in option 3. Focus on the words "1 day postoperative." This should assist in eliminating option 4. Review care of a child following surgical repair of a cleft lip if you had difficulty with this question.

References
Hockenberry, M., Wilson, D., & Winkelstein, M. (2005). *Wong's essentials of pediatric nursing* (7th ed., p. 876). St. Louis: Mosby.
Wong, D., Hockenberry, M., Perry, S., Lowdermilk, D., & Wilson, D. (2006). *Maternal-child nursing care* (3rd ed., p. 1527). St. Louis: Mosby.

---

145. A client is in ventricular tachycardia and the physician orders intravenous (IV) lidocaine (Xylocaine). The nurse plans to dilute the concentrated solution of lidocaine with:
1 Lactated Ringer's
2 Normal saline 0.9%
3 5% Dextrose in water
4 Normal saline 0.45%

Level of Cognitive Ability: Application
Client Needs: Physiological Integrity
Integrated Process: Nursing Process/ Implementation
Content Area: Adult Health/Cardiovascular

Answer: 3
Rationale: Lidocaine for IV administration is dispensed in concentrated and dilute formulations. The concentrated formulation must be diluted with 5% dextrose in water.

Test-Taking Strategy: Use the process of elimination. Eliminate options 2 and 4 first because they are similar solutions. From the remaining options, it is necessary to know that the concentrated formulation must be diluted with 5% dextrose in water. Review the procedure for administering this medication if you had difficulty with this question.

References
Gahart, B., & Nazareno, A. (2006). *2006 Intravenous medications* (22nd ed., p. 759). St. Louis: Mosby.
Hodgson, B., & Kizior, R. (2007). *Saunders nursing drug handbook 2007* (p. 690). Philadelphia: Saunders.

---

146. A client receiving parenteral nutrition (PN) via a central venous catheter (CVC) is scheduled to receive an intravenous (IV) antibiotic. Which should the nurse implement before administering the antibiotic?
1 Turn off the PN for 30 minutes.
2 Ensure a separate IV access route.
3 Check for compatibility with PN.
4 Flush the CVC with normal saline.

Answer: 2
Rationale: The PN line is used only for the administration of the PN solution to prevent crystallization in the CVC tubing and disruption of the PN infusion. Any other IV medication must be administered through a separate IV access site including a separate infusion port of the CVC catheter. Therefore, options 1, 3, and 4 are incorrect actions.

Test-Taking Strategy: Use the process of elimination. Eliminate options 1, 3, and 4 because they are comparable or alike in that they involve using the PN line for the administration of the antibiotic. Review care of the client receiving parenteral nutrition if you had difficulty with this question.

Level of Cognitive Ability: Application
Client Needs: Physiological Integrity
Integrated Process: Nursing Process/
Implementation
Content Area: Fundamental Skills

References
Ignatavicius, D., & Workman, M. (2006) *Medical-surgical nursing: Critical thinking for collaborative care* (5th ed., p. 1434). Philadelphia: Saunders.
Lewis, S., Heitkemper, M., Dirksen, S., O'Brien, P., & Bucher, L. (2007). *Medical-surgical nursing: Assessment and management of clinical problems* (7th ed., p. 990). St. Louis: Mosby.
Potter, P., & Perry, A. (2005). *Fundamentals of nursing* (6th ed., pp. 1161). St. Louis: Mosby.

---

147. A nurse is inserting an indwelling urinary catheter into a male client. As the nurse inflates the balloon with a syringe, the client complains of discomfort. The nurse should:
1 Administer pain medication.
2 Remove the syringe from the balloon.
3 Deflate the balloon and advance the catheter.
4 Remove the catheter and reinsert a new catheter.

Level of Cognitive Ability: Application
Client Needs: Physiological Integrity
Integrated Process: Nursing Process/
Implementation
Content Area: Fundamental Skills

Answer: 3
Rationale: Pain elicited during urinary catheter insertion is usually caused by balloon inflation within the urethra and can result in urethral trauma and pain. If pain occurs, the nurse aspirates fluid from the balloon and then inserts the catheter a little farther so the balloon can inflate in the bladder. Removing and reinserting the catheter is unnecessary, wasteful, and increases the risk of infection for the client. Administering pain medication is inappropriate.

Test-Taking Strategy: Note the subject—client's complaint of discomfort on balloon inflation. Use the process of elimination and attempt to visualize the procedure. This will direct you to option 3. Review the complications associated with insertion of a urinary catheter if you had difficulty with this question.

Reference
Potter, P., & Perry, A. (2005). *Fundamentals of nursing* (6th ed., pp. 1355-1356). St. Louis: Mosby.

---

148. A client with acquired immunodeficiency syndrome (AIDS) who has cytomegalovirus retinitis (CMV) is receiving ganciclovir sodium (Cytovene). The nurse implements which of the following in the care of this client?
1 Monitors blood glucose levels for elevation
2 Applies pressure to venipuncture sites for 2 minutes
3 Administers the medication on an empty stomach only
4 Tells the client to use a soft toothbrush and an electric razor

Level of Cognitive Ability: Application
Client Needs: Physiological Integrity
Integrated Process: Nursing Process/
Implementation
Content Area: Adult Health/Immune

Answer: 4
Rationale: Ganciclovir causes neutropenia and thrombocytopenia as the most frequent side effects. For this reason, the nurse monitors the client for signs and symptoms of bleeding and implements the same precautions that are used for a client receiving anticoagulant therapy. Thus, venipuncture sites should be held for approximately 10 minutes. The medication does not have to be taken on an empty stomach. The medication may cause hypoglycemia, but not hyperglycemia.

Test-Taking Strategy: Use the process of elimination. Recalling that this medication causes thrombocytopenia will direct you to option 4. Review the nursing considerations related to this medication if you had difficulty with this question.

References
Hodgson, B., & Kizior, R. (2007). *Saunders nursing drug handbook 2007* (p. 531). Philadelphia: Saunders.
Kee, J., Hayes, E., & McCuistion, L. (2006). *Pharmacology: A nursing process approach* (5th ed., p. 477). Philadelphia: Saunders.

149. A client without history of respiratory disease has experienced sudden onset of chest pain and dyspnea and is diagnosed with pulmonary embolus. The nurse immediately implements which expected order prescribed for this client?

1 Semi-Fowler's position, oxygen, and morphine sulfate intravenously (IV)
2 Supine position, oxygen, and meperidine hydrochloride (Demerol) intramuscularly (IM)
3 High Fowler's position, oxygen, and meperidine hydrochloride (Demerol) intravenously (IV)
4 High Fowler's position, oxygen, and two tablets of acetaminophen with codeine (Tylenol #3)

Level of Cognitive Ability: Application
Client Needs: Physiological Integrity
Integrated Process: Nursing Process/ Implementation
Content Area: Adult Health/Respiratory

Answer: 1
Rationale: Standard therapeutic intervention for the client with pulmonary embolus includes proper positioning, oxygen, and intravenous analgesics. The head of the bed is placed in semi-Fowler's position. High Fowler's is avoided because extreme hip flexure slows venous return from the legs and increases the risk of new thrombi. The supine position will increase the dyspnea that occurs with pulmonary embolism. The usual analgesic of choice is morphine sulfate administered IV. This medication reduces pain, alleviates anxiety, and can diminish congestion of blood in the pulmonary vessels because it causes peripheral venous dilation.

Test-Taking Strategy: Use the process of elimination. Eliminate option 2 first because a supine position will exacerbate the dyspnea. From the remaining options, recall that a high Fowler's position is avoided because extreme hip flexure slows venous return from the legs and increases the risk of new thrombi. This will assist in eliminating options 3 and 4. Review immediate care of the client with pulmonary embolus if you had difficulty with this question.

References
Black, J., & Hawks, J. (2005). *Medical-surgical nursing: Clinical management for positive outcomes* (7th ed., pp. 1832-1833). Philadelphia: Saunders.
Ignatavicius, D., & Workman, M. (2006). *Medical-surgical nursing: Critical thinking for collaborative care* (5th ed., p. 650). Philadelphia: Saunders.

---

150. A client who recently experienced a myocardial infarction is scheduled to have a percutaneous transluminal coronary angioplasty (PTCA). The nurse plans to teach the client that, during this procedure, a balloon-tipped catheter will:

1 Inflate a meshlike device that will spring open.
2 Be used to compress the plaque against the coronary blood vessel wall.
3 Cut away the plaque from the coronary vessel wall using a cutting blade.
4 Be positioned in a coronary artery to take pressure measurements in the vessel.

Level of Cognitive Ability: Application
Client Needs: Physiological Integrity
Integrated Process: Teaching and Learning
Content Area: Adult Health/Cardiovascular

Answer: 2
Rationale: In PTCA, a balloon-tipped catheter is used to compress the plaque against the coronary blood vessel wall. Option 3 describes coronary atherectomy, option 1 describes placement of a coronary stent, and option 4 describes part of the process used in cardiac catheterization.

Test-Taking Strategy: Look at the name of the procedure. "Angioplasty" refers to repair of a blood vessel; this will assist in eliminating options 1 and 4. From the remaining options, recalling that a procedure that cuts something away would have the suffix "-ectomy" will assist in eliminating option 3. Review this procedure if you had difficulty with this question.

Reference
Ignatavicius, D., & Workman, M. (2006). *Medical-surgical nursing: Critical thinking for collaborative care* (5th ed., pp. 796-797). Philadelphia: Saunders.

---

151. A nurse is caring for a client who has been placed in Buck's extension traction. The nurse provides for countertraction to reduce shear and friction by:

1 Using a footboard
2 Providing an overhead trapeze
3 Slightly elevating the foot of the bed
4 Slightly elevating the head of the bed

Answer: 3
Rationale: The part of the bed under an area in traction is usually elevated to aid in countertraction. For the client in Buck's extension traction (which is applied to a leg), the foot of the bed is elevated. An overhead trapeze or footboard is not used to provide countertraction. Option 3 provides a force that opposes the traction force effectively without harming the client.

Level of Cognitive Ability: Application
Client Needs: Physiological Integrity
Integrated Process: Nursing Process/
  Implementation
Content Area: Adult Health/Musculoskeletal

Test-Taking Strategy: Use the process of elimination. Eliminate option 4, recalling that Buck's extension traction is applied to the leg. From the remaining options, focus on the subject—providing countertraction—to eliminate options 1 and 2. Review Buck's extension traction if you had difficulty with this question.

Reference
Ignatavicius, D., & Workman, M. (2006). *Medical-surgical nursing: Critical thinking for collaborative care* (5th ed., pp. 1200-1201). Philadelphia: Saunders.

---

152. The nurse is preparing to initiate bolus enteral feedings via nasogastric (NG) tube to a client. Which of the following actions represents safe practice by the nurse?
    1 Checks the volume of the residual after administering the bolus feeding
    2 Aspirates gastric contents prior to initiating the feeding and assures that pH is > 9
    3 Elevates the head of the bed to 25 degrees and maintains for 30 minutes after instillation of feeding
    4 Measures the length of the tube from where it protrudes from the nose to the end and compares to previously documented measurements

Level of Cognitive Ability: Application
Client Needs: Physiological Integrity
Integrated Process: Nursing Process/
  Implementation
Content Area: Adult Health/Gastrointestinal

Answer: 4
Rationale: After initial radiographic confirmation of NG tube placement, methods used to verify nasogastric tube placement include measuring the length of the tube from the point it protrudes from the nose to the end; injecting 10 to 30 mL of air into the tube and auscultating over the left upper quadrant of the abdomen; and aspirating the secretions and checking to see if the pH is between 1 and 5. Fowler's position is recommended for bolus feedings, if permitted, and should be maintained for 1 hour after instillation. Residual should be assessed before administration of the next feeding.

Test-Taking Strategy: Focus on the strategic words "safe practice." Knowing that the pH of gastric contents should be between 1 and 5 will assist you to eliminate option 2. Option 3 can be eliminated because head of the bed elevation should be at a minimum of 30 degrees for all types of enteral feedings to prevent aspiration. From the remaining two options, use knowledge of when to check residuals to assist you in eliminating option 1. Review procedures related to administration of enteral feedings via nasogastric tube if you had difficulty with this question.

Reference
Monahan, F., Sands, J., Neighbors, M., Marek, J., & Green, C. (2007). *Phipps' medical-surgical nursing: Health and illness perspectives* (8th ed., p. 1233). St. Louis: Mosby.

---

153. A nurse has inserted a nasogastric (NG) tube to the level of the oropharynx and has repositioned the client's head in a flexed-forward position. The client has been asked to begin swallowing, and as the nurse starts to slowly advance the NG tube with each swallow, the client begins to gag. Which nursing action would least likely result in proper tube insertion and promote client relaxation?
    1 Pulling the tube back slightly
    2 Instructing the client to breathe slowly
    3 Continuing to advance the tube to the desired distance
    4 Checking the back of the pharynx using a tongue blade and flashlight

Answer: 3
Rationale: As the NG tube is passed through the oropharynx, the gag reflex is stimulated, which may cause gagging. Instead of passing through to the esophagus, the NG tube may coil around itself in the oropharynx, or it may enter the larynx and obstruct the airway. Because the tube may enter the larynx, advancing the tube may position it in the trachea. Slow breathing helps the client relax to reduce the gag response. The tube may be advanced after the client relaxes.

Test-Taking Strategy: Note the strategic words "least likely." Focusing on these strategic words and noting that the client is gagging will direct you to option 3. Review this procedure if you had difficulty with this question.

Level of Cognitive Ability: Application
Client Needs: Physiological Integrity
Integrated Process: Nursing Process/
  Implementation
Content Area: Adult Health/Gastrointestinal

Reference
Potter, P., & Perry, A. (2005). *Fundamentals of nursing* (6th ed., p. 1405). St. Louis: Mosby.

---

154. A nurse is planning care for the client with heart failure. The nurse asks the dietary department to remove which item from all meal trays before delivering them to the client?

1 1% Milk
2 Margarine
3 Salt packets
4 Decaffeinated tea

Level of Cognitive Ability: Application
Client Needs: Physiological Integrity
Integrated Process: Nursing Process/
  Implementation
Content Area: Adult Health/Cardiovascular

Answer: 3
Rationale: Sodium restriction reduces water retention and improves cardiac efficiency. A standard dietary modification for the client with heart failure is sodium restriction.

Test-Taking Strategy: Focusing on the client's diagnosis will assist in recalling the need for sodium restriction and direct you to option 3. Review care of the client with heart failure if you had difficulty with this question.

Reference
Lewis, S., Heitkemper, M., Dirksen, S., O'Brien, P., & Bucher, L. (2007). *Medical-surgical nursing: Assessment and management of clinical problems* (7th ed., p. 833). St. Louis: Mosby.

---

155. A nurse is caring for an infant with spina bifida cystica (meningomyelocele type) who had the sac surgically removed. The nurse plans which of the following in the postoperative period to maintain the infant's safety?

1 Covering the back dressing with a binder
2 Placing the infant in a head-down position
3 Strapping the infant in a baby seat sitting up
4 Elevating the head with the infant in the prone position

Level of Cognitive Ability: Application
Client Needs: Physiological Integrity
Integrated Process: Nursing Process/Planning
Content Area: Child Health

Answer: 4
Rationale: Elevating the head will decrease the chance of cerebrospinal fluid collecting in the cranial cavity. The infant needs to be prone for several days to decrease the pressure on the surgical site on the back. Binders and a baby seat should not be used because of the pressure they would exert on the surgical site.

Test-Taking Strategy: Use the process of elimination. Recall that preventing pressure on the surgical site and preventing intracranial cerebrospinal fluid collection are goals for the postoperative period. Options 1 and 3 would increase pressure on the surgical site, and option 2 would not promote drainage of cerebrospinal fluid from the cranial cavity. Review postoperative nursing care following this procedure if you had difficulty with this question.

Reference
Hockenberry, M., Wilson, D., & Winkelstein, M. (2005). *Wong's essentials of pediatric nursing* (7th ed., p. 1200). St. Louis: Mosby.

---

156. A client is experiencing signs and symptoms of acute iron intoxication. The nurse ensures that which medication is available to treat the intoxication?

1 Folic acid
2 Ferrous sulfate (Slow Fe)
3 Deferoxamine (Desferal)
4 Dirithromycin (Dynabac)

Answer: 3
Rationale: The antidote to iron dextran is deferoxamine, which is a heavy metal antagonist. This medication chelates unbound iron in the circulation and forms a water-soluble complex that can be eliminated by the kidneys. Dirithromycin is a macrolide anti-infective. Ferrous sulfate and folic acid are forms of iron supplements.

Level of Cognitive Ability: Application
Client Needs: Physiological Integrity
Integrated Process: Nursing Process/Planning
Content Area: Pharmacology

Test-Taking Strategy: Eliminate options 1 and 2 first because they are comparable or alike and are both iron supplements. From the remaining options, it is necessary to know that the antidote to iron dextran is deferoxamine. Review this antidote if you had difficulty with this question.

References

Mosby. (2007). *Mosby's nursing drug reference* (20th ed., p. 572). St. Louis: Mosby.
Lehne, R. (2007). *Pharmacology for nursing care* (6th ed., p. 635). Philadelphia: Saunders.

---

157. A client at risk for respiratory failure is receiving oxygen via nasal cannula at 6 L per minute. Arterial blood gas (ABG) results indicate: pH 7.29, P_{CO_2} 49 mm Hg, P_{O_2} 58 mm Hg, HCO_3 18 mEq/L. The nurse anticipates that the physician will order which of the following for respiratory support?

1 Intubation and mechanical ventilation
2 Adding a partial rebreather mask to the current order
3 Keeping the oxygen at 6 L per minute via nasal cannula
4 Lowering the oxygen to 4 L per minute via nasal cannula

Level of Cognitive Ability: Analysis
Client Needs: Physiological Integrity
Integrated Process: Nursing Process/Planning
Content Area: Adult Health/Respiratory

Answer: 1

Rationale: If respiratory failure occurs, endotracheal intubation and mechanical ventilation are necessary. The client is exhibiting respiratory acidosis, metabolic acidosis, and hypoxemia. Lowering or keeping the oxygen at the same liter flow will not improve the client's condition. A partial rebreather mask will raise CO_2 levels even further.

Test-Taking Strategy: Use the process of elimination, noting the ABG values. Noting that the oxygen level is low will eliminate options 3 and 4. Knowing that the P_{CO_2} is high will eliminate option 2, because a partial rebreather mask will raise CO_2 levels even further. Review ABG values and the treatment for respiratory failure if you had difficulty with this question.

References

Black, J., & Hawks, J. (2005). *Medical-surgical nursing: Clinical management for positive outcomes* (7th ed., pp. 1879-1880). Philadelphia: Saunders.
Monahan, F., Sands, J., Neighbors, M., Marek, J., & Green, C. (2007). *Phipps' medical-surgical nursing: Health and illness perspectives* (8th ed., p. 699). St. Louis: Mosby.

---

158. A nurse is preparing to assess the respirations of a newborn infant just admitted to the newborn nursery. The nurse performs the procedure and determines that the respiratory rate is normal if which of the following is noted?

1 A respiratory rate of 20 breaths per minute
2 A respiratory rate of 40 breaths per minute
3 A respiratory rate of 90 breaths per minute
4 A respiratory rate of 100 breaths per minute

Level of Cognitive Ability: Comprehension
Client Needs: Physiological Integrity
Integrated Process: Nursing Process/Assessment
Content Area: Maternity/Postpartum

Answer: 2

Rationale: Normal respiratory rate varies from 30 to 60 breaths per minute when the infant is not crying. Respirations should be counted for 1 full minute to ensure an accurate measurement because the newborn infant may be a periodic breather. Observing and palpating respirations while the infant is quiet promotes accurate assessment. Palpation aids observation in determining the respiratory rate. Option 1 indicates bradypnea, and options 3 and 4 indicate tachypnea.

Test-Taking Strategy: Use the process of elimination and knowledge regarding the normal respiratory rate for a newborn infant to answer this question. If you are unfamiliar with this normal finding, review this content.

References

McKinney, E., James, S., Murray, S., & Ashwill, J. (2005). *Maternal-child nursing* (2nd ed., p. 524). St. Louis: Saunders.
Murray, S., & McKinney, E. (2006). *Foundations of maternal-newborn nursing* (4th ed., p. 470). Philadelphia: Saunders.

159. During a routine prenatal visit, a client, in her second trimester of pregnancy, reports having frequent calf pain when she walks. The nurse checks for which sign to assist in identifying the origin of the discomfort?
  1 Kernig's sign
  2 Homans' sign
  3 Chadwick's sign
  4 Brudzinski's sign

Level of Cognitive Ability: Analysis
Client Needs: Physiological Integrity
Integrated Process: Nursing Process/Assessment
Content Area: Maternity/Antepartum

Answer: 2
Rationale: Homans' sign tests for venous thrombosis of the lower extremity. Pain in the calf during walking could indicate venous thrombosis. Chadwick's sign is a cervical change and is a probable sign of pregnancy. Brudzinski's sign and Kernig's sign test for meningeal irritability.

Test-Taking Strategy: Use the process of elimination. Eliminate options 1 and 4 first because they both test for meningeal irritation. From the remaining options, focus on the strategic words "frequent calf pain when she walks" to assist in directing you to option 2. Review the signs identified in the options if you had difficulty with this question.

Reference
McKinney, E., James, S., Murray, S., & Ashwill, J. (2005). *Maternal-child nursing* (2nd ed., p. 482). St. Louis: Saunders.

---

160. A nurse evaluates the patency of a peripheral intravenous (IV) site and suspects an infiltration. Which does the nurse implement to determine if the IV has infiltrated?
  1 Increases the infusion rate and observes for swelling
  2 Checks the regional tissue for redness and warmth
  3 Strips the tubing and assesses for a blood return
  4 Gently palpates regional tissue for edema and coolness

Level of Cognitive Ability: Application
Client Needs: Physiological Integrity
Integrated Process: Nursing Process/ Implementation
Content Area: Fundamental Skills

Answer: 4
Rationale: When assessing an IV for clinical indicators of infiltration, it is important to assess the site for edema and coolness, signifying leakage of the IV fluid into the surrounding tissues. Stripping the tubing will not cause a blood return but will force IV fluid into the vein or surrounding tissues that can increase the risk of tissue damage. Increasing the IV flow rate can further damage the tissues if the IV has infiltrated. Redness and warmth are more likely to indicate infection or phlebitis.

Test-Taking Strategy: Use the process of elimination, focusing on the subject—infiltration. Recalling that the site will feel cool will direct you to option 4. Review the signs of infiltration if you had difficulty with this question.

Reference
Potter, P., & Perry, A. (2005). *Fundamentals of nursing* (6th ed., p. 1189). St. Louis: Mosby.

---

161. A client who is unresponsive and pulseless and who has a possible neck injury is brought into the emergency department after a motor vehicle accident. Which method does the nurse use to open the client's airway?
  1 Insert oropharyngeal airway.
  2 Tilt the head and lift the chin.
  3 Place in the recovery position.
  4 Stabilize the skull and push up the jaw.

Level of Cognitive Ability: Application
Client Needs: Physiological Integrity
Integrated Process: Nursing Process/ Implementation
Content Area: Fundamental Skills

Answer: 4
Rationale: The health care team uses the jaw-thrust maneuver until a radiograph confirms that the client's cervical spine is stable to avoid potential aggravation of a cervical spine injury. Options 1 and 2 require manipulation of the spine to open the airway, and option 3 can be ineffective for opening the airway.

Test-Taking Strategy: Note the strategic words "possible neck injury." Recalling the principles related to airway management will assist in eliminating options 1 and 2. From the remaining options, visualize each and eliminate option 3 because this method can be ineffective if the client is unable to maintain the airway. Review basic life support measures if you had difficulty with this question.

References

Monahan, F., Sands, J., Neighbors, M., Marek, J., & Green, C. (2007). *Phipps' medical-surgical nursing: Health and illness perspectives* (8th ed., p. 800). St. Louis: Mosby.

Potter, P., & Perry, A. (2005). *Fundamentals of nursing* (6th ed., p. 890). St. Louis: Mosby.

---

162. A nurse is caring for a child with Reye's syndrome. The nurse monitors for signs of which major problem associated with this syndrome?
1 Protein in the urine
2 Symptoms of hyperglycemia
3 Increased intracranial pressure
4 A history of a staphylococcus infection

Level of Cognitive Ability: Application
Client Needs: Physiological Integrity
Integrated Process: Nursing Process/Assessment
Content Area: Child Health

Answer: 3

Rationale: Intracranial pressure and encephalopathy are major problems associated with Reye's syndrome. Protein is not present in the urine. Reye's syndrome is related to a history of viral infections, and hypoglycemia is a symptom of this disease.

Test-Taking Strategy: Use the process of elimination and note the strategic words "major problem." This will assist in directing you to option 3. Review the manifestations and problems associated with Reye's syndrome if you had difficulty with this question.

References

Hockenberry, M., Wilson, D., & Winkelstein, M. (2005). *Wong's essentials of pediatric nursing* (7th ed., p. 1651). St. Louis: Mosby.

Wong, D., Hockenberry, M., Perry, S., Lowdermilk, D., & Wilson, D. (2006). *Maternal-child nursing care* (3rd ed., p. 1702). St. Louis: Mosby.

---

163. A child is admitted to the hospital with a suspected diagnosis of pneumococcal pneumonia. The nurse prepares to implement which of the following?
1 Start antibiotic therapy immediately.
2 Monitor the child's respiratory rate and breath sounds.
3 Allow the child to go to the playroom to play with other children.
4 Have a chest radiograph done to determine how much consolidation there is in the lungs.

Level of Cognitive Ability: Application
Client Needs: Physiological Integrity
Integrated Process: Nursing Process/ Implementation
Content Area: Child Health

Answer: 2

Rationale: A complication of pneumococcal pneumonia is pleural effusion, so the respiratory status of the child needs to be monitored. Antibiotic therapy is not started until cultures are obtained. The child should not be allowed to be around other children at this time. A chest radiograph needs to be prescribed by the physician.

Test-Taking Strategy: Use the steps of the nursing process. Option 2 addresses assessment. This option also addresses the ABCs— airway, breathing, and circulation. Finally, this is the option that is directly related to the child's diagnosis. Review care of the child with pneumonia if you had difficulty with this question.

References

Hockenberry, M., & Wilson, D. (2007). *Nursing care of infants and children* (8th ed., p. 1339). St. Louis: Mosby.

Wong, D., Hockenberry, M., Perry, S., Lowdermilk, D., & Wilson, D. (2006). *Maternal-child nursing care* (3rd ed., p. 1443). St. Louis: Mosby.

164. A nurse admits a client to the hospital with a suspected diagnosis of bulimia nervosa. When performing the admission assessment, the nurse elicits data knowing that the client with bulimia:

1 Binge eats, then purges
2 Is accepting of body size
3 Overeats for the enjoyment of eating food
4 Overeats in response to losing control of diet

Level of Cognitive Ability: Analysis
Client Needs: Physiological Integrity
Integrated Process: Nursing Process/Assessment
Content Area: Mental Health

Answer: 1

Rationale: Individuals with bulimia nervosa develop cycles of binge eating, followed by purging. They seldom attempt to diet and have no sense of loss of control. Options 2, 3, and 4 are true of the obese person who may binge eat (not purge).

Test-Taking Strategy: Use the process of elimination. Eliminate options 3 and 4 because they are comparable or alike. From the remaining options, recalling the definition of bulimia will direct you to option 1. Review the characteristics associated with this disorder if you had difficulty with this question.

References

Stuart, G., & Laraia, M. (2005). *Principles and practice of psychiatric nursing* (8th ed., p. 527). St. Louis: Mosby.

Varcarolis, E., Carson, V., & Shoemaker, N. (2006). *Foundations of psychiatric mental health nursing* (5th ed., p. 303). Philadelphia: Saunders.

165. The nurse is caring for a client who develops compartment syndrome from a severely fractured arm. The client asks the nurse how this can happen. The nurse's response is based on the understanding that:

1 A bone fragment has injured the nerve supply in the area.
2 An injured artery causes impaired arterial perfusion through the compartment.
3 Bleeding and swelling cause increased pressure in an area that cannot expand.
4 The fascia expands with injury, causing pressure on underlying nerves and muscles.

Level of Cognitive Ability: Comprehension
Client Needs: Physiological Integrity
Integrated Process: Nursing Process/ Implementation
Content Area: Adult Health/Musculoskeletal

Answer: 3

Rationale: Compartment syndrome is caused by bleeding and swelling within a compartment, which is lined by fascia that does not expand. The bleeding and swelling place pressure on the nerves, muscles, and blood vessels in the compartment, triggering the symptoms.

Test-Taking Strategy: Use the process of elimination. Option 2 is eliminated first because this syndrome is not caused by an arterial injury. Knowing that the fascia cannot expand eliminates option 4. From the remaining options, it is necessary to know that bleeding and swelling (not a nerve injury) cause the symptoms. Review the physiology associated with compartment syndrome if you had difficulty with this question.

References

Black, J., & Hawks, J. (2005). *Medical-surgical nursing: Clinical management for positive outcomes* (7th ed., p. 628). Philadelphia: Saunders.

Monahan, F., Sands, J., Neighbors, M., Marek, J., & Green, C. (2007). *Phipps' medical-surgical nursing: Health and illness perspectives* (8th ed., pp. 1539-1540). St. Louis: Mosby.

166. A client has undergone fasciotomy to treat compartment syndrome of the leg. The nurse prepares to provide which type of wound care to the fasciotomy site?

1 Dry sterile dressings
2 Hydrocolloid dressings
3 Wet sterile saline dressings
4 One-half strength Betadine dressings

Level of Cognitive Ability: Application
Client Needs: Physiological Integrity
Integrated Process: Nursing Process/Planning
Content Area: Adult Health/Musculoskeletal

Answer: 3

Rationale: The fasciotomy site is not sutured but is left open to relieve pressure and edema. The site is covered with wet sterile saline dressings. After 3 to 5 days, when perfusion is adequate and edema subsides, the wound is debrided and closed. A hydrocolloid dressing is not indicated for use with clean, open incisions. The incision is clean, not dirty, so there should be no reason to require Betadine. Additionally, Betadine can be irritating to normal tissues.

Test-Taking Strategy: Use the process of elimination and knowledge of what a fasciotomy involves and the basics of wound care. Recall that the skin is not sutured closed but left open for pressure relief. Remembering that moist tissue needs to remain moist will direct you to option 3. Review care of a fasciotomy site if you had difficulty with this question.

References
Ignatavicius, D., & Workman, M. (2006). *Medical-surgical nursing: Critical thinking for collaborative care* (5th ed., pp. 1634-1635). Philadelphia: Saunders.
Monahan, F., Sands, J., Neighbors, M., Marek, J., & Green, C. (2007). *Phipps' medical-surgical nursing: Health and illness perspectives* (8th ed., p. 1542). St. Louis: Mosby.

---

167. A nurse is caring for a female client who was recently admitted to the hospital with a diagnosis of anorexia nervosa. When the nurse enters the room, the client is engaged in rigorous push-ups. Which nursing action would be therapeutic?

1 Allow the client to complete the exercise program.
2 Interrupt the client and weigh the client immediately.
3 Interrupt the client and offer to take the client for a walk.
4 Tell the client that she is not allowed to exercise rigorously.

Level of Cognitive Ability: Application
Client Needs: Physiological Integrity
Integrated Process: Nursing Process/ Implementation
Content Area: Mental Health

Answer: 3
Rationale: Clients with anorexia nervosa are frequently preoccupied with rigorous exercise and push themselves beyond normal limits to work off caloric intake. The nurse must provide for appropriate exercise as well as place limits on rigorous activities.

Test-Taking Strategy: Use the process of elimination, noting the strategic word "therapeutic." Focus on the need for the nurse to set firm limits with clients who have this disorder. Also, recalling that the nurse needs to provide and guide the client to perform appropriate exercise will direct you to option 3. Review interventions for clients with this disorder if you had difficulty with this question.

Reference
Stuart, G., & Laraia, M. (2005). *Principles and practice of psychiatric nursing* (8th ed., p. 530). St. Louis: Mosby.

---

168. The nurse assesses a peripheral intravenous (IV) dressing and notes that it is damp and the tape is loose. The best nursing action is to:

1 Stop the infusion immediately.
2 Apply a sterile, occlusive dressing.
3 Remove the IV and insert a new IV.
4 Ensure tight IV tubing connections.

Level of Cognitive Ability: Application
Client Needs: Physiological Integrity
Integrated Process: Nursing Process/ Implementation
Content Area: Fundamental Skills

Answer: 4
Rationale: To determine subsequent nursing interventions, the nurse checks all connections to ensure tight seals while the IV infuses to help locate the source of the leak. If the leak is at the insertion site, the nurse stops the infusion, discontinues the old IV, and inserts a new IV catheter. The nurse applies a fresh dressing after resolving the source of the leak.

Test-Taking Strategy: Note the strategic word "best" and recall that the nurse needs to determine the cause of the leaking. Use the steps of the nursing process and remember that assessment is the first step; however, analyze the options to determine which option indicates assessment to direct you to option 4. Review care of the client with an IV if you had difficulty with this question.

Reference
Potter, P., & Perry, A. (2005). *Fundamentals of nursing* (6th ed., pp. 1180-1181). St. Louis: Mosby.

169. The nurse assists the physician with the removal of a chest tube. During removal of the chest tube, the nurse instructs the client to perform which of the following?
1 Breathe in deeply.
2 Breathe normally.
3 Breathe out forcefully.
4 Exhale and bear down.

Level of Cognitive Ability: Application
Client Needs: Physiological Integrity
Integrated Process: Nursing Process/
  Implementation
Content Area: Adult Health/Respiratory

Answer: 4
Rationale: The client is instructed to perform the Valsalva maneuver (take a deep breath, exhale, and bear down) for chest tube removal. This maneuver will increase intrathoracic pressure, thereby lessening the potential for air to enter the pleural space. Options 1, 2, and 3 are incorrect.

Test-Taking Strategy: Use the process of elimination. Eliminate options 1 and 2 because they are comparable or alike in that breathing will cause air to enter the pleural space. From the remaining options, eliminate option 3 because of the word "forcefully." Review the procedure for the removal of chest tubes if you had difficulty with this question.

Reference
Potter, P., & Perry, A. (2005). *Fundamentals of nursing* (6th ed., p. 870). St. Louis: Mosby.

---

170. The nurse assesses the water seal chamber of a closed chest drainage system and notes fluctuations in the chamber. The nurse determines that this finding indicates that:
1 The tubing is kinked.
2 An air leak is present.
3 The lung has reexpanded.
4 The system is functioning as expected.

Level of Cognitive Ability: Analysis
Client Needs: Physiological Integrity
Integrated Process: Nursing Process/Analysis
Content Area: Adult Health/Respiratory

Answer: 4
Rationale: Fluctuations (tidaling) in the water seal chamber are normal during inhalation and exhalation until the lung reexpands and the client no longer requires chest drainage. If fluctuations are absent, it could indicate occlusion of the tubing or that the lung has re-expanded.

Test-Taking Strategy: Note the strategic words "water seal chamber" and "fluctuations." Recalling the normal expectations related to the functioning of chest tube drainage systems will direct you to option 4. Review care of the client with a chest tube if you had difficulty with this question.

Reference
Black, J., & Hawks, J. (2005). *Medical-surgical nursing: Clinical management for positive outcomes* (7th ed., p. 1863). Philadelphia: Saunders.

---

171. A nurse is caring for a client with depression who has not responded to antidepressant medication. The nurse anticipates that what treatment modality may be prescribed?
1 Psychosurgery
2 Short-term seclusion
3 Neuroleptic medication
4 Electroconvulsive therapy

Level of Cognitive Ability: Analysis
Client Needs: Physiological Integrity
Integrated Process: Nursing Process/Analysis
Content Area: Mental Health

Answer: 4
Rationale: Electroconvulsive therapy is an effective treatment for depression that has not responded to medication. Psychosurgery is invasive, rarely performed, and would not treat depression. Seclusion is not used to treat depression. Neuroleptics are not effective in the treatment of depression.

Test-Taking Strategy: Use the process of elimination. Eliminate option 1 first because it is the most invasive of the options given. Next, eliminate option 2 because seclusion would isolate the client and further exacerbate the client's feelings of depression. From the remaining options, recalling that neuroleptics are not used to treat depression will direct you to option 4. Review treatment measures for depression if you had difficulty with this question.

Reference
Varcarolis, E., Carson, V., & Shoemaker, N. (2006). *Foundations of psychiatric mental health nursing* (5th ed., pp. 351-352). Philadelphia: Saunders.

172. A client arrives in the emergency department after being in an automobile accident. The client was physically unharmed yet was hyperventilating and complaining of dizziness and nausea. In addition, the client appeared confused and had difficulty focusing on what was going on. The nurse assesses the client's level of anxiety as:

1 Mild
2 Panic
3 Severe
4 Moderate

Level of Cognitive Ability: Analysis
Client Needs: Physiological Integrity
Integrated Process: Nursing Process/Assessment
Content Area: Mental Health

Answer: 3
Rationale: The person whose anxiety is assessed as severe is unable to solve problems and has difficulty focusing on what is happening in the environment. Somatic symptoms are usually present. The individual with mild anxiety is only mildly uncomfortable and may even find performance enhanced. The individual with moderate anxiety grasps less information about a situation and has some difficulty with problem solving. The individual in panic will demonstrate markedly disturbed behavior and may lose touch with reality.

Test-Taking Strategy: Use the process of elimination. Focus on the signs and symptoms presented in the question to eliminate options 1 and 2. Noting the fact that the client is exhibiting somatic symptoms should direct you to option 3 from the remaining options. Review the characteristics related to the levels of anxiety if you had difficulty with this question.

Reference
Stuart, G., & Laraia, M. (2005). *Principles and practice of psychiatric nursing* (8th ed., p. 261). St. Louis: Mosby.

---

173. A child is admitted to the hospital with a diagnosis of rheumatic fever. The nurse reviews the blood laboratory findings, knowing that which of the following will confirm the likelihood of this disorder?

1 Increased leukocyte count
2 Decreased hemoglobin count
3 Increased antistreptolysin-O (ASO)
4 Decreased erythrocyte sedimentation rate

Level of Cognitive Ability: Analysis
Client Needs: Physiological Integrity
Integrated Process: Nursing Process/Assessment
Content Area: Child Health

Answer: 3
Rationale: Children suspected of having rheumatic fever are tested for streptococcal antibodies. The most reliable and best standardized test to confirm the diagnosis is the ASO titer. An elevated level indicates the presence of rheumatic fever.

Test-Taking Strategy: Use the process of elimination and note the strategic word "confirm." Focusing on the diagnosis will assist in eliminating options 2 and 4. From the remaining options, recall that an increased leukocyte count indicates the presence of infection but is not specific in confirming a particular diagnosis. Review the diagnostic tests for rheumatic fever if you had difficulty with this question.

Reference
Hockenberry, M., Wilson, D., & Winkelstein, M. (2005). *Wong's essentials of pediatric nursing* (7th ed., p. 923). St. Louis: Mosby.

---

174. A 5-year-old child is admitted to the hospital for heart surgery to repair the tetralogy of Fallot. The nurse reviews the child's record and notes that the child has clubbed fingers. The nurse understands that the clubbing is most likely caused by:

1 Tissue hypoxia
2 Chronic hypertension
3 Delayed physical growth
4 Destruction of bone marrow

Answer: 1
Rationale: Clubbing, a thickening and flattening of the tips of the fingers and toes, is thought to occur because of a chronic tissue hypoxia and polycythemia. Options 2, 3, and 4 do not cause clubbing.

Test-Taking Strategy: Use the ABCs—airway, breathing, and circulation. Hypoxia relates to oxygenation, which is a concern with this disorder. Review the manifestations associated with tetralogy of Fallot if you had difficulty with this question.

Level of Cognitive Ability: Analysis
Client Needs: Physiological Integrity
Integrated Process: Nursing Process/Analysis
Content Area: Child Health

References
Hockenberry, M., Wilson, D., & Winkelstein, M. (2005). *Wong's essentials of pediatric nursing* (7th ed., p. 902). St. Louis: Mosby.
McKinney, E., James, S., Murray, S., & Ashwill, J. (2005). *Maternal-child nursing* (2nd ed., pp. 1260, 1276). St. Louis: Saunders.
Wong, D., Hockenberry, M., Perry, S., Lowdermilk, D., & Wilson, D. (2006). *Maternal-child nursing care* (3rd ed., p. 1566). St. Louis: Mosby.

---

175. An older client admitted to the hospital with a hip fracture is placed in Buck's extension traction. The nurse plans to frequently monitor which specific item?

1 Temperature
2 Mental state
3 Neurovascular status
4 Range of motion ability

Level of Cognitive Ability: Application
Client Needs: Physiological Integrity
Integrated Process: Nursing Process/Assessment
Content Area: Adult Health/Musculoskeletal

Answer: 3
Rationale: The neurovascular status of the extremity of the client in Buck's extension traction must be assessed frequently. Older clients are especially at risk for neurovascular compromise because many older clients already have disorders that affect the peripheral vascular system. Although the client's temperature is monitored, it is not specific to the use of Buck's extension traction. Although clients in some types of traction do become depressed after a few days or weeks, Buck's extension traction is usually used preoperatively, which typically involves a few hours or 1 to 2 days, at the most. Range of motion of the involved leg is contraindicated in hip fractures.

Test-Taking Strategy: Use the process of elimination, focusing on the subject—Buck's extension traction. Recalling the purpose of this traction and visualizing its use will direct you to option 3. Also, use of the ABCs—airway, breathing, and circulation—will direct you to option 3. Review nursing care of the client in Buck's extension traction if you had difficulty with this question.

Reference
Ignatavicius, D., & Workman, M. (2006). *Medical-surgical nursing: Critical thinking for collaborative care* (5th ed., p. 1201). Philadelphia: Saunders.

---

176. A client who has a renal mass asks the nurse why an ultrasound has been scheduled, as opposed to other diagnostic tests that may be ordered. The nurse formulates a response based on the understanding that:

1 All other tests are more invasive than an ultrasound.
2 All other tests require more elaborate postprocedure care.
3 An ultrasound can differentiate a solid mass from a fluid-filled cyst.
4 An ultrasound is much more cost effective than other diagnostic tests.

Level of Cognitive Ability: Application
Client Needs: Physiological Integrity
Integrated Process: Nursing Process/Implementation
Content Area: Adult Health/Renal

Answer: 3
Rationale: A significant advantage of an ultrasound is that it can differentiate a solid mass from a fluid-filled cyst. It is noninvasive and does not require any special aftercare. Other diagnostic tests, such as magnetic resonance imaging and computed tomography scanning, are also noninvasive (unless contrast is used) and require no special aftercare, either. However, the ultrasound can discriminate between solid and fluid masses most optimally.

Test-Taking Strategy: Eliminate options 1 and 2 first because of the close-ended word "all." From the remaining options, focus on the client's diagnosis to direct you to option 3. Review the purpose of an ultrasound if you had difficulty with this question.

References
Ignatavicius, D., & Workman, M. (2006). *Medical-surgical nursing: Critical thinking for collaborative care* (5th ed., pp. 1670, 1673). Philadelphia: Saunders.
Lewis, S., Heitkemper, M., Dirksen, S., O'Brien, P., & Bucher, L. (2007). *Medical-surgical nursing: Assessment and management of clinical problems* (7th ed., p. 1148). St. Louis: Mosby.

177. A client has been admitted to the hospital with a diagnosis of acute glomerulonephritis. During history-taking the nurse first asks the client about a recent history of:
1 Bleeding ulcer
2 Deep vein thrombosis
3 Myocardial infarction
4 Streptococcal infection

Level of Cognitive Ability: Application
Client Needs: Physiological Integrity
Integrated Process: Nursing Process/Assessment
Content Area: Adult Health/Renal

Answer: 4
Rationale: The predominant cause of acute glomerulonephritis is infection with beta hemolytic *Streptococcus* 3 weeks before the onset of symptoms. In addition to bacteria, other infectious agents that could trigger the disorder include viruses, fungi, and parasites. Bleeding ulcer, deep vein thrombosis, and myocardial infarction are not precipitating causes.

Test-Taking Strategy: Use the process of elimination. Recalling that infection is a common trigger for glomerulonephritis assists in eliminating options 1, 2, and 3. It is also necessary to know that streptococcal infections are a common cause of this problem. Review the causes of acute glomerulonephritis if you had difficulty with this question.

Reference
Black, J., & Hawks, J. (2005). *Medical-surgical nursing: Clinical management for positive outcomes* (7th ed., p. 927). Philadelphia: Saunders.

178. A client has just been admitted to the emergency department with chest pain. Serum enzyme levels are drawn, and the results indicate an elevated serum creatine kinase (CK)-MB isoenzyme, troponin T, and troponin I. The nurse concludes that these results are compatible with:
1 Stable angina
2 Unstable angina
3 Prinzmetal's angina
4 New-onset myocardial infarction (MI)

Level of Cognitive Ability: Analysis
Client Needs: Physiological Integrity
Integrated Process: Nursing Process/Analysis
Content Area: Adult Health/Cardiovascular

Answer: 4
Rationale: Creatine kinase (CK)-MB isoenzyme is a sensitive indicator of myocardial damage. Levels begin to rise 3 to 6 hours after the onset of chest pain, peak at approximately 24 hours, and return to normal in about 3 days. Troponin is a regulatory protein found in striated muscle (skeletal and myocardial). Increased amounts of troponins are released into the bloodstream when an infarction causes damage to the myocardium. Therefore, the client's results are compatible with new-onset MI. Options 1, 2, and 3 all refer to angina. These levels would not be elevated in angina.

Test-Taking Strategy: Use the process of elimination. Eliminate options 1, 2, and 3 because they are comparable or alike and all refer to angina. Review the diagnostic laboratory values related to MI if you had difficulty with this question.

Reference
Black, J., & Hawks, J. (2005). *Medical-surgical nursing: Clinical management for positive outcomes* (7th ed., p. 1709). Philadelphia: Saunders.

179. As part of cardiac assessment, the nurse palpates the apical pulse. To perform this assessment, the nurse places the fingertips at which of the following locations?
1 At the left midclavicular line at the fifth intercostal space
2 At the left midclavicular line at the third intercostal space
3 To the right of the midclavicular line at the fifth intercostal space
4 To the right of the midclavicular line at the third intercostal space

Answer: 1
Rationale: The point of maximal impulse (PMI), where the apical pulse is palpated, is normally located in the fourth or fifth intercostal space, at the left midclavicular line.

Test-Taking Strategy: Use the process of elimination. Recalling that the PMI corresponds to the left ventricular apex and visualizing each position in the options will direct you to option 1. Review thoracic and cardiac landmarks if you had difficulty with this question.

Level of Cognitive Ability: Application
Client Needs: Health Promotion and
  Maintenance
Integrated Process: Nursing Process/
  Implementation
Content Area: Adult Health/Cardiovascular

Reference
Jarvis, C. (2004). *Physical examination and health assessment* (4th ed., p. 504). Philadelphia: Saunders.

---

180. A nurse is caring for a client receiving bolus feedings via a Levin-type nasogastric tube (NGT). Which position does the nurse use to administer the feeding?
  1 Supine
  2 Semi-Fowler's
  3 Trendelenberg's
  4 Lateral recumbent

Level of Cognitive Ability: Application
Client Needs: Physiological Integrity
Integrated Process: Nursing Process/
  Implementation
Content Area: Fundamental Skills

Answer: 2
Rationale: Clients are at high risk of aspiration during an NGT feeding because the tube bypasses a protective mechanism, the gag reflex. The head of the bed is elevated 35 to 40 degrees to prevent this complication by facilitating gastric emptying. The remaining options increase the risk of aspiration by blunting the effect of gravity on gastric emptying.

Test-Taking Strategy: Use the process of elimination. Eliminate options 1, 3, and 4 because these increase the risk of aspiration. Review care of the client receiving tube feedings if you had difficulty with this question.

Reference
Ignatavicius, D., & Workman, M. (2006). *Medical-surgical nursing: Critical thinking for collaborative care* (5th ed., p. 1431). Philadelphia: Saunders.

---

181. A nurse is caring for a client with acute pancreatitis who has a history of alcoholism. The nurse closely monitors the client for paralytic ileus, knowing that which assessment data indicate this complication of pancreatitis?
  1 Inability to pass flatus
  2 Loss of anal sphincter control
  3 Severe, constant pain with rapid onset
  4 Firm, nontender mass palpable at the lower right costal margin

Level of Cognitive Ability: Application
Client Needs: Physiological Integrity
Integrated Process: Nursing Process/Assessment
Content Area: Adult Health/Gastrointestinal

Answer: 1
Rationale: An inflammatory reaction such as acute pancreatitis can cause paralytic ileus, the common form of nonmechanical obstruction. Inability to pass flatus is a clinical manifestation of paralytic ileus. Option 4 is the description of the physical finding of liver enlargement. The liver is usually enlarged in the client with cirrhosis or hepatitis. Although this client may have an enlarged liver, an enlarged liver is not a sign of paralytic ileus. Pain is associated with paralytic ileus, but the pain usually presents as a more constant generalized discomfort. Pain that is severe, constant, and rapid in onset is more likely caused by strangulation of the bowel. Loss of sphincter control is not a sign of paralytic ileus.

Test-Taking Strategy: Focus on the subject—a sign of paralytic ileus. Recalling the definition of this complication will direct you to option 1. Review the signs of paralytic ileus if you had difficulty with this question.

References
Black, J., & Hawks, J. (2005). *Medical-surgical nursing: Clinical management for positive outcomes* (7th ed., p. 845). Philadelphia: Saunders.
Ignatavicius, D., & Workman, M. (2006). *Medical-surgical nursing: Critical thinking for collaborative care* (5th ed., p. 1327). Philadelphia: Saunders.

182. After performing an initial abdominal assessment on a client with a diagnosis of cholelithiasis, the nurse documents that the bowel sounds are normal. Which of the following descriptions best describes this assessment finding?

1 Waves of loud gurgles auscultated in all four quadrants
2 Soft gurgling or clicking sounds auscultated in all four quadrants
3 Low-pitched swishing sounds auscultated in one or two quadrants
4 Very high-pitched loud rushes auscultated especially in one or two quadrants

Level of Cognitive Ability: Analysis
Client Needs: Health Promotion and Maintenance
Integrated Process: Nursing Process/Assessment
Content Area: Adult Health/Gastrointestinal

Answer: 2
Rationale: Although frequency and intensity of bowel sounds will vary depending on the phase of digestion, normal bowel sounds are relatively soft gurgling or clicking sounds that occur irregularly 5 to 35 times per minute. Loud gurgles (borborygmi) indicate hyperperistalsis. Bowel sounds will be higher pitched and loud (hyperresonance) when the intestines are under tension, such as in intestinal obstruction. A swishing or buzzing sound represents turbulent blood flow associated with a bruit. No aortic bruits should be heard.

Test-Taking Strategy: Use the process of elimination. Normally, bowel sounds should be audible in all four quadrants; therefore, options 3 and 4 can be eliminated. From the remaining options, select option 2 because of the word "soft" in this option. Review normal abdominal assessment findings if you had difficulty with this question.

Reference
Potter, P., & Perry, A. (2005). *Fundamentals of nursing* (6th ed., p. 743). St. Louis: Mosby.

---

183. A nurse is assigned to care for a client with nephrotic syndrome. The nurse assesses which important parameter on a daily basis?

1 Weight
2 Albumin levels
3 Activity tolerance
4 Blood urea nitrogen (BUN) level

Level of Cognitive Ability: Application
Client Needs: Physiological Integrity
Integrated Process: Nursing Process/Assessment
Content Area: Adult Health/Renal

Answer: 1
Rationale: The client with nephrotic syndrome typically presents with edema, hypoalbuminemia, and proteinuria. The nurse carefully assesses the fluid balance of the client, which includes daily monitoring of weight, intake and output, edema, and girth measurements. Albumin levels are monitored as they are prescribed, as are the BUN and creatinine levels. The client's activity level is adjusted according to the amount of edema and water retention. As edema increases, the client's activity level should be restricted.

Test-Taking Strategy: Use the process of elimination, noting the strategic words "daily basis." Recalling the typical signs of nephrotic syndrome will direct you to option 1. Review these signs if you had difficulty with this question.

Reference
Black, J., & Hawks, J. (2005). *Medical-surgical nursing: Clinical management for positive outcomes* (7th ed., p. 926). Philadelphia: Saunders.

---

184. A client is being admitted to the hospital with a diagnosis of urolithiasis and ureteral colic. The nurse assesses the client for pain that is:

1 Dull and aching in the costovertebral area
2 Aching and cramplike throughout the abdomen
3 Sharp and radiating posteriorly to the spinal column
4 Excruciating, wavelike, and radiating toward the genitalia

Answer: 4
Rationale: The pain of ureteral colic is caused by movement of a stone through the ureter and is sharp, excruciating, and wavelike, radiating to the genitalia and thigh. The stone causes reduced flow of urine, and the urine also contains blood because of its abrasive action on urinary tract mucosa. Stones in the renal pelvis cause pain that is a deep ache in the costovertebral area. Renal colic is characterized by pain that is acute, with tenderness over the costovertebral area.

Level of Cognitive Ability: Analysis
Client Needs: Physiological Integrity
Integrated Process: Nursing Process/Assessment
Content Area: Adult Health/Renal

Test-Taking Strategy: Use the process of elimination, focusing on the diagnosis—urolithiasis and ureteral colic. Recall the anatomical location of the kidneys and the ureters. Because the kidneys are located in the posterior abdomen near the ribcage, pain in the costovertebral area is more likely to be associated with stones in the renal pelvis. On the other hand, sharp wave-like pain that radiates toward the genitalia is more consistent with the location of the ureters in the abdomen. Review the assessment findings for this disorder if you had difficulty with this question.

Reference
Black, J., & Hawks, J. (2005). *Medical-surgical nursing: Clinical management for positive outcomes* (7th ed., p. 884). Philadelphia: Saunders.

---

185. A nurse is assessing the client with left-sided heart failure. The client states that he needs to use three pillows under the head and chest at night to be able to breathe comfortably while sleeping. The nurse documents that the client is experiencing:
    1 Orthopnea
    2 Dyspnea at rest
    3 Dyspnea on exertion
    4 Paroxysmal nocturnal dyspnea

Level of Cognitive Ability: Analysis
Client Needs: Physiological Integrity
Integrated Process: Communication and Documentation
Content Area: Adult Health/Cardiovascular

Answer: 1
Rationale: Dyspnea is a subjective complaint that can range from an awareness of breathing to physical distress and does not necessarily correlate with the degree of heart failure. Dyspnea can be exertional or at rest. Orthopnea is a more severe form of dyspnea, requiring the client to assume a "three-point" position while upright and use pillows to support the head and thorax at night. Paroxysmal nocturnal dyspnea is a severe form of dyspnea occurring suddenly at night because of rapid fluid reentry into the vasculature from the interstitium during sleep.

Test-Taking Strategy: Use the process of elimination and knowledge of the different degrees of dyspnea. Eliminate options 3 and 4 because the question mentions nothing about exertion or a sudden (paroxysmal) event. From the remaining options, select option 1 because the client is breathing "comfortably" with the use of pillows. Review the various descriptions of dyspnea if you had difficulty with this question.

References
Black, J., & Hawks, J. (2005). *Medical-surgical nursing: Clinical management for positive outcomes* (7th ed., p. 1563). Philadelphia: Saunders.
Monahan, F., Sands, J., Neighbors, M., Marek, J., & Green, C. (2007). *Phipps' medical-surgical nursing: Health and illness perspectives* (8th ed., p. 726). St. Louis: Mosby.

---

186. The nurse admits a client who is in sickle cell crisis. Which does the nurse prepare as the priority in the management of the client?
    1 Pain management
    2 Fluid administration
    3 Oxygen administration
    4 Red blood cell transfusion

Answer: 3
Rationale: The priority nursing intervention for a client in sickle cell crisis is to administer supplemental oxygen because the client is hypoxemic, and, as a result, the red blood cells change to the sickle shape. In addition, oxygen is the priority because airway and breathing are more important than circulatory needs. The nurse also plans for fluid therapy to promote hydration and reverse the agglutination of sickled cells, opioid analgesics for relief from severe pain, and, blood transfusions to increase the blood's oxygen-carrying capacity.

Level of Cognitive Ability: Analysis
Client Needs: Physiological Integrity
Integrated Process: Nursing Process/Planning
Content Area: Fundamental Skills

Test-Taking Strategy: Focus on the client's diagnosis. Recalling that clumping of sickled cells occurs when the sickle cell client is hypoxemic and that airway and breathing are the client's priority will direct you to option 3. Review the treatment for sickle cell crisis if you had difficulty with this question.

Reference

Black, J., & Hawks, J. (2005). *Medical-surgical nursing: Clinical management for positive outcomes* (7th ed., pp. 2297, 2299). Philadelphia: Saunders.

---

187. The nurse suspects that a client who had a myocardial infarction is developing cardiogenic shock. The nurse assesses for which peripheral vascular manifestation of this complication?

1 Flushed, dry skin with bounding pedal pulses
2 Warm, moist skin with irregular pedal pulses
3 Cool, clammy skin with weak or thready pedal pulses
4 Cool, dry skin with alternating weak and strong pedal pulses

Level of Cognitive Ability: Analysis
Client Needs: Physiological Integrity
Integrated Process: Nursing Process/Assessment
Content Area: Adult Health/Cardiovascular

Answer: 3

Rationale: Classic signs of cardiogenic shock include increased pulse (weak and thready), decreased blood pressure, decreasing urinary output, signs of cerebral ischemia (confusion, agitation), and cool, clammy skin.

Test-Taking Strategy: Use the process of elimination and recall the signs and symptoms of shock. The word "clammy" in option 3 should direct you to this option. Review the signs of cardiogenic shock if you had difficulty with this question.

Reference

Ignatavicius, D., & Workman, M. (2006). *Medical-surgical nursing: Critical thinking for collaborative care* (5th ed., p. 853). Philadelphia: Saunders.

---

188. The nurse is caring for a client who returns from cardiac surgery with chest tubes in place. The nurse assesses the drainage on an hourly basis and determines that the client is stable as long as drainage does not exceed how many milliliters over the first 24 hours?

1 100
2 200
3 500
4 1000

Level of Cognitive Ability: Analysis
Client Needs: Physiological Integrity
Integrated Process: Nursing Process/Analysis
Content Area: Adult Health/Cardiovascular

Answer: 3

Rationale: Chest tube drainage should not exceed 100 mL per hour during the first 2 hours postoperatively, and approximately 500 mL of drainage is expected in the first 24 hours after cardiac surgery. The nurse measures and records the drainage on an hourly basis. The drainage is initially dark red and becomes more serous over time.

Test-Taking Strategy: Focus on the subject, a postoperative client. Eliminate options 1 and 2 because the values are so small. From the remaining options, try converting the drainage to liters, recalling that 1000 mL equals 1 liter and 500 mL equals 1/2 liter. Knowing that there are only about 6 liters of blood circulating in the body will direct you to option 3. Review the expected postoperative findings following cardiac surgery if you had difficulty with this question.

References

Black, J., & Hawks, J. (2005). *Medical-surgical nursing: Clinical management for positive outcomes* (7th ed., p. 1862). Philadelphia: Saunders.

Monahan, F., Sands, J., Neighbors, M., Marek, J., & Green, C. (2007). *Phipps' medical-surgical nursing: Health and illness perspectives* (8th ed., p. 850). St. Louis: Mosby.

189. A client with renal cancer is being treated preoperatively with radiation therapy. The nurse evaluates that the client has an understanding of proper care of the skin over the treatment field if the client states to:
1 Wash the ink marks off the skin.
2 Avoid skin exposure to direct sunlight.
3 Apply perfumed lotion to the affected skin.
4 Wear tight clothing over the skin site to provide support.

Level of Cognitive Ability: Analysis
Client Needs: Physiological Integrity
Integrated Process: Nursing Process/Evaluation
Content Area: Adult Health/Oncology

Answer: 2
Rationale: The client undergoing radiation therapy should wash the site using mild soap and warm or cool water and pat the area dry. No lotions, creams, alcohol, perfumes, or deodorants should be placed on the skin over the treatment site. Lines or ink marks that are placed on the skin to guide the radiation therapy should be left in place. The affected skin should be protected from temperature extremes, direct sunlight, and chlorinated water (as from swimming pools). The client should wear cotton clothing over the skin site and guard against irritation from tight or rough clothing such as belts or bras.

Test-Taking Strategy: Use the process of elimination, noting the strategic words "understanding of proper care." Recalling that the goal of care is to prevent skin irritation will direct you to option 2. Review client teaching related to radiation therapy if you had difficulty with this question.

Reference
Ignatavicius, D., & Workman, M. (2006). *Medical-surgical nursing: Critical thinking for collaborative care* (5th ed., p. 491). Philadelphia: Saunders.

---

190. A client with renal failure is receiving epoetin alfa (Epogen) to support erythropoiesis. The nurse questions the client about compliance with taking which of the following medications that supports red blood cell (RBC) production?
1 Iron supplement
2 Zinc supplement
3 Calcium supplement
4 Magnesium supplement

Level of Cognitive Ability: Application
Client Needs: Physiological Integrity
Integrated Process: Nursing Process/Assessment
Content Area: Adult Health/Renal

Answer: 1
Rationale: Iron is needed for RBC production. Otherwise, the body cannot produce sufficient erythrocytes. In either case, the client is not receiving the full benefit of epoetin alfa therapy if iron is not taken. Options 2, 3, or 4 are not needed for RBC production.

Test-Taking Strategy: Use the process of elimination. Note the relationship of RBC production in the question and iron in the correct option. Review the concepts related to epoetin alfa and RBC production if you had difficulty with this question.

Reference
Hodgson, B., & Kizior, R. (2007). *Saunders nursing drug handbook 2007* (p. 424). Philadelphia: Saunders.

---

191. The home health nurse is performing an initial assessment on a client who has arrived home after insertion of a permanent pacemaker. Evaluation of the client's understanding of self-care is evident if the client reports which of the following?
1 "I will never be able to operate a microwave oven again."
2 "I should expect occasional feelings of dizziness and fatigue."
3 "I will take my pulse in the wrist or neck daily and record it in a log."
4 "Moving my arms and shoulders vigorously helps to check pacemaker functioning."

Answer: 3
Rationale: Clients with permanent pacemakers must be able to take their pulse in the wrist and/or neck accurately in order to note any variation in the pulse rate or rhythm that may need to be reported to the physician. Clients can safely operate most appliances and tools, such as microwave ovens, video recorders, AM-FM radios, electric blankets, lawn mowers, and leaf blowers, as long as the devices are grounded and in good repair. If the client experiences any feelings of dizziness, fatigue, or an irregular heartbeat, the physician is notified. The arms and shoulders should not be moved vigorously for 6 weeks after insertion.

Test-Taking Strategy: Use the process of elimination. Recalling that a pacemaker assists in controlling cardiac rate and rhythm will direct you to option 3. Review client teaching points related to a pacemaker if you had difficulty with this question.

Level of Cognitive Ability: Analysis
Client Needs: Physiological Integrity
Integrated Process: Nursing Process/Evaluation
Content Area: Adult Health/Cardiovascular

Reference
Black, J., & Hawks, J. (2005). *Medical-surgical nursing: Clinical management for positive outcomes* (7th ed., p. 1697). Philadelphia: Saunders.

---

192. A client with a severe major depressive episode is unable to address activities of daily living (ADL). The appropriate nursing intervention would be to:
  1 Have the client's peers confront the client about how noncompliance in addressing ADL affects the milieu.
  2 Structure the client's day so that adequate time can be devoted to the client's assuming responsibility for ADL.
  3 Offer the client choices and describe the consequences for the failure to comply with the expectation of maintaining his own ADL.
  4 Feed, bathe, and dress the client as needed until the client's condition improves so that he can perform these activities independently.

Level of Cognitive Ability: Application
Client Needs: Physiological Integrity
Integrated Process: Nursing Process/
  Implementation
Content Area: Mental Health

Answer: 4
Rationale: The symptoms of major depression include depressed mood, loss of interest or pleasure, changes in appetite and sleep patterns, psychomotor agitation or retardation, fatigue, feelings of worthlessness or guilt, diminished ability to think or concentrate, and recurrent thoughts of death. Often, the client does not have the energy or interest to complete activities of daily living. Option 1 will increase the client's feelings of poor self-esteem and of unworthiness. Option 2 is incorrect because the client still lacks the energy and motivation to do these independently. Option 3 may lead to increased feelings of worthlessness as the client fails to meet expectations.

Test Taking Strategy: Focus on the client's diagnosis and the subject of the question. Use Maslow's Hierarchy of Needs theory. Remember that physiological needs are the priority. Review care of the client with depression if you had difficulty with this question.

Reference
Stuart, G., & Laraia, M. (2005). *Principles and practice of psychiatric nursing* (8th ed., p. 358). St. Louis: Mosby

---

193. A pregnant client of 32 weeks' gestation is admitted to the obstetric unit for observation after an automobile accident. The client is experiencing slight vaginal bleeding and mild cramps. The nurse does which of the following to determine the viability of the fetus?
  1 Inserts an intravenous line and begins an infusion at 125 mL per hour
  2 Administers oxygen to the woman via a face mask at 7 to 10 liters per minute
  3 Positions and connects a spiral electrode to the fetal monitor for internal fetal monitoring
  4 Positions and connects the ultrasound transducer and the tocotransducer to the external fetal monitor

Level of Cognitive Ability: Application
Client Needs: Physiological Integrity
Integrated Process: Nursing Process/
  Implementation
Content Area: Maternity/Antepartum

Answer: 4
Rationale: External fetal monitoring will allow the nurse to determine any change in the fetal heart rate and rhythm that would indicate that the fetus is in jeopardy. Internal monitoring is contraindicated when there is vaginal bleeding, especially in preterm labor. Because fetal distress has not been determined at this time, oxygen administration is premature. The amount of bleeding described is insufficient to require intravenous fluid replacement.

Test-Taking Strategy: Focus on the subject—to determine viability of the fetus. Next, use the steps of the nursing process, and note that option 4 is an assessment and a noninvasive measure. Review fetal assessment techniques if you had difficulty with this question.

References
McKinney, E., James, S., Murray, S., & Ashwill, J. (2005). *Maternal-child nursing* (2nd ed., pp. 406, 414). St. Louis: Saunders.
Murray, S., & McKinney, E. (2006). *Foundations of maternal-newborn nursing* (4th ed., pp. 312-314). Philadelphia: Saunders.

194. A nurse is reviewing the results of a sweat test performed on a child with cystic fibrosis (CF). The nurse would expect to note which finding?

1 A sweat sodium concentration less than 40 mEq/L
2 A sweat potassium concentration less than 40 mEq/L
3 A sweat chloride concentration greater than 60 mEq/L
4 A sweat potassium concentration greater than 40 mEq/L

Level of Cognitive Ability: Analysis
Client Needs: Physiological Integrity
Integrated Process: Nursing Process/Analysis
Content Area: Child Health

Answer: 3
Rationale: A consistent finding of abnormally high sodium and chloride concentrations in the sweat is a unique characteristic of CF. Normally, the sweat chloride concentration is less than 40 mEq/L. A sweat chloride concentration greater than 60 mEq/L is diagnostic of CF. Potassium concentration is unrelated to the sweat test.

Test-Taking Strategy: Use the process of elimination. Eliminate options 2 and 4 first because the potassium level is unrelated to the sweat test. From the remaining options, note that option 3 indicates a "greater" value. Review this test if you had difficulty with this question.

Reference
Hockenberry, M., Wilson, D., & Winkelstein, M. (2005). *Wong's essentials of pediatric nursing* (7th ed., p. 825). St. Louis: Mosby.

---

195. The nurse is assessing a client with a Cantor tube. Which finding indicates correct placement of the tube?

1 A pH of aspirate less than 7.0
2 A pH of aspirate of 7.0 or greater
3 The auscultation of air when inserted into the abdomen
4 The presence of gastric contents when checking residuals

Level of Cognitive Ability: Analysis
Client Needs: Physiological Integrity
Integrated Process: Nursing Process/Analysis
Content Area: Adult Health/Gastrointestinal

Answer: 2
Rationale: The Cantor tube is an intestinal tube and is used for aspirating intestinal contents. For intestinal intubation the tube is threaded through the nose into the stomach and then through the pylorus, where peristaltic activity of the bowel carries it to the desired intestinal area. The nurse ensures intestinal placement by checking the pH of aspirate. A pH reading greater than 7 indicates intestinal contents; a reading less than 7 indicates gastric contents.

Test-Taking Strategy: Use the process of elimination. Recalling that the Cantor tube is an intestinal tube will assist in eliminating options 3 and 4. From the remaining options, recalling that intestinal fluid is alkaline will assist in directing you to option 2. Review the principles associated with the care of a client with a Cantor tube if you had difficulty with this question.

Reference
Potter, P., & Perry, A. (2005). *Fundamentals of nursing* (6th ed., pp. 1022-1023, 1309). St. Louis: Mosby.

---

196. The nurse performs a neurovascular assessment on a client with a newly applied cast. Close observation and further evaluation would be required if the nurse notes which of the following?

1 Palpable pulses distal to the cast
2 Capillary refill less than 6 seconds
3 Blanching of the nail bed when it is depressed
4 Sensation when the area distal to the cast is pinched

Level of Cognitive Ability: Analysis
Client Needs: Physiological Integrity
Integrated Process: Nursing Process/Assessment
Content Area: Adult Health/Neurological

Answer: 2
Rationale: To assess for adequate circulation, the nail bed of each finger or toe is depressed until it blanches, and then the pressure is released. Optimally, the color will change from white to pink rapidly (less than 3 seconds). If this does not occur, the toes or fingers will require close observation and further evaluation. Palpable pulses and sensations distal to the cast are expected. However, if pulses could not be palpated or if the client complained of numbness or tingling, the physician should be notified.

Test-Taking Strategy: Use the process of elimination. Note the strategic words "close observation and further evaluation." Eliminate options 1, 3, and 4 because these options identify normal expected findings. Option 2 identifies an abnormal or unexpected finding. Review assessment of capillary refill if you had difficulty with this question.

References

Black, J., & Hawks, J. (2005). *Medical-surgical nursing: Clinical management for positive outcomes* (7th ed., p. 633). Philadelphia: Saunders.

Monahan, F., Sands, J., Neighbors, M., Marek, J., & Green, C. (2007). *Phipps' medical-surgical nursing: Health and illness perspectives* (8th ed., p. 728). St. Louis: Mosby.

Wilson, S., & Giddens, J. (2005). *Health assessment for nursing practice* (3rd ed., p. 381). St. Louis: Mosby.

---

197. The nurse is caring for a client with a head injury and is monitoring the client for decerebrate posturing. Which of the following is characteristic of this type of posturing?

  1 Flexion of the extremities after a noxious stimulus

  2 Extension of the extremities after a noxious stimulus

  3 Upper extremity extension with lower extremity flexion

  4 Upper extremity flexion with lower extremity extension

Level of Cognitive Ability: Analysis
Client Needs: Physiological Integrity
Integrated Process: Nursing Process/Assessment
Content Area: Adult Health/Neurological

Answer: 2

Rationale: Decerebrate posturing, which can occur with upper brainstem injury, is the extension of the extremities after a noxious stimulus is applied. Options 1, 3, and 4 are incorrect descriptions of this type of posturing.

Test-Taking Strategy: Use the process of elimination. Remember that decerebrate may also be known as extension. Recalling this concept will direct you to option 2. Review posturing and its relationship to neurological disorders if you had difficulty with this question.

Reference

Ignatavicius, D., & Workman, M. (2006). *Medical-surgical nursing: Critical thinking for collaborative care* (5th ed., p. 939). Philadelphia: Saunders.

---

198. The nurse is caring for a client admitted to the surgical nursing unit following right modified radical mastectomy. The nurse includes which of the following in the nursing plan of care for this client?

  1 Take blood pressures in the right arm only.

  2 Draw serum laboratory samples from the right arm only.

  3 Position the client supine with right arm elevated on a pillow.

  4 Check the right posterior axilla area when assessing the surgical dressing.

Level of Cognitive Ability: Application
Client Needs: Physiological Integrity
Integrated Process: Nursing Process/Planning
Content Area: Adult Health/Oncology

Answer: 4

Rationale: If there is drainage or bleeding from the surgical site after mastectomy, gravity will cause the drainage to seep down and soak the posterior axillary portion of the dressing first. The nurse checks this area to detect early bleeding. The client should be positioned with the head in semi-Fowler's position and the arm elevated on pillows to decrease edema. Edema is likely to occur because lymph drainage channels have been resected during the surgical procedure. Blood pressure measurement, venipuncture, and IV sites should not involve use of the operative arm.

Test-Taking Strategy: Use the process of elimination. Eliminate options 1 and 2 first because of the words "right arm only." From the remaining options, use knowledge of the effects of gravity to direct you to option 4. Review care of the client following mastectomy if you had difficulty with this question.

Reference

Ignatavicius, D., & Workman, M. (2006). *Medical-surgical nursing: Critical thinking for collaborative care* (5th ed., p. 1805). Philadelphia: Saunders.

199. The nurse is assisting the client with hepatic encephalopathy to fill out the dietary menu. The nurse advises the client to avoid which of the following entree items that could aggravate the client's condition?

1 Tomato soup
2 Fresh fruit plate
3 Vegetable lasagna
4 Ground beef patty

Level of Cognitive Ability: Application
Client Needs: Physiological Integrity
Integrated Process: Nursing Process/ Implementation
Content Area: Adult Health/Gastrointestinal

Answer: 4
Rationale: Clients with hepatic encephalopathy have impaired ability to convert ammonia to urea and must limit intake of protein and ammonia-containing foods in the diet. The client should avoid foods such as chicken, beef, ham, cheese, buttermilk, onions, peanut butter, and gelatin.

Test-Taking Strategy: Use the process of elimination, focusing on the client's diagnosis and note the strategic word "avoid." Note that options 1, 2, and 3 are comparable or alike in that they address food items of a fruit and vegetable nature. Review dietary measures for the client with hepatic encephalopathy if you had difficulty with this question.

Reference
Ignatavicius, D., & Workman, M. (2006). *Medical-surgical nursing: Critical thinking for collaborative care* (5th ed., p. 1370). Philadelphia: Saunders.

200. A client with a colostomy is complaining of gas building up in the colostomy bag. The nurse instructs the client that which of the following food items can be consumed to best prevent this problem?

1 Yogurt
2 Broccoli
3 Cabbage
4 Cauliflower

Level of Cognitive Ability: Application
Client Needs: Physiological Integrity
Integrated Process: Teaching and Learning
Content Area: Adult Health/Gastrointestinal

Answer: 1
Rationale: Consumption of yogurt, crackers and toast can help to prevent gas. Gas-forming foods include broccoli, mushrooms, cauliflower, onions, peas, and cabbage. These should be avoided by the client with a colostomy until tolerance to them is determined.

Test-Taking Strategy: Focus on the subject, prevention of gas build-up in the colostomy bag. Note the similarity between options 2, 3, and 4 in terms of their food substance to assist you in eliminating these options. Review those food items that are gas-forming and those that help to prevent the problem if you had difficulty with this question.

References
Black, J., & Hawks, J. (2005). *Medical-surgical nursing: Clinical management for positive outcomes* (7th ed., p. 838). Philadelphia: Saunders.
Ignatavicius, D., & Workman, M. (2006). *Medical-surgical nursing: Critical thinking for collaborative care* (5th ed., p. 1325). Philadelphia: Saunders.

201. A client receiving parenteral nutrition (PN) complains of nausea, excessive thirst, and increased frequency of voiding. The nurse initially assesses which of the following client data?

1 Rectal temperature
2 Last serum potassium
3 Capillary blood glucose
4 Serum blood urea nitrogen and creatinine

Level of Cognitive Ability: Analysis
Client Needs: Physiological Integrity
Integrated Process: Nursing Process/Assessment
Content Area: Adult Health/Gastrointestinal

Answer: 3
Rationale: The symptoms exhibited by the client are consistent with hyperglycemia. The nurse would need to assess the client's blood glucose level to verify these data. Clients receiving PN are at risk for hyperglycemia related to the increased glucose load of the solution. The other options would not provide any information that would correlate with the client's symptoms.

Test-Taking Strategy: Focus on the client's symptoms and think about the complications of PN. Recalling that hyperglycemia is a complication will direct you to option 3. Review the complications associated with PN and the signs of hyperglycemia if you had difficulty with this question.

References

Ignatavicius, D., & Workman, M. (2006). *Medical surgical nursing: Critical thinking for collaborative care* (5th ed., p. 1433). Philadelphia: Saunders.

Lewis, S., Heitkemper, M., Dirksen, S., O'Brien, P., & Bucher, L. (2007). *Medical-surgical nursing: Assessment and management of clinical problems* (7th ed., p. 990). St. Louis: Mosby.

---

202. A client admitted to the hospital with a diagnosis of cirrhosis has massive ascites and difficulty breathing. The nurse performs which intervention as a priority measure to assist the client with breathing?
  1 Repositions side to side every 2 hours
  2 Elevates the head of the bed 60 degrees
  3 Auscultates the lung fields every 4 hours
  4 Encourages deep breathing exercises every 2 hours

Level of Cognitive Ability: Application
Client Needs: Physiological Integrity
Integrated Process: Nursing Process/ Implementation
Content Area: Delegating/Prioritizing

Answer: 2
Rationale: The client is having difficulty breathing because of upward pressure on the diaphragm from the ascitic fluid. Elevating the head of the bed enlists the aid of gravity in relieving pressure on the diaphragm. The other options are general measures to promote lung expansion in the client with ascites, but the priority measure is the one that relieves diaphragmatic pressure.

Test-Taking Strategy: Note the strategic words "priority measure" and the subject: assist with breathing. Recalling that elevating the head will provide immediate relief of symptoms will direct you to option 2. Review care of the client with ascites who is having difficulty breathing if you had difficulty with this question.

Reference
Ignatavicius, D., & Workman, M. (2006). Medical-surgical nursing: Critical thinking for collaborative care (5th ed., p. 1377). Philadelphia: Saunders.

---

203. The nurse provides dietary measures to a client with diverticulosis. The nurse encourages the client to eat foods that are:
  1 High in fat
  2 Low in fiber
  3 Low roughage
  4 High in fiber

Level of Cognitive Ability: Application
Client Needs: Physiological Integrity
Integrated Process: Nursing Process/ Implementation
Content Area: Adult Health/Gastrointestinal

Answer: 4
Rationale: Diverticulosis is managed by consumption of a high-fiber diet and prevention of constipation with bran and bulk laxatives. A diet high in fat should be avoided because high-fat foods tend to be low in fiber. A low-roughage diet is similar to a low-fiber diet.

Test-Taking Strategy: Use the process of elimination. Eliminate options 2 and 3 first because they are comparable or alike. From the remaining options, recalling that the goal in diverticulosis is to prevent constipation will direct you to option 4. Review the diet prescribed for this disorder if you had difficulty with this question.

Reference
Black, J., & Hawks, J. (2005). *Medical-surgical nursing: Clinical management for positive outcomes* (7th ed., p. 842). Philadelphia: Saunders.

204. A client with Cushing's disease is being admitted to the hospital after a stab wound to the abdomen. The nurse places highest priority on which of the following nursing diagnoses developed for this client?
1 Risk for infection
2 Disturbed body image
3 Risk for deficient fluid volume
4 Ineffective health maintenance

Level of Cognitive Ability: Analysis
Client Needs: Physiological Integrity
Integrated Process: Nursing Process/Analysis
Content Area: Adult Health/Endocrine

Answer: 1
Rationale: The client with a stab wound has a break in the body's first line of defense against infection. The client with Cushing's disease is at great risk for infection caused by *excess* cortisol secretion, subsequent impaired antibody function, and decreased proliferation of lymphocytes. The client may also have Ineffective health maintenance and Disturbed body image, but these are not the highest priority at this time. The client would be at risk for Excess fluid volume, not Deficient fluid volume, with Cushing's disease.

Test-Taking Strategy: Note the strategic words "highest priority." Use Maslow's Hierarchy of Needs theory to eliminate options 2 and 4. From the remaining options, focus on the client's diagnosis. Eliminate option 3, which it is the opposite of what is expected with this disorder. Review the needs of a client with Cushing's disease if you had difficulty with this question.

Reference
Black, J., & Hawks, J. (2005). *Medical-surgical nursing: Clinical management for positive outcomes* (7th ed., p. 1222). Philadelphia: Saunders.

205. A female adolescent client is admitted to the mental health unit after medical stabilization for an overdose of acetaminophen (Tylenol). The client's boyfriend broke up with her 2 weeks ago and the client stopped eating at that time and has lost 15 pounds. The nurse avoids which intervention when caring for the client?
1 Offer frequent, nutritious snacks.
2 Offer bland, easily digestible foods.
3 Stand the client in front of a mirror to show her how thin she is.
4 Provide meals on an isolation tray that contains no glass or metal utensils.

Level of Cognitive Ability: Application
Client Needs: Physiological Integrity
Integrated Process: Nursing Process/ Implementation
Content Area: Mental Health

Answer: 3
Rationale: The client has been denying herself food as a means of self-harm. Reinforcing her success at this is not therapeutic. Meeting her nutritional needs is the nursing care priority. Options 1 and 2 meet the client's nutritional needs. Option 4 is a necessary safety measure.

Test-Taking Strategy: Note the strategic word "avoids." This word indicates a negative event query and the need to select the option that is an incorrect nursing action. Use Maslow's Hierarchy of Needs theory. Options 1 and 2 address a physiological need. Option 4 addresses both a physiological and safety need. Option 3 addresses a psychosocial need. Review care of the client at risk for self-harm if you had difficulty with this question.

Reference
Stuart, G., & Laraia, M. (2005). *Principles and practice of psychiatric nursing* (8th ed., pp. 372, 436-437). St. Louis: Mosby.

206. The nurse evaluates a client following treatment for carbon monoxide poisoning. The nurse would document that the treatment was effective if which of the following were present?
1 Client is sleeping soundly.
2 Client is awake and talking.
3 Heart monitor shows sinus tachycardia.
4 Carboxyhemoglobin levels are less than 5%.

Answer: 4
Rationale: Normal carboxyhemoglobin levels are less than 5% for an adult (0.05% to 2.5% for a nonsmoker and 5% to 10% for a heavy smoker). Clients can be awake and talking with abnormally high levels. The symptoms of carbon monoxide poisoning are tachycardia, tachypnea, and central nervous system depression.

Test-Taking Strategy: Note the relationship between the words "carbon monoxide poisoning" in the question and option 4. Option 4 is the only option that specifically addresses this subject. Review the normal carboxyhemoglobin levels if you had difficulty with this question.

Level of Cognitive Ability: Analysis
Client Needs: Physiological Integrity
Integrated Process: Nursing Process/Evaluation
Content Area: Adult Health/Respiratory

References
Black, J., & Hawks, J. (2005). *Medical-surgical nursing: Clinical management for positive outcomes* (7th ed., pp. 1906-1907). Philadelphia: Saunders.
Chernecky, C., & Berger, B. (2008). *Laboratory tests and diagnostic procedures* (5th ed., pp. 292-293). Philadelphia: Saunders.

---

207. A nurse instructs a preoperative client in the proper use of an incentive spirometer. Which does the nurse use to determine that the client is using the IS effectively?
1 Cloudy sputum
2 Shallow breathing
3 Unilateral wheezing
4 Productive coughing

Level of Cognitive Ability: Analysis
Client Needs: Physiological Integrity
Integrated Process: Nursing Process/Evaluation
Content Area: Fundamental Skills

Answer: 4
Rationale: Incentive spirometry helps reduce atelectasis, open airways, stimulate coughing, and help mobilize secretions for expectoration, via vital client participation in recovery. Cloudy sputum, shallow breathing, and wheezing indicate that the incentive spirometry is not effective because they indicate infection, counterproductive depth of breathing, and bronchoconstriction, respectively.

Test-Taking Strategy: Focus on the subject, the effectiveness of an incentive spirometer. Eliminate options 1, 2, and 3 that indicate abnormal findings. Review the purpose of an incentive spirometer if you had difficulty with this question.

References
Ignatavicius, D., & Workman, M. (2006). *Medical-surgical nursing: Critical thinking for collaborative care* (5th ed., p. 309). Philadelphia: Saunders.
Potter, P., & Perry, A. (2005). *Fundamentals of nursing* (6th ed., pp. 1109, 1117, 1671). St. Louis: Mosby.

---

208. A client is to be started on prazosin hydrochloride (Minipress). The client asks the nurse why the first dose must be taken at bedtime. The nurse's response is based on the understanding that during early use, prazosin:
1 Results in extreme drowsiness
2 Can cause significant dependent edema
3 Should be taken when the stomach is empty
4 Can cause dizziness, lightheadedness, or possible syncope

Level of Cognitive Ability: Application
Client Needs: Physiological Integrity
Integrated Process: Teaching and Learning
Content Area: Pharmacology

Answer: 4
Rationale: Prazosin is an alpha-adrenergic blocking agent. "First-dose hypotensive reaction" may occur during early therapy, which is characterized by dizziness, lightheadedness, and possible loss of consciousness. This can also occur when the dosage is increased. This effect usually disappears with continued use or when the dosage is decreased. Options 1, 2, and 3 are not characteristics of the medication.

Test-Taking Strategy: Note the name of the medication, Mini*press*. This will assist in determining that the medication is an antihypertensive agent. Recalling that orthostatic hypotension occurs with the use of antihypertensives will direct you to option 4. Review the effects of this medication if you had difficulty with this question.

Reference
Hodgson, B., & Kizior, R. (2007). *Saunders nursing drug handbook 2007* (p. 954). Philadelphia: Saunders.

209. The nurse has applied the prescribed dressing to the leg of a client with an ischemic arterial leg ulcer. The nurse should use which of the following methods to cover the dressing?
1 Apply a Kerlix roll and tape it to the skin.
2 Apply a large, soft pad, and tape it to the skin.
3 Apply small Montgomery straps and tie the edges together.
4 Apply a Kling roll and tape the edge of the roll onto the bandage.

Level of Cognitive Ability: Application
Client Needs: Physiological Integrity
Integrated Process: Nursing Process/ Implementation
Content Area: Adult Health/Cardiovascular

Answer: 4
Rationale: With an arterial leg ulcer, the nurse applies tape only to the bandage. Tape is never used directly on the skin because it could cause further tissue damage. For the same reason, Montgomery straps could not be applied to the skin (although these are generally intended for use on abdominal wounds, anyway). Standard dressing technique includes the use of Kling rolls on circumferential dressings.

Test-Taking Strategy: Use the process of elimination, noting that options 1, 2, and 3 are comparable or alike. Eliminate options 1 and 2, recalling that tape is not applied to the skin. For the same reason, eliminate option 3, because the Montgomery straps would need to be adhered to the skin as well. Review care of the client with an arterial leg ulcer if you had difficulty with this question.

References
Black, J., & Hawks, J. (2005). *Medical-surgical nursing: Clinical management for positive outcomes* (7th ed., p. 1528). Philadelphia: Saunders.
Ignatavicius, D., & Workman, M. (2006). *Medical-surgical nursing: Critical thinking for collaborative care* (5th ed., p. 795). Philadelphia: Saunders.
Potter, P., & Perry, A. (2005). *Fundamentals of nursing* (6th ed., pp. 1537, 1542). St. Louis: Mosby.

---

210. A child is admitted to the pediatric unit with a diagnosis of celiac disease. Based on this diagnosis, the nurse expects that the child's stools will be:
1 Malodorous
2 Dark in color
3 Unusually hard
4 Abnormally small in amount

Level of Cognitive Ability: Analysis
Client Needs: Physiological Integrity
Integrated Process: Nursing Process/Assessment
Content Area: Child Health

Answer: 1
Rationale: The stools of a child with celiac disease are characteristically malodorous, pale, large (bulky), and soft (loose). Excessive flatus is common, and bouts of diarrhea may occur.

Test-Taking Strategy: Use the process of elimination. Thinking about the pathophysiology that occurs in celiac disease will direct you to option 1. Review these manifestations if you had difficulty with this question.

Reference
Hockenberry, M., Wilson, D., & Winkelstein, M. (2005). *Wong's essentials of pediatric nursing* (7th ed., p. 886). St. Louis: Mosby.

---

211. A clinic nurse is caring for a client with a suspected diagnosis of gestational hypertension (GH). The nurse assesses the client, expecting to note which of the following if GH is present?
1 Edema, ketonuria, and obesity
2 Edema, tachycardia, and ketonuria
3 Glycosuria, hypertension, and obesity
4 Hypertension, edema, and proteinuria

Level of Cognitive Ability: Analysis
Client Needs: Physiological Integrity
Integrated Process: Nursing Process/Assessment
Content Area: Maternity/Antepartum

Answer: 4
Rationale: Gestational hypertension is the most common hypertensive disorder in pregnancy. It is characterized by the development of hypertension, proteinuria, and edema. Glycosuria and ketonuria occur in diabetes mellitus. Tachycardia and obesity are not specifically related to diagnosing GH.

Test-Taking Strategy: Use the process of elimination. Eliminate options 1 and 2 because they do not address hypertension. From the remaining options, recalling that glycosuria is an indication of diabetes mellitus will assist in directing you to option 4. Review the clinical manifestations associated with GH if you had difficulty with this question.

Reference
Wong, D., Hockenberry, M., Perry, S., Lowdermilk, D., & Wilson, D. (2006). *Maternal-child nursing care.* (3rd ed., pp. 371-372). St. Louis: Mosby.

---

212. A client who undergoes a gastric resection is at risk for developing dumping syndrome. The nurse monitors the client for:
1 Dizziness
2 Bradycardia
3 Constipation
4 Extreme thirst

Level of Cognitive Ability: Analysis
Client Needs: Physiological Integrity
Integrated Process: Nursing Process/Assessment
Content Area: Adult Health/Gastrointestinal

Answer: 1
Rationale: Early manifestations of dumping syndrome occur 5 to 30 minutes after eating. Symptoms include vasomotor disturbances such as dizziness, tachycardia, syncope, sweating, pallor, palpitations, and the desire to lie down.

Test-Taking Strategy: Use the process of elimination. Recalling that the symptoms of this disorder are vasomotor in nature will direct you to option 1. Review this disorder and the appropriate treatment measures if you had difficulty with this question.

Reference
Ignatavicius, D., & Workman, M. (2006). *Medical-surgical nursing: Critical thinking for collaborative care* (5th ed., p. 1303). Philadelphia: Saunders.

---

213. The nurse is caring for a client who had a craniotomy (supratentorial surgery). When assessing the client for the major postoperative complication following craniotomy, the nurse monitors for:
1 Bleeding
2 Restlessness
3 Hypotension
4 Narrowed pulse pressure

Level of Cognitive Ability: Analysis
Client Needs: Physiological Integrity
Integrated Process: Nursing Process/Assessment
Content Area: Adult Health/Neurological

Answer: 2
Rationale: The major postoperative complication following craniotomy (supratentorial surgery) is increased intracranial pressure (ICP) from cerebral edema, hemorrhage, or obstruction of the normal flow of cerebrospinal fluid (CSF). Symptoms of increased ICP include: severe headache, signs of deteriorating level of consciousness, such as restlessness and irritability, and dilated or pinpoint pupils that are slow to react or nonreactive to light. Without prompt recognition and treatment, herniation syndromes develop and death can occur. Options 1, 3, and 4 are not associated with increased ICP

Test-Taking Strategy: Note the client's diagnosis. Always monitor the neurological client for increased ICP. Remember that changes in the level of consciousness is the first key indicator of increased ICP. Option 2 is the only option that addresses level of consciousness. Review the signs of increased ICP and postoperative complications following craniotomy if you had difficulty with this question.

References
Ignatavicius, D., & Workman, M. (2006). *Medical-surgical nursing: Critical thinking for collaborative care* (5th ed., pp. 1060, 1064). Philadelphia: Saunders.
Monahan, F., Sands, J., Neighbors, M., Marek, J., & Green, C. (2007). *Phipps' medical-surgical nursing: Health and illness perspectives* (8th ed., pp. 1407-1408). St. Louis: Mosby.

214. Buck's extension traction is applied to an older client following a hip fracture. The nurse explains to the client that this type of traction is:
  1 Traction involving the use of a cast
  2 Skeletal traction involving the use of surgically inserted pins
  3 Circumferential traction involving the use of a belt around the body
  4 Skin traction involving the use of traction attached to the skin and soft tissues

Level of Cognitive Ability: Application
Client Needs: Physiological Integrity
Integrated Process: Nursing Process/ Implementation
Content Area: Adult Health/Musculoskeletal

Answer: 4
Rationale: Buck's extension traction is a form of skin traction and involves the use of a belt or boot that is attached to the skin and soft tissues. The purpose of this type of traction is to decrease painful muscle spasms that accompany fractures. The weight that is used as a pulling force is limited (usually 5 to 10 pounds) to prevent injury to the skin. Options 1, 2, and 3 are incorrect descriptions.

Test-Taking Strategy: Recalling that Buck's extension traction is a skin traction will assist in eliminating options 1, 2, and 3. Review the purpose and principles related to this type of traction if you had difficulty with this question.

References
Black, J., & Hawks, J. (2005). *Medical-surgical nursing: Clinical management for positive outcomes* (7th ed., p. 628). Philadelphia: Saunders.
Ignatavicius, D., & Workman, M. (2006). *Medical-surgical nursing: Critical thinking for collaborative care* (5th ed., pp. 1200-1201). Philadelphia: Saunders.
Monahan, F., Sands, J., Neighbors, M., Marek, J., & Green, C. (2007). *Phipps' medical-surgical nursing: Health and illness perspectives* (8th ed., pp. 1527-1528, 1535). St. Louis: Mosby.

---

215. A client is taking docusate calcium (Surfak). The nurse tells the client that which of the following may be experienced as a side effect of this medication?
  1 Abdominal cramps
  2 Peptic ulcer disease
  3 Partial bowel obstruction
  4 Gastrointestinal (GI) bleeding

Level of Cognitive Ability: Application
Client Needs: Physiological Integrity
Integrated Process: Teaching and Learning
Content Area: Pharmacology

Answer: 1
Rationale: Surfak is a laxative that causes nausea and abdominal cramps as the most frequent side effects. The problems identified in options 2, 3, and 4 are not side effects of this medication.

Test-Taking Strategy: Use the process of elimination. Remember that options that are comparable or alike are not likely to be correct. Therefore, eliminate options 2, 3, and 4 because they are GI disorders. Also recalling that this medication is a laxative and that laxatives can cause cramping will direct you to option 1. Review the action and side effects of this medication if you had difficulty with this question.

Reference
Hodgson, B., & Kizior, R. (2007). *Saunders nursing drug handbook 2007* (p. 192). Philadelphia: Saunders.

---

216. Skin closure with heterograft will be performed on a client with a burn injury, and the client asks the nurse about the meaning of a heterograft. The nurse tells the client that a heterograft is skin from:
  1 A cadaver
  2 Another species
  3 The burned client
  4 A synthetic source

Level of Cognitive Ability: Application
Client Needs: Physiological Integrity
Integrated Process: Nursing Process/ Implementation
Content Area: Adult Health/Integumentary

Answer: 2
Rationale: Biologic dressings are usually heterograft or homograft material. Heterograft is skin from another species. The most commonly used type of heterograft is pig skin because of its availability and its relative compatibility with human skin. Homograft is skin from another human, which is usually obtained from a cadaver and is provided through a skin bank. Autograft is skin from the client. Synthetic dressings are also available for covering burn wounds.

Test-Taking Strategy: Focus on the strategic word "heterograft." Also, options 1 and 3 are comparable or alike and relate to grafts from human skin. Review the various types of skin closure grafts if you had difficulty with this question.

Reference
Ignatavicius, D., & Workman, M. (2006). *Medical-surgical nursing: Critical thinking for collaborative care* (5th ed., pp. 1641-1642). Philadelphia: Saunders.

217. The nurse is caring for a client admitted to the hospital after sustaining a head injury. In which of the following positions should the nurse place the client to prevent increased intracranial pressure (ICP)?

1 In left Sims' position
2 In reverse Trendelenburg
3 With the head elevated on a pillow
4 With the head of the bed elevated at least 30 degrees

Level of Cognitive Ability: Application
Client Needs: Physiological Integrity
Integrated Process: Nursing Process/ Implementation
Content Area: Adult Health/Neurological

Answer: 4
Rationale: The client with a head injury is positioned to avoid extreme flexion or extension of the neck and to maintain the head in the midline, neutral position. The client is logrolled when turned to avoid extreme hip flexion. The head of the bed is elevated to at least 30 degrees or as recommended by the health care provider. All of these measures are used to enhance venous drainage, which helps prevent increased ICP.

Test-Taking Strategy: Use the process of elimination, recalling that the client with a head injury is at risk for increased ICP. Bearing this in mind and considering the principles of gravity will direct you to option 4. Review care of the client following a head injury if you had difficulty with this question.

Reference
Ignatavicius, D., & Workman, M. (2006). *Medical-surgical nursing: Critical thinking for collaborative care* (5th ed., p. 1051). Philadelphia: Saunders.

218. A newborn infant is diagnosed with esophageal atresia. The nurse assesses the infant, knowing that a typical finding in this disorder is:

1 Slowed reflexes
2 Continuous drooling
3 Diaphragmatic breathing
4 Passage of large amounts of frothy stool

Level of Cognitive Ability: Analysis
Client Needs: Physiological Integrity
Integrated Process: Nursing Process/Assessment
Content Area: Child Health

Answer: 2
Rationale: Esophageal atresia prevents the passage of swallowed mucus and saliva into the stomach. After fluid has accumulated in the pouch, it flows from the mouth and the infant then drools continuously. The inability to swallow amniotic fluid in utero prevents the accumulation of normal meconium, and lack of stools results. Responsiveness of the infant to stimulus would depend on the overall condition of the infant and is not considered a classic sign of esophageal atresia. Diaphragmatic breathing is not associated with this disorder.

Test-Taking Strategy: Focus on the anatomical location of the disorder to eliminate options 1 and 4 first. From the remaining options, recalling the pathophysiology associated with esophageal atresia and recalling that the word "atresia" indicates narrowing will direct you to option 2. Review the manifestations associated with this disorder if you had difficulty with this question.

Reference
Hockenberry, M., Wilson, D., & Winkelstein, M. (2005). *Wong's essentials of pediatric nursing* (7th ed., p. 878). St. Louis: Mosby.

219. The nurse is determining the need for suctioning in a client with an endotracheal (ET) tube attached to a mechanical ventilator. Which observation by the nurse indicates this need?
  1 Clear breath sounds
  2 Visible mucus bubbling in the ET tube
  3 Apical pulse rate of 72 beats per minute
  4 Low peak inspiratory pressure on the ventilator

Level of Cognitive Ability: Analysis
Client Needs: Physiological Integrity
Integrated Process: Nursing Process/Assessment
Content Area: Adult Health/Respiratory

Answer: 2
Rationale: Indications for suctioning include moist, wet respirations, restlessness, rhonchi on auscultation of the lungs, visible mucus bubbling in the ET tube, increased pulse and respiratory rates, and increased peak inspiratory pressures on the ventilator. A low peak inspiratory pressure would indicate a leak in the mechanical ventilation system.

Test-Taking Strategy: Focus on the subject, the need for suctioning. Eliminate options 1 and 3 first because they are normal findings. From the remaining options, focus on the subject and note the word "mucus" in option 2. Review assessment of the client being mechanically ventilated and the indications for the need for suctioning if you had difficulty with this question.

References
Black, J., & Hawks, J. (2005). *Medical-surgical nursing: Clinical management for positive outcomes* (7th ed., p. 1888). Philadelphia: Saunders.
Lewis, S., Heitkemper, M., Dirksen, S., O'Brien, P., & Bucher, L. (2007). *Medical-surgical nursing: Assessment and management of clinical problems* (7th ed., pp. 1778-1779). St. Louis: Mosby.

---

220. A client is intubated and receiving mechanical ventilation. The physician has added 7 cm of positive end expiratory pressure (PEEP) to the ventilator settings of the client. The nurse assesses for which of the following expected but adverse effects of PEEP?
  1 Decreased peak pressure on the ventilator
  2 Increased temperature from 98°F to 100°F rectally
  3 Decreased heart rate from 78 to 64 beats per minute
  4 Systolic blood pressure decrease from 122 to 98 mm Hg

Level of Cognitive Ability: Analysis
Client Needs: Physiological Integrity
Integrated Process: Nursing Process/Assessment
Content Area: Adult Health/Respiratory

Answer: 4
Rationale: PEEP leads to increased intrathoracic pressure, which in turn leads to decreased cardiac output. This is manifested in the client by decreased blood pressure and increased pulse (compensatory). Peak pressures on the ventilator should not be affected, although the pressure at the end of expiration remains positive at the level set for the PEEP. Fever would indicate respiratory infection or infection from another source.

Test-Taking Strategy: Note the strategic words "expected but adverse." Knowing that PEEP increases intrathoracic pressure leads you to look for the option that reflects a consequence of this event. Fever is irrelevant, and option 2 is eliminated first. From the remaining options, think about the effects of PEEP to direct you to option 4. Review the effects of PEEP if you had difficulty with this question.

Reference
Ignatavicius, D., & Workman, M. (2006). *Medical-surgical nursing: Critical thinking for collaborative care* (5th ed., p. 665). Philadelphia: Saunders.

---

221. The nurse is assessing the respiratory status of the client following thoracentesis. The nurse would become most concerned with which of the following assessment findings?
  1 Equal bilateral chest expansion
  2 Respiratory rate of 22 breaths per minute
  3 Diminished breath sounds on affected side
  4 Few scattered wheezes, unchanged from baseline

Answer: 3
Rationale: Following thoracentesis, the nurse assesses vital signs and breath sounds. The nurse especially notes increased respiratory rates, dyspnea, retractions, diminished breath sounds, or cyanosis, which could indicate pneumothorax. Any of these signs should be reported to the physician. Options 1 and 2 are normal findings. Option 4 indicates a finding that is unchanged from the baseline.

Level of Cognitive Ability: Analysis
Client Needs: Physiological Integrity
Integrated Process: Nursing Process/Analysis
Content Area: Adult Health/Respiratory

Test-Taking Strategy: Use the process of elimination, noting the strategic words "most concerned." Eliminate options 1 and 2 first because they are normal findings. Option 4 is an abnormality, but note that the wheezes are unchanged from the client's baseline. Option 3 is the abnormal finding. Review the signs of complications following a thoracentesis if you had difficulty with this question.

Reference
Ignatavicius, D., & Workman, M. (2006). *Medical-surgical nursing: Critical thinking for collaborative care* (5th ed., p. 542). Philadelphia: Saunders.

---

222. The nurse is preparing to administer a Mantoux skin test to a client. The nurse determines that which area is most appropriate for injection of the medication?
1 Dorsal aspect of the upper arm near a mole
2 Inner aspect of the forearm that is close to a burn scar
3 Inner aspect of the forearm that is not heavily pigmented
4 Dorsal aspect of the upper arm that has a small amount of hair

Level of Cognitive Ability: Application
Client Needs: Physiological Integrity
Integrated Process: Nursing Process/Assessment
Content Area: Adult Health/Respiratory

Answer: 3
Rationale: Intradermal injections are most commonly given in the inner surface of the forearm. Other sites include the dorsal area of the upper arm or the upper back beneath the scapulae. The nurse finds an area that is not heavily pigmented and is clear of hairy areas or lesions that could interfere with reading the results.

Test-Taking Strategy: Use the process of elimination. Note that options 1, 2, and 4 are comparable or alike in that they indicate areas that are not clear of lesions or hair. Review the basics of intradermal injection techniques if you had difficulty with this question.

References
Chernecky, C., & Berger, B. (2008). *Laboratory tests and diagnostic procedures* (5th ed., pp. 758-759). Philadelphia: Saunders.
Potter, P., & Perry, A. (2005). *Fundamentals of nursing* (6th ed., p. 884). St. Louis: Mosby.

---

223. The home care nurse is planning therapeutic measures for the client who experienced a rib fracture 2 days earlier. The nurse tells the client to avoid which of the following?
1 Analgesics
2 Ambulation
3 Strapping the ribs
4 Coughing and deep breathing

Level of Cognitive Ability: Application
Client Needs: Physiological Integrity
Integrated Process: Nursing Process/ Implementation
Content Area: Adult Health/Respiratory

Answer: 3
Rationale: Fractured ribs are treated with good pulmonary therapy techniques such as coughing and deep breathing, rapid mobilization, and adequate pain control. Strapping of the ribs is not a treatment measure because it restricts deep breathing and can increase the incidence of atelectasis and pneumonia.

Test-Taking Strategy: Use the process of elimination, focusing on the client's injury and noting the strategic word "avoid." Recalling that rib strapping restricts deep breathing will direct you to option 3. Review client teaching points related to measures in treating a rib fracture if you had difficulty with this question.

References
Black, J., & Hawks, J. (2005). *Medical-surgical nursing: Clinical management for positive outcomes* (7th ed., p. 1901). Philadelphia: Saunders.
Ignatavicius, D., & Workman, M. (2006). *Medical-surgical nursing: Critical thinking for collaborative care* (5th ed., p. 670). Philadelphia: Saunders.

224. A hospitalized client is dyspneic and has been diagnosed with left tension pneumothorax by chest X-ray after insertion of a central venous catheter. Which of the following observed by the nurse indicates that the pneumothorax is rapidly worsening?

1 Hypertension
2 Pain with respiration
3 Tracheal deviation to the left
4 Tracheal deviation to the right

Level of Cognitive Ability: Analysis
Client Needs: Physiological Integrity
Integrated Process: Nursing Process/Assessment
Content Area: Adult Health/Respiratory

Answer: 4
Rationale: A tension pneumothorax is characterized by distended neck veins, displaced point of maximal impulse (PMI), tracheal deviation to the unaffected side, asymmetry of the thorax, decreased to absent breath sounds on the affected side, and worsening cyanosis. The client could have pain with respiration. The increased intrathoracic pressure would cause the blood pressure to fall, not rise.

Test-Taking Strategy: Focus on the client's diagnosis and the strategic words "rapidly worsening." Pain and hypertension are the least specific indicators and are eliminated first. From the remaining options, remember that a tension pneumothorax causes the trachea to be pushed in the opposite direction, to the unaffected side. Review the complications of pneumothorax if you had difficulty with this question.

References
Ignatavicius, D., & Workman, M. (2006). *Medical-surgical nursing: Critical thinking for collaborative care* (5th ed., p. 670). Philadelphia: Saunders.
Lewis, S., Heitkemper, M., Dirksen, S., O'Brien, P., & Bucher, L. (2007). *Medical-surgical nursing: Assessment and management of clinical problems* (7th ed., pp. 586-587). St. Louis: Mosby.
Monahan, F., Sands, J., Neighbors, M., Marek, J., & Green, C. (2007). *Phipps' medical-surgical nursing: Health and illness perspectives* (8th ed., p. 668). St. Louis: Mosby.

---

225. A client is admitted to the hospital with a diagnosis of right lower lobe pneumonia. The nurse auscultates the right lower lobe, expecting to note which of the following types of breath sounds?

1 Absent
2 Vesicular
3 Bronchial
4 Bronchovesicular

Level of Cognitive Ability: Analysis
Client Needs: Physiological Integrity
Integrated Process: Nursing Process/Assessment
Content Area: Adult Health/Respiratory

Answer: 3
Rationale: Bronchial sounds are normally heard over the trachea. The client with pneumonia will have bronchial breath sounds over area(s) of consolidation, because the consolidated tissue carries bronchial sounds to the peripheral lung fields. The client may also have crackles in the affected area resulting from fluid in the interstitium and alveoli. Absent breath sounds are not likely to occur unless a serious complication of the pneumonia occurs. Bronchovesicular sounds are normally heard over the main bronchi. Vesicular sounds are normally heard over the lesser bronchi, bronchioles, and lobes.

Test-Taking Strategy: Use the process of elimination. Recalling that bronchovesicular sounds are normally heard over the main bronchi and vesicular breath sounds are normal in the lung periphery helps eliminate options 2 and 4. From the remaining options, recall that the pneumonia transmits bronchial breath sounds, so they are heard over the area of consolidation. Review assessment findings in pneumonia if you had difficulty with this question.

Reference
Ignatavicius, D., & Workman, M. (2006). *Medical-surgical nursing: Critical thinking for collaborative care* (5th ed., p. 635). Philadelphia: Saunders.

226. The nurse assesses the client with acquired immunodeficiency syndrome (AIDS) for early signs of Kaposi's sarcoma. The nurse observes the client for lesion(s) that are:
1 Unilateral, raised, and bluish-purple in color
2 Unilateral, red, raised, and resembling a blister
3 Bilateral, flat, and brownish and scaly in appearance
4 Bilateral, flat, and pink, turning to dark violet or black in color

Level of Cognitive Ability: Analysis
Client Needs: Physiological Integrity
Integrated Process: Nursing Process/Assessment
Content Area: Adult Health/Immune

Answer: 4
Rationale: Kaposi's sarcoma generally starts with an area that is flat and pink that changes to a dark violet or black color. The lesions are usually present bilaterally. They may appear in many areas of the body and are treated with radiation, chemotherapy, and cryotherapy.

Test-Taking Strategy: Use the process of elimination. Recalling that Kaposi's sarcoma occurs in a bilateral pattern eliminates options 1 and 2. From the remaining options, recalling the character of the lesions will direct you to option 4. Review the characteristics of this disorder if you had difficulty with this question.

Reference
Black, J., & Hawks, J. (2005). *Medical-surgical nursing: Clinical management for positive outcomes* (7th ed., p. 2393). Philadelphia: Saunders.

227. A client is suspected of having a pleural effusion. The nurse assesses the client for which typical manifestations of this respiratory problem?
1 Dyspnea at rest and moist, productive cough
2 Dyspnea at rest and dry, nonproductive cough
3 Dyspnea on exertion and moist, productive cough
4 Dyspnea on exertion and dry, nonproductive cough

Level of Cognitive Ability: Application
Client Needs: Physiological Integrity
Integrated Process: Nursing Process/Assessment
Content Area: Adult Health/Respiratory

Answer: 4
Rationale: Typical assessment findings in the client with a pleural effusion include dyspnea, which usually occurs with exertion, and a dry, nonproductive cough. The cough is caused by bronchial irritation and possible mediastinal shift.

Test-Taking Strategy: Use the process of elimination. Recalling that a pleural effusion is in the pleural space and not the airway helps to eliminate options 1 and 3. Remembering that dyspnea occurs on exertion before it occurs at rest will direct you to option 4 from the remaining options. Review the manifestations of pleural effusion if you had difficulty with this question.

Reference
Black, J., & Hawks, J. (2005). *Medical-surgical nursing: Clinical management for positive outcomes* (7th ed., p. 1873). Philadelphia: Saunders.

228. A client with pleural effusion had a thoracentesis, and a sample of fluid was sent to the laboratory. Analysis of the fluid reveals a high red blood cell count. The nurse interprets that this result is most consistent with:
1 Trauma
2 Infection
3 Liver failure
4 Heart failure

Answer: 1
Rationale: Pleural effusion that has a high red blood cell count may result from trauma and may be treated with placement of a chest tube for drainage. Other causes of pleural effusion include infection, heart failure, liver or renal failure, malignancy, or inflammatory processes. Infection would be accompanied by white blood cells. The fluid portion of the serum would accumulate with liver failure and heart failure.

Test-Taking Strategy: Use the process of elimination. Noting the strategic words "red blood cell count" will direct you to option 1. Review the causes of pleural effusion if you had difficulty with this question.

Level of Cognitive Ability: Analysis
Client Needs: Physiological Integrity
Integrated Process: Nursing Process/Analysis
Content Area: Adult Health/Respiratory

References
Black, J., & Hawks, J. (2005). *Medical-surgical nursing: Clinical management for positive outcomes* (7th ed., p. 1873). Philadelphia: Saunders.
Chernecky, C., & Berger, B. (2008). *Laboratory tests and diagnostic procedures* (5th ed., pp. 1063-1064). Philadelphia: Saunders.

---

229. A nurse is scheduling a client for diagnostic studies of the gastrointestinal (GI) system. Which of the following studies, if ordered, should the nurse schedule last?
 1 Ultrasound
 2 Colonoscopy
 3 Barium enema
 4 Computed tomography

Level of Cognitive Ability: Application
Client Needs: Physiological Integrity
Integrated Process: Nursing Process/Planning
Content Area: Delegating/Prioritizing

Answer: 3
Rationale: When barium is instilled into the lower GI tract, it may take up to 72 hours to clear the GI tract. The presence of barium could cause interference with obtaining clear visualization and accurate results of the other tests listed, if performed before the client has fully excreted the barium. For this reason, diagnostic studies that involve barium contrast are scheduled at the conclusion of other medical imaging studies.

Test-Taking Strategy: Use the process of elimination. Note the strategic word "last." Recall that barium shows up on X-ray as opaque and that this substance would impair visualization during other tests. Review the requirements for the successful completion of the medical imaging diagnostic modalities listed in the options if you had difficulty with this question.

References
Chernecky, C., & Berger, B. (2008). *Laboratory tests and diagnostic procedures* (5th ed., p. 185). Philadelphia: Saunders.
Monahan, F., Sands, J., Neighbors, M., Marek, J., & Green, C. (2007). *Phipps' medical-surgical nursing: Health and illness perspectives* (8th ed., p. 1178). St. Louis: Mosby.

---

230. The nurse is caring for a client who is scheduled to have a liver biopsy. Before the procedure, it is most important for the nurse to assess the client's:
 1 Tolerance for pain
 2 Allergy to iodine or shellfish
 3 History of nausea and vomiting
 4 Ability to lie still and hold the breath

Level of Cognitive Ability: Application
Client Needs: Physiological Integrity
Integrated Process: Nursing Process/Assessment
Content Area: Adult Health/Gastrointestinal

Answer: 4
Rationale: It is most important for the nurse to assess the client's ability to lie still and hold the breath for the procedure. This helps the physician avoid complications, such as puncturing the lung or other organs. Assessment of allergy to iodine or shellfish is unnecessary for this procedure, because no contrast dye is used. Knowledge of the history related to nausea and vomiting is generally a part of assessment of the gastrointestinal system but has no relationship to the procedure. The client's tolerance for pain is a useful item to know. However, the area will receive a local anesthetic.

Test-Taking Strategy: Use the process of elimination. Visualizing this procedure and thinking about its complications will direct you to option 4. Review this procedure if you had difficulty with this question.

References
Black, J., & Hawks, J. (2005). *Medical-surgical nursing: Clinical management for positive outcomes* (7th ed., pp. 1185-1186). Philadelphia: Saunders.
Chernecky, C., & Berger, B. (2008). *Laboratory tests and diagnostic procedures* (5th ed., p. 722). Philadelphia: Saunders.

231. The nurse is caring for a client diagnosed with pneumonia. The nurse plans which of the following as the best time to take the client for a short walk?

1 After the client eats lunch
2 After the client has a brief nap
3 After the client uses the metered-dose inhaler
4 After recording oxygen saturation on the bedside flow sheet

Level of Cognitive Ability: Application
Client Needs: Physiological Integrity
Integrated Process: Nursing Process/Planning
Content Area: Adult Health/Respiratory

Answer: 3

Rationale: The nurse should schedule activities for the client with pneumonia after the client has received respiratory treatments or medications. After the administration of bronchodilators (often administered by metered-dose inhaler), the client has the best oxygen exchange possible and would tolerate the activity best. Still, the nurse implements activity cautiously, so as not to increase the client's dyspnea. The client would become fatigued after eating; therefore, this is not a good time to ambulate the client. Although the client may be rested somewhat after a nap, from the options provided this is not the best time to ambulate. Option 4 is unrelated to the client's ability to tolerate ambulation.

Test-Taking Strategy: Note the strategic word "best." Use the ABCs—airway, breathing, and circulation. The use of bronchodilator medication would widen the air passages, allowing for more air to enter the client's lungs. Review care of the client with pneumonia if you had difficulty with this question.

References

Black, J., & Hawks, J. (2005). *Medical-surgical nursing: Clinical management for positive outcomes* (7th ed., pp. 1842-1843). Philadelphia: Saunders.
Monahan, F., Sands, J., Neighbors, M., Marek, J., & Green, C. (2007). *Phipps' medical-surgical nursing: Health and illness perspectives* (8th ed., pp. 625-626). St. Louis: Mosby.

232. A nurse inserts an indwelling Foley catheter into the bladder of a postoperative client who has not voided for 8 hours and has a distended bladder. After the tubing is secured and the collection bag is hung on the bed frame, the nurse notices that 800 mL of urine has drained into the collection bag. The appropriate nursing action for the safety of the client is to:

1 Check the specific gravity of the urine.
2 Clamp the tubing for 30 minutes and then release.
3 Provide suprapubic pressure to maintain a steady flow of urine.
4 Raise the collection bag high enough to slow the rate of drainage.

Level of Cognitive Ability: Application
Client Needs: Physiological Integrity
Integrated Process: Nursing Process/ Implementation
Content Area: Fundamental Skills

Answer: 2

Rationale: Rapid emptying of a large volume of urine may cause engorgement of pelvic blood vessels and hypovolemic shock. Clamping the tubing for 30 minutes allows for equilibration to prevent complications. Option 1 is an assessment and would not affect the flow of urine or prevent possible hypovolemic shock. Option 3 would increase the flow of urine, which would lead to hypovolemic shock. Option 4 could cause backflow of urine. Infection is likely to develop if urine is allowed to flow back into the bladder.

Test-Taking Strategy: Note the strategic words "800 mL." Recall the physiology of the hemodynamic changes following the rapid collapse of an overdistended bladder. Eliminate options 3 and 4, because slowing the rate of urine drainage is the subject. Note that option 1 is an assessment action rather than an action that affects the amount of urine drainage. Review the complications associated with inserting a Foley catheter in a client with a distended bladder if you had difficulty with this question.

References

Black, J., & Hawks, J. (2005). *Medical-surgical nursing: Clinical management for positive outcomes* (7th ed., p. 906). Philadelphia: Saunders.
Potter, P., & Perry, A. (2005). *Fundamentals of nursing* (6th ed., p. 1357). St. Louis: Mosby.

233. The nurse has an order to administer amphotericin B (Fungizone) intravenously to the client with histoplasmosis. The nurse plans to do which of the following during administration of the medication?

1 Monitor for hypothermia.
2 Assess the intravenous infusion site.
3 Monitor for an excessive urine output.
4 Administer a concurrent fluid challenge.

Level of Cognitive Ability: Application
Client Needs: Physiological Integrity
Integrated Process: Nursing Process/Planning
Content Area: Adult Health/Immune

Answer: 2
Rationale: Amphotericin B is a toxic medication, which can produce symptoms during administration such as chills, fever (hyperthermia), headache, vomiting, and impaired renal function (decreased urine output). The medication is also very irritating to the IV site, commonly causing thrombophlebitis. The nurse administering this medication monitors for these complications. Administering a concurrent fluid challenge is not necessary.

Test-Taking Strategy: Use the process of elimination, recalling the toxic effects of this medication. Knowing that fever and chills can occur eliminates option 1. Recalling that the medication can be toxic to the kidneys eliminates option 3. From the remaining options, knowing that there is no rationale for giving concurrent fluids will direct you to option 2. Review nursing care related to the administration of this medication if you had difficulty with this question.

References
Gahart, B., & Nazareno, A. (2006). *2006 Intravenous medications* (22nd ed., p. 95). St. Louis: Mosby.
Hodgson, B., & Kizior, R. (2007). *Saunders nursing drug handbook 2007* (p. 68). Philadelphia: Saunders.

---

234. A client who experiences repeated pleural effusions from inoperable lung cancer is to undergo pleurodesis. The nurse plans to assist with which of the following after the physician injects the sclerosing agent through the chest tube?

1 Ambulate the client.
2 Clamp the chest tube.
3 Ask the client to cough and deep breathe.
4 Ask the client to remain in one position only.

Level of Cognitive Ability: Application
Client Needs: Physiological Integrity
Integrated Process: Nursing Process/Planning
Content Area: Adult Health/Respiratory

Answer: 2
Rationale: After injection of the sclerosing agent, the chest tube is clamped to prevent the agent from draining back out of the pleural space. A repositioning schedule is used by some physicians, but its usefulness in dispersing the substance is controversial. Ambulation, coughing, and deep breathing have no specific purpose in the immediate period after injection.

Test-Taking Strategy: Note that the client is having a pleurodesis. This will assist in eliminating option 1. Eliminate option 4 because of the word "only." From the remaining options, recall the purpose of the procedure. It is most reasonable to clamp the chest tube so that the sclerosing agent cannot flow back out of the tube. Coughing and deep breathing have no specific purpose in this situation. Review this procedure if you had difficulty with this question.

Reference
Black, J., & Hawks, J. (2005). *Medical-surgical nursing: Clinical management for positive outcomes* (7th ed., pp. 1873-1874). Philadelphia: Saunders.

---

235. A client with a posterior wall bladder injury has had surgical repair and placement of a suprapubic catheter. The nurse plans to do which of the following to prevent complications with the use of this catheter?

1 Monitor urine output every shift.
2 Measure specific gravity once a shift.
3 Encourage a high intake of oral fluids.
4 Prevent kinking of the catheter tubing.

Answer: 4
Rationale: A complication after surgical repair of the bladder is disruption of sutures caused by tension on them from urine buildup. The nurse prevents this from happening by ensuring that the catheter is able to drain freely. This involves basic catheter care, including keeping the tubing free from kinks, keeping the tubing below the level of the bladder, and monitoring the flow of urine frequently. Measurement of urine specific gravity and a high oral fluid intake do not prevent complications of bladder surgery. Monitoring urine output every shift is insufficient to detect decreased flow from catheter kinking.

Level of Cognitive Ability: Application
Client Needs: Physiological Integrity
Integrated Process: Nursing Process/Planning
Content Area: Adult Health/Renal

Test-Taking Strategy: Use the process of elimination. Eliminate option 2 first because specific gravity measurement is not a preventive action. Eliminate option 1 next, because once-a-shift measurement is not a preventive action and is also insufficient in frequency. From the remaining options, knowing that a high oral fluid intake will not prevent complications with the catheter directs you to option 4. Review care of the client with a suprapubic catheter if you had difficulty with this question.

Reference
Black, J., & Hawks, J. (2005). *Medical-surgical nursing: Clinical management for positive outcomes* (7th ed., p. 894). Philadelphia: Saunders.

---

236. A client with benign prostatic hyperplasia undergoes transurethral resection of the prostate (TURP). The nurse orders which of the following solutions from the pharmacy so it is available postoperatively for continuous bladder irrigation (CBI)?
1 Sterile water
2 Sterile normal saline
3 Sterile Dakin's solution
4 Sterile water with 5% dextrose

Level of Cognitive Ability: Application
Client Needs: Physiological Integrity
Integrated Process: Nursing Process/
 Implementation
Content Area: Adult Health/Renal

Answer: 2
Rationale: Continuous bladder irrigation is done following TURP using sterile normal saline, which is isotonic. Sterile water is not used because the solution could be absorbed systemically, precipitating hemolysis and possibly renal failure. Dakin's solution contains hypochlorite and is used only for wound irrigation in selected circumstances. Solutions containing dextrose are not introduced into the bladder.

Test-Taking Strategy: Use the process of elimination, noting the subject, a continuous bladder irrigation. Recalling that normal saline is isotonic will direct you to option 2. Review the procedure for CBI if you had difficulty with this question.

Reference
Ignatavicius, D., & Workman, M. (2006). *Medical-surgical nursing: Critical thinking for collaborative care* (5th ed., p. 1069). Philadelphia: Saunders.

---

237. A client with acquired immunodeficiency syndrome (AIDS) is being admitted to the hospital for treatment of *Pneumocystis jiroveci* infection. Which of the following activities does the nurse plan to include in the care of this client that assists in maintaining comfort?
1 Monitor vital signs.
2 Evaluate arterial blood gas results.
3 Keep the head of the bed elevated.
4 Assess respiratory rate, rhythm, depth, and breath sounds.

Level of Cognitive Ability: Application
Client Needs: Physiological Integrity
Integrated Process: Nursing Process/Planning
Content Area: Adult Health/Immune

Answer: 3
Rationale: Clients with respiratory difficulties are often more comfortable with the head of the bed elevated. Options 1, 2, and 4 are appropriate measures to evaluate respiratory function and to avoid complications. Option 3 is the only option that addresses planning for client comfort.

Test-Taking Strategy: Use the process of elimination. Focusing on the subject, maintaining comfort, will direct you to option 3. Also, note that options 1, 2, and 4 are comparable or alike and are all measures to evaluate respiratory function. Review measures to promote comfort in a client with a respiratory infection if you had difficulty with this question.

Reference
Ignatavicius, D., & Workman, M. (2006). *Medical-surgical nursing: Critical thinking for collaborative care* (5th ed., p. 603). Philadelphia: Saunders.

238. A client with significant flail chest has arterial blood gases (ABGs) that reveal a Pao_2 of 68 and a $Paco_2$ of 51. Two hours ago the Pao_2 was 82 and the $Paco_2$ was 44. Based on these changes, the nurse obtains which of the following items?

1 Intubation tray
2 Chest tube insertion set
3 Portable chest X-ray machine
4 Injectable lidocaine (Xylocaine)

Level of Cognitive Ability: Application
Client Needs: Physiological Integrity
Integrated Process: Nursing Process/
    Implementation
Content Area: Adult Health/Respiratory

Answer: 1
Rationale: The client with flail chest has painful, rapid, shallow respirations while experiencing severe dyspnea. The effort of breathing and the paradoxical chest movement have the net effect of producing hypoxia and hypercapnia. The client develops respiratory failure and requires intubation and mechanical ventilation, usually with positive end expiratory pressure (PEEP). Therefore, an intubation tray is necessary.

Test-Taking Strategy: Use the process of elimination, noting the changes in the ABG values. Recall that a falling arterial oxygen level and a rising carbon dioxide level indicate respiratory failure. The usual treatment for respiratory failure is intubation, which makes option 1 correct. Review the complications of flail chest and the signs of respiratory failure if you had difficulty with this question.

References
Black, J., & Hawks, J. (2005). *Medical-surgical nursing: Clinical management for positive outcomes* (7th ed., pp. 2492-2493). Philadelphia: Saunders.
Ignatavicius, D., & Workman, M. (2006). *Medical-surgical nursing: Critical thinking for collaborative care* (5th ed., p. 670). Philadelphia: Saunders.

239. A client with empyema is to have a thoracentesis performed at the bedside. The nurse plans to have which of the following available in the event that the procedure is not effective?

1 Code cart
2 A small-bore needle
3 Extra-large drainage bottle
4 Chest tube and drainage system

Level of Cognitive Ability: Application
Client Needs: Physiological Integrity
Integrated Process: Nursing Process/Planning
Content Area: Adult Health/Respiratory

Answer: 4
Rationale: If the exudate is too thick for drainage via thoracentesis, the client may require placement of a chest tube to adequately drain the purulent effusion. A small-bore needle would not effectively allow exudate to drain. Options 1 and 3 are also unnecessary.

Test-Taking Strategy: Note the client's diagnosis. In this condition, the exudate is often very thick. Recalling that the purpose of thoracentesis is to provide drainage of the pleura will direct you to option 4. Review care of the client undergoing a thoracentesis if you had difficulty with this question.

References
Ignatavicius, D., & Workman, M. (2006). *Medical-surgical nursing: Critical thinking for collaborative care* (5th ed., pp. 540-541). Philadelphia: Saunders.
Lewis, S., Heitkemper, M., Dirksen, S., O'Brien, P., & Bucher, L. (2007). *Medical-surgical nursing: Assessment and management of clinical problems* (7th ed., pp. 528, 596). St. Louis: Mosby.

240. A nurse is preparing to administer an opioid to a client via an epidural catheter. Before administering the medication, the nurse aspirates and obtains 5 mL of clear fluid. The nurse takes which action?

1 Injects the opioid slowly
2 Notifies the anesthesiologist
3 Flushes the catheter with 6 mL of sterile water before injecting the opioid
4 Injects the aspirate (6 mL of clear fluid) back into the catheter and administers the opioid

Answer: 2
Rationale: Aspiration of clear fluid of less than 1 mL is indicative of epidural catheter placement. More than 1 mL of clear fluid or bloody return means that the catheter may be in the subarachnoid space or in a vessel. Therefore, the nurse would not inject the medication and would notify the anesthesiologist. Options 1, 3, and 4 are incorrect actions.

Test-Taking Strategy: Use the process of elimination, focusing on the strategic word "epidural." Eliminate options 1, 3, and 4 because they are comparable or alike and indicate administering the opioid. Review the procedure for administering medication through an epidural catheter if you had difficulty with this question.

Level of Cognitive Ability: Application
Client Needs: Physiological Integrity
Integrated Process: Nursing Process/
Implementation
Content Area: Pharmacology

References

Ignatavicius, D., & Workman, M. (2006). *Medical-surgical nursing: Critical thinking for collaborative care* (5th ed., pp. 1053-1054). Philadelphia: Saunders.

Lewis, S., Heitkemper, M., Dirksen, S., O'Brien, P., & Bucher, L. (2007). *Medical-surgical nursing: Assessment and management of clinical problems* (7th ed., pp. 392-393). St. Louis: Mosby.

---

241. A nurse is planning care for a client with a chest tube attached to a Pleur-Evac drainage system. The nurse avoids which of the following activities to prevent a tension pneumothorax?
1 Clamping the chest tube
2 Adding water to the suction control chamber as it evaporates
3 Maintaining the collection chamber below the client's waist
4 Taping the connection between the chest tube and the drainage system

Level of Cognitive Ability: Application
Client Needs: Physiological Integrity
Integrated Process: Nursing Process/
Implementation
Content Area: Adult Health/Respiratory

Answer: 1

Rationale: To prevent a tension pneumothorax, the nurse avoids clamping the chest tube, unless specifically ordered. In many facilities, clamping of the chest tube is contraindicated by agency policy. Adding water to the suction control chamber is an appropriate nursing action and is done as needed to maintain the full suction level ordered. Taping the connection between the chest tube and system is also indicated to prevent accidental disconnection. Maintaining the system below waist level is indicated to prevent fluid from reentering the pleural space.

Test-Taking Strategy: Use the process of elimination, noting the strategic word "avoids." This word indicates a negative event query and the need to select the option that is an incorrect nursing action. Recall that tension pneumothorax occurs when air is trapped in the pleural space and has no exit. Therefore, it is necessary to evaluate each of the options in terms of relative risk for air trapping in the pleural space. Clamping the chest tube could trap air in the pleural space. Review the causes of tension pneumothorax and care of the client with a chest tube if you had difficulty with this question.

Reference

Lewis, S., Heitkemper, M., Dirksen, S., O'Brien, P., & Bucher, L. (2007). *Medical-surgical nursing: Assessment and management of clinical problems* (7th ed., p. 588). St. Louis: Mosby.

---

242. A nurse is assisting a client with a chest tube to get out of bed, and the chest tubing accidentally gets caught in the bed rail and disconnects. While trying to reestablish the connection, the Pleur-Evac drainage system falls over and cracks. The nurse takes which immediate action?
1 Calls the physician
2 Clamps the chest tube
3 Applies a petrolatum gauze over the end of the chest tube
4 Immerses the chest tube in a bottle of sterile normal saline

Level of Cognitive Ability: Application
Client Needs: Physiological Integrity
Integrated Process: Nursing Process/
Implementation
Content Area: Adult Health/Respiratory

Answer: 4

Rationale: If a chest tube accidentally disconnects from the tubing of the drainage apparatus, the nurse should first reestablish an underwater seal to prevent tension pneumothorax and mediastinal shift. This can be accomplished by reconnecting the chest tube, or in this case, immersing the end of the chest tube in a bottle of sterile normal saline or water. The physician should be notified after taking corrective action. If the physician is called first, tension pneumothorax has time to develop. Clamping the chest tube could also cause tension pneumothorax. A petrolatum gauze would be applied to the skin over the chest tube insertion site if the entire chest tube was accidentally removed from the chest.

Test-Taking Strategy: Use the process of elimination, noting the strategic word "immediate." Eliminate option 3 as too time consuming to be the "immediate" action. Option 2 would create a tension pneumothorax, because this action does not reestablish an underwater seal. From the remaining options, noting that an underwater seal must be established will direct you to option 4. Review care of the client with a chest tube if you had difficulty with this question.

References

Black, J., & Hawks, J. (2005). *Medical-surgical nursing: Clinical management for positive outcomes* (7th ed., p. 1865). Philadelphia: Saunders.

Perry, A., & Potter, P. (2006). *Clinical nursing skills & techniques* (6th ed., p. 868). St. Louis: Mosby.

---

243. A nurse is caring for a client with a diagnosis of Cushing's syndrome. The nurse plans which of these measures to prevent complications from this medical condition?

1 Monitoring glucose levels
2 Encouraging daily jogging
3 Monitoring epinephrine levels
4 Encouraging visits from friends

Level of Cognitive Ability: Analysis
Client Needs: Physiological Integrity
Integrated Process: Nursing Process/Planning
Content Area: Adult Health/Endocrine

Answer: 1

Rationale: In the client with Cushing's syndrome, increased levels of glucocorticoids can result in hyperglycemia and signs and symptoms of diabetes mellitus. Epinephrine levels are not affected. Clients experience activity intolerance related to muscle weakness and fatigue, therefore option 2 is incorrect. Visitors should be limited because of the client's impaired immune response.

Test-Taking Strategy: Focus on complications of Cushing's syndrome. Recalling that increased levels of glucocorticoids can result in hyperglycemia will direct you to option 1. Review the clinical manifestations associated with Cushing's syndrome if you had difficulty with this question.

Reference

Ignatavicius, D., & Workman, M. (2006). *Medical-surgical nursing: Critical thinking for collaborative care* (5th ed., p. 1474). Philadelphia: Saunders.

---

244. A client with a central venous catheter who is receiving parenteral nutrition (PN) suddenly becomes short of breath, complains of chest pain, and is tachycardic, pale, and anxious. The nurse, suspecting an air embolism, places the client in lateral Trendelenburg position on the left side and:

1 Monitors vital signs every 30 minutes
2 Clamps the catheter and notifies the physician
3 Slows the rate of the PN after checking the lines for air
4 Boluses the client with 500 mL normal saline to break up the air embolus

Level of Cognitive Ability: Application
Client Needs: Physiological Integrity
Integrated Process: Nursing Process/Implementation
Content Area: Adult Health/Renal

Answer: 2

Rationale: If the client experiences air embolus, the nurse should clamp the catheter and notify the physician. The client is also placed in the lateral Trendelenburg position on the left side to trap the air in the right atrium. A fluid bolus would cause the air embolus to travel. Vital signs are monitored continuously.

Test-Taking Strategy: Note the strategic words "suspecting an air embolism." Recall that air embolism is a life-threatening condition and that the physician needs to be notified if a life-threatening condition exists. This will direct you to option 2. Review the interventions for an air embolism if you had difficulty with this question.

Reference

Ignatavicius, D., & Workman, M. (2006). *Medical-surgical nursing: Critical thinking for collaborative care* (5th ed., p. 263). Philadelphia: Saunders.

---

245. A nurse notes on the cardiac monitor that a client with aldosteronism is experiencing a dysrhythmia. The nurse immediately assesses the client's:

1 Peripheral pulses
2 Intake and output
3 Superficial reflexes
4 Plasma potassium level

Answer: 4

Rationale: Aldosteronism can lead to hypokalemia, which in turn can cause life-threatening dysrhythmias. Options 1, 2, and 3 are not immediate priorities for this client.

Level of Cognitive Ability: Application
Client Needs: Physiological Integrity
Integrated Process: Nursing Process/
Implementation
Content Area: Adult Health/Endocrine

Test-Taking Strategy: Note the strategic word "immediately." Recalling the complications associated with this disorder and that altered potassium levels can cause dysrhythmias will direct you to option 4. Review the complications of aldosteronism if you had difficulty with this question.

References
Lewis, S., Heitkemper, M., Dirksen, S., O'Brien, P., & Bucher, L. (2007). *Medical-surgical nursing: Assessment and management of clinical problems* (7th ed., pp. 326-327). St. Louis: Mosby.
Monahan, F., Sands, J., Neighbors, M., Marek, J., & Green, C. (2007). *Phipps' medical-surgical nursing: Health and illness perspectives* (8th ed., pp. 1100-1101). St. Louis: Mosby.

246. A nurse is monitoring the results of serial arterial blood gases for the client who has been diagnosed with carbon monoxide poisoning and is asking for the oxygen mask to be removed. The nurse determines that the oxygen may be safely removed once the carboxyhemoglobin level decreases to less than:

1 5%
2 10%
3 15%
4 25%

Level of Cognitive Ability: Analysis
Client Needs: Physiological Integrity
Integrated Process: Teaching and Learning
Content Area: Adult Health/Respiratory

Answer: 1
Rationale: Oxygen may be removed safely from the client with carbon monoxide poisoning once carboxyhemoglobin levels are less than 5%. Options 2, 3, and 4 are elevated levels.

Test-Taking Strategy: Focus on the subject, safely removing the oxygen. If you are unsure, it would be best to select the lowest level as identified in option 1. Review the normal carboxyhemoglobin levels if you had difficulty with this question.

References
Chernecky, C., & Berger, B. (2008). *Laboratory tests and diagnostic procedures* (5th ed., pp. 292-293). Philadelphia: Saunders.
Ignatavicius, D., & Workman, M. (2006). *Medical-surgical nursing: Critical thinking for collaborative care* (5th ed., pp. 1628-1629). Philadelphia: Saunders.

247. A nurse is teaching a pregnant client about nutrition. The nurse includes which information in the client's teaching plan?

1 Calcium is not important until the third trimester.
2 All mothers are at high risk for nutritional deficiencies.
3 Iron supplements are not necessary unless the mother has iron deficiency anemia.
4 The nutritional status of the mother significantly influences fetal growth and development.

Level of Cognitive Ability: Application
Client Needs: Physiological Integrity
Integrated Process: Nursing Process/
Implementation
Content Area: Maternity/Antepartum

Answer: 4
Rationale: Poor nutrition during pregnancy can negatively influence fetal growth and development. Although pregnancy poses some nutritional risk for the mother, not all clients are at high risk. Calcium is critical during the third trimester but must be increased from the onset of pregnancy. Intake of dietary iron is insufficient for the majority of pregnant women, and iron supplements are routinely prescribed.

Test-Taking Strategy: Use the process of elimination. Option 2 uses the close-ended word "all"; therefore, eliminate this option. Options 1 and 3 offer specific time frames or conditions for interventions; therefore, eliminate these options. Option 1 is also a general statement that is true for any stage of pregnancy. Review the importance of nutrition during pregnancy if you had difficulty with this question.

Reference
Wong, D., Hockenberry, M., Perry, S., Lowdermilk, D., & Wilson, D. (2006). *Maternal-child nursing care.* (3rd ed., pp. 326-327). St. Louis: Mosby.

248. A nurse is formulating a plan of care for a client receiving enteral feedings. The nurse identifies which nursing diagnosis as the highest priority for this client?
   1 Diarrhea
   2 Risk for aspiration
   3 Risk for deficient fluid volume
   4 Imbalanced nutrition, less than body requirements

Level of Cognitive Ability: Analysis
Client Needs: Physiological Integrity
Integrated Process: Nursing Process/Analysis
Content Area: Delegating/Prioritizing

Answer: 2
Rationale: Any condition in which gastrointestinal motility is slowed or esophageal reflux is possible places a client at risk for aspiration. Although options 1, 3, and 4 may be a concern, these are not the priority.

Test-Taking Strategy: Note the strategic words "highest priority." Use the ABCs—airway, breathing, and circulation. Option 2 addresses airway management. Options 1, 3, and 4 are possible problems, but not as high a priority as airway maintenance. Review care of the client receiving enteral feedings if you had difficulty with this question.

Reference
Ignatavicius, D., & Workman, M. (2006). *Medical-surgical nursing: Critical thinking for collaborative care* (5th ed., pp. 1430-1432). Philadelphia: Saunders.

---

249. A client is admitted to the hospital with a diagnosis of Cushing's syndrome. The nurse monitors the client for which of the following that is most likely to occur in this client?
   1 Hypovolemia
   2 Hypoglycemia
   3 Mood disturbances
   4 Deficient fluid volume

Level of Cognitive Ability: Application
Client Needs: Physiological Integrity
Integrated Process: Nursing Process/Assessment
Content Area: Adult Health/Endocrine

Answer: 3
Rationale: When Cushing's syndrome develops, the normal function of the glucocorticoids becomes exaggerated and the classic picture of the syndrome emerges. This exaggerated physiological action can cause mood disturbances, including memory loss, poor concentration and cognition, euphoria, and depression. It can also cause persistent hyperglycemia along with sodium and water retention, producing edema and hypertension.

Test-Taking Strategy: Use the process of elimination. Eliminate options 1 and 4 first because they are comparable or alike. Recalling that hyperglycemia rather than hypoglycemia occurs in this condition will direct you to option 3. Review the manifestations of Cushing's syndrome if you had difficulty with this question.

Reference
Ignatavicius, D., & Workman, M. (2006). *Medical-surgical nursing: Critical thinking for collaborative care* (5th ed., p. 1475). Philadelphia: Saunders.

---

250. A physician is performing indirect visualization of the larynx on a client to assess the function of the vocal cords. The nurse tells the client to do which of the following during the procedure?
   1 Try to swallow.
   2 Hold the breath.
   3 Breathe normally.
   4 Roll the tongue to the back of the mouth.

Answer: 3
Rationale: Indirect laryngoscopy is done to assess the function of the vocal cords or to obtain tissue for biopsy. Observations are made during rest and phonation by using a laryngeal mirror, head mirror, and light source. The client is placed in an upright position to facilitate passage of the laryngeal mirror into the mouth and is instructed to breathe normally. The tongue cannot be moved back because it would occlude the airway. Swallowing cannot be done with the mirror in place. The procedure takes longer than the time the client would be able to hold the breath, and this action is ineffective, anyway.

Level of Cognitive Ability: Application
Client Needs: Physiological Integrity
Integrated Process: Nursing Process/
  Implementation
Content Area: Adult Health/Respiratory

Test-Taking Strategy: Use the process of elimination. Option 4 is eliminated first because it is not possible to move the tongue back with the mirror in place. It would also cause the airway to become occluded. Given the length of time needed to do the procedure, the client could not realistically hold the breath, so option 2 is eliminated next. Trying to swallow would actually cause the larynx to move against the mirror and could cause gagging. Review care of the client during indirect laryngoscopy if you had difficulty with this question.

Reference
Ignatavicius, D., & Workman, M. (2006). *Medical-surgical nursing: Critical thinking for collaborative care* (5th ed., p. 574). Philadelphia: Saunders.

---

251. The nurse is caring for a client scheduled for a bilateral adrenalectomy for treatment of an adrenal tumor that is producing excessive aldosterone (primary hyperaldosteronism). The nurse appropriately tells the client which of the following?
  1 "You will need to wear an abdominal binder after surgery."
  2 "You will most likely need to undergo chemotherapy after surgery."
  3 "You will need to take hormone replacements for the rest of your life."
  4 "You will not require any special long-term treatment after surgery."

Level of Cognitive Ability: Application
Client Needs: Physiological Integrity
Integrated Process: Nursing Process/
  Implementation
Content Area: Adult Health/Endocrine

Answer: 3
Rationale: The major cause of primary hyperaldosteronism is an aldosterone-secreting tumor called an *aldosteronoma*. Surgery is the treatment of choice. Clients undergoing a bilateral adrenalectomy will need permanent replacement of adrenal hormones. Options 1, 2, and 4 are inaccurate.

Test-Taking Strategy: Note the strategic word "bilateral." Recalling the function of the adrenal glands and that glucocorticoids and mineralocorticoids are essential to sustain life will direct you to option 3. Review care following bilateral adrenalectomy if you had difficulty with this question.

Reference
Ignatavicius, D., & Workman, M. (2006). *Medical-surgical nursing: Critical thinking for collaborative care* (5th ed., p. 1476). Philadelphia: Saunders.

---

252. The nurse is caring for a client who is scheduled for an adrenalectomy. The nurse plans to administer which medication in the preoperative period to prevent Addison's crisis?
  1 Prednisone (Deltasone) orally
  2 Fludrocortisone (Florinef) subcutaneously
  3 Spironolactone (Aldactone) intramuscularly
  4 Methylprednisolone sodium succinate (Solu-Medrol) intravenously

Answer: 4
Rationale: A glucocorticoid preparation will be administered intravenously or intramuscularly in the immediate preoperative period to a client scheduled for an adrenalectomy. Methylprednisolone sodium succinate protects the client from developing acute adrenal insufficiency (Addison's crisis) that occurs as a result of the adrenalectomy. Aldactone is a potassium-sparing diuretic. Prednisone is an oral corticosteroid. Fludrocortisone is a mineralocorticoid.

Test-Taking Strategy: Focus on the subject, preventing Addison's crisis in a client scheduled for adrenalectomy. Recalling the function of the adrenals will assist in eliminating options 2 and 3. From the remaining options, select option 4 because the client is preoperative and should receive medications via routes other than orally. Review preoperative care for the client scheduled for adrenalectomy if you had difficulty with this question.

Level of Cognitive Ability: Analysis
Client Needs: Physiological Integrity
Integrated Process: Nursing Process/Planning
Content Area: Adult Health/Endocrine

Reference
Ignatavicius, D., & Workman, M. (2006). *Medical-surgical nursing: Critical thinking for collaborative care* (5th ed., p. 1476). Philadelphia: Saunders.

---

253. The nurse is preparing a client with Graves' disease to receive radioactive iodine therapy. The nurse tells the client which of the following about the therapy?

1 Following the initial dose, subsequent treatments must continue lifelong.

2 The radioactive iodine is designed to destroy the entire thyroid gland with just one dose.

3 It takes 6 to 8 weeks after treatment to experience relief from the symptoms of the disease.

4 The high levels of radioactivity prohibit contact with family for 4 weeks after initial treatment.

Level of Cognitive Ability: Application
Client Needs: Physiological Integrity
Integrated Process: Nursing Process/ Implementation
Content Area: Adult Health/Endocrine

Answer: 3
Rationale: Following treatment with radioactive iodine therapy, a decrease in thyroid hormone level should be noted, which would help alleviate symptoms. Relief of symptoms does not occur until 6 to 8 weeks after initial treatment. This form of therapy is not designed to destroy the entire gland; rather, some of the cells that synthesize thyroid hormone will be destroyed by the local radiation. The nurse needs to reassure the client and family that unless the dosage is extremely high, clients are not required to observe radiation precautions. The rationale for this is that the radioactivity quickly dissipates. Occasionally, a client may require a second or third dose, but treatments are not lifelong.

Test-Taking Strategy: Use the process of elimination and knowledge regarding this treatment. Note the close-ended words "entire," "prohibit," and "must" in the incorrect options. Review this treatment if you had difficulty with this question.

Reference
Ignatavicius, D., & Workman, M. (2006). *Medical-surgical nursing: Critical thinking for collaborative care* (5th ed., pp. 1486-1487). Philadelphia: Saunders.

---

254. A client arrives at the emergency department with upper gastrointestinal (GI) bleeding and is in moderate distress. The priority nursing action is to:

1 Obtain vital signs.

2 Complete an abdominal physical assessment.

3 Ask the client about the precipitating events.

4 Insert a nasogastric (NG) tube and Hematest the emesis.

Level of Cognitive Ability: Application
Client Needs: Physiological Integrity
Integrated Process: Nursing Process/ Implementation
Content Area: Delegating/Prioritizing

Answer: 1
Rationale: The priority action is to obtain vital signs to determine whether the client is in shock from blood loss and to obtain a baseline by which to monitor the progress of treatment. The client may not be able to provide subjective data until the immediate physical needs are met. Insertion of an NG tube may be prescribed but is not the priority action. A complete abdominal physical assessment needs to be performed but is not the priority.

Test-Taking Strategy: Use the process of elimination, noting the strategic word "priority." Recall that the client with a GI bleed is at risk for shock. Also, option 1 addresses the ABCs—airway, breathing, and circulation. Review care of the client with a GI bleed if you had difficulty with this question.

Reference
Black, J., & Hawks, J. (2005). *Medical-surgical nursing: Clinical management for positive outcomes* (7th ed., pp. 208, 744). Philadelphia: Saunders.

255. A client with acute renal failure is ordered to be on a fluid restriction of 1500 mL per day. The nurse best plans to assist the client with maintaining the restriction by:
1 Removing the water pitcher from the bedside
2 Using mouthwash with alcohol for mouth care
3 Prohibiting beverages with sugar to minimize thirst
4 Asking the client to calculate the IV fluids into the total daily allotment

Level of Cognitive Ability: Application
Client Needs: Physiological Integrity
Integrated Process: Nursing Process/
  Implementation
Content Area: Adult Health/Renal

Answer: 1
Rationale: The nurse can help the client maintain fluid restriction through a variety of means. One way is to provide frequent mouth care; however, alcohol-based products should be avoided because they are drying to mucous membranes. The use of ice chips and lip ointments is another intervention that may be helpful to the client on fluid restriction. Beverages that the client enjoys are provided and are not restricted based on sugar content. The client is not asked to keep track of IV fluid intake; this is the nurse's responsibility. The water pitcher should be removed from the bedside to aid in compliance.

Test-Taking Strategy: Use the process of elimination. Eliminate option 4 because this is a nursing responsibility. Eliminate option 2 next, because alcohol-based products are drying to oral mucous membranes and could exacerbate thirst. From the remaining options, focus on the strategic word "best" to direct you to option 1. Review measures to promote compliance with fluid restrictions if you had difficulty with this question.

References

Black, J., & Hawks, J. (2005). *Medical-surgical nursing: Clinical management for positive outcomes* (7th ed., pp. 216-217). Philadelphia: Saunders.
Ignatavicius, D., & Workman, M. (2006). *Medical-surgical nursing: Critical thinking for collaborative care* (5th ed., p. 1748). Philadelphia: Saunders.
Potter, P., & Perry, A. (2005). *Fundamentals of nursing* (6th ed., p. 1159). St. Louis: Mosby.

256. A nurse has administered approximately half of a high cleansing enema when the client complains of pain and cramping. Which nursing action is appropriate?
1 Reassuring the client and continuing the flow
2 Discontinuing the enema and notifying the physician
3 Raising the enema bag so that the solution can be completed quickly
4 Clamping the tubing for 30 seconds and restarting the flow at a slower rate

Level of Cognitive Ability: Application
Client Needs: Physiological Integrity
Integrated Process: Nursing Process/
  Implementation
Content Area: Fundamental Skills

Answer: 4
Rationale: The enema fluid should be administered slowly. If the client complains of pain or cramping, the flow is stopped for 30 seconds and restarted at a slower rate. Slow enema administration and stopping the flow temporarily, if necessary, will decrease the likelihood of intestinal spasm and premature ejection of the solution. The higher the solution container is held above the rectum, the faster the flow and the greater the force in the rectum. There is no need to discontinue the enema and notify the physician at this time.

Test-Taking Strategy: Use the process of elimination, focusing on the subject: alleviating pain and cramping. Eliminate options 1 and 3 first because they are comparable or alike. From the remaining options, noting that there is no need to notify the physician will direct you to option 4. Review the procedure for enema administration if you had difficulty with this question.

Reference

Potter, P., & Perry, A. (2005). *Fundamentals of nursing* (6th ed., pp. 1400-1401). St. Louis: Mosby.

257. The client with chronic renal failure who is scheduled for hemodialysis this morning is due to receive a daily dose of enalapril (Vasotec). The nurse plans to administer this medication:
1 During dialysis
2 Just before dialysis
3 The day after dialysis
4 Upon return from dialysis

Level of Cognitive Ability: Application
Client Needs: Physiological Integrity
Integrated Process: Nursing Process/Planning
Content Area: Pharmacology

Answer: 4
Rationale: Antihypertensive medications, such as enalapril, are administered to the client following hemodialysis. This prevents the client from becoming hypotensive during dialysis and also from having the medication removed from the bloodstream by dialysis. There is no rationale for waiting a full day to resume the medication. This would lead to ineffective control of the blood pressure.

Test-Taking Strategy: Use the process of elimination. Think about the effects of an antihypertensive medication on the blood pressure when fluid is being removed from the body. Because hypotension is much more likely to occur in this circumstance, eliminate options 1 and 2. Most clients are hemodialyzed three times a week, so if the medication were held for dialysis until the following day, the client would miss three of the seven doses that would usually be given in a week. This would lead to ineffective blood pressure control. Therefore, eliminate option 3. Review the procedure for preparing a client for dialysis if you had difficulty with this question.

References
Black, J., & Hawks, J. (2005). *Medical-surgical nursing: Clinical management for positive outcomes* (7th ed., p. 961). Philadelphia: Saunders.
Hodgson, B., & Kizior, R. (2007). *Saunders nursing drug handbook 2007* (pp. 408-409). Philadelphia: Saunders.

258. Which client position does the nurse use to administer a cleansing enema?
1 Dorsal recumbent position
2 Supine position with the legs elevated
3 Left lateral position with flexed right knee
4 Right lateral position with flexed left knee

Level of Cognitive Ability: Application
Client Needs: Physiological Integrity
Integrated Process: Nursing Process/ Implementation
Content Area: Fundamental Skills

Answer: 3
Rationale: The sigmoid and descending colon are located on the left side. Therefore, the left lateral position uses gravity to facilitate the flow of solution into the sigmoid and descending colon. Acute flexion of the right leg allows for adequate exposure of the anus. Options 1, 2, and 4 are incorrect positions because they fail to adequately expose the anus or facilitate infusion of the enema solution.

Test-Taking Strategy: Use the process of elimination. Visualize this procedure and think about the anatomy of the colon to direct you to option 3. Review this procedure if you had difficulty with this question.

Reference
Potter, P., & Perry, A. (2005). *Fundamentals of nursing* (6th ed., p. 1399). St. Louis: Mosby.

259. The nurse is preparing to care for a client returning from the operating room following a subtotal thyroidectomy. The nurse anticipates the need for which of the following items to be placed at the bedside?
1 Hypothermia blanket
2 Emergency tracheostomy kit
3 Magnesium sulfate in a ready-to-inject vial
4 Ampule of saturated solution of potassium iodide (SSKI)

Level of Cognitive Ability: Application
Client Needs: Physiological Integrity
Integrated Process: Nursing Process/Planning
Content Area: Adult Health/Endocrine

Answer: 2
Rationale: Respiratory distress can occur following thyroidectomy as a result of swelling in the tracheal area. The nurse would ensure that an emergency tracheostomy kit is available. Surgery on the thyroid does not alter the heat control mechanism of the body. Magnesium sulfate would not be indicated because the incidence of hypomagnesemia is not a common problem post-thyroidectomy. SSKI is typically administered preoperatively to block thyroid hormone synthesis and release, as well as to place the client in a euthyroid state.

Test-Taking Strategy: Recall the anatomical location of the thyroid gland to direct you to option 2. Also, use the ABCs—airway, breathing, and circulation. Maintaining a patent airway is critical. Review care of the client following thyroidectomy if you had difficulty with this question.

Reference
Ignatavicius, D., & Workman, M. (2006). *Medical-surgical nursing: Critical thinking for collaborative care* (5th ed., p. 1487). Philadelphia: Saunders.

260. Sodium nitroprusside is prescribed for a client with a diagnosis of cardiogenic shock. The nurse plans to do which of the following when preparing to administer this medication?
1 Protect the solution from light.
2 Add potassium to the infusion bag.
3 Obtain a baseline thiocyanate level.
4 Administer only through a central venous line.

Level of Cognitive Ability: Application
Client Needs: Physiological Integrity
Integrated Process: Nursing Process/Planning
Content Area: Pharmacology

Answer: 1
Rationale: Sodium nitroprusside becomes unstable when exposed to light and must be protected. No other medications are added to the infusion bag. It can be given through a peripheral line. The level of thiocyanate (a nitroprusside metabolite similar to cyanide) is usually drawn if the client is maintained on this therapy for several days.

Test-Taking Strategy: Use the process of elimination and knowledge of the principles related to administering IV medications. Options 2 and 4 can be eliminated even without knowledge of this medication using these basic principles. Usually, levels of any medication or its by-products are drawn after administration has been ongoing, so eliminate option 3. Review this medication if you had difficulty with this question.

Reference
Skidmore-Roth, L. (2008). *Mosby's nursing drug reference* (21st ed., p. 744). St. Louis: Mosby.

261. The nurse is encouraging the client to cough and deep breathe after cardiac surgery. The nurse ensures that which of the following items is available to maximize the effectiveness of this procedure?
1 Nebulizer
2 Ambu bag
3 Suction equipment
4 Incisional splinting pillow

Answer: 4
Rationale: The use of an incisional splint such as a "cough pillow" can ease discomfort during coughing and deep breathing. The client who is comfortable will do more effective deep breathing and coughing exercises. Use of an incentive spirometer is also indicated. Options 1, 2, and 3 will not encourage the client to cough and deep breathe.

Level of Cognitive Ability: Application
Client Needs: Physiological Integrity
Integrated Process: Nursing Process/
    Implementation
Content Area: Adult Health/Respiratory

Test-Taking Strategy: Use the process of elimination. Focus on the subject, an item that will maximize effectiveness. This subject eliminates options 2 and 3, which are items used by the nurse. A nebulizer (option 1) is used to deliver medication. Review measures that will assist the postoperative client to cough and deep breathe if you had difficulty with this question.

References
Monahan, F., Sands, J., Neighbors, M., Marek, J., & Green, C. (2007). *Phipps' medical-surgical nursing: Health and illness perspectives* (8th ed., pp. 255-256). St. Louis: Mosby.
Potter, P., & Perry, A. (2005). *Fundamentals of nursing* (6th ed., p. 1616). St. Louis: Mosby.

---

262. A nurse is preparing to administer an intermittent tube feeding through a nasogastric (NG) tube. The nurse assesses gastric residual volume before administering the tube feeding to:
  1 Confirm proper NG tube placement.
  2 Determine the client's nutritional status.
  3 Assess client's fluid and electrolyte status.
  4 Evaluate the adequacy of gastric emptying.

Level of Cognitive Ability: Comprehension
Client Needs: Physiological Integrity
Integrated Process: Nursing Process/Assessment
Content Area: Fundamental Skills

Answer: 4
Rationale: All stomach contents are aspirated and measured before administering a tube feeding to determine the gastric residual volume. If the stomach fails to empty and propel its contents forward, the tube feeding accumulates in the stomach and increases the client's risk of aspiration. If the aspirated gastric contents exceed the predetermined limit, the nurse withholds the tube feeding and collaborates with the provider on a plan of care. Assessing residual does not confirm placement or assess fluid and electrolyte status. The nurse uses clinical indicators including serum albumin levels to determine the client's nutritional status.

Test-Taking Strategy: Focus on the subject, the purpose for assessing the residual. Note the relationship between the subject and option 4. Review the purpose of assessing residual if you had difficulty with this question.

Reference
Ignatavicius, D., & Workman, M. (2006). *Medical-surgical nursing: Critical thinking for collaborative care* (5th ed., pp. 1430-1431). Philadelphia: Saunders.

---

263. The nurse is caring for a client scheduled to undergo a renal biopsy. To minimize the risk of postprocedure complications, the nurse reports which of the following laboratory results to the physician before the procedure?
  1 Potassium: 3.8 mEq/L
  2 Serum creatinine: 1.2 mg/dL
  3 Prothrombin time: 15 seconds
  4 Blood urea nitrogen (BUN): 18 mg/dL

Answer: 3
Rationale: Postprocedure hemorrhage is a complication after renal biopsy. Because of this, prothrombin time is assessed before the procedure. The normal prothrombin time range is 11 to 12.5 seconds. The nurse ensures that these results are available and reports abnormalities promptly. Options 1, 2, and 4 identify normal values. The normal BUN is 5 to 20 mg/dL, the normal serum creatinine is 0.6 to 1.3 mg/dL, and the normal potassium is 3.5 to 5.1 mEq/L.

Test-Taking Strategy: When a client is to have a biopsy, remember that bleeding is a concern. This will direct you to option 3. Also note that options 1, 2, and 4 identify normal values. Review the complications of renal biopsy and normal laboratory values if you had difficulty with this question.

Level of Cognitive Ability: Analysis
Client Needs: Physiological Integrity
Integrated Process: Nursing Process/
   Implementation
Content Area: Adult Health/Renal

References
Chernecky, C., & Berger, B. (2008). *Laboratory tests and diagnostic procedures* (5th ed., pp. 690-691). Philadelphia: Saunders.
Pagana, K., & Pagana, T. (2005). *Mosby's diagnostic and laboratory test reference* (7th ed., p. 794). St. Louis: Mosby.

264. A client involved in a house fire is experiencing respiratory distress, and an inhalation injury is suspected. The nurse monitors which of the following for the presence of carbon monoxide poisoning?
   1 Pulse oximetry
   2 Urine myoglobin
   3 Sputum carbon levels
   4 Serum carboxyhemoglobin levels

Level of Cognitive Ability: Application
Client Needs: Physiological Integrity
Integrated Process: Nursing Process/Assessment
Content Area: Adult Health/Respiratory

Answer: 4
Rationale: Serum carboxyhemoglobin levels are the most direct measure of carbon monoxide poisoning, provide the level of poisoning, and thus determine the appropriate treatment measures. The carbon monoxide molecule has a 200 times greater affinity for binding with hemoglobin than an oxygen molecule, causing decreased availability of oxygen to the cells. Clients are treated with 100% oxygen. Options 1, 2, and 3 would not identify carbon monoxide poisoning.

Test-Taking Strategy: Use the process of elimination. Note the relationship between "carbon monoxide" and option 4. Review carbon monoxide poisoning if you had difficulty with this question.

References
Black, J., & Hawks, J. (2005). *Medical-surgical nursing: Clinical management for positive outcomes* (7th ed., p. 1906). Philadelphia: Saunders.
Chernecky, C., & Berger, B. (2008). *Laboratory tests and diagnostic procedures* (5th ed., pp. 292-293). Philadelphia: Saunders.

265. A nurse is assigned to care for a client with hypertonic labor contractions. The nurse plans to conserve the client's energy and promote rest by:
   1 Assisting the client with breathing and relaxation techniques
   2 Keeping the television (TV) or radio on to provide distraction
   3 Keeping the room brightly lit so the client can watch her monitor
   4 Avoiding uncomfortable procedures such as intravenous infusions or epidural anesthesia

Level of Cognitive Ability: Application
Client Needs: Physiological Integrity
Integrated Process: Nursing Process/Planning
Content Area: Maternity/Antepartum

Answer: 1
Rationale: Breathing and relaxation techniques aid the client in coping with the discomfort of labor and in conserving energy. Intravenous or epidural pain relief can be useful. Intravenous hydration can increase perfusion and oxygenation of maternal and fetal tissues and provide glucose for energy needs. Noise from a TV or radio and light stimulation does not promote rest. A quiet, dim environment would be more advantageous.

Test-Taking Strategy: Focus on the subject, conserving energy and promoting rest for the client. Noting the strategic word "assisting" in option 1 will direct you to this option. Review care of the client with hypertonic labor contractions if you had difficulty with this question.

Reference
Wong, D., Hockenberry, M., Perry, S., Lowdermilk, D., & Wilson, D. (2006). *Maternal-child nursing care.* (3rd ed., pp. 556-557). St. Louis: Mosby.

266. A client with acute pyelonephritis has nausea and is vomiting and is scheduled for an intravenous pyelogram. The nurse places highest priority on which action?

1 Ask the client to sign the informed consent.
2 Explain the procedure thoroughly to the client.
3 Place the client on hourly intake and output measurements.
4 Request an order for an intravenous infusion from the physician.

Level of Cognitive Ability: Application
Client Needs: Physiological Integrity
Integrated Process: Nursing Process/ Implementation
Content Area: Adult Health/Renal

Answer: 4
Rationale: The highest priority of the nurse would be to request an order for an intravenous infusion. This is needed to replace fluid lost with vomiting, will be necessary for dye injection for the procedure, and will assist with the elimination of the dye following the procedure. The intake and output should be measured, but this will not assist in preventing dehydration. Explanation of the procedure and obtaining the signed informed consent are done once the client's physiological needs are met.

Test-Taking Strategy: Using Maslow's Hierarchy of Needs theory will assist in eliminating options 1 and 2. From the remaining options, noting that the client is vomiting will direct you to option 4. Review care of the client who is vomiting if you had difficulty with this question.

References
Chernecky, C., & Berger, B. (2008). *Laboratory tests and diagnostic procedures* (5th ed., p. 682). Philadelphia: Saunders.
Ignatavicius, D., & Workman, M. (2006). *Medical-surgical nursing: Critical thinking for collaborative care* (5th ed., pp. 1713-1714). Philadelphia: Saunders.
Lewis, S., Heitkemper, M., Dirksen, S., O'Brien, P., & Bucher, L. (2007). *Medical-surgical nursing: Assessment and management of clinical problems* (7th ed., p. 1164). St. Louis: Mosby.

267. The nurse is planning care for a client with a T3 spinal cord injury. The nurse includes which intervention in the plan to prevent autonomic hyperreflexia?

1 Administer dexamethasone (Decadron) as per physician's order.
2 Assess vital signs and observe for hypotension, tachycardia, and tachypnea.
3 Teach the client that this condition is relatively minor with few symptoms.
4 Assist the client to develop a daily bowel routine to prevent constipation.

Level of Cognitive Ability: Application
Client Needs: Physiological Integrity
Integrated Process: Nursing Process/Planning
Content Area: Adult Health/Neurological

Answer: 4
Rationale: Autonomic hyperreflexia is a potentially life-threatening condition and may be triggered by bladder distention, bowel distention, visceral distention, or stimulation of pain receptors in the skin. A daily bowel program eliminates this trigger. A client with autonomic hyperreflexia would be hypertensive and bradycardic. Removal of the stimuli results in prompt resolution of the signs and symptoms. Option 1 is unrelated to this specific condition.

Test-Taking Strategy: Focus on the strategic word "prevent" to eliminate options 2 and 3. From the remaining options, remembering that this condition may be triggered by bowel distention will direct you to option 4. Review the causes of autonomic hyperreflexia if you are unfamiliar with this syndrome.

References
Black, J., & Hawks, J. (2005). *Medical-surgical nursing: Clinical management for positive outcomes* (7th ed., p. 904). Philadelphia: Saunders.
Ignatavicius, D., & Workman, M. (2006). *Medical-surgical nursing: Critical thinking for collaborative care* (5th ed., pp. 987-988). Philadelphia: Saunders.

268. A client in cardiogenic shock has an order for an intravenous (IV) nitroglycerin (Nitrostat) drip for control of chest pain and to increase myocardial tissue perfusion. The nurse understands that the nitroglycerin must be prepared by mixing the medication:

1 Under a laminar flow hood
2 In a solution that is in a plastic bag
3 In a solution that is in a glass bottle
4 Every hour because of its unstable chemical structure

Level of Cognitive Ability: Analysis
Client Needs: Physiological Integrity
Integrated Process: Nursing Process/ Implementation
Content Area: Pharmacology

Answer: 3
Rationale: IV nitroglycerin is prepared only in glass bottles, using the administration sets provided. Standard plastic (polyvinyl chloride) tubing will absorb the nitroglycerin, thus reducing the potency and reliability of the medication. It should also be protected from extremes of light and temperature. It should be remixed every 4 hours. It does not require mixture under a laminar flow hood.

Test-Taking Strategy: Use the process of elimination. Eliminate option 4 because "every hour" is much too frequent. From the remaining options, note that options 2 and 3 provide opposite methods of administration. This should provide a clue that one of these methods may be accurate. Remember that standard plastic will absorb the nitroglycerin. Review the procedure for preparing IV nitroglycerin if you had difficulty with this question.

Reference
Gahart, B., & Nazareno, A. (2006). *2006 Intravenous medications* (22nd ed., p. 898). St. Louis: Mosby.

269. A client has a left pleural effusion that has not yet been treated. The nurse plans to have which of the following items available for immediate use?

1 Intubation tray
2 Paracentesis tray
3 Thoracentesis tray
4 Central venous line insertion tray

Level of Cognitive Ability: Application
Client Needs: Physiological Integrity
Integrated Process: Nursing Process/Planning
Content Area: Adult Health/Respiratory

Answer: 3
Rationale: The client with a significant pleural effusion is usually treated by thoracentesis. This procedure allows drainage of the fluid, which may then be analyzed to determine the precise cause of the effusion. The nurse ensures that a thoracentesis tray is readily available in case the client's symptoms should rapidly become more severe. A paracentesis tray is needed for the removal of abdominal effusion. Options 1 and 4 are not specifically indicated for this procedure.

Test-Taking Strategy: Use the process of elimination and knowledge regarding the usual treatment for pleural effusion. Note the relationship between the word "pleural" in the question and "thoracentesis" in the correct option. Review the treatment for pleural effusion if you had difficulty with this question.

Reference
Black, J., & Hawks, J. (2005). *Medical-surgical nursing: Clinical management for positive outcomes* (7th ed., p. 1873). Philadelphia: Saunders.

270. A client has been taking procainamide. The nurse knows the priority intervention before administering the medication is to:

1 Check the blood pressure and pulse.
2 Administer the medication as ordered.
3 Obtain a complete blood cell count and liver function studies.
4 Schedule the client for a drug level to be drawn 1 hour after the dose.

Answer: 1
Rationale: Procainamide is an antidysrhythmic medication. Before the medication is administered, the client's blood pressure and pulse are checked. This medication can cause toxic effects, and serum blood levels would be checked before administering the medication (therapeutic serum level is 3 to 10 mcg/mL). Obtaining a complete blood cell count and liver function studies is unnecessary.

Level of Cognitive Ability: Application
Client Needs: Physiological Integrity
Integrated Process: Nursing Process/
  Implementation
Content Area: Pharmacology

Test-Taking Strategy: Use the steps of the nursing process. This will direct you to option 1 because it is the only assessment action. Also recalling that this medication is an antidysrhythmic will direct you to the correct option. Review this medication if you had difficulty with this question.

Reference
Hodgson, B., & Kizior, R. (2007). *Saunders nursing drug handbook 2007* (pp. 965-966). Philadelphia: Saunders.

---

271. A client with urolithiasis is being evaluated to determine the type of stone that is being formed. The nurse plans to keep which of the following items available in the client's room to assist in this process?
1 A strainer
2 A calorie count sheet
3 A vital signs graphic sheet
4 An intake and output record

Level of Cognitive Ability: Application
Client Needs: Physiological Integrity
Integrated Process: Nursing Process/Planning
Content Area: Adult Health/Renal

Answer: 1
Rationale: The urine is strained until the stone is passed and obtained and analyzed. Straining the urine will catch small stones that may be sent to the laboratory for analysis. Once the type of stone is determined, an individualized plan of care for prevention and treatment is developed. Options 2, 3, and 4 are unrelated to the question.

Test-Taking Strategy: Focus on the subject, an item that will help determine the type of stone. Eliminate options 2, 3, and 4 because these items give information about food intake, vital signs, and fluid balance, but will not provide data that will help determine the type of stone. Review care of the client with urolithiasis if you had difficulty with this question.

Reference
Black, J., & Hawks, J. (2005). *Medical-surgical nursing: Clinical management for positive outcomes* (7th ed., p. 887). Philadelphia: Saunders.

---

272. A client develops bilateral wheezes, crackles from bases to apices, orthopnea, and tachypnea, and the nurse notes the presence of +2 pitting edema. The nurse suspects pulmonary edema and notifies the physician. While awaiting the physician's arrival, the nurse avoids which action?
1 Elevating the client's legs
2 Preparing to administer IV morphine sulfate
3 Preparing to administer IV furosemide (Lasix)
4 Placing the client in the high Fowler's position

Level of Cognitive Ability: Application
Client Needs: Physiological Integrity
Integrated Process: Nursing Process/
  Implementation
Content Area: Adult Health/Cardiovascular

Answer: 1
Rationale: Elevating the client's legs would rapidly increase venous return to the right side of the heart and worsen the client's condition. The feet should be in the horizontal position, or the client could dangle at the bedside if the client's condition permits. Anxiety causes an increase in the oxygen demands on the heart. Morphine sulfate reduces anxiety and causes peripheral vasodilation and is likely to be prescribed. Furosemide will be prescribed because of its diuretic action. A high Fowler's position increases the thoracic capacity, allowing for improved ventilation.

Test-Taking Strategy: Use the process of elimination and note the strategic word "avoids." This word indicates a negative event query and the need to select the option that is an incorrect nursing action. Recalling that the pulmonary system is congested will direct you to option 1 because this action would cause further congestion of the pulmonary system. Review care of the client with pulmonary edema if you had difficulty with this question.

Reference
Black, J., & Hawks, J. (2005). *Medical-surgical nursing: Clinical management for positive outcomes* (7th ed., p. 1880). Philadelphia: Saunders.

273. The nurse is preparing to care for a client following ureterolithotomy who has a ureteral catheter in place. The nurse plans to implement which action in the management of this catheter when the client arrives from the recovery room?
1 Clamps the catheter
2 Places tension on the catheter
3 Checks the drainage from the catheter
4 Irrigates the catheter using 10 mL sterile normal saline

Level of Cognitive Ability: Application
Client Needs: Physiological Integrity
Integrated Process: Nursing Process/
Implementation
Content Area: Adult Health/Renal

Answer: 3
Rationale: Drainage from the ureteral catheter should be checked when the client returns from the recovery room and at least every 1 to 2 hours thereafter. The catheter drains urine from the renal pelvis, which has a capacity of 3 to 5 mL. If the volume of urine or fluid in the renal pelvis increases, tissue damage to the pelvis will result from pressure. Therefore, the ureteral tube is never clamped. Additionally, irrigation is not performed unless there is a specific physician's order to do so.

Test-Taking Strategy: Focus on the subject, a ureteral catheter, and think about the anatomy of the kidney. Recalling that the ureteral catheter is placed in the renal pelvis and recalling the anatomy of this anatomical location will assist in eliminating options 1, 2, and 4. Review care of the client with a ureteral catheter if you had difficulty with this question.

Reference
Black, J., & Hawks, J. (2005). *Medical-surgical nursing: Clinical management for positive outcomes* (7th ed., p. 889). Philadelphia: Saunders.

274. Before administering an intermittent tube feeding, the nurse aspirates 40 mL of undigested formula from the client's nasogastric tube. Which should the nurse implement as a result of this finding?
1 Discard the aspirate and record as client output.
2 Mix with new formula to administer the feeding.
3 Dilute with water and inject into the nasogastric tube.
4 Reinstill the aspirate through the nasogastric tube via gravity using a syringe.

Level of Cognitive Ability: Application
Client Needs: Physiological Integrity
Integrated Process: Nursing Process/
Implementation
Content Area: Fundamental Skills

Answer: 4
Rationale: After checking residual feeding contents, the nurse reinstills the gastric contents into the stomach by removing the syringe bulb or plunger and pouring the gastric contents via the syringe into the nasogastric tube. Gastric contents should be reinstilled (unless they exceed an amount of 100 mL or as defined by agency policy) in order to maintain the client's fluid and electrolyte balance. The nurse avoids mixing gastric aspirate with fresh formula to prevent contamination. Because the gastric aspirate is a small volume, it should be reinstilled; however, mixing the formula with water can, also, disrupt the client's fluid and electrolyte balance unless the nurse determines that the client is dehydrated.

Test-Taking Strategy: Use the process of elimination. Eliminate option 1 because it increases the risk of dehydration. Remembering that the removal of the gastric contents can disturb the client's fluid and electrolyte balance will assist in eliminating options 2 and 3. Also, recalling that aspirated gastric contents are not mixed with formula will assist in directing you to the correct option. Review this procedure if you had difficulty with this question.

References
Black, J., & Hawks, J. (2005). *Medical-surgical nursing: Clinical management for positive outcomes* (7th ed., p. 746). Philadelphia: Saunders.
Monahan, F., Sands, J., Neighbors, M., Marek, J., & Green, C. (2007). *Phipps' medical-surgical nursing: Health and illness perspectives* (8th ed., p. 1233). St. Louis: Mosby.

275. In order to increase medication effectiveness, the nurse should instruct the client taking oral bisacodyl (Dulcolax) to take the medication:
1 At bedtime
2 With a large meal
3 With a glass of milk
4 On an empty stomach

Level of Cognitive Ability: Application
Client Needs: Physiological Integrity
Integrated Process: Teaching and Learning
Content Area: Pharmacology

Answer: 4
Rationale: The most rapid effect from bisacodyl occurs when it is taken on an empty stomach. It will not have a rapid effect if taken with a large meal. If it is taken at bedtime, the client will have a bowel movement in the morning. Taking the medication with a glass of milk will not speed up its effect.

Test-Taking Strategy: Focus on the subject, achieving a rapid effect. Recalling that medications generally are more effective if taken on an empty stomach will direct you to option 4. Review the concepts related to administering this medication if you had difficulty with this question.

Reference
Hodgson, B., & Kizior, R. (2007). *Saunders nursing drug handbook 2007* (p. 140). Philadelphia: Saunders.

---

276. A client with acute respiratory distress syndrome has an order to be placed on a continuous positive airway pressure (CPAP) face mask. The nurse implements which of the following for this procedure to be most effective?
1 Obtains baseline arterial blood gases
2 Obtains baseline pulse oximetry levels
3 Applies the mask to the face with a snug fit
4 Encourages the client to remove the mask frequently for coughing and deep breathing exercises

Level of Cognitive Ability: Application
Client Needs: Physiological Integrity
Integrated Process: Nursing Process/ Implementation
Content Area: Adult Health/Respiratory

Answer: 3
Rationale: The face mask must be applied over the nose and mouth with a snug fit, which is necessary to maintain positive pressure in the client's airways. The nurse obtains baseline respiratory assessments and arterial blood gases to evaluate the effectiveness of therapy, but these are not done to increase the effectiveness of the procedure. A disadvantage of the CPAP face mask is that the client must remove it for coughing, eating, or drinking. This removes the benefit of positive pressure in the airway each time it is removed.

Test-Taking Strategy: Focus on the subject, a nursing action that will make the procedure most effective. Options 1 and 2 do not make the therapy more effective and are eliminated. From the remaining options, knowing that positive pressure must be maintained to be effective will direct you to option 3. Review care of the client with a CPAP face mask if you had difficulty with this question.

Reference
Perry, A., & Potter, P. (2006). *Clinical nursing skills & techniques* (6th ed., p. 779). St. Louis: Mosby.

---

277. The nurse is caring for a client scheduled to undergo a cardiac catheterization for the first time. The nurse tells the client that the:
1 Procedure is performed in the operating room.
2 Initial catheter insertion is quite painful; after that, there is little or no pain.
3 Client may feel fatigue and have various aches, because it is necessary to lie quietly on a hard X-ray table for about 4 hours.
4 Client may feel certain sensations at various points during the procedure, such as a fluttery feeling, flushed warm feeling, desire to cough, or palpitations.

Answer: 4
Rationale: Preprocedure teaching points include that the procedure is done in a darkened cardiac catheterization room and that ECG leads are attached to the client. A local anesthetic is used so there is little to no pain with catheter insertion. The X-ray table is hard and may be tilted periodically. The procedure may take up to 2 hours, and the client may feel various sensations with catheter passage and dye injection.

Test-Taking Strategy: Use the process of elimination. The location (operating room) elimenates option 1. The duration of the procedure, 4 hours, eliminates option 3. From the remaining options, noting the words "quite painful" in option 2 will assist in eliminating this option. Review client preparation for this procedure if you had difficulty with this question.

Level of Cognitive Ability: Application
Client Needs: Physiological Integrity
Integrated Process: Nursing Process/
   Implementation
Content Area: Adult Health/Cardiovascular

Reference
Ignatavicius, D., & Workman, M. (2006). *Medical-surgical nursing: Critical thinking for collaborative care* (5th ed., pp. 697-698). Philadelphia: Saunders.

---

278. A client with acquired immunodeficiency syndrome (AIDS) will be receiving aerosolized pentamidine isethionate (NebuPent) prophylactically once every 4 weeks. The home health nurse visits and instructs the client about the medication. Which statement by the client indicates a need for further teaching?

1 "There are no known side effects of this therapy."
2 "I may experience some nausea with the inhalation therapy."
3 "If I have any visual disturbances, I need to let the doctor know."
4 "If I develop a cough or shortness of breath after receiving the inhalation therapy, I need to let a doctor or nurse know."

Level of Cognitive Ability: Analysis
Client Needs: Physiological Integrity
Integrated Process: Teaching and Learning
Content Area: Adult Health/Immune

Answer: 1

Rationale: Side effects associated with this aerosolized therapy include nausea, visual disturbances, and shortness of breath. The client needs to inform the health care provider if these side effects occur.

Test-Taking Strategy: Note the strategic words "indicates a need for further teaching." These words indicate a negative event query and the need to select an option that is an incorrect client statement. Noting the words "no known side effects" in option 1 will direct you to this option. Review this medication if you had difficulty with this question.

Reference
Hodgson, B., & Kizior, R. (2007). *Saunders nursing drug handbook 2007* (p. 915). Philadelphia: Saunders.

---

279. A nurse admits a client with myocardial infarction (MI) to the coronary care unit (CCU). The nurse plans to do which of the following in delivering care to this client?

1 Begin thrombolytic therapy.
2 Place the client on continuous cardiac monitoring.
3 Infuse intravenous (IV) fluid at a rate of 150 mL per hour.
4 Administer oxygen at a rate of 6 liters per minute by nasal cannula.

Level of Cognitive Ability: Application
Client Needs: Physiological Integrity
Integrated Process: Nursing Process/Planning
Content Area: Adult Health/Cardiovascular

Answer: 2

Rationale: Standard interventions upon admittance to the CCU as they relate to this question include continuous cardiac monitoring, administering oxygen at a rate of 2 to 4 liters per minute unless otherwise ordered, and ensuring an adequate IV line insertion of an intermittent lock. If an IV infusion is administered, it is maintained at a keep vein open rate to prevent fluid overload and heart failure. Thrombolytic therapy may or may not be prescribed by the physician. Thrombolytic agents are most effective if administered within the first 6 hours of the coronary event.

Test-Taking Strategy: Use the process of elimination. Eliminate options 3 and 4 because the values related to the rates of oxygen and IV fluid are high. From the remaining options, note the relationship between the client's diagnosis and option 2. Review care of the client following MI if you had difficulty with this question.

References
Black, J., & Hawks, J. (2005). *Medical-surgical nursing: Clinical management for positive outcomes* (7th ed., p. 1720). Philadelphia: Saunders.
Ignatavicius, D., & Workman, M. (2006). *Medical-surgical nursing: Critical thinking for collaborative care* (5th ed., pp. 845-846). Philadelphia: Saunders.

280. The nurse is analyzing an ECG rhythm strip on an assigned client. The nurse notes that there are three small boxes from the beginning of the "P" wave to "R" wave. The nurse records that the client's PR interval is:

1 0.12 second
2 0.20 second
3 0.24 second
4 0.40 second

Level of Cognitive Ability: Application
Client Needs: Physiological Integrity
Integrated Process: Nursing Process/ Implementation
Content Area: Adult Health/Cardiovascular

Answer: 1
Rationale: Standard ECG graph paper measurements are 0.04 second for each small box on the horizontal axis (measuring time) and 1 mm (measuring voltage) for each small box on the vertical axis.

Test-Taking Strategy: Knowledge regarding ECG basics is necessary to answer this question. Knowing that each small box is equal to 0.04 second and that there are three small boxes will direct you to option 1. Review ECG basics because they will be helpful in answering questions related to dysrhythmias.

Reference
Black, J., & Hawks, J. (2005). *Medical-surgical nursing: Clinical management for positive outcomes* (7th ed., pp. 1583-1584). Philadelphia: Saunders.

---

281. The nurse is applying ECG electrodes to a diaphoretic client. The nurse does which of the following to keep the electrodes from coming loose?

1 Secures the electrodes with adhesive tape
2 Places clear, transparent dressings over the electrodes
3 Applies lanolin to the skin before applying the electrodes
4 Cleanses the skin with alcohol before applying the electrodes

Level of Cognitive Ability: Application
Client Needs: Physiological Integrity
Integrated Process: Nursing Process/ Implementation
Content Area: Adult Health/Cardiovascular

Answer: 4
Rationale: Alcohol defats the skin and will help the electrodes adhere to the skin. Placing adhesive tape or a clear dressing over the electrodes will not help the adhesive gel of the actual electrode to make better contact with the diaphoretic skin. Lanolin or any other lotion makes the skin slippery and prevents good initial adherence.

Test-Taking Strategy: Use the process of elimination. Note that options 1 and 2 are comparable or alike in that they both provide an external form of providing security of the electrodes. From the remaining options, note that option 4 addresses cleansing the skin. Review the procedure for attaching ECG electrodes if you had difficulty with this question.

References
Black, J., & Hawks, J. (2005). *Medical-surgical nursing: Clinical management for positive outcomes* (7th ed., p. 1583). Philadelphia: Saunders.
Chernecky, C., & Berger, B. (2008). *Laboratory tests and diagnostic procedures* (5th ed., p. 461). Philadelphia: Saunders.

---

282. The nurse has developed a plan of care for a client with a diagnosis of anterior cord syndrome. Which intervention should the nurse include in the plan of care?

1 Remind the client to change positions slowly.
2 Assess the client for decreased sensation to touch.
3 Assess the client for decreased sensation to vibration.
4 Teach the client about loss of motor function and decreased pain sensation.

Answer: 4
Rationale: Clinical findings related to anterior cord syndrome include loss of motor function and decreased pain sensation below the level of injury. The syndrome does not affect sensations of touch, motion, position, and vibration.

Test-Taking Strategy: Specific knowledge of anterior cord syndrome is necessary to answer this question. Eliminate option 1 first, knowing that motor function is affected below the level of injury. Eliminate options 2 and 3 knowing that in anterior cord syndrome sensations of touch and vibration remain intact. Remember that this type of injury involves complete motor function loss and decreased pain sensation, directing you to option 4. If you are unfamiliar with this syndrome, review the nursing interventions related to the disorder.

Level of Cognitive Ability: Application
Client Needs: Physiological Integrity
Integrated Process: Nursing Process/Planning
Content Area: Adult Health/Neurological

References
Black, J., & Hawks, J. (2005). *Medical-surgical nursing: Clinical management for positive outcomes* (7th ed., p. 2215). Philadelphia: Saunders.
Ignatavicius, D., & Workman, M. (2006). *Medical-surgical nursing: Critical thinking for collaborative care* (5th ed., p. 985). Philadelphia: Saunders.

283. The nurse is caring for a client with a thoracic spinal cord injury. As part of the nursing care plan, the nurse monitors for spinal shock. In the event that spinal shock occurs, the nurse anticipates that the most likely intravenous (IV) fluid to be prescribed would be:

1 Dextran
2 0.9% normal saline
3 5% dextrose in water
4 5% dextrose in 0.9% normal saline

Level of Cognitive Ability: Analysis
Client Needs: Physiological Integrity
Integrated Process: Nursing Process/Planning
Content Area: Adult Health/Neurological

Answer: 2
Rationale: Normal saline 0.9% is an isotonic solution that primarily remains in the intravascular space, increasing intravascular volume. This IV fluid would increase the client's blood pressure. Dextran is rarely used in spinal shock because isotonic fluid administration is usually sufficient. Additionally, Dextran has potentially serious side effects. Dextrose 5% in water is a hypotonic solution that pulls fluid out of the intravascular space and is not indicated for shock. Dextrose 5% in normal saline 0.9% is hypertonic and indicated for shock resulting from hemorrhage or burns.

Test-Taking Strategy: Focus on the subject, spinal shock. Knowledge of the treatment for spinal shock and the purpose of the various IV fluids will direct you to option 2. Review the IV therapy associated with this disorder if you had difficulty with this question.

Reference
Lewis, S., Heitkemper, M., Dirksen, S., O'Brien, P., & Bucher, L. (2007). *Medical-surgical nursing: Assessment and management of clinical problems* (7th ed., pp 1783-1784). St. Louis: Mosby.

284. The nurse prepares to teach a client to ambulate with a cane. Before teaching cane-assisted ambulation, the priority nursing assessment is to determine that the client has:

1 Self-consciousness about using a cane
2 Full range of motion in lower extremities
3 An adequate level of stamina and energy
4 Balance, muscle strength, and confidence

Level of Cognitive Ability: Analysis
Client Needs: Physiological Integrity
Integrated Process: Nursing Process/Assessment
Content Area: Fundamental Skills

Answer: 4
Rationale: Assessing the client's balance, strength, and confidence helps determine if the cane is a suitable assistive device for the client. Although body image (self-consciousness) is a component of the assessment, it is not the priority. Full range of motion and a high level of stamina are not needed for walking with a cane.

Test-Taking Strategy: Note the strategic word "priority." Eliminate options 1 and 2 first because they are not required for the use of a cane. Use Maslow's Hierarchy of Needs theory to assist in directing you to option 4. Review teaching points related to the use of a cane if you had difficulty with this question.

References
Ignatavicius, D., & Workman, M. (2006). *Medical-surgical nursing: Critical thinking for collaborative care* (5th ed., p. 125). Philadelphia: Saunders.
Potter, P., & Perry, A. (2005). *Fundamentals of nursing* (6th ed., pp. 948-949). St. Louis: Mosby.

285. A client has Buck's extension traction applied to the right leg. The nurse plans which of the following interventions to prevent complications from the device?
1 Provide pin care once a shift.
2 Massage the skin of the right leg with lotion every 8 hours.
3 Inspect the skin on the right leg at least once every 8 hours.
4 Release the weights on the right leg for range of motion exercises daily.

Level of Cognitive Ability: Application
Client Needs: Physiological Integrity
Integrated Process: Nursing Process/Planning
Content Area: Adult Health/Musculoskeletal

Answer: 3
Rationale: Buck's extension traction is a type of skin traction. The nurse inspects the skin of the limb in traction at least once every 8 hours for irritation or inflammation. Massaging the skin with lotion is not indicated. The nurse never releases the weights of traction unless specifically ordered by the physician. There are no pins to care for with skin traction.

Test-Taking Strategy: Focus on the subject, Buck's extension traction. Recalling that there are no pins in Buck's traction and that the nurse never removes weights without a specific order to do so eliminates options 1 and 4. From the remaining options, noting that the device would have to be removed to apply lotion will direct you to option 3. Also, use of the nursing process will direct you to option 3 because it is the only assessment action. Review care of the client in Buck's extension traction if you had difficulty with this question.

Reference
Ignatavicius, D., & Workman, M. (2006). *Medical-surgical nursing: Critical thinking for collaborative care* (5th ed., p. 1201). Philadelphia: Saunders.

286. A nurse is assessing a client with cardiac disease at the 30-week gestation antenatal visit. The nurse assesses lung sounds in the lower lobes following a routine blood pressure screening. The nurse performs this assessment to:
1 Identify mitral valve prolapse.
2 Identify cardiac dysrhythmias.
3 Rule out the possibility of pneumonia.
4 Assess for early signs of congestive heart failure (CHF).

Level of Cognitive Ability: Analysis
Client Needs: Physiological Integrity
Integrated Process: Nursing Process/Assessment
Content Area: Maternity/Antepartum

Answer: 4
Rationale: Fluid volume during pregnancy peaks between 18 and 32 weeks' gestation. During this period, it is essential to observe and record maternal data that would indicate further signs of cardiac decompensation or CHF in the pregnant client with cardiac disease. By assessing lung sounds, the nurse may identify early symptoms of diminished oxygen exchange and potential CHF. Options 1, 2, and 3 are not related to the subject of the question.

Test-Taking Strategy: Focus on the data provided in the question. Note the relationship between cardiac disease and lung sounds in the question and the words "congestive heart failure" in the correct option. Review the complications associated with pregnancy in the client with cardiac disease if you had difficulty with this question.

References
McKinney, E., James, S., Murray, S., & Ashwill, J. (2005). *Maternal-child nursing* (2nd ed., p. 655). St. Louis: Saunders.
Wong, D., Hockenberry, M., Perry, S., Lowdermilk, D., & Wilson, D. (2006). *Maternal-child nursing care*. (3rd ed., pp. 349, 355). St. Louis: Mosby.

287. The nurse is caring for a client with a newly applied leg cast. The nurse prevents the development of compartment syndrome by:
1 Elevating the limb and applying ice to the affected leg
2 Elevating the limb and covering the limb with bath blankets
3 Keeping the leg horizontal and applying ice to the affected leg
4 Placing the leg in a slightly dependent position and applying ice

Level of Cognitive Ability: Application
Client Needs: Physiological Integrity
Integrated Process: Nursing Process/ Implementation
Content Area: Adult Health/Musculoskeletal

Answer: 1
Rationale: Compartment syndrome is prevented by controlling edema. This is achieved most optimally with the use of elevation and the application of ice. The use of bath blankets or a dependent or horizontal leg position will not prevent this syndrome.

Test-Taking Strategy: Use the process of elimination. Recalling that edema is controlled or prevented with limb elevation helps eliminate options 3 and 4. From the remaining options, think about the effects of ice versus bath blankets. Ice will further control edema, whereas bath blankets will produce heat and prevent air circulation needed for the cast to dry. Review interventions to prevent complications following cast application if you had difficulty with this question.

Reference
Ignatavicius, D., & Workman, M. (2006). *Medical-surgical nursing: Critical thinking for collaborative care* (5th ed., pp. 1191-1192). Philadelphia: Saunders.

---

288. A client is undergoing hemodialysis and becomes hypotensive. The nurse avoids taking which of the following contraindicated actions?
1 Raising the client's legs and feet
2 Preparing to administer a 250 mL normal saline bolus
3 Increasing the blood flow from the client into the dialyzer
4 Checking the client's weight and reassessing blood pressure

Level of Cognitive Ability: Application
Client Needs: Physiological Integrity
Integrated Process: Nursing Process/ Implementation
Content Area: Adult Health/Renal

Answer: 3
Rationale: To treat hypotension during hemodialysis, the nurse raises the client's feet and legs to enhance cardiac return. A normal saline bolus of up to 500 mL may be given to increase circulating volume. The nurse would check the client's weight and reassess the blood pressure. Finally, the transmembrane hydrostatic pressure or the blood flow rate into the dialyzer may be decreased. All of these measures should improve the circulating volume and blood pressure.

Test-Taking Strategy: Note the strategic word "avoids." This word indicates a negative event query and the need to select the option that is an incorrect nursing action. Focus on the subject, hypotension, and note that the client is being dialyzed. Thinking about each action in the options and how it may affect the blood pressure will direct you to option 3. Review the treatment for this complication of dialysis if you had difficulty with this question.

References
Ignatavicius, D., & Workman, M. (2006). *Medical-surgical nursing: Critical thinking for collaborative care* (5th ed., pp. 1755-1756). Philadelphia: Saunders.
Lewis, S., Heitkemper, M., Dirksen, S., O'Brien, P., & Bucher, L. (2007). *Medical-surgical nursing: Assessment and management of clinical problems* (7th ed., p. 1223). St. Louis: Mosby.

289. The nurse is preparing a client for cardioversion using anterolateral paddle placement. The nurse places the conductive gel pads at which areas on the client's chest in preparation for this procedure?
1 Left fourth intercostal space and left fifth intercostal space at midaxillary line
2 Left second intercostal space and left fifth intercostal space at midaxillary line
3 Right fourth intercostal space and left fifth intercostal space at anterior axillary line
4 Right second intercostal space and left fifth intercostal space at anterior axillary line

Level of Cognitive Ability: Application
Client Needs: Physiological Integrity
Integrated Process: Nursing Process/ Implementation
Content Area: Adult Health/Cardiovascular

Answer: 4
Rationale: Anterolateral paddle placement for external countershock involves placing one paddle at the right second intercostal space and the other at the fifth intercostal space at the anterior axillary line.

Test-Taking Strategy: Use the process of elimination. Remember that the paddles are positioned so the electric shock travels through as much myocardium as possible. Visualize each of the placements as described and use knowledge of cardiothoracic landmarks, remembering the position of the heart in the chest. This will direct you to option 4. Review the procedure for cardioversion if you had difficulty with this question.

Reference
Black, J., & Hawks, J. (2005). *Medical-surgical nursing: Clinical management for positive outcomes* (7th ed., p. 1689). Philadelphia: Saunders.

---

290. A client is hospitalized with a diagnosis of thrombophlebitis and is being treated with heparin infusion therapy. About 24 hours after the infusion has begun, the nurse notes that the client's partial thromboplastin time (PTT) is 65 seconds with a control of 30 seconds. What is the appropriate initial nursing action?
1 Discontinue the heparin infusion.
2 Prepare to administrate protamine sulfate.
3 Notify the physician of the laboratory results.
4 Do nothing because the client is adequately anticoagulated.

Level of Cognitive Ability: Application
Client Needs: Physiological Integrity
Integrated Process: Nursing Process/ Implementation
Content Area: Pharmacology

Answer: 4
Rationale: The effectiveness of heparin therapy is monitored by the results of the partial thromboplastin time (PTT). Desired range for therapeutic anticoagulation is 1.5 to 2.5 times the control. A PTT of 65 seconds is within the therapeutic range.

Test-Taking Strategy: Use the process of elimination. Remember that the desired range for therapeutic anticoagulation is 1.5 to 2.5 times the control. Noting that the control is 30 and that 1.5 to 2.5 times the control is a range of 45 to 75 will direct you to option 4. Review care of the client receiving a heparin infusion if you had difficulty with this question.

References
Gahart, B., & Nazareno, A. (2006). *2006 Intravenous medications* (22nd ed., p. 637). St. Louis: Mosby.
McKenry, L., Tressier, E., & Hogan, M. (2006). *Mosby's pharmacology in nursing* (22nd ed., p. 611). St. Louis: Mosby.

291. A man is brought to the emergency department complaining of chest pain. His vital signs are blood pressure (BP) 150/90 mm Hg, pulse (P) 88 beats per minute (BPM), and respirations (R) 20 breaths per minute. The nurse administers nitroglycerin 0.4 mg sublingually. To evaluate the effectiveness of this medication, the nurse assesses for the relief of chest pain and expects to note which of the following changes in the vital signs?

1 BP 150/90 mm Hg, P 70 BPM, R 24 breaths per minute
2 BP 100/60 mm Hg, P 96 BPM, R 20 breaths per minute
3 BP 100/60 mm Hg, P 70 BPM, R 24 breaths per minute
4 BP 160/100 mm Hg, P 120 BPM, R 16 breaths per minute

Level of Cognitive Ability: Analysis
Client Needs: Physiological Integrity
Integrated Process: Nursing Process/Evaluation
Content Area: Pharmacology

Answer: 2
Rationale: Nitroglycerin dilates both arteries and veins, causing blood to pool in the periphery. This causes a reduced preload and therefore a drop in cardiac output. This vasodilation causes the blood pressure to fall. The drop in cardiac output causes the sympathetic nervous system to respond and attempt to maintain cardiac output by increasing the pulse. Beta-blockers, such as propranolol (Inderal), are often used in conjunction with nitroglycerin to prevent this rise in heart rate.

Test-Taking Strategy: Use the process of elimination. Knowing that nitroglycerin is a vasodilator and that it causes the BP to drop will assist in eliminating options 1 and 4. Next recall that if chest pain is reduced and cardiac workload is reduced, the client will be more comfortable; therefore, a rise in respirations should not be seen. This assists in eliminating option 3. Review the effects of nitroglycerin if you had difficulty with this question.

Reference
Skidmore-Roth, L. (2008). *Mosby's nursing drug reference* (21st ed., pp. 743-744). St. Louis: Mosby.

---

292. A client who has had an abdominal aortic aneurysm repair is 1 day postoperative. The nurse performs an abdominal assessment and notes the absence of bowel sounds. The nurse should:

1 Feed the client.
2 Call the physician immediately.
3 Remove the nasogastric (NG) tube.
4 Document the finding and continue to assess for bowel sounds.

Level of Cognitive Ability: Application
Client Needs: Physiological Integrity
Integrated Process: Nursing Process/ Implementation
Content Area: Adult Health/Gastrointestinal

Answer: 4
Rationale: Bowel sounds may be absent for 3 to 4 days postoperative due to bowel manipulation during surgery. The nurse should document the finding and continue to monitor the client. The NG tube should stay in place if present, and the client is kept NPO until after the onset of bowel sounds. There is no need to call the physician immediately at this time.

Test-Taking Strategy: Use the process of elimination. Note the strategic words "1 day postoperative." Eliminate option 3 because there are no data in the question regarding the presence of an NG tube. Additionally, an NG tube would not be removed (option 3) and the client would not be fed (option 1) if bowel sounds were absent. Recalling that bowel sounds may not return for 3 to 4 days postoperative will direct you to option 4 from the remaining options. Review normal postoperative assessment findings if you had difficulty with this question.

References
Ignatavicius, D., & Workman, M. (2006). *Medical-surgical nursing: Critical thinking for collaborative care* (5th ed., pp. 345, 807-808). Philadelphia: Saunders.
Lewis, S., Heitkemper, M., Dirksen, S., O'Brien, P., & Bucher, L. (2007). *Medical-surgical nursing: Assessment and management of clinical problems* (7th ed., p. 897). St. Louis: Mosby.

293. A nurse is caring for a client with gestational hypertension (GH) who is in labor. The nurse monitors the client closely for which complication of GH?
1 Seizures
2 Placenta previa
3 Hallucinations
4 Altered respiratory status

Level of Cognitive Ability: Analysis
Client Needs: Physiological Integrity
Integrated Process: Nursing Process/Assessment
Content Area: Maternity/Intrapartum

Answer: 1
Rationale: The major complication of GH is seizures. Placenta previa, hallucinations, and altered respiratory status are not directly associated with GH.

Test-Taking Strategy: Use the process of elimination. Remember that seizures are a concern with GH to direct you to option 1. Review the complications associated with GH if you had difficulty with this question.

Reference
McKinney, E., James, S., Murray, S., & Ashwill, J. (2005). *Maternal-child nursing* (2nd ed., pp. 633-634). St. Louis: Saunders.

---

294. The nurse is evaluating the outcomes of care for a client who experienced an acute myocardial infarction. Which of the following findings indicate that an expected outcome for the nursing diagnosis of Decreased cardiac output has been met?
1 The client complains of symptoms that require immediate action.
2 The client reports absence of dyspnea and anginal pain with activity.
3 Cardiac output is 3 liters per minute when measured with a pulmonary artery catheter.
4 Cardiac monitor shows a heart rate of 50 beats per minute after the client has eaten dinner.

Level of Cognitive Ability: Analysis
Client Needs: Physiological Integrity
Integrated Process: Nursing Process/Evaluation
Content Area: Adult Health/Cardiovascular

Answer: 2
Rationale: Dyspnea and angina are signs of altered cardiac output. The absence of these with activity indicates that cardiac output is adequate. Normal adult cardiac output is 4 to 8 liters per minute. A low heart rate affects cardiac output. The client's heart rate should be between 60 and 100 beats per minute. Complaints of symptoms that require immediate action are not an expected outcome.

Test-Taking Strategy: Focus on the subject, an expected outcome. Use the ABCs—airway, breathing, and circulation. Option 3 identifies a low cardiac output reading, so it can be eliminated. Next eliminate option 4 because the heart rate is less than the expected normal values. Also note the strategic words "absence of dyspnea and anginal pain" in the correct option. Review normal cardiac output and heart rate if you had difficulty with this question.

References
Black, J., & Hawks, J. (2005). *Medical-surgical nursing: Clinical management for positive outcomes* (7th ed., pp. 1720-1721). Philadelphia: Saunders.
Monahan, F., Sands, J., Neighbors, M., Marek, J., & Green, C. (2007). *Phipps' medical-surgical nursing: Health and illness perspectives* (8th ed., pp. 400, 720). St. Louis: Mosby.

---

295. During an initial prenatal visit a hemoglobin level is obtained on a client in her first trimester of pregnancy. The nurse reviews the results and determines the findings to be abnormal and indicative of iron deficiency anemia. The nurse performs an assessment on the client expecting to note which of the following in this type of anemia?
1 Pink, mucous membranes
2 Increased vaginal secretions
3 Complaints of headaches and fatigue
4 Complaints of increased frequency of voiding

Answer: 3
Rationale: Iron deficiency anemia is described as a hemoglobin blood concentration of less than 10.5 to 11.0 g/dL. Complaints of headaches and fatigue are abnormal findings and may reflect complications of this type of anemia caused by the decreased oxygen supply to vital organs. Options 1, 2, and 4 are normal findings in the first trimester of pregnancy.

Level of Cognitive Ability: Analysis
Client Needs: Physiological Integrity
Integrated Process: Nursing Process/Assessment
Content Area: Maternity/Antepartum

Test-Taking Strategy: Note the strategic words "first trimester of pregnancy" in the question. Options 1, 2, and 4 are normal findings during the first trimester of pregnancy. Option 3 is abnormal and may reflect complications caused by the decreased oxygen supply to vital organs. Review the clinical manifestations associated with anemia if you had difficulty with this question.

Reference

McKinney, E., James, S., Murray, S., & Ashwill, J. (2005). *Maternal-child nursing* (2nd ed., p. 657). St. Louis: Saunders.

---

296. The nurse is caring for a client with multiple myeloma who is receiving intravenous hydration at 100 mL per hour. Which finding indicates a positive response to the treatment plan?
1 Creatinine of 1.0 mg/dL
2 Weight increase of 1 kilogram
3 White blood cell count of 6000/mm³
4 Respirations of 18 breaths per minute

Level of Cognitive Ability: Analysis
Client Needs: Physiological Integrity
Integrated Process: Nursing Process/Evaluation
Content Area: Adult Health/Oncology

Answer: 1

Rationale: Renal failure is a concern in the client with multiple myeloma. In multiple myeloma, hydration is essential to prevent renal damage resulting from precipitation of protein in the renal tubules and from excessive calcium and uric acid in the blood. Creatinine is the most accurate measure of renal status. Options 3 and 4 are unrelated to the subject of hydration. Weight gain is not a positive sign when concerned with renal status.

Test-Taking Strategy: Use the process of elimination and focus on the subject, hydration status. Recalling that renal failure is a concern in multiple myeloma will direct you to option 1. Review care of the client with multiple myeloma if you had difficulty with this question.

Reference

Ignatavicius, D., & Workman, M. (2006). *Medical-surgical nursing: Critical thinking for collaborative care* (5th ed., p. 1664). Philadelphia: Saunders.

---

297. A nurse provides discharge instructions to a client with testicular cancer who had testicular surgery. The nurse tells the client:
1 To avoid driving a car for at least 8 weeks
2 Not to be fitted for a prosthesis for at least 6 months
3 To avoid sitting for long periods for at least 6 weeks
4 To report any elevation in temperature to the physician

Level of Cognitive Ability: Application
Client Needs: Physiological Integrity
Integrated Process: Teaching and Learning
Content Area: Adult Health/Oncology

Answer: 4

Rationale: For the client who has had testicular surgery, the nurse should emphasize the importance of notifying the physician if chills, fever, drainage, redness, or discharge occurs. These symptoms may indicate the presence of an infection. One week after testicular surgery, the client may drive. Often, a prosthesis is inserted during surgery. Sitting needs to be avoided with prostate surgery because of the risk of hemorrhage, but this risk is not as high with testicular surgery.

Test-Taking Strategy: Use Maslow's Hierarchy of Needs theory and principles related to prioritizing. Infection is a priority. After any surgical procedure, elevation of temperature could signal an infection and should be reported. Also note the lengthy time periods in options 1, 2, and 3. These will assist in eliminating these options. Review post-testicular surgical teaching points if you had difficulty with this question.

References
Black, J., & Hawks, J. (2005). *Medical-surgical nursing: Clinical management for positive outcomes* (7th ed., p. 1038). Philadelphia: Saunders.
Ignatavicius, D., & Workman, M. (2006). *Medical-surgical nursing: Critical thinking for collaborative care* (5th ed., pp. 1874-1875). Philadelphia: Saunders.

298. A multidisciplinary team is working with the spouse of a home care client who has end-stage liver failure and is teaching the spouse about pain management. Which statement by the spouse indicates the need for further teaching?

1 "My husband can use breathing exercises to control pain."
2 "I will help to prevent constipation with increased fluids."
3 "The opioid causes very deep sleep that my husband needs."
4 "If the pain increases, I will report it to the nurse promptly."

Level of Cognitive Ability: Analysis
Client Needs: Physiological Integrity
Integrated Process: Teaching and Learning
Content Area: Fundamental Skills

Answer: 3
Rationale: A decreased level of consciousness is a potential clinical indicator of opioid overdose, as well as fluid, electrolyte, and oxygenation deficiencies; thus, the nurse teaches the client's spouse about the differences between sleep related to pain relief and a deteriorating change in neurological status. Options 1, 2, and 4 all indicate an understanding of suitable steps to be taken in pain management.

Test-Taking Strategy: Use the process of elimination and note the strategic words "need for further teaching." These words indicate a negative event query and the need to select the option that is an incorrect statement. Note that the client has end-stage liver disease meaning that the opioid analgesics take longer to metabolize so the dosage is likely to have a greater and longer effect than a client without liver disease. Focusing on the subject, pain management, will direct you to option 3. Review pain management if you had difficulty with this question.

References
Ignatavicius, D., & Workman, M. (2006). *Medical-surgical nursing: Critical thinking for collaborative care* (5th ed., pp. 86-87). Philadelphia: Saunders.
Lehne. R. (2007). *Pharmacology for nursing care* (6th ed., pp. 262, 280) Philadelphia: Saunders.

299. A nurse is reviewing the antenatal history of a client in early labor. The nurse recognizes which of the following factors documented in the history as having the greatest potential for causing neonatal sepsis following delivery?

1 Adequate prenatal care
2 History of substance abuse during pregnancy
3 Appropriate maternal nutrition and weight gain
4 Spontaneous rupture of membranes 2 hours ago

Level of Cognitive Ability: Analysis
Client Needs: Physiological Integrity
Integrated Process: Nursing Process/Assessment
Content Area: Maternity/Intrapartum

Answer: 2
Rationale: Risk factors for neonatal sepsis can arise from maternal, intrapartal, or neonatal conditions. Maternal risk factors before delivery include low socioeconomic status, poor prenatal care and nutrition, and a history of substance abuse during pregnancy. Premature rupture of the membranes or prolonged rupture of membranes greater than 18 hours before birth is also a risk factor for neonatal acquisition of infection.

Test-Taking Strategy: Use the process of elimination. Options 1 and 3 are optimal findings and can be eliminated. From the remaining options, note the strategic words "2 hours ago" to assist in eliminating option 4. Review potential maternal physiological and psychosocial risk factors that may cause neonatal infections if you had difficulty with this question.

Reference
McKinney, E., James, S., Murray, S., & Ashwill, J. (2005). *Maternal-child nursing* (2nd ed., pp. 753, 755). St. Louis: Saunders.

300. A nurse performs a prenatal assessment on a client in the first trimester of pregnancy and discovers that the client frequently consumes beverages containing alcohol. The nurse initiates interventions to assist the client to avoid alcohol consumption in order to:

1 Reduce the potential for fetal growth restriction in utero.
2 Promote the normal psychosocial adaptation of the mother to pregnancy.
3 Minimize the potential for placental abruptions during the intrapartum period.
4 Reduce the risk of teratogenic effects to developing fetal organs, tissues, and structures.

Level of Cognitive Ability: Application
Client Needs: Physiological Integrity
Integrated Process: Teaching and Learning
Content Area: Maternity/Antepartum

Answer: 4
Rationale: The first trimester, "organogenesis," is characterized by the differentiation and development of fetal organs, systems, and structures. The effects of alcohol on the developing fetus during this critical period depend not only on the amount of alcohol consumed but also on the interaction of quantity, frequency, type of alcohol, and other drugs that may be abused during this period by the pregnant woman. Eliminating consumption of alcohol during this time may promote normal fetal organ development.

Test-Taking Strategy: Use the process of elimination and focus on the strategic words "first trimester." Recall that during this trimester, development of fetal organs, tissues, and structures take place. Review the effects of alcohol on the fetus in the first trimester of pregnancy if you had difficulty with this question.

Reference
McKinney, E., James, S., Murray, S., & Ashwill, J. (2005). *Maternal-child nursing* (2nd ed., pp. 602-603). St. Louis: Saunders.

---

301. The nurse is admitting a client with a diagnosis of myxedema to the hospital. The nurse performs which of the following that will provide data related to this diagnosis?

1 Inspects facial features
2 Auscultates lung sounds
3 Percusses the thyroid gland
4 Palpates the adrenal glands

Level of Cognitive Ability: Application
Client Needs: Physiological Integrity
Integrated Process: Nursing Process/Assessment
Content Area: Adult Health/Endocrine

Answer: 1
Rationale: Inspection of facial features will reveal the characteristic coarse features, presence of edema around the eyes and face, and the blank expression that are characteristic of myxedema. The assessment techniques in options 2, 3, and 4 will not reveal information related to the diagnosis of myxedema.

Test-Taking Strategy: Use the process of elimination. Eliminate options 2 and 4 because they do not relate to the thyroid gland. From the remaining options, recall that palpation, rather than percussion, of the thyroid is the assessment technique used to evaluate the thyroid gland. Review the clinical manifestations associated with myxedema if you had difficulty with this question.

Reference
Ignatavicius, D., & Workman, M. (2006). *Medical-surgical nursing: Critical thinking for collaborative care* (5th ed., p. 1489). Philadelphia: Saunders.

---

302. The nurse is teaching a client with chronic obstructive pulmonary disease (COPD) how to do pursed-lip breathing. Evaluation of understanding is evident if the client demonstrates which of the following?

1 Breathes in and then holds the breath for 30 seconds
2 Loosens the abdominal muscles while breathing out
3 Breathes so that expiration is three times as long as inspiration
4 Inhales with pursed lips and exhales with the mouth open wide

Answer: 3
Rationale: Prolonging expiration time reduces air trapping caused by airway narrowing that occurs in COPD. Tightening (not loosening) the abdominal muscles aids in expelling air. Exhaling through pursed lips (not with the mouth wide open) increases the intraluminal pressure and prevents the airways from collapsing. The client is not instructed to breathe in and hold the breath for 30 seconds; this action has no useful purpose for the client with COPD.

Level of Cognitive Ability: Comprehension
Client Needs: Physiological Integrity
Integrated Process: Nursing Process/Evaluation
Content Area: Adult Health/Respiratory

Test-Taking Strategy: Focus on the subject, pursed-lip breathing, and visualize each of the actions in the options. Recalling that a major purpose of pursed-lip breathing is to prevent air trapping during exhalation will direct you to option 3. Review the principles of pursed-lip breathing if you are unfamiliar with this technique.

References

Black, J., & Hawks, J. (2005). *Medical-surgical nursing: Clinical management for positive outcomes* (7th ed., p. 1812). Philadelphia: Saunders.

Lewis, S., Heitkemper, M., Dirksen, S., O'Brien, P., & Bucher, L. (2007). *Medical-surgical nursing: Assessment and management of clinical problems* (7th ed., p. 646). St. Louis: Mosby.

---

303. A nurse is caring for a pregnant client with a history of human immunodeficiency virus (HIV). Which nursing diagnosis formulated by the nurse has the highest priority for this client?
1 Self-care deficit
2 Risk for infection
3 Activity intolerance
4 Imbalanced nutrition

Level of Cognitive Ability: Analysis
Client Needs: Physiological Integrity
Integrated Process: Nursing Process/Analysis
Content Area: Maternity/Antepartum

Answer: 2
Rationale: Clients with HIV often show some evidence of immune dysfunction and may have increased vulnerability to common infections. HIV infection impairs cellular and humoral immune function; therefore, individuals with HIV are vulnerable to common bacterial infections. Not every client with HIV will have problems with activity, self-care, or nutrition. Although nutritional deficit is a concern, infection is specifically related to HIV and is a priority because it is more life-threatening.

Test-Taking Strategy: Use the process of elimination, noting the strategic words "highest priority." Focus on the physiology related to HIV to direct you to option 2. Also, recall that infection is a life-threatening condition in the client with HIV. Review the risks associated with HIV infection if you had difficulty with this question.

References

McKinney, E., James, S., Murray, S., & Ashwill, J. (2005). *Maternal-child nursing* (2nd ed., p. 665). St. Louis: Saunders.

Murray, S., & McKinney, E. (2006). *Foundations of maternal-newborn nursing* (4th ed., pp. 689-690). Philadelphia: Saunders.

---

304. A client is taking lithium carbonate (Lithium) for the treatment of bipolar disorder. Which assessment question would the nurse ask the client to determine signs of early lithium toxicity?
1 "Do you have frequent headaches?"
2 "Have you noted excessive urination?"
3 "Have you been experiencing leg aches over the past few days?"
4 "Have you been experiencing any nausea, vomiting, or diarrhea?"

Level of Cognitive Ability: Analysis
Client Needs: Physiological Integrity
Integrated Process: Nursing Process/Assessment
Content Area: Pharmacology

Answer: 4
Rationale: One of the most common early signs of lithium toxicity is gastrointestinal (GI) disturbances such as nausea, vomiting, or diarrhea. The assessment questions in options 1, 2, and 3 are unrelated to the findings in lithium toxicity.

Test-Taking Strategy: Use the process of elimination and knowledge regarding the "early" signs of toxicity. Recalling that GI disturbances are early manifestations will direct you to option 4. Review these signs if you had difficulty with this question.

Reference

Skidmore-Roth, L. (2008). *Mosby's nursing drug reference* (21st ed., p. 621). St. Louis: Mosby.

305. A postpartum nurse is caring for a client who delivered a viable newborn infant 2 hours ago. The nurse palpates the fundus and notes the character of the lochia. Which characteristic of the lochia would the nurse expect to note at this time?

1 Pink-colored lochia
2 White-colored lochia
3 Serosanguineous lochia
4 Dark red–colored lochia

Level of Cognitive Ability: Analysis
Client Needs: Physiological Integrity
Integrated Process: Nursing Process/Assessment
Content Area: Maternity/Antepartum

Answer: 4

Rationale: When checking the perineum, the lochia is monitored for amount, color, and the presence of clots. The color of the lochia during the fourth stage of labor (the first 1 to 4 hours after birth) is a dark red color. Options 1, 2, and 3 are not the expected characteristics of lochia at this time period.

Test-Taking Strategy: Use the process of elimination. Noting that the question refers to a client who delivered 2 hours ago will direct you to option 4. Review postpartum assessments if you had difficulty with this question.

References

McKinney, E., James, S., Murray, S., & Ashwill, J. (2005). *Maternal-child nursing* (2nd ed., pp. 386, 480). St. Louis: Saunders.
Murray, S., & McKinney, E. (2006). *Foundations of maternal-newborn nursing* (4th ed., pp. 300, 395-396, 409). Philadelphia: Saunders.

---

306. A nurse is performing a prenatal examination on a client in the third trimester. The nurse begins an abdominal examination and performs Leopold maneuvers. The nurse determines which of the following after performing the first maneuver?

1 Fetal descent
2 Placenta previa
3 Fetal lie and presentation
4 Strength of uterine contractions

Level of Cognitive Ability: Analysis
Client Needs: Physiological Integrity
Integrated Process: Nursing Process/Assessment
Content Area: Maternity/Antepartum

Answer: 3

Rationale: The first maneuver determines the contents of the fundus (either the fetal head or breech) and thereby the fetal lie. Leopold maneuvers are not performed during a contraction. Placenta previa is diagnosed by ultrasound and not by palpation. Fetal descent is determined with the fourth maneuver.

Test-Taking Strategy: Use the process of elimination. Recalling the purpose and procedure of Leopold maneuvers will assist in eliminating options 2 and 4. From the remaining options, it is necessary to know that the first maneuver determines fetal lie. Review Leopold maneuvers if you had difficulty with this question.

Reference

McKinney, E., James, S., Murray, S., & Ashwill, J. (2005). *Maternal-child nursing* (2nd ed., pp. 366-367). St. Louis: Saunders.

---

307. The nurse is caring for a client with a spinal cord injury who has spinal shock. The nurse performs an assessment on the client, knowing that which assessment will provide the best information about recovery from spinal shock?

1 Reflexes
2 Pulse rate
3 Temperature
4 Blood pressure

Level of Cognitive Ability: Analysis
Client Needs: Physiological Integrity
Integrated Process: Nursing Process/Assessment
Content Area: Adult Health/Neurological

Answer: 1

Rationale: Areflexia characterizes spinal shock. Therefore, reflexes would provide the best information about recovery. Vital sign changes (options 2, 3, and 4) are not consistently affected by spinal shock. Because vital signs are affected by many factors, they do not give reliable information about spinal shock recovery. Blood pressure would provide good information about recovery from other types of shock, but not spinal shock.

Test-Taking Strategy: Use the process of elimination. Note that options 2, 3, and 4 are comparable or alike and are all vital signs. Therefore, eliminate these options. Review spinal shock if you are unfamiliar with this content.

References

Ignatavicius, D., & Workman, M. (2006). *Medical-surgical nursing: Critical thinking for collaborative care* (5th ed., p. 987). Philadelphia: Saunders.
Lewis, S., Heitkemper, M., Dirksen, S., O'Brien, P., & Bucher, L. (2007). *Medical-surgical nursing: Assessment and management of clinical problems* (7th ed., p. 1590). St. Louis: Mosby.

308. A client is admitted to the hospital for repair of an unruptured cerebral aneurysm. Before surgery, the nurse performs frequent assessments on the client. Which assessment finding would be noted first if the aneurysm ruptures?

1 Widened pulse pressure
2 Unilateral motor weakness
3 Unilateral slowing of pupil response
4 A decline in the level of consciousness

Level of Cognitive Ability: Analysis
Client Needs: Physiological Integrity
Integrated Process: Nursing Process/Assessment
Content Area: Adult Health/Neurological

Answer: 4
Rationale: Rupture of a cerebral aneurysm usually results in increased intracranial pressure (ICP). The first sign of pressure in the brain is a change in the level of consciousness. This change in consciousness can be as subtle as drowsiness or restlessness. Because centers that control blood pressure are located lower in the brain than those that control consciousness, pulse pressure alteration is a later sign. Slowing of pupil response and motor weakness are also late signs.

Test-Taking Strategy: Note the strategic word "first." Remember that changes in level of consciousness are the first indication of increased ICP. Review the clinical manifestations associated with a cerebral aneurysm and increased ICP if you had difficulty with this question.

Reference
Ignatavicius, D., & Workman, M. (2006). *Medical-surgical nursing: Critical thinking for collaborative care* (5th ed., p. 1064). Philadelphia: Saunders.

---

309. An emergency department staff member calls the mental health unit and tells the nurse that a severely depressed client is being transported to the unit. The nurse in the mental health unit expects to note which of the following on assessment of this client?

1 Reports of weight gain, hypersomnia, and a blunted affect
2 Reports of crying spells, normal weight and sleep patterns
3 Reports of a reluctance to participate in activities, but a normal affect
4 Reports of substantial weight loss, insomnia, and decreased crying spells

Level of Cognitive Ability: Analysis
Client Needs: Physiological Integrity
Integrated Process: Nursing Process/Assessment
Content Area: Mental Health

Answer: 4
Rationale: In the severely depressed client, loss of weight is typical, while the mildly depressed client may experience a gain in weight. Sleep is generally affected in a similar way, with hypersomnia in the mildly depressed client and insomnia in the severely depressed client. The severely depressed client may report that no tears are left for crying.

Test-Taking Strategy: Use the process of elimination and note the strategic words "severely depressed." Options 2 and 3 identify some degree of normalcy and can be eliminated. From the remaining options, focusing on the strategic words will direct you to option 4. Review assessment findings associated with the severely depressed client if you had difficulty with this question.

References
Stuart, G., & Laraia, M. (2005). *Principles and practice of psychiatric nursing* (8th ed., p. 334). St. Louis: Mosby.
Varcarolis, E., Carson, V., & Shoemaker, N. (2006). *Foundations of psychiatric mental health nursing* (5th ed., p. 330). Philadelphia: Saunders.

310. A client with a history of suicide attempts is admitted to the mental health unit with the diagnosis of depression. Upon the client's arrival, the client's therapist reports to the nurse that the client had telephoned the therapist earlier in the evening and reported having overwhelming suicidal thoughts. Keeping this information in mind, the priority of the nurse is to assess for:

1 Interaction with peers
2 The presence of suicidal thoughts
3 The amount of food intake for the past 24 hours
4 Information regarding the past medication regimen

Level of Cognitive Ability: Analysis
Client Needs: Physiological Integrity
Integrated Process: Nursing Process/Assessment
Content Area: Delegating/Prioritizing

Answer: 2
Rationale: The critical information from the therapist is that the client is having thoughts of self-harm; therefore, the nurse needs further information about present thoughts of suicide so that the treatment plan may be as appropriate as possible. The nurse must make sure the client is safe. The items in options 1, 3, and 4 should be assessed; however, evaluation for suicide potential is most important.

Test-Taking Strategy: Use the process of elimination and note the strategic word "priority." Note the relationship between "overwhelming suicidal thoughts" in the question and in the correct option. Review assessment of the client at risk for self-harm if you had difficulty with this question.

Reference
Stuart, G., & Laraia, M. (2005). *Principles and practice of psychiatric nursing* (8th ed., p. 348). St. Louis: Mosby.

---

311. A home care nurse finds a client in the bedroom, unconscious, with a pill bottle in hand. The pill bottle had contained the selective serotonin reuptake inhibitor, sertraline (Zoloft). The nurse immediately assesses the client's:

1 Pulse
2 Respirations
3 Blood pressure
4 Urinary output

Level of Cognitive Ability: Analysis
Client Needs: Physiological Integrity
Integrated Process: Nursing Process/Assessment
Content Area: Delegating/Prioritizing

Answer: 2
Rationale: In an emergency situation, the nurse should determine breathlessness first, then pulselessness. Blood pressure would be assessed after these assessments were determined. Urinary output is also important but is not the priority at this time.

Test-Taking Strategy: Use the ABCs—airway, breathing, and circulation—as the guide for answering this question. Respirations specifically relate to breathing and airway. Review priority assessments in an unconscious client suspected of an overdose from selective serotonin reuptake inhibitors if you had difficulty with this question.

Reference
Kee, J., Hayes, E., & McCuistion, L. (2006). *Pharmacology: A nursing process approach.* (5th ed., p. 398). Philadelphia: Saunders.

---

312. A nurse checks a unit of blood received from the blood bank and notes the presence of gas bubbles in the bag. Which should the nurse implement?

1 Return the bag to the blood bank.
2 Infuse the blood using filter tubing.
3 Add 10 mL normal saline to the bag.
4 Agitate the bag to mix contents gently.

Level of Cognitive Ability: Application
Client Needs: Physiological Integrity
Integrated Process: Nursing Process/Implementation
Content Area: Fundamental Skills

Answer: 1
Rationale: The nurse should return the unit of blood to the blood bank because the gas bubbles in the bag indicate possible contamination. If the nurse were going to administer the blood, the nurse would use filter tubing to trap particulate matter. Normal saline or any other substance should never be mixed with the blood in a blood bag. The bag should not be agitated because this can harm red blood cells.

Test-Taking Strategy: Use the process of elimination. Recalling that the presence of gas bubbles indicates potential bacterial growth directs you to option 1. Remember that, when in doubt, consult with the blood bank. Review concepts related to transfusion of blood if you had difficulty with this question.

Reference
Ignatavicius, D., & Workman, M. (2006). *Medical-surgical nursing: Critical thinking for collaborative care* (5th ed., p. 913). Philadelphia: Saunders.

---

313. The nurse checks the gauge of the client's intravenous catheter. Which is the smallest gauge catheter that the nurse can use to administer blood?
1 14-gauge
2 19-gauge
3 22-gauge
4 24-gauge

Level of Cognitive Ability: Application
Client Needs: Physiological Integrity
Integrated Process: Nursing Process/ Implementation
Content Area: Fundamental Skills

Answer: 2
Rationale: An intravenous catheter used to infuse blood should be at least 19-gauge or larger to help prevent additional hemolysis of red blood cells and to allow infusion of the blood without occluding the IV catheter. A 22-gauge or 24-gauge catheter is too small to infuse blood.

Test-Taking Strategy: Focus on the subject, infusion of blood. This focus will assist in eliminating options 3 and 4. From the remaining options, think about the gauge of IV catheters to direct you to option 2. Review IV catheter sizes and blood transfusions if you had difficulty with this question.

References
Ignatavicius, D., & Workman, M. (2006). *Medical-surgical nursing: Critical thinking for collaborative care* (5th ed., p. 913). Philadelphia: Saunders.
Potter, P., & Perry, A. (2005). *Fundamentals of nursing* (6th ed., p. 1190). St. Louis: Mosby.

---

314. A client began receiving an intravenous (IV) infusion of packed red blood cells 30 minutes ago. The client turns on the nurse call light and describes difficulty breathing, itching, and a tight sensation in the chest. Which of the following is the first action of the nurse?
1 Call the physician.
2 Stop the transfusion.
3 Check the client's temperature.
4 Recheck the unit of blood for compatibility.

Level of Cognitive Ability: Application
Client Needs: Physiological Integrity
Integrated Process: Nursing Process/ Implementation
Content Area: Delegating/Prioritizing

Answer: 2
Rationale: The symptoms reported by the client indicate that the client is experiencing a transfusion reaction. The first action of the nurse when a transfusion reaction is observed is to discontinue the transfusion. The IV line is kept open with normal saline and the physician is notified. The nurse then checks the client's vital signs, temperature, pulse, and respirations and then rechecks the unit of blood as appropriate for infusion into the client. Depending on agency protocol, the nurse may also obtain a urinalysis, draw a sample of blood, and return the unit of blood and tubing to the blood bank. The nurse also institutes supportive care for the client, which may include administration of antihistamines, crystalloids, epinephrine, or vasopressors as prescribed.

Test-Taking Strategy: Focus on the data in the question to determine that the client is experiencing a transfusion reaction. Noting that the question asks for the "first action" will direct you to option 2. Review the nursing actions when a transfusion reaction occurs if you had difficulty with this question.

References
Ignatavicius, D., & Workman, M. (2006). *Medical-surgical nursing: Critical thinking for collaborative care* (5th ed., pp. 914-915). Philadelphia: Saunders.
Potter, P., & Perry, A. (2005). *Fundamentals of nursing* (6th ed., p. 1193). St. Louis: Mosby.

315. A client has not eaten or had anything to drink for 4 hours following two episodes of nausea and vomiting. Which of the following items would be best to offer the client who is ready to try resuming oral intake?
1 Toast
2 Gelatin
3 Dry cereal
4 Ginger ale

Level of Cognitive Ability: Application
Client Needs: Physiological Integrity
Integrated Process: Nursing Process/ Implementation
Content Area: Adult Health/Gastrointestinal

Answer: 4
Rationale: Clear liquids are best tolerated first after episodes of nausea and vomiting. If the client tolerates sips (20 to 30 mL at a time) of clear liquids, such as water or ginger ale (with the carbonation removed if better tolerated), then the amounts may be increased and gelatin, tea, and broth may be added. Once these are tolerated, solid foods such as toast, cereal, chicken, and other easily digested foods may be tried.

Test-Taking Strategy: Use the process of elimination. Begin to answer this question by eliminating options 1 and 3, which identify solid foods and are less well tolerated than liquids. Choose ginger ale over gelatin because it is a liquid at all temperatures. Review care to the client with nausea and vomiting if you had difficulty with this question.

Reference
Monahan, F., Sands, J., Neighbors, M., Marek, J., & Green, C. (2007). *Phipps' medical-surgical nursing: Health and illness perspectives* (8th ed., p. 1229). St. Louis: Mosby.

316. A client has just undergone an upper gastrointestinal (GI) series. The nurse provides which of the following upon the client's return to the unit as an important part of routine postprocedure care?
1 Bland diet
2 NPO status
3 Mild laxative
4 Decreased fluids

Level of Cognitive Ability: Application
Client Needs: Physiological Integrity
Integrated Process: Nursing Process/ Implementation
Content Area: Adult Health/Gastrointestinal

Answer: 3
Rationale: Barium sulfate, which is used as a contrast material during an upper GI series, is constipating. If it is not eliminated from the GI tract, it can cause obstruction. Therefore, laxatives or cathartics are administered as part of routine postprocedure care. Increased (not decreased) fluids are also helpful but do not act in the same way as a laxative to eliminate the barium. Options 1 and 2 are not routine postprocedure measures.

Test-Taking Strategy: Focus on the diagnostic test and the strategic words "routine postprocedure." Recalling that barium is used in this diagnostic test will direct you to option 3. Review postprocedure care following an upper GI series if you had difficulty with this question.

Reference
Chernecky, C., & Berger, B. (2008). *Laboratory tests and diagnostic procedures* (5th ed., p. 1133). Philadelphia: Saunders.

317. The nurse prepares the client for the removal of a nasogastric tube. During the tube removal, the nurse instructs the client to:
1 Inhale deeply.
2 Exhale slowly.
3 Hold a deep breath in.
4 Pause between breaths.

Level of Cognitive Ability: Application
Client Needs: Physiological Integrity
Integrated Process: Nursing Process/ Implementation
Content Area: Fundamental Skills

Answer: 3
Rationale: Just before removing the tube, the client is asked to take a deep breath and hold it because breath-holding minimizes the risk of aspirating gastric contents spilled from the tube during removal. The maneuver partially occludes the airway during tube removal; afterward, the client exhales as soon as the tube is out and, thus, avoids drawing the gastric contents into the trachea. The nurse pulls the tube out steadily and smoothly while the client holds the breath. The remaining options are incorrect because options 1 and 2 increase the risk of aspiration, and option 4 is ineffective.

Test-Taking Strategy: Use the process of elimination and visualize this procedure. Recalling that the airway is partially occluded during tube removal will direct you to option 3. Review this procedure if you had difficulty with this question.

Reference
Potter, P., & Perry, A. (2005). *Fundamentals of nursing* (6th ed., p. 1407). St. Louis: Mosby.

---

318. A nurse is caring for a client who is receiving total parenteral nutrition and has a prescription for an intravenous intralipid infusion. Which does the nurse implement before hanging the intralipid infusion?
1 Refrigerate the bottle of solution.
2 Place an in-line filter on the administration tubing.
3 Add 100 mL normal saline to the infusion bottle.
4 Check the solution for separation or an oily residue.

Level of Cognitive Ability: Application
Client Needs: Physiological Integrity
Integrated Process: Nursing Process/
   Implementation
Content Area: Fundamental Skills

Answer: 4
Rationale: The nurse checks the solution for separation or an oily appearance because this can indicate a spoiled or contaminated solution. Refrigeration renders the intralipid solution too thick to administer. Because they can affect the stability of the solution, the nurse avoids injecting additives into the intralipid infusion. Further, an in-line filter is not used because it can disrupt the flow of solution by becoming clogged.

Test-Taking Strategy: Use the process of elimination and focus on the name of the solution: intralipids. Think about the consistency of this solution to direct you to option 4. Review this content if you are unfamiliar with the procedure for infusing intralipid solutions.

Reference
Gahart, B., & Nazareno, A. (2006). *2006 Intravenous medications* (22nd ed., p. 538). St. Louis: Mosby.

---

319. The nurse administers a continuous tube feeding to a client. Which should the nurse implement as routine care for this client?
1 Check the residual in the stomach every 4 hours.
2 Change the feeding bag and tubing every 48 hours.
3 Withhold the feeding if residual is greater than 200 mL.
4 Leave at least 25 mL of formula in the feeding bag when adding additional formula to the bag.

Level of Cognitive Ability: Application
Client Needs: Physiological Integrity
Integrated Process: Nursing Process/
   Implementation
Content Area: Fundamental Skills

Answer: 1
Rationale: The residual volume is checked at least every 4 hours during continuous tube feedings and before intermittent feedings and medications. If the residual exceeds 100 mL (or the volume determined by agency policy), the nurse withholds the feeding to reduce the risk of aspiration. The bag and tubing are replaced every 24 hours, and the bag should be rinsed before adding new formula to reduce the risk of infection.

Test-Taking Strategy: Note the strategic words "continuous tube feedings." Use the steps of the nursing process to answer the question. Option 1 is the only option that addresses an assessment, the first step in the nursing process. Review the nursing care associated with this procedure if you had difficulty with this question.

Reference
Lewis, S., Heitkemper, M., Dirksen, S., O'Brien, P., & Bucher, L. (2007). *Medical-surgical nursing: Assessment and management of clinical problems* (7th ed., pp. 962-963). St. Louis: Mosby.

320. A physician is inserting a chest tube. The nurse selects which of the following materials to be used as the first layer of the dressing at the chest tube insertion site?

1 Sterile 4 × 4 gauze pad
2 Petrolatum jelly gauze
3 Absorbent gauze dressing
4 Gauze impregnated with povidone-iodine

Level of Cognitive Ability: Application
Client Needs: Physiological Integrity
Integrated Process: Nursing Process/ Implementation
Content Area: Adult Health/Respiratory

Answer: 2
Rationale: The first layer of the chest tube dressing is petrolatum gauze, which allows for an occlusive seal at the chest tube insertion site. Additional layers of gauze cover this layer, and the dressing is secured with a strong adhesive tape or Elastoplast tape.

Test-Taking Strategy: Use the process of elimination noting the strategic words "first layer." Recall that an occlusive seal at the site is needed and think about which dressing material will help achieve this seal. Review care of the client requiring chest tube insertion if you had difficulty with this question.

Reference
Perry, A., & Potter, P. (2006). *Clinical nursing skills & techniques* (6th ed., p. 862). St. Louis: Mosby.

---

321. A client being seen in the physician's office for follow-up 2 weeks after pneumonectomy complains of numbness and tenderness at the surgical site. The nurse tells the client that this is:

1 Not likely to be permanent, but may last for some months
2 A severe problem and the client will probably be rehospitalized
3 Probably caused by permanent nerve damage as a result of surgery
4 Often the first sign of a wound infection and checks the client's temperature

Level of Cognitive Ability: Application
Client Needs: Physiological Integrity
Integrated Process: Nursing Process/ Implementation
Content Area: Adult Health/Respiratory

Answer: 1
Rationale: Clients who undergo pneumonectomy may experience numbness, altered sensation, or tenderness in the area that surrounds the incision. These sensations may last for months. It is not considered to be a severe problem and is not indicative of a wound infection.

Test-Taking Strategy: Use the process of elimination. Eliminate option 2 because of the word "severe." Eliminate option 3 because of the word "permanent." Eliminate option 4 because numbness and tenderness are not signs of infection. Review this surgical procedure and the expected postoperative occurrences if you are not familiar with it.

Reference
Ignatavicius, D., & Workman, M. (2006). *Medical-surgical nursing: Critical thinking for collaborative care* (5th ed., p. 625). Philadelphia: Saunders.

---

322. A client scheduled for pneumonectomy tells the nurse that a friend of his had lung surgery and had chest tubes. The client asks the nurse about how long his chest tubes will be in place after surgery. The nurse responds that:

1 They will be removed after 3 to 4 days.
2 They will be in place for 24 to 48 hours.
3 They usually remain in place for a full week after surgery.
4 Most likely, there will be no chest tubes in place after surgery.

Answer: 4
Rationale: Pneumonectomy involves removal of the entire lung, usually caused by extensive disease such as bronchogenic carcinoma, unilateral tuberculosis, or lung abscess. Chest tubes are not inserted because the cavity is left to fill with serosanguineous fluid, which later solidifies. Therefore, options 1, 2, and 3 are incorrect.

Test-Taking Strategy: Focus on the surgical procedure. Recall that the entire lung is removed with this procedure. This would guide you to reason that chest tubes are unnecessary, because there is no lung remaining to reinflate to fill the pleural space (option 4). Review care of the client following pneumonectomy if you had difficulty with this question.

Level of Cognitive Ability: Application
Client Needs: Physiological Integrity
Integrated Process: Nursing Process/
    Implementation
Content Area: Adult Health/Respiratory

References
Black, J., & Hawks, J. (2005). *Medical-surgical nursing: Clinical management for positive outcomes* (7th ed., p. 1905). Philadelphia: Saunders.
Ignatavicius, D., & Workman, M. (2006). *Medical-surgical nursing: Critical thinking for collaborative care* (5th ed., p. 624). Philadelphia: Saunders.

---

323. The nurse is caring for the client with a dissecting abdominal aortic aneurysm. The nurse avoids which of the following while caring for the client?

1 Performs deep palpation of the abdomen
2 Auscultates the abdominal mass for bruits
3 Tells the client to report abdominal or back pain
4 Turns the client to the side to look for ecchymoses on the lower back

Level of Cognitive Ability: Application
Client Needs: Physiological Integrity
Integrated Process: Nursing Process/
    Implementation
Content Area: Adult Health/Cardiovascular

Answer: 1
Rationale: The nurse avoids deep palpation in the client in which a dissecting abdominal aortic aneurysm is known or suspected. Doing so could place the client at risk for rupture. The nurse looks for ecchymoses on the lower back to determine if the aneurysm is leaking and tells the client to report abdominal pain, or back pain, which may radiate to the groin, buttocks, or legs. The nurse should auscultate for bruits.

Test-Taking Strategy: Note the strategic word "avoids" in the question. This indicates a negative event query and tells you that the correct option will be an incorrect nursing action or one that is contraindicated. With the diagnosis presented, the only option that could cause harm is the option related to deep palpation (option 1). Review care of the client with a dissecting abdominal aortic aneurysm if you had difficulty with this question.

References
Black, J., & Hawks, J. (2005). *Medical-surgical nursing: Clinical management for positive outcomes* (7th ed., p. 1531). Philadelphia: Saunders.
Ignatavicius, D., & Workman, M. (2006). *Medical-surgical nursing: Critical thinking for collaborative care* (5th ed., pp. 807-808). Philadelphia: Saunders.

---

324. A client has undergone angioplasty of the iliac artery. Which of the following techniques should the nurse perform to best detect bleeding from the angioplasty in the region of the iliac artery?

1 Palpate the pedal pulses.
2 Measure the abdominal girth.
3 Ask the client about mild pain in the area.
4 Auscultate over the iliac area with a Doppler device.

Level of Cognitive Ability: Analysis
Client Needs: Physiological Integrity
Integrated Process: Nursing Process/
    Implementation
Content Area: Adult Health/Cardiovascular

Answer: 2
Rationale: Bleeding after iliac artery angioplasty causes blood to accumulate in the retroperitoneal area. This can most directly be detected by measuring abdominal girth. Palpation and auscultation of pulses determine patency. Assessment of pain is routinely done, and mild regional discomfort is expected.

Test-Taking Strategy: Use the process of elimination. Focus on the strategic words "bleeding" and "iliac artery." Select the option that addresses an abdominal assessment because the iliac arteries are located in the peritoneal cavity. This will direct you to option 2. Review this procedure if you had difficulty with this question.

Reference
Ignatavicius, D., & Workman, M. (2006). *Medical-surgical nursing: Critical thinking for collaborative care* (5th ed., p. 698). Philadelphia: Saunders.

325. A client is scheduled for a right femoral-popliteal bypass graft. The client has a nursing diagnosis of Ineffective tissue perfusion. The nurse takes which of the following actions before surgery to address this nursing diagnosis?
1 Completes a preoperative checklist
2 Helps the client void before surgery
3 Marks the location of pedal pulses on the right leg
4 Checks the results of any baseline coagulation studies

Level of Cognitive Ability: Application
Client Needs: Physiological Integrity
Integrated Process: Nursing Process/ Implementation
Content Area: Adult Health/Cardiovascular

Answer: 3
Rationale: A nursing diagnosis of Ineffective tissue perfusion in the client scheduled for femoral-popliteal bypass grafting indicates that the client is likely to have diminished peripheral pulses. It is important to mark the location of any pulses that are palpated or auscultated. This provides a baseline for comparison in the postoperative period. The other options are part of routine preoperative care.

Test-Taking Strategy: Note the strategic words "to address this nursing diagnosis." In this case, each of the incorrect options is an action that is part of routine preoperative care and is not specific to this nursing diagnosis. Review care of the client with ineffective tissue perfusion if you had difficulty with this question.

References
Ignatavicius, D., & Workman, M. (2006). *Medical-surgical nursing: Critical thinking for collaborative care* (5th ed., p. 756). Philadelphia: Saunders.
Lewis, S., Heitkemper, M., Dirksen, S., O'Brien, P., & Bucher, L. (2007). *Medical-surgical nursing: Assessment and management of clinical problems* (7th ed., pp. 907-908). St. Louis: Mosby.

---

326. A client who underwent peripheral arterial bypass surgery 16 hours ago complains of increasing pain in the leg at rest, which worsens with movement and is accompanied by paresthesias. The nurse should take which of the following actions?
1 Call the physician.
2 Administer an opioid analgesic.
3 Apply warm moist heat for comfort.
4 Apply ice to minimize any developing swelling.

Level of Cognitive Ability: Application
Client Needs: Physiological Integrity
Integrated Process: Nursing Process/ Implementation
Content Area: Adult Health/Cardiovascular

Answer: 1
Rationale: The classic signs of compartment syndrome are pain at rest that intensifies with movement and the development of paresthesias. Compartment syndrome is characterized by increased pressure within a muscle compartment caused by bleeding or excessive edema. It compresses the nerves in the area and can cause vascular compromise. The physician is notified immediately because the client could require an emergency fasciotomy. Options 2, 3, and 4 are incorrect actions.

Test-Taking Strategy: Use the process of elimination. Note the strategic words "increasing pain." Also note that the surgery was 16 hours ago. The signs and symptoms described indicate a new problem. These factors should indicate that the physician needs to be notified. Review the complications of this type of surgery if you had difficulty with this question.

Reference
Black, J., & Hawks, J. (2005). *Medical-surgical nursing: Clinical management for positive outcomes* (7th ed., p. 1518). Philadelphia: Saunders.

---

327. The nurse in an ambulatory care clinic takes a client's blood pressure (BP) in the left arm; it is 200/118 mm Hg. Which action should the nurse implement next?
1 Notify the physician.
2 Inquire about the presence of kidney disorders.
3 Check the client's blood pressure in the right arm.
4 Recheck the pressure in the same arm within 30 seconds.

Answer: 3
Rationale: When a high BP reading is noted, the nurse takes the pressure in the opposite arm to see if the blood pressure is elevated in one extremity only. The nurse would also recheck the blood pressure in the same arm, but would wait at least 2 minutes between readings. The nurse would inquire about the presence of kidney disorders that could contribute to the elevated blood pressure. The nurse would notify the physician because immediate treatment may be required, but this would not be done without obtaining verification of the elevation.

Level of Cognitive Ability: Application
Client Needs: Physiological Integrity
Integrated Process: Nursing Process/
  Implementation
Content Area: Adult Health/Cardiovascular

Test-Taking Strategy: Use the process of elimination. Eliminate option 4 first because of the time frame, 30 seconds. From the remaining options, select option 3 because it provides verification of the initial reading. Review the procedures for BP measurement if you had difficulty with this question.

References
Monahan, F., Sands, J., Neighbors, M., Marek, J., & Green, C. (2007). *Phipps' medical-surgical nursing: Health and illness perspectives* (8th ed., pp. 859-860). St. Louis: Mosby.
Potter, P., & Perry, A. (2005). *Fundamentals of nursing* (6th ed., p. 660). St. Louis: Mosby.

---

328. A new prenatal client is 6 months pregnant. On the first prenatal visit, the nurse notes that the client is gravida 4, para 0, aborta 3. The client is 5′ 6″ tall, weighs 130 pounds, and is 25 years old. The client states, "I get really tired after working all day and I can't keep up with my housework." Which factor in the above data would lead the nurse to suspect gestational diabetes?
1 Fatigue
2 Obesity
3 Maternal age
4 Previous fetal demise

Level of Cognitive Ability: Analysis
Client Needs: Physiological Integrity
Integrated Process: Nursing Process/Analysis
Content Area: Maternity/Antepartum

Answer: 4
Rationale: Fatigue is a normal occurrence during pregnancy. Five feet, six inches tall and 130 pounds does not meet the criteria of 20% over ideal weight. Therefore, the client is not obese. To be at high risk for gestational diabetes, the maternal age should be greater than 30 years. A previous history of unexplained stillbirths or miscarriages puts the client at high risk for gestational diabetes.

Test-Taking Strategy: Use the process of elimination. Option 1 can be eliminated because fatigue is a normal occurrence during pregnancy. Recalling the risk factors associated with gestational diabetes will indicate that options 2 and 3 do not apply to this client. Review the risk factors associated with gestational diabetes if you had difficulty with this question.

References
McKinney, E., James, S., Murray, S., & Ashwill, J. (2005). *Maternal-child nursing* (2nd ed., pp. 650-651). St. Louis: Saunders.
Murray, S., & McKinney, E. (2006). *Foundations of maternal-newborn nursing* (4th ed., p. 667). Philadelphia: Saunders.

---

329. A nurse is caring for a client with preeclampsia. The nurse develops a plan of care knowing that if the client progresses from preeclampsia to eclampsia, the nurse's first action is to:
1 Administer oxygen by face mask.
2 Clear and maintain an open airway.
3 Assess the maternal blood pressure and fetal heart tones.
4 Administer an intravenous infusion of magnesium sulfate.

Level of Cognitive Ability: Application
Client Needs: Physiological Integrity
Integrated Process: Nursing Process/
  Implementation
Content Area: Delegating/Prioritizing

Answer: 2
Rationale: It is important as a first action to keep an open airway and prevent injuries to the client. Options 1, 3, and 4 are all procedures that should be done but are not the first action.

Test-Taking Strategy: Note the strategic words "first action." Use the ABCs—airway, breathing, and circulation—to direct you to option 2. Review care of the client with preeclampsia or eclampsia if you had difficulty with this question.

Reference
McKinney, E., James, S., Murray, S., & Ashwill, J. (2005). *Maternal-child nursing* (2nd ed., pp. 637-638). St. Louis: Saunders.

330. A nurse in the emergency department admits a client who is bleeding freely from a scalp laceration obtained during a fall from a stepladder when the client was doing outdoor home repair. The nurse takes which of the following actions first in the care of this wound?
  1 Prepares for suturing the area
  2 Administers a prophylactic antibiotic
  3 Cleanses the wound with sterile normal saline
  4 Asks the client about timing of the last tetanus vaccination

Level of Cognitive Ability: Application
Client Needs: Physiological Integrity
Integrated Process: Nursing Process/ Implementation
Content Area: Delegating/Prioritizing

Answer: 3
Rationale: The initial nursing action is to cleanse the wound thoroughly with sterile normal saline. This action removes dirt or foreign matter in the wound and allows visualization of the size of the wound. Direct pressure is also applied as needed to control bleeding. If suturing is necessary, the surrounding hair may be shaved. Prophylactic antibiotics are often prescribed. The date of the client's last tetanus shot is determined, and prophylaxis is given if needed.

Test-Taking Strategy: Use the process of elimination. Note the strategic words "first" and "care of this wound." The strategic word "first" implies that more than one or all of the options may be partially or totally correct. Focusing on the subject, care to the wound, will direct you to option 3. Review care of the client with a laceration if you had difficulty with this question.

References
Ignatavicius, D., & Workman, M. (2006). *Medical-surgical nursing: Critical thinking for collaborative care* (5th ed., p. 350). Philadelphia: Saunders.
Potter, P., & Perry, A. (2005). *Fundamentals of nursing* (6th ed., pp. 1506-1507, 1518). St. Louis: Mosby.

---

331. A client was admitted to the nursing unit with a closed head injury 6 hours ago. During initial assessment, the nurse finds that the client has vomited, is confused, and complains of dizziness and headache. Which of the following is the most important nursing action?
  1 Notify the physician.
  2 Administer an antiemetic.
  3 Reorient the client to surroundings.
  4 Change the client's gown and bed linens.

Level of Cognitive Ability: Application
Client Needs: Physiological Integrity
Integrated Process: Nursing Process/ Implementation
Content Area: Delegating/Prioritizing

Answer: 1
Rationale: The client with a closed head injury is at risk of developing increased intracranial pressure (ICP). Increased ICP is evidenced by signs and symptoms such as headache, dizziness, confusion, weakness, and vomiting. Because of the implications of the client's manifestations, the most important nursing action is to notify the physician. Other nursing actions that are appropriate include physical care of the client and reorientation to surroundings.

Test-Taking Strategy: Use the process of elimination. Note the strategic words "most important." This directs you to prioritize the possible nursing actions. Considering the client's diagnosis, a closed head injury, and the signs and symptoms, the nurse should suspect increased ICP. The physician needs to be notified. Review care of a client with increased ICP if you had difficulty with this question.

Reference
Ignatavicius, D., & Workman, M. (2006). *Medical-surgical nursing: Critical thinking for collaborative care* (5th ed., pp. 1045, 1064). Philadelphia: Saunders.

---

332. A client is being brought into the emergency department after suffering a head injury. The first action by the nurse is to determine the client's:
  1 Level of consciousness
  2 Pulse and blood pressure
  3 Respiratory rate and depth
  4 Ability to move extremities

Answer: 3
Rationale: The first action of the nurse is to ensure that the client has an adequate airway and respiratory status. In rapid sequence, the client's circulatory status is evaluated (option 2), followed by evaluation of the neurological status (options 1 and 4).

Level of Cognitive Ability: Application
Client Needs: Physiological Integrity
Integrated Process: Nursing Process/
  Implementation
Content Area: Delegating/Prioritizing

Test-Taking Strategy: In emergency situations, use the ABCs—airway, breathing, and circulation. The correct option will most often be the option that deals with the client's airway. Respiratory rate and depth supports this action. Review initial care of the client who sustains a head injury if you had difficulty with this question.

Reference
Ignatavicius, D., & Workman, M. (2006). *Medical-surgical nursing: Critical thinking for collaborative care* (5th ed., pp. 1048-1051). Philadelphia: Saunders.

---

333. A client with a spinal cord injury is at risk of developing footdrop. The nurse uses which of the following as the effective preventive measure?
  1 Foot board
  2 Heel protectors
  3 Posterior splints
  4 Pneumatic boots

Level of Cognitive Ability: Application
Client Needs: Physiological Integrity
Integrated Process: Nursing Process/
  Implementation
Content Area: Adult Health/Neurological

Answer: 3
Rationale: The effective means of preventing footdrop is the use of posterior splints or high-top sneakers. A foot board prevents plantar flexion but also places the client more at risk for developing pressure ulcers of the feet. Pneumatic boots prevent deep vein thrombosis, but not footdrop. Heel protectors protect the skin, but do not prevent footdrop.

Test-Taking Strategy: Note that the subject of the question is "prevention" of footdrop. This guides you to select the option that immobilizes the foot in a functional position while protecting the skin of the extremities. This will direct you to option 3. Review the purposes of the devices identified in the options if you had difficulty with this question.

Reference
Black, J., & Hawks, J. (2005). *Medical-surgical nursing: Clinical management for positive outcomes* (7th ed., p. 2225). Philadelphia: Saunders.

---

334. A client is ambulatory and wearing a halo vest after a cervical spine fracture. The nurse tells the client to avoid which of the following because the client has a risk for injury?
  1 Using a walker
  2 Bending at the waist
  3 Scanning the environment
  4 Wearing rubber-soled shoes

Level of Cognitive Ability: Application
Client Needs: Physiological Integrity
Integrated Process: Teaching and Learning
Content Area: Adult Health/Neurological

Answer: 2
Rationale: The client with a halo vest should avoid bending at the waist because the halo vest is heavy, and the client's trunk is limited in flexibility. It is helpful for the client to scan the environment visually because the client's peripheral vision is diminished from keeping the neck in a stationary position. Use of a walker and rubber-soled shoes may help prevent falls and injury and are therefore also helpful.

Test-Taking Strategy: Use the process of elimination and note the strategic word "avoid." This indicates a negative event query and guides you to look for an action that could place the client at risk for injury. Visualize each of the items or actions in the options to assist in identifying how injury could be prevented. Review teaching points for a client with a halo vest if you had difficulty with this question.

References
Black, J., & Hawks, J. (2005). *Medical-surgical nursing: Clinical management for positive outcomes* (7th ed., p. 2221). Philadelphia: Saunders.
Ignatavicius, D., & Workman, M. (2006). *Medical-surgical nursing: Critical thinking for collaborative care* (5th ed., p. 994). Philadelphia: Saunders.

335. A nurse is caring for a client who has undergone transphenoidal resection of a pituitary adenoma. The nurse measures which of the following to detect occurrence of a common complication of this type of surgery?

1 Pulse rate
2 Temperature
3 Urine output
4 Oxygen saturation

Level of Cognitive Ability: Analysis
Client Needs: Physiological Integrity
Integrated Process: Nursing Process/Assessment
Content Area: Adult Health/Neurological

Answer: 3

Rationale: A common complication of surgery on the pituitary gland is temporary diabetes insipidus. This results from a deficiency in antidiuretic hormone (ADH) secretion as a result of surgical trauma. The nurse measures the client's urine output to determine whether this complication is occurring. Options 1, 2, and 4 are not specifically related to a common complication following this surgery.

Test-Taking Strategy: Use the process of elimination. Recalling that the pituitary gland is responsible for the production of ADH will direct you to option 3. Review the complications of this surgical procedure if you had difficulty with this question.

Reference
Ignatavicius, D., & Workman, M. (2006). *Medical-surgical nursing: Critical thinking for collaborative care* (5th ed., p. 1465). Philadelphia: Saunders.

---

336. A nurse is preparing to check the fetal heart rate of a pregnant woman who is at gestational week 16. Which piece of equipment will the nurse appropriately use to check the fetal heart rate?

1 Fetal heart monitor
2 An adult stethoscope
3 Bell of a stethoscope
4 Ultrasound fetoscope

Level of Cognitive Ability: Application
Client Needs: Health Promotion and Maintenance
Integrated Process: Nursing Process/Assessment
Content Area: Maternity/Antepartum

Answer: 4

Rationale: Toward the end of the first trimester, the fetal heart tones can be heard with an ultrasound fetoscope. Options 2 and 3 will not adequately assess the fetal heart rate. A fetal heart monitor is used during labor or in other situations when the fetal heart rate needs continuous monitoring.

Test-Taking Strategy: Use the process of elimination. Eliminate options 2 and 3 first because they are comparable or alike. Recalling that a fetal heart monitor is used for continuous monitoring will direct you to option 4. Review fetal heart assessment if you had difficulty with this question.

Reference
McKinney, E., James, S., Murray, S., & Ashwill, J. (2005). *Maternal-child nursing* (2nd ed., p. 393). St. Louis: Saunders.

---

337. A nurse is preparing postoperative discharge instructions for a client who had one adrenal gland removed. The nurse includes which of the following in the instructions?

1 The reason for maintaining a diabetic diet
2 Teaching proper application of an ostomy pouch
3 Instructions about early signs of a wound infection
4 The need for lifelong replacement of all adrenal hormones

Answer: 3

Rationale: A client who had a unilateral adrenalectomy will be placed on corticosteroids temporarily to avoid a cortisol deficiency. These medications will be gradually weaned in the postoperative period until they are discontinued. Also, because of the anti-inflammatory properties of corticosteroids produced by the adrenals, clients who undergo an adrenalectomy are at increased risk of developing wound infections. Because of this increased risk of infection, it is important for the client to know measures to prevent infection, early signs of infection, and what to do if an infection seems to be present. The client does not need to maintain a diabetic diet, and the client will not have an ostomy following this surgery.

Level of Cognitive Ability: Application
Client Needs: Physiological Integrity
Integrated Process: Nursing Process/
   Implementation
Content Area: Adult Health/Endocrine

Test-Taking Strategy: Use the process of elimination. Note the strategic words "one adrenal gland removed." Recalling that the hormones from the adrenal glands are needed for proper immune system function will eliminate options 1 and 2. From the remaining options, recalling that one gland can take over the function of two adrenal glands will direct you to option 3. Review care of the client following a unilateral adrenalectomy if you had difficulty with this question.

Reference
Black, J., & Hawks, J. (2005). *Medical-surgical nursing: Clinical management for positive outcomes* (7th ed., p. 1227). Philadelphia: Saunders.

---

338. The nurse is caring for a client who has undergone transphenoidal surgery for a pituitary adenoma. In the postoperative period, the nurse teaches the client to:
1 Cough and deep breathe hourly.
2 Remove the nasal packing after 48 hours.
3 Report frequent swallowing or postnasal drip.
4 Take acetaminophen (Tylenol) for severe headache.

Level of Cognitive Ability: Application
Client Needs: Physiological Integrity
Integrated Process: Nursing Process/
   Implementation
Content Area: Adult Health/Neurological

Answer: 3
Rationale: The client should report frequent swallowing or postnasal drip after transphenoidal surgery because it could indicate cerebrospinal fluid (CSF) leakage. The surgeon removes the nasal packing, usually after 24 hours. The client should deep breathe, but coughing is contraindicated because it could cause increased intracranial pressure. The client should also report severe headache because it could indicate increased intracranial pressure.

Test-Taking Strategy: Think about the anatomical location of this surgical procedure. Recalling that the concern is increased intracranial pressure and CSF leakage will direct you to option 3. Review care of the client following transphenoidal surgery if you had difficulty with this question.

References
Ignatavicius, D., & Workman, M. (2006). *Medical-surgical nursing: Critical thinking for collaborative care* (5th ed., p. 1464). Philadelphia: Saunders.
Monahan, F., Sands, J., Neighbors, M., Marek, J., & Green, C. (2007). *Phipps' medical-surgical nursing: Health and illness perspectives* (8th ed., pp. 1064-1065). St. Louis: Mosby.

---

339. A client is receiving desmopressin (DDAVP) intranasally for management of diabetes insipidus. The nurse assesses the client, knowing that which of the following measurements would assist in determining the effectiveness of this medication?
1 Daily weight
2 Temperature
3 Apical heart rate
4 Pupillary response

Level of Cognitive Ability: Analysis
Client Needs: Physiological Integrity
Integrated Process: Nursing Process/Assessment
Content Area: Pharmacology

Answer: 1
Rationale: DDAVP is an analog of vasopressin (antidiuretic hormone). It is used in the management of diabetes insipidus. The nurse monitors the client's fluid balance to determine the effectiveness of the medication. Fluid status can be evaluated by noting intake and urine output, daily weight, and the presence of edema.

Test-Taking Strategy: Focus on the subject, effectiveness of the medication. Noting the client's diagnosis and recalling the pathophysiology associated with this diagnosis will direct you to option 1. Review this medication if you had difficulty with this question.

Reference
Skidmore-Roth, L. (2008). *Mosby's nursing drug reference* (21st ed., p. 342). St. Louis: Mosby.

340. As the nurse brings the 10:00 AM doses of furosemide (Lasix) and nifedipine (Procardia) into the room of an assigned client, the client asks the nurse for a dose of aluminum hydroxide (Amphojel), which is ordered on a prn basis for dyspepsia. Which of the following actions by the nurse would be best?

1 Administer all three medications at the same time.
2 Administer the nifedipine and aluminum hydroxide, then the furosemide 1 hour later.
3 Administer the furosemide and aluminum hydroxide, then the nifedipine 1 hour later.
4 Ask the client if it would be possible to wait 1 hour before taking the aluminum hydroxide.

Level of Cognitive Ability: Application
Client Needs: Physiological Integrity
Integrated Process: Nursing Process/ Implementation
Content Area: Pharmacology

Answer: 4

Rationale: Antacids such as aluminum hydroxide often interfere with the absorption of other medications. For this reason, antacids should be separated from other medications by at least 1 hour. Because of the diuretic action of the furosemide and the antihypertensive action of the nifedipine, it is more important to administer them on time, if the client can tolerate waiting for the aluminum hydroxide.

Test-Taking Strategy: Note the strategic word "best." Recalling that antacids interfere with absorption of other medications will assist in eliminating option 1. From the remaining options, knowledge that the diuretic and antihypertensive medication should be administered on time will assist in directing you to option 4. Review these medications if you had difficulty with this question.

Reference

Skidmore Roth, L. (2008). *Mosby's nursing drug reference* (21st ed., pp. 497-498). St. Louis: Mosby.

---

341. The nurse monitors the client taking amitriptyline for which common side effect of this medication?

1 Diarrhea
2 Drowsiness
3 Hypertension
4 Increased salivation

Level of Cognitive Ability: Application
Client Needs: Physiological Integrity
Integrated Process: Nursing Process/Assessment
Content Area: Pharmacology

Answer: 2

Rationale: Common side effects of amitriptyline (a tricyclic antidepressant) include the central nervous system effects of drowsiness, fatigue, lethargy, and sedation. Other common side effects include dry mouth or eyes, blurred vision, hypotension, and constipation. The nurse monitors the client for these side effects.

Test-Taking Strategy: Use the process of elimination. Recalling that amitriptyline is an antidepressant will lead you to option 2. Review this medication if you had difficulty with this question.

Reference

Hodgson, B., & Kizior, R. (2007). *Saunders nursing drug handbook 2007* (p. 61). Philadelphia: Saunders.

---

342. A client has been admitted to the mental health unit on a voluntary basis. The client has reported a history of depression over the past 5 years. Which of the following questions by the nurse would elicit the most thorough assessment data regarding the client's recent sleeping patterns?

1 "Are you sleeping well at home?"
2 "Did you get much sleep last night?"
3 "Tell me about your sleeping patterns."
4 "You look as if you could use some sleep."

Answer: 3

Rationale: Option 3 is an open-ended question and provides the client the opportunity to express thoughts and feelings. Options 1 and 2 could lead to a one-word answer that would not provide thorough assessment data. Additionally, one night of sleep may not tell the nurse how the pattern has been over time. Anyone may or may not sleep well for one night, and that sleep or loss of sleep does not indicate a problem. Option 4 could be interpreted by the depressed person as a negative statement and could block communication needed for a thorough assessment.

Level of Cognitive Ability: Application
Client Needs: Physiological Integrity
Integrated Process: Nursing Process/Assessment
Content Area: Mental Health

Test-Taking Strategy: Use the therapeutic communication techniques. Select the option that allows the client to take the lead in the conversation. This will direct you to option 3. Review therapeutic communication techniques if you had difficulty with this question.

Reference
Stuart, G., & Laraia, M. (2005). *Principles and practice of psychiatric nursing* (8th ed., pp. 29, 336). St. Louis: Mosby.

---

343. A client is admitted to the emergency department with drug-induced anxiety related to overingestion of prescribed antipsychotic medication. The most important piece of information the nurse should obtain initially is the:

1 Name of the nearest relative and their phone number
2 Name of the ingested medication and the amount ingested
3 Cause of the attempt and if the client plans another attempt
4 Length of time on the medication and any noted side effects

Level of Cognitive Ability: Application
Client Needs: Physiological Integrity
Integrated Process: Nursing Process/Assessment
Content Area: Mental Health

Answer: 2
Rationale: In an emergency, lifesaving facts are obtained first. The name of and the amount of medication ingested is of utmost importance in treating this potentially life-threatening situation. The relatives and the reason for the suicide attempt are not the most important initial assessment. The length of time on the medication is also not the priority in this situation.

Test-Taking Strategy: Note the strategic words "initially" and "overingestion." Lifesaving treatment cannot begin until the medication and amount are identified. Review care of the client with a drug overdose if you had difficulty with this question.

References
Kee, J., Hayes, E., & McCuistion, L. (2006). *Pharmacology: A nursing process approach.* (5th ed., p. 151). Philadelphia: Saunders.
Stuart, G., & Laraia, M. (2005). *Principles and practice of psychiatric nursing* (8th ed., pp. 498-499). St. Louis: Mosby.

---

344. A nurse determines that a client understands the purpose of a vitamin K (phytonadione) injection for her newborn if the client states that vitamin K is administered because newborns:

1 Lack vitamins.
2 Have low blood levels.
3 Lack intestinal bacteria.
4 Cannot produce vitamin K in the liver.

Level of Cognitive Ability: Analysis
Client Needs: Physiological Integrity
Integrated Process: Teaching and Learning
Content Area: Maternity/Postpartum

Answer: 3
Rationale: The absence of normal flora needed to synthesize vitamin K in the normal newborn gut results in low levels of vitamin K and creates a transient blood coagulation deficiency between the second and fifth day of life. From a low point at about 2 to 3 days after birth, these coagulation factors rise slowly, but do not approach normal adult levels until 9 months of age or later. Increasing levels of these vitamin K–dependent factors indicate a response to dietary intake and bacterial colonization of the intestines. An injection is administered prophylactically on the day of birth to combat the deficiency. Options 1, 2, and 4 are incorrect.

Test-Taking Strategy: Recalling the physiology associated with the synthesis of vitamin K in the newborn will direct you to option 3. Review the purpose of administering vitamin K to the newborn if you had difficulty with this question.

Reference
McKinney, E., James, S., Murray, S., & Ashwill, J. (2005). *Maternal-child nursing* (2nd ed., p. 554). St. Louis: Saunders.

345. A nurse is assigned to give a child a tepid tub bath to treat hyperthermia. Following the bath, the nurse plans to:
1 Leave the child uncovered for 15 minutes.
2 Assist the child to put on a cotton sleep shirt.
3 Take the child's axillary temperature in 2 hours.
4 Place the child in bed and cover the child with a blanket.

Level of Cognitive Ability: Application
Client Needs: Physiological Integrity
Integrated Process: Nursing Process/Planning
Content Area: Child Health

Answer: 2
Rationale: Cotton is a lightweight material that will protect the child from becoming chilled after the bath. Option 1 is incorrect because the child should not be left uncovered. Option 3 is incorrect because the child's temperature should be reassessed a half hour after the bath. Option 4 is incorrect because a blanket is heavy and may increase the child's body temperature and further increase metabolism.

Test-Taking Strategy: Use the process of elimination, focusing on the subject: to treat hyperthermia. Eliminate option 1 because of the word "uncovered." Eliminate option 3 because of the time frame. Eliminate option 4 because of the word "blanket." Review care of a child with hyperthermia if you had difficulty with this question.

References
Hockenberry, M., & Wilson, D. (2007). *Nursing care of infants and children* (8th ed., p. 1105). St. Louis: Mosby.
Hockenberry, M., Wilson, D., & Winkelstein, M. (2005). *Wong's essentials of pediatric nursing* (7th ed., p. 733). St. Louis: Mosby.
McKinney, E., James, S., Murray, S., & Ashwill, J. (2005). *Maternal-child nursing* (2nd ed., p. 510). St. Louis: Saunders.

346. A nurse is caring for an infant who has diarrhea. The nurse monitors the infant for which early sign of dehydration?
1 Cool extremities
2 Gray, mottled skin
3 Capillary refill of 2 seconds
4 Apical pulse rate of 200 beats per minute

Level of Cognitive Ability: Analysis
Client Needs: Physiological Integrity
Integrated Process: Nursing Process/Assessment
Content Area: Child Health

Answer: 4
Rationale: Dehydration causes interstitial fluid to shift to the vascular compartment in an attempt to maintain fluid volume. When the body is unable to compensate for fluid lost, circulatory failure occurs. The blood pressure will decrease and the pulse rate will increase. This will be followed by peripheral symptoms. Options 1, 2, and 3 are incorrect, and these assessment findings relate to peripheral circulatory status.

Test-Taking Strategy: Note the strategic word "early" and think about the physiology that occurs in dehydration. Also, note that options 1, 2, and 3 are comparable or alike and relate directly to peripheral circulatory status. Review the signs of dehydration if you had difficulty with this question.

References
Hockenberry, M., Wilson, D., & Winkelstein, M. (2005). *Wong's essentials of pediatric nursing* (7th ed., pp. 840-842). St. Louis: Mosby.
McKinney, E., James, S., Murray, S., & Ashwill, J. (2005). *Maternal-child nursing* (2nd ed., pp. 726-727). St. Louis: Saunders.

347. Acetylsalicylic acid (aspirin) is prescribed for a client with coronary artery disease before a percutaneous transluminal coronary angioplasty (PTCA). The nurse administers the medication, knowing that it is prescribed to:

1 Relieve postprocedure pain.
2 Prevent thrombus formation.
3 Prevent postprocedure hyperthermia.
4 Prevent inflammation of the puncture site.

Level of Cognitive Ability: Application
Client Needs: Physiological Integrity
Integrated Process: Nursing Process/ Implementation
Content Area: Adult Health/Cardiovascular

Answer: 2
Rationale: Before PTCA, the client is usually given an anticoagulant, commonly aspirin, to help reduce the risk of occlusion of the artery during the procedure because the aspirin inhibits platelet aggregation. Options 1, 3, and 4 are unrelated to the purpose of administering aspirin to this client.

Test-Taking Strategy: Use the process of elimination. Think about the potential complications of a PTCA and the action and properties of aspirin to direct you to option 2. Review the action and uses of aspirin and the complications associated with PTCA if you had difficulty with this question.

References
Hodgson, B., & Kizior, R. (2007). *Saunders nursing drug handbook 2007* (pp. 93-94). Philadelphia: Saunders.
Ignatavicius, D., & Workman, M. (2006). *Medical-surgical nursing: Critical thinking for collaborative care* (5th ed., p. 851). Philadelphia: Saunders.

---

348. A nurse reviews a physician's orders and notes that a topical nitrate is prescribed. The nurse notes that acetaminophen (Tylenol) is also prescribed to be administered before the nitrate. The nurse plans to implement the order, knowing that the acetaminophen is prescribed because:

1 Headache is a common side effect of nitrates.
2 Fever usually accompanies myocardial infarction.
3 Acetaminophen potentiates the therapeutic effect of nitrates.
4 Acetaminophen does not interfere with platelet action as acetylsalicylic acid (aspirin) does.

Level of Cognitive Ability: Application
Client Needs: Physiological Integrity
Integrated Process: Nursing Process/Planning
Content Area: Pharmacology

Answer: 1
Rationale: Headache occurs as a side effect of nitrates in many clients. Acetaminophen may be administered before nitrates to prevent headaches or to minimize the discomfort from the headaches. Options 2, 3, and 4 are incorrect.

Test-Taking Strategy: Use the process of elimination and focus on the subject. Recall that headache is a common side effect of nitrates. Eliminate option 3 first because this is an incorrect statement. Whereas options 2 and 4 are true statements, they do not address the subject of the question. Review the side effects of nitrates and the purpose of administering acetaminophen before these medications if you had difficulty with this question.

References
Ignatavicius, D., & Workman, M. (2006). *Medical-surgical nursing: Critical thinking for collaborative care* (5th ed., p. 855). Philadelphia: Saunders.
Kee, J., Hayes, E., & McCuistion, L. (2006). *Pharmacology: A nursing process approach* (5th ed., p. 613). Philadelphia: Saunders.

---

349. The nurse develops a plan of care for a client admitted to the hospital with a diagnosis of an acute myocardial infarction (MI). The priority nursing diagnosis in the acute phase would be:

1 Anxiety
2 Pain, acute
3 Powerlessness
4 Interrupted family processes

Answer: 2
Rationale: Pain is the prevailing symptom of acute MI. Relief of pain is a priority. Pain stimulates the autonomic nervous system, increasing myocardial oxygen demand. Although options 1, 3, and 4 may also be appropriate nursing diagnoses, the presence of pain impacts on these additional nursing diagnoses.

Test-Taking Strategy: Use Maslow's Hierarchy of Needs theory. Physiological needs are the priority; therefore, options 1, 3, and 4 can be eliminated. Review care of a client with an MI if you had difficulty with this question.

Level of Cognitive Ability: Analysis
Client Needs: Physiological Integrity
Integrated Process: Nursing Process/Analysis
Content Area: Adult Health/Cardiovascular

Reference
Black, J., & Hawks, J. (2005). *Medical-surgical nursing: Clinical management for positive outcomes* (7th ed., pp. 1719-1727). Philadelphia: Saunders.

---

350. A nurse is caring for a client with a diagnosis of urolithiasis. The nurse instructs the client that it is most important to perform which of the following activities?
  1 Record weight every day.
  2 Restrict physical activities.
  3 Strain all urine from each voiding.
  4 Turn, cough, and deep breathe every 2 hours.

Level of Cognitive Ability: Application
Client Needs: Physiological Integrity
Integrated Process: Teaching and Learning
Content Area: Adult Health/Renal

Answer: 3
Rationale: Obstruction of the urinary tract is the primary problem associated with urolithiasis. Stones recovered from straining urine can be analyzed and can provide direction for prevention of further stone formation. Activities should not be restricted. Options 1 and 4 are not specifically related to the client's diagnosis.

Test-Taking Strategy: Focus on the client's diagnosis. Recalling that urolithiasis relates to urinary tract stones will direct you to option 3. Review care of the client with urolithiasis if you had difficulty with this question.

Reference
Black, J., & Hawks, J. (2005). *Medical-surgical nursing: Clinical management for positive outcomes* (7th ed., p. 887). Philadelphia: Saunders.

---

351. A nurse is caring for a newly delivered breast-feeding infant. Which intervention performed by the nurse would best prevent jaundice in this infant?
  1 Placing the infant under phototherapy
  2 Keeping the infant NPO until the second period of reactivity
  3 Encouraging the mother to breast-feed the infant every 2 to 3 hours
  4 Encouraging the mother to offer a formula supplement after each breast-feeding session

Level of Cognitive Ability: Application
Client Needs: Health Promotion and Maintenance
Integrated Process: Nursing Process/ Implementation
Content Area: Maternity/Postpartum

Answer: 3
Rationale: To help prevent jaundice, the mother should feed the infant frequently in the immediate birth period because colostrum is a natural laxative and helps promote the passage of meconium. Offering the infant a formula supplement will cause nipple confusion and decrease the amount of milk produced by the mother. Breast-feeding should begin as soon as possible after birth while the infant is in the first period of reactivity. Delaying breast-feeding decreases the production of prolactin, which decreases the mother's milk production. Phototherapy requires a physician's order and is not implemented until bilirubin levels are 12 mg/dL or higher in the healthy term infant.

Test-Taking Strategy: Use the process of elimination. Recalling the physiology associated with jaundice and noting the strategic words "best prevent" will assist in eliminating options 1 and 2. From the remaining options, select option 3 because option 4 will cause nipple confusion. Review the interventions to prevent jaundice if you had difficulty with this question.

Reference
McKinney, E., James, S., Murray, S., & Ashwill, J. (2005). *Maternal-child nursing* (2nd ed., pp. 514, 584). St. Louis: Saunders.

352. A nurse is caring for a client scheduled for an arthroscopy. The nurse develops a post-operative plan of care and includes which priority nursing action in the plan?
  1 Monitor intake and output.
  2 Assess the tissue at the surgical site.
  3 Monitor the area for numbness or tingling.
  4 Assess the complete blood cell count results.

Level of Cognitive Ability: Application
Client Needs: Physiological Integrity
Integrated Process: Nursing Process/Planning
Content Area: Delegating/Prioritizing

Answer: 3
Rationale: The priority nursing action is to monitor the affected area for numbness or tingling. Options 1, 2, and 4 are also a component of postoperative care, but, from the options presented, are not the priority.

Test-Taking Strategy: Use the ABCs—airway, breathing, and circulation—to answer the question. Option 3 relates to circulation. Review nursing care following arthroscopy if you had difficulty with this question.

References
Black, J., & Hawks, J. (2005). *Medical-surgical nursing: Clinical management for positive outcomes* (7th ed., p. 577). Philadelphia: Saunders.
Ignatavicius, D., & Workman, M. (2006). *Medical-surgical nursing: Critical thinking for collaborative care* (5th ed., p. 1154). Philadelphia: Saunders.

---

353. A nurse is caring for a client with active tuberculosis who has started medication therapy that includes rifampin (Rifadin). The nurse instructs the client to expect which side effect of this medication?
  1 Bilious urine
  2 Yellow sclera
  3 Orange secretions
  4 Clay-colored stools

Level of Cognitive Ability: Application
Client Needs: Physiological Integrity
Integrated Process: Nursing Process/ Implementation
Content Area: Adult Health/Respiratory

Answer: 3
Rationale: Secretions will become orange in color as a result of the rifampin. The client should be instructed that this side effect will likely occur and should be told that soft contact lenses, if used by the client, will become permanently discolored. Options 1, 2, and 4 are not expected effects.

Test-Taking Strategy: Use the process of elimination and knowledge of the side effects of rifampin to answer this question. Eliminate options 1, 2, and 4 because they are comparable or alike in that they are all symptoms of intrahepatic obstruction as seen in viral hepatitis. Review the side effects of this medication if you had difficulty with this question.

Reference
Hodgson, B., & Kizior, R. (2007). *Saunders nursing drug handbook 2007* (p. 1021). Philadelphia: Saunders.

---

354. The nurse sends a sputum specimen to the laboratory for culture from a client with suspected active tuberculosis (TB). The results report that *Mycobacterium tuberculosis* is cultured. How would the nurse correctly analyze these results?
  1 Results are positive for active tuberculosis.
  2 Results indicate a less virulent strain of tuberculosis.
  3 Results are inconclusive until a repeat sputum is sent.
  4 Results are unreliable unless the client has also had a positive Mantoux test.

Answer: 1
Rationale: Culture of *Mycobacterium tuberculosis* from sputum or other body secretions or tissue is the only method of confirming the diagnosis. Options 2 and 3 are incorrect statements. The Mantoux test is performed to assist in diagnosing TB but does not confirm active disease.

Test-Taking Strategy: Use the process of elimination. Recall that culture of the bacteria from sputum confirms the diagnosis. Because tuberculosis affects the respiratory system, it would make sense that the bacteria would be found in the sputum if the client had active disease, therefore confirming the diagnosis. Review the diagnostic tests associated with active TB if you had difficulty with this question.

Level of Cognitive Ability: Analysis
Client Needs: Physiological Integrity
Integrated Process: Nursing Process/Analysis
Content Area: Adult Health/Respiratory

Reference
Black, J., & Hawks, J. (2005). *Medical-surgical nursing: Clinical management for positive outcomes* (7th ed., pp. 1846-1847). Philadelphia: Saunders.

355. A coronary care unit (CCU) nurse is caring for a client admitted with acute myocardial infarction (MI). The nurse monitors for which most common complication of MI?

1 Cardiogenic shock
2 Cardiac dysrhythmias
3 Congestive heart failure
4 Recurrent myocardial infarction

Level of Cognitive Ability: Application
Client Needs: Physiological Integrity
Integrated Process: Nursing Process/ Implementation
Content Area: Adult Health/Cardiovascular

Answer: 2
Rationale: Dysrhythmias are the most common complication and cause of death after an MI. Cardiogenic shock, congestive heart failure, and recurrent MI are also complications but occur less frequently.

Test-Taking Strategy: Use the process of elimination. Noting the strategic words "most common" and knowledge of the complications of MI will direct you to option 2. Review these complications if you had difficulty with this question.

References
Black, J., & Hawks, J. (2005). *Medical-surgical nursing: Clinical management for positive outcomes* (7th ed., pp. 1671, 1716). Philadelphia: Saunders.
Ignatavicius, D., & Workman, M. (2006). *Medical-surgical nursing: Critical thinking for collaborative care* (5th ed., pp. 735-736). Philadelphia: Saunders.

356. A nurse in the newborn nursery is planning for the admission of a large for gestational age (LGA) infant. In preparing to care for this infant, the nurse obtains equipment to perform which diagnostic test?

1 Serum insulin level
2 Heelstick blood glucose
3 Rh and ABO blood typing
4 Indirect and direct bilirubin levels

Level of Cognitive Ability: Application
Client Needs: Physiological Integrity
Integrated Process: Nursing Process/Planning
Content Area: Maternity/Postpartum

Answer: 2
Rationale: After birth, the most common problem in the LGA infant is hypoglycemia, especially if the mother is diabetic. At delivery, when the umbilical cord is clamped and cut, maternal blood glucose supply is lost. The newborn continues to produce large amounts of insulin, which depletes the infant's blood glucose within the first hours after birth. If immediate identification and treatment of hypoglycemia is not performed, the newborn may suffer central nervous system damage caused by inadequate circulation of glucose to the brain. Indirect and direct bilirubin levels are usually ordered after the first 24 hours, because jaundice is usually seen at 48 to 72 hours after birth. There is no rationale for ordering an Rh and ABO blood type unless the maternal blood type is "O" or "Rh negative." Serum insulin levels are not helpful, because there is no intervention to decrease these levels to prevent hypoglycemia.

Test-Taking Strategy: Focus on the subject, an LGA infant. Recalling that hypoglycemia is the concern will direct you to option 2. Review care of the LGA infant if you had difficulty with this question.

References
McKinney, E., James, S., Murray, S., & Ashwill, J. (2005). *Maternal-child nursing* (2nd ed., pp. 742, 757). St. Louis: Saunders.
Wong, D., Hockenberry, M., Perry, S., Lowdermilk, D., & Wilson, D. (2006). *Maternal-child nursing care.* (3rd ed., pp. 821-824). St. Louis: Mosby.

357. A nurse is caring for a 30-week gestation client in preterm labor, and the physician orders betamethasone (Celestone) intramuscularly. The client asks the nurse why she is receiving corticosteroids. The nurse tells the client that the betamethasone will:
1 Help stop the labor contractions.
2 Help the baby's lungs mature faster.
3 Prevent the membranes from rupturing.
4 Decrease the incidence of fetal infection.

Level of Cognitive Ability: Application
Client Needs: Physiological Integrity
Integrated Process: Nursing Process/ Implementation
Content Area: Maternity/Intrapartum

Answer: 2
Rationale: Respiratory distress syndrome (RDS) is the most common cause of morbidity and mortality in preterm infants. Betamethasone, a corticosteroid, is administered to enhance fetal lung maturity. The medication's optimal benefits begin 24 hours after initial therapy. Betamethasone does not prevent rupture of the membranes. Betamethasone does not decrease the incidence of fetal infection and can mask signs of infection when the client has premature rupture of the membranes with preterm labor. Even though betamethasone may be given during the time that tocolytic agents are administered, it does not inhibit preterm labor.

Test-Taking Strategy: Use the process of elimination, recalling that betamethasone is a corticosteroid. Noting the strategic word "preterm" may assist in recalling that this medication is administered to enhance fetal lung maturity. Review the action of this medication if you had difficulty with this question.

Reference
McKinney, E., James, S., Murray, S., & Ashwill, J. (2005). *Maternal-child nursing* (2nd ed., pp. 689, 690). St. Louis: Saunders.

---

358. A client receiving parenteral nutrition (PN) through a subclavian catheter suddenly develops dyspnea, tachycardia, cyanosis, and decreased level of consciousness. Which is the best intervention for the nurse to implement for the client?
1 Turn to left side in Trendelenburg's.
2 Obtain a stat oxygen saturation level.
3 Examine the insertion site for redness.
4 Perform a stat fingerstick glucose level.

Level of Cognitive Ability: Analysis
Client Needs: Physiological Integrity
Integrated Process: Nursing Process/Analysis
Content Area: Fundamental Skills

Answer: 1
Rationale: Clinical indicators of air embolism include chest pain, tachycardia, dyspnea, anxiety, feelings of impending doom, cyanosis, and hypotension. Positioning the client in Trendelenburg's and on the left side helps to isolate the air embolism in the right atrium and prevent a thromboembolic event in a vital organ. Monitoring the oxygen saturation is a reasonable nursing response to the client's condition; however, acting to prevent a deterioration in the client's condition is more important than obtaining additional client data. Options 3 and 4 are unrelated to the symptoms identified in the question.

Test-Taking Strategy: Focus on the assessment findings in the question and recall that the signs of air embolism are similar to those experienced with pulmonary embolism. Then analyze the options to determine the option that is the best in this situation, which will direct you to option 1. Review the signs of air embolism if you had difficulty with this question.

Reference
Ignatavicius, D., & Workman, M. (2006). *Medical-surgical nursing: Critical thinking for collaborative care* (5th ed., p. 263). Philadelphia: Saunders.

359. A client has a nursing diagnosis of Excess fluid volume listed on the care plan. Which of the following assessment findings supports continued use of this nursing diagnosis?
1 Weak pulse
2 Bibasilar crackles
3 Decreased blood pressure
4 Flat neck veins with the head of the bed at 45 degrees

Level of Cognitive Ability: Analysis
Client Needs: Physiological Integrity
Integrated Process: Nursing Process/Analysis
Content Area: Adult Health/Cardiovascular

Answer: 2
Rationale: Signs of excess fluid volume include bounding pulse, elevated blood pressure, crackles or other adventitious breath sounds, edema of the sacrum or lower extremities, and neck vein distention with the head of the bed positioned at a 45-degree angle. Other signs may include changes in level of consciousness if fluids shifts are occurring.

Test-Taking Strategy: Focus on the subject, excess fluid volume. Note the strategic words in the question "supports continued use." This tells you that the correct option will be consistent with excess fluid volume. Use basic nursing knowledge of the effects of volume on the cardiovascular and respiratory systems to eliminate options 1, 3, and 4. Review the signs of excess fluid volume if you had difficulty with this question.

References
Black, J., & Hawks, J. (2005). *Medical-surgical nursing: Clinical management for positive outcomes* (7th ed., p. 2496). Philadelphia: Saunders.
Ignatavicius, D., & Workman, M. (2006). *Medical-surgical nursing: Critical thinking for collaborative care* (5th ed., p. 223). Philadelphia: Saunders.

360. A client is experiencing acute cardiac and cerebral symptoms related to excess fluid volume. The nurse implements which of the following measures to increase the client's comfort until specific therapy is ordered by the physician?
1 Measures urine output on an hourly basis
2 Measures intravenous and oral fluid intake
3 Elevates the client's head to at least 45 degrees
4 Administers oxygen at 4 liters per minute by nasal cannula

Level of Cognitive Ability: Application
Client Needs: Physiological Integrity
Integrated Process: Nursing Process/ Implementation
Content Area: Adult Health/Cardiovascular

Answer: 3
Rationale: Elevating the head of the bed to 45 degrees decreases venous return to the heart from the lower body, thus reducing the volume of blood that has to be pumped by the heart. It also promotes venous drainage from the brain, reducing cerebral symptoms. Oxygen is a medication and is not administered without an order. Intake and output should be monitored and recorded to provide current information about the client's volume status. Options 1, 2, and 4 are important measures, although they do not improve the client's comfort.

Test-Taking Strategy: Use the process of elimination, focusing on the subject "increase the client's comfort." This tells you that the correct option is one that directly involves care delivery to the client. With this in mind, eliminate options 1 and 2 because they are assessment measures and will not improve the condition of the client. From the remaining options, note that option 3 identifies the nursing measure. Review care of the client with excess fluid volume if you had difficulty with this question.

Reference
Black, J., & Hawks, J. (2005). *Medical-surgical nursing: Clinical management for positive outcomes* (7th ed., p. 1659). Philadelphia: Saunders.

361. A nurse notes that a client's urinalysis report contains a notation of positive red blood cells (RBCs). The nurse interprets that this finding is unrelated to which of the following items that is part of the client's clinical picture?

1 Diabetes mellitus
2 History of kidney stones
3 Concurrent anticoagulant therapy
4 History of recent blow to the right flank

Level of Cognitive Ability: Analysis
Client Needs: Physiological Integrity
Integrated Process: Nursing Process/Analysis
Content Area: Adult Health/Renal

Answer: 1

Rationale: Hematuria can be caused by trauma to the kidney, such as with blunt trauma to the lower posterior trunk or flank. Kidney stones can cause hematuria because they scrape the endothelial lining of the urinary system. Anticoagulant therapy can cause hematuria as an adverse effect. Diabetes mellitus does not cause hematuria, although it can lead to renal failure from prerenal causes.

Test-Taking Strategy: Use the process of elimination, noting the strategic word "unrelated." Eliminate options 3 and 4, which are most likely to cause RBCs in the urine. From the remaining options, recalling that the scraping of the stones against mucosa could cause minor trauma and bleeding will assist you to eliminate option 2 as well. Thus, diabetes mellitus is the item unrelated to positive RBCs in the urine. Review these causes if you had difficulty with this question.

References

Black, J., & Hawks, J. (2005). *Medical-surgical nursing: Clinical management for positive outcomes* (7th ed., p. 796). Philadelphia: Saunders.

Ignatavicius, D., & Workman, M. (2006). *Medical-surgical nursing: Critical thinking for collaborative care* (5th ed., pp. 1665, 1667). Philadelphia: Saunders.

362. The nurse has an order to ambulate a client with a nephrostomy tube in the hall four times a day. The nurse determines that the safest way to accomplish this while maintaining the integrity of the nephrostomy tube is to:

1 Change the drainage bag to a leg collection bag.
2 Tie the drainage bag to the client's waist while ambulating.
3 Use a walker to hang the drainage bag from while ambulating.
4 Tell the client to hold the drainage bag higher than the level of the bladder.

Level of Cognitive Ability: Analysis
Client Needs: Physiological Integrity
Integrated Process: Nursing Process/Analysis
Content Area: Adult Health/Renal

Answer: 1

Rationale: The safest approach to protect the integrity and safety of the nephrostomy tube with a mobile client is to attach the tube to a leg collection bag. This allows for greater freedom of movement, while preventing accidental disconnection or dislodgment. The drainage bag is kept below the level of the bladder. Option 3 presents the risk of tension or pulling on the nephrostomy tube by the client during ambulation.

Test-Taking Strategy: Use the process of elimination. Note that options 2, 3, and 4 are comparable or alike because they all indicate placing the drainage bag above the level of the bladder. Review care of the client with a nephrostomy tube if you had difficulty with this question.

References

Black, J., & Hawks, J. (2005). *Medical-surgical nursing: Clinical management for positive outcomes* (7th ed., p. 879). Philadelphia: Saunders.

Potter, P., & Perry, A. (2005). *Fundamentals of nursing* (6th ed., pp. 1357-1358). St. Louis: Mosby.

363. A client newly diagnosed with polycystic kidney disease has just finished speaking with the physician about the disorder. The client asks the nurse to explain again what the most serious complication of the disorder might be. In formulating a response, the nurse incorporates the understanding that the most serious complication is:

1 Diabetes insipidus
2 End-stage renal disease (ESRD)
3 Chronic urinary tract infection (UTI)
4 Syndrome of inappropriate antidiuretic hormone secretion (SIADH)

Level of Cognitive Ability: Application
Client Needs: Physiological Integrity
Integrated Process: Nursing Process/Implementation
Content Area: Adult Health/Renal

Answer: 2
Rationale: The most serious complication of polycystic kidney disease is ESRD, which would be managed with dialysis or transplant. There is no reliable way to predict who will ultimately progress to ESRD. Chronic UTIs are the most common complication because of the altered anatomy of the kidney and from development of resistant strains of bacteria. Diabetes insipidus and SIADH secretion are unrelated disorders.

Test-Taking Strategy: Use the process of elimination, noting the strategic words "most serious." Eliminate options 1 and 4 because these imbalances are usually temporary and are amenable to treatment; additionally, they are unrelated to polycystic kidney disease. From the remaining options, focusing on the strategic words will direct you to option 2. Also recalling that ESRD is life-threatening and requires dialysis for treatment will direct you to the correct option. Review the complications of polycystic kidney disease if you had difficulty with this question.

References
Black, J., & Hawks, J. (2005). *Medical-surgical nursing: Clinical management for positive outcomes* (7th ed., p. 938). Philadelphia: Saunders.
Lewis, S., Heitkemper, M., Dirksen, S., O'Brien, P., & Bucher, L. (2007). *Medical-surgical nursing: Assessment and management of clinical problems* (7th ed., p. 1176). St. Louis: Mosby.

364. A nurse is assigned to care for a client who has returned to the nursing unit following left nephrectomy. The nurse places highest priority on obtaining which of the following assessments?

1 Temperature
2 Hourly urine output
3 Ability to turn side to side
4 Tolerance for sips of clear liquids

Level of Cognitive Ability: Application
Client Needs: Physiological Integrity
Integrated Process: Nursing Process/Assessment
Content Area: Adult Health/Renal

Answer: 2
Rationale: Following nephrectomy, it is imperative to measure the urine output on an hourly basis. This is done to monitor the effectiveness of the remaining kidney and to detect renal failure early, if it should occur. The client may also experience significant pain after this surgery, which could impact on the client's ability to reposition, cough, and deep breathe. Therefore, the next most important measurements are vital signs (including temperature), pain level, and bed mobility. Clear liquids are not given until the client has bowel sounds.

Test-Taking Strategy: Use the process of elimination, noting the strategic words "highest priority." Note the relationship between "nephrectomy" in the question and "urine output" in the correct option. Review care of the client following nephrectomy if you had difficulty with this question.

References
Black, J., & Hawks, J. (2005). *Medical-surgical nursing: Clinical management for positive outcomes* (7th ed., p. 930). Philadelphia: Saunders.
Ignatavicius, D., & Workman, M. (2006). *Medical-surgical nursing: Critical thinking for collaborative care* (5th ed., p. 1726). Philadelphia: Saunders.

365. A client with a history of respiratory disease is ambulating with the nurse to the doorway of the hospital room. The client becomes pale and dyspneic. The nurse has the client sit and takes the client's vital signs. The client's respiratory rate is 32 breaths per minute, oxygen saturation is 90%, and the heart rate has increased from 76 to 98 beats per minute. The nurse interprets that this client is experiencing:

1 Activity intolerance
2 Impaired physical mobility
3 Ineffective airway clearance
4 Ineffective breathing pattern

Level of Cognitive Ability: Analysis
Client Needs: Physiological Integrity
Integrated Process: Nursing Process/Analysis
Content Area: Adult Health/Respiratory

Answer: 1
Rationale: Activity intolerance is characterized by exertional dyspnea, adverse changes in blood pressure or heart rate with activity, and fatigue. Ineffective breathing pattern occurs when the rate, timing, depth, or rhythm of breathing is insufficient to maintain optimal ventilation. Ineffective airway clearance occurs when the client is unable to clear his or her own secretions from the airway. Impaired physical mobility occurs when the client is limited in physical movement and has limited muscle strength, range of motion, or coordination.

Test-Taking Strategy: Use the process of elimination and focus on the data in the question. The question does not mention information about the pattern of breathing or secretions, so eliminate options 3 and 4 first. From the remaining options, noting that the item triggering the dyspnea is ambulation guides you to select Activity intolerance over Impaired physical mobility. Review the characteristics of Activity intolerance if you had difficulty with this question.

References
Black, J., & Hawks, J. (2005). *Medical-surgical nursing: Clinical management for positive outcomes* (7th ed., p. 1825). Philadelphia: Saunders.
Ignatavicius, D., & Workman, M. (2006). *Medical-surgical nursing: Critical thinking for collaborative care* (5th ed., pp. 606-607). Philadelphia: Saunders.

---

366. A client with cancer is receiving cisplatin. On assessment of the client, which of the following findings indicates that the client is having an adverse reaction to the medication?

1 Tinnitus
2 Increased appetite
3 Excessive urination
4 Yellow halos in front of the eyes

Level of Cognitive Ability: Analysis
Client Needs: Physiological Integrity
Integrated Process: Nursing Process/Assessment
Content Area: Pharmacology

Answer: 1
Rationale: An adverse reaction related to the administration of cisplatin, an antineoplastic medication, is ototoxicity with hearing loss. The nurse should assess for this adverse reaction when administering this medication. Options 2, 3, and 4 are not adverse reactions to this medication.

Test-Taking Strategy: Focus on the subject, an adverse reaction. Recalling that ototoxicity is an adverse effect will direct you to option 1. Review the effects of this medication and the nursing responsibilities during its administration if you had difficulty with this question.

Reference
Skidmore-Roth, L. (2008). *Mosby's nursing drug reference* (21st ed., pp. 278-279). St. Louis: Mosby.

---

367. A nurse is caring for a client diagnosed as having a psychomotor retarded depression. In this condition, the nurse would expect to note which of the following behaviors in the client?
1 Slowed walking and talking
2 Rapid pacing back and forth
3 Verbalization of increasingly angry feelings
4 Standing statue-like for long periods of time

Answer: 1
Rationale: Slowed walking and talking is a characteristic behavior of a psychomotor retarded depression. The physical symptoms may be explained by the person's pessimistic view of the future, leading to the psychomotor inhibition or vegetative signs typically seen with depressed clients. Options 2 and 3 may occur in any agitated state. Option 4 is behavior more likely seen in schizophrenia.

Level of Cognitive Ability: Analysis
Client Needs: Physiological Integrity
Integrated Process: Nursing Process/Assessment
Content Area: Mental Health

Test-Taking Strategy: Use the process of elimination. The words "psychomotor retarded depression" should assist in eliminating options 2 and 3. From the remaining options, recalling that option 4 is most likely seen in the client with schizophrenia will direct you to option 1. Review the characteristics of this disorder if you had difficulty with this question.

Reference

Varcarolis, E., Carson, V., & Shoemaker, N. (2006). *Foundations of psychiatric mental health nursing* (5th ed., pp. 334, 336). Philadelphia: Saunders.

---

368. It has been 12 hours since the client's delivery of a newborn. The nurse assesses the client for the process of involution and documents that it is progressing normally when palpation of the client's fundus is noted:
1 At the level of the umbilicus
2 One finger breadth below the umbilicus
3 Two finger breadths below the umbilicus
4 Midway between the umbilicus and the symphysis pubis

Level of Cognitive Ability: Application
Client Needs: Physiological Integrity
Integrated Process: Communication and Documentation
Content Area: Maternity/Postpartum

Answer: 1

Rationale: The term "involution" is used to describe the rapid reduction in size and the return of the uterus to a normal condition similar to its nonpregnant state. Immediately following the delivery of the placenta, the uterus contracts to the size of a large grapefruit. The fundus is situated in the midline between the symphysis pubis and the umbilicus. Within 6 to 12 hours after birth, the fundus of the uterus rises to the level of the umbilicus. The top of the fundus remains at the level of the umbilicus for about a day and then descends into the pelvis approximately one finger breadth on each succeeding day.

Test-Taking Strategy: Focus on the subject, 12 hours after birth. Attempt to visualize the process of assessment of involution and the expected finding at this time to answer the question. Review this process if you had difficulty with this question.

Reference

Wong, D., Hockenberry, M., Perry, S., Lowdermilk, D., & Wilson, D. (2006). *Maternal-child nursing care.* (3rd ed., pp. 590-591). St. Louis: Mosby.

---

369. A client with a gastric tumor is scheduled for a subtotal gastrectomy (Billroth II procedure). The nurse explains the procedure to the client and tells the client that the:
1 Proximal end of the distal stomach is anastomosed to the duodenum
2 Entire stomach is removed and the esophagus is anastomosed to the duodenum
3 Lower portion of the stomach is removed and the remainder is anastomosed to the jejunum
4 Antrum of the stomach is removed with the remaining portion anastomosed to the duodenum

Level of Cognitive Ability: Application
Client Needs: Physiological Integrity
Integrated Process: Nursing Process/Implementation
Content Area: Adult Health/Gastrointestinal

Answer: 3

Rationale: In the Billroth II procedure, the lower portion of the stomach is removed and the remainder is anastomosed to the jejunum. The duodenal stump is preserved to permit bile flow to the jejunum. Options 1, 2, and 4 are incorrect descriptions.

Test-Taking Strategy: Use the process of elimination. The word "gastrectomy" indicates removal of the stomach. This should assist in eliminating option 1. From the remaining options, note the word "subtotal," which indicates "lower and a part of." This should direct you to option 3. Review this surgical procedure if you had difficulty with this question.

References

Black, J., & Hawks, J. (2005). *Medical-surgical nursing: Clinical management for positive outcomes* (7th ed., p. 758). Philadelphia: Saunders.
Ignatavicius, D., & Workman, M. (2006). *Medical-surgical nursing: Critical thinking for collaborative care* (5th ed., p. 1298). Philadelphia: Saunders.

370. A client with diabetes mellitus receives Humulin Regular insulin 8 units subcutaneously at 7:30 AM. The nurse would be most alert to signs of hypoglycemia at what time during the day?

1 1:30 PM to 3:30 PM
2 3:30 PM to 5:30 PM
3 11:30 AM to 1:30 PM
4 9:30 AM to 11:30 AM

Level of Cognitive Ability: Analysis
Client Needs: Physiological Integrity
Integrated Process: Nursing Process/Assessment
Content Area: Pharmacology

Answer: 4

Rationale: Humulin Regular insulin is a short-acting insulin. Its onset of action occurs in a half hour and peaks in 2 to 4 hours. Its duration of action is 4 to 6 hours. A hypoglycemic reaction will most likely occur at peak time, which, in this situation, is between 9:30 AM and 11:30 AM.

Test-Taking Strategy: Use the process of elimination and knowledge regarding the onset, peak, and duration of action of Regular insulin to answer this question. Recalling that Regular insulin is a short-acting insulin will direct you to option 4. Review both NPH and Regular insulin if you had difficulty with this question.

Reference
Hodgson, B., & Kizior, R. (2007). *Saunders nursing drug handbook 2007* (pp. 620-622). Philadelphia: Saunders.

371. A nursing student prepares a postoperative plan of care for a client scheduled for hypophysectomy. The registered nurse reviews the plan and informs the nursing student that the plan needs to be corrected if which of the following was noted?

1 Obtain daily weights.
2 Administer mouth care.
3 Monitor intake and output.
4 Encourage coughing and deep breathing.

Level of Cognitive Ability: Application
Client Needs: Physiological Integrity
Integrated Process: Teaching and Learning
Content Area: Leadership/Management

Answer: 4

Rationale: Toothbrushing, sneezing, coughing, nose blowing, and bending are activities that should be avoided postoperatively in the client who underwent a hypophysectomy. These activities interfere with the healing of the incision and can disrupt the graft. Options 1, 2, and 3 are appropriate postoperative interventions.

Test-Taking Strategy: Note the strategic words "the plan needs to be corrected." These words indicate a negative event query and the need to select the option that is an incorrect part of the nursing care plan. Consider the anatomical location of the surgical procedure. Although coughing and deep breathing are usually a normal component of postoperative care, in this situation, coughing is contraindicated. Review care following a hypophysectomy if you had difficulty with this question.

Reference
Ignatavicius, D., & Workman, M. (2006). *Medical-surgical nursing: Critical thinking for collaborative care* (5th ed., p. 1465). Philadelphia: Saunders.

372. A client undergoes a thyroidectomy and the nurse monitors the client for signs of damage to the parathyroid glands postoperatively. Which of the following findings would indicate damage to the parathyroid glands?

1 Neck pain
2 Hoarseness
3 Respiratory distress
4 Tingling around the mouth

Answer: 4

Rationale: The parathyroid glands can be damaged or their blood supply impaired during thyroid surgery. Hypocalcemia and tetany result when parathyroid hormone (PTH) levels decrease. The nurse monitors for complaints of tingling around the mouth or of the toes or fingers and muscular twitching because these are signs of calcium deficiency. Additional later signs of hypocalcemia are positive Chvostek's and Trousseau's signs. Hoarseness and neck pain are expected findings postoperatively. Respiratory distress indicates a complication but is not a sign of damage to the parathyroid glands.

Level of Cognitive Ability: Analysis
Client Needs: Physiological Integrity
Integrated Process: Nursing Process/Assessment
Content Area: Adult Health/Endocrine

Test-Taking Strategy: Focus on the subject, damage to the parathyroid glands. Recalling that hoarseness and neck pain are expected findings postoperatively will assist in eliminating options 1 and 2. From the remaining options, focusing on the subject will assist in eliminating option 3. Also, recalling that hypocalcemia results when PTH levels decrease will assist in directing you to the correct option. Review postoperative care following thyroidectomy and the signs of parathyroid damage if you had difficulty with this question.

Reference
Ignatavicius, D., & Workman, M. (2006). *Medical-surgical nursing: Critical thinking for collaborative care* (5th ed., p. 1487). Philadelphia: Saunders.

---

373. The nurse is performing an admission assessment for a client admitted to the hospital with a diagnosis of Raynaud's disease. The nurse assesses for the symptoms associated with Raynaud's disease by:

1 Checking for a rash on the digits
2 Observing for softening of the nails or nail beds
3 Palpating for a rapid or irregular peripheral pulse
4 Palpating for diminished or absent peripheral pulses

Level of Cognitive Ability: Application
Client Needs: Physiological Integrity
Integrated Process: Nursing Process/Assessment
Content Area: Adult Health/Cardiovascular

Answer: 4
Rationale: Raynaud's disease produces closure of the small arteries in the distal extremities in response to cold, vibration, or external stimuli. Palpation for diminished or absent peripheral pulses checks for interruption of circulation. The nails grow slowly, become brittle or deformed, and heal poorly around the nail beds when infected. Skin changes include hair loss, thinning or tightening of the skin, and delayed healing of cuts or injuries. Although palpation of peripheral pulses is correct, a rapid or irregular pulse would not be noted. Peripheral pulses may be normal, absent, or diminished.

Test-Taking Strategy: Recall the physiological occurrences in Raynaud's disease. Use the ABCs—airway, breathing, and circulation—to direct you to option 4. Review the manifestations associated with this disorder if you had difficulty with this question.

Reference
Ignatavicius, D., & Workman, M. (2006). *Medical-surgical nursing: Critical thinking for collaborative care* (5th ed., p. 811). Philadelphia: Saunders.

---

374. A nurse teaches a postpartum client about observation of lochia. The nurse determines the client's understanding when the client says that on the second day postpartum, the lochia should be:
1 Red
2 Pink
3 White
4 Yellow

Level of Cognitive Ability: Analysis
Client Needs: Health Promotion and Maintenance
Integrated Process: Nursing Process/Evaluation
Content Area: Maternity/Postpartum

Answer: 1
Rationale: The uterus rids itself of the debris that remains after birth through a discharge called "lochia," which is classified according to its appearance and contents. Lochia rubra is dark red in color. It occurs from delivery to 3 days postpartum and contains epithelial cells, erythrocytes, leukocytes, shreds of decidua, and occasionally fetal meconium, lanugo, and vernix caseosa. Lochia serosa is a brownish pink discharge that occurs from days 4 to 10. Lochia alba is a white discharge that occurs from days 10 to 14. Lochia should not be yellow in color or contain large clots; if it does, the cause should be investigated without delay.

Test-Taking Strategy: Use knowledge regarding the characteristics of lochia. Noting the words "second day postpartum" will direct you to option 1. Review the normal postpartum assessment findings if you had difficulty with this question.

Reference
Wong, D., Hockenberry, M., Perry, S., Lowdermilk, D., & Wilson, D. (2006). *Maternal-child nursing care.* (3rd ed., pp. 591-592). St. Louis: Mosby.

375. A nurse is caring for a client with depression who is being treated with a monoamine oxidase inhibitor (MAOI). The nurse who is monitoring the client for hypertensive crisis ensures that which medication is available for administration if a crisis occurs?

1 Furosemide (Lasix)
2 Phentolamine mesylate
3 Metoprolol tartrate (Lopressor)
4 Prazosin hydrochloride (Minipress)

Level of Cognitive Ability: Application
Client Needs: Physiological Integrity
Integrated Process: Nursing Process/Planning
Content Area: Pharmacology

Answer: 2
Rationale: Although all of the medications identified in the options decrease blood pressure, phentolamine acts quickly and is administered intravenously to treat a hypertensive crisis.

Test-Taking Strategy: Use the process of elimination and knowledge of the action and use of these medications. Recalling that phentolamine is rapid-acting will direct you to option 2. Review MAOIs and hypertensive crisis if you had difficulty with this question.

References
Kee, J., Hayes, E., & McCuistion, L. (2006). *Pharmacology: A nursing process approach.* (5th ed., pp. 276, 648). Philadelphia: Saunders.
Skidmore-Roth, L. (2008). *Mosby's nursing drug reference* (21st ed., pp. 278-279). St. Louis: Mosby.

376. A nurse is performing an admission assessment on a newborn infant admitted to the nursery with the diagnosis of subdural hematoma following a difficult vaginal delivery. The nurse assesses for major symptoms associated with subdural hematoma when the nurse:

1 Monitors the urine for blood
2 Monitors the urinary output pattern
3 Tests for contractures of the extremities
4 Tests for equality of extremities when stimulating reflexes

Level of Cognitive Ability: Analysis
Client Needs: Physiological Integrity
Integrated Process: Nursing Process/Assessment
Content Area: Child Health

Answer: 4
Rationale: A subdural hematoma can cause pressure on a specific area of the cerebral tissue. This can cause changes in the stimuli responses in the extremities on the opposite side of the body, especially if the infant is actively bleeding. Option 3 is incorrect because contractures would not occur this soon after delivery. Options 1 and 2 are incorrect. After delivery, an infant would normally be incontinent of urine. Blood in the urine would indicate abdominal trauma and would not be a result of the hematoma.

Test-Taking Strategy: Note the strategic words "major symptoms." Eliminate options 1 and 2 because they are similar assessments. Remember: the method of assessing for complications and active bleeding into the cranial cavity would be a neurological assessment. Checking newborn reflexes is a neurological assessment. Although contractures of extremities could occur as residual effects, this would not occur immediately. Review the signs of subdural hematoma in the newborn infant if you had difficulty with this question.

Reference
Wong, D., Hockenberry, M., Perry, S., Lowdermilk, D., & Wilson, D. (2006). *Maternal-child nursing care.* (3rd ed., p. 832). St. Louis: Mosby.

377. A client has received atropine sulfate pre-operatively. The nurse monitors the client for which of the following effects of the medication in the immediate postoperative period?
1 Diarrhea
2 Bradycardia
3 Urinary retention
4 Excessive salivation

Level of Cognitive Ability: Application
Client Needs: Physiological Integrity
Integrated Process: Nursing Process/ Implementation
Content Area: Pharmacology

Answer: 3
Rationale: Atropine sulfate is an anticholinergic medication that causes tachycardia, drowsiness, blurred vision, dry mouth, constipation, and urinary retention. The nurse monitors the client for any of these effects in the immediate postoperative period.

Test-Taking Strategy: Use the process of elimination. Recalling that atropine sulfate is an anticholinergic will direct you to option 3. Review the side effects of this medication if you had difficulty with this question.

Reference
Skidmore-Roth, L. (2008). *Mosby's nursing drug reference* (21st ed., p. 164). St. Louis: Mosby.

---

378. A client with a fractured femur who has had an open reduction–internal fixation is receiving ketorolac (Toradol). The nurse evaluates the effectiveness of the medication by monitoring the client's:
1 Pain rating
2 Temperature
3 Serum calcium level
4 White blood cell count

Level of Cognitive Ability: Analysis
Client Needs: Physiological Integrity
Integrated Process: Nursing Process/Evaluation
Content Area: Pharmacology

Answer: 1
Rationale: Ketorolac is a nonopioid analgesic and nonsteroidal anti-inflammatory drug (NSAID). It acts by inhibiting prostaglandin synthesis and produces analgesia that is peripherally mediated. The nurse evaluates the effectiveness of this medication by using the pain rating scale with the client. Options 2, 3, and 4 are not related to the action of this medication.

Test-Taking Strategy: Noting the diagnosis of the client, fractured femur, may provide you with the clue that this medication is an analgesic. Review this medication if you had difficulty with this question.

References
Hodgson, B., & Kizior, R. (2007) (p. 660). *Saunders nursing drug handbook 2007.* Philadelphia: Saunders.
Kee, J., Hayes, E., & McCuistion, L. (2006). *Pharmacology: A nursing process approach.* (5th ed., pp. 327, 408). Philadelphia: Saunders.

---

379. A nurse is conducting a health history on a client with hyperparathyroidism. Which of the following questions asked of the client would elicit information about this condition?
1 "Do you have tremors in your hands?"
2 "Are you experiencing pain in your joints?"
3 "Have you had problems with diarrhea lately?"
4 "Do you notice any swelling in your legs at night?"

Answer: 2
Rationale: Hyperparathyroidism causes an oversecretion of parathyroid hormone (PTH), which causes excessive osteoblast growth and activity within the bones. When bone reabsorption is increased, calcium is released from the bones into the blood, causing hypercalcemia. The bones suffer demineralization as a result of calcium loss, leading to bone and joint pain, and pathological fractures. Options 1 and 3 relate to assessment of hypoparathyroidism. Option 4 is unrelated to hyperparathyroidism.

Level of Cognitive Ability: Analysis
Client Needs: Physiological Integrity
Integrated Process: Nursing Process/Assessment
Content Area: Adult Health/Endocrine

Test-Taking Strategy: Knowledge regarding the pathophysiology associated with hyperparathyroidism is required to answer the question. Eliminate options 1 and 3 first because these options provide information about hypoparathyroidism. From the remaining options, it is necessary to know the relationship between hyperparathyroidism, PTH, and joint pain to direct you to option 2. Review this disorder if you had difficulty with this question.

References

Ignatavicius, D., & Workman, M. (2006). *Medical-surgical nursing: Critical thinking for collaborative care* (5th ed., pp. 1493-1494). Philadelphia: Saunders.
Lewis, S., Heitkemper, M., Dirksen, S., O'Brien, P., & Bucher, L. (2007). *Medical-surgical nursing: Assessment and management of clinical problems* (7th ed., p. 1310). St. Louis: Mosby.

---

380. An 18-year-old client seeks medical attention for intermittent episodes in which the fingers of both hands become cold, pale, and numb, followed by redness and swelling and throbbing, achy pain. Raynaud's disease is suspected. The nurse further assesses the client to see if these episodes occur with:
1 Exposure to heat
2 Being in a relaxed environment
3 Ingestion of coffee or chocolate
4 Prolonged episodes of inactivity

Level of Cognitive Ability: Analysis
Client Needs: Physiological Integrity
Integrated Process: Nursing Process/Assessment
Content Area: Adult Health/Cardiovascular

Answer: 3

Rationale: Raynaud's disease is a bilateral form of intermittent arteriolar spasm, which can be classified as obstructive or vasospastic. Episodes are characterized by pallor, cold, numbness, and possible cyanosis of the fingers, followed by erythema, tingling, and aching pain. Attacks are triggered by exposure to cold, nicotine, caffeine, trauma to the fingertips, and stress. Prolonged episodes of inactivity are unrelated to these episodes.

Test-Taking Strategy: Use the process of elimination, focusing on the symptoms identified in the question. Recalling that symptoms occur with vasoconstriction will assist in eliminating options 1, 2, and 4 because these events are unlikely to cause vasoconstriction. Review the characteristics associated with Raynaud's disease if you had difficulty with this question.

Reference

Black, J., & Hawks, J. (2005). *Medical-surgical nursing: Clinical management for positive outcomes* (7th ed., p. 1534). Philadelphia: Saunders.

---

381. The nurse is measuring the vital signs of a client with increased intracranial pressure (ICP). The respirations have a variable rate. The cycle of respirations begins shallowly with an increasing depth to hyperventilation and then decreases in depth to apnea. The cycle then repeats itself. The nurse documents that the client is exhibiting what type of respirations?
1 Bradypnea
2 Tachypnea
3 Kussmaul's respirations
4 Cheyne-Stokes respirations

Answer: 4

Rationale: The client with increased ICP may exhibit Cheyne-Stokes respirations. These types of respirations have a variable rate. The cycle of respirations begins shallowly and then increases in depth to hyperventilation, followed by a decrease in depth to apnea. The cycle then repeats itself. Bradypnea indicates that the rate of breathing is regular but abnormally slow. Tachypnea indicates that the rate of breathing is regular but abnormally rapid (greater than 20 breaths per minute). Kussmaul's respirations are abnormally deep, regular, and increased in rate.

Level of Cognitive Ability: Analysis
Client Needs: Physiological Integrity
Integrated Process: Nursing Process/Assessment
Content Area: Adult Health/Neurological

Test-Taking Strategy: Focus on the description of the respiratory pattern in the question. This will assist in eliminating options 1 and 2. From the remaining options, eliminate option 3, recalling that Kussmaul's respirations are usually noted in diabetic ketoacidosis. Review these types of respiratory pattern if you had difficulty with this question.

References

Black, J., & Hawks, J. (2005). *Medical-surgical nursing: Clinical management for positive outcomes* (7th ed., p. 2192). Philadelphia: Saunders.

Potter, P., & Perry, A. (2005). *Fundamentals of nursing* (6th ed., p. 650). St. Louis: Mosby.

---

382. The ambulatory care nurse is assessing a client with chronic sinusitis. The nurse determines that which manifestation reported by the client is unrelated to this problem?
1 Anosmia
2 Chronic cough
3 Purulent nasal discharge
4 Headache more pronounced in the evening

Level of Cognitive Ability: Analysis
Client Needs: Physiological Integrity
Integrated Process: Nursing Process/Assessment
Content Area: Adult Health/Respiratory

Answer: 4

Rationale: Chronic sinusitis is characterized by persistent purulent nasal discharge, a chronic cough resulting from nasal discharge, anosmia (loss of smell), nasal stuffiness, and headache that is worse upon arising after sleep.

Test-Taking Strategy: Note the strategic word "unrelated." This word indicates that this is a negative event query and the need to select the option that is not a manifestation of chronic sinusitis. Recalling these signs and symptoms will direct you to option 4. Review the manifestations of chronic sinusitis if you had difficulty with this question.

Reference

Ignatavicius, D., & Workman, M. (2006). *Medical-surgical nursing: Critical thinking for collaborative care* (5th ed., pp. 629-630). Philadelphia: Saunders.

---

383. A client who just underwent a tonsillectomy is becoming slightly restless, has an increased pulse rate, and exhibits slight pallor. The nurse notes that the client is swallowing frequently. Which of the following interpretations most appropriately describes the cause of the manifestations noted by the nurse?
1 The client needs pain medication.
2 This is an expected postoperative finding.
3 The client has some mild postoperative edema.
4 The client may have postoperative bleeding or hemorrhage.

Level of Cognitive Ability: Analysis
Client Needs: Physiological Integrity
Integrated Process: Nursing Process/Assessment
Content Area: Adult Health/Respiratory

Answer: 4

Rationale: Signs of postoperative hemorrhage include pallor, restlessness, frequent swallowing, large amounts of bloody drainage or vomitus, an increasing pulse rate, and a falling blood pressure. These signs should be reported to the surgeon. Although restlessness and an increased pulse could result from the presence of pain, these signs along with the others identified in the question indicate postoperative bleeding. These signs are not expected postoperative findings and are not related to the presence of edema.

Test-Taking Strategy: Focus on the signs and symptoms identified in the question to assist in eliminating options 2 and 3. From the remaining options, noting the words "swallowing frequently" will direct you to option 4. Review postoperative complications following tonsillectomy if you had difficulty with this question.

Reference

Black, J., & Hawks, J. (2005). *Medical-surgical nursing: Clinical management for positive outcomes* (7th ed., p. 1799). Philadelphia: Saunders.

384. A client has Impaired verbal communication as a result of a temporary tracheostomy following a laryngectomy. In planning for communication with this client, the nurse would avoid which of the following methods because it would be least helpful for this particular client?
1 Use of a picture board
2 Use of a pencil and paper
3 Use of hand or finger signals
4 Nodding and shaking the head for "yes" and "no"

Level of Cognitive Ability: Application
Client Needs: Physiological Integrity
Integrated Process: Communication and Documentation
Content Area: Adult Health/Respiratory

Answer: 4
Rationale: Following laryngectomy, the client should not be asked to nod or shake the head because it is painful for the client. The use of eye blink or hand or finger signals is acceptable. Other helpful methods include the use of a pencil and paper, a word or picture board, flash cards, or a magic slate.

Test-Taking Strategy: Note the strategic words "avoid" and "least helpful." These strategic words indicate a negative event query and the need to select the option that could be potentially harmful to the client. Eliminate options 1, 2, and 3 because they are comparable or alike and because these client actions involve the use of the hands. Also focusing on the diagnosis and surgical procedure will direct you to option 4. Review care of the client following laryngectomy if you had difficulty with this question.

References
Black, J., & Hawks, J. (2005). *Medical-surgical nursing: Clinical management for positive outcomes* (7th ed., pp. 1788, 1793). Philadelphia: Saunders.
Lewis, S., Heitkemper, M., Dirksen, S., O'Brien, P., & Bucher, L. (2007). *Medical-surgical nursing: Assessment and management of clinical problems* (7th ed., p. 554). St. Louis: Mosby.

---

385. A client with pneumonia has anorexia caused by the effort required for eating while dyspneic and decreased taste sensation. Which of the following actions by the nurse would be most helpful in increasing the client's appetite?
1 Keep fresh water at the bedside
2 Provide three large meals daily
3 Provide mouth care before meals
4 Encourage drinking fluids up to 3 liters per day

Level of Cognitive Ability: Application
Client Needs: Physiological Integrity
Integrated Process: Nursing Process/ Implementation
Content Area: Adult Health/Respiratory

Answer: 3
Rationale: The client with pneumonia may experience decreased taste sensation as a result of sputum expectoration. To minimize this adverse effect, the nurse should provide oral hygiene before meals. The client should also have small, frequent meals because of dyspnea. Increased oral fluids and keeping water at the bedside are good measures to prevent fluid deficit associated with pneumonia, but they do nothing to alleviate anorexia.

Test-Taking Strategy: Use the process of elimination, focusing on the subject—increasing the client's appetite. Eliminate options 1 and 4 because they are comparable or alike and will not increase the client's appetite. From the remaining options, focusing on the subject will direct you to option 3. Review measures that will increase appetite if you had difficulty with this question.

References
Black, J., & Hawks, J. (2005). *Medical-surgical nursing: Clinical management for positive outcomes* (7th ed., p. 1844). Philadelphia: Saunders.
Lewis, S., Heitkemper, M., Dirksen, S., O'Brien, P., & Bucher, L. (2007). *Medical-surgical nursing: Assessment and management of clinical problems* (7th ed., p. 567). St. Louis: Mosby.

---

386. The clinic nurse notes that a large number of clients whose chief complaint is the presence of flulike symptoms are being seen in the clinic. Which of the following recommendations by the nurse is least helpful for these clients?
1 Get plenty of rest.
2 Increase intake of liquids.
3 Get a flu shot immediately.
4 Take antipyretics for fever.

Answer: 3
Rationale: Immunizations against influenza are a prophylactic measure and are not used to treat flu symptoms. Treatment for the flu includes getting rest, drinking fluids, and taking in nutritious foods and beverages. Medications such as antipyretics and analgesics may also be used for symptom management.

Level of Cognitive Ability: Application
Client Needs: Physiological Integrity
Integrated Process: Nursing Process/
   Implementation
Content Area: Adult Health/Respiratory

Test-Taking Strategy: Use the process of elimination, noting the strategic words "least helpful." These words indicate that this is a negative event query and you need to select the option that is an incorrect recommendation. Recalling that a flu shot is a prophylactic measure will assist in directing you to the correct option. Review measures for the client with flu-like symptoms if you had difficulty with this question.

Reference
Ignatavicius, D., & Workman, M. (2006). *Medical-surgical nursing: Critical thinking for collaborative care* (5th ed., p. 633). Philadelphia: Saunders.

---

387. The nurse is beginning to ambulate a client with a nursing diagnosis of Activity intolerance who was admitted to the hospital for bacterial endocarditis. The nurse evaluates that the client is best tolerating the exercise if which of the following parameters is noted by the nurse?
1 Mild dyspnea after walking 10 feet
2 Minimal chest pain rated "1" on the pain scale
3 Pulse rate that increases from 68 to 98 beats per minute
4 Blood pressure that increases from 114/82 to 118/86 mm Hg

Level of Cognitive Ability: Analysis
Client Needs: Physiological Integrity
Integrated Process: Nursing Process/Evaluation
Content Area: Adult Health/Cardiovascular

Answer: 4
Rationale: General indicators that a client is tolerating exercise include an absence of chest pain or dyspnea, a pulse rate increase of less than 20 beats per minute, and a blood pressure change of less than 10 mm Hg.

Test-Taking Strategy: Use the process of elimination, noting the subject—best tolerating the exercise. Eliminate options 1 and 2 first because they represent abnormal data. From the remaining options, note that option 4 reflects the least physiological change as a result of the exercise. Review the defining characteristics of Activity intolerance if you had difficulty with this question.

Reference
Ignatavicius, D., & Workman, M. (2006). *Medical surgical nursing. Critical thinking for collaborative care* (5th ed., p. 760). Philadelphia: Saunders.

---

388. Cardiac monitoring leads are placed on a client who is at risk for premature ventricular contractions (PVCs). The nurse assesses the client's rhythm to detect PVCs by looking for:
1 Wide and bizarre QRS complexes
2 A P wave preceding every QRS complex
3 QRS complexes that are short and narrow
4 Inverted P waves before the QRS complexes

Level of Cognitive Ability: Analysis
Client Needs: Physiological Integrity
Integrated Process: Nursing Process/Assessment
Content Area: Adult Health/Cardiovascular

Answer: 1
Rationale: PVCs are abnormal ectopic beats originating in the ventricles. They are characterized by an absence of P waves, wide and bizarre QRS complexes, and a compensatory pause that follows the ectopy.

Test-Taking Strategy: Use the process of elimination. Remember that PVCs are characterized by wide and bizarre QRS complexes. Review the characteristics of a PVC if you had difficulty with this question.

Reference
Ignatavicius, D., & Workman, M. (2006). *Medical-surgical nursing: Critical thinking for collaborative care* (5th ed., p. 758). Philadelphia: Saunders.

389. A client with angina pectoris is receiving isosorbide mononitrate (Imdur) to promote vasodilation. The client states a dislike for the medication because it causes a headache. The nurse makes which of the following interpretations about the client's statement?

1 This is a common but unhealthy response to the medication.
2 This response is caused by cerebral hypoxia induced by the medication.
3 This is an extremely adverse reaction and should be reported to the physician.
4 This is a common response that will diminish as tolerance to nitroglycerin increases.

Level of Cognitive Ability: Analysis
Client Needs: Physiological Integrity
Integrated Process: Nursing Process/Analysis
Content Area: Adult Health/Cardiovascular

Answer: 4
Rationale: Headache is a common side effect of nitroglycerin because of its vasodilator properties. The incidence of headache diminishes over time as the client develops tolerance to the medication. The client should be encouraged to continue its use as needed and to take acetaminophen (Tylenol) or aspirin for headache, according to the preference of the prescribing physician.

Test-Taking Strategy: Use the process of elimination. Eliminate options 2 and 3 first because of the words "hypoxia" and "extremely adverse." Remember that oral nitrates such as Imdur will dilate vessels and relieve hypoxia to the cardiac tissue. From the remaining options, eliminate option 1 because of the word "unhealthy." Review the side effects related to nitroglycerin if you had difficulty with this question.

Reference
Ignatavicius, D., & Workman, M. (2006). *Medical-surgical nursing: Critical thinking for collaborative care* (5th ed., pp. 263, 855). Philadelphia: Saunders.

---

390. A client is experiencing pulmonary edema as an exacerbation of chronic left-sided heart failure. The nurse assesses the client for which of the following manifestations?

1 Weight loss
2 Bilateral crackles
3 Distended neck veins
4 Peripheral pitting edema

Level of Cognitive Ability: Analysis
Client Needs: Physiological Integrity
Integrated Process: Nursing Process/Assessment
Content Area: Adult Health/Cardiovascular

Answer: 2
Rationale: The client with pulmonary edema presents primarily with symptoms that are respiratory in nature, because the blood flow is stagnant in the lungs, which lie behind the left side of the heart from a circulatory standpoint. The client would experience weight gain from fluid retention, not weight loss. Distended neck veins and peripheral pitting edema are classic signs of right-sided heart failure.

Test-Taking Strategy: Focus on the subject and note the words "left-sided heart failure." Knowing that blood flow is stagnant behind the area of failure allows you to eliminate each of the incorrect options. With heart failure, to remember the signs and symptoms, remember "left, lungs" and "right, systemic." Option 2 relates to the lungs. Review the signs of left– and right–sided heart failure if you had difficulty with this question.

References
Black, J., & Hawks, J. (2005). *Medical-surgical nursing: Clinical management for positive outcomes* (7th ed., p. 1831). Philadelphia: Saunders.
Ignatavicius, D., & Workman, M. (2006). *Medical-surgical nursing: Critical thinking for collaborative care* (5th ed., pp. 748, 750, 761). Philadelphia: Saunders.

---

391. The nurse assesses a client with a triple-lumen catheter. Which is the nurse most likely to observe in a client with an air embolism?

1 Bilateral basilar crackles
2 Diminished breath sounds
3 Systolic click at right sternal border
4 Churning sound over right ventricle

Answer: 4
Rationale: Clients with triple-lumen catheters are at risk for air embolism. Because an air embolism can be fatal, the nurse monitors for chest pain, coughing, hypotension, cyanosis, and hypoxia. In addition, if the client does have an air embolism, auscultation over the right ventricle may reveal a "churning" sound indicating the location of the embolism. Options 1, 2, and 3 are uncharacteristic of an air embolism.

Level of Cognitive Ability: Analysis
Client Needs: Physiological Integrity
Integrated Process: Nursing Process/Assessment
Content Area: Fundamental Skills

Test-Taking Strategy: Use the process of elimination. Note that the subject of the question is "air" embolism. Remembering that fluid (not air) will produce crackles heard in the lung bases will assist you in eliminating option 1. From the remaining options, think about the signs of an embolism to direct you to option 4. Review the signs of an air embolism if you had difficulty with this question.

Reference
Black, J., & Hawks, J. (2005). *Medical-surgical nursing: Clinical management for positive outcomes* (7th ed., p. 1833). Philadelphia: Saunders.

---

392. When administering an intramuscular injection in the dorsogluteal muscle, the nurse places the client in which position to relax the muscle?
   1 Standing at the bedside
   2 Prone with a toe-in position
   3 Side-lying with a toe-in position
   4 Lateral while flexing the lower most leg

Level of Cognitive Ability: Application
Client Needs: Physiological Integrity
Integrated Process: Nursing Process/
   Implementation
Content Area: Fundamental Skills

Answer: 2
Rationale: A prone toe-in position promotes internal rotation of the hip, relaxes the muscle, and makes the injection less painful. The client can also be positioned on the side with the top leg flexed and in front of the lower leg. Options 1, 3, and 4 are incorrect positions for administering an intramuscular injection because they do not promote muscle relaxation.

Test-Taking Strategy: Note the strategic words "relax the muscle." Visualize each position described in the options to direct you to option 2. Review this procedure if you are unfamiliar with the position for administering intramuscular medications.

Reference
Perry, A., & Potter, P. (2006). *Clinical nursing skills & techniques* (6th ed., p. 728). St. Louis: Mosby.

---

393. The nurse prepares to administer an intravenous (IV) medication when the nurse notes that the medication is incompatible with the IV solution. Which is the best intervention for the nurse to implement for safe medication administration?
   1 Ask the provider to prescribe a compatible IV solution.
   2 Start a new IV catheter for the incompatible medication.
   3 Collaborate with provider for a new administration route.
   4 Flush tubing before and after the medication with normal saline.

Level of Cognitive Ability: Application
Client Needs: Physiological Integrity
Integrated Process: Nursing Process/
   Implementation
Content Area: Fundamental Skills

Answer: 4
Rationale: When giving a medication intravenously, if the medication is incompatible with the IV solution, the tubing is flushed before and after the medication with infusions of normal saline to prevent in-line precipitation of the incompatible agents. Starting a new IV, changing the solution, or changing the administration route are unnecessary because a simpler, less risky, viable option exists.

Test-Taking Strategy: Use the process of elimination. You can eliminate options 1, 2, and 3 because they are unnecessary; in addition, option 2 increases the risk of infection and is likely to cause the client discomfort. Remember that normal saline is physiologically similar to body fluid. Review the procedures for administering IV medications if you had difficulty with this question.

Reference
Potter, P., & Perry, A. (2005). *Fundamentals of nursing* (6th ed., p. 898). St. Louis: Mosby.

394. A nurse is preparing to administer ear-drops to an infant. The nurse plans to:

1 Pull down and back on the auricle and direct the solution onto the eardrum.
2 Pull up and back on the earlobe and direct the solution toward the wall of the ear canal.
3 Pull up and back on the auricle and direct the solution toward the wall of the ear canal.
4 Pull down and back on the earlobe and direct the solution toward the wall of the ear canal.

Level of Cognitive Ability: Application
Client Needs: Physiological Integrity
Integrated Process: Nursing Process/
 Implementation
Content Area: Pharmacology

Answer: 4
Rationale: The infant should be turned on the side with the affected ear uppermost. With the nondominant hand, the nurse pulls down and back on the earlobe. The wrist of the dominant hand is rested on the infant's head. The medication is administered by aiming it at the wall of the ear canal rather than directly onto the eardrum. The infant should be held or positioned with the affected ear uppermost for 10 to 15 minutes to retain the solution. In the adult, the auricle is pulled up and back to straighten the auditory canal.

Test-Taking Strategy: Basic safety principles related to the administration of ear medications should assist in eliminating option 1. Option 2 is eliminated because it is the adult procedure. It would be difficult to pull up and back on an earlobe; therefore, eliminate option 3. Review the procedure for administering ear medications in an infant and adult if you had difficulty with this question.

References
Hockenberry, M. & Wilson, D. (2007). *Nursing care of infants and children* (8th ed., pp. 1129-1130). St. Louis: Mosby.
Hodgson, B., & Kizior, R. (2007). *Saunders nursing drug handbook 2007* (p. 1304). Philadelphia: Saunders.
Wong, D., Hockenberry, M., Perry, S., Lowdermilk, D., & Wilson, D. (2006). *Maternal-child nursing care.* (3rd ed., pp. 1402-1403). St. Louis: Mosby.

---

395. A client seeks treatment in an ambulatory clinic for a complaint of hoarseness that has persisted for 8 weeks. Based on the symptom, the nurse interprets that the client is at risk of having:

1 Thyroid cancer
2 Acute laryngitis
3 Laryngeal cancer
4 Bronchogenic cancer

Level of Cognitive Ability: Analysis
Client Needs: Physiological Integrity
Integrated Process: Nursing Process/Analysis
Content Area: Adult Health/Respiratory

Answer: 3
Rationale: Hoarseness is a common early sign of laryngeal cancer, but not of bronchogenic or thyroid cancer. Hoarseness that persists for 8 weeks is not associated with an acute problem, such as laryngitis.

Test-Taking Strategy: Use the process of elimination. Begin to answer this question by eliminating option 2, because an acute problem would not generally last for 8 weeks. From the remaining options, recalling that the vocal cords are in the larynx makes option 3 preferable to any of the other options. Review the signs of laryngeal cancer if you had difficulty with this question.

Reference
Ignatavicius, D., & Workman, M. (2006). *Medical-surgical nursing: Critical thinking for collaborative care* (5th ed., p. 572). Philadelphia: Saunders.

---

396. A client is admitted to the cardiac intensive care unit following cardiac surgery. The nurse notes that in the first hour after admission, the mediastinal chest tube drainage was 75 mL. During the second hour, the drainage has dropped to 5 mL. The nurse interprets that:

1 This is normal.
2 The tube may be occluded.
3 The lung has fully reexpanded.
4 The client needs to cough and deep breathe.

Answer: 2
Rationale: Chest tube drainage should not exceed 100 mL per hour during the first 2 hours postoperatively, and approximately 500 mL of drainage is expected in the first 24 hours after cardiac surgery. The sudden drop in drainage between the first and second hour indicates that the tube is possibly occluded and requires further assessment by the nurse. Options 1, 3, and 4 are incorrect interpretations.

Level of Cognitive Ability: Analysis
Client Needs: Physiological Integrity
Integrated Process: Nursing Process/Analysis
Content Area: Adult Health/Cardiovascular

Test-Taking Strategy: Use the process of elimination. Eliminate option 3 first because the mediastinal chest tubes remove fluid from the mediastinum and are unrelated to restoration of negative pleural pressure. Needing to cough and deep breathe is a response that is unrelated to the client's problem, so option 4 is eliminated next. From the remaining options, knowing that the drainage would not drop so radically in 1 hour in the immediate postoperative period directs you to option 2. Review the concepts related to chest tube drainage systems in the postoperative cardiac surgery client if you had difficulty with this question.

References

Black, J., & Hawks, J. (2005). *Medical-surgical nursing: Clinical management for positive outcomes* (7th ed., pp. 308-309). Philadelphia: Saunders.

Ignatavicius, D., & Workman, M. (2006). *Medical-surgical nursing: Critical thinking for collaborative care* (5th ed., p. 346). Philadelphia: Saunders.

---

397. The nurse is auscultating the chest of a client who was diagnosed with pleurisy 48 hours ago. The client does not have a pleural friction rub, which was auscultated the previous day. The nurse interprets that this is most likely the result of:
1 Effectiveness of medication therapy
2 Deep breaths that the client is taking
3 Decreased inflammatory reaction at the site
4 Accumulation of pleural fluid in the inflamed area

Level of Cognitive Ability: Analysis
Client Needs: Physiological Integrity
Integrated Process: Nursing Process/Analysis
Content Area: Adult Health/Respiratory

Answer: 4

Rationale: Pleural friction rub is auscultated early in the course of pleurisy, before pleural fluid accumulates. Once fluid accumulates in the inflamed area, there is less friction between the visceral and parietal lung surfaces, and the pleural friction rub disappears. Options 1, 2, and 3 are incorrect interpretations.

Test-Taking Strategy: Use the process of elimination. Eliminate option 2 first, because it would intensify the pain. Options 1 and 3 are comparable or alike, and because the question states that the problem was diagnosed 48 hours ago, these should be eliminated next. Remember that fluid accumulation in the area provides a buffer between the lung and chest wall surfaces, which eliminates the friction rub. Review assessment findings in the client with pleurisy if you had difficulty with this question.

References

Black, J., & Hawks, J. (2005). *Medical-surgical nursing: Clinical management for positive outcomes* (7th ed., pp. 1564-1565, 1756, 1872). Philadelphia: Saunders.

Ignatavicius, D., & Workman, M. (2006). *Medical-surgical nursing: Critical thinking for collaborative care* (5th ed., pp. 635-636). Philadelphia: Saunders.

---

398. A client is admitted to the nursing unit with a diagnosis of pleurisy. The nurse assesses the client for which characteristic symptom of this disorder?
1 Early morning fatigue
2 Dyspnea that is relieved by lying flat
3 Pain that worsens when the breath is held
4 Knifelike pain that worsens on inspiration

Answer: 4

Rationale: A typical symptom of pleurisy is knifelike pain that worsens on inspiration caused by the friction created by the rubbing together of inflamed pleural surfaces. This pain usually disappears when the breath is held, because these surfaces stop moving. The client does not experience early morning fatigue or dyspnea relieved by lying flat.

Level of Cognitive Ability: Application
Client Needs: Physiological Integrity
Integrated Process: Nursing Process/Assessment
Content Area: Adult Health/Respiratory

Test-Taking Strategy: Use the process of elimination. Option 2 is eliminated first because dyspnea is not relieved by lying flat. Option 1 is eliminated next because fatigue, if it were to occur, would not be present in the morning when the client is most well rested. From the remaining options, keep in mind that pleurisy results from inflammation of the pleura. Because the visceral and parietal lung pleura glide over one another with respiration, it is expected that chest movement precipitates or intensifies the pain. Review the symptoms associated with pleurisy if you had difficulty with this question.

References
Ignatavicius, D., & Workman, M. (2006). *Medical-surgical nursing: Critical thinking for collaborative care* (5th ed., p. 636). Philadelphia: Saunders.
Lewis, S., Heitkemper, M., Dirksen, S., O'Brien, P., & Bucher, L. (2007). *Medical-surgical nursing: Assessment and management of clinical problems* (7th ed., p. 597). St. Louis: Mosby.

---

399. A client has frequent runs of ventricular tachycardia, and the physician prescribes flecainide (Tambocor). Because of the effects of the medications, the nurse does which of the following?
1 Monitors the client's urinary output
2 Assesses the client for neurological problems
3 Ensures that the bed rails remain in the up position
4 Monitors the client's vital signs (BP) and ECG frequently

Level of Cognitive Ability: Analysis
Client Needs: Physiological Integrity
Integrated Process: Nursing Process/ Implementation
Content Area: Pharmacology

Answer: 4
Rationale: Flecainide is an antidysrhythmic medication that slows conduction and decreases excitability, conduction velocity, and automaticity. The nurse needs to monitor for the development of a new or a worsening dysrhythmia. Options 1, 2, and 3 are components of standard care but are not specific to this medication.

Test-Taking Strategy: Use the process of elimination. Note the relation of the information in the question (client has a dysrhythmia) and the nursing action in the correct option. Option 4 is the only option that relates to cardiac status monitoring. Review this medication if you had difficulty with this question.

References
Kee, J., Hayes, E., & McCuistion, L. (2006). *Pharmacology: A nursing process approach.* (5th ed., pp. 620, 623). Philadelphia: Saunders.
Lehne, R. (2007). *Pharmacology for nursing care* (6th ed., p. 536). Philadelphia: Saunders.

---

400. The nurse is performing an assessment on a client with the diagnosis of Brown-Séquard syndrome. Which finding should the nurse expect to note?
1 Bilateral loss of pain and temperature sensation
2 Ipsilateral paralysis and loss of touch and vibration
3 Contralateral paralysis and loss of touch sensation and vibration
4 Complete paraplegia or quadriplegia, depending on the level of injury

Answer: 2
Rationale: Brown-Séquard syndrome results from hemisection of the spinal cord, resulting in ipsilateral paralysis and loss of touch, pressure, vibration, and proprioception. Contralaterally, pain and temperature sensation is lost because these fibers decussate after entering the cord. Options 1, 3, and 4 are not assessment findings in this syndrome.

Test-Taking Strategy: Recalling that Brown-Séquard syndrome results from hemisection of the spinal cord will assist in eliminating options 1 and 4. From the remaining options, it is necessary to know that it results in ipsilateral paralysis and loss of touch, pressure, vibration, and proprioception. Review the assessment findings and the nursing care if you are unfamiliar with this syndrome.

Level of Cognitive Ability: Analysis
Client Needs: Physiological Integrity
Integrated Process: Nursing Process/Assessment
Content Area: Adult Health/Neurological

Reference
Ignatavicius, D., & Workman, M. (2006). *Medical-surgical nursing: Critical thinking for collaborative care* (5th ed., p. 985). Philadelphia: Saunders.

---

401. A nurse is performing an assessment on a client who has a suspected spinal cord injury. Which of the following is the priority nursing assessment?
1 Pain level
2 Mobility level
3 Respiratory status
4 Pupillary response

Level of Cognitive Ability: Application
Client Needs: Physiological Integrity
Integrated Process: Nursing Process/Assessment
Content Area: Delegating/Prioritizing

Answer: 3
Rationale: All of these assessments would be performed on a client with a suspected spinal cord injury. However, respiratory status is the priority.

Test-Taking Strategy: Use the ABCs—airway, breathing, and circulation—to answer the question. Option 3 addresses airway. Review care of the client with a suspected spinal cord injury if you had difficulty with this question.

Reference
Ignatavicius, D., & Workman, M. (2006). *Medical-surgical nursing: Critical thinking for collaborative care* (5th ed., pp. 987-988). Philadelphia: Saunders.

---

402. The nurse is caring for a client who is newly diagnosed with a spinal cord injury. The nurse would anticipate that the most likely medication to be prescribed would be:
1 Morphine sulfate
2 Furosemide (Lasix)
3 Propranolol (Inderal)
4 Methylprednisolone sodium succinate (Solu-Medrol)

Level of Cognitive Ability: Analysis
Client Needs: Physiological Integrity
Integrated Process: Nursing Process/Analysis
Content Area: Adult Health/Neurological

Answer: 4
Rationale: The most likely medication to be prescribed for a client with a newly diagnosed spinal cord injury is methylprednisolone sodium succinate (Solu-Medrol). This medication is a short-acting glucocorticoid and would be administered to reduce traumatic edema. If administered, it should be given within 8 hours of injury. The use of morphine sulfate (an opioid analgesic), furosemide (a diuretic), or propranolol (a beta-blocker) would not be indicated based on the information in this question.

Test-Taking Strategy: Note the strategic words "newly diagnosed" and the diagnosis "spinal cord injury." Recalling the association between injury and edema and that methylprednisolone sodium succinate is used to reduce traumatic edema will assist you in answering the question. Review this content if you are unfamiliar with these medications or the treatment for spinal cord injury.

References
Black, J., & Hawks, J. (2005). *Medical-surgical nursing: Clinical management for positive outcomes* (7th ed., p. 1165). Philadelphia: Saunders.
Hodgson, B., & Kizior, R. (2007). *Saunders nursing drug handbook 2007* (p. 334). Philadelphia: Saunders.
Ignatavicius, D., & Workman, M. (2006). *Medical-surgical nursing: Critical thinking for collaborative care* (5th ed., p. 1052). Philadelphia: Saunders.

403. The nurse is admitting a client with a diagnosis of acquired immunodeficiency syndrome (AIDS) to the medical-surgical unit. The nurse most importantly assesses for which of the following?
1 Bradypnea
2 Jaundiced skin
3 Urine specific gravity of 1.010
4 White patches in the oral cavity

Level of Cognitive Ability: Analysis
Client Needs: Physiological Integrity
Integrated Process: Nursing Process/Assessment
Content Area: Adult Health/Immune

Answer: 4
Rationale: Clients with AIDS frequently develop opportunistic infections. *Candida albicans*, the causative organism of thrush, is a common opportunistic infection. Thrush presents as white patches in the oral cavity. Hairy leukoplakia also presents as white patches in the oral cavity. Clients with AIDS frequently acquire pneumonia and may present with tachypnea, not bradypnea. Jaundice is a symptom of hepatic disease. Clients with AIDS frequently have inadequate nutrition and hydration and may present with dehydration, resulting in a high specific gravity rather than a low specific gravity.

Test-Taking Strategy: Focus on the client's diagnosis. Recalling that the client with AIDS is at risk for developing an infection will direct you to option 4. Review the manifestations associated with AIDS if you had difficulty with this question.

References
Black, J., & Hawks, J. (2005). *Medical-surgical nursing: Clinical management for positive outcomes* (7th ed., pp. 1419, 2389). Philadelphia: Saunders.
Ignatavicius, D., & Workman, M. (2006). *Medical-surgical nursing: Critical thinking for collaborative care* (5th ed., pp. 1248-1249). Philadelphia: Saunders.

404. The nurse assesses a client who was involved in a motor vehicle accident. The nurse determines the need to prepare for chest tube insertion if the client exhibits:
1 Chest pain and shortness of breath
2 Peripheral cyanosis and hypotension
3 Shortness of breath and tracheal deviation
4 Decreasing oxygen saturation and bradypnea

Level of Cognitive Ability: Analysis
Client Needs: Physiological Integrity
Integrated Process: Nursing Process/Analysis
Content Area: Adult Health/Respiratory

Answer: 3
Rationale: Shortness of breath and tracheal deviation result when lung tissue and alveoli have collapsed. The trachea deviates to the unaffected side in the presence of a tension pneumothorax. Air entering the pleural cavity causes the lung to lose its normal negative pressure. The increasing pressure in the affected side displaces contents to the unaffected side. Shortness of breath results from a decreased area available for diffusion of gases. Chest pain and shortness of breath are more commonly associated with myocardial ischemia or infarction. Clients requiring chest tubes exhibit decreasing oxygen saturation but will more likely experience tachypnea related to the hypoxia. Peripheral cyanosis is caused by circulatory disorders. Hypotension may be a result of tracheal shift and impedance of venous return to the heart. However, it may also be the result of other problems such as a failing heart.

Test-Taking Strategy: Focus on the subject—preparation for chest tube insertion. Recalling the signs of a tension pneumothorax and noting the words "tracheal deviation" will direct you to option 3. Review the signs associated with tension pneumothorax and the conditions that require chest tube drainage if you had difficulty with this question.

Reference
Black, J., & Hawks, J. (2005). *Medical-surgical nursing: Clinical management for positive outcomes* (7th ed., p. 1904). Philadelphia: Saunders.

405. A nurse is admitting a client to the mental health unit who has a diagnosis of bipolar disorder, manic phase. In assessing the client regarding sleep patterns and the need for rest, the nurse knows that the most reliable information may be obtained by:
1 Asking the client how he slept last night
2 Observing the facial appearance of the client
3 Asking the significant other about sleep patterns
4 Asking the client to describe in detail his level of fatigue

Level of Cognitive Ability: Analysis
Client Needs: Physiological Integrity
Integrated Process: Nursing Process/Assessment
Content Area: Mental Health

Answer: 3

Rationale: Option 3 would provide the most reliable information because the client may not be able to report sleep patterns accurately. The client may report that sleep has not been a problem when in fact only 3 hours of sleep have been obtained for the last several days. Rest needs are very important because the manic client may be at the point of exhaustion by the time hospitalization occurs. Facial expressions may be an indicator of fatigue, but they are not quantifiable. The client may not be able to describe the level of fatigue accurately.

Test-Taking Strategy: Use the process of elimination, focusing on the words "most reliable." Eliminate options 1 and 4 because they are comparable or alike and require data collection from the client. From the remaining options, focus on the strategic words. In this situation, the significant other is the only one who can provide accurate information. Review assessment of the client with bipolar disorder if you had difficulty with this question.

Reference

Stuart, G., & Laraia, M. (2005). *Principles and practice of psychiatric nursing* (8th ed., pp. 244, 347). St. Louis: Mosby.

---

406. The parents of a male newborn who is not circumcised request information on how to clean the newborn's penis. The nurse tells the parents to:
1 Retract the foreskin and cleanse the glans with every diaper change.
2 Retract the foreskin and cleanse the glans when bathing the newborn.
3 Avoid retracting the foreskin to cleanse the glans because this may cause adhesions.
4 Retract the foreskin no farther than it will go and replace it over the glans after cleaning.

Level of Cognitive Ability: Application
Client Needs: Physiological Integrity
Integrated Process: Teaching and Learning
Content Area: Child Health

Answer: 3

Rationale: In newborn males, prepuce is continuous with the epidermis of the glans and is nonretractable. Forced retraction may cause adhesions to develop. It is best to allow separation to occur naturally, which will happen between 3 years and puberty. Most foreskins are retractable by 3 years of age and should be pushed back gently for cleaning once a week. Therefore, option 3 is correct.

Test-Taking Strategy: Eliminate options 1, 2, and 4 because they are comparable or alike and are incorrect because retracting the foreskin is not recommended in an uncircumcised newborn male. Option 3 is the different option, stating that the foreskin should not be retracted. Review parent teaching points related to the care of an uncircumcised newborn if you had difficulty with this question.

Reference

McKinney, E., James, S., Murray, S., & Ashwill, J. (2005). *Maternal-child nursing* (2nd ed., p. 564). St. Louis: Saunders.

407. The client who has been receiving intravenous (IV) theophylline has been prescribed an immediate-release oral form of the medication. The IV medication is to be discontinued. The nurse should administer the first dose of the oral medication:

1 Just after the next meal
2 Just before the next meal
3 Immediately upon discontinuing the IV form
4 In 4 to 6 hours after discontinuing the IV form

Level of Cognitive Ability: Application
Client Needs: Physiological Integrity
Integrated Process: Nursing Process/
   Implementation
Content Area: Pharmacology

Answer: 4
Rationale: With an immediate-release preparation, the oral theophylline should be administered in 4 to 6 hours after discontinuing the IV form of the medication. If the sustained-release form is used, the first oral dose should be administered immediately upon discontinuation of the IV infusion.

Test-Taking Strategy: Use the process of elimination. Eliminate options 1 and 2 because they do not provide information about when the client will eat his or her next meal. Next, note the strategic words "immediate-release." It then makes sense to wait 4 to 6 hours before administration of the oral form. Review this medication and its methods of administration if you had difficulty with this question.

Reference
Lehene, R. (2007). *Pharmacology for nursing care* (6th ed., pp. 873, 882). Philadelphia: Saunders.

---

408. A nurse finds that the client's serum sodium level is 129 mEq/L. Which does the nurse implement to restore the client's fluid and electrolyte balance gradually?

1 Administer a loop diuretic.
2 Provide a 2-gram sodium diet.
3 Provide a 4-gram sodium diet.
4 Place client on fluid restriction.

Level of Cognitive Ability: Application
Client Needs: Physiological Integrity
Integrated Process: Nursing Process/
   Implementation
Content Area: Fundamental Skills

Answer: 4
Rationale: A serum sodium level of less than 135 mEq/L means that the client is hyponatremic; when it is due to hypervolemia, hyponatremia is the result of hemodilution. Thus, a fluid restriction is indicated to restore fluid and electrolyte balance gradually by increasing the relative serum sodium level as the client excretes water. Option 1 is unlikely to restore fluid and electrolyte balance because loop diuretics excrete sodium and water; in addition, the fluid shifts are likely to occur within hours instead of gradually. A 2-gram sodium diet is a sodium-restricted diet and a 4-gram sodium diet is a no-added-salt diet; both diets are unlikely to increase the serum sodium.

Test-Taking Strategy: Use the process of elimination. Note that the serum sodium level is below normal and the strategic word "gradually." With this in mind, eliminate options 2 and 3. Next, eliminate option 1 because the action of a loop diuretic is fairly rapid. Knowing that hypervolemia causes hemodilution of the serum sodium would guide you to select option 4. Review treatment measures for hyponatremia if you had difficulty with this question.

References
Black, J., & Hawks, J. (2005). *Medical-surgical nursing: Clinical management for positive outcomes* (7th ed., p. 226). Philadelphia: Saunders.
Monahan, F., Sands, J., Neighbors, M., Marek, J., & Green, C. (2007). *Phipps' medical-surgical nursing: Health and illness perspectives* (8th ed., pp. 371-374). St. Louis: Mosby.

409. The nurse is planning care for a client whose oxygenation is being monitored by a pulse oximeter. The nurse includes which intervention in the plan to ensure accurate monitoring of the client's oxygenation status?
1 Instruct the client not to move the sensor.
2 Tape the sensor tightly to the client's finger.
3 Place the sensor on a finger below the blood pressure cuff.
4 Notify the physician immediately of O_2 saturation less than 90%.

Level of Cognitive Ability: Application
Client Needs: Physiological Integrity
Integrated Process: Nursing Process/Planning
Content Area: Adult Health/Respiratory

Answer: 1
Rationale: The pulse oximeter passes a beam of light through the tissue, and a sensor attached to the fingertip, toe, or earlobe measures the amount of light absorbed by the oxygen-saturated hemoglobin. The oximeter then gives a reading of the percentage of hemoglobin that is saturated with oxygen (Sao_2). Motion at the sensor site changes light absorption. The motion mimics the pulsatile motion of blood, and because the detector cannot distinguish between movement of blood and movement of the finger, results can be inaccurate. The sensor should not be placed distal to blood pressure cuffs, pressure dressings, arterial lines, or any invasive catheters. The sensor should not be taped to the client's finger. If values fall below preset norms (usually 90%), the client should be instructed to deep breathe, if this is appropriate. It is not necessary to call the physician immediately unless measures such as deep breathing do not raise the level back to normal.

Test-Taking Strategy: Focus on the subject—to ensure accurate monitoring. Eliminate option 4 because of the word "immediately." Additionally, option 4 is unrelated to ensuring accurate monitoring with a pulse oximeter. Option 3 is inappropriate; therefore, eliminate this option. From the remaining options, recalling that motion at the sensor site changes light absorption and noting the word "tightly" in option 2 will direct you to the correct option. Review the principles associated with pulse oximetry if you had difficulty with this question.

Reference
Potter, P., & Perry, A. (2005). *Fundamentals of nursing* (6th ed., pp. 651-652). St. Louis: Mosby.

---

410. The nurse teaches a client with thromboangiitis obliterans (Buerger's disease) about measures to control the disease process. The nurse determines that the client needs further instructions about these measures if the client states which of the following?
1 "I need to stop smoking immediately."
2 "I need to keep my legs and arms cool."
3 "I will need to take nifedipine (Procardia) as directed."
4 "I need to watch for signs and symptoms of skin breakdown."

Level of Cognitive Ability: Analysis
Client Needs: Physiological Integrity
Integrated Process: Teaching and Learning
Content Area: Adult Health/Cardiovascular

Answer: 2
Rationale: Interventions are directed at preventing the progression of thromboangiitis obliterans and include conveying the need for immediate smoking cessation, providing medications prescribed for vasodilation, such as nifedipine (Procardia), a calcium channel blocker, or prazosin (Minipress), an α-adrenergic blocker. The client should maintain warmth to the extremities, especially by avoiding exposure to cold. The client should inspect the extremities and report signs of infection or ulceration.

Test-Taking Strategy: Note the strategic words "needs further instructions." These words indicate a negative event query and the need to select the option that is an incorrect client statement. Because the goals of care for thromboangiitis obliterans are the same as for peripheral arterial disease, the answer to this question is the one that does not promote vasodilation, option 2. Review home care measures for the client with thromboangiitis obliterans if you had difficulty with this question.

References
Black, J., & Hawks, J. (2005). *Medical-surgical nursing: Clinical management for positive outcomes* (7th ed., p. 1534). Philadelphia: Saunders.
Ignatavicius, D., & Workman, M. (2006). *Medical-surgical nursing: Critical thinking for collaborative care* (5th ed., p. 810). Philadelphia: Saunders.

411. A client has been admitted to the mental health unit with a diagnosis of social phobia disorder. Which behavior would the nurse expect the client to report during the assessment?

1 Panic attack when leaving the house
2 Shortness of breath when riding the elevator
3 Persistent handwashing before and after eating
4 Fear of embarrassing himself in front of others

Level of Cognitive Ability: Analysis
Client Needs: Physiological Integrity
Integrated Process: Nursing Process/Assessment
Content Area: Mental Health

Answer: 4
Rationale: A social phobia is characterized by a fear of appearing incompetent in the presence of others and of doing something embarrassing. Thus, the client becomes anxious when the attention is on him. Option 1 identifies agoraphobia. Option 2 identifies claustrophobia. Option 3 identifies obsessive-compulsive behavior.

Test-Taking Strategy: Focus on the strategic words "social phobia." Note the relationship between these words and option 4. Review the characteristics of the various phobias if you had difficulty with this question.

Reference
Stuart, G., & Laraia, M. (2005). *Principles and practice of psychiatric nursing* (8th ed., p. 271). St. Louis: Mosby.

---

412. A nurse is caring for a client with Parkinson's disease who is taking benztropine mesylate (Cogentin) orally daily. The nurse does which of the following to assess for a side effect of the medication?

1 Checks pupillary response
2 Monitors intake and output
3 Monitors the prothrombin time (PT)
4 Checks the partial thromboplastin time (PTT)

Level of Cognitive Ability: Application
Client Needs: Physiological Integrity
Integrated Process: Nursing Process/Assessment
Content Area: Pharmacology

Answer: 2
Rationale: Urinary retention is a side effect of benztropine mesylate. The nurse needs to monitor the client's intake and output and observe for dysuria, distended abdomen, infrequent voiding of small amounts, and overflow incontinence. Options 1, 3, and 4 are unrelated to the side effects of this medication.

Test-Taking Strategy: Use the process of elimination. Eliminate options 3 and 4 first because they are comparable or alike. From the remaining options, it is necessary to know that urinary retention is a concern with this medication. Review this medication and its side effects if you had difficulty with this question.

Reference
Skidmore-Roth, L. (2008). *Mosby's nursing drug reference* (21st ed., p. 178). St. Louis: Mosby.

---

413. The home care nurse is assessing a client who has begun using peritoneal dialysis. The nurse determines that which manifestation noted in the client would most likely indicate the onset of peritonitis?

1 Cloudy dialysate output
2 Temperature of 99.0°F oral
3 Presence of crystals in dialysate output
4 History of gastrointestinal (GI) upset 1 week ago

Level of Cognitive Ability: Analysis
Client Needs: Physiological Integrity
Integrated Process: Nursing Process/Assessment
Content Area: Adult Health/Renal

Answer: 1
Rationale: Typical symptoms of peritonitis include fever, nausea, malaise, rebound abdominal tenderness, and cloudy dialysate output. The very slight temperature elevation in option 2 is not the clearest indicator of infection. Peritonitis would cause cloudy dialysate but would not cause crystals to appear in the dialysate. The complaint of GI upset is too vague to indicate peritonitis.

Test-Taking Strategy: Note the strategic words "most likely" and the subject—indicator of peritonitis. Begin to answer this question by eliminating options 2 and 4 because both of these manifestations are nonspecific. From the remaining options, recall that infection would cause white blood cells to be present in the dialysate, which would yield cloudiness, not crystals, in the dialysate output. Review the signs of peritonitis in the client receiving peritoneal dialysis if you had difficulty with this question.

Reference
Ignatavicius, D., & Workman, M. (2006). *Medical-surgical nursing: Critical thinking for collaborative care* (5th ed., p. 1758). Philadelphia: Saunders.

---

414. The nurse working on a medical-surgical nursing unit is caring for several clients with renal failure. The nurse interprets that which of the following clients is best suited for peritoneal dialysis as a treatment option?
  1 A client with severe congestive heart failure
  2 A client with a history of ruptured diverticula
  3 A client with a history of herniated lumbar disk
  4 A client with a history of three previous abdominal surgeries

Level of Cognitive Ability: Analysis
Client Needs: Physiological Integrity
Integrated Process: Nursing Process/Analysis
Content Area: Adult Health/Renal

Answer: 1
Rationale: Peritoneal dialysis may be the treatment option of choice for clients with severe cardiac disease because there is less cardiac stress with this treatment. Severe cardiac disease can be worsened by the rapid shifts in fluid, electrolytes, urea, and glucose that occur with hemodialysis. For the same reason, peritoneal dialysis may be indicated for the client with diabetes mellitus. Contraindications to peritoneal dialysis include diseases of the abdomen such as ruptured diverticula or malignancies; extensive abdominal surgeries; history of peritonitis; obesity; and those with a history of back problems, which could be aggravated by the fluid weight of the dialysate. Severe disease of the vascular system may also be a contraindication.

Test-Taking Strategy: Note the subject—the client who would be the best candidate for peritoneal dialysis. Eliminate options 2 and 4 first because they are comparable or alike and indicate clients with an abdominal condition. From the remaining options, recall the concepts related to fluid shifts in the body to direct you to option 1. Review the indications for peritoneal dialysis if you had difficulty with this question.

Reference
Black, J., & Hawks, J. (2005). *Medical-surgical nursing: Clinical management for positive outcomes* (7th ed., p. 956). Philadelphia: Saunders.

---

415. A client undergoing long-term peritoneal dialysis at home is currently experiencing a problem with reduced outflow from the dialysis catheter. The home care nurse inquires whether the client has had a recent problem with which of the following?
  1 Diarrhea
  2 Vomiting
  3 Flatulence
  4 Constipation

Level of Cognitive Ability: Analysis
Client Needs: Physiological Integrity
Integrated Process: Nursing Process/Assessment
Content Area: Adult Health/Renal

Answer: 4
Rationale: Reduced outflow may be caused by catheter position and adherence to the omentum, infection, or constipation. Constipation may contribute to reduced outflow in part because peristalsis seems to aid in drainage. For this reason, bisacodyl (Dulcolax) suppositories are sometimes used prophylactically, even without a history of constipation. The other options are unrelated to impaired catheter drainage.

Test-Taking Strategy: Use the process of elimination and focus on the subject—reduced outflow. Evaluate each option in terms of its effect on gut motility, which affects catheter outflow. Each of the incorrect options involves hypermotility of the gastrointestinal tract, which should theoretically facilitate outflow. Constipation is related to decreased gut motility, which could then impair fluid drainage. Review the causes of reduced outflow in peritoneal dialysis if you had difficulty with this question.

Reference
Black, J., & Hawks, J. (2005). *Medical-surgical nursing: Clinical management for positive outcomes* (7th ed., p. 958). Philadelphia: Saunders.

416. A client with a history of heart failure who is undergoing peritoneal dialysis has developed crackles in the lower lung fields. The nurse interprets that this finding is most likely related to:

1 Natural progression of the renal failure
2 Compliance with dietary sodium restriction
3 Intake greater than output on the dialysis record
4 Adherence to digoxin (Lanoxin) therapy schedule

Level of Cognitive Ability: Analysis
Client Needs: Physiological Integrity
Integrated Process: Nursing Process/Analysis
Content Area: Adult Health/Renal

Answer: 3
Rationale: Crackles in the lung fields of the peritoneal dialysis client result from overhydration or from insufficient fluid removal during dialysis. An intake that is greater than the output of peritoneal dialysis fluid would overhydrate the client, resulting in lung crackles. Adherence to medication and diet therapy should control this sign, not exacerbate it. If dialysis is effective, there is no connection between the progression of renal failure and the development of signs of overhydration.

Test-Taking Strategy: Note the strategic words "developed crackles." Begin to answer this question by eliminating options 2 and 4. Because adherence to standard therapy should control the signs of heart failure, not exacerbate them, these options are incorrect. From the remaining options, recalling that crackles is caused by excess fluid in the body directs you to option 3. Review complications of peritoneal dialysis if you had difficulty with this question.

Reference
Black, J., & Hawks, J. (2005). *Medical-surgical nursing: Clinical management for positive outcomes* (7th ed., p. 958). Philadelphia: Saunders.

417. The nurse is teaching the client with asthma how to perform a peak expiratory flow rate measurement. The nurse tells the client to:

1 Inhale an average-size breath.
2 Blow out as slowly as possible.
3 Record the final position of the indicator.
4 Form a loose seal with the mouth around the mouthpiece.

Level of Cognitive Ability: Application
Client Needs: Physiological Integrity
Integrated Process: Teaching and Learning
Content Area: Adult Health/Respiratory

Answer: 3
Rationale: A peak expiratory flow rate meter is used to provide an objective measure of the client's peak expiratory flow. The client is instructed to take the deepest possible breath, form a tight seal around the mouthpiece with the lips, and exhale forcefully and rapidly. The final position of the indicator on the meter is recorded.

Test-Taking Strategy: Visualizing this piece of equipment and how it is used will assist in directing you to option 3. Remember that the final position of the indicator on the meter is recorded. Review this commonly used device, which may be used to determine when medication adjustments are needed, if you had difficulty with this question.

Reference
Black, J., & Hawks, J. (2005). *Medical-surgical nursing: Clinical management for positive outcomes* (7th ed., p. 1762). Philadelphia: Saunders.

418. The nurse is teaching the client taking medications by inhalation about the advantages of a newly prescribed spacer device. The nurse determines the need for further teaching if the client states that the spacer device:

1 Disperses medication more deeply and uniformly
2 Reduces the frequency of medication to only once per day
3 Reduces the need to coordinate timing between pressing the inhaler and inspiration
4 Reduces the chance of yeast infection because large drops aren't deposited on the oral tissues

Level of Cognitive Ability: Analysis
Client Needs: Physiological Integrity
Integrated Process: Teaching and Learning
Content Area: Adult Health/Respiratory

Answer: 2
Rationale: There are key advantages to the use of a spacer device for medications administered by inhalation. One is that it reduces the incidence of yeast infections, because large medication droplets are not deposited on oral tissues. The medication is also dispersed more deeply and uniformly than without a spacer. There is less need to coordinate the effort of inhalation with pressing on the canister of the inhaler. Finally, the use of a spacer may decrease either the number or the volume of the puffs taken. Option 2 is too absolute and limiting by description.

Test-Taking Strategy: Use the process of elimination and note the strategic words "the need for further teaching." These words indicate a negative event query and that you need to select the client statement that is incorrect. Note the close-ended word "only" in option 2. The use of close-ended words such as "only" is likely to make the option incorrect. Review the advantages of the use of the spacer device with inhaled medications if you had difficulty with this question.

References
Perry, A., & Potter, P. (2006). *Clinical nursing skills & techniques* (6th ed., pp. 673-674). St. Louis: Mosby.
Potter, P., & Perry, A. (2005). *Fundamentals of nursing* (6th ed., p. 867). St. Louis: Mosby.

---

419. The nurse is assessing a client with a suspected diagnosis of pulmonary emphysema. The nurse assesses the client for which sign that distinguishes emphysema from chronic bronchitis?

1 Marked dyspnea
2 Minimal weight loss
3 Copious sputum production
4 Cough that began before the onset of dyspnea

Level of Cognitive Ability: Analysis
Client Needs: Physiological Integrity
Integrated Process: Nursing Process/Assessment
Content Area: Adult Health/Respiratory

Answer: 1
Rationale: Key features of pulmonary emphysema include dyspnea that is often marked, late cough (after the onset of dyspnea), scant mucus production, and marked weight loss. By contrast, chronic bronchitis is characterized by early onset of cough (before dyspnea), copious purulent sputum production, minimal weight loss, and milder severity of dyspnea.

Test-Taking Strategy: Focus on the subject—the differences between these two respiratory disorders and their associated manifestations. Recalling that marked dyspnea is associated with emphysema will direct you to option 1. Review the manifestations of emphysema and chronic bronchitis if you had difficulty with this question.

References
Black, J., & Hawks, J. (2005). *Medical-surgical nursing: Clinical management for positive outcomes* (7th ed., p. 1819). Philadelphia: Saunders.
Ignatavicius, D., & Workman, M. (2006). *Medical-surgical nursing: Critical thinking for collaborative care* (5th ed., pp. 646-647). Philadelphia: Saunders.

420. A client with late-stage emphysema becomes confused and is experiencing tremors. The nurse interprets that these symptoms are indicative of which complication of emphysema?
1 Encephalopathy
2 Cerebral embolism
3 Carbon dioxide narcosis
4 Carbon monoxide poisoning

Level of Cognitive Ability: Analysis
Client Needs: Physiological Integrity
Integrated Process: Nursing Process/Analysis
Content Area: Adult Health/Respiratory

Answer: 3
Rationale: With late-stage emphysema, the retention of carbon dioxide can lead to carbon dioxide narcosis. This is manifested by headache, drowsiness, inability to concentrate, confusion, tremors, and possible coma if the carbon dioxide level reaches 70 mm Hg or higher.

Test-Taking Strategy: Focus on the subject, a complication of emphysema, and on the client's complaints. Recalling that emphysema is characterized by high carbon dioxide levels will direct you to option 3. Review the manifestations and complications associated with emphysema if you had difficulty with this question.

References
Lewis, S., Heitkemper, M., Dirksen, S., O'Brien, P., & Bucher, L. (2007). *Medical-surgical nursing: Assessment and management of clinical problems* (7th ed., pp. 643-644). St. Louis: Mosby.
Mosby's dictionary of medicine, nursing & health professions (2006). (7th ed., pp. 296-297). St. Louis: Mosby.

---

421. The nurse witnesses an accident whereby a pedestrian is hit by an automobile. The nurse stops at the scene and assesses the victim and notes that the client is responsive and has suffered a flail chest involving at least three ribs. The nurse does which of the following to assist the client's respiratory status until help arrives?
1 Removes the victim's shirt
2 Assists the victim to sit up
3 Turns the client onto the side with the flail chest
4 Applies firm but gentle pressure with the hands to the flail segment

Level of Cognitive Ability: Application
Client Needs: Physiological Integrity
Integrated Process: Nursing Process/ Implementation
Content Area: Adult Health/Respiratory

Answer: 4
Rationale: If flail chest is present, the nurse applies firm yet gentle pressure to the flail segments of the ribs to stabilize the chest wall, which will ultimately help the client's respiratory status. The nurse does not move an injured person because of the risk of worsening an undetected spinal cord injury. Removing the victim's shirt is of no value in this situation and could in fact chill the victim, which is counterproductive. Injured persons should be kept warm until help arrives at the scene.

Test-Taking Strategy: Use knowledge of the principles of respiration and emergency nursing to answer this question. Eliminate options 2 and 3 because the client should not be moved. From the remaining options, recalling that the client should be kept warm will direct you to option 4. Review emergency care of the client with flail chest if you had difficulty with this question.

References
Black, J., & Hawks, J. (2005). *Medical-surgical nursing: Clinical management for positive outcomes* (7th ed., pp. 2492-2493). Philadelphia: Saunders.
Ignatavicius, D., & Workman, M. (2006). *Medical-surgical nursing: Critical thinking for collaborative care* (5th ed., p. 670). Philadelphia: Saunders.

---

422. A mental health nurse is assigned to care for a manic client. The nurse reviews the activity schedule for the day and determines that the best activity this client could participate in is:
1 Reading a book on the Civil War
2 Playing tetherball in the gym with staff
3 Working alone on a paint-by-number activity
4 Attending a deep breathing progressive relaxation group

Answer: 2
Rationale: A person who is experiencing mania is overactive, full of energy, lacks concentration, and has poor impulse control. The client needs an activity that will allow him to use excess energy, yet not endanger others during the process. Options 1, 3, and 4 are relatively sedate activities that require concentration, a quality that is lacking in the manic state. Such activities may lead to increased frustration and anxiety for the client. Tetherball is an exercise that uses the large muscle groups of the body and is a great way to expend the increased energy this client is experiencing.

Level of Cognitive Ability: Analysis
Client Needs: Physiological Integrity
Integrated Process: Nursing Process/Planning
Content Area: Mental Health

Test-Taking Strategy: Use the process of elimination and focus on the diagnosis of the client. Eliminate options 1, 3, and 4 because they are comparable or alike and are sedate activities. Review care of the client with mania if you had difficulty with this question.

Reference
Stuart, G., & Laraia, M. (2005). *Principles and practice of psychiatric nursing* (8th ed., p. 355). St. Louis: Mosby.

---

423. A client is brought to the emergency department by the police after having seriously lacerated both wrists. The initial action that the nurse will take is to:
 1 Assess and treat the wound sites.
 2 Secure and record a detailed history.
 3 Encourage the client to ventilate feelings.
 4 Administer a dose of an antianxiety agent.

Level of Cognitive Ability: Application
Client Needs: Physiological Integrity
Integrated Process: Nursing Process/
  Implementation
Content Area: Mental Health

Answer: 1
Rationale: The initial action when a client has attempted suicide is to assess and treat any injuries. Although options 2, 3, and 4 may be appropriate at some point, the initial action would be to treat the wounds.

Test-Taking Strategy: Use Maslow's Hierarchy of Needs theory to prioritize. Physiological needs come first. Option 1 is the only option that addresses a physiological need. Review initial care of the client who has attempted suicide if you had difficulty with this question.

References
Stuart, G., & Laraia, M. (2005). *Principles and practice of psychiatric nursing* (8th ed., p. 367). St. Louis: Mosby.
Varcarolis, E., Carson, V., & Shoemaker, N. (2006). *Foundations of psychiatric mental health nursing* (5th ed., p. 479). Philadelphia: Saunders.

---

424. The nurse notes bilateral +2 edema in the lower extremities of a client with known coronary artery disease who was admitted to the hospital 2 days ago. The nurse plans to do which of the following next after noting this finding?
 1 Order daily weights starting on the following morning.
 2 Review the intake and output records for the last 2 days.
 3 Request a sodium restriction of 1 g per day from the physician.
 4 Change the time of diuretic administration from morning to evening.

Level of Cognitive Ability: Application
Client Needs: Physiological Integrity
Integrated Process: Nursing Process/Planning
Content Area: Adult Health/Cardiovascular

Answer: 2
Rationale: Edema is the accumulation of excess fluid in the interstitial spaces, which can be measured by intake greater than output and by a sudden increase in weight (2.2 pounds = 1 kilogram). Obtaining a weight on the following day does not provide the nurse with immediate information. In addition, the nurse would need to evaluate serial weights for comparison. Strict sodium restrictions are reserved for clients with severe symptoms. Diuretics should be administered in the morning whenever possible to avoid nocturia.

Test-Taking Strategy: Note the strategic word "next" and use the steps of the nursing process. Option 2 can give the nurse immediate information about fluid balance. Review the manifestations associated with the complications of coronary artery disease if you had difficulty with this question.

Reference
Ignatavicius, D., & Workman, M. (2006). *Medical-surgical nursing: Critical thinking for collaborative care* (5th ed., pp. 754, 853). Philadelphia: Saunders.

425. The nurse in the emergency department is assessing a client with chest pain. Which finding helps determine that the pain is caused by myocardial infarction (MI)?
  1 The client experienced no nausea or vomiting.
  2 The pain was described as burning and gnawing.
  3 The client reports that the pain began while pushing a lawnmower.
  4 The pain, unrelieved by nitroglycerin, was relieved with morphine sulfate.

Level of Cognitive Ability: Analysis
Client Needs: Physiological Integrity
Integrated Process: Nursing Process/Analysis
Content Area: Adult Health/Cardiovascular

Answer: 4
Rationale: The pain of angina may radiate to the left arm, is often precipitated by exertion or stress, has few associated symptoms, and is relieved by rest and nitroglycerin. The pain of MI may radiate to the left arm, shoulder, jaw, and neck. It typically begins spontaneously, lasts longer than 30 minutes, is frequently accompanied by associated symptoms (nausea, vomiting, dyspnea, diaphoresis, anxiety), and requires opioid analgesics for relief. A burning and gnawing pain is more likely noted in an upper gastrointestinal disorder.

Test-Taking Strategy: Note the subject: pain caused by an MI. Recall that a classic hallmark of the pain from MI is that it is unrelieved by rest and nitroglycerin. Review the differences between angina and MI if you had difficulty with this question.

References
Black, J., & Hawks, J. (2005). *Medical-surgical nursing: Clinical management for positive outcomes* (7th ed., pp. 1706-1707). Philadelphia: Saunders.
Ignatavicius, D., & Workman, M. (2006). *Medical-surgical nursing: Critical thinking for collaborative care* (5th ed., pp. 844, 845). Philadelphia: Saunders.

---

426. The nurse is assessing a client who has been hospitalized with acute pericarditis. The nurse monitors the client for cardiac tamponade, knowing that which of the following is a manifestation of this complication of pericarditis?
  1 Bradycardia
  2 Paradoxical pulse
  3 Flattened jugular veins
  4 Bounding heart sounds

Level of Cognitive Ability: Analysis
Client Needs: Physiological Integrity
Integrated Process: Nursing Process/Assessment
Content Area: Adult Health/Cardiovascular

Answer: 2
Rationale: Assessment findings with cardiac tamponade include tachycardia, distant or muffled heart sounds, jugular vein distention, and a falling blood pressure (BP), accompanied by paradoxical pulse (a drop in inspiratory BP by greater than 10 mm Hg).

Test-Taking Strategy: Use the process of elimination. Think of the consequences of the pressure dynamics in the chest when the pericardial sac is rapidly filling with blood or fluid. This will assist in directing you to option 2. Review the signs of cardiac tamponade if you had difficulty with this question.

Reference
Black, J., & Hawks, J. (2005). *Medical-surgical nursing: Clinical management for positive outcomes* (7th ed., p. 1623). Philadelphia: Saunders.

---

427. The nurse is assisting with positioning the client for pericardiocentesis to treat cardiac tamponade. How should the nurse position the client?
  1 Supine with slight Trendelenburg's position
  2 Lying on right side with a pillow under the head
  3 Lying on left side with a pillow under the chest wall
  4 Supine with the head of bed elevated at a 30- to 60-degree angle

Answer: 4
Rationale: The client undergoing pericardiocentesis is positioned supine with the head of the bed raised to a 30- to 60-degree angle. This places the heart in proximity to the chest wall for easier insertion of the needle into the pericardial sac. Options 1, 2, and 3 are incorrect positions.

Test-Taking Strategy: If you are uncertain how to proceed with this question, visualize each of the positions described. Evaluate how the heart is sitting in the chest with each position and how easily the pericardial sac could be accessed with a needle. This will direct you to option 4. Review this procedure if you had difficulty with this question.

Level of Cognitive Ability: Application
Client Needs: Physiological Integrity
Integrated Process: Nursing Process/
  Implementation
Content Area: Adult Health/Cardiovascular

References
Chernecky, C., & Berger, B. (2008). *Laboratory tests and diagnostic procedures* (5th ed., p. 862). Philadelphia: Saunders.
Ignatavicius, D., & Workman, M. (2006). *Medical-surgical nursing: Critical thinking for collaborative care* (5th ed., p. 771). Philadelphia: Saunders.

---

428. A client with multiple sclerosis is treated with baclofen (Lioresal) for painful muscle spasms. The nurse assesses the client for side effects of the medication and monitors the client for:
1 Sedation
2 Headache
3 Urinary frequency
4 Increased salivation

Level of Cognitive Ability: Analysis
Client Needs: Physiological Integrity
Integrated Process: Nursing Process/
  Assessment
Content Area: Pharmacology

Answer: 1
Rationale: Baclofen is a centrally acting skeletal muscle relaxant. Sedation is a common side effect. Options 2, 3, and 4 are not side effects.

Test-Taking Strategy: Use the process of elimination. Recalling that diazepam is used for muscle spasms will direct you to think that this medication relaxes muscles. The only option that directly relates to this medication action is option 1. Review the action and side effects of this medication if you had difficulty with this question.

Reference
Lehne, R. (2007). *Pharmacology for nursing care* (6th ed., p. 238). Philadelphia: Saunders.

---

429. A client with epilepsy is taking the prescribed dose of phenytoin (Dilantin) to control seizures. A phenytoin (Dilantin) blood level is drawn, and the results reveal a level of 35 mcg/mL. Which effect(s) would the nurse expect based on this laboratory finding?
1 Diarrhea
2 Nystagmus
3 Tachycardia
4 No effects because this is a therapeutic phenytoin (Dilantin) level

Level of Cognitive Ability: Analysis
Client Needs: Physiological Integrity
Integrated Process: Nursing Process/Assessment
Content Area: Pharmacology

Answer: 2
Rationale: The therapeutic phenytoin (Dilantin) level is 10 to 20 mcg/mL. Blood levels above 30 mcg/mL produce nystagmus. Options 1, 3, and 4 are incorrect.

Test-Taking Strategy: Knowledge regarding the therapeutic phenytoin (Dilantin) level and the signs that occur in the client when the level rises is required to answer this question. Review the signs associated with an elevated level if you had difficulty with this question.

Reference
Hodgson, B., & Kizior, R. (2007). *Saunders nursing drug handbook 2007* (p. 929). Philadelphia: Saunders.

---

430. A nurse is caring for a child following cleft palate repair. To reduce the risk of aspiration after feeding the child, the nurse places the child in which best position?
1 Sims'
2 Prone
3 Supine
4 Right side in semi-Fowler's

Answer: 4
Rationale: The child with cleft palate repair is placed on the right side in a semi-Fowler's position after feeding to reduce the chance of aspirating regurgitated formula. Options 1, 2, and 3 are positions that would place the child at risk for aspiration.

Level of Cognitive Ability: Application
Client Needs: Physiological Integrity
Integrated Process: Nursing Process/
   Implementation
Content Area: Child Health

Test-Taking Strategy: Visualize the anatomical location of the stomach in answering this question and focus on the subject— to reduce the risk of aspiration. Eliminate options 1, 2, and 3 because they are comparable or alike and are flat positions. Also remember that positioning on the right side will aid in absorption and reduce the risk of aspiration. Review care of the child following cleft palate repair if you had difficulty with this question.

References
Hockenberry, M., & Wilson, D. (2007). *Nursing care of infants and children* (8th ed., p. 466). St. Louis: Mosby.
Hockenberry, M., Wilson, D., & Winkelstein, M. (2005). *Wong's essentials of pediatric nursing* (7th ed., p. 876). St. Louis: Mosby.

---

431. The nurse is monitoring drainage from a nasogastric (NG) tube in a client who had a gastric resection. No drainage is noted during the past 4 hours, and the client complains of severe nausea. Which of the following is an appropriate nursing action?
  1 Irrigate the tube.
  2 Reposition the tube.
  3 Notify the physician.
  4 Medicate for nausea.

Level of Cognitive Ability: Application
Client Needs: Physiological Integrity
Integrated Process: Nursing Process/
   Implementation
Content Area: Adult Health/Gastrointestinal

Answer: 3
Rationale: Nausea and vomiting should not occur if the NG tube is patent. The NG tube should not be repositioned or irrigated after gastric surgery because it is placed directly over the suture line. The NG tube is irrigated gently with normal saline only with a physician's order. The client may need medication for the nausea, but, in this situation, the physician should be notified.

Test-Taking Strategy: Note that the client had a surgical procedure that involved the gastric area and that an NG tube is placed in this surgical area. This will assist in eliminating options 1 and 2. From the remaining options, noting the strategic words "severe nausea" should alert you that the physician needs to be notified. Review postoperative nursing care following gastric surgery if you had difficulty with this question.

References
Black, J., & Hawks, J. (2005). *Medical-surgical nursing: Clinical management for positive outcomes* (7th ed., p. 760). Philadelphia: Saunders.
Ignatavicius, D., & Workman, M. (2006). *Medical-surgical nursing: Critical thinking for collaborative care* (5th ed., p. 345). Philadelphia: Saunders.

---

432. A nurse explains to a mother that her newborn infant is being admitted to the neonatal intensive care unit with a probable diagnosis of fetal alcohol syndrome (FAS). The nurse explains the expected effects of FAS to the mother and tells the mother that:
  1 Mental retardation is unlikely to happen.
  2 Withdrawal symptoms will occur after 6 days.
  3 Withdrawal symptoms include tremors, crying, seizures, and abnormal reflexes.
  4 The reason the newborn infant is so large is because of the fetal alcohol syndrome.

Answer: 3
Rationale: The long-term prognosis for newborns with FAS is poor. Symptoms of withdrawal include tremors, sleeplessness, seizures, abdominal distention, hyperactivity, abnormal reflexes, and uncontrollable crying. Central nervous system (CNS) disorders are the most common problems associated with FAS. Because of the CNS disorders, children born with FAS are often hyperactive and have a high incidence of speech and language disorders. Symptoms of withdrawal often occur within 6 to 12 hours after birth or, at the latest, within the first 3 days of life. Most neonates with FAS are mildly to severely mentally retarded. The newborn is usually growth deficient at birth.

Level of Cognitive Ability: Analysis
Client Needs: Physiological Integrity
Integrated Process: Nursing Process/
  Implementation
Content Area: Maternity/Postpartum

Test-Taking Strategy: Use the process of elimination. Focus on the diagnosis to eliminate options 1 and 4. From the remaining options, eliminate option 2 because of the words "after 6 days." Remember that withdrawal symptoms can appear within 6 to 12 hours after birth or, at the latest, within the first 3 days of life. Review the manifestations associated with FAS if you had difficulty with this question.

Reference
Wong, D., Hockenberry, M., Perry, S., Lowdermilk, D., & Wilson, D. (2006). *Maternal-child nursing care.* (3rd ed., pp. 842-844). St. Louis: Mosby.

---

433. A client who has type 1 diabetes mellitus is at 10 weeks' gestation and is receiving prenatal care at a high-risk clinic. The nurse tells the client about the early signs of hyperglycemia and determines that the client understands if the client states that an early sign of hyperglycemia is:
 1 Hunger
 2 Shakiness
 3 Nervousness
 4 Increased urination

Level of Cognitive Ability: Analysis
Client Needs: Physiological Integrity
Integrated Process: Teaching and Learning
Content Area: Maternity/Antepartum

Answer: 4
Rationale: Polyuria (increased urination) is an early sign of hyperglycemia. Other signs can include polydipsia, dry mouth, fatigue, nausea, hot flushed skin, rapid deep breathing, abdominal cramps, acetone breath, headache, drowsiness, depressed reflexes, stupor, and coma.

Test-Taking Strategy: Use the process of elimination. Options 2 and 3 are comparative or alike and are eliminated first. From the remaining options, recalling that hunger is a sign of hypoglycemia will assist in eliminating option 1. Review the signs of both hypoglycemia and hyperglycemia if you had difficulty with this question.

Reference
McKinney, E., James, S., Murray, S., & Ashwill, J. (2005). *Maternal-child nursing* (2nd ed., pp. 653-654). St. Louis: Saunders.

---

434. A client recovering from a craniotomy complains of a "runny nose." Which of the following nursing actions should be immediately implemented?
 1 Notify the physician.
 2 Provide the client with soft tissues.
 3 Monitor the client for signs of a cold.
 4 Tell the client to use soft tissues to soak up the drainage.

Level of Cognitive Ability: Application
Client Needs: Physiological Integrity
Integrated Process: Nursing Process/
  Implementation
Content Area: Adult Health/Neurological

Answer: 1
Rationale: If the client has sustained a craniocerebral injury or is recovering from a craniotomy, careful observation of any drainage from the eyes, ears, nose, or traumatic area is critical because this may indicate leakage of cerebrospinal fluid. Cerebrospinal fluid is colorless and generally nonpurulent, and its presence indicates a serious breach of cranial integrity. Any suspicious drainage should be reported to the physician immediately.

Test-Taking Strategy: Note the strategic words "immediately implemented." This should provide you with the clue that there is a serious nature to the situation presented. Eliminate options 2 and 4 first because they are comparable or alike. From the remaining options, recalling the signs of complications associated with craniotomy will direct you to option 1. Review postoperative nursing care following craniotomy if you had difficulty with this question.

References
Ignatavicius, D., & Workman, M. (2006). *Medical-surgical nursing: Critical thinking for collaborative care* (5th ed., pp. 1058, 1064). Philadelphia: Saunders.
Lewis, S., Heitkemper, M., Dirksen, S., O'Brien, P., & Bucher, L. (2007). *Medical-surgical nursing: Assessment and management of clinical problems* (7th ed., pp. 1491, 1493). St. Louis: Mosby.

435. The nurse is caring for a client who has returned from the postanesthesia care unit following prostatectomy. The client has a three-way Foley catheter with infusion of continuous bladder irrigation solution. The nurse assesses that the flow rate is adequate if the color of the urinary drainage is:

1 Clear as water
2 Dark cherry colored
3 Pale yellow or slightly pink
4 Concentrated yellow with small clots

Level of Cognitive Ability: Analysis
Client Needs: Physiological Integrity
Integrated Process: Nursing Process/Assessment
Content Area: Adult Health/Renal

Answer: 3
Rationale: The infusion of bladder irrigant is not at a preset rate, but rather it is increased or decreased to maintain urine that is a clear, pale yellow color or that has just a slight pink tinge. The infusion rate should be increased if the drainage is cherry colored or if clots are seen. Correspondingly, the rate can be slowed down slightly if the returns are as clear as water.

Test-Taking Strategy: Use the process of elimination. Eliminate option 4 as the least realistic or expected occurrence of all the urine characteristics described in the options. Next, eliminate options 1 and 2 as reflecting excessive or inadequate flow, respectively. With proper flow rate of bladder irrigant, the urine should be pale yellow or slightly pink. Review care of the client following prostatectomy if you had difficulty with this question.

Reference
Ignatavicius, D., & Workman, M. (2006). *Medical-surgical nursing: Critical thinking for collaborative care* (5th ed., p. 1863). Philadelphia: Saunders.

---

436. The nurse is assessing a client who is at risk of developing acute renal failure (ARF). The nurse would become most concerned if which of the following assessments was made?

1 Urine output 60 mL/hr for the last 3 hours, BUN 40 mg/dL, creatinine 1.1 mg/dL
2 Urine output 40 mL/hr for the last 3 hours, BUN 15 mg/dL, creatinine 0.8 mg/dL
3 Urine output 20 mL/hr for the last 3 hours, BUN 35 mg/dL, creatinine 2.1 mg/dL
4 Urine output 30 mL/hr for the last 3 hours, BUN 10 mg/dL, creatinine 1.2 mg/dL

Level of Cognitive Ability: Analysis
Client Needs: Physiological Integrity
Integrated Process: Nursing Process/Assessment
Content Area: Adult Health/Renal

Answer: 3
Rationale: With acute renal failure, the client is often oliguric or anuric, although the client may have nonoliguric renal failure. The BUN and serum creatinine levels also rise, indicating impaired kidney function. Normal serum BUN levels are usually 5 to 20 mg/dL. Normal creatinine levels range from 0.6 to 1.3 mg/dL. The client who has the greatest abnormality in urine output and laboratory values is the client in option 3. This is the client who is most at risk for developing renal failure.

Test-Taking Strategy: Focus on the subject—developing renal failure. Recalling the normal BUN and creatinine levels and that the minimum required hourly urine output is 30 mL will direct you to option 3. Review these normal values and the signs of renal failure if you had difficulty with this question.

Reference
Black, J., & Hawks, J. (2005). *Medical-surgical nursing: Clinical management for positive outcomes* (7th ed., pp. 944, 949). Philadelphia: Saunders.

---

437. A client with acute renal failure has been treated with sodium polystyrene sulfonate (Kayexalate) by mouth. The nurse would evaluate this therapy as effective if which of the following values was noted on follow-up laboratory testing?

1 Calcium: 9.8 mg/dL
2 Sodium: 142 mEq/L
3 Potassium: 4.9 mEq/L
4 Phosphorus: 3.9 mg/dL

Answer: 3
Rationale: Of all the electrolyte imbalances that accompany renal failure, hyperkalemia is the most dangerous because it can lead to cardiac dysrhythmias and death. If the potassium level rises too high, sodium polystyrene sulfonate (Kayexalate) may be administered to cause excretion of potassium through the gastrointestinal tract. Each of the electrolyte levels noted in the options falls within the normal reference range for that electrolyte. The potassium level, however, is measured following administration of this medication to note the extent of its effectiveness.

Level of Cognitive Ability: Analysis
Client Needs: Physiological Integrity
Integrated Process: Nursing Process/Evaluation
Content Area: Adult Health/Renal

Test-Taking Strategy: Use the process of elimination. Note the name of the medication (Kayexalate) and its relationship to the laboratory test in option 3. Review this medication if you had difficulty with this question.

References

Lewis, S., Heitkemper, M., Dirksen, S., O'Brien, P., & Bucher, L. (2007). *Medical-surgical nursing: Assessment and management of clinical problems* (7th ed., p. 1202). St. Louis: Mosby.

Pagana, K., & Pagana, T. (2005). *Mosby's diagnostic and laboratory test reference* (7th ed., p. 733). St. Louis: Mosby.

---

438. The nurse is admitting a client with chronic renal failure to the nursing unit. The nurse assesses for which most frequent cardiovascular sign that occurs in the client with chronic renal failure?
1 Bradycardia
2 Tachycardia
3 Hypotension
4 Hypertension

Level of Cognitive Ability: Analysis
Client Needs: Physiological Integrity
Integrated Process: Nursing Process/Assessment
Content Area: Adult Health/Renal

Answer: 4

Rationale: Hypertension is the most common cardiovascular finding in the client with chronic renal failure. It is caused by several mechanisms, including volume overload, renin-angiotensin system stimulation, vasoconstriction from sympathetic stimulation, and the absence of prostaglandins. Hypertension may also be the cause of the renal failure. It is an important item to assess because hypertension can lead to heart failure in the chronic renal failure client, because of increased cardiac workload in conjunction with fluid overload. The client may experience tachycardia or bradycardia or may have a normal pulse rate; these cardiovascular manifestations will depend on a variety of physiological events such as fluid overload, fluid deficit, or normal fluid volume.

Test-Taking Strategy: Use the process of elimination. Recalling that the blood pressure is the key item to assess helps you eliminate options 1 and 2. From the remaining options, recall the functions of the renal system and the kidneys to direct you to option 4. Review the manifestations of chronic renal failure if you had difficulty with this question.

Reference

Black, J., & Hawks, J. (2005). *Medical-surgical nursing: Clinical management for positive outcomes* (7th ed., p. 953). Philadelphia: Saunders.

---

439. A client has sustained a closed fracture and has just had a cast applied to the affected arm. The client is complaining of intense pain. The nurse has elevated the limb, applied an ice bag, and administered an analgesic, which has provided very little pain relief. The nurse interprets that this pain may be caused by:
1 Infection under the cast
2 The anxiety of the client
3 Impaired tissue perfusion
4 The newness of the fracture

Answer: 3

Rationale: Most pain associated with fractures can be minimized with rest, elevation, application of cold, and administration of analgesics. Pain that is not relieved from these measures should be reported to the physician, because it may be caused by impaired tissue perfusion, tissue breakdown, or necrosis. Because this is a new closed fracture and cast, infection would not have had time to set in.

Level of Cognitive Ability: Analysis
Client Needs: Physiological Integrity
Integrated Process: Nursing Process/Analysis
Content Area: Adult Health/Musculoskeletal

Test-Taking Strategy: Use the process of elimination. Focus on the information in the question to eliminate options 2 and 4. Because the fracture and cast are so new, it is extremely unlikely that infection could have possibly set in. Therefore, eliminate option 1. Review the complications associated with a casted extremity if you had difficulty with this question.

References
Black, J., & Hawks, J. (2005). *Medical-surgical nursing: Clinical management for positive outcomes* (7th ed., pp. 633, 635-636). Philadelphia: Saunders.
Ignatavicius, D., & Workman, M. (2006). *Medical-surgical nursing: Critical thinking for collaborative care* (5th ed., pp. 1191-1192). Philadelphia: Saunders.

---

440. The client with a fractured femur experiences sudden dyspnea. A set of arterial blood gases reveal the following: pH is 7.32, $Paco_2$ is 43, Pao_2 is 58, and HCO_3 is 20. Which of the following components of the ABG results supports the nurse's suspicion of fat embolus?

1 pH
2 Pao_2
3 $Paco_2$
4 HCO_3

Level of Cognitive Ability: Analysis
Client Needs: Physiological Integrity
Integrated Process: Nursing Process/Analysis
Content Area: Adult Health/Musculoskeletal

Answer: 2
Rationale: A key feature of fat embolism is a significant degree of hypoxemia with a Pao_2 often less than 60 mm Hg. Other features that distinguish fat embolism from pulmonary embolism are an elevated temperature and the presence of fat in the blood with fat embolus.

Test-Taking Strategy: Use the process of elimination. Recalling that fat embolus causes significant hypoxemia will direct you to option 2. Review the manifestations associated with this disorder if you had difficulty with this question.

References
Black, J., & Hawks, J. (2005). *Medical-surgical nursing: Clinical management for positive outcomes* (7th ed., pp. 629-630, 633, 635). Philadelphia: Saunders.
Ignatavicius, D., & Workman, M. (2006). *Medical-surgical nursing: Critical thinking for collaborative care* (5th ed., pp. 650, 1192-1193). Philadelphia: Saunders.
Lewis, S., Heitkemper, M., Dirksen, S., O'Brien, P., & Bucher, L. (2007). *Medical-surgical nursing: Assessment and management of clinical problems* (7th ed., p. 1651). St. Louis: Mosby.

---

441. Mannitol (Osmitrol) is administered intravenously to a client admitted to the hospital with loss of consciousness and a closed head injury. The nurse determines that the medication achieved its priority effect if which of the following outcomes was noted?

1 Weight loss of 1 kg and a serum creatinine of 0.8 mg/dL
2 Serum creatinine of 1.2 mg/dL and normal intracranial pressure
3 Improved level of consciousness and normal intracranial pressure
4 Diuresis of 500 mL in 2 hours and a blood urea nitrogen (BUN) of 15 mg/dL

Answer: 3
Rationale: Mannitol (Osmitrol) is an osmotic diuretic that can be administered parenterally to treat cerebral edema. Lowering of intracranial pressure occurs within 15 minutes of administration, and diuresis occurs within 1 to 3 hours. Expected effects of the medication include rapid diuresis and fluid loss. For the client with cerebral edema (as in closed head injury), effectiveness is measured by assessing neurological status and intracranial pressure readings.

Test-Taking Strategy: Note the strategic words "priority effect" in the query of the question. This tells you that more than one option is partially or totally correct. Next, note the strategic words "loss of consciousness and a closed head injury." Note the relationship between these words and the correct option. Review this medication and its expected effect if you had difficulty with this question.

Level of Cognitive Ability: Analysis
Client Needs: Physiological Integrity
Integrated Process: Nursing Process/Evaluation
Content Area: Pharmacology

References
Gahart, B., & Nazareno, A. (2006). *2006 Intravenous medications* (22nd ed., p. 781). St. Louis: Mosby.
Skidmore-Roth, L. (2008). *Mosby's nursing drug reference* (21st ed., pp. 636-637). St. Louis: Mosby.

442. A client with a history of renal insufficiency is having captopril (Capoten) added to the medication regimen. Before administering the first dose, the nurse reviews the medical record for the results of the urinalysis, especially noting for the presence of:

1 Casts
2 Protein
3 Red blood cells (RBCs)
4 White blood cells (WBCs)

Level of Cognitive Ability: Analysis
Client Needs: Physiological Integrity
Integrated Process: Nursing Process/Assessment
Content Area: Pharmacology

Answer: 2
Rationale: Captopril is an angiotensin-converting enzyme (ACE) inhibitor, which may be used for clients who do not respond to first-line antihypertensive agents. ACE inhibitors are used cautiously in clients with renal impairment. Before beginning treatment, baseline assessment of blood pressure, complete white cell count, and urine protein are performed. Clients with renal insufficiency may develop nephrotic syndrome, so the client may be monitored for proteinuria on a monthly basis for 9 months and periodically, afterward.

Test-Taking Strategy: Note the information in the question. The question tells you that the client has renal insufficiency and directs you to look at urinalysis results. RBCs and WBCs could be indications of trauma and/or infection, so these options can be eliminated first. Eliminate option 1 because casts are mineral deposits that form along the renal tubules and occasionally appear in the urine. Normally the kidneys conserve large protein molecules, which makes the presence of protein in the urine abnormal. Review this medication if you had difficulty with this question.

Reference
Hodgson, B., & Kizior, R. (2007). *Saunders nursing drug handbook 2007* (p. 182). Philadelphia: Saunders.

443. The nurse assesses a client with chronic arterial insufficiency. The client complains of leg pain and cramping after walking three blocks, which is relieved when the client stops and rests. How should the nurse correctly document this on the client record?

1 Venous insufficiency
2 Deep vein thrombosis
3 Arterial-venous shunting
4 Intermittent claudication

Level of Cognitive Ability: Application
Client Needs: Physiological Integrity
Integrated Process: Communication and Documentation
Content Area: Adult Health/Cardiovascular

Answer: 4
Rationale: Intermittent claudication is a classic symptom of peripheral vascular disease, also known by other names, including peripheral arterial disease and chronic arterial insufficiency. Intermittent claudication is described as a cramp-like pain that occurs with exercise and is relieved by rest. Intermittent claudication is caused by ischemia and is reproducible; that is, a predictable amount of exercise causes the pain each time. Options 1, 2, and 3 are incorrect.

Test-Taking Strategy: Use the process of elimination. Note that the question indicates that the client has an arterial disorder. This eliminates options 1 and 2. From the remaining options, noting the relationship between the timing in the question and the word "intermittent" in option 4 will direct you to this option. Review intermittent claudication if you had difficulty with this question.

References

Ignatavicius, D., & Workman, M. (2006). *Medical-surgical nursing: Critical thinking for collaborative care* (5th ed., p. 794). Philadelphia: Saunders.

Lewis, S., Heitkemper, M., Dirksen, S., O'Brien, P., & Bucher, L. (2007). *Medical-surgical nursing: Assessment and management of clinical problems* (7th ed., pp. 767, 900). St. Louis: Mosby.

---

444. A nurse is caring for a client with cancer who is receiving daunorubicin (Cerubidine) intravenously. The nurse monitors the client for which side effect of the medication?

1 Hypertension
2 Hypovolemia
3 Polycythemia
4 Nausea and vomiting

Level of Cognitive Ability: Application
Client Needs: Physiological Integrity
Integrated Process: Nursing Process/Assessment
Content Area: Pharmacology

Answer: 4

Rationale: Daunorubicin is an antineoplastic medication. The major gastrointestinal (GI) side effects include nausea, vomiting, stomatitis, and esophagitis. Cardiovascular side effects include congestive heart failure and dysrhythmias. Other frequently occurring side effects are alopecia and bone marrow depression. Options 1, 2, and 3 are not side effects of this medication.

Test-Taking Strategy: Focusing on the client's diagnosis will assist in determining that the medication is an antineoplastic. Recalling that antineoplastics commonly cause GI side effects will direct you to option 4. Review the side effects of this medication if you had difficulty with this question.

Reference

Skidmore-Roth, L. (2008). *Mosby's nursing drug reference* (21st ed., pp. 332-333). St. Louis: Mosby.

---

445. A home care nurse is visiting a client who was discharged to home with orders for continued administration of enoxaparin sodium (Lovenox) 30 mg twice daily subcutaneously. The priority assessment involves questioning the client about:

1 Constipation
2 Rashes or itching
3 Nausea or vomiting
4 Bleeding gums or bruising

Level of Cognitive Ability: Application
Client Needs: Physiological Integrity
Integrated Process: Nursing Process/Assessment
Content Area: Pharmacology

Answer: 4

Rationale: Enoxaparin sodium is an anticoagulant. A common side effect of anticoagulant therapy is bleeding. Because of this, the nurse questions the client about symptoms that could indicate bleeding, such as bleeding gums, bruising, hematuria, or dark tarry stools.

Test-Taking Strategy: Use the process of elimination. Recalling that this medication is an anticoagulant will assist in eliminating options 1 and 3 first. From the remaining options, noting the strategic word "priority" will direct you to option 4. Review this medication if you had difficulty with this question.

Reference

Skidmore-Roth, L. (2008). *Mosby's nursing drug reference* (21st ed., p. 952). St. Louis: Mosby.

446. A client has been given a prescription for sulfasalazine (Azulfidine) for the treatment of ulcerative colitis. Before teaching the client about the medication, the nurse asks the client about a history of allergy to:
1 Sulfonamides or salicylates
2 Salicylates or acetaminophen
3 Shellfish or calcium channel blockers
4 Histamine receptor antagonists or beta-blockers

Level of Cognitive Ability: Application
Client Needs: Physiological Integrity
Integrated Process: Nursing Process/Assessment
Content Area: Pharmacology

Answer: 1
Rationale: The client who has been prescribed sulfasalazine should be checked for history of allergy to either sulfonamides or salicylates because the chemical composition of sulfasalazine and these medications is similar or alike. The other options are incorrect.

Test-Taking Strategy: Focus on the subject—history of allergy. Note the relationship of "sulfasalazine" in the question and "sulfonamides" in the correct option. Review information about this medication if you had difficulty with this question.

Reference
Skidmore-Roth, L. (2008). *Mosby's nursing drug reference* (21st ed., p. 949). St. Louis: Mosby.

---

447. A nurse is caring for a client with a nursing diagnosis of Impaired oral mucous membranes. The nurse would avoid using which of the following items when giving mouth care to this client?
1 Lip moistener
2 Soft toothbrush
3 Lemon-glycerin swabs
4 Nonalcoholic mouthwash

Level of Cognitive Ability: Application
Client Needs: Physiological Integrity
Integrated Process: Nursing Process/Implementation
Content Area: Fundamental Skill

Answer: 3
Rationale: The nurse avoids using lemon-glycerin swabs for the client with impaired oral mucous membranes because they dry the membranes further and could cause pain. Items that are helpful include a soft toothbrush to prevent trauma, lip moistener to prevent lip cracking, and soothing cleansing rinses, such as nonalcoholic mouthwash or a saline and hydrogen peroxide mixture.

Test-Taking Strategy: Note the strategic word "avoid." This indicates a negative event query and the need to select the option that is an incorrect item to use for mouth care. Focus on the nursing diagnosis and evaluate each item in the options in terms of the likelihood of causing trauma to the oral mucous membranes. This will direct you to option 3. Review care of the client with impaired oral mucous membranes if you had difficulty with this question.

Reference
Ignatavicius, D., & Workman, M. (2006). *Medical-surgical nursing: Critical thinking for collaborative care* (5th ed., pp. 220-221). Philadelphia: Saunders.

---

448. A nurse has an order to administer 20 mEq of potassium to a client with a potassium level of 3.0 mEq/L. The nurse draws up this medication knowing it will be administered:
1 Intramuscularly
2 Subcutaneously
3 Directly by IV push
4 After dilution in an intravenous solution

Answer: 4
Rationale: Potassium chloride may be administered by the intravenous route when the client has moderate to severe hypokalemia. It is always diluted in an intravenous solution; administration by IV push could cause death by cardiac arrest. It is not administered intramuscularly or subcutaneously. Intravenous potassium should be administered through an infusion pump. A cardiac monitor should also be in use when administering intravenous potassium.

Level of Cognitive Ability: Application
Client Needs: Physiological Integrity
Integrated Process: Nursing Process/
   Implementation
Content Area: Pharmacology

Test-Taking Strategy: Use basic knowledge of electrolyte replacement and medication administration to answer this question. Recalling the physiology of the cardiac conduction system and the effects of potassium on the heart will direct you to the correct option. Review the procedure for administering potassium if you had difficulty with this question.

Reference
Skidmore-Roth, L. (2008). *Mosby's nursing drug reference* (21st ed., p. 833). St. Louis: Mosby.

---

449. The nurse has an order to administer two ophthalmic medications to the client who has undergone eye surgery. The nurse waits how many minutes after administering the first medication before giving the second?
   1 1 to 2
   2 3 to 5
   3 8 to 10
   4 It is not necessary to wait; the second medication can be administered immediately.

Level of Cognitive Ability: Application
Client Needs: Physiological Integrity
Integrated Process: Nursing Process/
   Implementation
Content Area: Adult Health/Eye

Answer: 2
Rationale: The nurse waits 3 to 5 minutes between administration of the two separate ophthalmic medications. This allows for adequate ocular absorption of the medication and prevents the second medication from flushing out the first.

Test-Taking Strategy: Use the process of elimination. Eliminate option 3 because of the lengthy time frame. Next, eliminate option 4 because it does not address the subject of the question. From the remaining options, recalling that time is needed for ocular absorption of the medication will direct you to option 2. If needed, review the principles of ocular medication administration.

Reference
Potter, P., & Perry, A. (2005). *Fundamentals of nursing* (6th ed., p. 862). St. Louis: Mosby.

---

450. A client has a pH of 7.51 with a bicarbonate level of 32 mEq/L. The nurse prepares to administer which of the following medications as a treatment for this acid-base disorder?
   1 Furosemide (Lasix)
   2 Sodium bicarbonate
   3 Acetazolamide (Diamox)
   4 Spironolactone (Aldactone)

Level of Cognitive Ability: Analysis
Client Needs: Physiological Integrity
Integrated Process: Nursing Process/Planning
Content Area: Pharmacology

Answer: 3
Rationale: Acetazolamide is a diuretic used in the treatment of metabolic alkalosis. This medication causes excretion of sodium, potassium, bicarbonate, and water by inhibiting the action of carbonic anhydrase. Administration of sodium bicarbonate would aggravate the already existing condition and is contraindicated. Furosemide and spironolactone are loop and potassium-sparing diuretics, respectively. These are of no value when there is a need to excrete bicarbonate.

Test-Taking Strategy: Begin to answer this question by interpreting that the acid-base disorder is metabolic alkalosis. Eliminate option 2 first, based on this interpretation. From the remaining options, it is necessary to know which diuretic is used to treat metabolic alkalosis. Review the treatment for this acid-base disorder if you had difficulty with this question.

Reference
Skidmore-Roth, L. (2008). *Mosby's nursing drug reference* (21st ed., p. 78). St. Louis: Mosby.

451. A client is admitted to the hospital in metabolic acidosis caused by diabetic ketoacidosis (DKA). The nurse prepares to administer which of the following medications as a primary initial treatment for this problem?
1 Potassium
2 Regular insulin
3 Calcium gluconate
4 Sodium bicarbonate

Level of Cognitive Ability: Analysis
Client Needs: Physiological Integrity
Integrated Process: Nursing Process/Planning
Content Area: Adult Health/Endocrine

Answer: 2
Rationale: The primary treatment for any acid-base imbalance is the treatment of the underlying disorder that caused the problem. In this case, the underlying cause of the metabolic acidosis is anaerobic metabolism caused by the lack of the ability by the body to use circulating glucose. The administration of insulin corrects this problem. Potassium may be added to the treatment regimen if serum potassium levels indicate it is necessary. Options 3 and 4 would not be used in the treatment of this disorder.

Test-Taking Strategy: Focus on the client's diagnosis—diabetic ketoacidosis. Noting both the diagnosis and the strategic words "primary initial treatment" will direct you to option 2. Review the treatment for DKA if you had difficulty with this question.

Reference
Black, J., & Hawks, J. (2005). *Medical-surgical nursing: Clinical management for positive outcomes* (7th ed., p. 1277). Philadelphia: Saunders.

452. A client is diagnosed with respiratory alkalosis induced by gram-negative sepsis. The nurse prepares to implement which prescribed measure as the most effective means to treat the problem?
1 Administer prn antipyretics.
2 Administer prescribed antibiotics.
3 Have the client breathe into a paper bag.
4 Place for a partial rebreather oxygen mask on the client.

Level of Cognitive Ability: Analysis
Client Needs: Physiological Integrity
Integrated Process: Nursing Process/Planning
Content Area: Adult Health/Immune

Answer: 2
Rationale: The most effective way to treat an acid-base disorder is to treat the underlying cause of the disorder. In this case, the problem is sepsis, which is most effectively treated with antibiotic therapy. Antipyretics will control fever secondary to sepsis but do nothing to treat the acid-base balance. The paper bag and partial rebreather mask will assist the client to rebreathe exhaled carbon dioxide, but again, these do not treat the primary cause of the imbalance.

Test-Taking Strategy: Note the strategic words "sepsis" and "most effective." Recalling that the most effective treatment of acid-base imbalances involves treatment of the primary cause will direct you to option 2. Remember that sepsis is a systemic infection and is treated with antibiotics. Review the treatment for respiratory alkalosis and sepsis if you had difficulty with this question.

References
Black, J., & Hawks, J. (2005). *Medical-surgical nursing: Clinical management for positive outcomes* (7th ed., pp. 2500-2501). Philadelphia: Saunders.
Ignatavicius, D., & Workman, M. (2006). *Medical-surgical nursing: Critical thinking for collaborative care* (5th ed., pp. 287-288). Philadelphia: Saunders.

453. The nurse notes that a client receiving lithium therapy is drowsy, has slurred speech, and is experiencing muscle twitching and impaired coordination. The nurse takes which of the following actions?

1 Holds one dose of lithium
2 Calls the health care provider
3 Doubles the next lithium dose
4 Increases fluids to 2000 mL per day

Level of Cognitive Ability: Application
Client Needs: Physiological Integrity
Integrated Process: Nursing Process/
   Implementation
Content Area: Pharmacology

Answer: 2
Rationale: Signs and symptoms of lithium toxicity include vomiting and diarrhea, as well as nervous system changes such as slurred speech, incoordination, drowsiness, muscle weakness, and twitching. Before administering any further doses, the nurse should notify the health care provider. As long as there are no contraindications, the client should routinely take in between 2000 and 3000 mL of fluid per day while taking this medication.

Test-Taking Strategy: Use the process of elimination. Eliminate options 1 and 3 first because it is not common practice to either hold one dose or double a medication dose without a specific order to do so. From the remaining options, focusing on the client's symptoms will direct you to option 2. Review the signs of toxicity of this medication if you had difficulty with this question.

Reference
Skidmore-Roth, L. (2008). *Mosby's nursing drug reference* (21st ed., p. 620). St. Louis: Mosby.

454. A client has been started on the medication metoclopramide (Reglan). The nurse monitors which item to determine effectiveness of therapy?

1 Urine output
2 Breath sounds
3 Episodes of vomiting
4 Complaints of headache

Level of Cognitive Ability: Analysis
Client Needs: Physiological Integrity
Integrated Process: Nursing Process/Evaluation
Content Area: Pharmacology

Answer: 3
Rationale: Metoclopramide is an antiemetic. The nurse would monitor to see whether the client has experienced a decrease or absence of vomiting to determine the effectiveness of therapy. Options 1, 2, and 4 are unrelated to the action of this medication.

Test-Taking Strategy: Use the process of elimination. Recalling that metoclopramide is an antiemetic will direct you to option 3. Review the action of this medication if you had difficulty with this question.

Reference
Skidmore-Roth, L. (2008). *Mosby's nursing drug reference* (21st ed., p. 673). St. Louis: Mosby.

455. A nurse is preparing to administer an intramuscular (IM) injection to a 2-year-old child. The best site to select for the injection is the:

1 Deltoid muscle
2 Dorsal gluteal muscle
3 Ventral gluteal muscle
4 Vastus lateralis muscle

Level of Cognitive Ability: Application
Client Needs: Physiological Integrity
Integrated Process: Nursing Process/
   Implementation
Content Area: Fundamental Skills

Answer: 4
Rationale: The vastus lateralis muscle, located on the anterior thigh, is well developed at birth. It is the best muscle for an IM injection for all age groups because it is able to tolerate larger volumes and is not located near vital structures such as nerves and blood vessels; as well, the vastus lateralis should always be used in children younger than 3 years of age. The deltoid is a much smaller muscle in a 2-year-old child, which increases the risk of injury. The dorsal and ventral gluteal muscles are also less developed than the vastus lateralis muscle and thus increase the risk of injury to adjacent structures and nerves.

Test-Taking Strategy: Use the process of elimination. Eliminate options 1, 2, and 3 because the locations present a risk of injury to a 2-year-old child. Review the procedure for administering intramuscular injections in a 2-year-old child if you had difficulty with this question.

Reference
Hockenberry, M., Wilson, D., & Winkelstein, M. (2005). *Wong's essentials of pediatric nursing* (7th ed., p. 753). St. Louis: Mosby.

---

456. A nurse is developing a plan of care for a school-age child with a knowledge deficit related to the use of inhalers and peak flow meters. The best expected outcome to be included in the plan of care is that the child will:

1 Deny shortness of breath or difficulty breathing.
2 Have regular respirations at a rate of 18 to 22 breaths per minute.
3 Watch the educational video and read printed information provided.
4 Express feelings of mastery and competence with the breathing devices.

Level of Cognitive Ability: Analysis
Client Needs: Physiological Integrity
Integrated Process: Nursing Process/Planning
Content Area: Child Health

Answer: 4
Rationale: School-age children strive for mastery and competence to achieve the developmental task of industry and accomplishment. Options 1 and 2 do not relate to the knowledge deficit. Option 3 may be a component of the teaching-learning process, but it is a passive process. Option 4 indicates more active participation on the part of the child, and expressing feelings of mastery and competence with the breathing devices indicates that learning took place.

Test-Taking Strategy: Focus on the subject, the best expected outcome. Eliminate options 1 and 2 first because they are comparable or alike. From the remaining options, focus on the subject and eliminate option 3 because it does not indicate that learning took place. Also noting that the child is school-age will direct you to option 4. Review development tasks of the school-age child if you had difficulty with this question.

Reference
Hockenberry, M., Wilson, D., & Winkelstein, M. (2005). *Wong's essentials of pediatric nursing* (7th ed., pp. 479-480). St. Louis: Mosby.

---

457. The lithium level results for a client receiving lithium carbonate (Eskalith) is 2.0 mEq/L. The nurse correctly analyzes these results as:

1 Insignificant
2 Within normal limits
3 Lower than normal limits
4 Higher than normal limits indicating toxicity

Level of Cognitive Ability: Analysis
Client Needs: Physiological Integrity
Integrated Process: Nursing Process/Analysis
Content Area: Pharmacology

Answer: 4
Rationale: The therapeutic level for lithium for the treatment of acute mania is 0.8 to 1.6 mEq/L. A level of 2.0 mEq/L indicates toxicity and requires that the medication be withheld and the blood work repeated. The physician also needs to be notified.

Test-Taking Strategy: Use the process of elimination. Eliminate options 1 and 2 first because they are comparable or alike. From the remaining options, recalling the therapeutic lithium level will direct you to option 4. Review this content if you are unfamiliar with this level.

Reference
Skidmore-Roth, L. (2008). *Mosby's nursing drug reference* (21st ed., p. 622). St. Louis: Mosby.

458. A client calls the ambulatory care clinic and tells the nurse that she found an area that looks like the peel of an orange when performing breast self-examination (BSE), but found no other changes. The nurse should:

1 Tell the client there is nothing to worry about.
2 Arrange for the client to be seen at the clinic as soon as possible.
3 Tell the client to take her temperature and call back if she has a fever.
4 Tell the client to point the area out to the physician at her next regularly scheduled appointment.

Level of Cognitive Ability: Application
Client Needs: Physiological Integrity
Integrated Process: Nursing Process/
   Implementation
Content Area: Adult Health/Oncology

Answer: 2
Rationale: Peau d'orange or the orange peel appearance of the skin over the breast is associated with late breast cancer. Therefore, the nurse would arrange for the client to come to the clinic at the earliest time possible. Peau d'orange is not indicative of an infection.

Test-Taking Strategy: Use the process of elimination. Eliminate options 1 and 4 because they are comparable or alike. From the remaining options, focus on the client's description to direct you to option 2. Review the signs of breast cancer if you had difficulty with this question.

Reference
Ignatavicius, D., & Workman, M. (2006). *Medical-surgical nursing: Critical thinking for collaborative care* (5th ed., p. 1800). Philadelphia: Saunders.

---

459. The nurse instructs a 60-years-old client about performing breast self-examination (BSE). Which client statement indicates a need for further instruction?

1 "I don't need to do that at my age."
2 "I examine my breasts in the shower."
3 "I lie on my back to examine my breasts."
4 "I do BSE on the first day of every month."

Level of Cognitive Ability: Analysis
Client Needs: Physiological Integrity
Integrated Process: Teaching and Learning
Content Area: Fundamental Skills

Answer: 1
Rationale: Women should continue to perform BSE on a regular schedule after menopause because breast cancer occurs in all age groups. Although the risk of breast cancer increases with age, malignant breast tumors in older clients are less aggressive than tumors in young breast cancer clients. Options 2, 3, and 4 identify correct components of performing BSE for a 60-year-old client.

Test-Taking Strategy: Use the process of elimination, noting the strategic words "need for further instruction." You need to select the client statement that does not comply with screening guidelines of the American Cancer Association. Recalling that breast cancer occurs in all age groups will direct you to option 1. Review this content if you had difficulty with this question or are unfamiliar with this procedure.

References
Ignatavicius, D., & Workman, M. (2006). *Medical-surgical nursing: Critical thinking for collaborative care* (5th ed., pp. 1796-1797). Philadelphia: Saunders.
Potter, P., & Perry, A. (2005). *Fundamentals of nursing* (6th ed., pp. 735-737). St. Louis: Mosby.

---

460. A client with Cushing's syndrome is being instructed by the nurse on follow-up care. Which statement by the client would indicate a need for further instructions?

1 "I should avoid contact sports."
2 "I should check my ankles for swelling."
3 "I need to avoid foods high in potassium."
4 "I need to check my blood glucose regularly."

Answer: 3
Rationale: Hypokalemia is a common characteristic of Cushing's syndrome, and the client is instructed to consume foods high in potassium. Clients also experience activity intolerance, osteoporosis, and frequent bruising. Excess fluid volume results from water and sodium retention. Hyperglycemia is caused by an increased cortisol secretion.

Level of Cognitive Ability: Analysis
Client Needs: Physiological Integrity
Integrated Process: Teaching and Learning
Content Area: Adult Health/Endocrine

Test-Taking Strategy: Note the strategic words "need for further instructions." This indicates a negative event query and the need to select the option that indicates an incorrect client statement. Thinking about the pathophysiology associated with Cushing's syndrome and recalling that hypokalemia is a concern will direct you to option 3. Review this disorder if you had difficulty with this question.

References
Black, J., & Hawks, J. (2005). *Medical-surgical nursing: Clinical management for positive outcomes* (7th ed., p. 1222). Philadelphia: Saunders.
Ignatavicius, D., & Workman, M. (2006). *Medical-surgical nursing: Critical thinking for collaborative care* (5th ed., pp. 1474-1475). Philadelphia: Saunders.

---

461. A client with hyperaldosteronism is being treated with spironolactone (Aldactone). Which of the following indicates to the nurse that the medication is effective?
1 A decrease in blood pressure
2 A decrease in sodium excretion
3 A decrease in body metabolism
4 A decrease in plasma potassium

Level of Cognitive Ability: Analysis
Client Needs: Physiological Integrity
Integrated Process: Nursing Process/Evaluation
Content Area: Adult Health/Endocrine

Answer: 1
Rationale: Aldactone antagonizes the effect of aldosterone and decreases circulating volume by inhibiting tubular reabsorption of sodium and water. Thus, it produces a decrease in blood pressure. It increases the excretion of sodium and water and increases potassium retention. It has no effect on body metabolism.

Test-Taking Strategy: Note the strategic words "medication is effective." Think about the action of this medication. Recalling that this medication is also used in hypertensive conditions will direct you to option 1. Review the effects of this medication if you had difficulty with this question.

Reference
Hodgson, B., & Kizior, R. (2007). *Saunders nursing drug handbook 2007* (p. 1074). Philadelphia: Saunders.

---

462. A nurse caring for a client with neuroleptic malignant syndrome that resulted from the use of antipsychotic medications would expect to note:
1 Dysphagia
2 Bradycardia
3 Hypotension
4 Hyperpyrexia

Level of Cognitive Ability: Analysis
Client Needs: Physiological Integrity
Integrated Process: Nursing Process/Assessment
Content Area: Pharmacology

Answer: 4
Rationale: Hyperpyrexia up to 107° F may be present in neuroleptic malignant syndrome. Symptoms develop suddenly and may include respiratory distress and muscle rigidity. As the condition progresses, there is evidence of tachycardia, hypertension, increasing respiratory distress, confusion, and delirium. The presence and severity of symptoms are compounded when two or more antipsychotics are taken concurrently.

Test-Taking Strategy: Consider the physiological responses that occur in neuroleptic malignant syndrome to answer this question. Recalling that an elevated temperature occurs in this disorder will direct you to the correct option. Review the physiological manifestations that occur in neuroleptic malignant syndrome if you had difficulty with this question.

Reference
Kee, J., Hayes, E., & McCuistion, L. (2006). *Pharmacology: A nursing process approach.* (5th ed., pp. 379, 381, 383). Philadelphia: Saunders.

463. A client with cancer who is receiving chemotherapy tells the nurse that the food on the meal tray "tastes funny." Which intervention by the nurse is appropriate?
 1 Keep the client NPO.
 2 Provide oral hygiene care.
 3 Administer an antiemetic as ordered.
 4 Obtain an order for parenteral nutrition (PN).

Level of Cognitive Ability: Application
Client Needs: Physiological Integrity
Integrated Process: Nursing Process/
  Implementation
Content Area: Adult Health/Oncology

Answer: 2
Rationale: Cancer treatments may cause distortion of taste. Frequent oral hygiene aids in preserving taste function. Keeping a client NPO increases nutritional risks. Antiemetics are used when nausea and vomiting are a problem. PN is used when oral intake is not possible.

Test-Taking Strategy: Focus on the subject, taste sensation. Only option 2 addresses this subject. Also note the relationship between the words "tastes" in the question and "oral hygiene care" in the correct option. Review the effects of cancer treatments and the appropriate nursing interventions if you had difficulty with this question.

References
Black, J., & Hawks, J. (2005). *Medical-surgical nursing: Clinical management for positive outcomes* (7th ed., p. 370). Philadelphia: Saunders.
Gulanick, M., & Myers, J. (2007). *Nursing care plans: Nursing diagnosis and intervention* (6th ed., pp. 815-818.). St. Louis: Mosby.
Ignatavicius, D., & Workman, M. (2006). *Medical-surgical nursing: Critical thinking for collaborative care* (5th ed., pp. 494, 496). Philadelphia: Saunders.

464. The nurse notes redness, warmth, and purulent drainage at the insertion site of a central venous catheter (CVC) in a client receiving parenteral nutrition (PN). The nurse collaborates with the provider about this finding because:
 1 The client is not tolerating the PN solution.
 2 The client is allergic to the dressing material.
 3 The CVC is infiltrated and should be stopped.
 4 Infections of a CVC site can lead to septicemia.

Level of Cognitive Ability: Application
Client Needs: Physiological Integrity
Integrated Process: Nursing Process/
  Implementation
Content Area: Fundamental Skills

Answer: 4
Rationale: Redness, warmth, and purulent drainage are signs of an infection, not an indication of intolerance to the solution or an allergic reaction. All clients who have an infected IV insertion site are at risk of septicemia because the potential source of the infection is already in a vessel. Additionally, clients with a CVC are at high risk for septicemia because the CVC is very close to the heart. Infiltration of a CVC is unlikely because the catheters are usually threaded into the vena cava or right atrium; besides, the surrounding tissue is more likely to become cool and pale with infiltration.

Test-Taking Strategy: Note the strategic words "redness, warmth, and a purulent drainage" and focus on the subject, clinical indicators of infection. Eliminate options 1, 2, and 3 because the client's assessment findings are inconsistent with these issues. Conversely, note that option 4 addresses septicemia, which can have devastating results or be life-threatening to the client. Review nursing interventions related to monitoring for complications of PN if you had difficulty with this question.

References
Ignatavicius, D., & Workman, M. (2006). *Medical-surgical nursing: Critical thinking for collaborative care* (5th ed., pp. 260-264, 832, 1433). Philadelphia: Saunders.
Potter, P., & Perry, A. (2005). *Fundamentals of nursing* (6th ed., p. 1315). St. Louis: Mosby.

465. The nurse is performing a health history on a client with chronic calcifying pancreatitis. The nurse expects to most likely note which of the following when obtaining information regarding the client's health history?

1 Weight gain
2 History of smoking
3 Chronic use of alcohol
4 Abdominal pain relieved with food or antacids

Level of Cognitive Ability: Analysis
Client Needs: Physiological Integrity
Integrated Process: Nursing Process/Assessment
Content Area: Adult Health/Gastrointestinal

Answer: 3
Rationale: Chronic use of alcohol is the most frequent cause of chronic calcifying pancreatitis. Abstinence from alcohol is important to prevent the client from developing chronic pancreatitis. Clients usually experience malabsorption with weight loss. Smoking is associated with cancer of the pancreas. Pain will not be relieved with food or antacids.

Test-Taking Strategy: Focus on the subject, the cause of chronic calcifying pancreatitis. Recalling the relationship between alcohol use and pancreatitis will direct you to option 3. Review the causes of pancreatitis if you had difficulty with this question.

Reference

Black, J., & Hawks, J. (2005). *Medical-surgical nursing: Clinical management for positive outcomes* (7th ed., p. 1297). Philadelphia: Saunders.

466. A client has been taking the glucocorticoid prednisone (Deltasone) control rheumatoid arthritis. The nurse monitors the client for which adverse effect of this pharmacological therapy?

1 Increased serum glucose
2 Decreased serum sodium
3 Elevated serum potassium
4 Increased white blood cells

Level of Cognitive Ability: Analysis
Client Needs: Physiological Integrity
Integrated Process: Nursing Process/Analysis
Content Area: Pharmacology

Answer: 1
Rationale: Glucocorticoids have three primary uses: replacement therapy for adrenal insufficiency, immunosuppressive therapy, and anti-inflammatory therapy. Exogenous glucocorticoids cause the same effects on cellular activity as the naturally produced glucocorticoids; however, exogenous glucocorticoids may produce undesired effects. The glucocorticoids stimulate appetite and increase caloric intake. They also increase the availability of glucose for energy. These combined effects cause the blood glucose levels to rise, making the client prone to hyperglycemia. Options 2, 3, and 4 do not occur as a result of the use of glucocorticoids.

Test-Taking Strategy: Use the process of elimination. First, eliminate options 2 and 3 because they are comparable or alike in that they both relate to electrolytes. From the remaining options, recalling that glucocorticoids increase the availability of glucose for energy will direct you to option 1. Review this content if you are unfamiliar with these type of medications, their uses, side effects and adverse effects, and contraindications.

Reference

Skidmore-Roth, L. (2008). *Mosby's nursing drug reference* (21st ed., p. 843). St. Louis: Mosby.

467. A client with a diagnosis of Cushing's syndrome is undergoing a dexamethasone suppression test. The nurse plans to implement which steps during this test?

1 Collect a 24-hour urine specimen to measure serum cortisol levels.

2 Administer 1 mg of dexamethasone orally at night and obtain serum cortisol levels the next morning.

3 Draw blood samples before and after exercise to evaluate the effect of exercise on serum cortisol levels.

4 Administer an injection of adrenocorticotropic hormone (ACTH) 30 minutes before drawing blood to measure serum cortisol levels.

Level of Cognitive Ability: Application
Client Needs: Physiological Integrity
Integrated Process: Nursing Process/Planning
Content Area: Adult Health/Endocrine

Answer: 2
Rationale: The dexamethasone suppression test is performed to evaluate the function of the adrenal cortex. The procedure for this test is to administer 1 mg of dexamethasone at 11:00 PM to suppress ACTH formation and then to obtain 8:00 AM serum cortisol levels on the following day.

Test-Taking Strategy: Recall that Cushing's syndrome is a disorder caused by excessive amounts of cortisol. Because the test is a dexamethasone suppression test, you would expect that something is given to suppress cortisol production. Keeping this in mind, options 1 and 3 can be eliminated. From the remaining options, focusing on the description of Cushing's syndrome and the purpose of this test will direct you to option 2. Review this test if you had difficulty with this question.

Reference
Chernecky, C., & Berger, B. (2008). *Laboratory tests and diagnostic procedures* (5th ed., pp. 434-435). Philadelphia: Saunders.

---

468. The nurse is performing an abdominal assessment on a client. The nurse determines that which of the following findings should be reported to the physician?

1 Absence of a bruit

2 Concave, midline umbilicus

3 Pulsation between the umbilicus and pubis

4 Bowel sound frequency of 15 sounds per minute

Level of Cognitive Ability: Analysis
Client Needs: Physiological Integrity
Integrated Process: Nursing Process/Assessment
Content Area: Adult Health/Gastrointestinal

Answer: 3
Rationale: The presence of pulsation between the umbilicus and the pubis could indicate abdominal aortic aneurysm and should be reported to the physician. Bruits are not normally present. The umbilicus should be in the midline, with a concave appearance. Bowel sounds vary according to the timing of the last meal and usually range in frequency from 5 to 35 per minute.

Test-Taking Strategy: Use basic nursing knowledge related to physical assessment to answer this question. Note that the wording of the question guides you to look for an abnormal finding. This will direct you to option 3. Review abdominal assessment if you had difficulty with this question.

References
Ignatavicius, D., & Workman, M. (2006). *Medical-surgical nursing: Critical thinking for collaborative care* (5th ed., pp. 1238-1240). Philadelphia: Saunders.
Jarvis, C. (2004). *Physical examination and health assessment* (4th ed., pp. 578-581). Philadelphia: Saunders.

---

469. The nurse is performing a cardiovascular assessment on a client. Which of the following items would the nurse assess to gain the best information about the client's left-sided heart function?

1 Breath sounds

2 Peripheral edema

3 Hepatojugular reflux

4 Jugular vein distention

Answer: 1
Rationale: The client with heart failure may present with different symptoms depending on whether the right or the left side of the heart is failing. Peripheral edema, hepatojugular reflux, and jugular vein distention are all indicators of right-sided heart function. Breath sounds are an accurate indicator of left-sided heart function.

Test-Taking Strategy: Focus on the subject—left-sided heart failure. Remember: "left and lungs." Left-sided heart failure leads to respiratory signs and symptoms. Review the signs of right- and left-sided heart failure if you had difficulty with this question.

Level of Cognitive Ability: Application
Client Needs: Physiological Integrity
Integrated Process: Nursing Process/Assessment
Content Area: Adult Health/Respiratory

Reference
Ignatavicius, D., & Workman, M. (2006). *Medical-surgical nursing: Critical thinking for collaborative care* (5th ed., pp. 752-753). Philadelphia: Saunders.

---

470. The nurse is caring for the following group of clients on the clinical nursing unit. The nurse interprets that which of these clients is most at risk for the development of pulmonary embolism?

1 A 25-year-old woman with diabetic ketoacidosis
2 A 65-year-old man out of bed 1 day after prostate resection
3 A 73-year-old woman who has just had a pinning of a hip fracture
4 A 38-year-old man with a closed pneumothorax after an auto accident

Level of Cognitive Ability: Analysis
Client Needs: Physiological Integrity
Integrated Process: Nursing Process/Assessment
Content Area: Adult Health/Respiratory

Answer: 3
Rationale: Clients frequently at risk for pulmonary embolism include those who are immobilized, especially postoperative clients. Other causes include those with conditions that are characterized by hypercoagulability, endothelial disease, and advancing age.

Test-Taking Strategy: The options can best be compared by evaluating the degree of immobility that each client has, and also the age of the client, which is provided in each option. The clients in options 1 and 2 have the least long-term anticipated immobility and, therefore, should be eliminated first. From the remaining options, the younger client with the closed pneumothorax with the presence of chest tubes would be expected to be less immobile than the older woman with a hip fracture. Review the causes of pulmonary embolism if you had difficulty with this question.

References
Ignatavicius, D., & Workman, M. (2006). *Medical-surgical nursing: Critical thinking for collaborative care* (5th ed., p. 650). Philadelphia: Saunders.
Meiner, S., & Leuckenotte, A. (2006). *Gerontologic nursing* (3rd ed., p. 178). St. Louis: Mosby.

---

471. A graduate nurse is assigned to admit a client with a diagnosis of anorexia nervosa to the nursing unit. The nurse preceptor would remind the graduate nurse that assessment findings may indicate:

1 Low blood urea nitrogen
2 Elevated potassium levels
3 Weight loss of 4% of original weight over a short period
4 That the client is knowledgeable about the caloric value of food

Level of Cognitive Ability: Analysis
Client Needs: Physiological Integrity
Integrated Process: Nursing Process/Assessment
Content Area: Mental Health

Answer: 4
Rationale: The potassium level is usually low and the blood urea nitrogen is usually high in clients with anorexia nervosa. These clients lose at least 15% of their original body weight in a short period of time. They are very knowledgeable about nutrition and the caloric value of food.

Test-Taking Strategy: Use the process of elimination, focusing on the client's diagnosis. Option 3 is eliminated because the small amount of weight loss (4% of original weight) is not a concern or typical of anorexia nervosa. Eliminate options 1 and 2 because these findings do not occur in starvation or in the fluid or electrolyte deficiency typical of anorexia nervosa. Review the typical assessment findings in the client with anorexia nervosa if you had difficulty with this question.

Reference
Stuart, G., & Laraia, M. (2005). *Principles and practice of psychiatric nursing* (8th ed., p. 520). St. Louis: Mosby.

472. A physician has inserted a nasointestinal tube into a client. Following insertion, the nurse tells the client to lie in which position to help the tube advance into the duodenum, past the pyloric sphincter?
1 On the left side
2 Supine with the head of the bed flat
3 On the right side with the head elevated
4 Supine with the head elevated 30 degrees

Level of Cognitive Ability: Application
Client Needs: Physiological Integrity
Integrated Process: Nursing Process/ Implementation
Content Area: Adult Health/Gastrointestinal

Answer: 3
Rationale: Following insertion of a nasointestinal tube, the client is instructed to lie on the right side with the head elevated to aid in the passage of the tube from the stomach into the duodenum, past the pyloric sphincter. Options 1, 2, and 4 are incorrect positions.

Test-Taking Strategy: Use knowledge of basic anatomy and the position of the stomach in the abdomen to help eliminate options 1, 2, and 4. Knowledge of this position can be applied to the management of a client with any type of nasointestinal tube. Review care of the client with a nasointestinal tube if you had difficulty with this question.

References
Ignatavicius, D., & Workman, M. (2006). *Medical-surgical nursing: Critical thinking for collaborative care* (5th ed., p. 1329). Philadelphia: Saunders.
Lewis, S., Heitkemper, M., Dirksen, S., O'Brien, P., & Bucher, L. (2007). *Medical-surgical nursing: Assessment and management of clinical problems* (7th ed., p. 962). St. Louis: Mosby.
Perry, A., & Potter, P. (2006). *Clinical nursing skills & techniques* (6th ed., p. 1020). St. Louis: Mosby.

---

473. A client with coronary artery disease suddenly complains of palpitations and an irregular heartbeat. The nurse would assess for which of the following to determine if the client is experiencing an inadequate stroke volume?
1 Pulse deficit
2 Pulse pressure
3 Pulsus alternans
4 Water hammer pulse

Level of Cognitive Ability: Analysis
Client Needs: Physiological Integrity
Integrated Process: Nursing Process/Assessment
Content Area: Adult Health/Cardiovascular

Answer: 1
Rationale: Palpitations are often a subjective complaint that accompanies dysrhythmias. Irregular rhythms produce varying strengths of stroke volume because of irregular ventricular filling times, and therefore arterial pulsations may become weakened or intermittently absent. The nurse determines this by assessing an apical-radial pulse. An apical rate that is greater than the radial rate is called a "pulse deficit." The pulse pressure is the difference between the systolic and diastolic blood pressures. Pulsus alternans has a regular rhythm accompanied by pulse volume that alternates strong with weak. A water hammer pulse (Corrigan's pulse) is a bounding pulse in which a great surge is felt, followed by a sudden and complete absence of force or fullness in the artery. This type of pulse is associated with aortic regurgitation.

Test-Taking Strategy: Use the process of elimination. Remember that "stroke volume X heart rate = cardiac output." Measures that give a general indication of cardiac output are not specific enough to answer this question, therefore eliminate options 2 and 4. Pulsus alternans (option 3) occurs with a regular rhythm so it can also be eliminated. Review the definition of pulse deficit if you had difficulty with this question.

References
Ignatavicius, D., & Workman, M. (2006). *Medical-surgical nursing: Critical thinking for collaborative care* (5th ed., pp. 692, 845). Philadelphia: Saunders.
Mosby. (2006). *Mosby's dictionary of medicine, nursing & health professions.* (7th ed., pp. 467, 1564-1565). St. Louis: Mosby.
Potter, P., & Perry, A. (2005). *Fundamentals of nursing* (6th ed., p. 725). St. Louis: Mosby.

474. The nurse is listening to the client's breath sounds and hears a creaking, grating sound on inspiration and expiration over the posterior right lower lobe. How should the nurse correctly document this on the client record?

1 Crackles auscultated
2 Rhonchi auscultated
3 Wheezes auscultated
4 Pleural friction rub auscultated

Level of Cognitive Ability: Analysis
Client Needs: Physiological Integrity
Integrated Process: Communication and Documentation
Content Area: Adult Health/Respiratory

Answer: 4
Rationale: The nurse is hearing a pleural friction rub, which is characterized by sounds that are described as creaking, groaning, or grating in quality. The sounds are localized over an area of inflammation of the pleura and may be heard in both the inspiratory and expiratory phases of the respiratory cycle. Crackles have the sound that is heard when a few strands of hair are rubbed together near the ear and indicate fluid in the alveoli. Wheezes are musical noises heard on inspiration, expiration, or both. They are the result of narrowed air passages. Rhonchi are usually heard on expiration when there is excessive production of mucus, which accumulates in the air passages.

Test-Taking Strategy: Note the strategic words "creaking, grating sound." The image called to mind by these sounds is most compatible with the words "friction rub," and that may be sufficient to help you answer the question correctly. In addition, knowing that these sounds are not the classic descriptors for crackles, wheezes, or rhonchi helps you eliminate each of the other options. Review the characteristics of a pleural friction rub if you had difficulty with this question.

References
Black, J., & Hawks, J. (2005). *Medical-surgical nursing: Clinical management for positive outcomes* (7th ed., p. 1757). Philadelphia: Saunders.
Potter, P., & Perry, A. (2005). *Fundamentals of nursing* (6th ed., p. 721). St. Louis: Mosby.

475. The nurse is assessing the renal function of a client. After directly noting urine volume and characteristics, the nurse assesses which item as the best indirect indicator of renal function?

1 Pulse rate
2 Blood pressure
3 Bladder distention
4 Level of consciousness

Level of Cognitive Ability: Application
Client Needs: Physiological Integrity
Integrated Process: Nursing Process/Assessment
Content Area: Adult Health/Renal

Answer: 2
Rationale: The kidneys normally receive 20% to 25% of the cardiac output, even under conditions of rest. In order for kidney function to be optimal, adequate renal perfusion is necessary. Perfusion can best be estimated by the blood pressure, which is an indirect reflection of the adequacy of cardiac output. The pulse rate affects the cardiac output, but it can be altered by factors unrelated to kidney function. Bladder distention reflects a problem or obstruction that is most often distal to the kidneys. Level of consciousness is an unrelated item.

Test-Taking Strategy: Focus on the subject—renal function. Eliminate option 4 first as the item most unrelated to kidney function. Because bladder distention can be affected by several other factors besides renal function, this is eliminated next. From the remaining options, remember that the cardiac output equals heart rate times stroke volume. The cardiac output overall helps determine the blood pressure and renal perfusion. Thus, blood pressure is the more comprehensive option and the one more directly related to kidney perfusion. Review assessment of renal function if you had difficulty with this question.

References
Black, J., & Hawks, J. (2005). *Medical-surgical nursing: Clinical management for positive outcomes* (7th ed., pp. 767, 914). Philadelphia: Saunders.
Ignatavicius, D., & Workman, M. (2006). *Medical-surgical nursing: Critical thinking for collaborative care* (5th ed., p. 1662). Philadelphia: Saunders.

476. The nurse notes that the infusion bag of a client receiving parenteral nutrition (PN) has become empty. The nurse calls the pharmacy, but the next bag will not be delivered for another 30 minutes. The nurse hangs which of the following solutions until the PN arrives?

1 5% dextrose in water
2 10% dextrose in water
3 50% dextrose in saline
4 5% dextrose in 0.45% saline

Level of Cognitive Ability: Application
Client Needs: Physiological Integrity
Integrated Process: Nursing Process/
Implementation
Content Area: Adult Health/Gastrointestinal

Answer: 2
Rationale: If a PN solution bag becomes empty, the nurse should hang an infusion of 10% dextrose in water until another bag of PN solution is available. This minimizes the chance of the client developing hypoglycemia, because the body produces more insulin in the presence of the high PN glucose load.

Test-Taking Strategy: Use the process of elimination, recalling that the glucose concentration of PN is high. Eliminate option 3 because there is no such solution of this type. Remember that options that are comparable or alike are not likely to be correct. This guides you to eliminate options 1 and 4, because the percentage of dextrose is the same. Review care of the client receiving PN if you had difficulty with this question.

Reference
Ignatavicius, D., & Workman, M. (2006). *Medical-surgical nursing: Critical thinking for collaborative care* (5th ed., p. 1433). Philadelphia: Saunders.

---

477. A client seen in the ambulatory care clinic has ascites and slight jaundice. The nurse assesses the client for a history of chronic use of which of the following medications?

1 Ranitidine (Zantac)
2 Acetaminophen (Tylenol)
3 Docusate sodium (Colace)
4 Acetylsalicylic acid (aspirin)

Level of Cognitive Ability: Analysis
Client Needs: Physiological Integrity
Integrated Process: Nursing Process/Assessment
Content Area: Adult Health/Gastrointestinal

Answer: 2
Rationale: Acetaminophen is a potentially hepatotoxic medication. Use of this medication and other hepatotoxic agents should be investigated whenever a client presents with symptoms compatible with liver disease (such as ascites and jaundice). Hepatotoxicity is not an adverse effect of the medications identified in options 1, 3, and 4.

Test-Taking Strategy: Focus on the signs noted in the question and recall that these symptoms are compatible with liver disease. With this in mind, evaluate each of the options in relation to their relative ability to be toxic to the liver. Recalling that acetaminophen is hepatotoxic will direct you to option 2. Review these medications if you are unfamiliar with them.

Reference
Kee, J., Hayes, E., & McCuistion, L. (2006). *Pharmacology: A nursing process approach.* (5th ed., p. 324). Philadelphia: Saunders.

---

478. The nurse is assigned to care for a client who has just undergone cataract surgery. The nurse plans to instruct the client that which of the following activities is permitted in the postoperative period?

1 Bending over
2 Lifting objects
3 Coughing exercises
4 Watching television

Answer: 4
Rationale: The client is taught to avoid activities that raise intraocular pressure and could cause complications in the postoperative period. The client is also taught to avoid activities that cause rapid eye movements that are irritating in the presence of postoperative inflammation. For these reasons, the client is taught to avoid bending over, lifting heavy objects, straining, sneezing, coughing, making sudden movements, or reading. Watching television is permissible because the eye does not need to move rapidly with this activity, and it does not increase the intraocular pressure.

Level of Cognitive Ability: Application
Client Needs: Physiological Integrity
Integrated Process: Nursing Process/Planning
Content Area: Adult Health/Eye

Test-Taking Strategy: Focus on the subject of intraocular pressure when answering this question. Eliminate options 1, 2, and 3 because they increase intraocular pressure. Select option 4 because it is the least taxing activity on the eyes. Review postoperative client instructions following eye surgery if you had difficulty with this question.

Reference
Ignatavicius, D., & Workman, M. (2006). *Medical-surgical nursing: Critical thinking for collaborative care* (5th ed., p. 1095). Philadelphia: Saunders.

---

479. The nurse is listening to the lungs of a client who has left lower lobe pneumonia. The nurse interprets that the pneumonia is resolving if which of the following is heard over the affected lung area?
1 Egophony
2 Bronchophony
3 Vesicular breath sounds
4 Whispered pectoriloquy

Level of Cognitive Ability: Analysis
Client Needs: Physiological Integrity
Integrated Process: Nursing Process/Evaluation
Content Area: Adult Health/Respiratory

Answer: 3
Rationale: Vesicular breath sounds are normal sounds that are heard over peripheral lung fields where the air enters the alveoli. A return of breath sounds to normal is consistent with a resolving pneumonia. Egophony occurs when the sound of the letter "e" is heard as an "a" with auscultation and also indicates lung consolidation. Bronchophony is an abnormal finding indicative of lung consolidation and is identified if the nurse can clearly hear the client say "ninety-nine" through the stethoscope when auscultating the lungs. (Normally the client's words are unintelligible if heard through a stethoscope.) Finally, whispered pectoriloquy is present if the nurse hears the client when "one-two-three" is whispered. This is an abnormal finding, again heard over an area of consolidation. Consolidation typically occurs with pneumonia.

Test-Taking Strategy: Use knowledge regarding respiratory assessment findings to answer the question. Knowing the anatomical areas where bronchial, vesicular, and bronchovesicular breath sounds are heard will direct you to option 3. Review these types of breath sounds if you had difficulty with this question.

References
Black, J., & Hawks, J. (2005). *Medical-surgical nursing: Clinical management for positive outcomes* (7th ed., p. 1755). Philadelphia: Saunders.
Ignatavicius, D., & Workman, M. (2006). *Medical-surgical nursing: Critical thinking for collaborative care* (5th ed., pp. 633, 635). Philadelphia: Saunders.
Wilson, S., & Giddens, J. (2005). *Health assessment for nursing practice* (3rd ed., pp. 347-348). St. Louis. Mosby.

---

480. A female client with a history of chronic infection of the urinary system complains of burning and urinary frequency. To determine whether the current problem is of renal origin, the nurse would assess whether the client has pain or discomfort in the:
1 Urinary meatus
2 Suprapubic area
3 Pain in the labium
4 Right or left costovertebral angle

Answer: 4
Rationale: Pain or discomfort from a problem that originates in the kidney is felt at the costovertebral angle on the affected side. Bladder infection is often accompanied by suprapubic pain and pain or burning at the urinary meatus when voiding. Ureteral pain is felt in the ipsilateral labium in the female client or the ipsilateral scrotum in the male client.

Test-Taking Strategy: Focus on the subject, a renal problem. Note the similarity between options 1, 2, and 3 in that they relate to the lower urinary tract. Recalling that the kidneys sit higher than the level of the bladder and retroperitoneally will also direct you to option 4. Review the signs of both renal and bladder infections if you had difficulty with this question.

Level of Cognitive Ability: Analysis
Client Needs: Physiological Integrity
Integrated Process: Nursing Process/Assessment
Content Area: Adult Health/Renal

References
Ignatavicius, D., & Workman, M. (2006). *Medical-surgical nursing: Critical thinking for collaborative care* (5th ed., pp. 1680-1681). Philadelphia: Saunders.
Wilson, S., & Giddens, J. (2005). *Health assessment for nursing practice* (3rd ed., pp. 450-451). St. Louis: Mosby.

---

481. During a routine visit to the physician's office for monitoring of diabetic control, an older client with diabetes mellitus complains to the nurse of vision changes. The client describes blurring of the vision with difficulty in reading and with driving at night. Given the client's history, the nurse interprets that the client is probably developing:

1 Cataracts
2 Glaucoma
3 Papilledema
4 Detached retina

Answer: 1
Rationale: Although the incidence of cataracts increases with age, the older client with diabetes mellitus is at greater risk for developing cataracts. The most frequent complaint is blurred vision that is not accompanied by pain. The client may also experience difficulty with reading, night driving, and glare. Options 2, 3, and 4 are not directly associated with this client's history or complaints.

Test-Taking Strategy: Note that the client has diabetes mellitus. Use knowledge related to the risks for and signs and symptoms of common eye disorders to answer this question. Review the signs and symptoms of cataracts and the associated risk factors if you had difficulty with this question.

Level of Cognitive Ability: Analysis
Client Needs: Physiological Integrity
Integrated Process: Nursing Process/Analysis
Content Area: Adult Health/Eye

Reference
Ignatavicius, D., & Workman, M. (2006). *Medical-surgical nursing: Critical thinking for collaborative care* (5th ed., p. 1093). Philadelphia: Saunders.

---

482. The nurse inquires about a smoking history while conducting a hospital admission assessment for a client with coronary artery disease (CAD). Which of the following is the most important item for the nurse to assess?

1 Number of pack-years
2 Desire to quit smoking
3 Brand of cigarettes used
4 Number of past attempts to quit smoking

Answer: 1
Rationale: The number of cigarettes smoked daily and the duration of the habit are used to calculate the number of pack-years, which is the standard method of documenting smoking history. The brand of cigarettes may give a general indication of tar and nicotine levels, but the information has no immediate clinical use. Desire to quit and number of past attempts to quit smoking may be useful when the nurse develops a smoking cessation plan with the client.

Test-Taking Strategy: Note the strategic words "most important item." The option that would most closely predict the degree of added risk of CAD is the number of pack-years. Review the technique to assess smoking history if you had difficulty with this question.

Level of Cognitive Ability: Analysis
Client Needs: Physiological Integrity
Integrated Process: Nursing Process/Assessment
Content Area: Adult Health/Cardiovascular

Reference
Ignatavicius, D., & Workman, M. (2006). *Medical-surgical nursing: Critical thinking for collaborative care* (5th ed., p. 529). Philadelphia: Saunders.

483. The client with open-angle glaucoma who is taking timolol maleate (Timoptic) drops asks the nurse how this medication works. The nurse responds correctly by telling the client that the medication lowers intraocular pressure by:

1 Constricting the pupil
2 Reducing intracranial pressure
3 Increasing contractions of the ciliary muscle
4 Decreasing the production of aqueous humor

Level of Cognitive Ability: Application
Client Needs: Physiological Integrity
Integrated Process: Teaching and Learning
Content Area: Pharmacology

Answer: 4
Rationale: Beta-adrenergic blocking agents, such as timolol acetate, reduce intraocular pressure by decreasing the production of aqueous humor. Miotic agents (such as pilocarpine) increase contractions of the ciliary muscle and constrict the pupil, thereby increasing the outflow of aqueous humor. This medication does not affect intracranial pressure.

Test-Taking Strategy: Specific knowledge about the action of this medication is needed to answer this question. Remember that beta-adrenergic blocking agents reduce intraocular pressure by decreasing the production of aqueous humor. Review the action of this medication if you are unfamiliar with it.

Reference
Skidmore-Roth, L. (2008). *Mosby's nursing drug reference* (21st ed., p. 897). St. Louis: Mosby.

---

484. The rehabilitation nurse is providing home care instruction for a client being discharged after above-the-knee amputation of the right lower limb with a fitted prosthesis. The nurse determines the client requires further teaching if the client makes which of the following statements?

1 "I will elevate the residual limb on a pillow."
2 "I will change the residual limb sock every day."
3 "I will check the residual limb for skin irritation daily."
4 "I will notify my prosthetist if my residual limb sock becomes stretched or ill-fitting."

Level of Cognitive Ability: Analysis
Client Needs: Physiological Integrity
Integrated Process: Teaching and Learning
Content Area: Adult Health/Musculoskeletal

Answer: 1
Rationale: Clients must avoid elevation of the residual limb to prevent flexion contractures of the right hip. Additionally, sitting in a chair should be limited to 1-hour intervals to avoid the same. If there is no contraindication, clients should lie in the prone position three to four times a day to promote hip extension. Limb socks should be removed daily, laundered in mild soap, and replaced with a clean sock. When the sock is removed, the residual limb should be inspected for erythema and excoriation. As the edema resolves, the residual limb shrinks and the sock may not fit properly, leading to skin irritation. The prosthetist should be notified of the ill-fitting sock.

Test-Taking Strategy: Focus on the words "requires further teaching." Eliminate options 2, 3, and 4 because they are focused on either maintenance of skin integrity or early identification of skin breakdown. Review care of the client with an amputation and prosthetic device if you had difficulty with this question.

Reference
Lewis, S., Heitkemper, M., Dirksen, S., O'Brien, P., & Bucher, L. (2007). *Medical surgical nursing: Assessment and management of clinical problems* (7th ed., p. 1661). St. Louis: Mosby.

---

485. A client arrives at the clinic complaining of knee pain. On assessment the nurse notes that the knee area is swollen. The nurse interprets that the client's signs and symptoms likely indicate:

1 Osteoporosis
2 A recent injury
3 Rheumatoid arthritis
4 Degenerative joint disease

Answer: 2
Rationale: Pain and swelling are associated with musculoskeletal inflammation, infection, or a recent injury. Degenerative joint disease, osteoporosis, and rheumatoid arthritis may be accompanied by pain, but swelling may or may not be present.

Level of Cognitive Ability: Analysis
Client Needs: Physiological Integrity
Integrated Process: Nursing Process/Analysis
Content Area: Adult Health/Musculoskeletal

Test-Taking Strategy: Focus on the signs and symptoms in the question and note the strategic words "likely," which indicates that more than one option may be correct. Swelling and pain are signs of injury or inflammation. This should direct you to option 2. Review the signs associated with a musculoskeletal injury and the signs of degenerative disease if you had difficulty with this question.

References
Black, J., & Hawks, J. (2005). *Medical-surgical nursing: Clinical management for positive outcomes* (7th ed., p. 653). Philadelphia: Saunders.
Ignatavicius, D., & Workman, M. (2006). *Medical-surgical nursing: Critical thinking for collaborative care* (5th ed., pp. 1224-1225). Philadelphia: Saunders.

---

486. A client seeks treatment in the emergency department for a lower leg injury. There is visible deformity to the lower aspect of the leg, and the injured leg appears shorter than the other leg. The area is painful, swollen, and beginning to become ecchymotic. The nurse interprets that this client has experienced a:
1 Strain
2 Sprain
3 Fracture
4 Contusion

Level of Cognitive Ability: Analysis
Client Needs: Physiological Integrity
Integrated Process: Nursing Process/Assessment
Content Area: Adult Health/Musculoskeletal

Answer: 3
Rationale: Typical signs and symptoms of fracture include pain, loss of function in the area, deformity, shortening of the extremity, crepitus, swelling, and ecchymosis. Not all fractures lead to the development of every sign. A strain results from a pulling force on the muscle. Symptoms include soreness and pain with muscle use. A sprain is an injury to a ligament caused by a wrenching or twisting motion. Symptoms include pain, swelling, and inability to use the joint or bear weight normally. A contusion results from a blow to soft tissue and causes pain, swelling, and ecchymosis.

Test-Taking Strategy: Use the process of elimination and focus on the signs and symptoms in the question. Within the list of signs and symptoms, note the one that states that one leg is shorter than another. Only a fractured bone (which shortens with displacement) could cause this sign. This makes it easy to eliminate each of the incorrect options. Review the signs and symptoms of a fracture if you had difficulty with this question.

Reference
Ignatavicius, D., & Workman, M. (2006). *Medical-surgical nursing: Critical thinking for collaborative care* (5th ed., pp. 1194-1195). Philadelphia: Saunders.

---

487. A client arrives at the emergency room with a chemical burn of the left eye. The nurse immediately:
1 Applies a light bandage to the eye
2 Performs an assessment on the client
3 Applies a cold compress to the injured eye
4 Flushes the eye continuously with a sterile solution

Level of Cognitive Ability: Application
Client Needs: Physiological Integrity
Integrated Process: Nursing Process/Implementation
Content Area: Adult Health/Eye

Answer: 4
Rationale: When the client has suffered a chemical burn of the eye, the nurse immediately flushes the site with a sterile solution continuously for 15 minutes. If a sterile eye irrigation solution is not available, running water may be used. Performing an assessment may be helpful but is not the priority action. Applying compresses or bandages is incorrect, because they do not rid the eye of the damaging chemical. Cold compresses are used for blows to the eye, whereas light bandages may be placed over cuts of the eye or eyelid.

Test-Taking Strategy: Focus on the injury described in the question: a chemical burn. Next, note the strategic word "immediately." This focus will direct you to option 4. Review emergency care related to chemical burns to the eye if you had difficulty with this question.

References

Black, J., & Hawks, J. (2005). *Medical-surgical nursing: Clinical management for positive outcomes* (7th ed., p. 1446) Philadelphia: Saunders.

Lewis, S., Heitkemper, M., Dirksen, S., O'Brien, P., & Bucher, L. (2007). *Medical-surgical nursing: Assessment and management of clinical problems* (7th ed., p. 421). St. Louis: Mosby.

---

488. A client tells the nurse about a pattern of getting a strong urge to void, which is followed by incontinence before the client can get to the bathroom. The nurse formulates which of the following nursing diagnoses for this client?

1 Urge urinary incontinence
2 Total urinary incontinence
3 Stress urinary incontinence
4 Reflex urinary incontinence

Level of Cognitive Ability: Analysis
Client Needs: Physiological Integrity
Integrated Process: Nursing Process/Analysis
Content Area: Adult Health/Renal

Answer: 1

Rationale: Urge incontinence occurs when the client has urinary incontinence soon after experiencing urgency. Stress incontinence occurs when the client voids in increments that are less than 50 mL and has increased abdominal pressure. Total incontinence occurs when there is an unpredictable and continuous loss of urine. Reflex incontinence occurs when incontinence occurs at rather predictable times that correspond to when a certain bladder volume is attained.

Test-Taking Strategy: Use the process of elimination. Eliminate option 3 first as having the least degree of relationship with the information in the question. Note that the question includes the word "urge." This will direct you to option 1 from the remaining options. Review nursing diagnoses related to incontinence if you had difficulty with this question.

References

Black, J., & Hawks, J. (2005). *Medical-surgical nursing: Clinical management for positive outcomes* (7th ed., p. 895). Philadelphia: Saunders.

Ignatavicius, D., & Workman, M. (2006). *Medical-surgical nursing: Critical thinking for collaborative care* (5th ed., pp. 1692-1693). Philadelphia: Saunders.

---

489. A 52-year-old male client is seen in the physician's office for a physical examination after experiencing unusual fatigue over the last several weeks. The client's height is 5 feet, 8 inches, and his weight is 220 pounds. Vital signs are temperature 98°F orally, pulse 86 beats per minute, and respirations 18 breaths per minute. The blood pressure (BP) is 184/100 mm Hg. Random blood glucose is 122 mg/dL. Which of the following questions should the nurse ask the client first?

1 "Do you exercise regularly?"
2 "Are you considering trying to lose weight?"
3 "Is there a history of diabetes mellitus in your family?"
4 "When was the last time you had your blood pressure checked?"

Level of Cognitive Ability: Analysis
Client Needs: Physiological Integrity
Integrated Process: Nursing Process/Assessment
Content Area: Delegating/Prioritizing

Answer: 4

Rationale: The client is hypertensive, which is a known major modifiable risk factor for coronary artery disease (CAD). The other major modifiable risk factors not exhibited by this client include smoking and hypercholesterolemia. The client is overweight, which is a contributing risk factor. The client's nonmodifiable risk factors are age and gender. Because the client presents with several risk factors, the nurse places priority of attention on the client's major modifiable risk factors.

Test-Taking Strategy: Use the process of elimination, noting the strategic word "first." Eliminate options 1 and 2 first because they are comparable or alike. From the remaining options, note the client's blood pressure and its relationship to option 4. Review the risk factors for CAD if you had difficulty with this question.

Reference

Ignatavicius, D., & Workman, M. (2006). *Medical-surgical nursing: Critical thinking for collaborative care* (5th ed., pp. 843, 845). Philadelphia: Saunders.

490. The nurse is instilling an otic solution into the adult client's left ear. The nurse avoids doing which of the following as part of this procedure?
1 Pulling the auricle backward and upward
2 Warming the solution to room temperature
3 Placing the tip of the dropper on the edge of the ear canal
4 Placing the client in a side-lying position with the ear facing up

Level of Cognitive Ability: Application
Client Needs: Physiological Integrity
Integrated Process: Nursing Process/ Implementation
Content Area: Adult Health/Ear

Answer: 3
Rationale: The dropper is not allowed to touch any object or any part of the client's skin. The solution is warmed before use. The client is placed on the side with the affected ear upward. The nurse pulls the auricle backward and upward and instills the medication by holding the dropper about 1 cm above the ear canal.

Test-Taking Strategy: Note the strategic word "avoids." This word indicates a negative event query and the need to select the option that is an incorrect nursing action. Basic knowledge of proper procedure for administering otic solutions and the principles related to aseptic technique will direct you to option 3. Review this basic nursing procedure if you had difficulty with this question.

References
Ignatavicius, D., & Workman, M. (2006). *Medical-surgical nursing: Critical thinking for collaborative care* (5th ed., pp. 1126-1127). Philadelphia: Saunders.
Potter, P., & Perry, A. (2005). *Fundamentals of nursing* (6th ed., pp. 862-863). St. Louis: Mosby.

491. Levothyroxine sodium (Synthroid) is administered to a hospitalized child with congenital hypothyroidism. The child vomits 10 minutes after administration of the dose. The best nursing action is to:
1 Contact the physician.
2 Hold the dose for today.
3 Repeat the prescribed dose.
4 Give two doses of the prescribed medicine on the next day.

Level of Cognitive Ability: Application
Client Needs: Physiological Integrity
Integrated Process: Nursing Process/ Implementation
Content Area: Child Health

Answer: 1
Rationale: Levothyroxine sodium (Synthroid) is the medication of choice for hypothyroidism. The most significant factor adversely affecting the eventual intelligence of children born with congenital hypothyroidism is inadequate treatment. Therefore, compliance with the medication regimen is essential. If the infant or child vomits after the administration of the medication, the physician is notified.

Test-Taking Strategy: Use the process of elimination. General principles related to medication administration will assist in eliminating option 4. Eliminate option 3 because this is not considered best practice. From the remaining options, recalling the importance of the medication to treat this disorder will allow you to eliminate option 2. Having knowledge of best practice with medication administration to children should direct you to option. 1. Review the administration of this medication in congenital hypothyroidism if you had difficulty with this question.

References
McKinney, E., James, S., Murray, S., & Ashwill, J. (2005). *Maternal-child nursing* (2nd ed., p. 1456). St. Louis: Saunders.
Wong, D., Hockenberry, M., Perry, S., Lowdermilk, D., & Wilson, D. (2006). *Maternal-child nursing care.* (3rd ed., p. 864). St. Louis: Mosby.

492. A client diagnosed as having catatonic excitement has been pacing rapidly non-stop for several hours and is not eating or drinking. The nurse recognizes that in this situation:

1 There is a need to encourage verbaliza-tion of feelings.
2 The client will soon demonstrate a catatonic stuporous.
3 There is an urgent need for physical and medical control.
4 There is an urgent need to obtain a physical restraint order.

Level of Cognitive Ability: Analysis
Client Needs: Physiological Integrity
Integrated Process: Nursing Process/Analysis
Content Area: Mental Health

Answer: 3
Rationale: Catatonic excitement is manifested by a state of extreme psychomotor agitation. Clients urgently require physical and medical control because they are often destructive and violent to others, and their excitement can cause them to injure themselves or to collapse from complete exhaustion. Options 1, 2, and 4 are incorrect.

Test-Taking Strategy: Use Maslow's Hierarchy of Needs theory to answer the question. Physiological needs are the priority. Noting the client's behavior described in the question will direct you to option 3. Review care of the client with catatonic excitement if you had difficulty with this question.

Reference
Varcarolis, E., Carson, V., & Shoemaker, N. (2006). *Foundations of psychiatric mental health nursing* (5th ed., pp. 394-395). Philadelphia: Saunders.

---

493. The nurse is caring for a client with type 1 diabetes mellitus. Which of the following laboratory results would indicate a poten-tial complication associated with this dis-order?

1 Ketonuria
2 Potassium: 4.2 mEq
3 Blood glucose: 112 mg/dL
4 Blood urea nitrogen (BUN): 18 mg/dL

Level of Cognitive Ability: Analysis
Client Needs: Physiological Integrity
Integrated Process: Nursing Process/Analysis
Content Area: Adult Health/Endocrine

Answer: 1
Rationale: Ketonuria is an abnormal finding in the client with dia-betes mellitus indicating ketosis. Ketosis is a metabolic effect from the lack of insulin on fat metabolism and occurs in type 1 diabetes mellitus. It is associated with the severe complication of diabetic ketoacidosis (hyperglycemia, ketosis, and acidosis). Options 2, 3, and 4 are all normal laboratory findings.

Test-Taking Strategy: Note the strategic words "indicate a poten-tial complication." Options 2, 3, and 4 are all normal values, so eliminate these options. Review the complications of type 1 diabetes mellitus and normal laboratory values if you had difficulty with this question.

References
Black, J., & Hawks, J. (2005). *Medical-surgical nursing: Clinical management for positive outcomes* (7th ed., pp. 1250,1252). Philadelphia: Saunders.
Ignatavicius, D., & Workman, M. (2006). *Medical-surgical nursing: Critical thinking for collaborative care* (5th ed., p. 1508). Philadelphia: Saunders.

---

494. The nurse employed in a diabetes melli-tus clinic is caring for a client on insulin pump therapy. Which statement by the client indicates that a knowledge deficit exists regarding insulin pump therapy?

1 "If my blood glucose is elevated, I can bolus myself with additional insulin as ordered."
2 "I'll need to check my blood glucose before meals in case I need a premeal insulin bolus."
3 "I still need to follow a diet and exer-cise plan even though I don't inject myself daily anymore."
4 "Now that I have this pump, I don't have to worry about insulin reactions or ketoacidosis ever happening again."

Answer: 4
Rationale: Hypoglycemic reactions can occur if there is an error in calculating the insulin dose or if the pump malfunctions. Ketoacidosis can occur if too little insulin is used or if there is an increase in metabolic need. The pump does not have a built-in blood glucose monitoring feedback system, so the client is subject to the usual complications associated with insulin administration without the use of a pump. Options 1, 2, and 3 are accurate regard-ing the use of the insulin pump.

Level of Cognitive Ability: Analysis
Client Needs: Physiological Integrity
Integrated Process: Teaching and Learning
Content Area: Adult Health/Endocrine

Test-Taking Strategy: Knowledge of the basics of insulin therapy is helpful to answer this question, even if you know little about insulin pump therapy. Options 1, 2, and 3 are logical statements regarding the use of endogenous insulin. Option 4, however, presumes a guarantee from a complication of insulin therapy. No biomedical equipment is capable of being 100% safe. Review the principles related to an insulin pump if you had difficulty with this question.

References
Black, J., & Hawks, J. (2005). *Medical-surgical nursing: Clinical management for positive outcomes* (7th ed., pp. 1255-1256). Philadelphia: Saunders.
Ignatavicius, D., & Workman, M. (2006). *Medical-surgical nursing: Critical thinking for collaborative care* (5th ed., p. 1521). Philadelphia: Saunders.

---

495. A client with Graves' disease has exophthalmos and is experiencing photophobia. Which of the following nursing interventions would best assist the client with this problem?
1 Obtain dark glasses for the client.
2 Lubricate the eyes with tap water every 2 to 4 hours.
3 Administer methimazole (Tapazole) every 8 hours around the clock.
4 Instruct the client to avoid straining or heavy lifting because this can increase eye pressure.

Level of Cognitive Ability: Application
Client Needs: Physiological Integrity
Integrated Process: Nursing Process/ Implementation
Content Area: Adult Health/Endocrine

Answer: 1
Rationale: Medical therapy for Graves' disease does not help alleviate the clinical manifestation of exophthalmos. Because photophobia (light intolerance) accompanies this disorder, dark glasses are helpful in alleviating the problem. Tap water, which is hypotonic, could actually cause more swelling around the eye because it could pull fluid into the interstitial space. In addition, the client is at risk for developing an eye infection because the solution is not sterile. Methimazole inhibits the synthesis of thyroid hormone and is used to treat hyperthyroidism but will not alleviate exophthalmos or photophobia. There is no need to avoid straining with exophthalmos.

Test-Taking Strategy: Focus on the subject, photophobia. Recalling the definition of photophobia will direct you to option 1. Review the measures to treat this problem if you had difficulty with this question.

References
Black, J., & Hawks, J. (2005). *Medical-surgical nursing: Clinical management for positive outcomes* (7th ed., pp. 1200, 1964-1965). Philadelphia: Saunders.
Ignatavicius, D., & Workman, M. (2006). *Medical-surgical nursing: Critical thinking for collaborative care* (5th ed., p. 1490). Philadelphia: Saunders.

---

496. The nurse is caring for a client with pneumonia who suddenly becomes restless and has a Pao_2 of 60 mm Hg. Which of the following nursing diagnoses would be most appropriate for this client?
1 Fatigue related to a debilitated state
2 Ineffective airway clearance related to pneumonia
3 Ineffective airway clearance related to dilated bronchioles
4 Impaired gas exchange related to effects of alveolar-capillary membrane changes

Answer: 4
Rationale: Restlessness and a low Pao_2 are hallmark signs of impaired gas exchange. Although many clients with pneumonia experience fatigue, this nursing diagnosis is not the most appropriate, based on the Pao_2 level. Pneumonia is a medical diagnosis. Dilated bronchioles would be a goal for treatment and not part of the nursing diagnosis.

Test-Taking Strategy: Eliminate option 2 first because this incorporates a medical diagnosis. Focus on the data in the question to eliminate option 1 next, because it is unrelated to these data. From the remaining options, recalling that the bronchioles are not dilated in pneumonia will direct you to option 4. Review care of the client with pneumonia if you had difficulty with this question.

Level of Cognitive Ability: Analysis
Client Needs: Physiological Integrity
Integrated Process: Nursing Process/Analysis
Content Area: Adult Health/Respiratory

Reference
Ignatavicius, D., & Workman, M. (2006). *Medical-surgical nursing: Critical thinking for collaborative care* (5th ed., pp. 637-638). Philadelphia: Saunders.

---

497. A client with tuberculosis (TB) is to be started on rifampin (Rifadin). The nurse should instruct the client:
1 That yellow-colored skin is common
2 To wear glasses instead of soft contact lenses
3 To always take the medication on an empty stomach
4 That, as soon as the cultures come back negative, the medication may be stopped

Level of Cognitive Ability: Application
Client Needs: Physiological Integrity
Integrated Process: Teaching and Learning
Content Area: Pharmacology

Answer: 2
Rationale: Soft contacts may be permanently damaged by the orange discoloration that rifampin causes in body fluids. Any sign of jaundice (yellow-colored skin) should always be reported. If rifampin is not tolerated on an empty stomach, it may be taken with food. The client may be on the medication for 12 months even if cultures are negative.

Test-Taking Strategy: Use the process of elimination. Eliminate option 3 because of the close-ended word "always." Eliminate option 1 because it is an indication of jaundice. From the remaining options, recalling the side effects of rifampin will direct you to option 2. Review this medication if you are unfamiliar with it.

Reference
Skidmore-Roth, L. (2008). *Mosby's nursing drug reference* (21st ed., pp. 278-279). St. Louis: Mosby.

---

498. The nurse reviews the physician's orders for a client with Guillain-Barré syndrome. Which order written by the physician should the nurse question?
1 Provide a clear liquid diet.
2 Assess vital signs frequently.
3 Obtain bilateral calf measurements daily.
4 Perform passive range of motion exercises three times daily.

Level of Cognitive Ability: Analysis
Client Needs: Physiological Integrity
Integrated Process: Nursing Process/ Implementation
Content Area: Adult Health/Neurological

Answer: 1
Rationale: Clients with Guillain-Barré syndrome have dysphagia. Clients with dysphagia are more likely to aspirate clear liquids than thick or semi-solid foods. Because clients with Guillain-Barré syndrome are at risk for hypotension or hypertension, bradycardia, and respiratory depression, frequent monitoring of vital signs is required. Passive range of motion exercises can help prevent contractures, and assessing calf measurements can help detect deep vein thrombosis, for which these clients are at risk.

Test-Taking Strategy: Use the process of elimination, recalling that the client with Guillain-Barré syndrome is at risk for dysphagia. Even if you are unaware that dysphagia is a problem, note that options 2, 3, and 4 are generally part of routine nursing care. Review the manifestations associated with this disorder if you had difficulty with this question.

References
Ignatavicius, D., & Workman, M. (2006). *Medical-surgical nursing: Critical thinking for collaborative care* (5th ed., pp. 1008-1009). Philadelphia: Saunders.
Lewis, S., Heitkemper, M., Dirksen, S., O'Brien, P., & Bucher, L. (2007). *Medical-surgical nursing: Assessment and management of clinical problems* (7th ed., p. 1586). St. Louis: Mosby.

499. A client with myasthenia gravis arrives at the emergency room and crisis is suspected. The physician plans to administer edrophonium chloride (Tensilon) to differentiate between myasthenic and cholinergic crisis. The nurse prepares to administer which medication if the client is in cholinergic crisis?
1 Atropine sulfate
2 Morphine sulfate
3 Isoproterenol (Isuprel)
4 Pyridostigmine bromide (Mestinon)

Level of Cognitive Ability: Application
Client Needs: Physiological Integrity
Integrated Process: Nursing Process/Planning
Content Area: Adult Health/Neurological

Answer: 1
Rationale: Clients with cholinergic crisis have experienced overdosage of medication. Tensilon will exacerbate symptoms in cholinergic crisis to the point where the client may need intubation and mechanical ventilation. Intravenous atropine sulfate is used to reverse the effects of these anticholinesterase medications. Morphine sulfate and pyridostigmine bromide would worsen the symptoms of cholinergic crisis. Isuprel is not indicated for cholinergic crisis.

Test-Taking Strategy: Focus on the subject, cholinergic crisis. Recalling the antidote for anticholinesterase medications will direct you to option 1. Memorize this antidote if you had difficulty with this question.

Reference
Ignatavicius, D., & Workman, M. (2006). *Medical-surgical nursing: Critical thinking for collaborative care* (5th ed., p. 1041). Philadelphia: Saunders.

---

500. The nurse is completing a health history on a client with diabetes mellitus who has been taking insulin for many years. At present the client states that he is experiencing periods of hypoglycemia followed by periods of hyperglycemia. The most likely cause for this occurrence is which of the following?
1 Eating snacks between meals
2 Initiating the use of the insulin pump
3 Injecting insulin at a site of lipodystrophy
4 Adjusting insulin according to blood glucose levels

Level of Cognitive Ability: Analysis
Client Needs: Physiological Integrity
Integrated Process: Nursing Process/Analysis
Content Area: Adult Health/Endocrine

Answer: 3
Rationale: Lipodystrophy, specifically lipohypertrophy, involves swelling of the fat at the site of repeated injections. This can interfere with the absorption of insulin, resulting in erratic blood glucose levels. Because the client has been on insulin for many years, this is the most likely cause of poor control. Options 1, 2, and 4 are appropriate techniques to use in order to regulate blood glucose levels.

Test-Taking Strategy: Note the strategic words "taking insulin for many years." This indicates that you must consider a long-term complication of insulin administration as the answer to the question. Options 1, 2, and 4 are eliminated because they are actually appropriate techniques to use in order to regulate blood glucose levels. Review lipodystrophy if you had difficulty with this question.

Reference
Ignatavicius, D., & Workman, M. (2006). *Medical-surgical nursing: Critical thinking for collaborative care* (5th ed., pp. 1519-1520). Philadelphia: Saunders.

---

501. A nurse receives a report at the beginning of the shift regarding a client with an intrauterine fetal demise. On assessment of the client, the nurse expects to note which of the following?
1 Intractable vomiting and dehydration
2 Elevated blood pressure, proteinuria, and edema
3 Uterine size greater than expected for gestational age
4 Regression of pregnancy symptoms and absence of fetal heart tones

Answer: 4
Rationale: Symptoms of a fetal demise include a decrease in fetal movement, no change or a decrease in fundal height, and absent fetal heart tones. Additionally, many symptoms of the pregnancy may diminish, such as breast size and tenderness. Option 2 is associated with preeclampsia. Option 1 is associated with hyperemesis gravidarum.

Test-Taking Strategy: Focus on the subject—intrauterine fetal demise. Recalling that fetal demise means fetal death will direct you to option 4. Review the signs associated with fetal demise if you had difficulty with this question.

Level of Cognitive Ability: Analysis
Client Needs: Physiological Integrity
Integrated Process: Nursing Process/Assessment
Content Area: Maternity/Intrapartum

Reference
Wong, D., Hockenberry, M., Perry, S., Lowdermilk, D., & Wilson, D. (2006). *Maternal-child nursing care.* (3rd ed., pp. 213-214). St. Louis: Mosby.

---

502. A client admitted to the nursing unit from the emergency department has a spinal cord injury at the level of the fourth cervical vertebra (C-4). Which assessment should the nurse perform first when admitting the client to the nursing unit?
1 Listen to breath sounds.
2 Observe for dyskinesias.
3 Take the client's temperature.
4 Assess extremity muscle strength.

Level of Cognitive Ability: Application
Client Needs: Physiological Integrity
Integrated Process: Nursing Process/Assessment
Content Area: Delegating/Prioritizing

Answer: 1
Rationale: Because compromise of respiration is a leading cause of death in cervical spinal cord injury, respiratory assessment is the highest priority. Assessment of temperature and strength can be done after adequate oxygenation is assured. Dyskinesias occur in cerebellar disorders, so they are not as important in spinal cord-injured clients, unless head injury accompanies the spinal cord injury.

Test-Taking Strategy: Remembering that a spinal cord injury, particularly at the level of C-4, can affect respiratory status will direct you to the correct option. Also, use of the ABCs—airway, breathing, and circulation—can guide assessment priorities in this situation. Breath sounds will be diminished if respiratory muscles are weakened or paralyzed. Review priority care of the client with a C-4 spinal cord injury if you had difficulty with this question.

References
Black, J., & Hawks, J. (2005). *Medical-surgical nursing: Clinical management for positive outcomes* (7th ed., pp. 2214, 2219). Philadelphia: Saunders.
Ignatavicius, D., & Workman, M. (2006). *Medical-surgical nursing: Critical thinking for collaborative care* (5th ed., pp. 987-988). Philadelphia: Saunders.

---

503. A nurse is assisting in positioning a client for a surgical procedure. The nurse knows that the respiratory system is vulnerable to which of the following positions?
1 Sims'
2 Lateral
3 Supine
4 Lithotomy

Level of Cognitive Ability: Analysis
Client Needs: Physiological Integrity
Integrated Process: Nursing Process/Analysis
Content Area: Fundamental Skills

Answer: 4
Rationale: The thoracic cage normally expands in all directions except posteriorly. In the lithotomy position, increased intraabdominal pressure restricts lung expansion at the lower margins, making full lung expansion very difficult and risky if accomplished with mechanical ventilation. Surgical anesthesia further impairs respiratory excursion with respiratory suppression and hypoventilation; thus, the client is at high risk for respiratory complications, especially atelectasis and pneumonia, because the volume of inspired air is compromised. The nurse continues to monitor postoperatively for respiratory complications because they are most likely to appear at that time. Options 1, 2, and 3 are not as likely to impair diaphragmatic excursion as the lithotomy position because they do not increase intraabdominal pressure.

Test-Taking Strategy: Use the process of elimination, noting that the lithotomy position is the only one listed that impairs diaphragmatic excursion. Review these positions if you had difficulty with this question.

Reference
Ignatavicius, D., & Workman, M. (2006). *Medical-surgical nursing: Critical thinking for collaborative care* (5th ed., p. 336). Philadelphia: Saunders.

504. A nurse is caring for a client who is receiving an intravenous infusion of theophylline. The nurse checks which of the following to determine medication effectiveness?

1 Pulse rate
2 Temperature
3 Lung sounds
4 Pupillary response

Level of Cognitive Ability: Analysis
Client Needs: Physiological Integrity
Integrated Process: Nursing Process/Evaluation
Content Area: Pharmacology

Answer: 3
Rationale: Theophylline is a bronchodilator used to treat bronchial asthma or to reverse bronchospasm caused by chronic bronchitis, emphysema, or chronic obstructive pulmonary disease. To determine medication effectiveness, the nurse would auscultate lung sounds for the absence of rhonchi, crackles, or wheezes. Although the client's temperature would be monitored for signs of respiratory infection in a client with a respiratory disorder, temperature is unrelated to medication effectiveness. Although the pulse rate would be monitored because tachycardia is a sign of toxicity, pulse rate is unrelated to medication effectiveness. Pupillary response is a neurological assessment and is unrelated to this medication.

Test-Taking Strategy: Note the strategic words "to determine medication effectiveness." Focus on the name of the medication and recall that medication names that end with "line" are bronchodilators. This will direct you to option 3. Also, use of the ABCs—airway, breathing, and circulation—will direct you to the correct option. Review the expected effects of this medication if you had difficulty with this question.

Reference
Skidmore-Roth, L. (2008). *Mosby's nursing drug reference* (21st ed., p. 984). St. Louis: Mosby.

---

505. A nurse monitoring a client with premature ventricular contractions (PVCs) greater than 6 per minute is preparing to administer a bolus of lidocaine (Xylocaine). Which of the following assessments takes priority after administration of the medication?

1 Skin temperature and neurological status
2 Vital signs, ECG, and neurological status
3 Visual changes and kidney and liver function
4 Kidney and liver function and neurological status

Level of Cognitive Ability: Analysis
Client Needs: Physiological Integrity
Integrated Process: Nursing Process/Assessment
Content Area: Pharmacology

Answer: 2
Rationale: Lidocaine can cause atrioventricular block with conduction defects. It can also cause paresthesia, numbness, disorientation, and agitation. Monitoring the vital signs, ECG, and neurological status is the priority.

Test-Taking Strategy: Focus on the client's diagnosis: premature ventricular contractions. Note that option 2 is the only option that addresses direct cardiac monitoring. Review this medication if you had difficulty with this question.

Reference
Hodgson, B., & Kizior, R. (2007). *Saunders nursing drug handbook 2007* (p. 691). Philadelphia: Saunders.

---

506. A nurse is caring for a client experiencing hypertensive crisis. The physician tells the nurse that medication will be prescribed to help reduce both preload and afterload. The nurse anticipates that the physician will prescribe which medication?

1 Morphine sulfate
2 Digoxin (Lanoxin)
3 Furosemide (Lasix)
4 Nitroprusside sodium

Answer: 4
Rationale: Intravenous nitroprusside is a potent vasodilator that reduces preload and afterload. Digoxin (Lanoxin) is a cardiac glycoside that increases cardiac contractility. Morphine sulfate is a opioid analgesic. Furosemide (Lasix) is a loop diuretic and can reduce preload by enhancing the renal excretion of sodium and water, which reduces circulating blood volume.

Level of Cognitive Ability: Analysis
Client Needs: Physiological Integrity
Integrated Process: Nursing Process/Analysis
Content Area: Pharmacology

Test-Taking Strategy: Focus on the subject—reducing preload and afterload and the client's diagnosis (hypertensive crisis). Use the process of elimination and recall that nitroprusside sodium is a vasodilator. Review the effects of the medications in the options if you had difficulty with this question.

Reference
Skidmore-Roth, L. (2008). *Mosby's nursing drug reference* (21st ed., p. 744). St. Louis: Mosby.

---

507. Streptokinase (Streptase) is being administered to a client following an acute inferior myocardial infarction. The nurse understands that the primary purpose of this medication is to:
1 Dissolve the thrombus.
2 Prevent platelet aggregation.
3 Inhibit further clot formation.
4 Reduce myocardial oxygen demand.

Level of Cognitive Ability: Analysis
Client Needs: Physiological Integrity
Integrated Process: Nursing Process/Analysis
Content Area: Pharmacology

Answer: 1
Rationale: Streptokinase is a thrombolytic medication that causes lysis of blood clots. Anticoagulants prevent further clot formation. Beta-blockers, nitrates, and calcium channel blockers are used to reduce myocardial oxygen demand. Streptokinase does not prevent platelet aggregation.

Test-Taking Strategy: Recalling that streptokinase is a thrombolytic medication and that these medications dissolve clots will direct you to option 1. Review this medication if you had difficulty with this question.

Reference
Skidmore-Roth, L. (2008). *Mosby's nursing drug reference* (21st ed., p. 943). St. Louis: Mosby.

---

508. The nurse is planning to care for a client with heart failure. The nurse establishes a goal to have the client participate in activities that reduce cardiac workload. The nurse identifies which client action as contributing to this goal?
1 Sleeping in the supine position
2 Elevating the legs when in bed
3 Using a bedside commode for stools
4 Using seasonings to improve the taste of food

Level of Cognitive Ability: Analysis
Client Needs: Physiological Integrity
Integrated Process: Nursing Process/Analysis
Content Area: Adult Health/Cardiovascular

Answer: 3
Rationale: Using a bedside commode decreases the work of getting to the bathroom or struggling to use the bedpan. Elevating the client's legs increases venous return to the heart, thus increasing cardiac workload. The supine position increases respiratory effort and decreases oxygenation. This increases cardiac workload. Seasonings are high in sodium.

Test-Taking Strategy: Use the process of elimination, focusing on the subject—reducing cardiac overload. Keeping this subject in mind will direct you to option 3. Review measures that will reduce cardiac workload if you had difficulty with this question.

References
Black, J., & Hawks, J. (2005). *Medical-surgical nursing: Clinical management for positive outcomes* (7th ed., pp. 1878-1880). Philadelphia: Saunders.
Ignatavicius, D., & Workman, M. (2006). *Medical-surgical nursing: Critical thinking for collaborative care* (5th ed., pp. 829-830). Philadelphia: Saunders.
Potter, P., & Perry, A. (2005). *Fundamentals of nursing* (6th ed., pp. 1394-1395). St. Louis: Mosby.

509. A child is sent to the school nurse by the teacher. On assessment, the school nurse notes that the child has a rash. The nurse suspects that the child has erythema infectiosum (fifth disease) because the skin assessment revealed a rash that is:

1 A discrete rose-pink maculopapular rash on the trunk
2 A highly pruritic, profuse macule to papule rash on the trunk
3 An erythema on the face that has a "slapped face" appearance
4 A discrete pinkish red maculopapular rash that is spreading to the trunk

Level of Cognitive Ability: Analysis
Client Needs: Physiological Integrity
Integrated Process: Nursing Process/Assessment
Content Area: Child Health

Answer: 3
Rationale: The classic rash of erythema infectiosum, or fifth disease, is the erythema on the face. The discrete rose-pink maculopapular rash is the rash of exanthema subitum (roseola). The highly pruritic, profuse macule to papule rash is the rash of varicella (chickenpox). The discrete pinkish red maculopapular rash is the rash of rubella (German measles).

Test-Taking Strategy: Knowledge regarding the characteristics associated with erythema infectiosum is required to answer the question. If you were unfamiliar with this disorder, note that in options 1, 2, and 4, a similarity exists in that the rash is on the trunk. Option 3 addresses a rash on the face. Review this disorder if you had difficulty with this question.

References
Hockenberry, M. & Wilson, D. (2007). *Nursing care of infants and children* (8th ed., pp. 668-669). St. Louis: Mosby.
Hockenberry, M., Wilson, D., & Winkelstein, M. (2005). *Wong's essentials of pediatric nursing* (7th ed., pp. 438-439). St. Louis: Mosby.

---

510. A client is taking a monoamine oxidase inhibitor (MAOI). The nurse assesses the client closely because:

1 Hypotension may indicate toxicity.
2 These medications increase the amount of MAOI in the liver.
3 Headache, hypertension, and nausea and vomiting may indicate toxicity.
4 Hypotensive crisis may be precipitated by foods rich in tyramine and tryptophan.

Level of Cognitive Ability: Application
Client Needs: Physiological Integrity
Integrated Process: Nursing Process/Assessment
Content Area: Pharmacology

Answer: 3
Rationale: Headache, hypertension, tachycardia, nausea, and vomiting are precursors to hypertensive crisis brought about by the ingestion of foods rich in tyramine and tryptophan while the client is taking an MAOI. These medications act by decreasing the amount of MAOI in the liver, which is necessary for the breakdown and utilization of tyramine and tryptophan. Hypertensive crisis may lead to circulatory collapse, intracranial hemorrhage, and death.

Test-Taking Strategy: Use the process of elimination. Eliminate options 1 and 4 first because they are comparable or alike. From the remaining options, recalling the relationship between MAOIs and toxicity will direct you to option 3. Review the actions and side effects of MAOIs if you had difficulty with this question.

Reference
Kee, J., Hayes, E., & McCuistion, L. (2006). *Pharmacology: A nursing process approach.* (5th ed., pp. 395, 398). Philadelphia: Saunders.

---

511. A client arrives in the postanesthesia recovery unit (PACU) in the supine position following an abdominal hysterectomy. Which is the best intervention for the nurse to implement to assess for hidden signs of postoperative bleeding?

1 Roll the client to one side.
2 Look at the surgical dressing.
3 Ask if the client feels moisture.
4 Check the client's perineal pad.

Answer: 1
Rationale: The nurse should roll the client to one side after checking the perineal pad and the abdominal dressing because this allows the nurse to check under the pelvic region. By lying supine, vaginal drainage can pool by gravity under the client and be invisible from above. The remaining options are reasonable nursing interventions for assessing the client for bleeding postoperatively.

Level of Cognitive Ability: Analysis
Client Needs: Physiological Integrity
Integrated Process: Nursing Process/Assessment
Content Area: Fundamental Skills

Test-Taking Strategy: Use the process of elimination. Eliminate option 3 first because it relies on the client; in the PACU, the client is likely to be sedated and unable to report. Then, eliminate options 2 and 4 because they are unlikely to uncover hidden bleeding. Note that option 1 addresses rolling the client. Review care of the client following hysterectomy if you had difficulty with this question.

Reference
Ignatavicius, D., & Workman, M. (2006). *Medical-surgical nursing: Critical thinking for collaborative care* (5th ed., pp. 1840-1841). Philadelphia: Saunders.

---

512. The nurse is caring for a client who returned to the nursing unit following suprapubic prostatectomy. The nurse monitors the continuous bladder irrigation to detect which of the following signs of catheter blockage?
  1 Drainage that is pale pink
  2 Drainage that is bright red
  3 True urine output of 50 mL/hr
  4 Urine leakage around the three-way catheter at the meatus

Level of Cognitive Ability: Analysis
Client Needs: Physiological Integrity
Integrated Process: Nursing Process/Assessment
Content Area: Adult Health/Renal

Answer: 4
Rationale: Catheter blockage or occlusion by clots following prostatectomy can result in urine backup and leakage around the urethral meatus. This would be accompanied by a stoppage of outflow through the catheter into the drainage bag. Drainage that is bright red indicates that the irrigant is running too slowly; drainage that is pale pink indicates sufficient flow. A true urine output of 50 mL per hour indicates catheter patency.

Test-Taking Strategy: Use the process of elimination, focusing on the subject—catheter blockage. Eliminate options 1 and 2 first because of the word "drainage." This implies catheter patency. From the remaining options, apply basic principles related to Foley catheter management. A leakage around the catheter at the meatus indicates blockage. Review care of the client following prostatectomy if you had difficulty with this question.

Reference
Ignatavicius, D., & Workman, M. (2006). *Medical-surgical nursing: Critical thinking for collaborative care* (5th ed., pp. 1863-1864). Philadelphia: Saunders.

---

513. The nurse is assigned to a client returning from the postanesthesia care unit following transurethral prostatectomy. The nurse avoids doing which of the following after this procedure?
  1 Reporting signs of confusion
  2 Monitoring hourly urine output
  3 Removing the traction tape on the three-way catheter
  4 Administering a B&O (belladonna and opium) suppository at room temperature

Level of Cognitive Ability: Application
Client Needs: Physiological Integrity
Integrated Process: Nursing Process/Implementation
Content Area: Adult Health/Renal

Answer: 3
Rationale: The nurse avoids removing the traction tape applied by the surgeon in the operating room. The purpose of this tape is to place pressure on the prostate and reduce hemorrhage. B&O suppositories, ordered on a prn basis for bladder spasm, should be warmed to room temperature before administration. The nurse routinely monitors hourly urine output because the client has a three-way bladder irrigation running. The nurse also assesses for confusion, which could result from hyponatremia secondary to the hypotonic irrigant used during the surgical procedure.

Test-Taking Strategy: Use the process of elimination, noting the strategic word "avoids." This word indicates a negative event query and the need to select the incorrect nursing action. Eliminate options 2 and 4 first because they are part of routine nursing care and would not be contraindicated in the care of this client. From the remaining options, recalling the need to reduce hemorrhage will direct you to option 3. Review care of the client following prostatectomy if you had difficulty with this question.

Reference
Ignatavicius, D., & Workman, M. (2006). *Medical-surgical nursing: Critical thinking for collaborative care* (5th ed., pp. 1863-1864). Philadelphia: Saunders.

---

514. A client is due for a dose of bumetanide (Bumex). The nurse would temporarily withhold the dose and notify the physician if which of the following laboratory results was noted?
  1 Sodium: 137 mEq/L
  2 Chloride: 106 mEq/L
  3 Potassium: 2.9 mEq/L
  4 Magnesium: 2.6 mg/dL

Level of Cognitive Ability: Application
Client Needs: Physiological Integrity
Integrated Process: Nursing Process/ Implementation
Content Area: Pharmacology

Answer: 3
Rationale: Bumetanide is a loop diuretic that is not potassium-sparing. The value given for potassium is below the therapeutic range of 3.5 to 5.1 mEq/L for this electrolyte. The nurse should notify the physician before giving the dose so that potassium may be ordered. Options 1, 2, and 4 identify normal values.

Test-Taking Strategy: Note the strategic words "notify the physician." Use the process of elimination and knowledge of the normal laboratory values. Option 3 is the only abnormal value. Review this medication if you had difficulty with this question.

Reference
Skidmore-Roth, L. (2008). *Mosby's nursing drug reference* (21st ed., p. 199). St. Louis: Mosby.

---

515. A client with heart failure is receiving furosemide (Lasix) and digoxin (Lanoxin) daily. When the nurse enters the room to administer the morning doses, the client complains of anorexia, nausea, and yellow vision. The nurse should do which of the following first?
  1 Give the digoxin only.
  2 Administer the medications.
  3 Check the morning serum digoxin level.
  4 Check the morning serum potassium level.

Level of Cognitive Ability: Application
Client Needs: Physiological Integrity
Integrated Process: Nursing Process/ Implementation
Content Area: Pharmacology

Answer: 3
Rationale: The nurse should check for the result of the digoxin level that was drawn, because the symptoms are compatible with digitalis toxicity. Knowing that a low potassium level may contribute to digitalis toxicity, checking the serum potassium level may give useful additive information, but the digoxin level is checked first. The digoxin should be withheld until the level is known, making options 1 and 2 incorrect.

Test-Taking Strategy: Note the strategic word "first." Eliminate options 1 and 2 first, because it is not prudent to administer the medication(s) without doing further investigation. From the remaining options, recalling the signs of digoxin toxicity will direct you to option 3. Review the signs of digoxin toxicity if you had difficulty with this question.

References
Hodgson, B., & Kizior, R. (2007). *Saunders nursing drug handbook 2007* (p. 358). Philadelphia: Saunders.
Kee, J., Hayes, E., & McCuistion, L. (2006). *Pharmacology: A nursing process approach.* (5th ed., pp. 608-609). Philadelphia: Saunders.

---

516. A nurse is administering an oral dose of erythromycin (E-Mycin) to an assigned client. The nurse administers this medication with a:
  1 Full glass of milk
  2 Full glass of water
  3 Sip of orange juice
  4 Any citrus beverage

Answer: 2
Rationale: Erythromycin is a macrolide antibiotic that should be taken with a full glass of water. Sufficient volume is needed to obtain the maximal effect of the medication. Depending on the specific type of erythromycin, it may need to be administered on an empty stomach, with meals, or regardless of timing of meals. The nurse should verify the best method of administration for the type of erythromycin ordered. Options 1, 3, and 4 are incorrect.

Level of Cognitive Ability: Application
Client Needs: Physiological Integrity
Integrated Process: Nursing Process/
  Implementation
Content Area: Pharmacology

Test-Taking Strategy: Use the process of elimination. Eliminate options 3 and 4 first because they are comparable or alike. From the remaining options, recalling that medication administered with milk affects absorption will direct you to option 2. Review this medication if you had difficulty with this question.

Reference
Skidmore-Roth, L. (2008). *Mosby's nursing drug reference* (21st ed., p. 429). St. Louis: Mosby.

---

517. A nurse has given the client a dose of intravenous hydralazine (Apresoline). The nurse evaluates the effectiveness of the medication by monitoring which of the following client parameters?
  1 Urine output
  2 Blood pressure
  3 Muscle strength
  4 Blood glucose level

Level of Cognitive Ability: Analysis
Client Needs: Physiological Integrity
Integrated Process: Nursing Process/Evaluation
Content Area: Pharmacology

Answer: 2
Rationale: Hydralazine is an antihypertensive medication used in the management of moderate to severe hypertension. It is a vasodilator medication that decreases afterload. The blood pressure needs to be monitored. Options 1, 3, and 4 are not specifically associated with the use of this medication.

Test-Taking Strategy: Use the process of elimination. Note the name of the medication, *Apresoline,* to assist you in determining that the medication is an antihypertensive. This will direct you to option 2. Review this medication if it is unfamiliar to you.

Reference
Skidmore-Roth, L. (2008). *Mosby's nursing drug reference* (21st ed., p. 530). St. Louis: Mosby.

---

518. A client arrives in the emergency room and carbon monoxide (CO) poisoning is suspected. The nurse expects the physician to prescribe which of the following to confirm the diagnosis?
  1 Pulse oximetry
  2 Carboxyhemoglobin level
  3 Complete blood cell count
  4 Computed tomography (CT) scan of the head

Level of Cognitive Ability: Analysis
Client Needs: Physiological Integrity
Integrated Process: Nursing Process/Assessment
Content Area: Adult Health/Respiratory

Answer: 2
Rationale: The diagnosis of carbon monoxide poisoning is confirmed by measurement of carboxyhemoglobin levels in the client's blood. Pulse oximetry readings are unreliable because of the detection of CO-hemoglobin as oxyhemoglobin. A complete blood cell count may provide useful information but will not confirm the diagnosis. The neurological system may be affected by carbon monoxide poisoning, but this will be detected by assessment of clinical manifestations. A CT scan of the head will not confirm the diagnosis or provide any useful information unless a structural defect or injury in the head is a concern.

Test-Taking Strategy: Note the strategic word "confirm." Note the relationship between the words "carbon monoxide (CO) poisoning" in the question and option 2. Review content related to carbon monoxide poisoning if you had difficulty with this question.

References
Black, J., & Hawks, J. (2005). *Medical-surgical nursing: Clinical management for positive outcomes* (7th ed., p. 1907). Philadelphia: Saunders.
Mosby. (2006). *Mosby's dictionary of medicine, nursing & health professions.* (7th ed., p. 297). St. Louis: Mosby.

519. A client receiving a dose of intravenous vancomycin (Vancocin) develops chills, tachycardia, syncope, and flushing of the face and trunk. The nurse interprets that:
1 The medication is infusing too rapidly.
2 The client is allergic to the medication.
3 The client is experiencing upper airway obstruction.
4 The medication has interacted with another medication that the client is receiving.

Level of Cognitive Ability: Analysis
Client Needs: Physiological Integrity
Integrated Process: Nursing Process/Analysis
Content Area: Pharmacology

Answer: 1
Rationale: The client is experiencing signs and symptoms of what is called "red man" or "red neck" syndrome. This is a response caused by histamine release that occurs with rapid or bolus injection. The client may experience chills, fever, flushing of the face and/or trunk, tachycardia, syncope, tingling, and an unpleasant taste in the mouth. The corrective action is to administer the medication more slowly. An antihistamine such as diphenhydramine (Benadryl) may be administered as well. Options 2, 3, and 4 are incorrect interpretations.

Test-Taking Strategy: This question may be difficult, and you may want to quickly select option 2. Remember that options that are comparable or alike are not likely to be correct. For this reason, begin to answer this question by eliminating options 2 and 3 first. From the remaining options, recalling the adverse effect of "red neck" syndrome associated with the use of this medication will direct you to option 1. Review the adverse effects of this medication if you had difficulty with this question.

Reference
Hodgson, B., & Kizior, R. (p. 1198). *Saunders nursing drug handbook 2007* (p. 1198). Philadelphia: Saunders.

---

520. A client has an order for beclomethasone dipropionate (Qvar) by the intranasal route. The client also has an order for a nasal decongestant. The nurse plans to:
1 Administer the beclomethasone 15 minutes before the decongestant.
2 Administer the decongestant 15 minutes before the beclomethasone.
3 Administer the decongestant immediately before the beclomethasone.
4 Administer the beclomethasone immediately before the decongestant.

Level of Cognitive Ability: Application
Client Needs: Physiological Integrity
Integrated Process: Nursing Process/ Implementation
Content Area: Pharmacology

Answer: 2
Rationale: The nasal decongestant should be administered 15 minutes before the beclomethasone (a glucocorticoid) to clear the nasal passages and enhance absorption of the glucocorticoid. Options 1, 3, and 4 are incorrect methods of administration.

Test-Taking Strategy: Use the same principles in answering this question that you would use when administering bronchodilators and corticosteroids (glucocorticoids) together. Remember that the glucocorticoid is administered last. Review the procedure for administering intranasal medications if you had difficulty with this question.

Reference
Lehne. R. (2007). *Pharmacology for nursing care* (6th ed., p. 885). Philadelphia: Saunders.

---

521. A client suddenly experiences a seizure, and the nurse notes that the client exhibits uncontrollable jerking movements. The nurse documents that the client experienced which type of seizure?
1 Tonic seizure
2 Clonic seizure
3 Absence seizure
4 Myoclonic seizure

Answer: 4
Rationale: A myoclonic seizure is characterized by sudden uncontrollable jerking movements of a single muscle group or multiple muscle groups. A clonic seizure is characterized by rhythmic muscular contraction and relaxation lasting several minutes. A tonic seizure is characterized by an abrupt increase in muscle tone and contraction and the presence of autonomic manifestations. Absence seizures occur in childhood and are characterized by a vacant facial expression or appearance of "day-dreaming".

Level of Cognitive Ability: Analysis
Client Needs: Physiological Integrity
Integrated Process: Nursing Process/Assessment
Content Area: Adult Health/Neurological

Test-Taking Strategy: Focus on the data in the question and use knowledge regarding the characteristics of the various types of seizures to answer this question. Review the types of seizures and their characteristics if you had difficulty with this question.

References
Black, J., & Hawks, J. (2005). *Medical-surgical nursing: Clinical management for positive outcomes* (7th ed., p. 2076). Philadelphia: Saunders.
Monahan, F., Sands, J., Neighbors, M., Marek, J., & Green, C. (2007). *Phipps' medical-surgical nursing: Health and illness perspectives* (8th ed., pp. 1398-1399). St. Louis: Mosby.

---

522. A client is receiving tobramycin (Tobrex). The nurse evaluates that the client is responding well to the medication therapy if which of the following laboratory results is noted?
1 Sodium of 145 mEq/L and chloride of 106 mEq/L
2 Sodium of 140 mEq/L and potassium of 3.9 mEq/L
3 WBC count of 15,000/mm³ and a blood urea nitrogen (BUN) of 38 mg/dL
4 White blood cell (WBC) count of 8,000/mm³ and creatinine level of 0.9 mg/dL

Level of Cognitive Ability: Analysis
Client Needs: Physiological Integrity
Integrated Process: Nursing Process/Evaluation
Content Area: Pharmacology

Answer: 4
Rationale: Tobramycin is an antibiotic (aminoglycoside) that causes nephrotoxicity and ototoxicity. The medication is therapeutic if the WBC count drops back into the normal range and the kidney function remains normal. Option 3 indicates an abnormal WBC count, and options 1 and 2 are not directly to the use of this medication.

Test-Taking Strategy: Use the process of elimination. Begin to answer this question by eliminating options 1 and 2 first, knowing that tobramycin is an antibiotic. Recalling that aminoglycosides cause nephrotoxicity, select option 4 using laboratory values as your guide. Review this medication and normal laboratory values if you had difficulty with this question.

Reference
Skidmore-Roth, L. (2008). *Mosby's nursing drug reference* (21st ed., p. 1007). St. Louis: Mosby.

---

523. A nurse is caring for a client who is taking a maintenance dosage of lithium carbonate (Eskalith). The nurse plans to:
1 Perform a weekly ECG.
2 Monitor intake and output.
3 Monitor daily serum lithium levels.
4 Observe for remission of depressive states.

Level of Cognitive Ability: Application
Client Needs: Physiological Integrity
Integrated Process: Nursing Process/Planning
Content Area: Pharmacology

Answer: 2
Rationale: Lithium is used to treat manic disorders, not depression. Side effects of lithium are nausea, tremors, polyuria, and polydipsia. Serum lithium concentration is assessed approximately every 2 to 4 days during initial therapy and at longer intervals thereafter. Toxic levels of lithium may induce ECG changes, but there is no need to perform weekly ECGs if maintenance levels are maintained.

Test-Taking Strategy: Use the process of elimination. Eliminate options 1 and 3 first because of the words "weekly" and "daily" in these options. From the remaining options, recalling that this medication is used to treat manic disorders will direct you to option 2. Review the nursing interventions associated with administering this medication if you had difficulty with this question.

Reference
Hodgson, B., & Kizior, R. (2007). *Saunders nursing drug handbook 2007* (p. 699). Philadelphia: Saunders.

524. A nurse is caring for a client with chronic obstructive pulmonary disease (COPD) who is receiving theophylline intravenously. A theophylline blood serum level is drawn on the client. The nurse monitors the results of this blood test and expects the findings to be at which therapeutic level?

1 5 mcg/mL
2 8 mcg/mL
3 18 mcg/mL
4 25 mcg/mL

Level of Cognitive Ability: Comprehension
Client Needs: Physiological Integrity
Integrated Process: Nursing Process/Assessment
Content Area: Pharmacology

Answer: 3
Rationale: Theophylline is a bronchodilator. The therapeutic serum level range of theophylline is 10 to 20 mcg/mL. It is critical that the nurse monitor theophylline blood serum levels daily when a client is on this medication to ensure that a therapeutic range is present and to monitor for the potential for toxicity. Options 1 and 2 indicate low levels. Option 4 is a toxic level, indicating the need to stop the medication and notify the physician.

Test-Taking Strategy: Specific knowledge of this medication and the therapeutic serum level range is required to answer this question. Remember that this therapeutic serum level range is the same as the therapeutic serum level range for phenytoin (Dilantin). Review this medication if you had difficulty with this question.

References
Chernecky, C., & Berger, B. (2008). *Laboratory tests and diagnostic procedures* (5th ed., pp. 1060-1061). Philadelphia: Saunders.
Hodgson, B., & Kizior, R. (2007). *Saunders nursing drug handbook 2007* (p. 57). Philadelphia: Saunders.

---

525. The nurse is caring for a client with a closed chest drainage system. On assessment of the client, the nurse notes a rise and fall (fluctuation) of fluid in the water seal chamber. Based on this finding, what action should the nurse take?

1 Contact the physician.
2 Add water to the water seal chamber.
3 Add water to the suction control chamber.
4 Document that the system is functioning accurately.

Level of Cognitive Ability: Analysis
Client Needs: Physiological Integrity
Integrated Process: Nursing Process/Implementation
Content Area: Adult Health/Respiratory

Answer: 4
Rationale: Fluid in the water seal compartment should rise with inspiration and fall with expiration (fluctuations). When fluctuations occur, the drainage tubes are patent and the apparatus is functioning properly. Fluctuations stop when the lung has reexpanded or if the chest drainage tubes are kinked or obstructed. Therefore, the nurse would document that the system is functioning accurately. There are no data in the question indicating the need to add fluid to the chambers. There is no need to call the physician because this is an expected finding.

Test-Taking Strategy: Focus on the nurse's assessment finding—a rise and fall (fluctuation) of fluid in the water seal chamber. Visualize the chest tube drainage system and think about the function of each chamber to assist in determining the nurse's action. Review the functioning of chest tube drainage systems if you had difficulty with this question.

Reference
Black, J., & Hawks, J. (2005). *Medical-surgical nursing: Clinical management for positive outcomes* (7th ed., p. 1863). Philadelphia: Saunders.

---

526. The nurse is performing an admission assessment on a client admitted to the hospital with a diagnosis of pheochromocytoma. The nurse prepares to implement what action to assess for the principal manifestation associated with this disorder?

1 Checks the client's pupils
2 Checks the peripheral pulses
3 Takes the client's blood pressure
4 Assesses for the presence of peripheral edema

Answer: 3
Rationale: Pheochromocytoma is a catecholamine-secreting tumor that is usually located in the adrenal medulla. Hypertension is the principal manifestation associated with pheochromocytoma, and it can be persistent, fluctuating, intermittent, or paroxysmal. The blood pressure status would be assessed by taking the client's blood pressure. The assessments in options 1, 2, and 4 are not associated with this disorder.

Level of Cognitive Ability: Application
Client Needs: Physiological Integrity
Integrated Process: Nursing Process/Assessment
Content Area: Adult Health/Endocrine

Test-Taking Strategy: Note the strategic words "principal manifestation." Recalling that pheochromocytoma is a tumor of the adrenal gland and recalling the function of the adrenal gland will direct you to option 3. Review the principal manifestations of pheochromocytoma if you had difficulty with this question.

Reference
Black, J., & Hawks, J. (2005). *Medical-surgical nursing: Clinical management for positive outcomes* (7th ed., p. 1231). Philadelphia: Saunders.

---

527. A client received a thermal burn caused by the inhalation of steam. The client's mouth is edematous and the nurse notes blisters in the client's mouth. The nurse first assesses which priority item(s)?
1 Neurological status
2 Level of consciousness
3 Temperature via the rectal route
4 Respiratory status and lung sounds

Level of Cognitive Ability: Analysis
Client Needs: Physiological Integrity
Integrated Process: Nursing Process/Assessment
Content Area: Delegating/Prioritizing

Answer: 4
Rationale: Thermal burns to the lower airways can occur with the inhalation of steam or explosive gases or with the aspiration of scalding liquids. Thermal burns to the upper airways are more common and generally appear erythematous and edematous with mucosal blisters or ulcerations. The mucosal edema can lead to upper airway obstruction, particularly during the first 24 to 48 hours after burn injury. Assessment of respiratory status is the priority. Although the nurse would check the client's temperature and the client's neurological status, respiratory status is the priority.

Test-Taking Strategy: Focus on the type of burn injury described in the question and note the strategic words "mouth is edematous." Eliminate options 1 and 2 first because they are comparable or alike. Use the ABCs—airway, breathing, and circulation—to assist you in answering this question. Review care of the client with a burn injury if you had difficulty with this question.

Reference
Black, J., & Hawks, J. (2005). *Medical-surgical nursing: Clinical management for positive outcomes* (7th ed., p. 1440). Philadelphia: Saunders.

---

528. A client with late-stage chronic obstructive pulmonary disease (COPD) is admitted to the hospital with acute exacerbation. Which of the following blood gas results would the nurse most likely expect to note?
1 Po_2 of 68 and Pco_2 of 40
2 Po_2 of 55 and Pco_2 of 40
3 Po_2 of 70 and Pco_2 of 50
4 Po_2 of 60 and Pco_2 of 50

Level of Cognitive Ability: Analysis
Client Needs: Physiological Integrity
Integrated Process: Nursing Process/Analysis
Content Area: Adult Health/Respiratory

Answer: 4
Rationale: During an acute exacerbation, the arterial blood gases deteriorate with a decreasing Po_2 and an increasing Pco_2. In early stages of COPD, arterial blood gases demonstrate mild to moderate hypoxemia with the Po_2 in the high 60s to high 70s and a normal arterial Pco_2. As the condition advances, hypoxemia increases and hypercapnia may result.

Test-Taking Strategy: Note the strategic words "acute exacerbation" and "most likely." Recall the physiological manifestations that occur in COPD. Remembering that in COPD a low Po_2 and an elevated Pco_2 are the likely occurrences, will direct you to the correct option. Review the clinical manifestations that are likely to occur in an acute exacerbation if you had difficulty with this question.

References

Black, J., & Hawks, J. (2005). *Medical-surgical nursing: Clinical management for positive outcomes* (7th ed., pp. 1819, 1822). Philadelphia: Saunders.

Monahan, F., Sands, J., Neighbors, M., Marek, J., & Green, C. (2007). *Phipps' medical-surgical nursing: Health and illness perspectives* (8th ed., p. 680). St. Louis: Mosby.

---

529. The nurse monitors the respiratory status of the client being treated for acute exacerbation of chronic obstructive pulmonary disease (COPD). Which assessment finding would indicate a deterioration in ventilation?

1 Cyanosis
2 Hyperinflated chest
3 Coarse crackles bilaterally
4 Rapid, shallow respirations

Level of Cognitive Ability: Analysis
Client Needs: Physiological Integrity
Integrated Process: Nursing Process/Assessment
Content Area: Adult Health/Respiratory

Answer: 4

Rationale: An increase in the rate of respirations and a decrease in the depth of respirations indicate a deterioration in ventilation. Cyanosis is not a good indicator of oxygenation in the client with COPD. Cyanosis may be present with some, but not all, clients. A hyperinflated chest (barrel-chest) and hypertrophy of the accessory muscles of the upper chest and neck may normally be found in clients with severe COPD. During an exacerbation, coarse crackles are expected to be heard bilaterally throughout the lungs but do not indicate deterioration in ventilation.

Test-Taking Strategy: Note the strategic words "deterioration in ventilation." Eliminate options 2 and 3, recalling the normal clinical signs seen in COPD and the signs of exacerbation. Because cyanosis is not a good indicator of oxygenation in the client with COPD, eliminate option 1. Review the clinical manifestations associated with COPD and a deterioration in ventilation if you had difficulty with this question.

Reference

Ignatavicius, D., & Workman, M. (2006). *Medical-surgical nursing: Critical thinking for collaborative care* (5th ed., pp. 597-598, 601). Philadelphia: Saunders.

---

530. A physician has prescribed atropine sulfate gr 1/100, intramuscularly. The nurse notes that the medication vial reads 0.4 mg/mL and administers how many milliliter(s) to the client?

1 0.5
2 1.0
3 1.5
4 2.0

Answer: 3

Rationale: In this medication problem, both the apothecary (grains) and the metric (milligrams) systems are involved. Because the medication preparation is in milligrams (as noted on the medication vial), it is necessary to convert grains (gr) to milligrams (mg).

Formula for converting grains to milligrams:
gr:mg :: gr:mg
$$1:60 :: 1/100:X$$
$$X = 60/100$$
$$X = 0.6 \text{ mg}$$

Formula:
$$\frac{\text{Desired} \times \text{mL}}{\text{Available}} = \text{mL per dose}$$

$$\frac{0.6 \text{ mg} \times 1 \text{ mL}}{0.4 \text{ mg}} = 1.5 \text{ mL}$$

Level of Cognitive Ability: Application
Client Needs: Physiological Integrity
Integrated Process: Nursing Process/
    Implementation
Content Area: Fundamental Skills

Test-Taking Strategy: Read the physician's order, noting that it is first necessary to convert grains to milligrams. Next, follow the formula for the calculation of the correct dose. Use a calculator to verify your answer and make sure that the answer makes sense. Review medication calculation problems if you had difficulty with this question.

Reference
Kee, J., & Marshall, S. (2004). *Clinical calculations: With applications to general and specialty areas* (5th ed.). Philadelphia: Saunders, pp. 84-85.

---

531. A nurse is preparing a client for venography. The nurse understands that which of the following is unnecessary before this procedure?
  1 Obtaining a signed informed consent
  2 Asking the client about allergies to iodine or shellfish
  3 Determining the location and strength of peripheral pulses
  4 Placing the client on NPO status after midnight on the night before the test

Level of Cognitive Ability: Application
Client Needs: Physiological Integrity
Integrated Process: Nursing Process/Planning
Content Area: Adult Health/Cardiovascular

Answer: 4
Rationale: Venography is similar to arteriography, except it evaluates the venous system. A radiopaque dye is injected into selected veins to evaluate patency and blood flow characteristics. The client signs an informed consent because it is an invasive procedure. Allergies to shellfish or iodine must be noted. Peripheral pulses are assessed so that comparisons can be made after the procedure. The client is usually given clear liquids for 3 to 4 hours before the procedure to help with dye excretion afterward.

Test-Taking Strategy: Use the process of elimination, noting the strategic word "unnecessary." Because venography is an invasive procedure using a contrast agent, options 1 and 2 are eliminated first, because they must be done. From the remaining options, recall that an NPO status will promote dehydration rather than dye clearance and that assessing peripheral pulses is necessary to identify potential complications. Review preprocedure care for venography if you had difficulty with this question.

References
Ignatavicius, D., & Workman, M. (2006). *Medical-surgical nursing: Critical thinking for collaborative care* (5th ed., p. 813). Philadelphia: Saunders.
Lewis, S., Heitkemper, M., Dirksen, S., O'Brien, P., & Bucher, L. (2007). *Medical-surgical nursing: Assessment and management of clinical problems* (7th ed., p. 755). St. Louis: Mosby.

---

532. A physician writes an order to obtain a 12-lead ECG on a client, and the nurse informs the client of the procedure. Which client statement indicates that the client understands the procedure?
  1 "I should not breathe while the ECG is running."
  2 "I need to lie still while the ECG is being done."
  3 "I must take a deep breath when the ECG begins."
  4 "If I move when the ECG begins, I will

Answer: 2
Rationale: Good contact between the skin and electrodes is necessary to obtain a clear 12-lead ECG tracing. Therefore, the electrodes are placed on the flat surfaces of the skin just above the ankles and wrists. Movement may cause a disruption in that contact. The client does not need to hold his breath or take a deep breath during the procedure. The client needs to be reassured that a shock will not be received. Options 1, 3, and 4 are incorrect client statements.

Test-Taking Strategy: Use the process of elimination, focusing on the subject—performing an ECG. Recalling that good contact is required to obtain a clear ECG will direct you to option 2. Review this procedure if you had difficulty with this question.

Level of Cognitive Ability: Analysis
Client Needs: Physiological Integrity
Integrated Process: Nursing Process/Evaluation
Content Area: Adult Health/Cardiovascular

Reference
Ignatavicius, D., & Workman, M. (2006). *Medical-surgical nursing: Critical thinking for collaborative care* (5th ed., p. 701). Philadelphia: Saunders.

---

533. A nurse is giving a bed bath to a client who is on bed rest. In order to increase venous return from the extremities, the nurse bathes the client's extremities by using:
  1 Long, firm strokes from distal to proximal areas
  2 Firm circular strokes from proximal to distal areas
  3 Short, patting strokes from distal to proximal areas
  4 Back and forth strokes from proximal to distal areas

Level of Cognitive Ability: Application
Client Needs: Physiological Integrity
Integrated Process: Nursing Process/
  Implementation
Content Area: Fundamental Skills

Answer: 1
Rationale: Long, firm strokes in the direction of venous flow promote venous return when bathing the extremities. Circular strokes are used on the face. Short, patting strokes and back and forth strokes are not as comfortable for the client and they do not promote venous return because the stroke direction inhibits venous return partially.

Test-Taking Strategy: Use the process of elimination, focusing on the subject: increase venous return. Eliminate options that are unlikely to facilitate venous return. The only bathing stroke that mimics the flow of venous blood is option 1. Review the principles related to a bed bath if you had difficulty with this question.

Reference
Potter, P., & Perry, A. (2005). *Fundamentals of nursing* (6th ed., pp. 1025, 1027). St. Louis: Mosby.

---

534. The nurse prepares to give an intramuscular injection using the Z-track technique. Which does the nurse implement to administer the medication?
  1 Pinches the site before piercing the skin with the needle
  2 Injects the medication quickly after the needle is inserted
  3 Selects a large deep muscle for the intramuscular injection site
  4 Withdraws and administers the medication with the same needle

Level of Cognitive Ability: Application
Client Needs: Physiological Integrity
Integrated Process: Nursing Process/
  Implementation
Content Area: Fundamental Skills

Answer: 3
Rationale: The nurse uses the Z-track method to administer an intramuscular injection that is highly irritating to subcutaneous and skin tissues. The nurse selects an intramuscular site for injection, preferably in a large deep muscle such as the ventrogluteal muscle to deposit the medication in an area that will self-seal after the injection. Pinching the skin is a technique used for subcutaneous injections. The medication is injected slowly after aspiration because the medication is usually thick, and the needle remains inserted for 10 seconds to allow the medication to disperse evenly. A sterile needle is used to withdraw the medication and a second needle to administer the medication to prevent medication adhering to the outside of the needle leading to tissue irritation. The nurse then releases the skin after withdrawing the needle.

Test-Taking Strategy: Focus on the subject—Z-track injection. Recalling the purpose of using the Z-track technique and noting that an irritating medication is administered with this technique directs you to option 3. Review this procedure for administering medications using the Z-track method if you had difficulty with this question.

Reference
Potter, P., & Perry, A. (2005). *Fundamentals of nursing* (6th ed., p. 890). St. Louis: Mosby.

535. The nurse needs to suction a client's tracheostomy. Which client position does the nurse use to promote deep breathing and coughing during suctioning?

1 Sims' position
2 Supine position
3 Side-lying position
4 Semi-Fowler's position

Level of Cognitive Ability: Application
Client Needs: Physiological Integrity
Integrated Process: Nursing Process/
  Implementation
Content Area: Fundamental Skills

Answer: 4
Rationale: If not contraindicated, before suctioning a tracheostomy, the client is placed in semi-Fowler's position to promote deep breathing, maximum lung expansion, and productive coughing. In this position, gravity pulls downward on the diaphragm, which allows greater chest expansion and lung volume. The lateral position, the supine position, or the Sims' position is unlikely to allow for easy visualization of the tracheostomy or easy access of the suction catheter; in addition, the supine position increases the risk of client aspiration.

Test-Taking Strategy: Use the process of elimination and focus on the subject—the position that will promote deep breathing and coughing during suctioning. Visualize each position and note that options 1, 2, and 3 are comparable or alike positions in that the client lies flat. The semi-Fowler's position promotes deep breathing, maximum lung expansion, and productive coughing. Review this procedure if you had difficulty with this question.

Reference
Potter, P., & Perry, A. (2005). *Fundamentals of nursing* (6th ed., p. 1102). St. Louis: Mosby.

---

536. A client is in labor is at 40 weeks' gestation. The nurse checks the fetal heart rate (FHR) for a baseline rate and tells the client that the baby's heart rate is within normal limits. The nurse then documents which FHR finding?

1 90 beats per minute
2 140 beats per minute
3 180 beats per minute
4 200 beats per minute

Level of Cognitive Ability: Application
Client Needs: Health Promotion and
  Maintenance
Integrated Process: Communication and
  Documentation
Content Area: Maternity/Intrapartum

Answer: 2
Rationale: The normal FHR ranges from 110 to 160 beats per minute; therefore, option 2 is the only correct option.

Test-Taking Strategy: Knowledge of the normal fetal heart rate is required to answer this question. Remember that the normal FHR ranges from 110 to 160 beats per minute. Review this normal rate if you are unfamiliar with it.

References
McKinney, E., James, S., Murray, S., & Ashwill, J. (2005). *Maternal-child nursing* (2nd ed., p. 399). St. Louis: Saunders.
Murray, S., & McKinney, E. (2006). *Foundations of maternal-newborn nursing* (4th ed., p. 269). Philadelphia: Saunders.

---

537. A client receiving chemotherapy has an infiltrated intravenous line and extravasation at the site. The nurse avoids doing which of the following in the management of this situation?

1 Applying direct manual pressure to the site
2 Stopping the administration of the medication
3 Administering an available antidote as prescribed
4 Leaving the needle in place and aspirating any residual medication

Answer: 1
Rationale: General recommendations for managing extravasation of a chemotherapeutic agent include stopping the infusion, leaving the needle in place and attempting to aspirate any residual medication from the site, administering an antidote if available, and assessing the site for complications. Direct pressure is not applied to the site because it could further injure tissues exposed to the chemotherapeutic agent.

Level of Cognitive Ability: Application
Client Needs: Physiological Integrity
Integrated Process: Nursing Process/
Implementation
Content Area: Adult Health/Oncology

Test-Taking Strategy: Use the process of elimination, noting the strategic word "avoids." This word indicates a negative event query and the need to select the option that is an incorrect nursing action. Noting that the client was receiving chemotherapy and recalling the damaging effects of extravasation will direct you to option 1. Review treatment measures for extravasation if you had difficulty with this question.

Reference
Black, J., & Hawks, J. (2005). *Medical-surgical nursing: Clinical management for positive outcomes* (7th ed., p. 374). Philadelphia: Saunders.

---

538. A nurse is suctioning the airway of a client with a tracheostomy. To properly perform the procedure, the nurse:
    1 Turns on the wall suction to 180 mm Hg
    2 Inserts the catheter until coughing or resistance is felt
    3 Withdraws the catheter while continuously suctioning
    4 Reenters the tracheostomy after suctioning the mouth

Level of Cognitive Ability: Application
Client Needs: Physiological Integrity
Integrated Process: Nursing Process/
Implementation
Content Area: Adult Health/Respiratory

Answer: 2
Rationale: The nurse inserts the catheter until resistance is felt and then withdraws it 1 cm to move away from mucosa. The wall suction unit is usually set to 80 to 120 mm Hg pressure. This allows adequate removal of secretions while protecting the airway from trauma. The nurse suctions intermittently during withdrawal of the catheter and does not reenter the tracheostomy after suctioning the client's mouth.

Test-Taking Strategy: Use the process of elimination. Eliminate option 4 because the trachea is not reentered and option 3 because of the word "continuously." From the remaining options, it is necessary to know that 180 mm Hg pressure would cause trauma to the mucosa. Review this procedure if you had difficulty with this question.

References
Lewis, S., Heitkemper, M., Dirksen, S., O'Brien, P., & Bucher, L. (2007). *Medical-surgical nursing: Assessment and management of clinical problems* (7th ed., p. 545). St. Louis: Mosby.
Potter, P., & Perry, A. (2005). *Fundamentals of nursing* (6th ed., p. 1103). St. Louis: Mosby.

---

539. The nurse has prepared a client for an intravenous pyelogram. The nurse determines that the client understands the procedure if the client states to report which sensation immediately, if it occurs during the procedure?
    1 Nausea
    2 Difficulty breathing
    3 Salty taste in the mouth
    4 Momentary episode of shivering

Level of Cognitive Ability: Analysis
Client Needs: Physiological Integrity
Integrated Process: Nursing Process/Evaluation
Content Area: Adult Health/Renal

Answer: 2
Rationale: Intravenous pyelography is a contrast study of the kidneys to determine a variety of disorders of the kidneys, ureters, and bladder. Normal sensations during injection of the iodine-based radiopaque dye include a warm, flushed feeling, salty taste in the mouth, and transient nausea. Difficulty breathing, wheezing, hives, or itching indicate an allergic response and should be reported to the physician immediately. This complication is prevented by inquiring about allergies to iodine or shellfish before the procedure.

Test-Taking Strategy: Use the process of elimination and recall that this diagnostic test may involve injection of iodine-based contrast medium. Use of the ABCs—airway, breathing, and circulation—will direct you to option 2. Review this diagnostic procedure if you had difficulty with this question.

References

Black, J., & Hawks, J. (2005). *Medical-surgical nursing: Clinical management for positive outcomes* (7th ed., p. 799). Philadelphia: Saunders.

Chernecky, C., & Berger, B. (2008). *Laboratory tests and diagnostic procedures* (5th ed., p. 682). Philadelphia: Saunders.

---

540. A 15-year-old pregnant client is being treated by a dermatologist for acne. The clinic nurse asks the client about the treatment prescribed for the acne, knowing that which treatment is contraindicated during pregnancy?

1 Exfoliation
2 Oral tetracycline
3 Topical erythromycin cream
4 Cleansing with antibacterial soap

Level of Cognitive Ability: Analysis
Client Needs: Physiological Integrity
Integrated Process: Nursing Process/Assessment
Content Area: Maternity/Antepartum

Answer: 2

Rationale: Tetracycline use during pregnancy may lead to discoloration of the child's teeth when they erupt. This treatment for acne is contraindicated during pregnancy. Options 1, 3, and 4 are appropriate treatments.

Test-Taking Strategy: Use the process of elimination. Focus on the safety factor for the unseen client (fetus) and note the strategic word "contraindicated." Eliminate options 1, 3, and 4 because they are comparable or alike and are all topical treatments. Review the concepts related to medications and safety during pregnancy if you had difficulty with this question.

References

Hodgson, B., & Kizior, R. (2007). *Saunders nursing drug handbook 2007* (p. 1118). Philadelphia: Saunders.

Murray, S., & McKinney, E. (2006). *Foundations of maternal-newborn nursing* (4th ed., p. 924). Philadelphia: Saunders.

---

541. A client with osteomyelitis is scheduled for indium imaging. Which does the nurse include in client teaching?

1 Indium collects in normal bone only.
2 Indium collects in infected bone only.
3 Leukocytes tagged with indium accumulate in normal bone.
4 Leukocytes tagged with indium accumulate in infected bone.

Level of Cognitive Ability: Application
Client Needs: Physiological Integrity
Integrated Process: Teaching and Learning
Content Area: Fundamental Skills

Answer: 4

Rationale: A sample of the client's blood is collected, and the leukocytes from the sample are tagged with indium. After injecting the leukocytes into the client, they accumulate in infected areas of bone and scanning detects the accumulation of indium, thus defining the infected bone. No special preparation or postprocedure care is necessary. Options 1, 2, and 3 are incorrect descriptions.

Test-Taking Strategy: Use the process of elimination, focusing on the information in the question. Note that the client has a bone infection. Recall that with any type of infection, leukocytes migrate to the area. This will direct you to option 4. Review this test if you had difficulty with this question.

Reference

Pagana, K., & Pagana, T. (2005). *Mosby's diagnostic and laboratory test reference* (7th ed., pp. 1000-1001). St. Louis: Mosby.

542. A client with repeated episodes of pulmonary emboli from thromboembolism is scheduled for insertion of an inferior vena cava filter (Greenfield filter). The nurse determines that the client has an adequate understanding of the procedure if the client makes which of the following statements?

1 "The filter will keep new blood clots from forming in my legs."
2 "It's too bad I have to continue anticoagulant therapy after the surgery."
3 "The filter will be like a catcher's mitt and keep the clots from going to my lungs."
4 "I don't mind having a filter in my artery if it means I won't have any more trouble."

Level of Cognitive Ability: Analysis
Client Needs: Physiological Integrity
Integrated Process: Nursing Process/Evaluation
Content Area: Adult Health/Cardiovascular

Answer: 3
Rationale: Insertion of an inferior vena cava filter is indicated for clients with recurrent deep vein thrombosis and/or pulmonary emboli who do not respond to medical therapy, and when anticoagulant therapy is ineffective or contraindicated. The filter device or "umbrella" is inserted percutaneously in the inferior vena cava, where it springs open and attaches to the vena caval wall. The device has holes to allow blood flow, but traps larger clots, thus preventing pulmonary emboli. The filter does not prevent blood clots from forming and is not placed in an artery. Vena cava filters are less effective than anticoagulation and may lead to deep vein thrombosis, so they are generally used only when anticoagulant therapy is ineffective or contraindicated.

Test-Taking Strategy: Specific knowledge regarding this filter is required to answer this question. Thinking about the purpose and the action of a filter will direct you to option 3. Review this content if you had difficulty with this question.

References
Black, J., & Hawks, J. (2005). *Medical-surgical nursing: Clinical management for positive outcomes* (7th ed., p. 1833). Philadelphia: Saunders.
Lewis, S., Heitkemper, M., Dirksen, S., O'Brien, P., & Bucher, L. (2007). *Medical-surgical nursing: Assessment and management of clinical problems* (7th ed., p. 915). St. Louis: Mosby.

---

543. A client is admitted to the hospital with a diagnosis of infective endocarditis from *Streptococcus viridans*. The client asks the nurse about the antibiotic therapy that will be given. Knowing that the client has no medication allergies, the nurse prepares the client to receive:

1 Amphotericin B (Fungizone) IV for 10 days, followed by oral doses for 3 weeks
2 Amphotericin B (Fungizone) IV for 4 to 6 weeks, continuing at home after hospital discharge
3 Penicillin G benzathine (Bicillin L-A) IV for 4 to 6 weeks, continuing at home after hospital discharge
4 Penicillin G benzathine (Bicillin L-A) intravenously (IV) for 10 days, followed by oral doses for 2 weeks

Level of Cognitive Ability: Analysis
Client Needs: Physiological Integrity
Integrated Process: Nursing Process/Planning
Content Area: Adult Health/Cardiovascular

Answer: 3
Rationale: Penicillin is frequently the medication of choice for treating endocarditis of bacterial origin. The standard duration of therapy is 4 to 6 weeks, with home care support after hospital discharge, which is usually in 7 to 10 days. Amphotericin B is an antifungal agent and would not be effective with this type of infection.

Test-Taking Strategy: Use the process of elimination. Recalling that amphotericin B is an antifungal agent eliminates options 1 and 2. From the remaining options, note that the severity and nature of the infection make continued IV therapy necessary; therefore, option 3 is the best option. Review the treatment for this disorder if you had difficulty with this question.

Reference
Black, J., & Hawks, J. (2005). *Medical-surgical nursing: Clinical management for positive outcomes* (7th ed., pp. 1618-1619). Philadelphia: Saunders.

544. A nurse is doing a dressing change on a venous stasis ulcer that is clean and has a growing bed of granulation tissue. The nurse avoids using which of the following dressing materials on this wound?

1 Hydrocolloid dressing
2 Vaseline gauze dressing
3 Wet-to-dry saline dressing
4 Wet-to-wet saline dressing

Level of Cognitive Ability: Application
Client Needs: Physiological Integrity
Integrated Process: Nursing Process/ Implementation
Content Area: Fundamental Skills

Answer: 3

Rationale: The use of wet-to-dry saline dressings provides a nonselective mechanical debridement, whereby both devitalized and viable tissue are removed. This method should not be used on a clean, granulating wound. Granulation tissue in a venous stasis ulcer is protected through the use of wet-to-wet saline dressings, Vaseline gauze, or moist occlusive dressings, such as hydrocolloid dressings.

Test-Taking Strategy: Use the process of elimination and note the strategic word "avoids." This word indicates a negative event query and that you need to select the option that is an incorrect dressing material. Note that the question specifically tells you that the wound is clean with granulation tissue (which needs protection). Next, look at the options and note that options 1, 2, and 4 are comparable or alike and have one thing in common: continuous moisture. The wet-to-dry saline dressing could disrupt the healing tissue. Review care of a venous stasis ulcer if you had difficulty with this question.

References
Black, J., & Hawks, J. (2005). *Medical-surgical nursing: Clinical management for positive outcomes* (7th ed., p. 1541). Philadelphia: Saunders.
Ignatavicius, D., & Workman, M. (2006). *Medical-surgical nursing: Critical thinking for collaborative care* (5th ed., pp. 1588-1589). Philadelphia: Saunders.

---

545. A nurse preparing to admit an older client with severe digitalis toxicity from accidental ingestion of a week's supply of the medication would anticipate the health care provider to order which of the following?

1 Protamine sulfate
2 Furosemide (Lasix)
3 Potassium chloride (K-Dur)
4 Digoxin immune Fab (Digibind)

Level of Cognitive Ability: Application
Client Needs: Physiological Integrity
Integrated Process: Nursing Process/ Implementation
Content Area: Pharmacology

Answer: 4

Rationale: Digoxin immune Fab is an antidote for severe digitalis toxicity. It contains an antibody produced in sheep, which antigenically binds any unbound digitalis in the serum and removes it. As more digoxin reenters the bloodstream from the tissues, it binds that also for excretion by the kidneys. Potassium chloride is a potassium supplement. Protamine sulfate is the antidote for heparin. Furosemide is a diuretic.

Test-Taking Strategy: Note the client's diagnosis and the names of the medications in the options. Noting the relationship between the diagnosis and option 4 will direct you to this option. Review the treatment for digitalis toxicity if you had difficulty with this question.

References
Hodgson, B., & Kizior, R. (2007). *Saunders nursing drug handbook 2007* (pp. 358-359). Philadelphia: Saunders.
McKenry, L., Tressier, E., & Hogan, M. (2006). *Mosby's pharmacology in nursing* (22nd ed, pp. 513-514.). St. Louis: Mosby.

546. The parents of a 6-month-old male report that the infant has been screaming and drawing the knees up to the chest and has passed stools mixed with blood and mucus that are jelly-like. A nurse recognizes these signs and symptoms as indicative of:

1 Peritonitis
2 Appendicitis
3 Intussusception
4 Hirschsprung's disease

Level of Cognitive Ability: Analysis
Client Needs: Physiological Integrity
Integrated Process: Nursing Process/Assessment
Content Area: Child Health

Answer: 3
Rationale: The classic signs and symptoms of intussusception are acute, colicky abdominal pain with currant jelly–like stools. Clinical manifestations of Hirschsprung's disease include constipation, abdominal distention, and ribbon-like, foul-smelling stools. Peritonitis is a serious complication that may follow intestinal obstruction and perforation. The most common symptom of appendicitis is colicky, periumbilical or lower abdominal pain in the right quadrant.

Test-Taking Strategy: Use the process of elimination. Eliminate options 1 and 2 because they are comparable or alike. Recalling that in Hirschsprung's disease the stools are ribbon-like will assist in eliminating option 4. Review the clinical manifestations of intussusception if you had difficulty with this question.

Reference
Hockenberry, M., Wilson, D., & Winkelstein, M. (2005). *Wong's essentials of pediatric nursing* (7th ed., pp. 882-883). St. Louis: Mosby.

---

547. A nurse is caring for a client who has been placed in seclusion. The nurse is documenting care provided to the client and addresses which items in the client's record?

1 Vital signs, reason for the procedure, and date and time
2 Vital signs, toileting, and checking the client based on protocol time frame, such as every 15 minutes
3 Ambulating, toileting, and checking the client based on protocol time frame, such as every 15 minutes
4 Vital signs, toileting, feeding and fluid intake, and checking the client based on protocol time frame, such as every 15 minutes

Level of Cognitive Ability: Application
Client Needs: Physiological Integrity
Integrated Process: Communication and Documentation
Content Area: Mental Health

Answer: 4
Rationale: The client in seclusion is assessed continuously or at least every 15 minutes, or according to agency protocol. Vital signs, food and fluid intake, and toileting needs are assessed. Option 1 contains client documentation that would precede seclusion. Options 2 and 3 are not complete in terms of identification of physiological needs.

Test-Taking Strategy: Use Maslow's Hierarchy of Needs theory and the process of elimination. Note that option 4 is complete in terms of the client's basic needs. Review care of the client in seclusion if you had difficulty with this question.

References
Stuart, G., & Laraia, M. (2005). *Principles and practice of psychiatric nursing* (8th ed., pp. 645-646). St. Louis: Mosby.
Varcarolis, E., Carson, V., & Shoemaker, N. (2006). *Foundations of psychiatric mental health nursing* (5th ed., p. 124). Philadelphia: Saunders.

---

548. During the admission assessment, the nurse asks the client to run the heel of one foot down the lower anterior surface of the other leg. The nurse notices rhythmic tremors of the leg being tested and concludes that the client has an alteration in the area of:

1 Sensation and reflexes
2 Balance and coordination
3 Bowel and bladder function
4 Muscle strength and flexibility

Answer: 2
Rationale: In this situation the nurse is performing one test of cerebellar function and is testing for ataxia. Alterations in the cerebellar function are noted by alterations in balance and coordination. Options 1, 3, and 4 are not associated with this assessment technique.

Level of Cognitive Ability: Analysis
Client Needs: Physiological Integrity
Integrated Process: Nursing Process/Assessment
Content Area: Adult Health/Neurological

Test-Taking Strategy: Use the process of elimination. Note the relationship between the word "tremors" in the question and "coordination" in option 2. Review assessment for cerebellar function and coordination if you had difficulty with this question.

Reference
Lewis, S., Heitkemper, M., Dirksen, S., O'Brien, P., & Bucher, L. (2007). *Medical-surgical nursing: Assessment and management of clinical problems* (7th ed., pp. 49, 1460). St. Louis: Mosby.

---

549. The nurse is monitoring the intracranial pressure (ICP) of a client with a head injury and notes that the ICP is averaging 25 mm Hg. How should the nurse correctly interpret this result?
1 The result is normal.
2 Compensation is occurring, indicating adequate brain adaptation.
3 ICP is increased, indicating a serious compromise in cerebral perfusion.
4 ICP is borderline in elevation, indicating the initial stage of decompensation.

Level of Cognitive Ability: Analysis
Client Needs: Physiological Integrity
Integrated Process: Nursing Process/Analysis
Content Area: Adult Health/Neurological

Answer: 3
Rationale: The normal intracranial pressure is 10 to 15 mm Hg. A pressure of 25 mm Hg is increased and may require intervention if this pressure is sustained.

Test-Taking Strategy: Use the process of elimination. Eliminate options 1 and 2 because they are comparable or alike. From the remaining options, focusing on the level identified in the question will direct you to option 3. Review normal values for intracranial pressure if you had difficulty with this question.

Reference
Ignatavicius, D., & Workman, M. (2006). *Medical-surgical nursing: Critical thinking for collaborative care* (5th ed., p. 1045). Philadelphia: Saunders.

---

550. A woman at 32 weeks' gestation is brought into the emergency department after an automobile accident. The client is bleeding vaginally and fetal assessment indicates moderate fetal distress. Which of the following should the nurse do first in an attempt to reduce the stress on the fetus?
1 Start intravenous (IV) fluids at a keep open rate.
2 Set up for an immediate cesarean section delivery.
3 Elevate the head of the bed to a semi-Fowler's position.
4 Administer oxygen via a face mask at 7 to 10 liters per minute.

Level of Cognitive Ability: Application
Client Needs: Physiological Integrity
Integrated Process: Nursing Process/Implementation
Content Area: Maternity/Antepartum

Answer: 4
Rationale: Administering oxygen will increase the amount of oxygen for transport to the fetus, partially compensating for the loss of circulating blood volume. This action is essential regardless of the cause or amount of bleeding. IV fluids will also be initiated. The client will be positioned per physician's order. Although a cesarean delivery may be needed, there are no data that indicate that it is necessary at this time.

Test-Taking Strategy: Note the strategic word "first." Using the ABCs—airway, breathing, and circulation—will direct you to option 4. Review care of the pregnant client when fetal distress occurs if you had difficulty with this question.

References
McKinney, E., James, S., Murray, S., & Ashwill, J. (2005). *Maternal-child nursing* (2nd ed., p. 406). St. Louis: Saunders.
Murray, S., & McKinney, E. (2006). *Foundations of maternal-newborn nursing* (4th ed., p. 325). Philadelphia: Saunders.

551. A physician has ordered a partial rebreather face mask for a client who has terminal lung cancer. The nurse prepares to implement the order knowing that the mask:

1 Delivers accurate fraction of inspired oxygen (FIO_2) to the client
2 Requires a low liter flow to prevent rebreathing of carbon dioxide
3 Conserves oxygen by having the client rebreathe his own exhaled air
4 Requires that the reservoir bag deflate during inspiration to work effectively

Level of Cognitive Ability: Application
Client Needs: Physiological Integrity
Integrated Process: Nursing Process/Planning
Content Area: Adult Health/Respiratory

Answer: 3
Rationale: Rebreathing masks have a reservoir bag that conserves oxygen and requires a high liter flow to achieve concentrations of 40% to 60%. They do not deliver accurate FIO_2 to the client. The bag should not deflate during inspiration. Rebreathing masks conserve oxygen by having the client rebreathe his own exhaled air.

Test-Taking Strategy: Use the process of elimination. Note the relationship between "partial rebreather" in the question and "rebreathe his own exhaled air" in the correct option. Review this oxygen delivery system if you had difficulty with this question.

References
Ignatavicius, D., & Workman, M. (2006). *Medical-surgical nursing: Critical thinking for collaborative care* (5th ed., pp. 548-549). Philadelphia: Saunders.
Lewis, S., Heitkemper, M., Dirksen, S., O'Brien, P., & Bucher, L. (2007). *Medical-surgical nursing: Assessment and management of clinical problems* (7th ed., p. 641). St. Louis: Mosby.

---

552. A client has a slow, regular pulse. On the monitor, the nurse notes regular QRS complexes with no P waves and a ventricular rate of 50 beats per minute. The nurse suspects that there is a problem at which part of the cardiac conduction system?

1 The left ventricle
2 The bundle of His
3 The sinoatrial (SA) node
4 The atrioventricular (AV) node

Level of Cognitive Ability: Analysis
Client Needs: Physiological Integrity
Integrated Process: Nursing Process/Analysis
Content Area: Adult Health/Cardiovascular

Answer: 3
Rationale: A normal P wave indicates that the impulse that depolarized the atrium was initiated in the SA node. A change in the form (inverted P wave) or the absence of a P wave can indicate a problem at this part of the conduction system, with the resulting impulse originating from an alternate site lower in the conduction pathway. Options 1, 2, and 4 are incorrect.

Test-Taking Strategy: Use the process of elimination. Option 1 can be eliminated first because it does not identify a mechanism of the conduction system. The question also identifies a regular QRS complex and a ventricular rate of 50 beats per minute, indicating an intact AV node; thus the problem lies higher in the conduction system. Correlate a P wave with the SA node. Review the conduction system of the heart if you had difficulty with this question.

Reference
Ignatavicius, D., & Workman, M. (2006). *Medical-surgical nursing: Critical thinking for collaborative care* (5th ed., pp. 679, 684). Philadelphia: Saunders.

ALTERNATE ITEM FORMATS

553. A client is admitted to the hospital with a diagnosis of acute bacterial pericarditis, and the nurse prepares to perform an assessment on the client. Which of the following findings are associated with this inflammatory heart odisease?
Select all that apply.

☐ **1** Fever
☐ **2** Leukopenia
☐ **3** Bradycardia
☐ **4** Pericardial friction rub
☐ **5** Decreased erythrocyte sedimentation rate
☐ **6** Severe precordial chest pain that intensifies when in the supine position

Level of Cognitive Ability: Analysis
Client Needs: Physiological Integrity
Integrated Process: Nursing Process/Assessment
Content Area: Adult Health/Cardiovascular

Answer: 1, 4, 6
Rationale: In acute bacterial pericarditis, the membranes surrounding the heart become inflamed and rub against each other, producing the classic pericardial friction rub. The client complains of severe precordial chest pain that intensifies when lying supine and decreases in a sitting position. The pain also intensifies when the client breathes deeply. Fever typically occurs and is accompanied by leukocytosis and an elevated erythrocyte sedimentation rate. Malaise, myalgias, and tachycardia are common.

Test-Taking Strategy: Focusing on the diagnosis will assist in determining that the client would have a fever (option 1); the compensatory response to fever is an increased metabolic rate and tachycardia. Also remember that when the client has an inflammatory disease, the erythrocyte sedimentation rate would increase, as would the white blood cell count (leukocytosis, not leukopenia). Lastly, focusing on the diagnosis will assist in determining that a pericardial friction rub and severe precordial chest pain will be present (options 4 and 6). Review the characteristics associated with acute bacterial pericarditis if you had difficulty with this question.

Reference
Ignatavicius, D., & Workman, M. (2006). *Medical-surgical nursing: Critical thinking for collaborative care* (5th ed., p. 770). Philadelphia: Saunders.

554. A nurse is assessing a client's cigarette smoking habit, and the client states that he has smoked three fourths of a pack per day over the last 10 years. The nurse calculates that the client has a smoking history of how many pack-years?
Answer: _____ pack years

Level of Cognitive Ability: Application
Client Needs: Physiological Integrity
Integrated Process: Nursing Process/Assessment
Content Area: Adult Health/Respiratory

Answer: 7.5
Rationale: The standard method for quantifying smoking history is to multiply the number of packs smoked per day by the number of years of smoking. The number is recorded as the number of pack-years. The calculation for the number of pack-years for the client who has smoked three fourths of a pack per day for 10 years is: 0.75 pack × 10 years = 7.5 pack-years.

Test-Taking Strategy: Focus on the information in the question and multiply the number of packs of cigarettes smoked per day by the number of years of smoking. Review this calculation if you had difficulty with this question.

Reference
Ignatavicius, D., & Workman, M. (2006). *Medical-surgical nursing: Critical thinking for collaborative care* (5th ed., pp. 529-530). Philadelphia: Saunders.

555. An adult client arrives in the emergency unit with burns to both legs and perineal area. Using the Rule of Nines, the nurse would determine that approximately what percentage of the client's body surface has been burned?

Answer: _____%

Level of Cognitive Ability: Analysis
Client Needs: Physiological Integrity
Integrated Process: Nursing Process/Assessment
Content Area: Adult Health/Integumentary

Answer: 37
Rationale: The most rapid method used to calculate the size of a burn injury in adult clients whose weights are in normal proportion to their heights is the Rule of Nines. This method divides the body into areas that are multiples of 9%, except for the perineum. Each leg is 18%, each arm is 9%, and the head is 9%. The trunk is 36%, and the perineal area is 1%. Both legs and perineal area equal 37%.

Test-Taking Strategy: Knowledge regarding the percentages associated with this method of calculating burn injuries is required to answer this question. Remember that each leg is 18%, each arm is 9%, the head is 9% the trunk is 36%, and the perineal area is 1%. Memorize these percentages if you had difficulty with this question.

Reference
Ignatavicius, D., & Workman, M. (2006). *Medical-surgical nursing: Critical thinking for collaborative care* (5th ed., pp. 1630-1631). Philadelphia: Saunders.

---

556. A client who works as a security guard at night in an industrial building is brought to the emergency room with suspected carbon monoxide poisoning. List in order of priority the actions that the nurse takes on arrival of the client. (Number 1 is the first action.)

—Administer 100% oxygen.
—Check the blood pressure and pulse.
—Check the client's airway for patency.
—Draw blood for carboxyhemoglobin levels.
—Document assessment findings, treatment, and client response.
—Notify the local health department and request an inspection at the industrial building.

Level of Cognitive Ability: Application
Client Needs: Physiological Integrity
Integrated Process: Nursing Process/Implementation
Content Area: Delegating/Prioritizing

Answer: 2, 3, 1, 4, 5, 6
Rationale: On arrival of the client, the nurse immediately checks the client's airway for patency and then quickly administers 100% oxygen at atmospheric pressure or hyperbaric pressure to speed up the elimination of carbon monoxide from the hemoglobin and to reverse hypoxia. The next most important action is assessment of the client's vital signs. Then blood is drawn (initially and serially) to monitor carboxyhemoglobin levels; once they drop below 5%, oxygen may be discontinued. Following assessment, treatment, and evaluation of the client's response, the nurse documents. If the episode was unintentional and precipitated by conditions in a dwelling, the health department is notified.

Test-Taking Strategy: Use the ABCs—airway, breathing, and circulation—to direct you to first checking the client's airway and then the action that indicates to administer 100% oxygen. Next, use the steps of the nursing process—finish the assessment of the client. From the remaining actions listed, use Maslow's Hierarchy of Needs theory, recalling that physiological needs are the priority. This will assist you in determining that drawing blood for carboxyhemoglobin levels is the next action, followed by documentation. Review care of the client with carbon monoxide poisoning if you had difficulty with this question.

References
Black, J., & Hawks, J. (2005). *Medical-surgical nursing: Clinical management for positive outcomes* (7th ed., 1906). Philadelphia: Saunders.
Chernecky, C., & Berger, B. (2008). *Laboratory tests and diagnostic procedures* (5th ed., pp. 292-293). Philadelphia: Saunders.

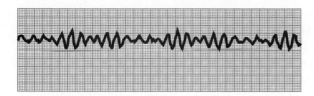

From Ignatavicius, D., & Workman, M. (2006). *Medical-surgical nursing: Critical thinking for collaborative care* (5th ed.). Philadelphia: Saunders.

557. The nurse is in the room of a client on a cardiac monitor who suddenly becomes unconscious and exhibits this cardiac rhythm (see figure above). The nurse calls for help, knowing that which of the following items will be needed immediately?

1 Ventilator
2 Defibrillator
3 Lidocaine (Xylocaine)
4 Pacemaker insertion tray

Level of Cognitive Ability: Application
Client Needs: Physiological Integrity
Integrated Process: Nursing Process/
   Implementation
Content Area: Adult Health/Cardiovascular

Answer: 2
Rationale: This cardiac rhythm indicates coarse ventricular fibrillation. A defibrillator is needed to correct ventricular fibrillation. Options 1 and 3 will do nothing to correct this rhythm. Lidocaine may be used to treat ventricular dysrhythmias; however, defibrillation would be the priority intervention in this situation.

Test-Taking Strategy: Focus on the cardiac rhythm, noting that the client is exhibiting ventricular fibrillation. Note the relationship between this cardiac rhythm and defibrillation in the correct option. Review the characteristics of and treatment for ventricular fibrillation if you had difficulty with this question.

References
Lewis, S., Heitkemper, M., Dirksen, S., O'Brien, P., & Bucher, L. (2007). *Medical-surgical nursing: Assessment and management of clinical problems* (7th ed., pp. 855-856). St. Louis: Mosby.
Monahan, F., Sands, J., Neighbors, M., Marek, J., & Green, C. (2007). *Phipps' medical-surgical nursing: Health and illness perspectives* (8th ed., pp. 786-787). St. Louis: Mosby.

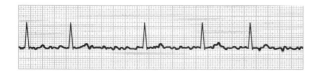

From Ignatavicius, D., & Workman, M. (2006). *Medical-surgical nursing: Critical thinking for collaborative care* (5th ed.). Philadelphia: Saunders.

558. A nurse analyzed an ECG strip (see figure above) for a client with left-sided heart failure, as follows: atrial rate: no identifiable P waves; ventricular rate: 110 beats per minute (BPM); ventricular rhythm: irregular; QRS: 0.08.
   The nurse interprets the rhythm strip as:

1 Atrial fibrillation
2 Sinus dysrhythmia
3 Ventricular fibrillation
4 Third-degree heart block

Level of Cognitive Ability: Analysis
Client Needs: Physiological Integrity
Integrated Process: Nursing Process/Analysis
Content Area: Adult Health/Cardiovascular

Answer: 1
Rationale: Atrial fibrillation is characterized by rapid, chaotic atrial depolarization. Ventricular rates may be less than 100 BPM (controlled) or greater than 100 BPM (uncontrolled). The ECG reveals chaotic or no identifiable P waves and an irregular ventricular rhythm. A sinus dysrhythmia has a normal P wave, PR interval, and QRS complex. In ventricular fibrillation, there are no identifiable P waves, QRS complexes, or T waves. In third-degree heart block, the atria and ventricles beat independently.

Test-Taking Strategy: Recall that in atrial fibrillation the P wave is absent or chaotic and the ventricular rhythm is irregular. This will direct you to option 1. Review this content if you are unfamiliar with the cardiac dysrhythmias identified in the options.

Reference
Monahan, F., Sands, J., Neighbors, M., Marek, J., & Green, C. (2007). *Phipps' medical-surgical nursing: Health and illness perspectives* (8th ed., pp. 782-783). St. Louis: Mosby.

559. The nurse is sending an arterial blood gas (ABG) specimen to the laboratory for analysis. Which of the following pieces of information should the nurse write on the laboratory requisition?
Select all that apply.
- ☐ **1** Ventilator settings
- ☐ **2** A list of client allergies
- ☐ **3** The client's temperature
- ☐ **4** The date and time the specimen was drawn
- ☐ **5** Any supplemental oxygen the client is receiving
- ☐ **6** Extremity from which the specimen was obtained

Level of Cognitive Ability: Application
Client Needs: Physiological Integrity
Integrated Process: Communication and Documentation
Content Area: Adult Health/Respiratory

Answer: 1, 3, 4, 5
Rationale: An ABG requisition usually contains information about the date and time the specimen was drawn, the client's temperature, whether the specimen was drawn on room air or using supplemental oxygen, and the ventilator settings if the client is on a mechanical ventilator. The client's allergies and the extremity from which the specimen was drawn do not have a direct bearing on the laboratory results.

Test-Taking Strategy: Review the pieces of information from the viewpoint of the relevance of the item to the client's airway status or oxygen utilization. The only pieces of information that do not relate to airway status or oxygen utilization are the client's allergies and the extremity from which the specimen was drawn. Review the procedure related to drawing ABGs if you had difficulty with this question.

Reference
Chernecky, C., & Berger, B. (2008). *Laboratory tests and diagnostic procedures* (5th ed., pp. 210-214). Philadelphia: Saunders.

---

560. A nurse witnesses a client going into pulmonary edema. The client exhibits respiratory distress, but the blood pressure is stable at this time. While waiting for help to arrive, the nurse performs the following actions in which order of priority? (Number 1 is the first action.)
- ___Rechecks the vital signs
- ___Places the client in high Fowler's position
- ___Calls the respiratory therapy department for a ventilator
- ___Places the client on a pulse oximeter and cardiac monitor
- ___Begins the client's prn oxygen at 2 liters by nasal cannula
- ___Administers the client's prn morphine sulfate intravenous injection

Level of Cognitive Ability: Application
Client Needs: Physiological Integrity
Integrated Process: Nursing Process/ Implementation
Content Area: Delegating/Prioritizing

Answer: 4, 1, 6, 3, 2, 5
Rationale: The client in pulmonary edema is immediately placed in high Fowler's position and an oxygen delivery apparatus is applied. The nurse would also place the client on a pulse oximeter and a cardiac monitor to monitor cardiopulmonary status. The nurse would also monitor the client's vital signs closely. Next, the nurse would administer the client's prn morphine sulfate. Because a ventilator may or may not be needed, calling the respiratory therapy department would be the final action from the actions provided. Additional interventions include the administration of diuretics and insertion of a Foley catheter. The nurse should have delegated the task of notifying to the client's physician when signs of pulmonary edema were initially observed.

Test-Taking Strategy: Remember that in a respiratory emergency situation, client positioning may be the first action because it will alleviate dyspnea. Application of nasal mask or cannula will improve the client's available ambient oxygen supply. Next use the ABCs—airway, breathing, and circulation—to determine that placing the client on a pulse oximeter and cardiac monitor would be the next action. From the remaining options, if the client is stable, the nurse administers morphine sulfate as ordered. Recall that mechanical ventilation may or may not be needed. This recollection will assist in determining that rechecking the vital signs would precede requests for ventilation equipment. Review the immediate nursing actions for a client in pulmonary edema if you had difficulty with this question.

Reference
Ignatavicius, D., & Workman, M. (2006). *Medical-surgical nursing: Critical thinking for collaborative care* (5th ed., p. 761). Philadelphia: Saunders.

561. A physician's order reads: acetaminophen (Tylenol) liquid, 450 mg PO every 4 hours prn for pain. The medication label reads: 160 mg/5 mL. The nurse prepares how many milliliters to administer one dose?
Answer: _____ mL

Level of Cognitive Ability: Application
Client Needs: Physiological Integrity
Integrated Process: Nursing Process/Planning
Content Area: Fundamental Skills

Answer: 14
Rationale: Use the formula for calculating medication dosages.

Formula:
$$\frac{\text{Desired} \times \text{Volume}}{\text{Available}} = \text{mL per dose}$$

$$\frac{450 \text{ mg} \times 5 \text{ mL}}{160 \text{ mg}} = 14 \text{ mL}$$

Test-Taking Strategy: Identify the strategic components of the question and what the question is asking. In this case, the question asks for mL per dose. Set up the formula knowing that the desired dose is 450 mg and that what is available is 160 mg per 5 mL. Verify the answer using a calculator. Review medication calculations if you had difficulty with this question.

Reference
Kee, J., & Marshall, S. (2004). *Clinical calculations: With applications to general and specialty areas* (4th ed., pp. 80-81). Philadelphia: Saunders.

REFERENCES

Black, J., & Hawks, J. (2005). *Medical-surgical nursing: Clinical management for positive outcomes* (7th ed.). Philadelphia: Saunders.

Chernecky, C., & Berger, B. (2008). *Laboratory tests and diagnostic procedures* (5th ed.). Philadelphia: Saunders.

Gahart, B., & Nazareno, A. (2006). *2006 Intravenous medications* (22nd ed.). St. Louis: Mosby.

Grodner, M., Long, S., & DeYoung, S. (2004). *Foundations and clinical applications of nutrition: A nursing approach.* (3rd ed.). St. Louis: Mosby.

Gulanick, M., & Myers, J. (2007). *Nursing care plans: Nursing diagnosis and intervention* (6th ed.). St. Louis: Mosby.

Hockenberry, M., Wilson, D., & Winkelstein, M. (2005). *Wong's essentials of pediatric nursing* (7th ed.). St. Louis: Mosby.

Hockenberry, M., & Wilson, D. (2007). *Nursing care of infants and children* (8th ed.). St. Louis: Mosby.

Hodgson, B., & Kizior, R. (2007). *Saunders nursing drug handbook 2007.* Philadelphia: Saunders.

Ignatavicius, D., & Workman, M. (2006). *Medical-surgical nursing: Critical thinking for collaborative care* (5th ed.). Philadelphia: Saunders.

Jarvis, C. (2004). *Physical examination and health assessment* (4th ed.). Philadelphia: Saunders.

Kee, J., Hayes, E., & McCuistion, L. (2006). *Pharmacology: A nursing process approach.* (5th ed.). Philadelphia: Saunders.

Kee, J., & Marshall, S. (2004). *Clinical calculations: With applications to general and specialty areas* (5th ed.). Philadelphia: Saunders.

Lehne, R. (2007). *Pharmacology for nursing care* (6th ed.). Philadelphia: Saunders.

Lewis, S., Heitkemper, M., Dirksen, S., O'Brien, P., & Bucher, L. (2007). *Medical-surgical nursing: Assessment and management of clinical problems* (7th ed.). St. Louis: Mosby.

Lowdermilk, D., & Perry, A. (2006). *Maternity nursing* (7th ed.). St. Louis: Mosby.

McKenry, L., Tressier, E., & Hogan, M. (2006). *Mosby's pharmacology in nursing* (22nd ed.). St. Louis: Mosby.

McKinney, E., James, S., Murray, S., & Ashwill, J. (2005). *Maternal-child nursing* (2nd ed.). St. Louis: Saunders.

Meiner, S., & Leuckenotte, A. (2006). *Gerontologic nursing* (3rd ed.). St. Louis: Mosby.

Monahan, F., Sands, J., Neighbors, M., Marek, J., & Green, C. (2007). *Phipps' medical-surgical nursing: Health and illness perspectives* (8th ed.). St. Louis: Mosby.

Mosby. (2007). *Mosby's nursing drug reference* (20th ed.). St. Louis: Mosby.

Mosby's dictionary of medicine, nursing & health professions (2006). (7th ed.). St. Louis: Mosby.

Murray, S., & McKinney, E. (2006). *Foundations of maternal-newborn nursing* (4th ed.). Philadelphia: Saunders

Nix, S. (2005). *Williams' basic nutrition & diet therapy* (12th ed.). St. Louis: Mosby

Pagana, K., & Pagana, T. (2005). *Mosby's diagnostic and laboratory test reference* (7th ed.). St. Louis: Mosby.

Perry, A., & Potter, P. (2006). *Clinical nursing skills & techniques* (6th ed.). St. Louis: Mosby.

Potter, P., & Perry, A. (2005). *Fundamentals of nursing* (6th ed.). St. Louis: Mosby.

Skidmore-Roth, L. (2008). *Mosby's nursing drug reference* (21st ed.). St. Louis: Mosby.

Stuart, G., & Laraia, M. (2005). *Principles and practice of psychiatric nursing* (8th ed.). St. Louis: Mosby.

Varcarolis, E., Carson, V., & Shoemaker, N. (2006). *Foundations of psychiatric mental health nursing* (5th ed., p. 304). Philadelphia: Saunders.

Wilson, S., & Giddens, J. (2005). *Health assessment for nursing practice* (3rd ed.). St. Louis: Mosby.

Wong, D., Hockenberry, M., Perry, S., Lowdermilk, D., & Wilson, D. (2006). *Maternal-child nursing care.* (3rd ed.). St. Louis: Mosby.

Safe and Effective Care Environment

562. A client diagnosed with tuberculosis (TB) is scheduled to go to the radiology department for a chest x-ray study. Which nursing intervention would be appropriate when preparing to transport the client?
1 Apply a mask to the client.
2 Apply a mask and gown to the client.
3 Apply a mask, gown, and gloves to the client.
4 Notify the x-ray department so that the personnel can be sure to wear a mask when the client arrives.

Level of Cognitive Ability: Application
Client Needs: Safe and Effective Care Environment
Integrated Process: Nursing Process/ Implementation
Content Area: Fundamental Skills

Answer: 1
Rationale: Clients known or suspected of having TB should wear a mask when out of the hospital room to prevent the spread of the infection to others. A gown or gloves are not necessary.

Test-Taking Strategy: Use the process of elimination. Recalling that the route of transmission of TB is airborne will direct you to option 1. Review the transmission associated with TB if you had difficulty with this question.

References
Ignatavicius, D., & Workman, M. (2006). *Medical-surgical nursing: Critical thinking for collaborative care* (5th ed., pp. 644-645). Philadelphia: Saunders.
Potter, P., & Perry, A. (2005). *Fundamentals of nursing* (6th ed., pp. 788, 797). St. Louis: Mosby.

---

563. A registered nurse (RN) is planning the assignments for the day and is leading a team composed of a licensed practical nurse (LPN) and a nursing assistant (NA). The nurse assigns which client to the LPN?
1 Client with dementia
2 A 1-day postoperative mastectomy client
3 A client who requires some assistance with bathing
4 A client who requires some assistance with ambulation

Answer: 2
Rationale: Assignment of tasks needs to be implemented based on the job description of the LPN and NA, the level of education and clinical competence, and state law. The 1-day postoperative mastectomy client will need care that requires the skill of a licensed nurse. The nursing assistant has the skills to care for a client with dementia, a client who requires some assistance with bathing, and a client who requires some assistance with ambulation.

Test-Taking Strategy: Focus on the clients identified in the options and the job description and level of education of the LPN and NA. Think about the needs of each client to assist in determining the assignment. Remember that the LPN will be performing at a higher skill level than the NA. Review the principles associated with delegating and assignment making if you had difficulty with this question.

Level of Cognitive Ability: Application
Client Needs: Safe and Effective Care
 Environment
Integrated Process: Nursing Process/Planning
Content Area: Delegating/Prioritizing

Reference
Potter, P., & Perry, A. (2005). *Fundamentals of nursing* (6th ed., pp. 42, 378-379, 418). St. Louis: Mosby.

---

564. A client requests pain medication and the nurse administers a ventrogluteal intramuscular injection. After administration of the injection, the nurse does which of the following first?
1 Washes the hands
2 Removes the gloves
3 Applies gentle pressure to the injection site
4 Places the syringe in the secure, puncture-resistant needle box container

Level of Cognitive Ability: Application
Client Needs: Safe and Effective Care
 Environment
Integrated Process: Nursing Process/
 Implementation
Content Area: Delegating/Prioritizing

Answer: 3
Rationale: Following administration of an intramuscular injection, the nurse would apply gentle pressure to the site to assist in medication absorption and prevent bleeding. Then, the nurse assists the client to a comfortable position. The uncapped needle and syringe are discarded in a secure, puncture-resistant container, gloves are removed, and the hands are washed. Of the options provided, the nurse would perform option 3 first.

Test-Taking Strategy: Note the strategic word "first." Visualize the procedure and read each option to identify the first action. Review this procedure if you had difficulty with this question.

Reference
Potter, P., & Perry, A. (2005). *Fundamentals of nursing* (6th ed., p. 729). St. Louis: Mosby.

---

565. A nurse is in the process of giving a client a bed bath. In the middle of the procedure, the unit secretary calls the nurse on the intercom to tell the nurse that there is an emergency phone call. The appropriate nursing action is to:
1 Finish the bath before answering the phone call.
2 Immediately walk out of the client's room and answer the phone call.
3 Cover the client, place the call light within reach, and answer the phone call.
4 Leave the client's door open so the client can be monitored and the nurse can answer the phone call.

Level of Cognitive Ability: Application
Client Needs: Safe and Effective Care
 Environment
Integrated Process: Nursing Process/
 Implementation
Content Area: Fundamental Skills

Answer: 3
Rationale: Because the telephone call is an emergency, the nurse may need to answer it. The other appropriate action is to ask another nurse to accept the call. This, however, is not one of the options. To maintain privacy and safety, the nurse covers the client and places the call light within the client's reach. Additionally, the client's door should be closed or the room curtains pulled around the bathing area.

Test-Taking Strategy: Use the process of elimination. Noting the strategic words "emergency phone call" will assist in eliminating option 1. From the remaining options, recalling the rights of the client and the principles related to safety will direct you to option 3. Review these guidelines for care if you had difficulty with this question.

Reference
Potter, P., & Perry, A. (2005). *Fundamentals of nursing* (6th ed., p. 1030). St. Louis: Mosby.

566. A nurse manager is reviewing with the nursing staff the purposes for applying wrist and ankle restraints (security devices) to a client. The nurse manager determines that further review is necessary when a nursing staff member states that an indication for the use of a restraint is to:

1 Limit movement of a limb.
2 Keep the client in bed at night.
3 Prevent the violent client from injuring self and others.
4 Prevent the client from pulling out intravenous lines and catheters.

Level of Cognitive Ability: Application
Client Needs: Safe and Effective Care Environment
Integrated Process: Teaching and Learning
Content Area: Leadership/Management

Answer: 2
Rationale: Wrist and ankle restraints are devices used to limit the client's movement in situations when it is necessary to immobilize a limb. They are applied to prevent the client from injuring self or others; from pulling out intravenous lines, catheters, or tubes; or from removing dressings. Restraints also may be used to keep children still and from injuring themselves during treatments and diagnostic procedures. Restraints are not applied to keep a client in bed at night and should never be used as a form of punishment.

Test-Taking Strategy: Note the strategic words "further review is necessary." These words indicate a negative event query and the need to select the option that identifies an inaccurate use for restraints. Eliminate options 1 and 4 first because they are comparable or alike. From the remaining options, read each option carefully. Recalling the guidelines for the use of restraints will direct you to option 2. Review these guidelines if you had difficulty with this question.

References
Ignatavicius, D., & Workman, M. (2006). *Medical-surgical nursing: Critical thinking for collaborative care* (5th ed., pp. 44-55). Philadelphia: Saunders.
Potter, P., & Perry, A. (2005). *Fundamentals of nursing* (6th ed., pp. 411, 981). St. Louis: Mosby.

---

567. A client has an order to receive valproic acid (Depakene) 250 mg once daily. To maximize the client's safety, the nurse schedules administration of the medication:

1 With lunch
2 With breakfast
3 Before breakfast
4 At bedtime with a snack

Level of Cognitive Ability: Application
Client Needs: Safe and Effective Care Environment
Integrated Process: Nursing Process/ Implementation
Content Area: Pharmacology

Answer: 4
Rationale: Valproic acid is an anticonvulsant that causes central nervous system (CNS) depression. For this reason, the side effects include sedation, dizziness, ataxia, and confusion. When the client is taking this medication as a single daily dose, administering it at bedtime negates the risk of injury from sedation and enhances client safety. Otherwise, it may be given after meals to avoid gastrointestinal upset.

Test-Taking Strategy: Note the strategic words "to maximize the client's safety." Recalling that this medication is an anticonvulsant with CNS depressant properties and that sedation is a side effect will direct you to option 4. Administration at bedtime allows the sedative effects of the medication to occur at a time when the client is sleeping. Also note that options 1, 2, and 3 are comparable or alike in that they indicate administering the medication with meals. Review the side effects of this medication if you had difficulty with this question.

References
Hodgson, B., & Kizior, R. (2007). *Saunders nursing drug handbook 2007.* (p. 1193). Philadelphia: Saunders.
Lehne, R. (2007). *Pharmacology for nursing care.* (6th ed., p. 235) St. Louis: Saunders.

568. A hospitalized client with a diagnosis of anorexia nervosa and in a state of starvation is in a two-bed hospital room. A newly admitted client will be assigned to this client's room. Which client would be inappropriate to assign to this two-bed room?

1 A client with pneumonia
2 A client who can perform self-care
3 A client with a fractured leg that is casted
4 A client who is scheduled for a diagnostic test

Level of Cognitive Ability: Application
Client Needs: Safe and Effective Care Environment
Integrated Process: Nursing Process/ Implementation
Content Area: Leadership/Management

Answer: 1
Rationale: The client in a state of starvation has a compromised immune system. Having a roommate with pneumonia would place the client at risk for infection. Options 2, 3, and 4 are appropriate roommates.

Test-Taking Strategy: Note the client's diagnosis and the strategic words "in a state of starvation." Also note the strategic word "inappropriate." This strategic word indicates a negative event query and the need to select the client who should not be assigned to the room of the client with anorexia nervosa. Thinking about the physiological risks for this client will direct you to option 1. Review care of the client with anorexia nervosa if you had difficulty with this question.

References
Stuart, G., & Laraia, M. (2005). *Principles and practice of psychiatric nursing* (8th ed., p. 522). St. Louis: Mosby.
Varcarolis, E., Carson, V., & Shoemaker, N. (2006). *Foundations of psychiatric mental health nursing* (5th ed., p. 304). Philadelphia: Saunders.

---

569. A nurse has an order to obtain a sputum culture from a client admitted to the hospital with a diagnosis of pneumonia. The nurse avoids which action when obtaining the specimen?

1 Obtaining the specimen early in the morning
2 Having the client brush his teeth before expectoration
3 Instructing the client to take deep breaths before coughing
4 Placing the lid of the culture container face down on the bedside table

Level of Cognitive Ability: Application
Client Needs: Safe and Effective Care Environment
Integrated Process: Nursing Process/ Implementation
Content Area: Fundamental Skills

Answer: 4
Rationale: Placing the lid face down on the bedside table contaminates the lid and could result in inaccurate findings. The specimen is obtained early in the morning whenever possible, because increased amounts of sputum collect in the airways during sleep. The client should rinse the mouth or brush the teeth before specimen collection to avoid contaminating the specimen. The client should take deep breaths before expectoration for best sputum production.

Test-Taking Strategy: Use the process of elimination, noting the strategic word "avoids." This strategic word indicates a negative event query and the need to select the option that indicates an incorrect nursing action. Begin by eliminating options 1 and 3, which are helpful in obtaining a specimen of sufficient volume. From the remaining options, using the basic principles of aseptic technique will direct you to option 4. Review the procedure for sputum collection if you had difficulty with this question.

References
Black, J., & Hawks, J. (2005). *Medical-surgical nursing: Clinical management for positive outcomes* (7th ed., pp. 92-94). Philadelphia: Saunders.
Chernecky, C., & Berger, B. (2008). *Laboratory tests and diagnostic procedures* (5th ed., pp. 1034-1035). Philadelphia: Saunders.

570. A multidisciplinary health care team is planning care for a client with hyperparathyroidism. The nurse identifies which client outcome to the health care team?

1 Describes how to take antacids
2 Restricts fluids to 1000 mL per day
3 Describes how to take antidiarrheal medications
4 Walks down the hall for 15 minutes, three times a day

Level of Cognitive Ability: Analysis
Client Needs: Safe and Effective Care Environment
Integrated Process: Nursing Process/Planning
Content Area: Leadership/Management

Answer: 4
Rationale: Mobility of the client with hyperparathyroidism should be encouraged as much as possible because of the calcium imbalance that occurs in this disorder and the predisposition to the formation of renal calculi. Fluids should not be restricted. Options 1 and 3 are not specifically associated with this disorder.

Test-Taking Strategy: Use the process of elimination. Eliminate options 1 and 3 first because they are comparable or alike. From the remaining options, recalling that the client is predisposed to the formation of renal calculi will direct you to option 4. Review care of the client with hyperparathyroidism if you had difficulty with this question.

Reference
Black, J., & Hawks, J. (2005). *Medical-surgical nursing: Clinical management for positive outcomes* (7th ed., p. 1211). Philadelphia: Saunders.

---

571. A nurse has inserted a nasogastric tube (NG) into the stomach of a client and prepares to check for accurate tube placement. The nurse avoids which least reliable method for checking tube placement?

1 Measuring the pH of gastric aspirate
2 Placing the end of the tube in water to check for bubbling
3 Aspirating the tube with a 50-mL syringe to obtain gastric contents
4 Instilling 10 to 20 mL of air into the tube while auscultating over the stomach

Level of Cognitive Ability: Application
Client Needs: Safe and Effective Care Environment
Integrated Process: Nursing Process/ Implementation
Content Area: Fundamental Skills

Answer: 2
Rationale: The least reliable method for determining accurate placement of the NG tube is to place the end of the tube in water to observe for bubbling. Options 1, 3, and 4 are accurate methods to determine placement. The best method, however, is to verify placement by x-ray study.

Test-Taking Strategy: Use the process of elimination. Note the strategic words "avoids" and "least reliable." These words indicate a negative event query and the need to select the option that is an unreliable method. Visualize this procedure and focus on the subject, accurate tube placement, to direct you to option 2. Review this procedure if you had difficulty with this question.

Reference
Ignatavicius, D., & Workman, M. (2006). *Medical-surgical nursing: Critical thinking for collaborative care* (5th ed., p. 1297). Philadelphia: Saunders.

---

572. A nurse employed in a preschool agency is planning a staff education program to prevent the spread of an outbreak of an intestinal parasitic disease. The nurse includes which priority prevention measure in the educational session?

1 All food will be cooked before eating.
2 Only bottled water will be used for drinking.
3 All toileting areas will be cleansed daily with soap and water.
4 Staff will practice standard precautions when changing diapers and assisting children with toileting.

Answer: 4
Rationale: The fecal-oral route is the mode of transmission of an intestinal parasitic disease. Standard precautions prevent the transmission of infection. Cleaning with soap and water is not as effective as the use of bleach. Water and fresh foods can be vehicles for transmission, but municipal water sources are usually safe. Some fresh foods do not need to be cooked as long as they are washed well and weren't grown in soil contaminated with human feces.

Level of Cognitive Ability: Application
Client Needs: Safe and Effective Care Environment
Integrated Process: Teaching and Learning
Content Area: Child Health

Test-Taking Strategy: Focus on the subject—preventing the spread of infection. Option 4 addresses the subject of the question and is the umbrella option, addressing standard precautions. Also, note that options 1, 2, and 3 contain the close-ended words "all" and "only." Review measures that will prevent the spread of an intestinal parasitic infection if you had difficulty with this question.

References

Hockenberry, M., & Wilson, D. (2007). *Nursing care of infants and children* (8th ed., pp. 679, 698). St. Louis: Mosby.

McKinney, E., James, S., Murray, S., & Ashwill, J. (2005). *Maternal-child nursing* (2nd ed., p. 1039). St. Louis: Saunders.

---

573. A client has arrived at the labor and delivery unit in active labor. The nursing assessment reveals a history of recurrent genital herpes and the presence of lesions in the genital tract. The nurse plans to:

1 Prepare the client for a cesarean delivery.

2 Limit visitors and maintain reverse isolation.

3 Prepare the client for a spontaneous vaginal delivery.

4 Rupture the membranes artificially, looking for meconium-stained fluid.

Level of Cognitive Ability: Application
Client Needs: Safe and Effective Care Environment
Integrated Process: Nursing Process/Planning
Content Area: Maternity/Intrapartum

Answer: 1

Rationale: A cesarean delivery can reduce the risk of neonatal infection with a mother in labor who has herpetic genital tract lesions. Intact membranes provide another barrier to transmitting the disease to the neonate. There is no need to limit visitors or maintain isolation, although standard precautions should be maintained.

Test-Taking Strategy: Use the process of elimination, focusing on the subject—presence of genital herpes lesions. Eliminate options 3 and 4 first because they are comparable or alike and would place the neonate in contact with the lesions. From the remaining options, consider the risks to the neonate to direct you to option 1. Review care of the client in labor who has genital herpes lesions if you had difficulty with this question.

Reference

Wong, D., Hockenberry, M., Perry, S., Lowdermilk, D., & Wilson, D. (2006). *Maternal-child nursing care.* (3rd ed., p. 129). St. Louis: Mosby..

---

574. The nurse prepares to insert an indwelling Foley catheter into a client. To maintain the integrity of the Foley catheter and client safety, the nurse avoids:

1 Placing the drainage bag lower than the bladder level

2 Inflating the balloon with 4 to 5 mL beyond its capacity

3 Testing the balloon for patency before catheter insertion

4 Advancing the catheter after urine appears in the tubing

Level of Cognitive Ability: Application
Client Needs: Safe and Effective Care Environment
Integrated Process: Nursing Process/Implementation
Content Area: Fundamental Skills

Answer: 2

Rationale: The nurse risks rupturing the catheter's balloon by overinflating it; thus the nurse inflates the balloon with the specified volume for the catheter. Best practice is to test the patency of the balloon before insertion to verify its integrity and reduce the risk of infection. Advancing the catheter 1 to 2 inches beyond the point where the flow of urine is first noted is also good practice because this ensures that the catheter balloon is completely in the bladder before it is inflated. The drainage bag is placed lower than bladder level to ensure drainage, prevent retrograde flow of urine, and reduce the risk of infection.

Test-Taking Strategy: Note the strategic word "avoids." This word indicates the need to select the incorrect nursing action. Visualize the procedure to assist in answering the question. Noting the words "beyond its capacity" in option 2 will direct you to this option. Review this procedure if you had difficulty with this question.

Reference
Potter, P., & Perry, A. (2005). *Fundamentals of nursing* (6th ed., pp. 1348-1350). St. Louis: Mosby.

575. A moderately depressed client who was admitted to the mental health unit 2 days ago suddenly begins smiling and reporting that the crisis is over. The client says to the nurse, "Call the doctor. I'm finally cured." The nurse interprets this behavior as a cue to modify the treatment plan by:

1 Allowing off-unit privileges prn
2 Suggesting a reduction of medication
3 Allowing increased "in-room" activities
4 Increasing the level of suicide precautions

Level of Cognitive Ability: Analysis
Client Needs: Safe and Effective Care Environment
Integrated Process: Nursing Process/Planning
Content Area: Mental Health

Answer: 4
Rationale: A client who is moderately depressed and has only been hospitalized 2 days is unlikely to have such a dramatic cure. When a mood suddenly lifts, it is likely that the client may have made the decision to harm himself. Suicide precautions are necessary to keep the client safe.

Test-Taking Strategy: Use the process of elimination, focusing on the data in the question and recalling that depression does not resolve in 2 days. Options 1 and 2 support the client's notion that a cure has occurred. Option 3 allows the client to increase isolation. Recalling that safety is of the utmost importance will direct you to option 4. Review care of the client with depression if you had difficulty with this question.

Reference
Stuart, G., & Laraia, M. (2005). *Principles and practice of psychiatric nursing* (8th ed., p. 348). St. Louis: Mosby.

576. A nurse is planning care for a suicidal client. The nurse implements additional precautions at which of the following times?

1 During the day shift
2 On weekday evenings
3 Between 8 AM and 10 AM
4 During the unit shift change

Level of Cognitive Ability: Application
Client Needs: Safe and Effective Care Environment
Integrated Process: Nursing Process/Planning
Content Area: Mental Health

Answer: 4
Rationale: At shift change, there is often less availability of staff. The psychiatric nurse and staff should increase precautions for suicidal clients at that time. Weekends are also high-risk times, not weekdays. The night shift also presents a high-risk time.

Test-Taking Strategy: Use the process of elimination. Options 1, 2, and 3 are comparable or alike and can be eliminated. Remember that the nurse could anticipate that times with less supervision of the client could be times of increased risks. Review care of the suicidal client if you had difficulty with this question.

Reference
Varcarolis, E., Carson, V., & Shoemaker, N. (2006). *Foundations of psychiatric mental health nursing* (5th ed., pp. 481-482). Philadelphia: Saunders.

577. The nurse assists with the transfer of a female client from the operating room table to a stretcher. To maintain client safety, the nurse:

1 Checks wheel locks of the operating room table
2 Applies a safety belt to the client after the transfer
3 Completes the client transfer as quickly as possible
4 Tells the client to move herself from table to stretcher

Answer: 2
Rationale: As part of a safe transfer of a client after a surgical procedure, the nurse secures the client with a safety belt because safety belts can prevent the client from falling off the stretcher. This is important because the client is likely to be sedated and unable to protect herself from falling. In addition, the nurse checks both the wheel locks of the table and the stretcher to prevent any movement during the transfer. The personnel avoid hurried movements and rapid changes in position because hurried movements predispose the client to hypotension; besides, secure, deliberate movement increases the security of the client. Because the client remains affected by anesthesia, the client should not move herself.

Level of Cognitive Ability: Application
Client Needs: Safe and Effective Care
Environment
Integrated Process: Nursing Process/
Implementation
Content Area: Fundamental Skillsa

Test-Taking Strategy: Use the process of elimination and focus on the subject—safety. Options 1 and 3 are likely to increase the risk of client injury. Option 4 is unsuitable because of the residual effects of anesthesia. Review care of the postoperative client if you had difficulty with this question.

References
Ignatavicius, D., & Workman, M. (2006). *Medical-surgical nursing: Critical thinking for collaborative care* (5th ed., p. 321). Philadelphia: Saunders.
Potter, P., & Perry, A. (2005). *Fundamentals of nursing* (6th ed., pp. 1467, 1472, 1630). St. Louis: Mosby.

---

578. A nurse is planning care for a hallucinating and delusional client who has been rescued from a suicide attempt. The nurse plans to:
  1 Check the client's location every 15 minutes.
  2 Begin suicide precautions with 30-minute checks.
  3 Initiate one-to-one suicide precautions immediately.
  4 Ask the client to report suicidal thoughts immediately.

Level of Cognitive Ability: Application
Client Needs: Safe and Effective Care
Environment
Integrated Process: Nursing Process/Planning
Content Area: Mental Health

Answer: 3
Rationale: One-to-one suicide precautions are required for the client rescued from a suicide attempt. In this situation, additional key information is that the client is delusional and hallucinating. Both of these factors increase the risk of unpredictable behavior, decreased judgment, and the risk of suicide. Options 1, 2, and 4 do not provide the constant supervision necessary for this client.

Test-Taking Strategy: Use the process of elimination. Focusing on the data in question will direct you to option 3, the intervention that will provide the most supervision. Review suicide precautions if you had difficulty with this question.

References
Stuart, G., & Laraia, M. (2005). *Principles and practice of psychiatric nursing* (8th ed., p. 379). St. Louis: Mosby.
Varcarolis, E., Carson, V., & Shoemaker, N. (2006). *Foundations of psychiatric mental health nursing* (5th ed., p. 481). Philadelphia: Saunders.

---

579. A nurse is developing a plan of care for a client receiving anticoagulant agents. The nurse identifies which priority nursing diagnosis for the client?
  1 Risk for injury
  2 Risk for infection
  3 Deficient fluid volume
  4 Risk for activity intolerance

Level of Cognitive Ability: Analysis
Client Needs: Safe and Effective Care
Environment
Integrated Process: Nursing Process/Analysis
Content Area: Pharmacology

Answer: 1
Rationale: Anticoagulant therapy predisposes the client to injury because of the agent's inhibitory effects on the body's normal blood-clotting mechanism. Bruising, bleeding, and hemorrhage may occur in the course of activities of daily living and with other activities. Options 2, 3, and 4 are unrelated to this form of therapy.

Test-Taking Strategy: Use the process of elimination. Recalling that anticoagulants present a risk for bleeding will assist in directing you to option 1. Review the effects of anticoagulants if you had difficulty with this question.

References
Ignatavicius, D., & Workman, M. (2006). *Medical-surgical nursing: Critical thinking for collaborative care* (5th ed., p. 654). Philadelphia: Saunders.
Kee, J., Hayes, E., & McCuistion, L. (2006). *Pharmacology: A nursing process approach.* (5th ed., pp. 662, 666). Philadelphia: Saunders.

580. A client being seen in the emergency department with complaints of abdominal pain has a diagnosis of acute abdomen and the cause has not been determined. The nurse would question an order for which of the following at this time?
1 Clear liquid diet only
2 Insertion of a nasogastric tube
3 Insertion of an intravenous (IV) line
4 Administration of an analgesic, such as ketorolac tromethamine (Toradol)

Level of Cognitive Ability: Application
Client Needs: Safe and Effective Care Environment
Integrated Process: Nursing Process/ Implementation
Content Area: Adult Health/Gastrointestinal

Answer: 1
Rationale: Until the cause of the acute abdomen is determined and a decision about the need for surgery is made, the nurse would question an order to give a clear liquid diet. The nurse can expect the client to be placed on NPO status and to have an IV line inserted. Insertion of a nasogastric tube may be helpful to provide decompression of the stomach. Pain management with medications that do not alter level of consciousness (e.g., ketorolac tromthamine) can decrease diffuse abdominal pain and rigidity, help with localizing the pain, and lead to more prompt diagnosis and treatment.

Test-Taking Strategy: Note the strategic words "cause has not been determined" and "would question an order." Think about the client's diagnosis. Recalling that surgery may be a necessary intervention should direct you to option 1. Review interventions for the client with acute abdomen if you had difficulty with this question.

References
Ignatavicius, D., & Workman, M. (2006). *Medical-surgical nursing: Critical thinking for collaborative care* (5th ed., p. 1242). Philadelphia: Saunders.
Lewis, S., Heitkemper, M., Dirksen, S., O'Brien, P., & Bucher, L. (2007). *Medical-surgical nursing: Assessment and management of clinical problems* (7th ed., p. 1044). St. Louis: Mosby.

581. A woman identifying herself as a family friend telephones the home health nurse to inquire if there is anything she can do, as a friend, to assist her neighbors, the parents of a newborn with congenital tracheoesophageal fistula. The parents had expressed nervousness about giving enteral feedings. The best nursing action is to:
1 Inform the friend to directly contact the family and offer her assistance to them.
2 Report the friend's telephone call to the nurse manager for referral to the client's social worker.
3 Request that the friend come to the client's home, where she can be taught to administer the feedings.
4 Inform the friend that the family has no need for assistance because the nurse is making daily visits.

Level of Cognitive Ability: Application
Client Needs: Safe and Effective Care Environment
Integrated Process: Caring
Content Area: Leadership/Management

Answer: 1
Rationale: A nurse must uphold the client's rights and does not give any information regarding a client's care needs to anyone who is not directly involved in the client's care. To request that the friend come for teaching is a direct violation of the client's right to privacy. There is no information in the question to indicate that the family desires assistance from the friend. To refer the call to the nurse manager and social worker again assumes that the friend's assistance and involvement are desired by the family. Informing the friend that the nurse is visiting daily is providing information that is considered confidential. Option 1 directly refers the friend to the family.

Test-Taking Strategy: Use the process of elimination and focus on the subject, confidentiality and the client's right to privacy. Option 1 is the only option that upholds the client's rights. Review these rights if you had difficulty with this question.

References
Huber, D. (2006). *Leadership and nursing care management* (3rd ed., p. 745). Philadelphia: Saunders.
Potter, P., & Perry, A. (2005). *Fundamentals of nursing* (6th ed., pp. 391-392). St. Louis: Mosby.

582. The nurse has been assigned to care for a young man recovering at home from a disabling lung infection. While obtaining a nursing history, the nurse learns that the infection is probably the result of human immunodeficiency virus (HIV). The nurse informs the client that she is morally opposed to homosexuality and cannot care for him. The nurse then leaves the client's home. Which of the following is true regarding the nurse's actions?

  1 The nurse has a legal right to inform the client of any barriers to providing care.
  2 The nurse has the right to refuse to care for any client without justifying that refusal.
  3 The nurse has a duty to protect self from client care situations that are morally repellent.
  4 The nurse has a duty to provide competent care to assigned clients in a nondiscriminatory manner.

Level of Cognitive Ability: Analysis
Client Needs: Safe and Effective Care Environment
Integrated Process: Caring
Content Area: Adult Health/Immune

Answer: 4

Rationale: The nurse has a duty to provide care to all clients in a nondiscriminatory manner. Personal autonomy does not apply if it interferes with the rights of the client. There is no legal obligation to inform the client of the nurse's personal objections to the client. Refusal to provide care may be acceptable if that refusal does not put the client's safety at risk and the refusal is primarily associated with religious objections, not personal objection to lifestyle or medical diagnosis. The nurse also has an obligation to observe the principle of nonmaleficence (neither causing nor allowing harm to befall the client).

Test-Taking Strategy: Use the process of elimination, thinking about the client's rights and the nurse's ethical and legal responsibilities. Note the strategic words "provide competent care" and "nondiscriminatory" in the correct option. Review client rights if you had difficulty with this question.

Reference
Potter, P., & Perry, A. (2005). *Fundamentals of nursing* (6th ed., pp. 391). St. Louis: Mosby.

---

583. A nurse is preparing to administer heparin sodium 5000 units subcutaneously. The nurse takes which action to safely administer the medication?

  1 Injects via an infusion device
  2 Injects within 1 inch of the umbilicus
  3 Massages the injection site following administration
  4 Changes the needle on the syringe after withdrawing the medication from the vial

Level of Cognitive Ability: Application
Client Needs: Safe and Effective Care Environment
Integrated Process: Nursing Process/ Implementation
Content Area: Pharmacology

Answer: 4

Rationale: The injection site is located in the abdominal fat layer. It is not injected within 2 inches of the umbilicus or into any scar tissue. The needle is withdrawn rapidly, pressure is applied, and the area is not massaged. Injection sites are rotated. Heparin administered subcutaneously does not require an infusion device. After withdrawal of heparin from the vial, the needle is changed before injection to prevent leakage of medication along the needle tract.

Test-Taking Strategy: Use the process of elimination. Noting the strategic word "subcutaneously" will assist in eliminating option 1. From the remaining options, recall that heparin is an anticoagulant. This will assist in eliminating options 2 and 3. Review this procedure if you had difficulty with this question.

Reference
Hodgson, B., & Kizior, R. (2007). *Saunders nursing drug handbook 2007.* (p. 571). Philadelphia: Saunders.

584. A client asks the nurse to act as a witness for an advanced directive. Which is the best intervention for the nurse to implement?
1 Decline the client's request politely.
2 Agree to sign the document as a witness.
3 Help client find an unrelated third party.
4 Notify the provider of the client's request.

Level of Cognitive Ability: Application
Client Needs: Safe and Effective Care Environment
Integrated Process: Nursing Process/ Implementation
Content Area: Fundamental Skills

Answer: 3
Rationale: An advanced directive addresses the withdrawal or withholding of life-sustaining interventions that can prolong life and identifies the person who will make care decisions if the client becomes incompetent. Two people unrelated to the client witness the client's signature and then sign the document signifying that the client signed the advanced directive authentically. Nurses or employees of a facility in which the client is receiving care and beneficiaries of the client should not serve as a witness because of conflict of interest concerns. There is no reason to call the provider unless the absence of the advanced directive interferes with client care.

Test-Taking Strategy: Use the process of elimination. Eliminate option 1 because it demonstrates lack of client advocacy. Examine the remaining options and recall the nurse's role as a witness of a legal document. Review the concepts surrounding an advanced directive if you are unfamiliar with them.

References
Ignatavicius, D., & Workman, M. (2006). *Medical-surgical nursing: Critical thinking for collaborative care* (5th ed., p. 106). Philadelphia: Saunders.
Potter, P., & Perry, A. (2005). *Fundamentals of nursing* (6th ed., pp. 409-410). St. Louis: Mosby.

---

585. A home care nurse visits a 3-year-old child with chickenpox. The child's mother tells the nurse that the child keeps scratching the skin at night and asks the nurse what to do. The nurse tells the mother to:
1 Place soft cotton gloves on the child's hands at night.
2 Apply generous amounts of a cortisone cream to prevent itching.
3 Give the child a glass of warm milk at bedtime to help the child to sleep.
4 Keep the child in a warm room at night so the covers will not cause the child to scratch.

Level of Cognitive Ability: Application
Client Needs: Safe and Effective Care Environment
Integrated Process: Teaching and Learning
Content Area: Child Health

Answer: 1
Rationale: Gloves will keep the child from scratching the open lesions from chickenpox. Generous amounts of any topical cream can lead to drug toxicity. A warm room will increase the child's skin temperature and make itching worse. Warm milk will have no effect on itching.

Test-Taking Strategy: Use the process of elimination. Eliminate option 4 first because this action will promote scratching and itching. Option 3 should be eliminated next because it is unrelated to scratching. From the remaining options, the words "generous amounts" in option 2 should provide you with the clue that this option is incorrect. Review home care measures for the child with chickenpox if you had difficulty with this question.

Reference
Hockenberry, M., Wilson, D., & Winkelstein, M. (2005). *Wong's essentials of pediatric nursing* (7th ed., p. 437). St. Louis: Mosby.

586. An older client has been identified as a victim of physical abuse. In planning care, the nurse places highest priority on:

1 Adhering to federal mandatory abuse reporting laws
2 Obtaining treatment for the abusing family member
3 Notifying the case worker to intervene in the family situation
4 Removing the client from any situation that presents immediate danger

Level of Cognitive Ability: Application
Client Needs: Safe and Effective Care Environment
Integrated Process: Nursing Process/Planning
Content Area: Mental Health

Answer: 4
Rationale: The priority nursing intervention is to remove the abused victim from the abusive environment. Options 1, 2, and 3 may be appropriate interventions but are not the priority.

Test-Taking Strategy: Note the strategic words "highest priority." Use Maslow's Hierarchy of Needs theory, remembering that if a physiological need is not present, then safety is the priority. Option 4 is the only option that directly addresses client safety. Review care of the abused older client if you had difficulty with this question.

Reference
Varcarolis, E., Carson, V., & Shoemaker, N. (2006). *Foundations of psychiatric mental health nursing* (5th ed., pp. 512, 521). Philadelphia: Saunders.

---

587. A client diagnosed with leukemia asks the nurse questions about preparing a living will. The nurse informs the client that the best method of preparing this document is to:

1 Talk to the hospital chaplain.
2 Obtain advice from an attorney.
3 Discuss the request with the provider.
4 Consult the American Cancer Society.

Level of Cognitive Ability: Application
Client Needs: Safe and Effective Care Environment
Integrated Process: Nursing Process/ Implementation
Content Area: Fundamental Skills

Answer: 3
Rationale: Living wills are legal documents known as advanced directives wherein the client delineates the withdrawal or withholding of treatment when the client is incompetent; it should not be confused with a will that bequeaths personal property and specifies other actions at the time of the client's death. The client starts the process of writing a living will by discussing treatment options and other related issues with the provider. As well, the client should discuss this issue with the family. Although options 1 and 2 may be helpful, contacting them is not the initial step because both professionals lack the medical information the client needs to make an informed decision; however, the lawyer may be involved following discussion with the provider and family. The American Cancer Society may have pertinent information on living wills; however, the information is not individualized to the client's needs.

Test-Taking Strategy: Use the process of elimination and note the strategic words "best method of preparing." This indicates an initial step. Remembering that the provider is the primary care person will assist in directing you to the correct option. Contacts addressed in options 1, 2, and 4 may follow the discussion with the provider. Review the concepts related to living wills if you had difficulty with this question.

References
Ignatavicius, D., & Workman, M. (2006). *Medical-surgical nursing: Critical thinking for collaborative care* (5th ed., p. 106). Philadelphia: Saunders.
Potter, P., & Perry, A. (2005). *Fundamentals of nursing* (6th ed., pp. 409-410). St. Louis: Mosby.

588. A hospitalized client becomes disoriented frequently. Which should the nurse implement to ensure client safety at all times?
1 Request that the family hire a sitter.
2 Check in with the client frequently.
3 Position the call bell within easy reach.
4 Keep all side rails in the raised position at all times.

Level of Cognitive Ability: Application
Client Needs: Safe and Effective Care Environment
Integrated Process: Nursing Process/ Implementation
Content Area: Fundamental Skills

Answer: 2
Rationale: Checking in with the client provides the nurse with an opportunity to interact with the client for assessment, reorientation, and verification of client safety and is one of several strategies the nurse can employ before asking the family to hire a sitter. The nurse implements call bell positioning for every client to prevent reaching, but this does not help a client who is out of the room. If the disoriented client is unaware of the call bell, the nurse can remind the client before leaving the room. Keeping all side rails in the raised position at all times is not appropriate.

Test-Taking Strategy: Focus on the subject—safety. Eliminate option 1 because the nurse has other methods to try before approaching the family. Eliminate option 3 because this cannot ensure client safety if the disoriented client is unaware of the call bell or out of the room. Eliminate option 4, noting the close-ended word "all" in this option. Review basic safety measures for the disoriented client if you had difficulty with this question.

Reference
Potter, P., & Perry, A. (2005). *Fundamentals of nursing* (6th ed., p. 990). St. Louis: Mosby.

---

589. A client with a subarachnoid hemorrhage secondary to ruptured cerebral aneurysm has been placed on aneurysm precautions. To provide a safe environment, the nurse ensures that the client is provided with which of the following?
1 Bright lights
2 Enemas as needed
3 Television and radio
4 Daily stool softeners

Level of Cognitive Ability: Application
Client Needs: Safe and Effective Care Environment
Integrated Process: Nursing Process/ Implementation
Content Area: Adult Health/Neurological

Answer: 4
Rationale: Aneurysm precautions include a variety of measures designed to decrease stimuli that could increase the client's intracranial pressure. These include instituting dim lighting and reducing environmental noise and stimuli. Enemas should be avoided, but stool softeners should be provided. Straining at stool is contraindicated because it increases intracranial pressure.

Test-Taking Strategy: Focus on the client's diagnosis and the need to reduce environmental stimuli and prevent increased intracranial pressure. Options 1 and 3 can be eliminated first because these items will stimulate the client. From the remaining options, eliminate option 2 because administration of an enema will increase intracranial pressure. Review the nursing interventions for the client with aneurysm precautions if you had difficulty with this question.

Reference
Monahan, F., Sands, J., Neighbors, M., Marek, J., & Green, C. (2007). *Phipps' medical-surgical nursing: Health and illness perspectives* (8th ed., p. 1441). St. Louis: Mosby.

---

590. A nurse is about to administer an intravenous dose of tobramycin (Tobrex) when the client complains of vertigo and ringing in the ears. The nurse should:
1 Hold the dose and call the physician.
2 Check the client's pupillary responses.
3 Hang the dose of medication immediately.
4 Give a dose of droperidol (Inapsine) with the tobramycin.

Answer: 1
Rationale: Ringing in the ears and vertigo are two symptoms that may indicate dysfunction of the eighth cranial nerve. Ototoxicity is a toxic effect of therapy with aminoglycosides and could result in permanent hearing loss. The nurse should hold the dose and notify the physician. Options 2, 3, and 4 are incorrect nursing actions.

Level of Cognitive Ability: Application
Client Needs: Safe and Effective Care
   Environment
Integrated Process: Nursing Process/
   Implementation
Content Area: Pharmacology

Test-Taking Strategy: Focus on the client's complaints and recall that ototoxicity can occur with this medication. Recalling that the physician is notified if toxicity is suspected will direct you to option 1. Review the toxic effects of this medication if you had difficulty with this question.

Reference
Skidmore-Roth, L. (2008). *Mosby's nursing drug reference* (21st ed., p. 1007). St. Louis: Mosby.

---

591. A nurse is preparing to administer amiodarone (Cordarone) intravenously. To provide a safe environment, the nurse ensures that which specific item is in place for the client before administering the medication?
   1 Oxygen therapy
   2 Oxygen saturation monitor
   3 Continuous cardiac monitoring
   4 Noninvasive blood pressure cuff

Level of Cognitive Ability: Application
Client Needs: Safe and Effective Care
   Environment
Integrated Process: Nursing Process/
   Implementation
Content Area: Pharmacology

Answer: 3
Rationale: Amiodarone is an antidysrhythmic used to treat life-threatening ventricular dysrhythmias. The client should have continuous cardiac monitoring in place, and the medication should be infused by intravenous pump. Although options 1, 2, and 4 may be in place for the client, they are not specific items needed for the administration of this medication.

Test-Taking Strategy: Focus on the name of the medication. Recalling that this medication is an antidysrhythmic will direct you to option 3. Review the classification of this medication and the nursing considerations when administering this medication if you had difficulty with this question.

References
Gahart, B., & Nazareno, A. (2006). *2006 Intravenous medications* (22nd ed., p. 89). St. Louis: Mosby.
Skidmore-Roth, L. (2008). *Mosby's nursing drug reference* (21st ed., pp. 120-121) St. Louis: Mosby.

---

592. During the admission process of a male client who is admitted to the hospital for surgery to remove a tumor, the client asks the nurse if his living will, prepared 3 years ago, remains in effect. Which response should the nurse provide to the client?
   1 "Yes, a living will never expires."
   2 "You need to speak with an attorney."
   3 "It needs renewal yearly with your provider."
   4 "I will call someone to answer your question."

Level of Cognitive Ability: Application
Client Needs: Safe and Effective Care
   Environment
Integrated Process: Nursing Process/
   Implementation
Content Area: Fundamental Skills

Answer: 3
Rationale: The client discusses the living will with the provider annually to ensure that it contains the client's current wishes and desires based on his current health status. Option 1 is incorrect. Although the client consults an attorney if the living will needs to be changed, the accurate nursing response is to tell the client that a living will should be reviewed annually. Option 4 is not at all helpful to the client and is, in fact, a communication block.

Test-Taking Strategy: Use the process of elimination. Eliminate options 1 and 4 first because they are nontherapeutic, close-ended statements, and they place the client's question "on hold." From the remaining options, it is necessary to know that the document is reviewed annually. Review the concepts related to living wills if you had difficulty with this question.

References
Black, J., & Hawks, J. (2005). *Medical-surgical nursing: Clinical management for positive outcomes* (7th ed., p. 63). Philadelphia: Saunders.
Ignatavicius, D., & Workman, M. (2006). *Medical-surgical nursing: Critical thinking for collaborative care* (5th ed., p. 106). Philadelphia: Saunders.
Monahan, F., Sands, J., Neighbors, M., Marek, J., & Green, C. (2007). *Phipps' medical-surgical nursing: Health and illness perspectives* (8th ed., p. 241). St. Louis: Mosby.

593. The nurse reviews wound culture results and learns that an assigned client has methicillin-resistant *Staphylococcus aureus* (MRSA) in a wound bed. Which type of transmission-based precautions does the nurse institute for this client?
1 Enteric precautions
2 Droplet precautions
3 Contact precautions
4 Airborne precautions

Level of Cognitive Ability: Application
Client Needs: Safe and Effective Care Environment
Integrated Process: Nursing Process/ Implementation
Content Area: Fundamental Skills

Answer: 3
Rationale: Contact precautions include standard precautions and require the use of barrier precautions such as gloves and goggles. Contact precautions are used for clients who have diarrhea, draining wounds not contained by a sterile dressing, or methicillin-resistant infections. The goal of these precautions is to eliminate disease transmission resulting either from direct contact with the client or from indirect contact through inanimate objects or surfaces that the pathogen has contaminated, such as instruments, linens, dressing materials, or hands. Enteric precautions are initiated if the organism is transmitted via the gastrointestinal tract. Airborne and droplet precautions are used if the organism is transmitted via the respiratory tract.

Test-Taking Strategy: Focus on the client's diagnosis—MRSA that can be transmitted by contact with the infecting organism. Note the location of the pathogen to decide how its transmission can be prevented to assist in answering the question. Using the process of elimination, recall that "enteric" refers to the gastrointestinal tract and eliminate option 1. Eliminate options 2 and 4 because they are comparable or alike and unrelated to a wound bed. Review contact precautions if you had difficulty with this question.

Reference
Potter, P., & Perry, A. (2005). *Fundamentals of nursing* (6th ed., p. 797). St. Louis: Mosby.

594. The nurse is caring for a client immediately following a bronchoscopy. The client received intravenous sedation and a topical anesthetic for the procedure. In order to provide a safe environment for the client at this time, the nurse plans to:
1 Place a padded tongue blade at the bedside in case of a seizure.
2 Connect the client to a bedside ECG to monitor for dysrhythmias.
3 Place a water-seal chest drainage set at the bedside in case of a pneumothorax.
4 Check the bedside to ensure that no food or fluid is within the client's reach to prevent aspiration.

Level of Cognitive Ability: Application
Client Needs: Safe and Effective Care Environment
Integrated Process: Nursing Process/Planning
Content Area: Adult Health/Respiratory

Answer: 4
Rationale: Following this procedure, the client remains NPO until the cough and swallow reflexes have returned, which is usually in 1 to 2 hours. Once the client can swallow, oral intake may begin with ice chips and small sips of water. No information in the question suggests that the client is at risk for a seizure. Even though the client is monitored for signs of any distress, seizures would not be anticipated, and therefore a padded tongue blade would not be placed at the bedside. A pneumothorax is a possible complication of this procedure, and the nurse should monitor the client for signs of distress. However, a water-seal chest drainage set would not be placed routinely at the bedside. No data are given to support that the client is at increased risk for cardiac dysrhythmias.

Test-Taking Strategy: Note the strategic words "immediately following a bronchoscopy" and "topical anesthetic." Use the ABCs—airway, breathing, and circulation—to direct you to option 4. Review postprocedure care for this procedure if you had difficulty with this question.

References
Black, J., & Hawks, J. (2005). *Medical-surgical nursing: Clinical management for positive outcomes* (7th ed., pp. 1768-1769). Philadelphia: Saunders.
Chernecky, C., & Berger, B. (2008). *Laboratory tests and diagnostic procedures* (5th ed., pp. 262-263). Philadelphia: Saunders.

595. A client with a history of silicosis is admitted to the hospital with respiratory distress and impending respiratory failure. To ensure a safe environment, the nurse plans to have which of the following items readily available at the client's bedside?
1 Code cart
2 Intubation tray
3 Thoracentesis tray
4 Chest tube and drainage system

Level of Cognitive Ability: Application
Client Needs: Safe and Effective Care Environment
Integrated Process: Nursing Process/Planning
Content Area: Adult Health/Respiratory

Answer: 2
Rationale: The client with impending respiratory failure may need intubation and mechanical ventilation. The nurse ensures that an intubation tray is readily available. The other items are not needed at the client's bedside.

Test-Taking Strategy: Focus on the client's diagnosis. Use the ABCs—airway, breathing, and circulation—to direct you to option 2. Review care of the client with impending respiratory failure if you had difficulty with this question.

Reference
Ignatavicius, D., & Workman, M. (2006). *Medical-surgical nursing: Critical thinking for collaborative care* (5th ed., pp. 657, 660). Philadelphia: Saunders.

---

596. A nurse is preparing to administer a first dose of pentamidine isethionate (Pentam-300) intravenously to a client. Before administering the dose, the nurse should place the client:
1 In a private room
2 In a supine position
3 In semi-Fowler's position
4 On respiratory precautions

Level of Cognitive Ability: Application
Client Needs: Safe and Effective Care Environment
Integrated Process: Nursing Process/Implementation
Content Area: Pharmacology

Answer: 2
Rationale: Pentamidine isethionate can cause severe and sudden hypotension, even with administration of a single dose. The client should be lying down during administration of this medication. The blood pressure is monitored frequently during administration. Options 1 and 4 are unnecessary. Option 3 is incorrect.

Test-Taking Strategy: Use the process of elimination. Note that both options 2 and 3 address a client position. This indicates that one of these options may be correct. Recalling that the medication causes hypotension will direct you to option 2. Review the nursing considerations related to this medication if you had difficulty with this question.

Reference
Skidmore-Roth, L. (2008). *Mosby's nursing drug reference* (21st ed., pp. 799-800). St. Louis: Mosby.

---

597. A nurse is administering a dose of intravenous hydralazine (Apresoline) to a client. To provide a safe environment, the nurse ensures that which item is in place before injecting the medication?
1 Central line
2 Foley catheter
3 Cardiac monitor
4 Noninvasive blood pressure cuff

Level of Cognitive Ability: Application
Client Needs: Safe and Effective Care Environment
Integrated Process: Nursing Process/Implementation
Content Area: Pharmacology

Answer: 4
Rationale: Hydralazine is an antihypertensive medication used in the management of moderate to severe hypertension. The blood pressure and pulse should be monitored frequently after administration, so a noninvasive blood pressure cuff is the item to have in place. Options 1, 2, and 3 are not necessary.

Test-Taking Strategy: Focus on the name of the medication. The name of the medication "*Apresoline*" may provide you with the clue that the medication is used to lower the blood pressure. This will direct you to option 4. Review the action of this medication if you had difficulty with this question.

Reference
Skidmore-Roth, L. (2008). *Mosby's nursing drug reference* (21st ed., p. 529). St. Louis: Mosby.

598. A nurse is preparing to care for a client who has undergone left pneumonectomy. The nurse plans to do which of the following immediately after transfer from the postanesthesia care unit?
1 Position the client supine.
2 Position the client on the left side.
3 Assist the client to sit in the bedside chair.
4 Place the client's intravenous (IV) fluid on a pump.

Level of Cognitive Ability: Application
Client Needs: Safe and Effective Care Environment
Integrated Process: Nursing Process/Planning
Content Area: Adult Health/Respiratory

Answer: 4
Rationale: Following pneumonectomy, the fluid status of the client is monitored closely to prevent fluid overload, because the size of the pulmonary vascular bed has been reduced as a result of the pneumonectomy. Complete lateral turning and positioning are avoided. The head of the bed should be elevated to promote lung expansion. The client should remain on bed rest in the immediate postoperative period.

Test-Taking Strategy: Use the process of elimination. Eliminate options 1 and 2 first, because the client should not lie flat and because lateral positioning is avoided. Eliminate option 3 next, because the client should not be sitting in a chair immediately after a surgical procedure such as this. Review postoperative care following pneumonectomy if you had difficulty with this question.

Reference
Black, J., & Hawks, J. (2005). *Medical-surgical nursing: Clinical management for positive outcomes* (7th ed., p. 1859). Philadelphia: Saunders.

---

599. A client being seen in the emergency department is being evaluated for possible pleurisy. The nurse preparing the client for a chest x-ray plans to:
1 Scrub the client's chest with Betadine.
2 Determine if the client has any metallic implants.
3 Ask the client about the time of last food intake.
4 Ask the client to remove a neck chain being worn.

Level of Cognitive Ability: Application
Client Needs: Safe and Effective Care Environment
Integrated Process: Nursing Process/Planning
Content Area: Adult Health/Respiratory

Answer: 4
Rationale: If a chest x-ray is prescribed, jewelry or metal objects that might obstruct the x-ray need to be removed. Skin preparation is not required, and the client does not need to have food or fluid restricted before a chest x-ray. Notation of metallic implants is required before a magnetic resonance imaging (MRI), but an MRI is not used to diagnose pleurisy.

Test-Taking Strategy: Use the process of elimination, noting the diagnostic test addressed in the question. Focus on the anatomical area of the x-ray and recall the principles related to client preparation to direct you to option 4. Review this diagnostic test if you had difficulty with this question.

Reference
Chernecky, C., & Berger, B. (2008). *Laboratory tests and diagnostic procedures* (5th ed., pp. 328-329). Philadelphia: Saunders.

---

600. A nurse has administered diazepam (Valium) 5 mg intravenously (IV) to a client. To ensure safety, the nurse plans to maintain the client on bed rest for at least:
1 1 hour
2 3 hours
3 8 hours
4 30 minutes

Answer: 2
Rationale: The client should remain in bed for at least 3 hours following a parenteral dose of diazepam. The medication is a centrally acting skeletal muscle relaxant and has antianxiety, sedative-hypnotic, and anticonvulsant properties. Cardiopulmonary side effects include apnea, hypotension, bradycardia, or cardiac arrest. For this reason, resuscitative equipment is also kept nearby.

Test-Taking Strategy: Think about the effects of diazepam administered intravenously to answer this question. Options 1 and 4 can be eliminated first because of the short time frames. From the remaining options, eliminate option 3 because of the lengthy time frame. Review the nursing considerations related to the administration of this medication if you had difficulty with this question.

Level of Cognitive Ability: Application
Client Needs: Safe and Effective Care
 Environment
Integrated Process: Nursing Process/Planning
Content Area: Pharmacology

References
Gahart, B., & Nazareno, A. (2006). *2006 Intravenous medications* (22nd ed., p. 395). St. Louis: Mosby.
Skidmore-Roth, L. (2008). *Mosby's nursing drug reference* (21st ed., p. 355). St. Louis: Mosby.

---

601. A nurse is caring for a hospitalized client who is having a prescribed dosage of clonazepam (Klonopin) adjusted. Because of the adjustment in the medication that is being made, the nurse plans to:
 1 Weigh the client daily.
 2 Observe for ecchymoses.
 3 Institute seizure precautions.
 4 Monitor blood glucose levels.

Level of Cognitive Ability: Application
Client Needs: Safe and Effective Care
 Environment
Integrated Process: Nursing Process/Planning
Content Area: Pharmacology

Answer: 3
Rationale: Clonazepam is a benzodiazepine that is used as an anticonvulsant. During initial therapy and during periods of dosage adjustment, the nurse should initiate seizure precautions for the client. Options 1, 2, and 4 are unrelated to the use of this medication.

Test-Taking Strategy: Focus on the name of the medication. Recalling that this medication is an anticonvulsant will direct you to option 3. Review the nursing considerations related to this medication if you had difficulty with this question.

Reference
Skidmore-Roth, L. (2008). *Mosby's nursing drug reference* (21st ed., p. 288). St. Louis: Mosby.

---

602. The nurse is planning to obtain an arterial blood gas (ABG) from a client with chronic obstructive pulmonary disease (COPD). To prevent bleeding following the procedure, the nurse plans time for which activity after the arterial blood is drawn?
 1 Holding a warm compress over the puncture site for 5 minutes
 2 Encouraging the client to open and close the hand rapidly for 2 minutes
 3 Applying pressure to the puncture site by applying a 2 × 2 gauze for 5 minutes
 4 Having the client keep the radial pulse puncture site in a dependent position for 5 minutes

Level of Cognitive Ability: Application
Client Needs: Safe and Effective Care
 Environment
Integrated Process: Nursing Process/Planning
Content Area: Adult Health/Respiratory

Answer: 3
Rationale: Applying pressure over the puncture site for 5 to 10 minutes reduces the risk of hematoma formation and damage to the artery. A cold compress would aid in limiting blood flow; a warm compress would increase blood flow. Keeping the extremity still and out of a dependent position will aid in the formation of a clot at the puncture site.

Test-Taking Strategy: Use the process of elimination. Focus on the subject, preventing bleeding. Eliminate options 1, 2, and 4 because they promote bleeding. Option 3 aids in the prevention of bleeding into the surrounding tissues. Review nursing responsibilities following ABGs if you had difficulty with this question.

Reference
Chernecky, C., & Berger, B. (2008). *Laboratory tests and diagnostic procedures* (5th ed., pp. 210-214). Philadelphia: Saunders.

603. The nurse is admitting to the nursing unit a client who has an arteriovenous (AV) fistula in the right arm for hemodialysis. The nurse plans to best prevent injury to the site by implementing which of the following?

1 Applying an allergy bracelet to the right arm
2 Putting a large note about the access site on the front of the medical record
3 Telling the client to inform all caregivers who enter the room about the presence of the access site
4 Placing a sign at the bedside that says "No blood pressure (BP) measurements or venipunctures in the right arm"

Level of Cognitive Ability: Application
Client Needs: Safe and Effective Care Environment
Integrated Process: Nursing Process/Planning
Content Area: Adult Health/Renal

Answer: 4
Rationale: There should be no venipunctures or blood pressure measurements in the extremity with a hemodialysis access device. This is commonly communicated to all caregivers by placing a sign at the client's bedside. Placing a note on the front of the medical record does not ensure that everyone caring for the client is aware of the access device. An allergy bracelet is placed on the client with an allergy. Some health care agencies, however, do have policies that require application of a wrist bracelet of some type to be placed on the client with a hemodialysis access device. The client should not be responsible for informing the caregivers.

Test-Taking Strategy: Use the process of elimination, noting the strategic word "best." Eliminate option 1 because an allergy bracelet is used for a client with an allergy. Eliminate option 3 next because this responsibility should not be placed on the client. From the remaining options, note that option 4 best informs those caring for the client of the presence of the fistula. Review care of the client with an AV fistula if you had difficulty with this question.

Reference
Ignatavicius, D., & Workman, M. (2006). *Medical-surgical nursing: Critical thinking for collaborative care* (5th ed., p. 1754). Philadelphia: Saunders.

604. Regular insulin by continuous intravenous (IV) infusion is prescribed for a client with a blood glucose level of 700 mg/dL. The nurse plans to:

1 Mix the solution in 5% dextrose.
2 Change the solution every 6 hours.
3 Infuse the medication via an electronic infusion pump.
4 Titrate the infusion according to the client's urine glucose levels.

Level of Cognitive Ability: Application
Client Needs: Safe and Effective Care Environment
Integrated Process: Nursing Process/Planning
Content Area: Adult Health/Endocrine

Answer: 3
Rationale: Insulin is administered via an infusion pump to prevent inadvertent overdose and subsequent hypoglycemia. There is no reason to change the solution every 6 hours. Dextrose is added to the IV infusion once the serum glucose level reaches 250 mg/dL to prevent the occurrence of hypoglycemia. Administering dextrose to a client with a serum glucose level of 700 mg/dL would counteract the beneficial effects of insulin in reducing the glucose level. Glycosuria is not a reliable indicator of the actual serum glucose levels because many factors affect the renal threshold for glucose loss in the urine.

Test-Taking Strategy: Use the process of elimination. Eliminate option 4, knowing that urine glucose levels do not provide an accurate indication of the client's status. Next, eliminate option 1, knowing that dextrose would not be administered to a client with a blood glucose of 700 mg/dL. From the remaining options, recalling the complications associated with a continuous infusion of insulin will direct you to option 3. Review nursing care of a client with a continuous IV infusion of insulin if you had difficulty with this question.

References
Black, J., & Hawks, J. (2005). *Medical-surgical nursing: Clinical management for positive outcomes* (7th ed., pp. 1255-1256). Philadelphia: Saunders.
Ignatavicius, D., & Workman, M. (2006). *Medical-surgical nursing: Critical thinking for collaborative care* (5th ed., p. 1521). Philadelphia: Saunders.

605. The nurse is developing a plan of care for a client with diabetic ketoacidosis (DKA). The nurse includes which intervention in the plan?
1 Assess for fluid overload.
2 Limit family visitation time.
3 Ambulate the client every 2 hours.
4 Maintain side rails in the upright position.

Level of Cognitive Ability: Application
Client Needs: Safe and Effective Care Environment
Integrated Process: Nursing Process/Planning
Content Area: Adult Health/Endocrine

Answer: 4
Rationale: The client with DKA may experience a decrease in the level of consciousness (LOC) secondary to acidosis. Safety becomes a priority for any client with a decreased LOC, thus requiring the use of side rails to prevent fall injuries. The client will experience fluid loss (dehydration) rather than overload and may be too ill to ambulate. Family visitation is helpful for both the client and family to assist with psychosocial adaptation.

Test-Taking Strategy: Focus on the client's diagnosis to eliminate options 2 and 3. From the remaining options, recalling that dehydration is an issue in DKA and that mental status changes occur will direct you to option 4. Review care of the client with DKA if you had difficulty with this question.

References
Black, J., & Hawks, J. (2005). *Medical-surgical nursing: Clinical management for positive outcomes* (7th ed., p. 1269). Philadelphia: Saunders.
Lewis, S., Heitkemper, M., Dirksen, S., O'Brien, P., & Bucher, L. (2007). *Medical-surgical nursing: Assessment and management of clinical problems* (7th ed., p. 1280). St. Louis: Mosby.

606. A clinic nurse wants to develop a diabetic teaching program. In order to meet the clients' needs, the nurse must first:
1 Assess the clients' functional abilities.
2 Ensure that insurance will pay for participation in the program.
3 Discuss the focus of the program with the multidisciplinary team.
4 Include everyone who comes into the clinic in the teaching sessions.

Level of Cognitive Ability: Application
Client Needs: Safe and Effective Care Environment
Integrated Process: Teaching and Learning
Content Area: Leadership/Management

Answer: 1
Rationale: Nurse-managed clinics focus on individualized disease prevention and health promotion and maintenance. Therefore the nurse must first assess the clients and their needs in order to effectively plan the program. Options 2, 3, and 4 do not address the clients' needs.

Test-Taking Strategy: Use the process of elimination and the steps of the nursing process. Remember that the first step is assessment. Option 1 reflects assessment. Review teaching and learning principles if you had difficulty with this question.

References
Ignatavicius, D., & Workman, M. (2006). *Medical-surgical nursing: Critical thinking for collaborative care* (5th ed., p. 8). Philadelphia: Saunders.
Potter, P., & Perry, A. (2005). *Fundamentals of nursing* (6th ed., pp. 451-454). St. Louis: Mosby.

607. A nurse notes that a postoperative client has not been obtaining relief from pain with the prescribed opioid analgesics when a particular licensed practical nurse (LPN) is assigned to the client. The appropriate action for the nurse to take is to:

1 Reassign the LPN to the care of clients not receiving opioids.
2 Notify the physician that the client needs an increase in opioid dosage.
3 Review the client's medication administration record immediately and discuss the observations with the nursing supervisor.
4 Confront the LPN with the information about the client having pain control problems and ask if the LPN is using the opioids personally.

Level of Cognitive Ability: Application
Client Needs: Safe and Effective Care Environment
Integrated Process: Nursing Process/ Implementation
Content Area: Leadership/Management

Answer: 3
Rationale: In this situation, the nurse has noted an unusual occurrence, but before deciding what action to take next, the nurse needs more data than just suspicion. This can be obtained by reviewing the client's record. State and federal labor and opioid regulations, as well as institutional policies and procedures, must be followed. It is therefore most appropriate that the nurse discuss the situation with the nursing supervisor before taking further action. The client does not need an increase in opioids. To reassign the LPN to clients not receiving opioids ignores the issue. A confrontation is not the most advisable action because it could result in an argumentative situation.

Test-Taking Strategy: Use the process of elimination and knowledge regarding the roles and responsibilities of the nurse and the organizational channels of communication. Option 3 is the only option that includes consultation with an authority figure, the nursing supervisor. Review the nurse's role when substance abuse in another nurse is suspected if you had difficulty with this question.

Reference
Ignatavicius, D., & Workman, M. (2006). *Medical-surgical nursing: Critical thinking for collaborative care* (5th ed., p. 93). Philadelphia: Saunders.

---

608. A medication nurse is supervising a newly hired licensed practical nurse (LPN) during the administration of oral pyridostigmine bromide (Mestinon) to a client with myasthenia gravis. Which observation by the medication nurse would indicate safe practice by the LPN?

1 Asking the client to take sips of water
2 Asking the client to lie down on his right side
3 Asking the client to look up at the ceiling for 30 seconds
4 Instructing the client to void before taking the medication

Level of Cognitive Ability: Analysis
Client Needs: Safe and Effective Care Environment
Integrated Process: Nursing Process/Evaluation
Content Area: Leadership/Management

Answer: 1
Rationale: Myasthenia gravis can affect the client's ability to swallow. The primary assessment is to determine the client's ability to handle oral medications or any oral substance. Options 2 and 3 are not appropriate. Option 2 could result in aspiration, and option 3 has no useful purpose. There is no specific reason for the client to void before taking this medication.

Test-Taking Strategy: Use the process of elimination. Recalling that myasthenia gravis affects the client's ability to swallow will direct you to option 1. Also, note the relation between the words "oral" in the question and "sips of water" in the correct option. Review nursing care of the client with myasthenia gravis if you had difficulty with this question.

Reference
Ignatavicius, D., & Workman, M. (2006). *Medical-surgical nursing: Critical thinking for collaborative care* (5th ed., p. 1013). Philadelphia: Saunders.

609. The nurse does not act when a client becomes hypotensive after surgery. The client requires emergency surgery to stop postoperative bleeding later that night. Which type of prosecution does the nurse potentially face for failing to act?
1 Feloney
2 Tort law
3 Statutory law
4 Misdemeanor

Level of Cognitive Ability: Analysis
Client Needs: Safe and Effective Care Environment
Integrated Process: Nursing Process/Analysis
Content Area: Fundamental Skills

Answer: 2
Rationale: Tort law deals with wrongful acts intentionally or unintentionally committed against a person or the person's property. The nurse commits a tort offense by failing to act when the client became hypotensive. Options 1 and 4 are offenses under criminal law. Option 3 describes laws enacted by state, federal, or local governments.

Test-Taking Strategy: Focus on the data in the question and the definition of the terms in the options. Recalling that a tort is a wrongful act will direct you to option 2. Review the definitions related to the various types of laws if you had difficulty with this question.

References
Huber, D. (2006). *Leadership and nursing care management* (3rd ed., p. 735). Philadelphia: Saunders.
Potter, P., & Perry, A. (2005). *Fundamentals of nursing* (6th ed., pp. 413-414). St. Louis: Mosby.

---

610. A well-known individual from the community is admitted to the hospital with a diagnosis of Parkinson's disease. The nurse gives medical information regarding the client's condition to a person who is assumed to be a family member. Later, the nurse discovers that this person is not a family member and realizes that she has violated which legal concept of the nurse-client relationship?
1 Client's right to privacy
2 Nurse's lack of experience
3 Teaching and learning principles
4 Performing focused physical assessment

Level of Cognitive Ability: Comprehension
Client Need: Safe and Effective Care Environment
Integrated Process: Nursing Process/ Implementation
Content Area: Adult Health/Neurological

Answer: 1
Rationale: Discussing a client's condition without client permission violates a client's rights and places the nurse in legal jeopardy. This action by the nurse is both an invasion of privacy and affects the confidentiality issue with client rights. Options 2, 3, and 4 do not represent violation of the situation presented.

Test-Taking Strategy: Focus on the information in the question. The subject of the question is related to sharing information, which constitutes an invasion of privacy. Review client rights and the situations that involve invasion of privacy if you had difficulty with this question.

Reference
Potter, P., & Perry, A. (2005). *Fundamentals of nursing* (6th ed., pp. 413-414). St. Louis: Mosby.

---

611. The clinic nurse is assessing a client for environmental risk factors related to neurological disorders. The nurse understands that which of the following is least likely associated with neurological disorders?
1 Exposure to pesticides
2 Ventilation in the work area
3 Number of windows in the work area
4 Exposure to fumes, such as paints or bonding agents (glue)

Answer: 3
Rationale: The nurse would assess for the risk of exposure to neurotoxic fumes and chemicals. These could include paint, bonding agents, pesticides, and many more substances. The nurse also inquires about the adequacy of ventilation in the home and work area. Many work spaces (e.g., factories, insurance companies, and operating rooms) are adequately ventilated without the use of windows.

Level of Cognitive Ability: Analysis
Client Needs: Safe and Effective Care Environment
Integrated Process: Nursing Process/Assessment
Content Area: Adult Health/Neurological

Test-Taking Strategy: Note the strategic words "least likely." Focusing on the subject—environmental risk factors—will direct you to option 3. Review environmental risk factors associated with neurological disorders if you had difficulty with this question.

References
Black, J., & Hawks, J. (2005). *Medical-surgical nursing: Clinical management for positive outcomes* (7th ed., pp. 13-15). Philadelphia: Saunders.
Ignatavicius, D., & Workman, M. (2006). *Medical-surgical nursing: Critical thinking for collaborative care* (5th ed., p. 473). Philadelphia: Saunders.
Monahan, F., Sands, J., Neighbors, M., Marek, J., & Green, C. (2007). *Phipps' medical-surgical nursing: Health and illness perspectives* (8th ed., pp. 515-516). St. Louis: Mosby.

---

612. A nurse performing an initial admission assessment notes that a client has been taking metoclopramide (Reglan) for a prolonged period. The nurse would immediately call the physician if which signs or symptoms were then noted by the nurse?
1 Anxiety or irritability
2 Excessive drowsiness
3 Uncontrolled rhythmic movements of the face or limbs
4 Dry mouth relieved with the use of sugar-free hard candy

Level of Cognitive Ability: Analysis
Client Needs: Safe and Effective Care Environment
Integrated Process: Communication and Documentation
Content Area: Pharmacology

Answer: 3
Rationale: If the client experiences tardive dyskinesia (rhythmic movements of the face or limbs), the nurse should call the physician because these side effects may be irreversible. The medication would be discontinued, and no further doses should be given by the nurse. Anxiety, irritability, and dry mouth are mild side effects that do not harm the client.

Test-Taking Strategy: Note that the question contains the strategic word "immediately," which guides you to select the most harmful option. Recalling that this medication causes tardive dyskinesia will direct you to option 3. Review the side effects of this medication and the signs of tardive dyskinesia if you had difficulty with this question.

References
Hodgson, B., & Kizior, R. (2007). *Saunders nursing drug handbook 2007* (p. 762). Philadelphia: Saunders.
Kee, J., Hayes, E., & McCuistion, L. (2006). *Pharmacology: A nursing process approach.* (5th ed., pp. 690-691). Philadelphia: Saunders.

---

613. The nurse is outside of a client's room and hears the provider tell the client that the nurse "doesn't know anything" in a derogatory manner. Which legal tort has the provider violated?
1 Libel
2 Battery
3 Assault
4 Slander

Level of Cognitive Ability: Analysis
Client Needs: Safe and Effective Care Environment
Integrated Process: Nursing Process/Analysis
Content Area: Fundamental Skills

Answer: 4
Rationale: Defamation takes place when a falsehood is said (slander) or written (libel) about a person that results in injury to that person's good name and reputation. An assault occurs when a person puts another person in fear of a harmful or offensive act. Battery involves offensive touching or the use of force by a perpetrator without the permission of the victim.

Test-Taking Strategy: Use the process of elimination and eliminate options 2 and 3 first because the nurse was neither threatened nor touched. From the remaining options, recall that slander constitutes verbal defamation to direct you to option 4. Review the torts identified in each option if you had difficulty with this question.

Reference
Potter, P., & Perry, A. (2005). *Fundamentals of nursing* (6th ed., p. 414). St. Louis: Mosby.

614. The nurse finds the client sitting on the floor, ensures the client's safety, completes an incident report, and notifies the provider of the incident. Which does the nurse implement next?

  1 Staple the incident report in the client's medical record.
  2 Document the client events and follow-up nursing actions.
  3 Provide a copy of the incident report to the provider and family.
  4 Document in the client's medical record that the nurse sent a copy of the report to risk management.

Level of Cognitive Ability: Application
Client Needs: Safe and Effective Care Environment
Integrated Process: Communication and Documentation
Content Area: Fundamental Skills

Answer: 2
Rationale: The nurse documents the incident completely and objectively in the client's record to communicate client data to the health care team. The incident report is a confidential, privileged, and internal document used to improve client safety and quality of care and, therefore, should not be copied, stapled, or placed in the chart. Furthermore, the nurse avoids referring to the incident report in the client's record, such as recording that the incident report has been sent to another department. These actions are necessary because any mention of an incident report in the medical record allows the plaintiff's attorney access to the document through discovery.

Test-Taking Strategy: Use the process of elimination and eliminate options 1 and 4 first because incident reports are neither stapled nor referred to in the medical record. From the remaining options, recall that an incident report is an internal, confidential document, is not intended for the family, and is never copied, to eliminate option 3. Review nursing responsibilities related to incident reports if you had difficulty with this question.

Reference
Potter, P., & Perry, A. (2005). *Fundamentals of nursing* (6th ed., pp. 419, 497) St. Louis: Mosby.

---

615. A client had a colon resection. A nasogastric tube was in place when a regular diet was brought to the client's room. The client did not want to eat solid food and asked that the physician be called. The nurse insisted that the solid food was the correct diet. The client ate and subsequently had additional surgery as a result of complications. The determination of negligence in this situation is based on:

  1 The nurse's persistence
  2 Not calling the physician
  3 A duty existed and it was breached
  4 The dietary department sending the wrong food

Level of Cognitive Ability: Analysis
Client Needs: Safe and Effective Care Environment
Integrated Process: Nursing Process/Analysis
Content Area: Fundamental Skills

Answer: 3
Rationale: For negligence to be proven, there must be a duty, and then a breach of duty; the breach of duty must cause the injury, and damages or injury must be experienced. Options 1, 2, and 4 do not fall under the criteria for negligence. Option 3 is the only option that fits the criteria of negligence.

Test-Taking Strategy: Use the process of elimination. Options 1, 2, and 4 do not directly support the subject of negligence because it would be difficult to determine that these elements caused injury. The focus relates to what the nurse is responsible for. Option 3 is an umbrella response to the question. Review the legal elements of nursing practice and criteria for negligence if you had difficulty with this question.

Reference
Potter, P., & Perry, A. (2005). *Fundamentals of nursing* (6th ed., p. 414). St. Louis: Mosby.

616. A nurse is caring for a child with intussusception. During care, the child passes a normal brown stool. The appropriate nursing action is to:

1 Note the child's physical symptoms.
2 Prepare the child for hydrostatic reduction.
3 Prepare the child and parents for the possibility of surgery.
4 Report the passage of a normal brown stool to the physician.

Level of Cognitive Ability: Application
Client Needs: Safe and Effective Care Environment
Integrated Process: Nursing Process/ Implementation
Content Area: Child Health

Answer: 4
Rationale: Passage of a normal brown stool usually indicates that the intussusception has reduced itself. This is immediately reported to the physician, who may choose to alter the diagnostic or therapeutic plan of care. Hydrostatic reduction and surgery may not be necessary. Although the nurse would note the child's physical symptoms, based on the data in the question, option 4 is the appropriate action.

Test-Taking Strategy: Use the process of elimination. Note the similarity between the information in the question and the correct option. Also, recalling the physiology associated with intussusception will direct you to option 4. Review care of the child with intussusception if you had difficulty with this question.

Reference
Hockenberry, M., & Wilson, D. (2007). *Nursing care of infants and children* (8th ed., pp. 882-883). St. Louis: Mosby.

---

617. During orientation, a graduate nurse learns that the nursing model of practice implemented in the facility is a primary nursing approach. When the nurse attends report on the medical unit, the nurse will verify with the staff which of the following characteristics of primary nursing?

1 Critical paths are used when providing client care.
2 The nurse manager assigns tasks to the staff members.
3 A registered nurse (RN) leads nursing staff in giving care to a group of clients.
4 A single RN is responsible for planning and providing individualized nursing care to clients.

Level of Cognitive Ability: Comprehension
Client Needs: Safe and Effective Care Environment
Integrated Process: Nursing Process/ Implementation
Content Area: Leadership/Management

Answer: 4
Rationale: Primary nursing is concerned with keeping the nurse at the bedside actively involved in direct care while planning goal-directed, individualized client care. Option 1 identifies a component of case management. Option 2 identifies functional nursing. Option 3 identifies team nursing.

Test-Taking Strategy: Note that the focus of the question relates to primary nursing. Keep this subject in mind and use the process of elimination. Option 4 is the only option that identifies the primary nursing approach. Review the various types of nursing delivery systems if you had difficulty with this question.

References
Huber, D. (2006). *Leadership and nursing care management* (3rd ed., pp. 569-570). Philadelphia: Saunders.
Potter, P., & Perry, A. (2005). *Fundamentals of nursing* (6th ed., p. 373). St. Louis: Mosby.

---

618. A client asks the nurse how to become an organ donor. Which does the nurse include in client teaching?

1 The client can donate with written consent.
2 A family member must witness the consent.
3 The donor must be older than 21 years of age.
4 A family member must be present when a client consents to organ donation.

Answer: 1
Rationale: The client has the right to donate her or his own organs for transplantation, and any person who is 18 years of age or older may become an organ donor by written consent without the permission or presence of the family. In the absence of suitable documentation, a family member or legal guardian can authorize donation of the decedent's organs.

Level of Cognitive Ability: Application
Client Needs: Safe and Effective Care Environment
Integrated Process: Nursing Process/Evaluation
Content Area: Fundamental Skills

Test-Taking Strategy: Use the process of elimination and focus on the issues related to client rights. This will direct you to option 1. Review the procedure for organ donation if you had difficulty with this question.

References
Lynch, V., & Duval, J. (2006). *Forensic nursing* (pp. 220-222). St. Louis: Mosby.
Potter, P., & Perry, A. (2005). *Fundamentals of nursing* (6th ed., p. 410). St. Louis: Mosby.

---

619. A registered nurse (RN) is providing post-mortem care for a deceased client whose eyes will be donated. Which nursing action is required to provide sound care of the client's body?
   1 Closes the eyes and places the bed flat
   2 Maintains the client in a supine position
   3 Irrigates the client's eyes with normal saline
   4 Places wet saline gauze pads on the eyelids and a small ice pack on the gauze pads

Level of Cognitive Ability: Application
Client Needs: Safe and Effective Care Environment
Integrated Process: Nursing Process/Implementation
Content Area: Fundamental Skills

Answer: 4
Rationale: When a corneal donor dies, the eyes are closed and gauze pads wet with saline are placed over them with a small ice pack. Within 2 to 4 hours the eyes are enucleated, and the corneas are usually transplanted within 24 to 48 hours. The head of the bed should be elevated. With the head of the bed elevated, the eyes will likely remain closed. Eye irrigations, if indicated, would be prescribed by the transplant surgeon.

Test-Taking Strategy: Note that the subject relates to donation of the eyes. Also note the strategic word "required" in the question. This strategic word indicates that a procedure specific to eye harvesting is necessary to preserve the cornea. Visualize each option and think about the subject of preserving the eyes. This will direct you to option 4. Review corneal transplantation and associated procedures if you had difficulty with this question.

Reference
Ignatavicius, D., & Workman, M. (2006). *Medical-surgical nursing: Critical thinking for collaborative care* (5th ed., p. 1092). Philadelphia: Saunders.

---

620. A clinical nurse manager conducts an in-service educational session for the staff nurses about case management. The clinical nurse manager determines that a review of the material needs to be done if a staff nurse stated that case management:
   1 Manages client care by managing the client care environment
   2 Maximizes hospital revenues while providing for optimal client care
   3 Represents a primary health prevention focus managed by a single case manager
   4 Is designed to promote appropriate use of hospital personnel and material resources

Level of Cognitive Ability: Comprehension
Client Needs: Safe and Effective Care Environment
Integrated Process: Teaching and Learning
Content Area: Leadership/Management

Answer: 3
Rationale: Case management represents an interdisciplinary health care delivery system to promote appropriate use of hospital personnel and material resources to maximize hospital revenues while providing for optimal client of care. It manages client care by managing the client care environment.

Test-Taking Strategy: Note the strategic words "a review of the material needs to be done." These strategic words indicate a negative event query and the need to select the option that is an incorrect characteristic of case management. Noting the word "single" in option 3 will direct you to this option. Review the characteristics of case management if you had difficulty with this question.

References
Ignatavicius, D., & Workman, M. (2006). *Medical-surgical nursing: Critical thinking for collaborative care* (5th ed., pp. 28-29). Philadelphia: Saunders.
Potter, P., & Perry, A. (2005). *Fundamentals of nursing* (6th ed., pp. 485, 487). St. Louis: Mosby.

621. A registered nurse is delegating activities to the nursing staff. Which activity is least appropriate for the nursing assistant?
  1 Collecting a urine specimen from a client
  2 Obtaining frequent oral temperatures on a client
  3 Accompanying a man being discharged to transportation home
  4 Assisting a postcardiac catheterization client who needs to lie flat to eat lunch

Level of Cognitive Ability: Application
Client Needs: Safe and Effective Care Environment
Integrated Process: Nursing Process/ Implementation
Content Area: Delegating/Prioritizing

Answer: 4
Rationale: Work that is delegated to others must be consistent with the individual's level of expertise and licensure, if any. Based on the options provided, the least appropriate activity for a nursing assistant would be assisting the postcardiac catheterization client. Because this client needs to eat while lying flat, the client is at risk for aspiration. The remaining three options do not include situations that indicate that these activities carry foreseeable risk.

Test-Taking Strategy: Note the strategic words "least appropriate." Use the ABCs—airway, breathing, and circulation—and recall the principles of delegation in answering the question. Review the principles of assignments and delegation if you had difficulty with this question.

References
Huber, D. (2006). *Leadership and nursing care management* (3rd ed., pp. 545-547). Philadelphia: Saunders.
Potter, P., & Perry, A. (2005). *Fundamentals of nursing* (6th ed., pp. 378, 418). St. Louis: Mosby.

---

622. A nurse manager is reviewing the critical paths of the clients on the nursing unit. The nurse manager collaborates with each nurse assigned to the clients and performs a variance analysis. Which of the following would indicate the need for further action and analysis?
  1 A client is performing his own colostomy care.
  2 A 1-day postoperative client has a temperature of 98.8° F.
  3 Purulent drainage is noted from a postoperative wound incision.
  4 A client newly diagnosed with diabetes mellitus is preparing his own insulin for injection.

Level of Cognitive Ability: Analysis
Client Needs: Safe and Effective Care Environment
Integrated Process: Nursing Process/Evaluation
Content Area: Leadership/Management

Answer: 3
Rationale: Variances are actual deviations or detours from the critical paths. Variances can be either positive or negative, or avoidable or unavoidable, and can be caused by a variety of things. Positive variance occurs when the client achieves maximum benefit and is discharged earlier than anticipated. Negative variance occurs when untoward events prevent a timely discharge. Variance analysis occurs continually in order to anticipate and recognize negative variance early so that appropriate action can be taken. Option 3 is the only option that identifies the need for further action.

Test-Taking Strategy: Use the process of elimination, identifying the negative variance. Options 1, 2, and 4 identify positive outcomes. Option 3 identifies a negative outcome. Review the purpose of variance analysis if you had difficulty with this question.

Reference
Potter, P., & Perry, A. (2005). *Fundamentals of nursing* (6th ed., p. 485). St. Louis: Mosby.

---

623. A nurse is planning the client assignments for the shift. Which client would the nurse assign to the nursing assistant?
  1 A client requiring dressing changes
  2 A client requiring frequent ambulation
  3 A client with diabetes mellitus requiring daily insulin and reinforcement of dietary measures
  4 A client on a bowel management program requiring rectal suppositories and a daily enema

Answer: 2
Rationale: Assignment of tasks to the nursing assistant needs to be made based on job description, level of clinical competence, and state law. Options 1, 3, and 4 involve care that requires the skill of a licensed nurse. The client described in option 2 has needs that can be met by a nursing assistant.

Level of Cognitive Ability: Application
Client Needs: Safe and Effective Care Environment
Integrated Process: Nursing Process/Planning
Content Area: Delegating/Prioritizing

Test-Taking Strategy: Focus on the subject—the assignment to a nursing assistant. Think about the tasks that the nursing assistant can safely perform and match the client's needs with these tasks. Eliminate options 1, 3, and 4 because these clients require care that needs to be provided by a licensed nurse. Review the guidelines regarding assignment making and delegating if you had difficulty with this question.

References

Huber, D. (2006). *Leadership and nursing care management* (3rd ed., pp. 315-317). Philadelphia: Saunders.

Potter, P., & Perry, A. (2005). *Fundamentals of nursing* (6th ed., pp. 42, 378-379, 418). St. Louis: Mosby.

---

624. A psychotic client is pacing, agitated, and presenting with aggressive gestures. The client's speech pattern is rapid, and the client's affect is belligerent. Based on these objective data, the immediate priority of care is to:

1 Provide safety for the client and other clients on the unit.
2 Bring the client to a less stimulated area to regain control.
3 Provide the clients on the unit with a sense of comfort and safety.
4 Assist the staff in caring for the client in a controlled environment.

Level of Cognitive Ability: Application
Client Needs: Safe and Effective Care Environment
Integrated Process: Nursing Process/Implementation
Content Area: Mental Health

Answer: 1

Rationale: If a client is exhibiting signs that indicate loss of control, the nurse's immediate priority is to ensure safety for all clients. Option 1 is the only option that addresses the client's and other clients' safety needs. Option 2 addresses the client's needs. Option 3 addresses other clients' needs. Option 4 is not client centered.

Test-Taking Strategy: Focus on the data in the question. Note the subject of the question, safety. Option 1 is an umbrella option and addresses the safety of all. Review nursing care for the client who is agitated and out of control if you had difficulty with this question.

Reference

Stuart, G., & Laraia, M. (2005). *Principles and practice of psychiatric nursing* (8th ed., pp. 378, 721). St. Louis: Mosby

---

625. A magnetic resonance imaging (MRI) test is prescribed for a client with Bell's palsy. Which nursing action is included in the client's plan of care to prepare for this test?

1 Keep the client NPO for 6 hours before the test.
2 Shave the groin for insertion of a femoral catheter.
3 Remove all metal-containing objects from the client.
4 Instruct the client in inhalation techniques for the administration of gas.

Level of Cognitive Ability: Application
Client Needs: Safe and Effective Care Environment
Integrated Process: Nursing Process/Planning
Content Area: Adult Health/Neurological

Answer: 3

Rationale: In an MRI scan, radiofrequency pulses in a magnetic field are converted into pictures. All metal objects, such as rings, bracelets, hairpins, and watches, should be removed. In addition, a history should be taken to ascertain whether the client has any internal metallic devices, such as orthopedic hardware, pacemakers, shrapnel, and the like. For an abdominal MRI, the client is usually NPO. An NPO status is not necessary for an MRI of the head. The groin may be shaved for an angiogram, and inhalation of gas may be prescribed for positron emission tomography study.

Test-Taking Strategy: Focus on the name of the test and the client's diagnosis. Note the relation between "magnetic" in the question and "metal" in the correct option. If you are unfamiliar with client preparation for an MRI scan, review this content.

Reference
Chernecky, C., & Berger, B. (2008). *Laboratory tests and diagnostic procedures* (5th ed., p. 750). Philadelphia: Saunders.

626. Based upon a request made by the client's spouse and children, a physician asks a nurse to discontinue the feeding tube in a client who is in a chronic debilitated and comatose state. The nurse understands the legal basis for carrying out the order and first checks the client's record for documentation of:

1 A court approval to discontinue the treatment
2 Approval by the institutional Ethics Committee
3 A written order by the physician to remove the tube
4 Authorization by the family to discontinue the treatment

Level of Cognitive Ability: Application
Client Needs: Safe and Effective Care Environment
Integrated Process: Communication and Documentation
Content Area: Leadership/Management

Answer: 4
Rationale: The family or a legal guardian can make treatment decisions for the client who is unable to do so. Once the decision is made, the physician writes the order. Generally, the family makes decisions in collaboration with physicians, other health care workers, and other trusted advisors. Although a written order by the physician is necessary, the nurse first checks for documentation of the family's request. Unless special circumstances exist, a court order is not necessary. Although some health care agencies may require reviewing such requests via the Ethics Committee, this is not the nurse's first action.

Test-Taking Strategy: Note the strategic word "first" to determine the sequence of decision making in this situation. No data in the question indicate the need for court approval. Therefore assessment for family authorization is the nurse's first action. Review these ethical and legal principles if you had difficulty with this question.

References
Huber, D. (2006). *Leadership and nursing care management* (3rd ed., p. 158). Philadelphia: Saunders.
Monahan, F., Sands, J., Neighbors, M., Marek, J., & Green, C. (2007). *Phipps' medical-surgical nursing: Health and illness perspectives* (8th ed., p. 241). St. Louis: Mosby.
Potter, P., & Perry, A. (2005). *Fundamentals of nursing* (6th ed., p. 416). St. Louis: Mosby.

627. A nurse is assisting the physician with the insertion of a Miller-Abbott tube. The nurse understands that the procedure puts the client at risk for aspiration and implements which action to decrease this risk?

1 Inserts the tube with the balloon inflated
2 Places the client in a high-Fowler's position
3 Instructs the client to cough when the tube reaches the nasal pharynx
4 Instructs the client to perform a Valsalva maneuver if the impulse to gag and vomit occurs

Level of Cognitive Ability: Application
Client Needs: Safe and Effective Care Environment
Integrated Process: Nursing Process/ Implementation
Content Area: Adult Health/Gastrointestinal

Answer: 2
Rationale: The Miller-Abbott tube is a nasoenteric tube that is used to decompress the intestine, as in correcting a bowel obstruction. Initial insertion of the tube is a physician responsibility. The tube is inserted with the balloon deflated in a manner similar to the proper procedure for inserting a nasogastric tube. The client is usually given water to drink to facilitate passage of the tube through the nasopharynx and esophagus. A high-Fowler's position decreases the risk of aspiration if vomiting occurs.

Test-Taking Strategy: Focus on the subject, decreasing the risk of aspiration for the client undergoing insertion of a Miller-Abbott tube. Option 1 can be eliminated because the balloon of a Miller-Abbott tube is inflated once the tube has reached the stomach. Eliminate option 3 because coughing can cause the tube to be expelled. A Valsalva maneuver is not used if the impulse to gag or vomit occurs. Review this procedure if you had difficulty with this question.

References
Black, J., & Hawks, J. (2005). *Medical-surgical nursing: Clinical management for positive outcomes* (7th ed., p. 745). Philadelphia: Saunders.
Ignatavicius, D., & Workman, M. (2006). *Medical-surgical nursing: Critical thinking for collaborative care* (5th ed., pp. 1329-1330). Philadelphia: Saunders.
Potter, P., & Perry, A. (2005). *Fundamentals of nursing* (6th ed., p. 1300). St. Louis: Mosby.

---

628. A nurse is caring for a client receiving parenteral nutrition (PN). Which does the nurse implement to decrease the risk of infection?
  1 Assesses vital signs at 4-hour intervals
  2 Administers prophylactic antimicrobial agents
  3 Checks the solution's label against the prescription
  4 Uses aseptic technique in handling the PN solution

Level of Cognitive Ability: Application
Client Needs: Safe and Effective Care Environment
Integrated Process: Nursing Process/ Implementation
Content Area: Fundamental Skills

Answer: 4
Rationale: Clients receiving PN are at high risk for developing infection because the concentrated glucose solutions are an excellent medium for bacterial growth. The nurse reduces the client's risk of infection by using aseptic technique when handling all equipment and solutions related to the PN infusion. Option 1 is a reasonable intervention for early detection of infection but does not prevent infection. Prophylactic antibiotics are not indicated for PN infusions and can contribute to the development of secondary infections. The nurse implements option 3 to ensure that the client receives the correct infusion.

Test-Taking Strategy: Note the strategic words "decrease the risk of infection." Option 1 relates to early detection of infection, option 2 is not indicated, and option 3 does not relate to the subject. Remember that aseptic technique is critical to prevent infection. Review care of the client receiving PN and the measures to prevent infection if you had difficulty with this question.

References
Black, J., & Hawks, J. (2005). *Medical-surgical nursing: Clinical management for positive outcomes* (7th ed., pp. 708-709). Philadelphia: Saunders.
Ignatavicius, D., & Workman, M. (2006). *Medical-surgical nursing: Critical thinking for collaborative care* (5th ed., p. 512). Philadelphia: Saunders.
Potter, P., & Perry, A. (2005). *Fundamentals of nursing* (6th ed., pp. 803-805). St. Louis: Mosby.

---

629. The home care nurse is assisting a client in managing cancer pain. To ensure that the client has adequate and safe pain control, the nurse plans to:
  1 Rely totally on prescription and over-the-counter medications to relieve pain.
  2 Keep a baseline level of pain so that the client does not become sedated or addicted.
  3 Try multiple medication modalities for pain relief to get the maximum pain relief effect.
  4 Start with low doses of medication and gradually increase to a dose that relieves pain, not exceeding the maximum daily dose.

Answer: 4
Rationale: Safe pain control includes starting with low doses and working up to a dose of medication that relieves the pain. Multiple medication modalities interventions can be unsafe and ineffective. Option 1 does not take into account other nursing interventions that may relieve pain, such as massage, therapeutic touch, or music. Maintaining a baseline level of pain to avoid sedation or addiction is not appropriate practice, unless the client requests this, and this information has not been provided in the case situation.

Test-Taking Strategy: Use the process of elimination and focus on safety issues. Option 1 uses the word "totally," and option 3 uses the word "multiple." Therefore, eliminate these options. Option 2 can be eliminated next because it is inaccurate information. Review safe pain control management if you had difficulty with this question.

Level of Cognitive Ability: Application
Client Needs: Safe and Effective Care
Environment
Integrated Process: Caring
Content Area: Adult Health/Oncology

References
Black, J., & Hawks, J. (2005). *Medical-surgical nursing: Clinical management for positive outcomes* (7th ed., pp. 450, 454, 460). Philadelphia: Saunders.
Monahan, F., Sands, J., Neighbors, M., Marek, J., & Green, C. (2007). *Phipps' medical-surgical nursing: Health and illness perspectives* (8th ed., pp. 322, 559-560). St. Louis: Mosby.

---

630. The home care nurse provides medication instructions to a male client. To ensure that the client self-administers his medications safely in the home, the nurse:
  1 Performs a pill count of each prescription bottle at every home visit
  2 Instructs the client to double up on a medication when a dose is missed
  3 Demonstrates the proper procedure for self-administration of medications
  4 Asks the client to explain and demonstrate self-administration procedures

Level of Cognitive Ability: Application
Client Needs: Safe and Effective Care
Environment
Integrated Process: Teaching and Learning
Content Area: Fundamental Skills

Answer: 4
Rationale: To ensure safe administration of medication, the nurse asks the client to explain and demonstrate correct self-administration of medication procedures because demonstrating the proper procedure for the client does not ensure that the client can safely perform any procedure. Usually, it is not acceptable to double up on missed medication, and conducting a pill count on each visit is unrealistic and disrespectful.

Test-Taking Strategy: Focus on the subject—safe administration of medication. Eliminate options 1 and 2 first because these are unlikely to ensure correct client practices. From the remaining options, note that option 4 is client-centered. Review the principles of teaching and learning and the methods of ensuring safe administration of medication if you had difficulty with this question.

Reference
Potter, P., & Perry, A. (2005). *Fundamentals of nursing* (6th ed., pp. 844-845). St. Louis: Mosby.

---

631. A client remains in atrial fibrillation with rapid ventricular response despite pharmacological intervention. Synchronous cardioversion is scheduled to convert the rapid rhythm. The nurse plans to implement which important action to ensure safety and prevent complications of this procedure?
  1 Cardiovert the client at 360 joules.
  2 Sedate the client before cardioversion.
  3 Ensure that emergency equipment is available.
  4 Ensure that the defibrillator is set on the synchronous mode.

Level of Cognitive Ability: Application
Client Needs: Safe and Effective Care
Environment
Integrated Process: Nursing Process/
Implementation
Content Area: Adult Health/Cardiovascular

Answer: 4
Rationale: Cardioversion is similar to defibrillation with two major exceptions: (1) the countershock is synchronized to occur during ventricular depolarization (QRS complex), and (2) less energy is used for the countershock. The rationale for delivering the shock during the QRS complex is to prevent the shock from being delivered during repolarization (T wave), often termed the "vulnerable period." If the shock is delivered during this period, the resulting complication is ventricular fibrillation. It is crucial that the defibrillator is set on the "synchronous" mode for a successful cardioversion. Options 2 and 3 will not prevent complications. Cardioversion usually begins with 50 to 100 joules.

Test-Taking Strategy: Focus on the subject—ensure safety and prevent complications. Noting the strategic word "synchronous" in the question will direct you to option 4. Review this procedure if you had difficulty with this question.

References
Ignatavicius, D., & Workman, M. (2006). *Medical-surgical nursing: Critical thinking for collaborative care* (5th ed., pp. 728, 739, 741). Philadelphia: Saunders.
Lewis, S., Heitkemper, M., Dirksen, S., O'Brien, P., & Bucher, L. (2007). *Medical-surgical nursing: Assessment and management of clinical problems* (7th ed., p. 857). St. Louis: Mosby.

632. A client with a diagnosis of thrombophlebitis is being treated with heparin sodium therapy. In planning a safe environment, the nurse ensures that which medication is available if the client develops a significant bleeding problem?
1 Protamine sulfate
2 Fresh frozen plasma
3 Streptokinase (Streptase)
4 Phytonadione (vitamin K)

Level of Cognitive Ability: Application
Client Needs: Safe and Effective Care Environment
Integrated Process: Nursing Process/Planning
Content Area: Pharmacology

Answer: 1
Rationale: Protamine sulfate is the antidote for heparin sodium. Phytonadione is the antidote for warfarin (Coumadin). Fresh frozen plasma may also be used for bleeding related to warfarin (Coumadin) therapy. Streptokinase is a thrombolytic agent used to dissolve blood clots.

Test-Taking Strategy: Focus on the subject—planning a safe environment—and note the name of the medication. Recalling that the antidote for heparin sodium is protamine sulfate will direct you to the correct option. Review the antidotes for commonly administered medications if you had difficulty with this question.

Reference
Skidmore-Roth, L. (2008). *Mosby's nursing drug reference* (21st ed., pp. 278-279). St. Louis: Mosby.

---

633. The nurse is teaching a client with cardiomyopathy about home care safety measures. The nurse provides instruction on which most important measure to ensure client safety?
1 Reporting pain
2 Taking vasodilators
3 Avoiding over-the-counter medications
4 Moving slowly from a sitting to a standing position

Level of Cognitive Ability: Application
Client Needs: Safe and Effective Care Environment
Integrated Process: Teaching and Learning
Content Area: Adult Health/Cardiovascular

Answer: 4
Rationale: Orthostatic changes can occur in the client with cardiomyopathy as a result of venous return obstruction. Sudden changes in blood pressure may lead to falls. Vasodilators are not normally prescribed for the client with cardiomyopathy. Options 1 and 3, although important, are not directly related to the issue of safety.

Test-Taking Strategy: Focus on the subject—to ensure client safety at home—and note the strategic words "most important." Recalling that blood pressure changes occur in cardiomyopathy will direct you to option 4. Review client teaching related to cardiomyopathy if you had difficulty with this question.

References
Black, J., & Hawks, J. (2005). *Medical-surgical nursing: Clinical management for positive outcomes* (7th ed., p. 1607). Philadelphia: Saunders.
Ignatavicius, D., & Workman, M. (2006). *Medical-surgical nursing: Critical thinking for collaborative care* (5th ed., pp. 772-773). Philadelphia: Saunders.

---

634. The nurse instructs a client with a diagnosis of atrial fibrillation to use an electric razor for shaving. The nurse tells the client that the importance of its use is that:
1 Cuts need to be avoided.
2 Any cut may cause infection.
3 Electric razors can be disinfected.
4 All straight razors contain bacteria.

Level of Cognitive Ability: Application
Client Needs: Safe and Effective Care Environment.
Integrated Process: Teaching and Learning
Content Area: Adult Health/Cardiovascular

Answer: 1
Rationale: Clients with atrial fibrillation are placed on anticoagulants to prevent thrombus formation and possible stroke. The importance of use of an electric razor is to prevent cuts and possible bleeding. Options 2, 3, and 4 are all unrelated to the subject of bleeding; rather, they relate to infection.

Test-Taking Strategy: Recalling that the client with atrial fibrillation will be prescribed anticoagulants will assist in answering the question. Note that options 2, 3, and 4 are comparable or alike and relate to infection. Option 1 relates to bleeding. Review care of the client with atrial fibrillation if you had difficulty with this question.

Reference
Ignatavicius, D., & Workman, M. (2006). *Medical-surgical nursing: Critical thinking for collaborative care* (5th ed., p. 767). Philadelphia: Saunders.

635. A cardiac catheterization, using the femoral artery approach, is performed to assess the degree of coronary artery thrombosis in a client. Which nursing action following the procedure is unsafe for the client?
   1 Encouraging the client to increase fluid intake
   2 Placing the client's bed in the Fowler's position
   3 Resuming prescribed precatheterization medications
   4 Instructing the client to move the toes when checking circulation, motion, and sensation

Level of Cognitive Ability: Application
Client Needs: Safe and Effective Care Environment
Integrated Process: Nursing Process/ Implementation
Content Area: Adult Health/Cardiovascular

Answer: 2
Rationale: Immediately following a cardiac catheterization with the femoral artery approach, the client should not flex or hyperextend the affected leg to avoid blood vessel occlusion or hemorrhage. Placing the client in the Fowler's position (flexion) increases the risk of occlusion or hemorrhage. Fluids are encouraged to assist in removing the contrast medium from the body. The precatheterization medications are needed to treat acute and chronic conditions. Asking the client to move the toes is done to assess motion, which could be impaired if a hematoma or thrombus was developing.

Test-Taking Strategy: Note the strategic word "unsafe." This strategic word indicates a negative event query and the need to select the option that indicates an incorrect nursing action. Also note the words "femoral artery approach." Recalling that flexion or hyperextension is avoided following this procedure will direct you to option 2. Review postcardiac catheterization care if you had difficulty with this question.

Reference
Ignatavicius, D., & Workman, M. (2006). *Medical-surgical nursing: Critical thinking for collaborative care* (5th ed., pp. 697-698). Philadelphia: Saunders.

636. A nurse plans to carry out a multidisciplinary research project on the effects of immobility on clients' stress levels. Of the following statements, which principle is most important when planning this project?
   1 Any client has the right to refuse to participate in research studies.
   2 Collaboration with other disciplines is essential to the successful practice of nursing.
   3 The cooperation of the physicians on staff must be ensured in order for the project to succeed.
   4 The corporate nurse executive should be consulted, because the project will take nursing time.

Level of Cognitive Ability: Application
Client Needs: Safe and Effective Care Environment
Integrated Process: Nursing Process/Planning
Content Area: Leadership/Management

Answer: 1
Rationale: The proposed project is research and includes human subjects. Although options 2, 3, and 4 need to be considered, they are all secondary to the overriding principle of the legal and ethical practice of nursing that any client has the right to refuse to participate in research using human subjects.

Test-Taking Strategy: Focus on the subject, the most important principle. Recalling that the client has the right to refuse to participate in research will direct you to option 1. Review the ethical and legal guidelines related to research if you had difficulty with this question.

References
Monahan, F., Sands, J., Neighbors, M., Marek, J., & Green, C. (2007). *Phipps' medical-surgical nursing: Health and illness perspectives* (8th ed., p. 6). St. Louis: Mosby.
Potter, P., & Perry, A. (2005). *Fundamentals of nursing* (6th ed., pp. 81-82). *Phipps',* St. Louis: Mosby.

637. A nurse manager has identified a problem on the nursing unit and holds unit meetings for all shifts. The nurse manager presents an analysis of the problem and proposals for actions to team members and invites the team members to comment and provide input. Which style of leadership is the nurse manager specifically employing?

1 Situational
2 Laissez faire
3 Participative
4 Authoritarian

Level of Cognitive Ability: Comprehension
Client Needs: Safe and Effective Care Environment
Integrated Process: Nursing Process/ Implementation
Content Area: Leadership/Management

Answer: 3
Rationale: Participative leadership demonstrates an "in-between" style, neither authoritarian nor democratic style. In participative leadership, the manager presents an analysis of problems and proposals for actions to team members, inviting critique and comments. The participative leader then analyzes the comments and makes the final decision. A laissez-faire leader abdicates leadership and responsibilities, allowing staff to work without assistance, direction, or supervision. The autocratic style of leadership is task oriented and directive. The situational leadership style utilizes a style depending on the situation and events.

Test-Taking Strategy: Focus on the data in the question. Noting the words "invites the team members to comment and provide input" will direct you to option 3. Review the various types of leadership styles if you had difficulty with this question.

Reference
Huber, D. (2006). *Leadership and nursing care management* (3rd ed., pp. 17-18). Philadelphia: Saunders.

---

638. A clinic nurse teaches a pregnant client with herpes genitalis about the measures that will be implemented during the pregnancy. Which statement by the client indicates that teaching was effective?

1 "I need to take sitz baths four times a day."
2 "I must continue to take my acyclovir (Zovirax)."
3 "I need to abstain from sexual intercourse during the entire pregnancy."
4 "I may need a cesarean section if the lesions are present at the time of labor."

Level of Cognitive Ability: Analysis
Client Needs: Safe and Effective Care Environment
Integrated Process: Teaching and Learning
Content Area: Maternity/Antepartum

Answer: 4
Rationale: For women with active lesions, either recurrent or primary, at the time of labor, delivery should be cesarean; therefore, option 4 is correct. Acyclovir is used with caution during pregnancy. Clients should be advised to abstain from sexual contact while the lesions are present. If it is an initial infection, they should continue to abstain until they become culture-negative because prolonged viral shedding may occur in such cases. Option 1 is incorrect. Keeping the genital area clean and dry will promote healing.

Test-Taking Strategy: Use the process of elimination and eliminate option 2 first because of the close-ended word "must." Next, eliminate option 3 because of the word "entire." Knowing that the genital area should remain clean and dry will assist in eliminating option 1. Review the health care measures related to herpes genitalis if you had difficulty with this question.

References
McKinney, E., James, S., Murray, S., & Ashwill, J. (2005). *Maternal-child nursing* (2nd ed., pp. 663-664). St. Louis: Saunders.
Wong, D., Hockenberry, M., Perry, S., Lowdermilk, D., & Wilson, D. (2006). *Maternal-child nursing care.* (3rd ed., p. 129). St. Louis: Mosby.

639. A client asks the home care nurse to witness the client's signature on a living will with the client's attorney in attendance. Which should the nurse implement?

1 Decline to witness the signature on the will.
2 Sign the will as a witness to the signature only.
3 Notify the supervisor that a living will is being witnessed.
4 Sign the will with identifying credentials and employment agency.

Level of Cognitive Ability: Application
Client Needs: Safe and Effective Care Environment
Integrated Process: Nursing Process/ Implementation
Content Area: Fundamental Skills

Answer: 1
Rationale: Living wills must be written documents and signed by the client. The client's signature either must be witnessed by nonagency individuals or notarized, thus the nurse should decline to sign the will to avoid a conflict of interest. The nurse's signature on the living will testifies to the validity of the client's signature. If the nurse contacts the supervisor, the supervisor should advise the nurse to decline.

Test-Taking Strategy: Use the process of elimination. Eliminate options 2, 3, and 4 because they are comparable or alike and indicate that the nurse will sign as a witness. Review legal implications associated with wills if you had difficulty with this question.

References
Ignatavicius, D., & Workman, M. (2006). *Medical-surgical nursing: Critical thinking for collaborative care* (5th ed., p. 106). Philadelphia: Saunders.
Potter, P., & Perry, A. (2005). *Fundamentals of nursing* (6th ed., pp. 409-410). St. Louis: Mosby.

---

640. The nurse notes old and new ecchymotic areas on an older client's arms and buttocks upon admission. The client tells the nurse in confidence that her daughter frequently hits her. Which statement should the nurse use in response?

1 "I have a legal obligation to report this type of abuse."
2 "Let's get these treated and I will maintain the confidence."
3 "If this happens again, you must call the emergency department."
4 "Let's talk about ways to prevent your daughter from hitting you."

Level of Cognitive Ability: Application
Client Needs: Safe and Effective Care Environment
Integrated Process: Nursing Process/ Implementation
Content Area: Fundamental Skills

Answer: 1
Rationale: The nurse should inform the client that nurses cannot maintain confidences about alleged abusive behavior and that the nurse must report situations related to abuse. The nurse avoids bargaining with the client about treatment to maintain a confidence that the nurse is legally bound to report. Options 3 and 4 delay protective action and place the client at risk for future abuse.

Test-Taking Strategy: Use the process of elimination. Option 2 can be eliminated first because this action does not protect the client from injury. Options 3 and 4 should be eliminated next because they place the client at risk for future abuse. Review the nursing responsibilities related to reporting obligations if you had difficulty with this question.

Reference
Ignatavicius, D., & Workman, M. (2006). *Medical-surgical nursing: Critical thinking for collaborative care* (5th ed., pp. 48-49). Philadelphia: Saunders.

641. A client receives cardiopulmonary resuscitation in the emergency department, but it is unsuccessful. The wife of the client indicates that the client is an organ donor and that they want to donate the client's eyes. Which should the nurse implement first to promote organ transplantation?

1 Confirm that the client is a valid donor with an organ registry.

2 Cover the eyes with wet saline gauze pads and small ice packs.

3 Place the client in a supine position with the head on one pillow.

4 Ask the wife to produce the legal documents supporting the donation.

Level of Cognitive Ability: Analysis
Client Needs: Safe and Effective Care Environment
Integrated Process: Nursing Process/ Implementation
Content Area: Fundamental Skills

Answer: 2
Rationale: When a corneal donor dies, the eyes are closed, covered with sterile gauze pads wet with saline, and cooled with small ice packs. Within 2 to 4 hours the eyes are harvested, and the cornea is usually transplanted within 24 to 48 hours after harvesting. The head of the bed is elevated 30 to 45 degrees to prevent edema and tissue damage. Calling an organ registry and asking the wife to produce documents does not promote organ transplantation.

Test-Taking Strategy: Note that the subject relates to donation of the eyes to assist in eliminating options. Eliminate option 1 because it is unnecessary and option 4 because the family can determine organ donation for the decedent; in addition, these actions do not contribute promoting organ transplantation. Eliminate option 3 because it can increase the risk of tissue damage. Review the procedure for caring for an eye donor if you had difficulty with this question.

Reference
Ignatavicius, D., & Workman, M. (2006). *Medical-surgical nursing: Critical thinking for collaborative care* (5th ed., p. 1092). Philadelphia: Saunders.

642. A client tells the home care nurse of a personal decision to refuse external cardiac resuscitation measures. Which of the following is the most appropriate initial nursing action?

1 Notify the physician of the client's request.

2 Discuss the client's request with the client's family.

3 Document the client's request in the home care nursing care plan.

4 Conduct a client conference with the home care staff to share the client's request.

Level of Cognitive Ability: Application
Client Needs: Safe and Effective Care Environment
Integrated Process: Nursing Process/ Implementation
Content Area: Delegating/Prioritizing

Answer: 1
Rationale: External cardiac resuscitation is a life-saving treatment that a client may refuse. The most appropriate initial nursing action is to notify the physician, because a written "do not resuscitate" (DNR) order from the physician is needed to ensure that the client's wishes are followed. The DNR order must be reviewed or renewed on a regular basis per agency policy. Although options 2, 3, and 4 may be appropriate, remember that obtaining a written physician's DNR order must be completed first.

Test-Taking Strategy: Use the process of elimination and prioritize the options. Note the strategic words "most appropriate initial." These strategic words indicate that more than one option may be correct. Although options 2, 3, and 4 may be appropriate, remember that first a written physician's order is necessary. Review DNR procedures if you had difficulty with this question.

References
Ignatavicius, D., & Workman, M. (2006). *Medical-surgical nursing: Critical thinking for collaborative care* (5th ed., pp. 106, 333). Philadelphia: Saunders.
Lewis, S., Heitkemper, M., Dirksen, S., O'Brien, P., & Bucher, L. (2007). *Medical-surgical nursing: Assessment and management of clinical problems* (7th ed., pp. 155-156). St. Louis: Mosby.

643. The nurse prepares a client for discharge who needs intermittent antibiotic infusions through a peripherally inserted central catheter (PICC) line. Which should the nurse include in client teaching about daily infusion care in the home?
1 Keep the affected arm immobilized.
2 Aspirate 3 mL of blood from the PICC line.
3 Maintain a continuous intravenous infusion.
4 Check the insertion site for redness and swelling.

Level of Cognitive Ability: Application
Client Needs: Safe and Effective Care Environment
Integrated Process: Nursing Process/Planning
Content Area: Fundamental Skills

Answer: 4
Rationale: A PICC is designed for long-term intravenous infusions and, usually, is inserted into the median cubital vein with the terminal end of the catheter in the superior vena cava. Although the risk of infection is less with a PICC line than with a central venous catheter, it is possible for phlebitis or infection to develop. Clients must inspect the insertion site and affected arm daily and report any discharge, redness, swelling, or pain to the nurse or provider immediately. A PICC line does not require the affected arm to be immobilized and can be used for intermittent or continuous fluid infusion. Although a PICC line can be used to obtain a blood specimen, the risk of occlusion from aspirating blood as part of the related daily care is greater than any potential benefit.

Test-Taking Strategy: Use the process of elimination and note the strategic words, "daily infusion care." Eliminate option 1 because this action can be suitable for a short-length peripheral intravenous catheter if placed in a movable or vulnerable spot (such as the wrist). Eliminate option 2 because it is contraindicated; the risks of aspirating blood from the catheter are greater than the potential benefit, and this practice is not recommended as a routine care. Because the nature of a PICC line allows for either continuous or intermittent infusions, option 3 is also incorrect. Basic principles of infection control could lead you to choose option 4. Additionally, option 4 represents the first step of the nursing process, assessment. Review home care instructions for a client with a PICC line if you had difficulty with this question.

References

Ignatavicius, D., & Workman, M. (2006). *Medical-surgical nursing: Critical thinking for collaborative care* (5th ed., pp. 250, 256-257). Philadelphia: Saunders.
Potter, P., & Perry, A. (2005). *Fundamentals of nursing* (6th ed., p. 927). St. Louis: Mosby.

644. The nurse is in orientation for a full-time position as a case manager. Which should the nurse implement related to professional liability insurance?
1 Obtain his own malpractice insurance.
2 Wait for six months to a year to decide.
3 Rely on the agency for liability insurance
4 Discontinue his own malpractice insurance.

Level of Cognitive Ability: Application
Client Needs: Safe and Effective Care Environment
Integrated Process: Teaching and Learning
Content Area: Fundamental Skills

Answer: 1
Rationale: Nurses need individual liability insurance policies for protection against malpractice lawsuits beginning on the first day of employment. Many agencies discourage nurses from obtaining professional malpractice insurance because, if a plaintiff brings a suit against the nurse or the hospital, the agency prefers to have their attorneys in control. However, this may not be in the best interests of an individual nurse, and, if the nurse breached any agency policy, the hospital can deny legal protection to the nurse. Still, nurses should be aware that carrying malpractice insurance increases the likelihood of being named in a suit at the onset of the case, especially when the plaintiff is seeking monetary compensation.

Test-Taking Strategy: Use the process of elimination. Eliminate options 3 and 4 because they refer to having no individual malpractice insurance. Eliminate option 2 because waiting to obtain mal practice insurance does not provide protection for the nurse. Review liability related to malpractice insurance if you had difficulty with this question.

Reference
Potter, P., & Perry, A. (2005). *Fundamentals of nursing* (6th ed., p. 418). St. Louis: Mosby.

645. A charge nurse observes that a staff nurse is not able to meet client needs in a reasonable time frame, does not problem-solve situations, and does not prioritize nursing care. The charge nurse has the responsibility to:
  1 Supervise the staff nurse more closely so that tasks are completed.
  2 Ask other staff members to help the staff nurse get the work done.
  3 Provide support and identify the underlying cause of the staff nurse's problem.
  4 Report the staff nurse to the supervisor so that something is done to resolve the problem.

Level of Cognitive Ability: Application
Client Needs: Safe and Effective Care Environment
Integrated Process: Nursing Process/ Implementation
Content Area: Leadership/Management

Answer: 3
Rationale: Option 3 empowers the charge nurse to assist the staff nurse while trying to identify and reduce the behaviors that make it difficult for the staff nurse to function. Options 1, 2, and 4 are punitive actions, shift the burden to other workers, and do not solve the problem.

Test-Taking Strategy: Remember that assessment is the first step of the nursing process. The charge nurse needs to gather information before making any decisions or deciding on a course of action. Identifying the underlying cause of the problem is a process of assessment. Review the leadership role of the nurse if you had difficulty with this question.

Reference
Potter, P., & Perry, A. (2005). *Fundamentals of nursing* (6th ed., pp. 384-385). St. Louis: Mosby.

646. A registered nurse is a preceptor for a new nursing graduate and is observing the new nursing graduate organize the client assignment and daily tasks. The registered nurse intervenes if the new nursing graduate does which of the following?
  1 Provides time for unexpected tasks
  2 Lists the supplies needed for a task
  3 Prioritizes client needs and daily tasks
  4 Plans to document task completion at the end of the day

Level of Cognitive Ability: Application
Client Needs: Safe and Effective Care Environment
Integrated Process: Nursing Process/ Implementation
Content Area: Leadership/Management

Answer: 4
Rationale: The nurse should document task completion continuously throughout the day. Options 1, 2, and 3 identify accurate components of time management.

Test-Taking Strategy: Note the strategic word "intervenes." This strategic word indicates a negative event query and the need to select the incorrect component of time management. Recalling that the nurse needs to document client data and task completion continuously throughout the day will direct you to option 4. Review time management principles and the principles related to documentation if you had difficulty with this question.

Reference
Potter, P., & Perry, A. (2005). *Fundamentals of nursing* (6th ed., pp. 480-483). St. Louis: Mosby.

647. A registered nurse is a preceptor for a new nursing graduate and is describing critical paths and variance analysis to the new nursing graduate. The registered nurse instructs the new nursing graduate that a variance analysis is performed on all clients:

1 Continuously
2 Daily during hospitalization
3 Every third day of hospitalization
4 Every other day of hospitalization

Level of Cognitive Ability: Application
Client Needs: Safe and Effective Care Environment
Integrated Process: Teaching and Learning
Content Area: Leadership/Management

Answer: 1
Rationale: Variance analysis occurs continually as the case manager and other caregivers monitor client outcomes against critical paths. The goal of critical paths is to anticipate and recognize negative variance early so that appropriate action can be taken. A negative variance occurs when untoward events preclude a timely discharge and the length of stay is longer than planned for a client on a specific critical path. Options 2, 3, and 4 are incorrect.

Test-Taking Strategy: Focus on the subject—critical paths and variance analysis. Recall that the goal of critical paths is to recognize negative variance early. This will direct you to option 1. Remember that it is best to monitor a client continuously. Review the characteristics of critical paths and variance analysis if you had difficulty with this question.

References
Cohen, E. & Cesta, T. (2005). *Nursing case management: From essentials to advanced practice applications* (4th ed., p. 473). St. Louis: Mosby.
Potter, P., & Perry, A. (2005). *Fundamentals of nursing* (6th ed., p. 485). St. Louis: Mosby.

---

648. When a nurse manager makes decisions regarding the management of the nursing unit without input from the staff, the type of leadership style that the nurse manager is demonstrating is:

1 Autocratic
2 Situational
3 Democratic
4 Laissez faire

Level of Cognitive Ability: Application
Client Needs: Safe and Effective Care Environment
Integrated Process: Nursing Process/ Implementation
Content Area: Leadership/Management

Answer: 1
Rationale: The autocratic style of leadership is task oriented and directive. The leader uses his or her power and position in an authoritarian manner to set and implement organizational goals. Decisions are made without input from the staff. Democratic styles best empower staff toward excellence because this style of leadership allows nurses to provide input regarding the decision-making process and an opportunity to grow professionally. The situational leadership style utilizes a style depending on the situation and events. The laissez-faire style allows staff to work without assistance, direction, or supervision.

Test-Taking Strategy: Use the process of elimination. Noting the strategic words "made without input from the staff" will assist in directing you to option 1. Review the various leadership styles if you had difficulty with this question.

Reference
Huber, D. (2006). *Leadership and nursing care management* (3rd ed., pp. 157, 569). Philadelphia: Saunders.

649. A hospital administrator has implemented a change in the method of assigning nurses to client care units. Nurses will now be required to work in other nursing departments and will not be specifically assigned to a client care unit. A group of registered nurses is resistant to the change, and the nursing administrator anticipates that the nurses will not facilitate the process of change. Which of the following would be the best approach on the part of the administrator in dealing with the resistance?

1 Ignore the resistance.
2 Exert coercion with the nurses.
3 Manipulate the nurses to participate in the change.
4 Confront the nurses to encourage verbalization of feelings regarding the change.

Level of Cognitive Ability: Application
Client Needs: Safe and Effective Care Environment
Integrated Process: Nursing Process/ Implementation
Content Area: Leadership/Management

650. A registered nurse (RN) in charge of the client care unit is preparing the assignments for the day. The RN assigns a nursing assistant to make beds and bathe one of the clients on the unit and assigns another nursing assistant to fill the water pitchers and serve juice to all of the clients. Another RN is assigned to administer all medications. Based on the assignments designed by the RN in charge, which type of nursing care is being implemented?

1 Team nursing
2 Primary nursing
3 Functional nursing
4 Exemplary nursing

Level of Cognitive Ability: Application
Client Needs: Safe and Effective Care Environment
Integrated Process: Nursing Process/ Implementation
Content Area: Leadership/Management

Answer: 4
Rationale: Confrontation is an important strategy to meet resistance head-on. Face-to-face meetings to confront the issue at hand will allow verbalization of feelings, identification of problems and issues, and the development of strategies to solve the problem. Option 1 will not address the problem. Option 2 may produce additional resistance. Option 3 may provide a temporary solution to the resistance but will not specifically address the concern.

Test-Taking Strategy: Use the process of elimination. Options 1 and 2 can be easily eliminated first because these actions do not address the problem and may produce additional resistance. From the remaining options, select option 4 because this option specifically addresses the subject and would provide problem-solving measures. Review the strategies associated with dealing with resistance to change if you had difficulty with this question.

References
Huber, D. (2006). *Leadership and nursing care management* (3rd ed., p. 527). Philadelphia: Saunders.
Potter, P., & Perry, A. (2005). *Fundamentals of nursing* (6th ed., p. 440). St. Louis: Mosby.

Answer: 1
Rationale: The functional model of care involves an assembly-line approach to client care, with major tasks being delegated by the charge nurse to individual staff members. Team nursing is characterized by a high degree of communication and collaboration between members. The team is generally led by a registered nurse, who is responsible for assessing, developing nursing diagnoses, planning, and evaluating each client's plan of care. In an exemplary model of team nursing, each staff member works fully within the realm of educational and clinical experience in an effort to provide comprehensive individualized client care. Each staff member is accountable for client care and outcomes of care. In primary nursing, concern is with keeping the nurse at the bedside actively involved in care, providing goal-directed and individualized client care.

Test-Taking Strategy: Focus on the information provided in the question to assist in directing you to the correct option. Noting that each staff member is assigned a specific task will direct you to option 1. Review the various nursing delivery systems if you had difficulty with this question.

Reference
Huber, D. (2006). *Leadership and nursing care management* (3rd ed., pp. 317, 321-322). Philadelphia: Saunders.

651. The nurse is receiving a client being transferred from the postanesthesia care unit following an above-the-knee amputation. The nurse should take which action to safely position the client at this time?
1 Elevate the foot of the bed.
2 Position the residual limb flat on the bed.
3 Put the bed in reverse Trendelenburg.
4 Keep the residual limb flat with the client lying on the operative side.

Level of Cognitive Ability: Application
Client Needs: Safe and Effective Care Environment
Integrated Process: Nursing Process/ Implementation
Content Area: Adult Health/Cardiovascular

Answer: 1
Rationale: Edema of the residual limb is controlled by elevating it on pillows or the foot of the bed for the first 24 hours only after surgery. Following the first 24 hours, the residual limb is usually placed flat on the bed to reduce hip contracture. Edema is also controlled by residual limb wrapping techniques. Reverse Trendelenburg does not provide direct limb elevation.

Test-Taking Strategy: Use the process of elimination. Eliminate options 2 and 4 first because they are similar positions. To select from the remaining options, note that the client has just returned from surgery. Using basic principles related to immediate postoperative care and preventing postoperative edema will assist in directing you to option 1. Review postoperative positioning following amputation if you had difficulty with this question.

Reference
Black, J., & Hawks, J. (2005). *Medical-surgical nursing: Clinical management for positive outcomes* (7th ed., p. 1524). Philadelphia: Saunders.

---

652. A charge nurse knows that drug and alcohol use by nurses is a reason for the increasing numbers of disciplinary cases by the Board of Nursing. The charge nurse understands that when dealing with a nurse with such an illness, it is most important to assess the impaired nurse to determine:
1 If falsification of client records occurred
2 The magnitude of drug diversion over time
3 The types of illegal activities related to the abuse
4 The physiological impact of the illness on practice

Level of Cognitive Ability: Analysis
Client Needs: Safe and Effective Care Environment
Integrated Process: Nursing Process/Analysis
Content Area: Leadership/Management

Answer: 4
Rationale: A nurse must be able to function at a level that does not affect the ability to provide safe, quality care. The highest priority is to determine how the illness affects the nurse's ability to practice. The other options will be addressed if an investigation is carried out.

Test-Taking Strategy: Use Maslow's Hierarchy of Needs theory. Option 4 addresses physiological integrity and also focuses on the client of the question: the impaired nurse. Review the concepts related to the impaired nurse if you had difficulty with this question.

References
Ignatavicius, D., & Workman, M. (2006). *Medical-surgical nursing: Critical thinking for collaborative care* (5th ed., p. 93). Philadelphia: Saunders.
Potter, P., & Perry, A. (2005). *Fundamentals of nursing* (6th ed., pp. 66, 93). St. Louis: Mosby.
Stuart, G., & Laraia, M. (2005). *Principles and practice of psychiatric nursing* (8th ed., pp. 510-511). St. Louis: Mosby.

653. A pregnant client tests positive for the hepatitis B virus. The client asks the nurse if she will be able to breast-feed the baby as planned after delivery. The nurse makes which response to the client?
1 "You will not be able to breast-feed the baby until 6 months after delivery."
2 "Breast-feeding is not advised, and you should seriously consider bottle-feeding the baby."
3 "Breast-feeding is not a problem, and you will be able to breast-feed immediately after delivery."
4 "Breast-feeding is allowed if the baby receives prophylaxis at birth and remains on the scheduled immunization."

Level of Cognitive Ability: Application
Client Needs: Safe and Effective Care Environment
Integrated Process: Teaching and Learning
Content Area: Maternity/Antepartum

Answer: 4
Rationale: The pregnant client who tests positive for hepatitis B virus should be reassured that breast-feeding is not contraindicated if the infant receives prophylaxis at birth and remains on the schedule for immunizations. Options 1, 2, and 3 are incorrect.

Test-Taking Strategy: Use the process of elimination. Eliminate options 1, 2, and 3 because of the close-ended word "not" in these options. Also use therapeutic communication techniques to direct you to option 4. Review the management of hepatitis B virus if you had difficulty with this question.

Reference
McKinney, E., James, S., Murray, S., & Ashwill, J. (2005). *Maternal-child nursing* (2nd ed., pp. 665, 1150). St. Louis: Saunders.

---

654. A nurse manager is planning to implement a change in the method of the documentation system for the nursing unit. Many problems have occurred as a result of the present documentation system, and the nurse manager determines that a change is required. The initial step in the process of change for the nurse manager is which of the following?
1 Plan strategies to implement the change.
2 Set goals and priorities regarding the change process.
3 Identify the inefficiency that needs improvement or correction.
4 Identify potential solutions and strategies for the change process.

Level of Cognitive Ability: Application
Client Needs: Safe and Effective Care Environment
Integrated Process: Nursing Process/Planning
Content Area: Leadership/Management

Answer: 3
Rationale: When beginning the change process, the nurse should identify and define the problem that needs improvement or correction. This important first step can prevent many future problems, because, if the problem is not correctly identified, a plan for change may be aimed at the wrong problem. This is followed by goal setting, prioritizing, and identifying potential solutions and strategies to implement the change.

Test-Taking Strategy: Use the steps of the nursing process and knowledge regarding the change process to answer this question. Option 3 is the only option that identifies an assessment step. Review the steps of the change process if you had difficulty with this question.

References
Huber, D. (2006). *Leadership and nursing care management* (3rd ed., pp. 812-814). Philadelphia: Saunders.
Potter, P., & Perry, A. (2005). *Fundamentals of nursing* (6th ed., pp. 266-267). St. Louis: Mosby.

655. A delivery room nurse is preparing a client for a cesarean delivery. The client is placed on the delivery room table and the nurse positions the client:

1 In the prone position
2 In semi-Fowler's position
3 In Trendelenburg's position
4 In the supine position with a wedge under the right hip

Level of Cognitive Ability: Application
Client Needs: Safe and Effective Care Environment
Integrated Process: Nursing Process/ Implementation
Content Area: Maternity/Intrapartum

Answer: 4
Rationale: Vena cava and descending aorta compression by the pregnant uterus impedes blood return from the lower trunk and extremities, therefore decreasing cardiac return, cardiac output, and blood flow to the uterus and subsequently the fetus. The best position to prevent this would be side-lying with the uterus displaced off the abdominal vessels. Positioning for abdominal surgery necessitates a supine position, so a wedge placed under the right hip provides displacement of the uterus. Trendelenburg positioning places pressure from the pregnant uterus on the diaphragm and lungs, decreasing respiratory capacity and oxygenation. A semi-Fowler's or prone position is not practical for this type of abdominal surgery.

Test-Taking Strategy: Use the process of elimination and visualize each of the positions in the options. Recalling the concern in the pregnant client related to vena cava and descending aorta compression will direct you to option 4. Review positioning concepts if you had difficulty with this question.

Reference
Wong, D., Hockenberry, M., Perry, S., Lowdermilk, D., & Wilson, D. (2006). *Maternal-child nursing care.* (3rd ed., p. 575). St. Louis: Mosby.

---

656. A nurse in the day care center is told that a child with autism will be attending the center. The nurse collaborates with the staff of the day care center and plans activities that will meet the child's needs. The priority consideration in planning activities for the child is to ensure:

1 Safety with activities
2 That activities provide verbal stimulation
3 Social interactions with other children in the same age group
4 Familiarity with all activities and providing orientation throughout the activities

Level of Cognitive Ability: Application
Client Needs: Safe and Effective Care Environment
Integrated Process: Nursing Process/Planning
Content Area: Child Health

Answer: 1
Rationale: Safety with activities is a priority in planning activities with the child. The child with autism is unable to anticipate danger, has a tendency for self-mutilation, and has sensory perceptual deficits. Although social interactions, verbal communications, and providing familiarity and orientation are also appropriate interventions, the priority is safety.

Test-Taking Strategy: Use Maslow's Hierarchy of Needs theory to answer this question. Physiological needs take priority. When a physiological need does not exist, safety needs are the priority. None of the options addresses a physiological need. Option 1 addresses the safety need. Options 2, 3, and 4 address psychosocial needs. Review care of the child with autism if you had difficulty with this question.

References
Hockenberry, M., Wilson, D., & Winkelstein, M. (2005). *Wong's essentials of pediatric nursing* (7th ed., p. 619). St. Louis: Mosby.
McKinney, E., James, S., Murray, S., & Ashwill, J. (2005). *Maternal-child nursing* (2nd ed., p. 1577). St. Louis: Saunders.

657. A registered nurse is reviewing a plan of care developed by a nursing student for a child who is being admitted to the pediatric unit with a diagnosis of seizures. The registered nurse determines that the student nurse needs to revise the plan of care if which incorrect intervention is documented?

1 Maintain the bed in a low position.
2 Restrain the child if a seizure occurs.
3 Pad the side rails of the bed with blankets.
4 Place the child in a side-lying lateral position if a seizure occurs.

Level of Cognitive Ability: Analysis
Client Needs: Safe and Effective Care Environment
Integrated Process: Teaching and Learning
Content Area: Child Health

Answer: 2

Rationale: Restraints are not to be applied to a child with a seizure because they could cause injury to the child. The side rails of the bed are padded with blankets, and the bed is maintained in low position to provide safety in the event that the child has a seizure. Positioning the child on his or her side will prevent aspiration as the saliva drains out of the child's mouth during the seizure.

Test-Taking Strategy: Note the strategic word "incorrect." This strategic word indicates a negative event query and the need to select the incorrect intervention. Focus on safety to eliminate the incorrect options and recall that restraints are not to be used. Review safety measures related to the child with seizures if you had difficulty with this question.

References

Hockenberry, M., & Wilson, D. (2007). *Nursing care of infants and children* (8th ed., p. 1667) St. Louis: Mosby.

Wong, D., Hockenberry, M., Perry, S., Lowdermilk, D., & Wilson, D. (2006). *Maternal-child nursing care* (3rd ed., p. 1709) St. Louis: Mosby.

---

658. In the role as a caregiver, the nurse's primary responsibility is to assess the client's ability to:

1 Protect self.
2 Set own goals.
3 Decide the best approach(es) for care.
4 Restore physical, emotional, and social well-being.

Level of Cognitive Ability: Application
Client Needs: Safe and Effective Care Environment
Integrated Process: Nursing Process/ Implementation
Content Area: Fundamental Skills

Answer: 4

Rationale: A primary role of the caregiver is to assess the client's ability to restore well-being. Options 1, 2, and 3 identify the nurse's role as a client advocate.

Test-Taking Strategy: Use the process of elimination. Focus on the strategic word "caregiver" to direct you to option 4. Options 1, 2, and 3 are comparable or alike and address the nurse's role as a client advocate. Review the roles and responsibilities of the nurse as a caregiver if you had difficulty with this question.

Reference

Potter, P., & Perry, A. (2005). *Fundamentals of nursing* (6th ed., p. 19). St. Louis: Mosby.

---

659. A nurse receives a telephone call from the emergency department and is told that a child with a diagnosis of tonic-clonic seizures will be admitted to the pediatric unit. The nurse prepares for the admission of the child and instructs the nursing assistant to place which items at the bedside?

1 A tracheotomy set and oxygen
2 Suction apparatus and an airway
3 An endotracheal tube and an airway
4 An emergency cart and laryngoscope

Level of Cognitive Ability: Application
Client Needs: Safe and Effective Care Environment
Integrated Process: Nursing Process/Planning
Content Area: Leadership/Management

Answer: 2

Rationale: Tonic-clonic seizures cause tightening of all body muscles followed by tremors. Obstructed airway and increased oral secretions are the major complications during and following a seizure. Suction is helpful to prevent choking and cyanosis. Options 1 and 3 are incorrect because inserting an endotracheal tube or a tracheostomy is not done. It is not necessary to have an emergency cart (which contains a laryngoscope) at the bedside, but a cart should be available in the treatment room or on the nursing unit.

Test-Taking Strategy: Use the process of elimination. Recalling that tonic-clonic seizures produce excessive oral secretions and airway obstruction will assist in selecting the correct option. Review the plan of care associated with seizure precautions if you had difficulty with this question.

References
Hockenberry, M., Wilson, D., & Winkelstein, M. (2005). *Wong's essentials of pediatric nursing* (7th ed., p. 1052). St. Louis: Mosby.
Wong, D., Hockenberry, M., Perry, S., Lowdermilk, D., & Wilson, D. (2006). *Maternal-child nursing care* (3rd ed., pp. 1708-1709). St. Louis: Mosby.

---

660. The nurse is admitting a 56-year-old male client with exacerbation of chronic obstructive pulmonary disease (COPD) to the hospital and questions the client as to whether he has received previous immunization for pneumococcal pneumonia. The client replies that he received the vaccine 6 years ago. Which of the following is essential to include in the plan of care during the client's hospital admission?

1 Offer revaccination to the client.
2 No further nursing action is needed.
3 Document the previous immunization on the client record.
4 Explain to the client that he can only be revaccinated during the fall months.

Level of Cognitive Ability: Application
Client Needs: Safe and Effective Care Environment
Integrated Process: Nursing Process/Planning
Content Area: Adult Health/Respiratory

Answer: 1
Rationale: During the history-taking of a client with a respiratory disorder, the nurse should ask the if the client had been previously vaccinated for influenza (flu) and had received pneumococcal pneumonia vaccine (Pneumovax). The pneumococcal pneumonia vaccine is administered any time during the year. Revaccination is currently advised in a client with COPD if the client received the vaccine more than 5 years previously and if the client was younger than 65 years of age at the time of vaccination. Options 2 and 4 are incorrect. Although documentation would be done, this is not the essential action.

Test-Taking Strategy: Use the process of elimination. Eliminate option 2 first, because the question indicates that an intervention is "essential." Eliminate option 4 next, knowing that pneumococcal pneumonia vaccine can be administered any time of the year. From the remaining options, select option 1 based on guidelines for administration of pneumococcal pneumonia vaccine and the fact that it is client focused. Review criteria for immunization with pneumococcal pneumonia vaccine if you had difficulty with this question.

Reference
Lewis, S., Heitkemper, M., Dirksen, S., O'Brien, P., & Bucher, L. (2007). *Medical-surgical nursing: Assessment and management of clinical problems* (7th ed., p. 519). St. Louis: Mosby.

---

661. The nurse in a well baby clinic is providing safety instructions to the mother of a 1-month-old infant. Which safety instruction is most appropriate at this age?

1 Lock up all poisons.
2 Cover electrical outlets.
3 Never shake the infant's head.
4 Remove hazardous objects from low places.

Level of Cognitive Ability: Application
Client Needs: Safe and Effective Care Environment
Integrated Process: Teaching and Learning
Content Area: Child Health

Answer: 3
Rationale: The age-appropriate instruction that is most important is to instruct the mother not to shake or vigorously jiggle the baby's head. Options 1, 2, and 4 are most important instructions to provide to the mother as the child reaches the age of 6 months and begins to explore the environment.

Test-Taking Strategy: Focus on the age of the infant to direct you to the correct option. A 1-month-old is not at a developmental level to explore the environment, which will assist in eliminating options 1, 2, and 4. Review age-appropriate safety measures if you had difficulty with this question.

References
Hockenberry, M., Wilson, D., & Winkelstein, M. (2005). *Wong's essentials of pediatric nursing* (7th ed., p. 463). St. Louis: Mosby.
Wong, D., Hockenberry, M., Perry, S., Lowdermilk, D., & Wilson, D. (2006). *Maternal-child nursing care.* (3rd ed., p. 1142). St. Louis: Mosby.

662. The nurse has an order to test a client's stools using Hemoccult slides. The nurse would question the order if the client was taking which medication that could cause a false-negative result?
1 Iodine
2 Colchicine
3 Ascorbic acid (vitamin C)
4 Acetylsalicylic acid (aspirin)

Level of Cognitive Ability: Application
Client Needs: Safe and Effective Care Environment
Integrated Process: Nursing Process/ Implementation
Content Area: Adult Health/Gastrointestinal

Answer: 3
Rationale: Ascorbic acid can interfere with the result of occult blood testing, causing false-negative findings. Colchicine and iodine can cause false-positive results. Acetylsalicylic acid would either have no effect on results or could cause a positive result, because aspirin is irritating to the stomach lining.

Test-Taking Strategy: Focus on the strategic words "false-negative results." Specific knowledge of the factors that interfere with occult blood testing is needed to answer this question accurately. Review the nursing considerations associated with this test if you had difficulty with this question.

Reference
Chernecky, C., & Berger, B. (2008). *Laboratory tests and diagnostic procedures* (5th ed., p. 817). Philadelphia: Saunders.

---

663. A community health nurse is providing instructions to a group of mothers regarding the safe use of car seats for toddlers. The nurse determines that the mother of a toddler understands the instructions if the mother states which of the following?
1 "The car seat should never be placed in a face-forward position."
2 "The car seat can be placed in a face-forward position at any time."
3 "The car seat is suitable for the toddler until the toddler reaches the weight of 40 pounds."
4 "The car seat can be placed in a face-forward position when the height of the toddler is 27 inches."

Level of Cognitive Ability: Analysis
Client Needs: Safe and Effective Care Environment
Integrated Process: Nursing Process/Evaluation
Content Area: Child Health

Answer: 3
Rationale: The transition point for switching to the forward-facing position is defined by the manufacturer of the safety seat but is generally at a body weight of 9 kg (20 pounds). The car safety seat should be used until the child weighs at least 40 pounds, regardless of age. Options 1, 2, and 4 are incorrect.

Test-Taking Strategy: Use the process of elimination and focus on the subject of the question. Eliminate options 1 and 2 first because of the close-ended words "never" and "any." From the remaining options, visualize each and use knowledge regarding car safety and the toddler to answer the question. Review these safety principles if you had difficulty with this question.

References
Hockenberry, M., & Wilson, D. (2007). *Nursing care of infants and children* (8th ed., p. 633) St. Louis: Mosby.
McKinney, E., James, S., Murray, S., & Ashwill, J. (2005). *Maternal-child nursing* (2nd ed., pp. 97, 118, 120). St. Louis: Saunders.

---

664. A home care nurse is providing instructions to the mother of a toddler regarding safety measures in the home to prevent an accidental burn injury. Which statement by the mother indicates a need for further instruction?
1 "I need to use the back burners for cooking."
2 "I need to remain in the kitchen when I prepare meals."
3 "I need to be sure to place my cup of coffee on the counter."
4 "I need to turn pot handles inward and to the middle of the stove."

Answer: 3
Rationale: Toddlers, with their increased mobility and developing motor skills, can reach hot water or hot objects placed on counters and open fires or burners on stoves above their eye level. Parents should be encouraged to remain in the kitchen when preparing a meal, to use the back burners on the stove, and to turn pot handles inward and toward the middle of the stove. Hot liquids should never be left unattended, and the toddler should always be supervised. The mother's statement in option 3 does not indicate an adequate understanding of the principles of safety.

Level of Cognitive Ability: Analysis
Client Needs: Safe and Effective Care
 Environment
Integrated Process: Teaching and Learning
Content Area: Child Health

Test-Taking Strategy: Use the process of elimination and note the strategic words "a need for further instruction." These strategic words indicate a negative event query and the need to select the option that identifies an incorrect statement by the mother. Options 1, 2, and 4 can be eliminated because they identify basic safety principles. Also recalling that the toddler is in the stage of developing motor skills will assist in directing you to option 3. Review these safety principles if you had difficulty with this question.

References
Hockenberry, M., & Wilson, D. (2007). *Nursing care of infants and children* (8th ed., p. 559) St. Louis: Mosby.
McKinney, E., James, S., Murray, S., & Ashwill, J. (2005). *Maternal-child nursing* (2nd ed., pp. 118-119). St. Louis: Saunders.

---

665. The nurse prepares a client who has a right pleural effusion for a thoracentesis; however, the client experiences severe dizziness when sitting upright. Into which alternate position does the nurse assist the client to maintain safety during the procedure?
1 Right side-lying with the head of the bed flat
2 Prone with the head turned toward the affected side
3 Sims' position with the head of the bed elevated 45 degrees
4 Left side-lying with the head of the bed elevated 45 degrees

Level of Cognitive Ability: Application
Client Needs: Safe and Effective Care
 Environment
Integrated Process: Nursing Process/
 Implementation
Content Area: Fundamental Skills

Answer: 4
Rationale: Positioning can help isolate the fluid in a pleural effusion; generally, the client sits at the edge of the bed, leaning over the bedside table, allowing the fluid to collect in a dependent body area. If the client is unable to sit up, the nurse turns the client to the unaffected side and elevates the head of the bed 30 to 45 degrees. Turning to the affected side, the prone, and the Sims' positions are unsuitable positions for this procedure because these do not facilitate fluid removal.

Test-Taking Strategy: Use the process of elimination. Eliminate option 1 because lying on the affected side makes it difficult to perform the procedure. Eliminate option 2 because prone positioning does not facilitate fluid removal, and eliminate option 3 because the Sims' position is used for rectal enemas or irrigations primarily. Review the procedure for a thoracentesis if you had difficulty with this question.

References
Ignatavicius, D., & Workman, M. (2006). *Medical-surgical nursing: Critical thinking for collaborative care* (5th ed., p. 542). Philadelphia: Saunders.
Pagana, K., & Pagana, T. (2005). *Mosby's diagnostic and laboratory test reference* (7th ed., p. 901). St. Louis: Mosby.

---

666. A physician has written an order to administer methylergonovine maleate (Methergine) to a postpartum client with uterine atony. The nurse would contact the physician to verify the order if which of the following conditions were present in the mother?
1 Hypertension
2 Excessive lochia
3 Difficulty locating the uterine fundus
4 Excessive bleeding and saturation of more than one peripad per hour

Answer: 1
Rationale: Methergine is contraindicated for the hypertensive woman, individuals with severe hepatic or renal disease, and during the third stage of labor. A uterine fundus that is difficult to locate, excessive bleeding, and excessive lochia are clinical manifestations of uterine atony indicating the need for methylergonovine.

Test-Taking Strategy: Use the process of elimination. Eliminate options 2, 3, and 4 because they are comparable or alike in that they are clinical manifestations of uterine atony. Review this content if you had difficulty with this question or are unfamiliar with the use of this medication and its contraindications.

Level of Cognitive Ability: Application
Client Needs: Safe and Effective Care Environment
Integrated Process: Nursing Process/ Implementation
Content Area: Maternity/Postpartum

Reference
Wong, D., Hockenberry, M., Perry, S., Lowdermilk, D., & Wilson, D. (2006). *Maternal-child nursing care* (3rd ed., p. 662). St. Louis: Mosby.

667. After receiving detailed information about a colonoscopy from the provider, the nurse asks the client to sign the informed consent form and discovers that the client cannot write. Which is the best intervention for the nurse to implement?
   1 Contact the provider to obtain informed consent.
   2 Obtain a verbal informed consent from the client.
   3 Have two nurses witness the client sign with an X.
   4 Clarify information to the client with another nurse.

Level of Cognitive Ability: Application
Client Needs: Safe and Effective Care Environment
Integrated Process: Nursing Process/ Implementation
Content Area: Fundamental Skills

Answer: 3
Rationale: Nurses are responsible to make sure the signed informed consent form is in the client's medical record prior to a procedure and for clarifying facts presented by the provider. Nonetheless, the person performing the procedure obtains informed consent and provides the explanations to the client. Informed consent can be obtained verbally, but that is also the responsibility of the provider. Clients who cannot write may sign an informed consent with an X in the presence of two witnesses. Nurses can serve as a witness to the client's signature but not to the fact that the client is informed.

Test-Taking Strategy: Use the process of elimination. Eliminate options 1, 2, and 4 because the provider has provided detailed information to the client. Review the principles related to informed consent if you had difficulty with this question.

Reference
Ignatavicius, D., & Workman, M. (2006). *Medical-surgical nursing: Critical thinking for collaborative care* (5th ed., p. 304). Philadelphia: Saunders.

668. A child with a brain tumor is admitted to the hospital for removal of the tumor. To ensure a safe environment for the child, the nurse includes which of the following in the plan of care?
   1 Initiating seizure precautions
   2 Using a wheelchair for out-of-bed activities
   3 Assisting the child with ambulation at all times
   4 Avoiding contact with other children on the nursing unit

Level of Cognitive Ability: Application
Client Needs: Safe and Effective Care Environment
Integrated Process: Nursing Process/Planning
Content Area: Child Health

Answer: 1
Rationale: Seizure precautions should be implemented for any child with a brain tumor, both preoperatively and postoperatively. Options 2 and 3 are not required unless functional deficits exist. Based on the child's diagnosis, option 4 is not necessary.

Test-Taking Strategy: Note the strategic words "safe environment." Eliminate options 2 and 3 first because they are comparable or alike. Additionally, note the close-ended word "all" in option 3. From the remaining options, eliminate option 4 because there is no reason for the child to avoid contact with other children. Review nursing interventions related to the child with a brain tumor if you had difficulty with this question.

Reference
McKinney, E., James, S., Murray, S., & Ashwill, J. (2005). *Maternal-child nursing* (2nd ed., p. 1347). St. Louis: Saunders.

669. A home care nurse provides instructions to the mother of a child with croup. The mother expresses concern regarding the occurrence of an acute spasmodic episode, and the nurse instructs the mother regarding management if an acute episode occurs. Which statement by the mother indicates a need for further instructions?

1 "I will place a steam vaporizer in my child's room."
2 "I will place a cool mist humidifier in my child's room."
3 "I will take my child outside to breathe the cool humid night air."
4 "I will place my child in a closed bathroom and allow my child to inhale steam from warm running water."

Level of Cognitive Ability: Analysis
Client Needs: Safe and Effective Care Environment
Integrated Process: Teaching and Learning
Content Area: Child Health

Answer: 1
Rationale: Steam from warm running water in a closed bathroom and cool mist from a bedside humidifier are effective in reducing mucosal edema. Cool mist humidifiers are recommended over steam vaporizers, which present a danger of scald burns. Taking the child outside to breathe the cool humid night air may also relieve mucosal swelling.

Test-Taking Strategy: Focus on the subject—to reduce mucosal edema and to provide a safe environment. Also note the strategic words "need for further instructions." These words indicate a negative event query and the need to select the incorrect statement or unsafe action. Option 1 would provide an unsafe environment for the child. Review management of acute spasmodic croup if you had difficulty with this question.

Reference
Hockenberry, M., Wilson, D., & Winkelstein, M. (2005). *Wong's essentials of pediatric nursing* (7th ed., p. 802). St. Louis: Mosby.

670. A nurse is reviewing the results of the rubella screening (titer) with a pregnant 24-year-old client. The test results are positive, and the client asks if it is safe for her toddler to receive the vaccine. The appropriate nursing response is:

1 "Most children do not receive the vaccine until they are 5 years of age."
2 "You are still susceptible to rubella, so your toddler should receive the vaccine."
3 "It is not advised for children of pregnant women to be vaccinated during their mother's pregnancy."
4 "Your titer supports your immunity to rubella, and it is safe for your toddler to receive the vaccine at this time."

Level of Cognitive Ability: Application
Client Needs: Safe and Effective Care Environment
Integrated Process: Nursing Process/ Implementation
Content Area: Maternity/Antepartum

Answer: 4
Rationale: All pregnant women should be screened for prior rubella exposure during pregnancy. All children of pregnant women should receive their immunizations according to schedule. Additionally, no definitive evidence suggests that the rubella vaccine virus is transmitted from person to person. A positive maternal titer further indicates that a significant antibody titer has developed in response to a prior exposure to the *Rubivirus*.

Test-Taking Strategy: Focus on the data in the question. Recalling that a positive titer indicates immunity will direct you to option 4. Review this important screening test if you had difficulty with this question.

References
McKinney, E., James, S., Murray, S., & Ashwill, J. (2005). *Maternal-child nursing* (2nd ed., p. 476). St. Louis: Saunders.
Wong, D., Hockenberry, M., Perry, S., Lowdermilk, D., & Wilson, D. (2006). *Maternal-child nursing care.* (3rd ed., pp. 617, 660). St. Louis: Mosby.

671. Following delivery, the postpartum nurse instructs the client with known cardiac disease to call for the nurse when she needs to get out of bed or when she plans to care for her newborn infant. The nurse informs the client that this is necessary to:

1 Help the mother assume the parenting role.

2 Minimize the potential of postpartum hemorrhage.

3 Provide an opportunity for the nurse to teach newborn infant care techniques.

4 Avoid maternal or infant injury caused by the potential for syncope or overexertion.

Level of Cognitive Ability: Application
Client Needs: Safe and Effective Care Environment
Integrated Process: Teaching and Learning
Content Area: Maternity/Postpartum

Answer: 4
Rationale: The immediate postpartum period is associated with increased risks for the cardiac client. Hormonal changes and fluid shifts from extravascular tissues to the circulatory system cause additional stress on cardiac functioning. Although options 1, 2, and 3 are appropriate nursing concerns during the postpartum period, the primary concern for the cardiac client is to maintain a safe environment because of the potential for cardiac compromise.

Test-Taking Strategy: Focus on the subject—safety—and use the process of elimination. Option 4 is the only option that relates directly to the subject of safety. Review the physiological manifestations that occur in a cardiac client following delivery and the need to implement safety precautions if you had difficulty with this question.

Reference
Wong, D., Hockenberry, M., Perry, S., Lowdermilk, D., & Wilson, D. (2006). *Maternal-child nursing care* (3rd ed., p. 353). St. Louis: Mosby.

672. The nurse is assessing a client who has just been measured and fitted for crutches. The nurse determines that the client's crutches are fitted correctly if:

1 The top of the crutch is even with the axilla.

2 The elbow is straight when the hand is on the handgrip.

3 The client's axilla is resting on the crutch pad during ambulation.

4 The elbow is at a 30-degree angle when the hand is on the handgrip.

Level of Cognitive Ability: Analysis
Client Needs: Safe and Effective Care Environment
Integrated Process: Nursing Process/Evaluation
Content Area: Adult Health/Musculoskeletal

Answer: 4
Rationale: For optimal upper extremity leverage, the elbow should be at approximately 30 degrees of flexion when the hand is resting on the handgrip. The top of the crutch needs to be two to three finger widths lower than the axilla. When crutch walking, all weight needs to be on the hands to prevent nerve palsy from pressure on the axilla.

Test-Taking Strategy: Use the process of elimination. Options 1 and 3 are comparable or alike and can be eliminated first. Visualize the mechanics of crutch walking to assist in selecting from the remaining options. If the weight should be resting on the hands, then there needs to be some flexion to push off from during ambulation. Review crutch walking and the safe and appropriate associated measures if you had difficulty with this question.

References
Ignatavicius, D., & Workman, M. (2006). *Medical-surgical nursing: Critical thinking for collaborative care* (5th ed., p. 1204). Philadelphia: Saunders.
Potter, P., & Perry, A. (2005). *Fundamentals of nursing* (6th ed., pp. 949-950). St. Louis: Mosby.

673. When assessing the client with the vest restraint (security device) at the beginning of day shift, which observation by the charge nurse would indicate that the nurse who placed the vest restraint on the client failed to follow safety guidelines?
1 A hitch knot was used to secure the restraint.
2 The call light was placed within reach of the client.
3 The restraint was applied tightly across the client's chest.
4 The client's record indicates that the restraint will be released every 2 hours.

Level of Cognitive Ability: Analysis
Client Needs: Safe and Effective Care Environment
Integrated Process: Nursing Process/Evaluation
Content Area: Leadership/Management

Answer: 3
Rationale: A vest restraint should never be applied tightly because it could impair respirations. A hitch knot may be used on the client because it can easily be released in an emergency. The call light must always be within the client's reach in case the client needs assistance. The Restraint wording needs to be released every 2 hours (or per agency policy) to provide movenent.

Test-Taking Strategy: Note the strategic words "failed to follow safety guidelines" in the question. This strategic word indicates a negative event query and the need to select the option that indicates an unsafe action. Noting the word "tightly" in option 3 will direct you to this option. Review the principles regarding the safe use of restraints if you had difficulty with this question.

Reference
Ignatavicius, D., & Workman, M. (2006). *Medical-surgical nursing: Critical thinking for collaborative care* (5th ed., pp. 44-45). Philadelphia: Saunders.

---

674. The nurse documents an entry regarding client care in the client's medical record. When checking the entry, the nurse notices some incorrect information. Which should the nurse implement?
1 Obliterate the incorrect information with a black marker.
2 Use correction fluid to cover up the incorrect information.
3 Erase the error completely and write in the correct information.
4 Draw a line through the incorrect information and initial the change.

Level of Cognitive Ability: Application
Client Needs: Safe and Effective Care Environment
Integrated Process: Communication and Documentation
Content Area: Fundamental Skills

Answer: 4
Rationale: To correct an error documented in a medical record, the nurse draws one line through the incorrect information and then initials the error. The information remains visible and properly labeled as incorrect. Errors are never erased, and correction fluid or black markers are never used on a legal document such as the medical record.

Test-Taking Strategy: Focus on the subject, correcting an error documented in a medical record. Note that options 1, 2, and 3 are comparable or alike in that they indicate complete covering up or eliminating the incorrect information. Review the principles of documentation if you are unfamiliar with them.

Reference
Ignatavicius, D., & Workman, M. (2006). *Medical-surgical nursing: Critical thinking for collaborative care* (5th ed., p. 16). Philadelphia: Saunders.

---

675. The nurse prepares to suction a client through a tracheostomy tube. Which should the nurse wear to perform this procedure?
1 Mask, gown, and a cap
2 Mask, sterile gloves, and a cap
3 Gown, mask, and sterile gloves
4 Goggles, mask, and sterile gloves

Answer: 4
Rationale: The nurse should wear a mask and goggles when suctioning the client. Sterile gloves are also worn unless suctioning is performed using a closed suctioning system. A mask offers full protection of the nurse's nose and mouth, and goggles protect the nurse's eyes from getting splashed with sputum. A gown protects the nurse's uniform, and a cap protects the nurse's hair, but these items are not required for suctioning a client.

Level of Cognitive Ability: Application
Client Needs: Safe and Effective Care
   Environment
Integrated Process: Nursing Process/
   Implementation
Content Area: Fundamental Skills

Test-Taking Strategy: Use the process of elimination. Visualize the suctioning procedure and the potential exposure of body fluids that this procedure could cause. This should direct you to option 4. Review standard precautions if you had difficulty with this question.

References

Monahan, F., Sands, J., Neighbors, M., Marek, J., & Green, C. (2007). *Phipps' medical-surgical nursing: Health and illness perspectives* (8th ed., pp. 112-115). St. Louis: Mosby.

Potter, P., & Perry, A. (2005). *Fundamentals of nursing* (6th ed., p. 797). St. Louis: Mosby.

---

676. The nurse instructs a client how to use crutches safely for ambulating at home. Which instruction should the nurse recommend to minimize the risk of falls?
   1 Remove all area rugs.
   2 Wear soft, slip-on shoes.
   3 Use the bathtub's grab bars.
   4 Remove pets from the home.

Level of Cognitive Ability: Application
Client Needs: Safe and Effective Care
   Environment
Integrated Process: Teaching and Learning
Content Area: Fundamental Skills

Answer: 1
Rationale: To reduce the risk of falls, the nurse recommends the removal of all obstacles and trip hazards from the home. Tie-on shoes with nonslip soles should be worn while crutch walking. Grab bars in the bath tub or shower will not necessarily assist the client while walking with crutches. Not all pets are trip hazards (e.g., fish, birds, guinea pigs).

Test-Taking Strategy: Focus on the subject, minimize the risk of falls when ambulating. Use the process of elimination and principles related to safety measures. Eliminate option 2 first because slip-on shoes can come off easily. Visualize the items identified in the remaining options to assist in directing you to option 1. Review home care measures related to safety and ambulation if you had difficulty with this question.

Reference

Potter, P., & Perry, A. (2005). *Fundamentals of nursing* (6th ed., pp. 978-980). St. Louis: Mosby.

---

677. The nurse observes that an older postoperative client has episodes of extreme agitation. Which is the best nursing measure to implement to help avoid episodes of agitation?
   1 Gently hold the client's hand while speaking.
   2 Wait until the client's agitation has subsided.
   3 Speak while moving slowly toward the client.
   4 Speak to the client from the entrance to the room.

Level of Cognitive Ability: Application
Client Needs: Safe and Effective Care
   Environment
Integrated Process: Nursing Process/
   Implementation
Content Area: Fundamental Skills

Answer: 3
Rationale: Speaking and moving slowly toward the client will prevent the client from becoming further agitated, because any sudden moves or speaking too quickly may cause the client to have a violent episode. Holding the client's hand can be misinterpreted by a client to mean restraint. If the client's agitation is not addressed, it is likely to increase; therefore, waiting for the agitation to subside is not a suitable option. Remaining at the entrance of the room can make the client feel alienated.

Test-Taking Strategy: Remember that one of the most basic principles in preventing episodes of agitation or violent episodes is to avoid further agitation. Remember to be empathetic to the client while avoiding actions that potentially startle the client. These principles will direct you to option 3. Review nursing interventions for the client who is agitated if you had difficulty with this question.

Reference

Ignatavicius, D., & Workman, M. (2006). *Medical-surgical nursing: Critical thinking for collaborative care* (5th ed., pp. 971). Philadelphia: Saunders.

678. A 17-year-old client is about to be discharged to home with her newborn baby, and the nurse provides information to the client about home safety for children. Which statement by the client would alert the nurse that further teaching is required regarding home safety?

1 "I keep all my pots and pans in my lower cabinets."
2 "I will not use the microwave oven to heat my baby's formula."
3 "I have locks on all my cabinets that contain my cleaning supplies."
4 "I have a car seat that I will put in the front seat to keep my baby safe."

Level of Cognitive Ability: Analysis
Client Needs: Safe and Effective Care Environment
Integrated Process: Teaching and Learning
Content Area: Child Health

Answer: 4
Rationale: A baby car seat should never be placed in the front seat because of the potential for injury on impact. Any cabinets that contain dangerous items that a baby or child could swallow should be locked. Microwave ovens should never be used to heat formula because the formula heats unevenly, and it could burn and even scald the baby's mouth. Even though the bottle may feel warm, it could contain hot spots that could severely damage the baby's mouth. It is perfectly safe to leave pots and pans in the lower cabinets for a child to investigate, as long as they are not made of glass, which would harm the baby if broken.

Test-Taking Strategy: Note the strategic words "further teaching is required." These words indicate a negative event query and the need to select the incorrect client statement. Remember that a baby car seat should never be placed in the front seat because of the potential for injury on impact. Review these safety principles if you had difficulty with this question.

References
Hockenberry, M., & Wilson, D. (2007). *Nursing care of infants and children* (8th ed., pp. 408-409). St. Louis: Mosby.
Wong, D., Hockenberry, M., Perry, S., Lowdermilk, D., & Wilson, D. (2006). *Maternal-child nursing care* (3rd ed., p.761). St. Louis: Mosby.

---

679. A nurse has administered an injection to a client. After the injection, the nurse accidentally drops the syringe on the floor. Which nursing action is appropriate in this situation?

1 Obtain a dust pan and mop to sweep up the syringe.
2 Call the housekeeping department to pick up the syringe.
3 Carefully pick up the syringe from the floor and gently recap the needle.
4 Carefully pick up the syringe from the floor and dispose of it in a sharps container.

Level of Cognitive Ability: Application
Client Needs: Safe and Effective Care Environment
Integrated Process: Nursing Process/ Implementation
Content Area: Fundamental Skills

Answer: 4
Rationale: Syringes should never be recapped, in any circumstances, because of the risk of getting pricked with a contaminated needle. Used syringes should always be placed in a sharps container immediately after use to avoid individuals from becoming injured. A syringe should not be swept up, because this action poses an additional risk for getting pricked. It is not the responsibility of the housekeeping department to pick up the syringe.

Test-Taking Strategy: Use the process of elimination and basic principles related to the safe disposal of syringes to answer the question. Remember that a needle is never recapped and is always disposed of in a sharps container. Review these safety principles if you had difficulty with this question.

Reference
Potter, P., & Perry, A. (2005). *Fundamentals of nursing* (6th ed., p. 891). St. Louis: Mosby.

680. The nurse is assigned to care for a client who is in traction. The nurse ensures a safe environment for the client by:

1 Making sure that the knots are at the pulleys
2 Checking the weights to be sure that they are off the floor
3 Making sure that the head of the bed is kept at a 90-degree angle
4 Monitoring the weights to be sure that they are resting on a firm surface

Level of Cognitive Ability: Application
Client Needs: Safe and Effective Care Environment
Integrated Process: Nursing Process/ Implementation
Content Area: Adult Health/Musculoskeletal

Answer: 2
Rationale: To achieve proper traction, weights need to be free-hanging, with knots kept away from the pulleys. Weights are not to be kept resting on a firm surface. The head of the bed is usually kept low to provide countertraction.

Test-Taking Strategy: Use the process of elimination. Visualize the traction, recalling that there must be weight to exert the pull from the traction setup. This concept will assist in eliminating options 1 and 4. Recalling that countertraction is needed will assist in eliminating option 3. Review care of the client in traction if you had difficulty with this question.

References
Ignatavicius, D., & Workman, M. (2006). *Medical-surgical nursing: Critical thinking for collaborative care* (5th ed., p. 1201). Philadelphia: Saunders.
Lewis, S., Heitkemper, M., Dirksen, S., O'Brien, P., & Bucher, L. (2007). *Medical-surgical nursing: Assessment and management of clinical problems* (7th ed., p. 1639). St. Louis: Mosby.

---

681. A nurse is observing a client using a walker. The nurse determines that the client is using the walker correctly if the client:

1 Puts weight on the hand pieces, moves the walker forward, and then walks into it
2 Puts weight on the hand pieces, slides the walker forward, and then walks into it
3 Puts all four points of the walker flat on the floor, puts weight on the hand pieces, and then walks into it
4 Walks into the walker, puts weight on the hand pieces, and then puts all four points of the walker flat on the floor

Level of Cognitive Ability: Analysis
Client Needs: Safe and Effective Care Environment
Integrated Process: Nursing Process/Evaluation
Content Area: Fundamental Skills

Answer: 3
Rationale: When the client uses a walker, the nurse stands adjacent to the affected side. The client is instructed to put all four points of the walker 2 feet forward flat on the floor before putting weight on the hand pieces. This will ensure client safety and prevent stress cracks in the walker. The client is then instructed to move the walker forward and walk into it.

Test-Taking Strategy: Visualize each of the options. Options 1 and 2 can be eliminated because putting weight on the hand pieces initially would cause an unsafe situation. From the remaining options, recalling that the walker is placed on all four points first will direct you to option 3. Review this procedure if you had difficulty with this question.

Reference
Ignatavicius, D., & Workman, M. (2006). *Medical-surgical nursing: Critical thinking for collaborative care* (5th ed., pp. 125, 1204). Philadelphia: Saunders.

---

682. The nurse observes clients to evaluate for the correct height of crutches. Which client is correctly fitted with crutches?

1 The client stands with the axillae on the top of the crutches.
2 The client keeps the arms straight when standing with crutches.
3 Two fingers fit between the client's axillae and the top of the crutches.
4 A pencil can slide between the client's axillae and the top of the crutches.

Answer: 3
Rationale: With the client's elbows flexed 20 to 30 degrees, the shoulders in a relaxed position, and the crutches placed approximately 15 cm (6 inches) anterolateral from the toes, the nurse should be able to place two fingers comfortably between the client's axillae and the axillary bars. The crutches are adjusted if there is too much or too little space at the axillary area. The client is advised to avoid resting the axillae on the axillary bars because this could injure the brachial plexus (the nerves in the axillae that supply the arm and shoulder area). The nurse should terminate ambulation and recheck the crutch height if the client complains of numbness or tingling in the hands or arms.

Level of Cognitive Ability: Analysis
Client Needs: Safe and Effective Care
Environment
Integrated Process: Nursing Process/Evaluation
Content Area: Fundamental Skills

Test-Taking Strategy: Focus on the subject—correct height of crutches—and visualize each of the options. This will direct you to option 3, because the remaining options are unsafe and can cause client injury. Review this procedure if you had difficulty with this question.

Reference
Perry, A., & Potter, P. (2006) *Clinical nursing skills & techniques* (6th ed., pp. 283, 286-287). St. Louis: Mosby.

---

683. A nurse is caring for an adolescent client with conjunctivitis. The nurse provides instructions to the client and tells the adolescent to:
1 Avoid using all eye makeup to prevent possible reinfection.
2 Apply warm compresses to decrease pain and lessen irritation.
3 Obtain a new set of contact lenses for use after the infection clears.
4 Stay home for 3 days after starting antibiotic eye drops to avoid the spread of infection.

Level of Cognitive Ability: Application
Client Needs: Safe and Effective Care
Environment
Integrated Process: Teaching and Learning
Content Area: Child Health

Answer: 3
Rationale: Eye makeup should be replaced but can still be worn. Cool compresses decrease pain and irritation. Isolation for 24 hours after antibiotics are initiated is necessary. A new set of contact lenses should be obtained.

Test-Taking Strategy: Use the process of elimination. Eliminate option 1 because of the close-ended word "all." Recalling the principles related to the effectiveness of antibiotics will assist in eliminating option 4. From the remaining options, recalling the effects related to cool and warm compresses will direct you to option 3. Review home care instructions for the client with conjunctivitis if you had difficulty with this question.

Reference
McKinney, E., James, S., Murray, S., & Ashwill, J. (2005). *Maternal-child nursing* (2nd ed., p. 1588). St. Louis: Saunders.

---

684. A client who has experienced a brain attack (stroke) has partial hemiplegia of the left leg. The straight-leg cane formerly used by the client is not sufficient to provide support. The nurse determines that the client could benefit from the somewhat greater support and stability provided by which of the following devices?
1 Quad-cane
2 Wheelchair
3 Wooden crutch
4 Lofstrand crutch

Level of Cognitive Ability: Analysis
Client Needs: Safe and Effective Care
Environment
Integrated Process: Nursing Process/Assessment
Content Area: Adult Health/Neurological

Answer: 1
Rationale: A quad-cane may be prescribed for the client who requires greater support and stability than is provided by a straight-leg cane. The quad-cane provides a four-point base of support and is indicated for use by clients with partial or complete hemiplegia. Neither crutches nor a wheelchair is indicated for use with a client such as described in this question. A Lofstrand crutch is useful for clients with bilateral weakness.

Test-Taking Strategy: Use the process of elimination. Providing a wheelchair to a client with partial hemiplegia is excessive and is eliminated first. Wooden crutches are not indicated, because there is no restriction in weight bearing. From the remaining options, recalling that a Lofstrand crutch is useful for bilateral weakness will direct you to option 1. Review the use of assistive devices for ambulation if you had difficulty with this question.

Reference
Perry, A., & Potter, P. (2006) *Clinical nursing skills & techniques* (6th ed., pp. 948-949). St. Louis: Mosby.

685. A postoperative client begins to drain small amounts of bright red blood from the tracheostomy tube 24 hours after a laryngectomy. The best nursing action is to:
1 Notify the surgeon.
2 Increase the frequency of suctioning.
3 Add moisture to the oxygen delivery system.
4 Document the character and amount of drainage.

Level of Cognitive Ability: Application
Client Needs: Safe and Effective Care Environment
Integrated Process: Nursing Process/ Implementation
Content Area: Adult Health/Respiratory

Answer: 1
Rationale: Immediately following laryngectomy, a small amount of bleeding occurs from the tracheostomy that resolves within the first few hours. Otherwise, bleeding that is bright red may be a sign of impending rupture of a vessel. The bleeding in this instance represents a potential life-threatening situation, and the surgeon is notified to further evaluate the client and suture or repair the bleed. The other options do not address the urgency of the problem. Failure to notify the surgeon places the client at risk.

Test-Taking Strategy: Note the strategic words "bright red blood" and "24 hours after." This should indicate that a potential complication exists and direct you to option 1. Review the complications following laryngectomy if you had difficulty with this question.

References
Ignatavicius, D., & Workman, M. (2006). *Medical-surgical nursing: Critical thinking for collaborative care* (5th ed., p. 576). Philadelphia: Saunders.
Lewis, S., Heitkemper, M., Dirksen, S., O'Brien, P., & Bucher, L. (2007). *Medical-surgical nursing: Assessment and management of clinical problems* (7th ed., p. 556). St. Louis: Mosby.

---

686. A client is at risk for infection following a radical vulvectomy. Which does the nurse implement when giving perineal care to this client?
1 Provides a sitz bath
2 Provides care twice a day
3 Applies a fresh sterile dressing
4 Cleanses using warm tap water

Level of Cognitive Ability: Application
Client Needs: Safe and Effective Care Environment
Integrated Process: Nursing Process/ Implementation
Content Area: Fundamental Skills

Answer: 1
Rationale: The nurse provides a sitz bath to soothe tissues and to stimulate healing by increasing the regional blood flow. Perineal care is provided at least twice a day and after each voiding and bowel movement. A dressing is not used for a vulvectomy. Sterile solutions are used for perineal care using a sterile syringe or water pick.

Test-Taking Strategy: Note the strategic word "vulvectomy." Focus on the subject—risk for infection. Use principles of asepsis and principles for perineal care. Eliminate option 2 because this care is required following every voiding or bowel movement. Eliminate option 3 because dressings are avoided with external female perineal surgery. Noting the words "tap water" in option 4 will assist in eliminating this option. Review these principles if you had difficulty with this question.

Reference
Ignatavicius, D., & Workman, M. (2006). *Medical-surgical nursing: Critical thinking for collaborative care* (5th ed., p. 1852). Philadelphia: Saunders.

687. A nurse prepares to assist a postoperative client to progress from a lying to a sitting position to prepare for ambulation. Which nursing action is appropriate to maintain the safety of the client?

1 Assess the client for signs of dizziness and hypotension.

2 Allow the client to rise from the bed to a standing position unassisted.

3 Elevate the head of the bed quickly to assist the client to a sitting position.

4 Assist the client to move quickly from the lying position to the sitting position.

Level of Cognitive Ability: Application
Client Needs: Safe and Effective Care Environment
Integrated Process: Nursing Process/ Implementation
Content Area: Fundamental Skills

Answer: 1
Rationale: Early ambulation should not exceed the client's tolerance. The client should be assessed before sitting. The client is assisted to rise from the lying position to the sitting position gradually until any evidence of dizziness, if present, has subsided. This position can be achieved by raising the head of the bed slowly. After sitting, the client may be assisted to a standing position. The nurse should be at the client's side to provide physical support and encouragement.

Test-Taking Strategy: Use the process of elimination. Eliminate options 3 and 4 because of the word "quickly" and option 2 because of the word "unassisted." Additionally, option 1 is the only option that reflects assessment, the first step of the nursing process. Review safety measures for ambulation if you had difficulty with this question.

References
Ignatavicius, D., & Workman, M. (2006). *Medical-surgical nursing: Critical thinking for collaborative care* (5th ed., pp. 311-312). Philadelphia: Saunders.
Potter, P., & Perry, A. (2005). *Fundamentals of nursing* (6th ed., p. 1638). St. Louis: Mosby.

---

688. A client has an order for a stool culture to be sent to the laboratory immediately when obtained. The nurse avoids doing which of the following when carrying out this order?

1 Using a sterile container

2 Refrigerating the specimen

3 Using a sterile tongue blade

4 Sending the specimen directly to the laboratory

Level of Cognitive Ability: Application
Client Needs: Safe and Effective Care Environment
Integrated Process: Nursing Process/ Implementation
Content Area: Adult Health/Gastrointestinal

Answer: 2
Rationale: Storing a stool specimen for culture in a refrigerator is not done because it can retard the growth of organisms. Refrigeration is only done if the specimen cannot be sent to the laboratory immediately (the nurse should always follow agency protocols). A stool specimen is obtained using a sterile tongue blade to place the specimen obtained from the bedpan or specimen hat into the sterile container. After obtaining the specimen, the stool is sent immediately to the laboratory.

Test-Taking Strategy: Note the strategic word "avoids." This strategic word indicates a negative event query and the need to select the action that is incorrect. Recalling that a culture is done to identify organisms will assist you in determining that options 1, 3, and 4 must be carried out to ensure accuracy of results. Review this procedure if you had difficulty with this question.

References
Black, J., & Hawks, J. (2005). *Medical-surgical nursing: Clinical management for positive outcomes* (7th ed., pp. 782-783). Philadelphia: Saunders.
Chernecky, C., & Berger, B. (2008). *Laboratory tests and diagnostic procedures* (5th ed., p. 1041). Philadelphia: Saunders.

689. Upon transfer from the postanesthesia care unit following spinal fusion with rod insertion, the nurse prepares to transfer the client from the stretcher to the bed by using which of the following techniques?
1 A transfer board and the assistance of two people
2 A bath blanket and the assistance of four people
3 A transfer board and the assistance of four people
4 A bath blanket and the assistance of three people

Level of Cognitive Ability: Application
Client Needs: Safe and Effective Care Environment
Integrated Process: Nursing Process/Planning
Content Area: Adult Health/Neurological

Answer: 3
Rationale: Following spinal fusion, with or without instrumentation, the client is transferred from the stretcher to the bed using a transfer board and the assistance of four people. This permits optimal stabilization and support of the spine, while allowing the client to be moved smoothly and gently.

Test-Taking Strategy: Use the process of elimination. Think about the level of comfort and stability provided to the client's spine with the amounts of assistance given in each option. Using this approach will assist in eliminating options 1, 2, and 4. Review care of the client following spinal fusion with rod insertion if you had difficulty with this question.

References
Black, J., & Hawks, J. (2005). *Medical-surgical nursing: Clinical management for positive outcomes* (7th ed., pp. 2144, 2146-2147). Philadelphia: Saunders.
Perry, A., & Potter, P. (2006) *Clinical nursing skills & techniques* (6th ed., pp. 236-237). St. Louis: Mosby.
Potter, P., & Perry, A. (2005). *Fundamentals of nursing* (6th ed., pp. 1472, 1475). St. Louis: Mosby.

---

690. The nurse is preparing to nasotracheally suction a client with acquired immunodeficiency syndrome (AIDS) who has had blood-tinged sputum with previous suctioning. The nurse plans to use which of the following items as part of standard precautions for this client?
1 Gloves, gown, and mask
2 Gown, mask, and protective eyewear
3 Gloves, mask, and protective eyewear
4 Gloves, gown, and protective eyewear

Level of Cognitive Ability: Application
Client Needs: Safe and Effective Care Environment
Integrated Process: Nursing Process/Planning
Content Area: Adult Health/Immune

Answer: 3
Rationale: Standard precautions include the use of gloves whenever there is actual or potential contact with blood or body fluids. During procedures that aerosolize blood, the nurse wears a mask and protective eyewear or a face shield. Impervious gowns are worn in those instances when it is anticipated that there will be contact with a large amount of blood.

Test-Taking Strategy: Focus on the data in the question. Note the subject, suctioning, so expect airborne secretions and possibly airborne particles of blood with this procedure. This will direct you to the option that includes a mask, protective eyewear, and gloves. Review standard precautions if you had difficulty this question.

References
Black, J., & Hawks, J. (2005). *Medical-surgical nursing: Clinical management for positive outcomes* (7th ed., pp. 428-429). Philadelphia: Saunders.
Ignatavicius, D., & Workman, M. (2006). *Medical-surgical nursing: Critical thinking for collaborative care* (5th ed., pp. 512-513). Philadelphia: Saunders.

---

691. The nurse inserts an indwelling urinary catheter into a male client. As the catheter moves into the bladder, urine begins to flow into the tubing. Which should the nurse implement next?
1 Inflate the balloon with water.
2 Insert the catheter 2.5 to 5 cm.
3 Secure the catheter to the client.
4 Measure the initial urine output.

Answer: 2
Rationale: The catheter's balloon is behind the opening at the insertion tip, so the nurse inserts the catheter 2.5 to 5 cm further after urine begins to flow in order to provide sufficient space to inflate the balloon. After the nurse secures the catheter to the client's leg, the nurse measures the initial urine output.

Level of Cognitive Ability: Application
Client Needs: Safe and Effective Care
  Environment
Integrated Process: Nursing Process/
  Implementation
Content Area: Fundamental Skills

Test-Taking Strategy: Note the strategic word "next." Visualize the procedure described in the question and the effects of each description in the options to direct you to option 2. Review the procedure for inserting a urinary catheter into a male if you had difficulty with this question.

Reference
Potter, P., & Perry, A. (2005). *Fundamentals of nursing* (6th ed., pp. 1356-1357). St. Louis: Mosby.

---

692. A nurse is preparing to administer oxygen to a client who has chronic obstructive pulmonary disease (COPD) and is at risk for carbon dioxide narcosis. The nurse checks to see that the oxygen flow rate is prescribed at:
  1 2 to 3 liters per minute
  2 4 to 5 liters per minute
  3 6 to 8 liters per minute
  4 8 to 10 liters per minute

Level of Cognitive Ability: Application
Client Needs: Safe and Effective Care
  Environment
Integrated Process: Nursing Process/
  Implementation
Content Area: Adult Health/Respiratory

Answer: 1
Rationale: In carbon dioxide narcosis, the central chemoreceptors lose their sensitivity to increased levels of carbon dioxide and no longer respond by increasing the rate and depth of respiration. For these clients, the stimulus to breathe is a decreased arterial oxygen concentration. In the client with COPD, a low arterial oxygen level is the client's primary drive for breathing. If high levels of oxygen are administered, the client loses the respiratory drive, and respiratory failure results. Thus the nurse checks the flow of oxygen to see that it does not exceed 2 to 3 liters per minute.

Test-Taking Strategy: Focus on the client's diagnosis. Recalling the pathophysiology that occurs in COPD and that a low arterial oxygen level is the client's primary drive for breathing will direct you to option 1, the lowest oxygen liter flow. Review the concerns related to the administration of oxygen to a client with COPD if you had difficulty with this question.

Reference
Ignatavicius, D., & Workman, M. (2006). *Medical-surgical nursing: Critical thinking for collaborative care* (5th ed., p. 600). Philadelphia: Saunders.

---

693. A client undergoes a subtotal thyroidectomy. The nurse ensures that which priority item is at the client's bedside upon arrival from the operating room?
  1 An apnea monitor
  2 A suction unit and oxygen
  3 A blood transfusion warmer
  4 An ampule of phytonadione (vitamin K)

Level of Cognitive Ability: Application
Client Needs: Safe and Effective Care
  Environment
Integrated Process: Nursing Process/Planning
Content Area: Adult Health/Endocrine

Answer: 2
Rationale: Following thyroidectomy, respiratory distress can occur from tetany, tissue swelling, or hemorrhage. It is important to have oxygen and suction equipment readily available and in working order if such an emergency were to arise. Apnea is not a problem associated with thyroidectomy, unless the client experienced a respiratory arrest. Blood transfusions can be administered without a warmer, if necessary. Vitamin K would not be administered for a client who is hemorrhaging, unless deficiencies in clotting factors warrant its administration.

Test-Taking Strategy: Recall the anatomic location of the thyroid gland and its proximity to the trachea. Use the ABCs—airway, breathing, and circulation—to direct you to option 2. Review postoperative care following thyroidectomy if you had difficulty with this question.

Reference
Ignatavicius, D., & Workman, M. (2006). *Medical-surgical nursing: Critical thinking for collaborative care* (5th ed., p. 1487). Philadelphia: Saunders.

694. The nurse places a hospitalized client with active tuberculosis in a private, well-ventilated isolation room. In addition, which critical action(s) should the nurse take before entering the client's room?
1 Wash the hands.
2 Wash the hands and wear a gown and gloves.
3 Wash the hands and place a high-efficiency particulate air (HEPA) respirator over the nose and mouth.
4 The nurse needs no special precautions, but the client is instructed to cover his or her mouth and nose when coughing or sneezing.

Level of Cognitive Ability: Application
Client Needs: Safe and Effective Care and Environment
Integrated Process: Nursing Process/ Implementation
Content Area: Adult Health/Respiratory

Answer: 3
Rationale: The nurse wears a HEPA respirator when caring for a client with active tuberculosis. Hands are always thoroughly washed before and after caring for the client. Option 1 is an incomplete action. Option 2 is also inaccurate and incomplete. Gowning is only indicated when there is a possibility of contaminating clothing. Option 4 is an incorrect statement because special precautions are needed.

Test-Taking Strategy: Use the process of elimination. Noting the client's diagnosis and recalling the need for respiratory precautions will direct you to option 3. Review these respiratory isolation precautions if you had difficulty with this question.

Reference
Ignatavicius, D., & Workman, M. (2006). *Medical-surgical nursing: Critical thinking for collaborative care* (5th ed., p. 644). Philadelphia: Saunders.

---

695. A nurse is assigned to care for a hospitalized toddler. The nurse plans care knowing that the highest priority should be directed toward:
1 Providing a consistent caregiver
2 Protecting the toddler from injury
3 Adapting the toddler to the hospital routine
4 Allowing the toddler to participate in play and diversional activities

Level of Cognitive Ability: Application
Client Needs: Safe and Effective Care Environment
Integrated Process: Nursing Process/Planning
Content Area: Child Health

Answer: 2
Rationale: The toddler is at high risk for injury as a result of developmental abilities and an unfamiliar environment. Whereas adaptation, diversion, and consistency are important, protection from injury is the highest priority.

Test Taking Strategy: Note the strategic words "highest priority." Use Maslow's Hierarchy of Needs theory. Physiological needs come first, followed by safety. Because no physiological needs are addressed, the safety option of preventing injury takes priority. Review care of the hospitalized toddler if you had difficulty with this question.

References
Hockenberry, M., Wilson, D., & Winkelstein, M. (2005). *Wong's essentials of pediatric nursing* (7th ed., pp. 641, 695). St. Louis: Mosby.
McKinney, E., James, S., Murray, S., & Ashwill, J. (2005). *Maternal-child nursing* (2nd ed., p. 890). St. Louis: Saunders.

---

696. A client is to undergo pleural biopsy at the bedside. Knowing the potential complications of the procedure, the nurse plans to have which of the following items available at the bedside?
1 Intubation tray
2 Morphine sulfate injection
3 Portable chest x-ray machine
4 Chest tube and drainage system

Answer: 4
Rationale: Complications following pleural biopsy include hemothorax, pneumothorax, and temporary pain from intercostal nerve injury. The nurse has a chest tube and drainage system available at the bedside for use if hemothorax or pneumothorax develops. An intubation tray is not indicated. The client should be premedicated before the procedure, or a local anesthetic is used. A portable chest x-ray machine would be called for to verify placement of a chest tube if one was inserted, but it is unnecessary to have at the bedside before the procedure.

Level of Cognitive Ability: Application
Client Needs: Safe and Effective Care
Environment
Integrated Process: Nursing Process/Planning
Content Area: Adult Health/Respiratory

Test-Taking Strategy: Note that the client is having a pleural biopsy. Recalling the complications of this procedure and noting the relation of this procedure to option 4 will direct you to this option. Review this procedure and its complications if you had difficulty with this question.

References
Black, J., & Hawks, J. (2005). *Medical-surgical nursing: Clinical management for positive outcomes* (7th ed., p. 1773). Philadelphia: Saunders.
Lewis, S., Heitkemper, M., Dirksen, S., O'Brien, P., & Bucher, L. (2007). *Medical-surgical nursing: Assessment and management of clinical problems* (7th ed., p. 588). St. Louis: Mosby.

---

697. The nurse manager of a hemodialysis unit is observing a new nurse preparing to begin hemodialysis on a client with renal failure. The nurse manager intervenes if the new nurse carries out which of the following actions?
1 Uses sterile technique for needle insertion
2 Wears full protective clothing such as goggles, mask, gown, and gloves
3 Covers the connection site with a bath blanket to enhance extremity warmth
4 Puts on a mask and gives one to the client to wear during connection to the machine

Level of Cognitive Ability: Application
Client Needs: Safe and Effective Care
Environment
Integrated Process: Nursing Process/
Implementation
Content Area: Adult Health/Renal

Answer: 3

Rationale: The connection site should not be covered, and it should be visible so that the nurse can assess for bleeding, ischemia, and infection at the site during the hemodialysis procedure. Infection is a major concern with hemodialysis. For that reason, the use of sterile technique and the application of a face mask for both the nurse and client are extremely important. It is also imperative that standard precautions be followed, which includes the use of goggles, mask, gloves, and a gown.

Test-Taking Strategy: Note the strategic word "intervenes." This strategic word indicates a negative event query and the need to select the option that indicates an incorrect nursing action. Eliminate options 1, 2, and 4 because they are comparable or alike in that they relate to infection control and standard precautions. Review the basic procedure related to hemodialysis if you had difficulty with this question.

References
Black, J., & Hawks, J. (2005). *Medical-surgical nursing: Clinical management for positive outcomes* (7th ed., pp. 958, 967). Philadelphia: Saunders.
Monahan, F., Sands, J., Neighbors, M., Marek, J., & Green, C. (2007). *Phipps', medical-surgical nursing: Health and illness perspectives* (8th ed., p. 1024). St. Louis: Mosby.

---

698. The nurse is going to suction an adult client with a tracheostomy who has copious amounts of respiratory secretions. The nurse does which of the following to perform this procedure safely?
1 Sets the suction pressure range between 160 to 180 mm Hg
2 Hyperoxygenates the client using a manual resuscitation bag
3 Applies continuous suction in the airway for up to 20 seconds
4 Occludes the Y-port of the suction catheter while advancing it into the tracheostomy

Answer: 2

Rationale: To perform suctioning, the nurse hyperoxygenates the client using a manual resuscitation bag or the sigh mechanism if the client is on a mechanical ventilator. The safe suction range for an adult is 100 to 120 mm Hg. The nurse advances the suction catheter into the tracheostomy without occluding the Y-port; suction is never applied while introducing the catheter, because it would traumatize mucosa and remove oxygen from the respiratory tract. The nurse uses intermittent suction in the airway for up to 10 to 15 seconds.

Level of Cognitive Ability: Application
Client Needs: Safe and Effective Care
  Environment
Integrated Process: Nursing Process/
  Implementation
Content Area: Adult Health/Respiratory

Test-Taking Strategy: Use the process of elimination and visualize this procedure. Recalling that suction is applied intermittently and on catheter withdrawal only will eliminate options 3 and 4. From the remaining options, use the ABCs—airway, breathing, and circulation—to direct you to option 2. Review this procedure if you had difficulty with this question.

References

Monahan, F., Sands, J., Neighbors, M., Marek, J., & Green, C. (2007). *Phipps', medical-surgical nursing: Health and illness perspectives* (8th ed., p. 703). St. Louis: Mosby.
Potter, P., & Perry, A. (2005). *Fundamentals of nursing* (6th ed., p. 1106). St. Louis: Mosby.

---

699. A nurse is collecting a sputum specimen for culture and sensitivity testing from a client who has a productive cough. The nurse plans to implement which intervention to obtain the specimen?
  1 Ask the client to obtain the specimen after breakfast.
  2 Use a sterile plastic container for obtaining the specimen.
  3 Provide tissues for expectoration and obtaining the specimen.
  4 Ask the client to expectorate a small amount of sputum into the emesis basin.

Level of Cognitive Ability: Application
Client Needs: Safe and Effective Care
  Environment
Integrated Process: Nursing Process/Planning
Content Area: Fundamental Skills

Answer: 2
Rationale: Sputum specimens for culture and sensitivity testing need to be obtained using sterile techniques, because the test is done to determine the presence of organisms. If the procedure for obtaining the specimen is not sterile, then the specimen would be contaminated and the results of the test would be invalid. A first morning specimen is preferred because it represents overnight secretions of the tracheobronchial tree.

Test-Taking Strategy: Note the strategic words "culture and sensitivity." This tells you that the test is being done to identify the presence of microorganisms. Recalling that microorganisms will multiply in the specimen and that accurate identification of organisms is needed to determine treatment will direct you to option 2. Also, noting the word "sterile" in option 2 will direct you to this option. Review the procedure for sputum collection if you had difficulty with this question.

Reference

Chernecky, C., & Berger, B. (2008). *Laboratory tests and diagnostic procedures* (5th ed., pp. 1034-1035). Philadelphia: Saunders.

---

700. The postmyocardial infarction client is scheduled for a technetium-99m ventriculography (multigated acquisition [MUGA] scan). The nurse ensures that which item is in place before the procedure?
  1 A Foley catheter
  2 Signed informed consent
  3 A central venous pressure (CVP) line
  4 Notation of allergies to iodine or shellfish

Level of Cognitive Ability: Application
Client Needs: Safe and Effective Care
  Environment
Integrated Process: Nursing Process/
  Implementation
Content Area: Adult Health/Cardiovascular

Answer: 2
Rationale: MUGA is a radionuclide study used to detect myocardial infarction, decreased myocardial blood flow, and left ventricular function. A radioisotope is injected intravenously. Therefore, a signed informed consent is necessary. A Foley catheter and CVP line are not required. The procedure does not use radiopaque dye; therefore allergy to iodine and shellfish is not a concern.

Test-Taking Strategy: Focus on the procedure. Recalling that the procedure involves injection of a radioisotope will direct you to option 2. Review preparation for this procedure if you had difficulty with this question.

References

Black, J., & Hawks, J. (2005). *Medical-surgical nursing: Clinical management for positive outcomes* (7th ed., pp. 1591-1592). Philadelphia: Saunders.
Ignatavicius, D., & Workman, M. (2006). *Medical-surgical nursing: Critical thinking for collaborative care* (5th ed., pp. 304-306, 755). Philadelphia: Saunders.

701. The nurse is developing a nursing care plan for a client with severe Alzheimer's disease. The nurse identifies which nursing diagnosis as the priority?
1 Risk for injury
2 Social isolation
3 Ineffective role performance
4 Impaired verbal communication

Level of Cognitive Ability: Analysis
Client Needs: Safe and Effective Care Environment
Integrated Process: Nursing Process/Analysis
Content Area: Adult Health/Neurological

Answer: 1
Rationale: Clients who have Alzheimer's disease have significant cognitive impairment and are therefore at risk for injury. It is critical for the nurse to maintain a safe environment, particularly as the client's judgment becomes increasingly impaired. Options 2, 3, and 4 may be appropriate, but the highest priority is directed toward safety.

Test-Taking Strategy: Use Maslow's Hierarchy of Needs theory. When a physiological need is not addressed, safety needs receive priority. This will direct you to option 1. Review care of the client with Alzheimer's disease if you had difficulty with this question.

References
Black, J., & Hawks, J. (2005). *Medical-surgical nursing: Clinical management for positive outcomes* (7th ed., pp. 2168-2169). Philadelphia: Saunders.
Monahan, F., Sands, J., Neighbors, M., Marek, J., & Green, C. (2007). *Phipps' medical-surgical nursing: Health and illness perspectives* (8th ed., pp. 26-27). St. Louis: Mosby.

---

702. A client with a diagnosis of recurrent major depression who is exhibiting psychotic behaviors is admitted to the psychiatric unit. In creating a safe environment for the client, the nurse most importantly develops a plan of care that deals specifically with the client's:
1 Disturbed thought processes
2 Bathing/hygiene self-care deficit
3 Knowledge deficient related to condition
4 Imbalanced nutrition: less than body requirements

Level of Cognitive Ability: Analysis
Client Needs: Safe and Effective Care Environment
Integrated Process: Nursing Process/Analysis
Content Area: Mental Health

Answer: 1
Rationale: Major depression, recurrent, with psychotic behaviors alerts the nurse that in addition to the criteria that designate the diagnosis of major depression, one must also deal with a client's psychosis. Psychosis is defined as a state in which a person's mental capacity to recognize reality and communicate and relate to others is impaired, thus interfering with the person's capacity to deal with life's demands. Disturbed thought processes generally indicate a state in which hallucinations and delusions prevail. Although options 2 and 4 are important, option 1 is specific to the client. Option 3 is not a priority at this time.

Test-Taking Strategy: Focus on the client's diagnosis and the strategic word "specifically." Recall that the client with psychotic behavior experiences disturbed thought processes, such as hallucinations and delusions, and that disturbed thought processes present a risk related to safety. Review care of the client with major depression and psychosis if you had difficulty with this question.

Reference
Varcarolis, E., Carson, V., & Shoemaker, N. (2006). *Foundations of psychiatric mental health nursing* (5th ed., pp. 396, 401, 403). Philadelphia: Saunders.

---

703. A client is being admitted to the hospital after receiving a radiation implant for cervical cancer. The nurse takes which priority action in the care of this client?
1 Encourages the family to visit
2 Admits the client to a private room
3 Places the client on reverse isolation
4 Encourages the client to take frequent rest periods

Answer: 2
Rationale: The client who has a radiation implant is placed in a private room and has limited visitors. This reduces the exposure of others to the radiation. Reverse isolation is unnecessary. Frequent rest periods are a helpful general intervention but are not a priority for the client in this situation.

Level of Cognitive Ability: Application
Client Needs: Safe and Effective Care Environment
Integrated Process: Nursing Process/ Implementation
Content Area: Adult Health/Oncology

Test-Taking Strategy: Note the strategic word "priority" and focus on the subject, radiation implant. Recalling the concepts related to environmental safety and that other individuals should have limited exposure to clients with radiation implants will direct you to option 2. Review care of the client with a radiation implant if you had difficulty with this question.

References
Black, J., & Hawks, J. (2005). *Medical-surgical nursing: Clinical management for positive outcomes* (7th ed., p. 363). Philadelphia: Saunders.
Monahan, F., Sands, J., Neighbors, M., Marek, J., & Green, C. (2007). *Phipps' medical-surgical nursing: Health and illness perspectives* (8th ed., p. 539). St. Louis: Mosby.

---

704. A client is to undergo weekly intravesical chemotherapy for bladder cancer for the next 8 weeks. The nurse interprets that the client understands how to manage the urine as a biohazard if the client states to:

1 Void into a bedpan and then empty the urine into the toilet.
2 Disinfect the urine and toilet with bleach for 6 hours following a treatment.
3 Purchase extra bottles of scented disinfectant for daily bathroom cleansing.
4 Have one bathroom strictly set aside for the client's use for the next 8 weeks.

Level of Cognitive Ability: Analysis
Client Needs: Safe and Effective Care Environment
Integrated Process: Nursing Process/Evaluation
Content Area: Adult Health/Oncology

Answer: 2
Rationale: After intravesical chemotherapy, the client treats the urine as a biohazard. This involves disinfecting the urine and the toilet with household bleach for 6 hours following a treatment. There is no value in using a bedpan for voiding. Scented disinfectants are of no particular use. The client does not need to have a separate bathroom for personal use.

Test-Taking Strategy: Use the process of elimination. Option 1 makes no sense and is eliminated first. Because scented disinfectants have no value, option 3 is eliminated next. Knowing that the urine and toilet need special treatment for 6 hours after each treatment directs you to option 2. Also, option 4 is unnecessary and may be unrealistic for many clients. Review care of the client receiving intravesical chemotherapy if you had difficulty with this question.

Reference
Black, J., & Hawks, J. (2005). *Medical-surgical nursing: Clinical management for positive outcomes* (7th ed., p. 871). Philadelphia: Saunders.

---

705. A male client who is admitted to the hospital for an unrelated medical problem is diagnosed with urethritis caused by chlamydial infection. The nursing assistant assigned to the client asks the nurse what measures are necessary to prevent contraction of the infection during care. The nurse tells the nursing assistant that:

1 Enteric precautions should be instituted for the client.
2 Gloves and mask should be used when in the client's room.
3 Contact isolation should be initiated, because the disease is highly contagious.
4 Standard precautions are sufficient, because the disease is transmitted sexually.

Answer: 4
Rationale: Chlamydia is a sexually transmitted disease. Caregivers cannot acquire the disease during administration of care, and standard precautions are the only measure that needs to be used.

Test-Taking Strategy: Use the process of elimination. Recall that this infection is sexually transmitted. Also, note that option 4 is the umbrella option. Review transmission of this disorder and standard precautions if you had difficulty with this question.

Level of Cognitive Ability: Application
Client Needs: Safe and Effective Care
  Environment
Integrated Process: Teaching and Learning
Content Area: Leadership/Management

References
Black, J., & Hawks, J. (2005). *Medical-surgical nursing: Clinical management for positive outcomes* (7th ed., p. 1131). Philadelphia: Saunders.
Lewis, S., Heitkemper, M., Dirksen, S., O'Brien, P., & Bucher, L. (2007). *Medical-surgical nursing: Assessment and management of clinical problems* (7th ed., pp. 1162-1163). St. Louis: Mosby.
Potter, P., & Perry, A. (2005). *Fundamentals of nursing* (6th ed., p. 797). St. Louis: Mosby.

706. A client is in extreme pain from scrotal swelling that is caused by epididymitis. The nurse administers a subcutaneous opioid analgesic in the left arm to relieve the pain. After administering the subcutaneous injection, the nurse takes which action next?
  1 Dims the lights in the room
  2 Puts the side rails up on the bed
  3 Checks the name bracelet of the client
  4 Tells the client to do range-of-motion (ROM) exercises with the left arm to absorb the medication into the bloodstream

Level of Cognitive Ability: Application
Client Needs: Safe and Effective Care
  Environment
Integrated Process: Nursing Process/
  Implementation
Content Area: Pharmacology

Answer: 2
Rationale: The client who receives an opioid analgesic should immediately have the side rails raised on the bed to prevent injury once the medication has taken effect. Dimming the light in the room is the next helpful action. The name bracelet should have been checked before administering the medication. It is unnecessary to do ROM exercises at the site of injection.

Test-Taking Strategy: Use the process of elimination. Eliminate option 3 first because this should have been done before administering the medication. Option 4 is not necessary and is eliminated next. From the remaining options, note the strategic word "next" to direct you to option 2. As part of protecting the client's safety after administration of an opioid analgesic, the nurse puts the side rails up. Review nursing interventions when administering an opioid analgesic if you had difficulty with this question.

Reference
Kee, J., Hayes, E., & McCuistion, L. (2006). *Pharmacology: A nursing process approach* (5th ed., pp. 334-335). Philadelphia: Saunders.

707. A nurse is preparing the client's morning NPH insulin dose and notices a clumpy precipitate inside the insulin vial. The nurse should:
  1 Draw the dose from a new vial.
  2 Draw up and administer the dose.
  3 Shake the vial in an attempt to disperse the clumps.
  4 Warm the bottle under running water to dissolve the clump.

Level of Cognitive Ability: Application
Client Needs: Safe and Effective Care
  Environment
Integrated Process: Nursing Process/
  Implementation
Content Area: Pharmacology

Answer: 1
Rationale: The nurse should always inspect the vial of insulin before use for solution changes that may signify loss of potency. NPH insulin is normally uniformly cloudy. Clumping, frosting, and precipitates are signs of insulin damage. In this situation, because potency is questionable, it is safer to discard the vial and draw up the dose from a new vial.

Test-Taking Strategy: Remember that NPH insulin is cloudy but not clumpy. This will direct you to option 1, the safest action. Remember that when in doubt, throw it out. Review the characteristics of NPH insulin if you had difficulty with this question.

References
Hodgson, B., & Kizior, R. (2007). *Saunders nursing drug handbook 2007.* (p. 621). Philadelphia: Saunders.
Lehne, R. (2007). *Pharmacology for nursing care.* (6th ed., pp. 604, 616). St. Louis: Saunders.

708. The nurse is preparing the bedside for a postoperative parathyroidectomy client who is expected to return to the nursing unit from the recovery room in 1 hour. The nurse ensures that which piece of medical equipment is at the client's bedside?
1 Cardiac monitor
2 Tracheotomy set
3 Intermittent gastric suction
4 Underwater seal chest drainage system

Level of Cognitive Ability: Application
Client Needs: Safe and Effective Care Environment
Integrated Process: Nursing Process/Planning
Content Area: Adult Health/Endocrine

Answer: 2
Rationale: Respiratory distress caused by hemorrhage and swelling and compression of the trachea is a primary concern for the nurse managing the care of a postoperative parathyroidectomy client. An emergency tracheotomy set is always routinely placed at the bedside of the client with this type of surgery, in anticipation of this potential complication. Options 1, 3, and 4 are not specifically needed with the surgical procedure.

Test-Taking Strategy: Use the process of elimination. Think about the location of the surgical incision and what potential problems might occur from that location. This will direct you to option 2. Review postoperative care following parathyroidectomy if you had difficulty with this question.

Reference
Ignatavicius, D., & Workman, M. (2006). *Medical-surgical nursing: Critical thinking for collaborative care* (5th ed., p. 1487). Philadelphia: Saunders.

---

709. The nurse has an order to administer foscarnet sodium (Foscavir) intravenously to a client with acquired immunodeficiency syndrome (AIDS). Before administering this medication, the nurse plans to:
1 Obtain a sputum culture.
2 Obtain folic acid (Folvite) as an antidote.
3 Place the solution on a controlled infusion pump.
4 Ensure that liver enzyme levels have been drawn as a baseline.

Level of Cognitive Ability: Application
Client Needs: Safe and Effective Care Environment
Integrated Process: Nursing Process/Planning
Content Area: Adult Health/Immune

Answer: 3
Rationale: Foscarnet sodium is an antiviral agent used to treat cytomegalovirus (CMV) retinitis in clients with AIDS. Because of the potential toxicity of the medication, it is administered with the use of a controlled infusion device. A sputum culture is not necessary. Folic acid is not an antidote. It is highly toxic to the kidneys, and serum creatinine levels are measured frequently during therapy.

Test-Taking Strategy: Use the process of elimination. Eliminate option 1 because the medication is usually indicated in the treatment of CMV retinitis, not respiratory infection. Additionally, no data in the question indicate the need for a sputum culture. Option 2 is eliminated next, because folic acid is not an antidote. From the remaining options, it is necessary to know that the medication can be toxic and cannot be infused too quickly. This will direct you to option 3. Also, recalling that the medication is toxic to the kidneys, not the liver, will direct you to the correct option. Review this medication if you had difficulty with this question.

References
Gahart, B., & Nazareno, A. (2006). *2006 Intravenous medications* (22nd ed., p. 580). St. Louis: Mosby.
Hodgson, B., & Kizior, R. (2007). *Saunders nursing drug handbook 2007.* (p. 515). Philadelphia: Saunders.

710. A client who is 40 years old has a severe mental impairment and is scheduled for gallbladder surgery. Which should the nurse implement about the informed consent first to facilitate the scheduled surgery?
1 Check for the identity of the client's legal guardian.
2 Inform the legal guardian about advanced directives.
3 Arrange for the surgeon to provide informed consent.
4 Ensure that the legal guardian signed the informed consent.

Level of Cognitive Ability: Application
Client Needs: Safe and Effective Care Environment
Integrated Process: Nursing Process/ Implementation
Content Area: Fundamental Skills

Answer: 1
Rationale: The client is not competent to sign an informed consent, so the nurse verifies the identity of the client's legal guardian to fulfill part of the nurse's duty in informed consent. This helps avoid improperly signed documents and to direct the surgeon to the legal representatives of the client's interests. Most states require client notification of advanced directives at admission.

Test-Taking Strategy: Note the strategic word "first" and focus on the subject, obtaining permission for the surgical procedure for a client who is "mentally impaired." To ensure safe, effective care, the nurse ensures the identity of the client's legal guardian before checking any other aspect of obtaining informed consent. Review the process of informed consent if you had difficulty with this question.

References
Ignatavicius, D., & Workman, M. (2006). *Medical-surgical nursing: Critical thinking for collaborative care* (5th ed., pp. 304, 857). Philadelphia: Saunders.
Potter, P., & Perry, A. (2005). *Fundamentals of nursing* (6th ed., pp. 416-417). St. Louis: Mosby.

---

711. A client with an acute respiratory infection is admitted to the hospital with a diagnosis of sinus tachycardia. The nurse develops a plan of care for the client and includes which intervention?
1 Limiting oral and intravenous fluids
2 Measuring the client's pulse once each shift
3 Providing the client with short, frequent walks
4 Eliminating sources of caffeine from meal trays

Level of Cognitive Ability: Application
Client Needs: Safe and Effective Care Environment
Integrated Process: Nursing Process/Planning
Content Area: Adult Health/Cardiovascular

Answer: 4
Rationale: Sinus tachycardia is often caused by fever, physical and emotional stress, heart failure, hypovolemia, certain medications, nicotine, caffeine, and exercise. Measuring the client's pulse during each shift will not decrease the heart rate. Additionally, the pulse should be taken more frequently than once each shift. Exercise and fluid restriction will not alleviate tachycardia.

Test-Taking Strategy: Use the process of elimination, focusing on the client's diagnosis. Recalling the causes of tachycardia will direct you to option 4. Remember that caffeine is a stimulant and will increase the heart rate. Review care of the client with tachycardia if you had difficulty with this question.

References
Black, J., & Hawks, J. (2005). *Medical-surgical nursing: Clinical management for positive outcomes* (7th ed., pp. 1557, 1570). Philadelphia: Saunders.
Ignatavicius, D., & Workman, M. (2006). *Medical-surgical nursing: Critical thinking for collaborative care* (5th ed., p. 720). Philadelphia: Saunders.

---

712. Which action does the nurse implement to obtain a urine specimen for a urinalysis from a female client with an indwelling urinary catheter?
1 Detach the tubing of the drainage bag.
2 Use a sterile container for the specimen.
3 Cleanse the perineum from front to back.
4 Aspirate the urine from the drainage bag port.

Answer: 4
Rationale: A specimen for urinalysis does not need to be sterile; however, the system must remain sterile to reduce the risk of infection. Therefore, the nurse obtains the specimen using sterile technique and obtains a fresh specimen by aspirating urine from the drainage bag port after sanitizing the port and inserting a sterile needle. The nurse avoids breaking the integrity of the urinary collection system to prevent contamination. The nurse also avoids taking urine from the urinary drainage bag because the urine is less likely to reflect the current client status and because urine undergoes chemical changes and particulate matter settles over time. A sterile container is unnecessary for a urinalysis, and, because the client has an indwelling catheter, perineal cleansing before obtaining a urine specimen is unnecessary.

Level of Cognitive Ability: Application
Client Needs: Safe and Effective Care Environment
Integrated Process: Nursing Process/ Implementation
Content Area: Fundamental Skills

Test-Taking Strategy: Use the process of elimination, focusing on the subject of obtaining a urine specimen for urinalysis. Basic principles of asepsis direct you to eliminate options 1 and 2. Eliminate option 3 because the client has an indwelling catheter. Review this procedure if you had difficulty with this question.

References

Ignatavicius, D., & Workman, M. (2006). *Medical-surgical nursing: Critical thinking for collaborative care* (5th ed., pp. 1666-1667). Philadelphia: Saunders.
Potter, P., & Perry, A. (2005). *Fundamentals of nursing* (6th ed., pp. 1356-1357). St. Louis: Mosby.

---

713. A nursing assistant is caring for an older male client with cystitis who has an indwelling urinary catheter. The registered nurse provides directions regarding urinary catheter care and ensures that the nursing assistant:

1 Loops the tubing under the client's leg
2 Places the tubing below the client's knee
3 Uses soap and water to cleanse the perineal area
4 Keeps the drainage bag above the level of the bladder

Level of Cognitive Ability: Application
Client Needs: Safe and Effective Care Environment
Integrated Process: Teaching and Learning
Content Area: Leadership/Management

Answer: 3

Rationale: Proper care of an indwelling urinary catheter is especially important to prevent prolonged infection or reinfection in the client with cystitis. The perineal area is cleansed thoroughly using mild soap and water at least twice a day and following a bowel movement. The drainage bag is kept below the level of the bladder to prevent urine from being trapped in the bladder, and, for the same reason, the drainage tubing is not placed or looped under the client's leg. The tubing must drain freely at all times.

Test-Taking Strategy: Use the process of elimination. Eliminate options 1 and 2 first because they are comparable or alike. From the remaining options, noting the word "above" in option 4 will assist in eliminating this option. Also, note that option 3 relates to preventing infection. Review care of the client with an indwelling urinary catheter if you had difficulty with this question.

References

Monahan, F., Sands, J., Neighbors, M., Marek, J., & Green, C. (2007). *Phipps' medical-surgical nursing: Health and illness perspectives* (8th ed., pp. 998-999). St. Louis: Mosby.
Potter, P., & Perry, A. (2005). *Fundamentals of nursing* (6th ed., p. 1349). St. Louis: Mosby.

---

714. A nurse is assigned to care for a client with preeclampsia. The nurse plans to initiate which action to provide a safe environment?

1 Maintain fluid and sodium restrictions.
2 Take the client's vital signs every 4 hours.
3 Turn off the room lights and draw the window shades.
4 Encourage visits from family and friends for psychosocial support.

Answer: 3

Rationale: Clients with preeclampsia are at risk of developing eclampsia (seizures). Bright lights and sudden loud noises may initiate seizures in this client. A woman with preeclampsia should be placed in a dimly lighted, quiet, private room. Visitors should be limited to allow for rest and to prevent overstimulation. Clients with preeclampsia have decreased plasma volume, and adequate fluid and sodium intake is necessary to maintain fluid volume and tissue perfusion. Vital signs need to be monitored more frequently than every 4 hours when preeclampsia is present.

Level of Cognitive Ability: Application
Client Needs: Safe and Effective Care Environment
Integrated Process: Nursing Process/Planning
Content Area: Maternity/Antepartum

Test-Taking Strategy: Use the process of elimination. Eliminate option 4 because it is not a physiological need. Eliminate option 2 next because vital signs need to be monitored more frequently than every 4 hours. From the remaining options, knowing that seizures may be precipitated by sudden loud noises and bright lights will assist in directing you to option 3. Review care of the client with preeclampsia if you had difficulty with this question.

Reference
Wong, D., Hockenberry, M., Perry, S., Lowdermilk, D., & Wilson, D. (2006). *Maternal-child nursing care* (3rd ed., p. 382). St. Louis: Mosby.

---

715. A client is scheduled for a bronchoscopy. The nurse plans to implement which priority measure?

1 Asking the client about allergies to shellfish
2 Obtaining informed consent for an invasive procedure
3 Restricting the diet to clear liquids on the day of the test
4 Administration of preprocedure antibiotics prophylactically

Level of Cognitive Ability: Application
Client Needs: Safe and Effective Care Environment
Integrated Process: Nursing Process/Planning
Content Area: Adult Health/Respiratory

Answer: 2
Rationale: Bronchoscopy requires that informed consent be obtained from the client before the procedure. It is unnecessary to inquire about allergies to shellfish before this procedure, because contrast dye is not injected. The client is kept NPO for at least 6 hours before the procedure. There is also no need for prophylactic antibiotics.

Test-Taking Strategy: Use the process of elimination. Recalling that bronchoscopy is an invasive procedure and requires an informed consent will direct you to option 2. Review preprocedure preparation for bronchoscopy if you had difficulty with this question.

References
Chernecky, C., & Berger, B. (2008). *Laboratory tests and diagnostic procedures* (5th ed., p. 262). Philadelphia: Saunders.
Lewis, S., Heitkemper, M., Dirksen, S., O'Brien, P., & Bucher, L. (2007). *Medical-surgical nursing: Assessment and management of clinical problems* (7th ed., p. 528). St. Louis: Mosby.

---

716. The nurse has given a subcutaneous injection to a client with acquired immunodeficiency syndrome (AIDS). The nurse disposes of the used needle and syringe by:

1 Breaking the needle before discarding it
2 Recapping the needle and discarding the syringe in a disposal unit
3 Placing the uncapped needle and syringe in a labeled cardboard box
4 Placing the uncapped needle and syringe in a labeled, rigid plastic container

Level of Cognitive Ability: Application
Client Needs: Safe and Effective Care Environment
Integrated Process: Nursing Process/Implementation
Content Area: Fundamental Skills

Answer: 4
Rationale: Standard precautions include specific guidelines for handling of needles. Needles should not be recapped, bent, broken, or cut after use. They should be disposed of in a labeled, impermeable container specific for this purpose. Needles should not be discarded in cardboard boxes, because these types of boxes are not impervious. Needles should never be left lying around after use.

Test-Taking Strategy: Use the process of elimination and focus on the guidelines related to standard precautions. Recalling that a needle should never be recapped or broken will eliminate options 1 and 2. From the remaining options, noting the strategic words "rigid plastic container" in option 4 will direct you to this option. Review the principles related to needle disposal if you had difficulty with this question.

Reference
Potter, P., & Perry, A. (2005). *Fundamentals of nursing* (6th ed., pp. 891-892). St. Louis: Mosby.

717. A nurse is planning care for a client with acute glomerulonephritis. The nurse instructs the nursing assistant to do which of the following in the care of the client?

1 Ambulate the client frequently.
2 Encourage a diet that is high in protein.
3 Monitor the temperature every 2 hours.
4 Remove the water pitcher from the bedside.

Level of Cognitive Ability: Application
Client Needs: Safe and Effective Care Environment
Integrated Process: Teaching and Learning
Content Area: Leadership/Management

Answer: 4

Rationale: A client with acute glomerulonephritis commonly experiences fluid volume excess and fatigue. Interventions include fluid restriction as well as monitoring weight and intake and output. The client may be placed on bed rest or at least encouraged to rest, because a direct correlation exists between proteinuria, hematuria, edema, and increased activity levels. The diet is high in calories but low in protein. It is unnecessary to monitor the temperature as frequently as every 2 hours.

Test-Taking Strategy: Use the process of elimination. Knowing that the client needs rest eliminates option 1. The question provides no information about the client's actual temperature, so option 3 is eliminated next. From the remaining options, it is necessary to know either that fluid is restricted or that protein is limited. Review interventions related to this condition if you had difficulty with this question.

References
Black, J., & Hawks, J. (2005). *Medical-surgical nursing: Clinical management for positive outcomes* (7th ed., pp. 926, 930). Philadelphia: Saunders.
Ignatavicius, D., & Workman, M. (2006). *Medical-surgical nursing: Critical thinking for collaborative care* (5th ed., pp. 1718-1719). Philadelphia: Saunders.

---

718. The nurse is caring for a client with a C-6 spinal cord injury during the spinal shock phase. The nurse implements which of the following when preparing the client to sit in a chair?

1 Applies knee splints to stabilize the joints during transfer
2 Teaches the client to lock the knees during the pivoting stage of the transfer
3 Administers a vasodilator in order to improve circulation of the lower limbs
4 Raises the head of the bed slowly to decrease orthostatic hypotensive episodes

Level of Cognitive Ability: Application
Client Needs: Safe and Effective Care Environment
Integrated Process: Nursing Process/ Implementation
Content Area: Adult Health/Neurological

Answer: 4

Rationale: Spinal shock is often accompanied by vasodilation in the lower limbs, which results in a fall in blood pressure upon rising. The client can have dizziness and feel faint. The nurse should provide for a gradual progression in head elevation while monitoring the blood pressure. A vasodilator would exacerbate the problem. Clients with cervical cord injuries cannot lock their knees, and the use of splints would impair the transfer.

Test-Taking Strategy: Use the process of elimination. Focusing on the client's diagnosis will assist in eliminating options 1 and 2. From the remaining options, recalling that spinal shock is accompanied by vasodilation will direct you to option 4. Review care of the client with spinal shock if you had difficulty with this question.

Reference
Ignatavicius, D., & Workman, M. (2006). *Medical-surgical nursing: Critical thinking for collaborative care* (5th ed., p. 987). Philadelphia: Saunders.

---

719. A nurse notes that a client's lithium level is 3.9 mEq/L. The nurse implements which priority intervention?

1 Determining visual acuity
2 Assisting with ambulation
3 Monitoring intake and output
4 Instituting seizure precautions

Answer: 4

Rationale: A therapeutic regimen is designed to attain a serum lithium level of 1.0 to 1.5 mEq/L during acute mania, and levels of 0.6 to 1.4 mEq/L for maintenance treatment. A level of 3.9 mEq/L is in the toxic range, and seizures may occur at levels of 3.5 mEq/L and higher. Options 1, 2, and 3 are appropriate interventions but are not the priority.

Level of Cognitive Ability: Application
Client Needs: Safe and Effective Care
  Environment
Integrated Process: Nursing Process/
  Implementation
Content Area: Pharmacology

Test-Taking Strategy: Use the process of elimination. Focusing on the word "priority" and recalling the manifestations that occur in a toxic level will direct you to option 4. Review toxicity related to lithium and the manifestations that occur as a result of toxicity if you had difficulty with this question.

Reference
Skidmore-Roth, L. (2008). *Mosby's nursing drug reference* (21st ed., p. 621). St. Louis: Mosby.

---

720. A hospitalized child develops exanthema (rash) that covers the trunk and the extremities. The nurse reviews the child's health history and notes that the child was exposed to varicella 2 weeks ago. The appropriate nursing intervention is to:
  1 Immediately admit the client to any available bed.
  2 Place the child in a private room on strict isolation.
  3 Assess the progression of the exanthema and report it to the physician.
  4 Allow the child to play in the playroom until the physician can be contacted.

Level of Cognitive Ability: Application
Client Needs: Safe and Effective Care
  Environment
Integrated Process: Nursing Process/
  Implementation
Content Area: Child Health

Answer: 2
Rationale: The child with undiagnosed exanthema needs to be placed on strict isolation. Varicella causes a profuse rash on the trunk with a sparse rash on the extremities. The incubation period is 14 to 21 days. It is important to prevent the spread of this communicable disease by placing the child in isolation until further diagnosis and treatment are made. Options 1 and 4 are inaccurate, and option 3 is not the most appropriate intervention.

Test-Taking Strategy: Use the process of elimination. Noting the strategic words "exposed to varicella" will direct you to option 2. This action will prevent exposure of this communicable disease to others. Review care of the child with varicella if you had difficulty with this question.

Reference
Hockenberry, M., Wilson, D., & Winkelstein, M. (2005). *Wong's essentials of pediatric nursing* (7th ed., p. 437). St. Louis: Mosby.

---

721. A nurse watches a second nurse performing hemodialysis on a client. The second nurse is drinking coffee and eating a doughnut next to the hemodialysis machine while talking with the client about the client's week. The first nurse should:
  1 Get a cup of coffee and join in on the conversation.
  2 Determine whether or not the client would like a cup of coffee.
  3 Admire the therapeutic relationship the second nurse has with the client.
  4 Ask the second nurse to refrain from eating and drinking in the client area.

Level of Cognitive Ability: Application
Client Needs: Safe and Effective Care
  Environment
Integrated Process: Nursing Process/
  Implementation
Content Area: Leadership/Management

Answer: 4
Rationale: A potential complication of hemodialysis is the acquisition of dialysis-associated hepatitis B. This is a concern for clients (who may carry the virus), client families (at risk from contact with the client and with environmental surfaces), and staff (who may acquire the virus from contact with the client's blood). This risk is minimized by the use of standard precautions, appropriate handwashing and sterilization procedures, and the prohibition of eating, drinking, or other hand-to-mouth activity in the hemodialysis unit. The first nurse should ask the second nurse to stop eating and drinking in the client area.

Test-Taking Strategy: Use the process of elimination and the principles related to standard precautions to direct you to option 4. Review infection control measures related to the client receiving hemodialysis if you had difficulty with this question.

References
Black, J., & Hawks, J. (2005). *Medical-surgical nursing: Clinical management for positive outcomes* (7th ed., pp. 959, 967). Philadelphia: Saunders.
Ignatavicius, D., & Workman, M. (2006). *Medical-surgical nursing: Critical thinking for collaborative care* (5th ed., pp. 756-757). Philadelphia: Saunders.

722. A nurse is caring for a client who is going to have an arthrogram using a contrast medium. Which preprocedure assessment would be of highest priority?
1 Allergy to iodine or shellfish
2 Whether the client wishes to void before the procedure
3 Ability of the client to remain still during the procedure
4 Whether the client has any remaining questions about the procedure

Level of Cognitive Ability: Analysis
Client Needs: Safe and Effective Care Environment
Integrated Process: Nursing Process/Assessment
Content Area: Delegating/Prioritizing

Answer: 1
Rationale: Because of the risk associated with allergy to contrast medium, the nurse places highest priority on assessing whether the client has an allergy to iodine or shellfish. The nurse also reinforces information about the test, tells the client about the need to remain still during the procedure, and encourages the client to void before the procedure for comfort.

Test-Taking Strategy: Note the strategic words "highest priority." This tells you that more than one or all of the options are correct. Although options 2, 3, and 4 all compete for priority, only option 1 could present a life-threatening situation. Review priority assessments of a client receiving a contrast medium if you had difficulty with this question.

References
Chernecky, C., & Berger, B. (2008). *Laboratory tests and diagnostic procedures* (5th ed., p. 169). Philadelphia: Saunders.
Pagana, K., & Pagana, T. (2005). *Mosby's diagnostic and laboratory test reference* (7th ed., p. 137). St. Louis: Mosby.

---

723. A client with a possible rib fracture has never had a chest x-ray. The nurse plans to tell the client which of the following about the procedure?
1 The x-ray stimulates a small amount of pain.
2 The x-ray technologist will stand next to the client during the x-ray.
3 The client will be asked to breathe in and out continuously during the x-ray.
4 It is necessary to remove jewelry and any other metal objects from the chest area.

Level of Cognitive Ability: Application
Client Needs: Safe and Effective Care Environment
Integrated Process: Nursing Process/ Implementation
Content Area: Adult Health/Musculoskeletal

Answer: 4
Rationale: An x-ray is a photographic image of a part of the body on a special film, which is used to diagnose a wide variety of conditions. Any radiopaque objects such as jewelry or other metal must be removed from the chest area because they will interfere with the interpretation of the results. The x-ray is painless, and any discomfort would arise from repositioning a painful part for filming. The nurse may premedicate a client, if prescribed, who is at risk for pain. The client is asked to breathe in deeply and then hold the breath while the chest x-ray is taken. To minimize the risk of radiation exposure, the x-ray technologist stands in a separate area protected by a lead wall. The client also wears a lead shield over the reproductive organs.

Test-Taking Strategy: Note the name of the diagnostic procedure and the relation between the procedure and option 4. Remember that any radiopaque objects such as jewelry or other metal must be removed from the chest area because they will interfere with the interpretation of the chest x-ray results. Review the procedure for a chest x-ray if you had difficulty with this question.

References
Chernecky, C., & Berger, B. (2008). *Laboratory tests and diagnostic procedures* (5th ed., pp. 328-329). Philadelphia: Saunders.
Lewis, S., Heitkemper, M., Dirksen, S., O'Brien, P., & Bucher, L. (2007). *Medical-surgical nursing: Assessment and management of clinical problems* (7th ed., p. 527). St. Louis: Mosby.

724. The nurse is planning a discharge teaching plan for a client with a spinal cord injury. To provide for a safe environment regarding home care, which of the following would be the priority in the discharge teaching plan?

1 What the physician has indicated needs to be taught
2 Assisting the client to deal with long-term care placement
3 Follow-up laboratory and diagnostic tests that need to be done
4 Including the client's significant others in the teaching session

Level of Cognitive Ability: Application
Client Needs: Safe and Effective Care Environment
Integrated Process: Teaching and Learning
Content Area: Adult Health/Neurological

Answer: 4
Rationale: Involving the client's significant others in discharge teaching is a priority in planning for the client with a spinal cord injury. The client will need the support of the significant others. Knowledge and understanding of what to expect will help both the client and significant others deal with the client's limitations. A physician's order is not necessary for discharge planning and teaching; this is an independent nursing action. Long-term placement is not the only option for a client with a spinal cord injury. Laboratory and diagnostic testing are not priority discharge instructions for this client.

Test-Taking Strategy: Use the process of elimination. Eliminate option 2 first because long-term placement is not the only option for a client with a spinal cord injury. Eliminate option 1 next, because, although the physician's orders need to be addressed, teaching is an independent nursing action. From the remaining options, focusing on the client's diagnosis will direct you to option 4. Remember that home care and support will be needed. Review care of the client with a spinal cord injury if you had difficulty with this question.

Reference
Ignatavicius, D., & Workman, M. (2006). *Medical-surgical nursing: Critical thinking for collaborative care* (5th ed., p. 995). Philadelphia: Saunders.

725. A nurse observes a client wringing her hands and looking frightened. The client reports to the nurse that she "feels out of control." Which approach by the nurse is most appropriate to maintain a safe environment?

1 Administer a prn antianxiety medication immediately.
2 Move the client to a quiet room and talk about her feelings.
3 Provide isolation for the client in the unit's "time-out" room.
4 Observe the client in an ongoing manner but do not intervene.

Level of Cognitive Ability: Application
Client Needs: Safe and Effective Care Environment
Integrated Process: Nursing Process/Implementation
Content Area: Mental Health

Answer: 2
Rationale: The anxiety symptoms demonstrated by this client require some form of intervention. Moving the client to a quiet room decreases environmental stimulus. Talking provides the nurse an opportunity to assess the cause of the client's feelings and to identify appropriate interventions. Isolation is appropriate if a client is a danger to self or others. Medication is used only when other noninvasive approaches have been unsuccessful.

Test-Taking Strategy: Use therapeutic communication techniques. Option 2 is the only option that addresses the client's feelings. Remember that a client's feelings are most important. Review therapeutic communication techniques if you had difficulty with this question.

References
Black, J., & Hawks, J. (2005). *Medical-surgical nursing: Clinical management for positive outcomes* (7th ed., p. 526). Philadelphia: Saunders.
Varcarolis, E., Carson, V., & Shoemaker, N. (2006). *Foundations of psychiatric mental health nursing* (5th ed., pp. 216-217). Philadelphia: Saunders.

726. A client with urolithiasis is scheduled for extracorporeal shock wave lithotripsy. The nurse ensures that the client understands the procedure and tells the client that:
1 There is no pain at all involved with this procedure.
2 He will be anesthetized and placed on a water cushion.
3 There are no side effects or complications associated with this procedure.
4 The procedure involves breaking up the stone by a vibrating needle that is inserted into the urinary tract.

Level of Cognitive Ability: Application
Client Needs: Safe and Effective Care Environment
Integrated Process: Nursing Process/ Implementation
Content Area: Adult Health/Renal

Answer: 2
Rationale: In extracorporeal shock wave lithotripsy, a noninvasive procedure, the client is anesthetized (spinal or general) and placed on a water cushion. Anesthesia is necessary to keep the client very still during the procedure. Shock waves are administered that shatter the stone without damaging the surrounding tissues. The stone is broken into fine sand, which is secreted into the client's urine within a few days after the procedure. Hematuria is common after the procedure. The presence of clots in the urine needs to be reported to the physician. Clots could indicate a complication such as a hematoma.

Test-Taking Strategy: Use the process of elimination. Eliminate options 1 and 3 first because of the close-ended word "no" in these options. From the remaining options, recalling that the procedure is noninvasive and is done via shock waves (not a vibrating needle) will direct you to option 2. Review this procedure if you had difficulty with this question.

References
Ignatavicius, D., & Workman, M. (2006). *Medical-surgical nursing: Critical thinking for collaborative care* (5th ed., p. 1699). Philadelphia: Saunders.
Monahan, F., Sands, J., Neighbors, M., Marek, J., & Green, C. (2007). *Phipps' medical-surgical nursing: Health and illness perspectives* (8th ed., p. 979). St. Louis: Mosby.

---

727. The nurse is assisting with cardiopulmonoary resuscitation and the physician is going to defibrillate the client. Of the following items, which is the only one that the nurse does not need to remove from the client just before the client is defibrillated?
1 Oxygen
2 Back board
3 Nitroglycerin patch
4 Pulse oximetry machine plugged into an electrical socket

Level of Cognitive Ability: Application
Client Needs: Safe and Effective Care Environment
Integrated Process: Nursing Process/ Implementation
Content Area: Adult Health/Cardiovascular

Answer: 2
Rationale: Flammable materials and metal devices or liquids (that are capable of carrying electricity) are removed from the client and bed before discharging the paddles of the defibrillator. The nitroglycerin patch may have a metallic backing and should be removed.

Test-Taking Strategy: Use the process of elimination. Note the strategic words "does not need to remove." Eliminate options 1 and 4 because they are comparable or alike. From the remaining options, recall that the back board is needed to resume cardiopulmonary resuscitation immediately if defibrillation is unsuccessful. Review procedures for defibrillation if you had difficulty with this question.

References
Black, J., & Hawks, J. (2005). *Medical-surgical nursing: Clinical management for positive outcomes* (7th ed., p. 1689). Philadelphia: Saunders.
Ignatavicius, D., & Workman, M. (2006). *Medical-surgical nursing: Critical thinking for collaborative care* (5th ed., p. 742). Philadelphia: Saunders.

728. A nurse is planning the discharge instructions from the emergency department for an adult client who is a victim of family violence. The nurse understands that the discharge plans must include:
   1 Instructions to call the police the next time the abuse occurs
   2 Exploration of the pros and cons of remaining with the abusive family member
   3 Specific information regarding "safe havens" or shelters in the client's neighborhood
   4 Specific information about available opportunities to enroll in local self-defense classes

Level of Cognitive Ability: Application
Client Needs: Safe and Effective Care Environment
Integrated Process: Nursing Process/Planning
Content Area: Mental Health

Answer: 3
Rationale: Any of the options might be included in the discharge plan at some point if long-term therapy or a long-term relationship with the nurse is established. The question refers to an emergency department setting. It is most important to assist victims of abuse with identifying a plan for how to remove self from harmful situations should they arise again. An abused person is usually reluctant to call the police. Teaching the victim to fight back (as in the use of self-defense) is not the best action when dealing with a violent person.

Test-Taking Strategy: Use Maslow's Hierarchy of Needs theory. Remember that if a physiological need is not present, then safety is the priority. This will direct you to option 3. Review care of the victim of abuse if you had difficulty with this question.

Reference
Stuart, G., & Laraia, M. (2005). *Principles and practice of psychiatric nursing* (8th ed., pp. 806, 812). St. Louis: Mosby.

---

729. During a code, a physician is about to defibrillate a client in ventricular fibrillation and says in a loud voice "CLEAR!" Which of the following should the nurse immediately perform?
   1 Shut off the mechanical ventilator.
   2 Shut off the intravenous infusion going into the client's arm.
   3 Place the conductive gel pads for defibrillation on the client's chest.
   4 Step away from the bed and make sure that all others have done the same.

Level of Cognitive Ability: Application
Client Needs: Safe and Effective Care Environment
Integrated Process: Nursing Process/ Implementation
Content Area: Adult Health/Cardiovascular

Answer: 4
Rationale: For the safety of all personnel, when the defibrillator paddles are being discharged, all personnel must stand back and be clear of all contact with the client or the client's bed. It is the primary responsibility of the person defibrillating to communicate the "clear" message loudly enough for all to hear and ensure their compliance. All personnel must immediately comply with this command. A ventilator is not in use during a code; rather an Ambu (resuscitation) bag is used. Shutting off the intravenous infusion has no useful purpose. The gel pads should have been placed on the client's chest before the defibrillator paddles were applied. Stepping back from the bed prevents the nurse or others from being defibrillated along with the client.

Test-Taking Strategy: Use the process of elimination, focusing on the subject—the procedure for defibrillation. Recalling the risks associated with this procedure and noting the word "CLEAR" in the question will direct you to option 4. Review the risks associated with this procedure if you had difficulty with this question.

Reference
Black, J., & Hawks, J. (2005). *Medical-surgical nursing: Clinical management for positive outcomes* (7th ed., p. 1689). Philadelphia: Saunders.

730. A client with chronic renal failure has an indwelling peritoneal catheter in the abdomen for peritoneal dialysis. While bathing, the client spills water on the abdominal dressing covering the abdomen. The nurse plans to immediately:
1 Change the dressing.
2 Reinforce the dressing.
3 Flush the peritoneal dialysis catheter.
4 Scrub the catheter with povidone-iodine.

Level of Cognitive Ability: Application
Client Needs: Safe and Effective Care Environment
Integrated Process: Nursing Process/Planning
Content Area: Adult Health/Renal

Answer: 1
Rationale: Clients with peritoneal dialysis catheters are at high risk for infection. A dressing that is wet is a conduit for bacteria to reach the catheter insertion site. The nurse ensures that the dressing is kept dry at all times. Reinforcing the dressing is not a safe practice to prevent infection in this circumstance. Flushing the catheter is not indicated. Scrubbing the catheter with povidone-iodine is done at the time of connection or disconnection of peritoneal dialysis.

Test-Taking Strategy: Focus on the subject—the dressing is wet. The correct option would focus on the dressing, not the catheter. Therefore, eliminate options 3 and 4. Knowing that it is better to change a wet dressing than reinforce it will direct you to option 1. Review care of the client with a peritoneal dialysis catheter if you had difficulty with this question.

Reference
Black, J., & Hawks, J. (2005). *Medical-surgical nursing: Clinical management for positive outcomes* (7th ed., pp. 958, 967). Philadelphia: Saunders.

731. A client is scheduled for elective cardioversion to treat chronic high-rate atrial fibrillation. The nurse determines that the client is not yet ready for the procedure after noting that the:
1 Client has received a dose of midazolam (Versed) intravenously.
2 Client's digoxin (Lanoxin) has been withheld for the last 48 hours.
3 Defibrillator has the synchronizer turned on and is set at 50 joules.
4 Client is wearing a nasal cannula delivering oxygen at 2 liters per minute.

Level of Cognitive Ability: Analysis
Client Needs: Safe and Effective Care Environment
Integrated Process: Nursing Process/Evaluation
Content Area: Adult Health/Cardiovascular

Answer: 4
Rationale: The client typically receives a dose of an intravenous sedative or antianxiety agent. Digoxin may be withheld for up to 48 hours before cardioversion because it increases ventricular irritability and may cause ventricular dysrhythmias post countershock. The defibrillator is switched to synchronizer mode to time the delivery of the electrical impulse to coincide with the QRS and avoid the T wave, which could cause ventricular fibrillation. Energy level is typically set at 50 to 100 joules. During the procedure, any oxygen is removed temporarily, because oxygen supports combustion, and a fire could result from electrical arcing.

Test-Taking Strategy: Use the process of elimination, noting the strategic words "not yet ready for the procedure." Think about the procedure and recall the concept related to oxygen combustion to direct you to option 4. Review this procedure if you had difficulty with this question.

References
Black, J., & Hawks, J. (2005). *Medical-surgical nursing: Clinical management for positive outcomes* (7th ed., p. 1678). Philadelphia: Saunders.
Ignatavicius, D., & Workman, M. (2006). *Medical-surgical nursing: Critical thinking for collaborative care* (5th ed., pp. 644, 741-742). Philadelphia: Saunders.

732. A nurse is planning activities for a depressed client who was just admitted to the hospital. The nurse plans to:

1 Provide an activity that is quiet and solitary in nature.

2 Plan nothing until the client asks to participate in the milieu.

3 Offer the client a menu of activities and insist that the client participate in all of them.

4 Provide a structured daily program of activities and encourage the client to participate.

Level of Cognitive Ability: Application
Client Needs: Safe and Effective Care Environment
Integrated Process: Nursing Process/Planning
Content Area: Mental Health

Answer: 4

Rationale: A depressed person is often withdrawn. Also, the person experiences difficulty concentrating, loss of interest or pleasure, low energy and fatigue, and feelings of worthlessness and poor self-esteem. The plan of care needs to provide stimulation in a structured environment. Options 1 and 2 are restrictive and offer little or no structure and stimulation. The nurse should not insist that a client participate in all activities.

Test-Taking Strategy: Use the process of elimination, focusing on the client's diagnosis. Eliminate option 3 first because of the word "insist" and the close-ended word "all." From the remaining options, noting the word "structured" in option 4 will direct you to this option. Review care of the client with depression if you had difficulty with this question.

Reference

Stuart, G., & Laraia, M. (2005). *Principles and practice of psychiatric nursing* (8th ed., p. 348). St. Louis: Mosby.

---

733. A client who is 85 years old had an open reduction with internal fixation (ORIF) for a hip fracture 4 days ago. Which does the nurse implement to provide safe, effective care?

1 Provide ice chips instead of drinking water.

2 Instruct the client to call for help before getting up.

3 Minimize opioid administration to prevent dizziness.

4 Tell the client to roll to the affected side first before getting up.

Level of Cognitive Ability: Application
Client Needs: Safe and Effective Care Environment
Integrated Process: Nursing Process/ Implementation
Content Area: Fundamental Skills

Answer: 2

Rationale: The nurse instructs the client to call for help before getting up because the client has multiple risk factors for falls, is of older age, has postoperative status, and is receiving opioid analgesia. Restricting fluid intake with ice chips is not indicated; besides, adequate hydration is important for maintaining cardiac output and renal function, for keeping respiratory secretions thin, and in preventing constipation. The nurse administers opioid analgesics as indicated and fulfills the nurse's duty owed to the client by acting to resolve pain. The nurse instructs the client to roll to the unaffected side to get up to prevent excessive stress on the fragile surgical wound.

Test-Taking Strategy: Focusing on the subject—preventing injury—will direct you to option 2. Restricting fluid, unresolved pain, and incomplete instructions prevent the nurse from fulfilling the duty owed to the client and prevent safe, effective care. Review measures to prevent injury if you had difficulty with this question.

References

Ignatavicius, D., & Workman, M. (2006). *Medical-surgical nursing: Critical thinking for collaborative care* (5th ed., pp. 1209-1215). Philadelphia: Saunders.

Meiner, S., & Leuckenotte, A. (2006). *Gerontologic nursing* (3rd ed., pp. 248-250). St. Louis: Mosby.

734. The nurse is assisting in the care of a client who is to be cardioverted. The nurse plans to set the monophasic defibrillator to which of the following starting energy range levels, depending on the specific physician order?
1 50 to 100 joules
2 150 to 200 joules
3 250 to 300 joules
4 350 to 400 joules

Level of Cognitive Ability: Application
Client Needs: Safe and Effective Care Environment
Integrated Process: Nursing Process/Planning
Content Area: Adult Health/Cardiovascular

Answer: 1
Rationale: When a client is cardioverted, the defibrillator is charged to the energy level ordered by the physician. Cardioversion is usually started at 50 to 100 joules. Options 2, 3, and 4 are incorrect and identify energy levels that are too high for cardioversion.

Test-Taking Strategy: Use the process of elimination. Remember that, in instances when cardioversion is used, an underlying cardiac rhythm needs to be converted to a better rhythm. So, lower voltages are used. Review this procedure if you had difficulty with this question.

References
Black, J., & Hawks, J. (2005). *Medical-surgical nursing: Clinical management for positive outcomes* (7th ed., p. 1678). Philadelphia: Saunders.
Lewis, S., Heitkemper, M., Dirksen, S., O'Brien, P., & Bucher, L. (2007). *Medical-surgical nursing: Assessment and management of clinical problems* (7th ed., p. 857). St. Louis: Mosby.

---

735. The nurse has an order to get the client out of bed to a chair on the first postoperative day following total knee replacement. The nurse plans to do which of the following to protect the knee joint?
1 Apply a compression dressing and put ice on the knee while sitting.
2 Obtain a walker to minimize weight-bearing by the client on the affected leg.
3 Lift the client to the bedside chair, leaving the continuous passive motion (CPM) machine in place.
4 Apply a knee immobilizer before getting the client up and elevate the client's surgical leg while sitting.

Level of Cognitive Ability: Application
Client Needs: Safe and Effective Care Environment
Integrated Process: Nursing Process/Planning
Content Area: Adult Health/Musculoskeletal

Answer: 4
Rationale: The nurse assists the client to get out of bed on the first postoperative day after putting a knee immobilizer on the affected joint to provide stability. The surgeon orders the weight-bearing limits on the affected leg. The leg is elevated while the client is sitting in the chair to minimize edema. Ice is not used unless prescribed. A compression dressing should already be in place on the wound. A CPM machine is used only while the client is in bed.

Test-Taking Strategy: Use the process of elimination. Note the relation between the subject "protect the knee joint" and "knee immobilizer" in option 4. Review postoperative care following total knee replacement if you had difficulty with this question.

References
Black, J., & Hawks, J. (2005). *Medical-surgical nursing: Clinical management for positive outcomes* (7th ed., p. 596). Philadelphia: Saunders.
Ignatavicius, D., & Workman, M. (2006). *Medical-surgical nursing: Critical thinking for collaborative care* (5th ed., p. 380). Philadelphia: Saunders.
Lewis, S., Heitkemper, M., Dirksen, S., O'Brien, P., & Bucher, L. (2007). *Medical-surgical nursing: Assessment and management of clinical problems* (7th ed., pp. 1640-1641). St. Louis: Mosby.

---

736. A client is admitted to the psychiatric unit following a suicide attempt by hanging. The nurse's most important aspect of care is to maintain client safety, and so the nurse plans to:
1 Assign a staff member who will remain with the client at all times.
2 Remove the client's personal clothing and replace them with a hospital gown.
3 Request that the client's peers arrange to remain with the client continuously.
4 Place the client in a seclusion room where all dangerous articles are removed.

Answer: 1
Rationale: Hanging is a serious suicide attempt. The plan of care must reflect the action that will promote the client's safety. Constant observation by a staff member is necessary. It is not a peer's responsibility to safeguard a client. Removing one's clothing does not maximize all possible safety strategies. Placing the client in seclusion further isolates the client.

Level of Cognitive Ability: Application
Client Needs: Safe and Effective Care
  Environment
Integrated Process: Nursing Process/Planning
Content Area: Mental Health

Test-Taking Strategy: Use the process of elimination, focusing on the subject—suicide attempt. Recalling that one-to-one supervision is necessary will direct you to option 1. Review suicide precautions if you had difficulty with this question.

References
Stuart, G., & Laraia, M. (2005). *Principles and practice of psychiatric nursing* (8th ed., p. 379). St. Louis: Mosby.
Varcarolis, E., Carson, V., & Shoemaker, N. (2006). *Foundations of psychiatric mental health nursing* (5th ed., p. 481). Philadelphia: Saunders.

---

737. A nurse receives a telephone call from a male client who states that he wants to kill himself and has a loaded gun on the table. The best nursing intervention is to:

1 Keep the client talking while encouraging him to ventilate his feelings.
2 Use therapeutic communication techniques, especially the reflection of feelings.
3 Tell the client that killing himself is not the way to deal with his problem.
4 Keep the client talking while another staff member contacts the police so that appropriate help can be sent.

Level of Cognitive Ability: Application
Client Needs: Safe and Effective Care
  Environment
Integrated Process: Nursing Process/
  Implementation
Content Area: Mental Health

Answer: 4
Rationale: In a crisis, the nurse must take an authoritative, active role to promote the client's safety. A loaded gun in the home of the client who says that he wants to kill himself is a crisis. The client's safety is of prime concern. Keeping the client on the phone and getting help to the client is the best intervention. Insisting on information may anger the client and he might hang up. Option 1 lacks the authoritative action stance of securing the client's safety. Using therapeutic communication techniques is important, but overuse of reflection may sound uncaring or superficial and is lacking direction and a solution to the immediate problem of the client's safety. Option 3 is not a helpful strategy and may block communication.

Test-Taking Strategy: Use the process of elimination and focus on the crisis—a potential for suicide. The only option that will provide direct help is option 4. Review crisis intervention for a client contemplating suicide if you had difficulty with this question.

References
Stuart, G., & Laraia, M. (2005). *Principles and practice of psychiatric nursing* (8th ed., p. 367). St. Louis: Mosby.
Keltner, N., Schwecke, Bostrom, C. (2007). *Psychiatric nursing* (5th ed., p. 390). St Louis Mosby.

---

738. The nurse needs to place a vest restraint (security device) on a client. The client tells the nurse that he does not want to wear the vest restraint. The best nursing action is to:

1 Sedate the client first.
2 Apply the vest restraint.
3 Contact the client's family.
4 Consider alternative measures.

Answer: 4
Rationale: Before applying restraints, the nurse must exhaust alternative measures to restraints such as a bed alarm, distraction, and a sitter. If the nurse determines that a restraint is necessary, its use the client is discussed with the family and a prescription is obtained from the provider. The nurse should explain carefully to the client and family the indications for the restraint, the type of restraint selected, and the anticipated duration its use. Sedation can be considered as a chemical restraint. The nurse avoids applying the restraint on a client who refused it to prevent client coercion and future charges of battery.

Level of Cognitive Ability: Application
Client Needs: Safe and Effective Care Environment
Integrated Process: Nursing Process/ Implementation
Content Area: Fundamental Skills

Test-Taking Strategy: Use the process of elimination and principles and concepts related to ethical and legal issues. Eliminate option 1 because, potentially, it is another type of restraint. Eliminate option 2 because the client refused and the nurse does not have the right to coerce a client. Eliminate option 3 because the nurse knows that alternative measures must be exhausted before using a restraint. Review the legal implications related to the use of restraints if you had difficulty with this question.

References

Ignatavicius, D., & Workman, M. (2006). *Medical-surgical nursing: Critical thinking for collaborative care* (5th ed., pp. 44-45). Philadelphia: Saunders.
Potter, P., & Perry, A. (2005). *Fundamentals of nursing* (6th ed., pp. 411, 980). St. Louis: Mosby.

---

739. The nurse prepares a client who is being discharged from the hospital to receive oxygen therapy at home. Which should the nurse include in client teaching about oxygen safety?

1 Hold the oxygen tank on your lap when traveling.
2 Light candles a few feet away from the oxygen tank.
3 Report low oxygen levels in the tank to the physician.
4 Check the oxygen level of the tank on a regular basis.

Level of Cognitive Ability: Analysis
Client Needs: Safe and Effective Care Environment
Integrated Process: Teaching and Learning
Content Area: Fundamental Skills

Answer: 4

Rationale: The nurse instructs the client and family to check the oxygen level in the tank on a regular basis to prevent the oxygen from running out. When traveling, the oxygen tank should be secured in place to prevent tank damage and a potentially devastating injury from a moving tank. Oxygen is a highly combustible gas, and, although it will not spontaneously burn or cause an explosion, it contributes to a fire if it contacts a spark from a cigarette, burning candle, or electrical equipment. The nurse instructs the client to contact the oxygen supplier about low oxygen levels in the tank; contacting the provider is likely to delay prompt replacement of the oxygen tank.

Test-Taking Strategy: Note the strategic words "oxygen safety." Use the process of elimination and eliminate option 1 by visualizing travel with an oxygen tank. A heavy, metal tank can cause an injury if it is not secured in place. Recall that oxygen is a highly combustible gas to direct you to eliminate option 2, and recall that oxygen is not supplied by the physician, to eliminate option 3. Review teaching points related to home care and oxygen if you had difficulty with this question.

References

Ignatavicius, D., & Workman, M. (2006). *Medical-surgical nursing: Critical thinking for collaborative care* (5th ed., pp. 551-552). Philadelphia: Saunders.
Potter, P., & Perry, A. (2005). *Fundamentals of nursing* (6th ed., p. 1122). St. Louis: Mosby.

---

740. Which should the nurse implement to ensure electrical safety for a home care client who needs to receive intravenous (IV) therapy via an IV pump?

1 Keep the pump on at all times.
2 Use an extension cord during ambulation.
3 Obtain a three-pronged grounded plug adapter.
4 Keep the pump plugged in the wall at all times.

Answer: 3

Rationale: Electrical equipment requires grounding to prevent static, sparks, and uninterrupted operation. Extension cords are never recommended; instead, the nurse suggests that the client sit close to a 3-pronged outlet during therapy. The pump should not be left "on" at all times, and plugging into wall power may be unnecessary because many pump batteries recharge during operation of the pump. Keeping the pump plugged into the wall can create a trip hazard.

Level of Cognitive Ability: Application
Client Needs: Safe and Effective Care
    Environment
Integrated Process: Nursing Process/
    Implementation
Content Area: Fundamental Skills

Reference
Potter, P., & Perry, A. (2005). *Fundamentals of nursing* (6th ed., p. 992). St. Louis: Mosby.

---

741. The home care nurse assesses the client's environment for potential hazards. Which observation requires the nurse to counsel the client and family about the potential for injury?
1 Fluorescent light bulbs in every table lamp
2 Trash can next to the client's favorite chair
3 Stairway with a landing that leads to bedrooms
4 Extension cord tucked away between the seating area and wall

Level of Cognitive Ability: Analysis
Client Needs: Safe and Effective Care
    Environment
Integrated Process: Nursing Process/Assessment
Content Area: Fundamental Skills

Answer: 3
Rationale: The stairway creates a potential hazard for the client, because stairs are associated with an increased risk of falls. Options 1 and 2 do not represent potential hazards for the client. An extension cord tucked away from a traffic area is not a potential hazard as long as a suitable electrical demand is drawn on the cord, the cord is grounded properly, and the cord does not traverse a pathway.

Test-Taking Strategy: Focus on the strategic words "potential hazards" in the environment. Recalling that stairs are associated with an increased risk of falls will direct you to option 3. Review these safety principles if you had difficulty with this question.

Reference
Potter, P., & Perry, A. (2005). *Fundamentals of nursing* (6th ed., p. 980). St. Louis: Mosby.

---

742. A hospitalized female client wants to leave the hospital before being discharged by the physician. Which is the priority nursing intervention?
1 Notify the nursing supervisor of the client's plans to leave.
2 Ask the client about transportation plans from the hospital.
3 Arrange medication prescriptions at her preferred pharmacy.
4 Discuss the potential consequences of her plans with the client.

Level of Cognitive Ability: Application
Client Needs: Safe and Effective Care
    Environment
Integrated Process: Nursing Process/
    Implementation
Content Area: Fundamental Skills

Answer: 1
Rationale: The nurse notifies the nursing supervisor of the client's plan to leave without the physician's approval to ensure client safety and to help the nurse manage the situation. This will help the nurse to manage the situation in a thoughtful, comprehensive manner and complete nursing interventions that include asking about transportation, arranging medication prescriptions, and discussing the risks and benefits of leaving or remaining in the hospital. The physician should be contacted and the client encouraged to remain until the physician arrives. The nurse avoids coercion, restraint, or security measures meant to prohibit the client's exit to prevent claims of false imprisonment.

Test-Taking Strategy: Note the strategic word "priority." You need to choose the most important intervention. Review the options for the choice that offers the most potential for a positive outcome. Note that option 1 offers the nurse assistance in a difficult situation involving client safety. Review the points related to false imprisonment if you had difficulty with this question.

Reference
Varcarolis, E., Carson, V., & Shoemaker, N. (2006). *Foundations of psychiatric mental health nursing* (5th ed., pp. 128-129). Philadelphia: Saunders.

743. The nurse is in the cafeteria and tells a physical therapist about a female client who is physically abused. During the client's next visit to physical therapy, she discovers that the nurse told the therapist about the abuse and is emotionally harmed. As a result of the events in the cafeteria, which legal ramification do the nurse and physical therapist potentially face?

1 They can be charged with libel.

2 They can be charged with slander.

3 None; both can receive privileged client data.

4 None, because no one overheard the conversation.

Level of Cognitive Ability: Analysis
Client Needs: Safe and Effective Care Environment
Integrated Process: Nursing Process/Analysis
Content Area: Fundamental Skills

Answer: 2

Rationale: Defamation of a client occurs when information is communicated to a third party that causes damage to the client's reputation either verbally (slander) or in writing (libel). In addition, this situation violates the client's right to confidentiality. Common examples of slander are discussing information about a client in public areas or speaking negatively about coworkers. Both the nurse and the therapist can receive privileged information about the client but not in this manner, because communicating aspects of the medical record should not occur in a public setting. The nurse and therapist do not know with certainty that the conversation was not overheard by another person.

Test-Taking Strategy: Use the process of elimination and focus on the subject—client rights and confidentiality—and the health care team's responsibilities with privileged information. This will assist in eliminating options 3 and 4 first. From the remaining options, recall that slander constitutes verbal discussion regarding a client. Review this legal responsibility if you had difficulty with this question.

Reference
Potter, P., & Perry, A. (2005). *Fundamentals of nursing* (6th ed., p. 414). St. Louis: Mosby.

744. A registered nurse (RN) asks a licensed practical nurse (LPN) to change the colostomy bag on a client. The LPN tells the RN that although attendance at the hospital inservice was completed regarding this procedure, the LPN has never performed a colostomy bag change on a client. The appropriate action by the RN is to:

1 Perform the procedure with the LPN

2 Request that the LPN observe another LPN perform the procedure.

3 Ask the LPN to review the materials from the in-service before performing the procedure.

4 Instruct the LPN to review the procedure in the hospital manual and take the written procedure into the client's room for reference.

Level of Cognitive Ability: Application
Client Needs: Safe and Effective Care Environment
Integrated Process: Teaching and Learning
Content Area: Delegating/Prioritizing

Answer: 1

Rationale: The RN must remember that, even though a task may be delegated to someone, the nurse who delegates maintains accountability for the overall nursing care of the client. Only the task, not the ultimate accountability, may be delegated to another. The RN is responsible for ensuring that competent and accurate care is delivered to the client. Requesting that the LPN observe another LPN perform the procedure does not ensure that the procedure will be done correctly. Because colostomy bag change is a new procedure for this LPN, the RN should accompany the LPN, provide guidance, and answer questions following the procedure. Although it is appropriate to review the in-service materials and the hospital procedure manual, it is best for the RN to accompany the LPN to perform the procedure.

Test-Taking Strategy: Use the process of elimination and eliminate options 3 and 4 first. Although it may be important for the LPN to review in-service materials and the hospital procedure manual, these options are not complete. From the remaining options, select option 1 because option 2 does not ensure that another LPN will perform this procedure appropriately. Additionally, it is the RN's responsibility to educate. Review the principles related to delegating and accountability if you had difficulty with this question.

References
Huber, D. (2006). *Leadership and nursing care management* (3rd ed., pp. 551-553). Philadelphia: Saunders.
Potter, P., & Perry, A. (2005). *Fundamentals of nursing* (6th ed., pp. 19, 42, 375). St. Louis: Mosby.

745. The nurse has applied the patch electrodes of an automatic external defibrillator (AED) to the chest of a client who is pulseless. The defibrillator has interpreted the rhythm to be ventricular fibrillation. The nurse then:

1 Administers rescue breathing during the defibrillation

2 Performs cardiopulmonary resuscitation (CPR) for 1 minute before defibrillating

3 Charges the machine and immediately pushes the "discharge" buttons on the console

4 Orders any personnel away from the client, charges the machine, and defibrillates through the console

Level of Cognitive Ability: Application
Client Needs: Safe and Effective Care Environment
Integrated Process: Nursing Process/ Implementation
Content Area: Adult Health/Cardiovascular

Answer: 4
Rationale: If the AED advises to defibrillate, the nurse or rescuer orders all persons away from the client, charges the machine, and pushes both of the "discharge" buttons on the console at the same time. The charge is delivered through the patch electrodes, and this method is known as "hands-off" defibrillation, which is safest for the rescuer. The sequence of charges (up to three consecutive attempts at 200, 300, and 360 joules) is similar to that of conventional defibrillation. Option 1 is contraindicated for the safety of any rescuer. Performing CPR delays the defibrillation attempt.

Test-Taking Strategy: Use the process of elimination and the guidelines related to defibrillation. Recalling the need to avoid contact with the client during this procedure will direct you to option 4. Review this procedure if you had difficulty with this question.

Reference
Ignatavicius, D., & Workman, M. (2006). *Medical-surgical nursing: Critical thinking for collaborative care* (5th ed., p. 742). Philadelphia: Saunders.

---

746. The nurse is planning care for a client diagnosed with deep vein thrombosis (DVT) of the left leg who is experiencing severe edema and pain in the affected extremity. Which intervention should the nurse avoid in the care of this client?

1 Elevate the left leg.

2 Apply moist heat to the left leg.

3 Administer acetaminophen (Tylenol).

4 Ambulate in the hall three times per shift.

Level of Cognitive Ability: Application
Client Needs: Safe and Effective Care Environment
Integrated Process: Nursing Process/ Implementation
Content Area: Adult Health/Cardiovascular

Answer: 4
Rationale: Management of the client with DVT who is experiencing severe edema and pain includes bed rest; limb elevation; relief of discomfort with warm moist heat and analgesics as needed; anticoagulant therapy; and monitoring for signs of pulmonary embolism. In current practice, activity restriction may not be ordered if the client is receiving low-molecular-weight heparin; however, some physicians may still prefer bed rest for the client.

Test-Taking Strategy: Use the process of elimination, noting the strategic word "avoid." This strategic word indicates a negative event query and the need to select the option that is an incorrect nursing action. Recalling that the client is experiencing severe edema and pain will direct you to option 4, since this activity will increase the client's symptoms. Review care of the client with DVT if you had difficulty with this question.

References
Black, J., & Hawks, J. (2005). *Medical-surgical nursing: Clinical management for positive outcomes* (7th ed., pp. 1540-1541). Philadelphia: Saunders.
Ignatavicius, D., & Workman, M. (2006). *Medical-surgical nursing: Critical thinking for collaborative care* (5th ed., pp. 813-814). Philadelphia: Saunders.

---

747. A nurse is caring for a pregnant client who is receiving an intravenous (IV) infusion of magnesium sulfate. To provide a safe environment, the nurse ensures that which priority item is at the bedside?

1 Tongue blade

2 Percussion hammer

3 Calcium gluconate injection

4 Potassium chloride injection

Answer: 3
Rationale: Toxic effects of magnesium sulfate may cause loss of deep tendon reflexes, heart block, respiratory paralysis, and cardiac arrest. The antidote for magnesium sulfate is calcium gluconate and should be available at the client's bedside. A percussion hammer may be important to assess reflexes but is not the priority item. An airway rather than a tongue blade is also an appropriate item. Potassium chloride is not related to the administration of magnesium sulfate.

Level of Cognitive Ability: Application
Client Needs: Safe and Effective Care
   Environment
Integrated Process: Nursing Process/
   Implementation
Content Area: Pharmacology

Test-Taking Strategy: Use the process of elimination. Note the strategic word "priority." This strategic word indicates that more than one or all of the options may be correct but that you need to identify the most important one. Remember that the percussion hammer would identify the decrease in deep tendon reflexes, but the calcium gluconate is required to treat the life-threatening condition that can occur. Review care of the client receiving IV magnesium sulfate if you had difficulty with this question.

References
Hodgson, B., & Kizior, R. (2007). *Saunders nursing drug handbook 2007.* (p. 720). Philadelphia: Saunders.
McKenry, L., Tressier, E., & Hogan, M. (2006). *Mosby's pharmacology in nursing* (22nd ed., pp. 925-926). St. Louis: Mosby.

---

748. A nurse administers digoxin (Lanoxin) 0.25 mg by mouth rather than the prescribed dose of 0.125 mg to the client. Which should the nurse implement first?
  1 Write an incident report.
  2 Tell the client about the medication error.
  3 Tell the client about the adverse effects of digoxin.
  4 Administer digoxin immune Fab (Digibind).

Level of Cognitive Ability: Application
Client Needs: Safe and Effective Care
   Environment
Integrated Process: Nursing Process/
   Implementation
Content Area: Fundamental Skills

Answer: 1
Rationale: According to agency policy, the nurse should file an incident report when a medication error occurs to accurately document the facts. The nurse should also contact the physican because the client received too much medication. The client should be informed of the error and the adverse effects in a professional manner to avoid alarm and concern. In many situations, the physician prefers to discuss this with the client. Digoxin immune Fab is reserved for extreme toxicity and requires a prescription; depending on the client's response and the serum digoxin level, Digibind is potentially not indicated.

Test-Taking Strategy: Note the strategic word "first." Eliminate options 2 and 3 because the physician usually prefers to inform the client of the error. Eliminate option 4 because a physician's order is needed for its administration. Remember to complete an incident report when an error occurs. Review the principles related to incident reports if you had difficulty with this question.

Reference
Potter, P., & Perry, A. (2005). *Fundamentals of nursing* (6th ed., pp. 419, 497). St. Louis: Mosby.

---

749. When planning the discharge of a client with chronic anxiety, the nurse develops goals to promote a safe environment at home. The appropriate maintenance goal for the client should focus on which of the following?
  1 Identifying anxiety-producing situations
  2 Maintaining contact with a crisis counselor
  3 Techniques for ignoring feelings of anxiety
  4 Eliminating all anxiety from daily situations

Answer: 1
Rationale: Recognizing situations that produce anxiety allows the client to prepare to cope with anxiety or avoid a specific stimulus. Counselors will not be available for all anxiety-producing situations. Additionally, this option does not encourage the development of internal strengths. Ignoring feelings will not resolve anxiety. It is impossible to eliminate all anxiety from life.

Level of Cognitive Ability: Application
Client Needs: Safe and Effective Care
   Environment
Integrated Process: Nursing Process/Planning
Content Area: Mental Health

Test-Taking Strategy: Use the process of elimination. Eliminate option 4 first because of the close-ended word "all." Eliminate option 3 next because feelings should not be ignored. From the remaining options, select option 1 because this option is more client-centered and provides preparation for the client to deal with anxiety if it occurs. Review goals of care for the client with anxiety if you had difficulty with this question.

References
Stuart, G., & Laraia, M. (2005). *Principles and practice of psychiatric nursing* (8th ed., pp. 279-280). St. Louis: Mosby.
Varcarolis, E., Carson, V., & Shoemaker, N. (2006). *Foundations of psychiatric mental health nursing* (5th ed., pp. 240, 243-244). Philadelphia: Saunders.

---

750. The nurse is planning to instruct a client with chronic vertigo about safety measures to prevent exacerbation of symptoms or injury. The nurse plans to teach the client that it is important to:
1 Turn the head slowly when spoken to.
2 Remove throw rugs and clutter in the home.
3 Drive at times when the client does not feel dizzy.
4 Go to the bedroom and lie down when vertigo is experienced.

Level of Cognitive Ability: Application
Client Needs: Safe and Effective Care
   Environment
Integrated Process: Teaching and Learning
Content Area: Adult Health/Ear

Answer: 2
Rationale: The client should maintain the home in a clutter-free state and have throw rugs removed, because the effort of trying to regain balance after slipping could trigger the onset of vertigo. The client with chronic vertigo should avoid driving and using public transportation. The sudden movements involved in each could precipitate an attack. To further prevent vertigo attacks, the client should change position slowly and should turn the entire body, not just the head, when spoken to. If vertigo does occur, the client should immediately sit down or grasp the nearest piece of furniture.

Test-Taking Strategy: Use the process of elimination, focusing on the subject—chronic vertigo and preventing injury. Eliminate options 3 and 4 first, because they put the client at greatest risk of injury secondary to vertigo. From the remaining options, recalling that the client is taught to turn the entire body, not just the head, will direct you to option 2. Review safety measures for the client with chronic vertigo if you had difficulty with this question.

References
Black, J., & Hawks, J. (2005). *Medical-surgical nursing: Clinical management for positive outcomes* (7th ed., pp. 1990-1991). Philadelphia: Saunders.
Ignatavicius, D., & Workman, M. (2006). *Medical-surgical nursing: Critical thinking for collaborative care* (5th ed., pp. 1131-1132). Philadelphia: Saunders.

---

751. A client receiving heparin therapy for acute myocardial infarction has an activated partial thromboplastin time (aPTT) value of 100 seconds. Before reporting the results to the physician, the nurse verifies that which of the following is available for use if prescribed?
1 Protamine sulfate
2 Phytonadione (vitamin K)
3 Methylene blue (Urolene Blue)
4 Cyanocobalamin (vitamin B_{12})

Answer: 1
Rationale: Therapeutic values of the aPTT for clients on heparin range between 60 and 70 seconds, depending on the control value. A value of 100 seconds indicates that the client has received too much heparin. The antidote for heparin overdosage is protamine sulfate. Vitamin K is the antidote for warfarin sodium (Coumadin) overdosage. Methylene blue is an antidote for cyanide poisoning. Vitamin B_{12} is used to treat clients with pernicious anemia.

Level of Cognitive Ability: Application
Client Needs: Safe and Effective Care
  Environment
Integrated Process: Nursing Process/
  Implementation
Content Area: Pharmacology

Test-Taking Strategy: Focus on the subject—heparin therapy—and note the strategic words "available for use." Recalling that protamine sulfate is the antidote for heparin will direct you to option 1. Review the normal aPTT and the antidote for heparin if you had difficulty with this question.

Reference
Skidmore-Roth, L. (2008). *Mosby's nursing drug reference* (21st ed., pp. 524-525). St. Louis: Mosby.

---

752. A suicidal client is being discharged home with his family. Which statement by a family member might constitute criteria for delaying discharge?
  1 The client's wife asks, "Does he know that I've already moved out and filed for a divorce?"
  2 The client's daughter states, "I've decided to postpone my wedding until Dad's feeling better."
  3 The client's son states, "One of his friends visited last week to tell us Dad's union is out on strike."
  4 The client's brother asks, "Will my brother be able to continue as executor of our parent's trust?"

Level of Cognitive Ability: Analysis
Client Needs: Safe and Effective Care
  Environment
Integrated Process: Nursing Process/Analysis
Content Area: Mental Health

Answer: 1
Rationale: Single, divorced, and widowed clients have suicide rates that are greater than those who are married. While the situation of the strike is stressful, the client will probably receive a portion of his wages and can derive hope and a sense of belonging from being a member of the union. While the client might feel responsible for his daughter's postponement of the wedding, if presented as an action to include him, the client will feel loved and cared for. While being suicidal may reduce the ability to concentrate, if the client perceives the executorship positively, taking the role away reinforces the client's low self-esteem and self-worth. This statement by the client's brother also indicates a need for the client's brother to be educated about depressive illness.

Test-Taking Strategy: Use the process of elimination and focus on the subject, delaying discharge. Recalling the risks associated with a suicide intent will direct you to option 1. Review these risks if you had difficulty with this question.

Reference
Stuart, G., & Laraia, M. (2005). *Principles and practice of psychiatric nursing* (8th ed., pp. 373-374). St. Louis: Mosby.

---

753. A nurse is preparing to ambulate a client with Parkinson's disease who has recently been started on L-dopa (levodopa). The nurse assesses which most important item before performing this activity with the client?
  1 The client's history of falls
  2 Assistive devices used by the client
  3 The client's postural (orthostatic) vital signs
  4 The degree of intention tremors exhibited by the client

Level of Cognitive Ability: Application
Client Needs: Safe and Effective Care
  Environment
Integrated Process: Nursing Process/Assessment
Content Area: Pharmacology

Answer: 3
Rationale: Clients with Parkinson's disease are at risk for postural (orthostatic) hypotension from the disease. This problem is exacerbated with the introduction of levodopa, which can also cause postural hypotension and increase the client's risk for falls. Although knowledge of the client's use of assistive devices and history of falls is helpful, it is not the most important piece of assessment data, based on the wording of this question. Clients with Parkinson's disease generally have resting, not intention, tremors.

Test-Taking Strategy: Focus on the strategic words "most important." Postural hypotension presents the greatest safety risk to the client. Also, use of the ABCs—airway, breathing, and circulation—will direct you to option 3. Checking postural vital signs is one way to assess circulation. Review the complications associated with Parkinson's disease and the effects of levodopa if you had difficulty with this question.

References

Kee, J., Hayes, E., & McCuistion, L. (2006). *Pharmacology: A nursing process approach* (5th ed., pp. 354-355). Philadelphia: Saunders.

Hodgson, B., & Kizior, R. (2007). *Saunders nursing drug handbook 2007.* (p. 186). Philadelphia: Saunders.

---

754. The nurse prepares to transfer a client who has right-sided weakness from the bed to the wheelchair. With the client dangling on the side of the bed, where should the nurse position the wheelchair?

1 Directly in front of the client
2 At a right angle to the client's left leg
3 Ninety degrees to the client's right leg
4 At a right angle to the client's right leg

Level of Cognitive Ability: Application
Client Needs: Safe and Effective Care Environment
Integrated Process: Nursing Process/ Implementation
Content Area: Fundamental Skills

Answer: 2

Rationale: When a client has a weakened lower extremity, movement should occur toward the client's unaffected (strong) side, the left side. This wheelchair position allows the client to use the unaffected leg effectively and safely to stand, pivot, and sit in the wheelchair. Placing the wheelchair in front of the client directly increases the risk to the client because the client must pivot 180 degrees to the wheelchair in this position.

Test-Taking Strategy: Use the process of elimination, focusing on the subject—a safe transfer technique with right-sided weakness. Visualize each option to direct you to option 2. Positioning the wheelchair next to the client's unaffected leg allows the client to use the stronger leg more effectively for a safe transfer. Review transfer techniques if you had difficulty with this question.

References

Monahan, F., Sands, J., Neighbors, M., Marek, J., & Green, C. (2007). *Phipps' medical-surgical nursing: Health and illness perspectives* (8th ed., p. 1426). St. Louis: Mosby.

Potter, P., & Perry, A. (2005). *Fundamentals of nursing* (6th ed., pp. 1469-1470). St. Louis: Mosby.

---

755. The nurse is caring for a client who has brain death and is a potential organ donor. Before approaching the family to discuss organ donation, the nurse reviews the client's medical record for potential contraindications to organ donation including:

1 Allergy to penicillin
2 Hepatitis B infection
3 Older than 35 years old
4 History of foreign travel

Level of Cognitive Ability: Comprehension
Client Needs: Safe and Effective Care Environment
Integrated Process: Nursing Process/Assessment
Content Area: Fundamental Skills

Answer: 2

Rationale: A decedent who had a hepatitis B infection cannot donate organs because the organ recipient will contract the infection. Contraindications to organ donation do not include penicillin allergies or foreign travel. Although foreign travel increases the risk of contracting certain communicable diseases, foreign travel alone does not constitute a contraindication. Age can be a contraindication depending on the organ involved; for example, age must not exceed 65 years for kidney donation, 55 years for pancreas or liver donation, or 40 years for heart donation.

Test-Taking Strategy: Focus on the subject—contraindications to organ donations. Noting the word "infection" in option 2 will direct you to this option. Review these contraindications if you had difficulty with this question.

References

Lewis, S., Heitkemper, M., Dirksen, S., O'Brien, P., & Bucher, L. (2007). *Medical-surgical nursing: Assessment and management of clinical problems* (7th ed., p. 1226). St. Louis: Mosby.

Lynch, V., & Duval, J. (2006). *Forensic nursing* (p. 223). St. Louis: Mosby.

756. The nurse monitors a client who has been diagnosed with brain death and is a potential organ donor. Which client assessment data indicate to the nurse that the standard of care as an organ donor has been maintained?

1 pH of arterial blood: 7.32
2 Urine output: 45 mL/hr
3 Capillary refill: 5 seconds
4 Blood pressure: 90/48 mm Hg

Level of Cognitive Ability: Analysis
Client Needs: Safe and Effective Care Environment
Integrated Process: Nursing Process/Evaluation
Content Area: Fundamental Skills

Answer: 2

Rationale: Urine output at 45 mL per hour indicates adequate renal perfusion and indicates that care standards as an organ donor are maintained. Clinical indicators of care below the standard include a pH of 7.32, indicating acidosis; capillary refill at 5 seconds, which is too slow; and hypotension, indicating an inadequate cardiac output.

Test-Taking Strategy: Use the process of elimination and eliminate options 1, 3, and 4 because they are below optimal values. Review normal values for physical assessment measurements and the criteria related to organ donation if you had difficulty with this question.

References

Black, J., & Hawks, J. (2005). *Medical-surgical nursing: Clinical management for positive outcomes* (7th ed., p. 2430). Philadelphia: Saunders.
Fultz, J., & Sturt, P. (2005). *Emergency nursing reference* (3rd ed., p. 47). St. Louis: Mosby.

---

757. A client who has been diagnosed with brain death had received vigorous treatment to control cerebral edema. Which intervention does the nurse plan to implement to maintain viability of the kidneys before organ donation?

1 Screen the donor for infection.
2 Administer intravenous (IV) fluids.
3 Maintain ventilation and oxygenation.
4 Administer vasopressors intravenously.

Level of Cognitive Ability: Application
Client Needs: Safe and Effective Care Environment
Integrated Process: Nursing Process/Planning
Content Area: Fundamental Skills

Answer: 2

Rationale: The kidneys require a minimum perfusion pressure of 80 mm Hg to produce urine and maintain renal function, and, because of the aggressive treatment for cerebral edema, the client is likely to have a fluid volume deficiency. Therefore, the nurse restores the intravascular blood volume to maintain the blood pressure and renal perfusion pressure. The nurse screens the donor for infections, because diseases such as hepatitis B and HIV contraindicate organ donation. Ventilation and oxygenation are important factors in tissue viability; however, the organ must be perfused adequately, first, to deliver any blood. The nurse administers vasopressors with caution to help maintain the donor's blood pressure; however, vasopressors potentially contribute to tissue destruction.

Test-Taking Strategy: Note the strategic words "treatment to control cerebral edema" and focus on the subject, maintaining viability of the kidneys. Use the process of elimination, noting the relation between the subject and option 2. Review the concepts related to organ donation of the kidneys if you had difficulty with this question.

Reference

Fultz, J., & Sturt, P. (2005). *Emergency nursing reference* (3rd ed., p. 47). St. Louis: Mosby.

758. A nurse is working in the emergency department of a small local hospital when a client with multiple gunshot wounds arrives by ambulance. Which of the following actions by the nurse is contraindicated in the handling legal evidence?
1 Initiate a chain of custody log.
2 Give clothing and wallet to the family.
3 Cut clothing along seams, avoiding bullet holes.
4 Place personal belongings in a labeled, sealed paper bag.

Level of Cognitive Ability: Application
Client Needs: Safe and Effective Care Environment
Integrated Process: Nursing Process/ Implementation
Content Area: Leadership/Management

Answer: 2
Rationale: Basic rules for handling evidence include limiting the number of people with access to the evidence, initiating a chain of custody log to track handling and movement of evidence, and carefully removing of clothing to avoid destroying evidence. This usually includes cutting clothes along seams, while avoiding areas where there are obvious holes or tears. Potential evidence is never released to the family to take home.

Test-Taking Strategy: Focus on the client situation, and note the strategic word "contraindicated." This strategic word indicates a negative event query and the need to select the option that identifies an incorrect nursing action. Use knowledge of basic emergency care principles related to a potential crime to eliminate each of the incorrect options. Remember that giving the client's belongings to the family may be giving up evidence. Review the legal principles related to care of a client with a gunshot wound if you had difficulty with this question.

Reference
Fultz, J., & Sturt, P. (2005). *Emergency nursing reference* (3rd ed., pp. 865-868). St. Louis: Mosby.

---

759. A nurse working on a medical nursing unit during an external disaster is called to assist with care for clients coming into the emergency department. Using principles of triage, the nurse initiates immediate care for a client with which of the following injuries?
1 Fractured tibia
2 Penetrating abdominal injury
3 Open massive head injury to deep coma
4 Bright red bleeding from a neck wound

Level of Cognitive Ability: Application
Client Needs: Safe and Effective Care Environment
Integrated Process: Nursing Process/ Implementation
Content Area: Delegating/Prioritizing

Answer: 4
Rationale: The client with bright red (arterial) bleeding from a neck wound is in "immediate" need of treatment to save the client's life. This client is classified as an emergent client and would wear a color tag of red from the triage process. The client with a penetrating abdominal injury would be tagged yellow and classified as "delayed," requiring intervention within 30 to 60 minutes. A green or "minimal" designation would be given to the client with a fractured tibia, who requires intervention but who can provide self-care if needed. A designation of "expectant" would be applied to the client with massive injuries and minimal chance of survival. This client would be color-coded "black" in the triage process. The client who is color-coded "black" is given supportive care and pain management but is given definitive treatment last.

Test-Taking Strategy: Use the process of elimination and focus on the strategic words "initiates immediate care." Use the principles of triage and prioritize. Noting the words "bright red" in option 4 will direct you to this option. Review disaster planning and the principles of triage if you had difficulty with this question.

References
Ignatavicius, D., & Workman, M. (2006). *Medical-surgical nursing: Critical thinking for collaborative care* (5th ed., pp. 167-168). Philadelphia: Saunders.
Lewis, S., Heitkemper, M., Dirksen, S., O'Brien, P., & Bucher, L. (2007). *Medical-surgical nursing: Assessment and management of clinical problems* (7th ed., pp. 1821-1822, 1842). St. Louis: Mosby.

760. A nurse working on an adult nursing unit is told to review the client census to determine which clients could be discharged if there are a large number of admissions from a newly declared disaster. The nurse determines that the client with which of the following problems would need to remain hospitalized?
1 Laparoscopic cholecystectomy
2 Fractured hip, pinned 5 days ago
3 Diabetes mellitus with blood glucose at 180 mg/dL
4 Ongoing ventricular dysrhythmias while receiving procainamide (Procanbid)

Level of Cognitive Ability: Analysis
Client Needs: Safe and Effective Care Environment
Integrated Process: Nursing Process/Analysis
Content Area: Delegating/Prioritizing

Answer: 4
Rationale: The client with ongoing ventricular dysrhythmias requires ongoing medical evaluation and treatment because of potentially lethal complications of the problem. Each of the other problems listed may be managed at home with appropriate agency referrals for home care services and support from the family at home.

Test-Taking Strategy: Use the principles of triage. Severity of illness usually guides the determination of who requires ongoing monitoring and care. Use of the ABCs—airway, breathing, and circulation—will direct you to option 4. Review the principles of triage and prioritizing if you had difficulty with this question.

Reference
Lewis, S., Heitkemper, M., Dirksen, S., O'Brien, P., & Bucher, L. (2007). *Medical-surgical nursing: Assessment and management of clinical problems* (7th ed., pp. 1822-1823). St. Louis: Mosby.

761. A registered nurse (RN) is orienting a nursing assistant to the clinical nursing unit. The RN would intervene if the nursing assistant did which of the following during a routine handwashing procedure?
1 Kept hands lower than elbows
2 Dried from forearm down to fingers
3 Washed continuously for 10 to 15 seconds
4 Used 3 to 5 mL of soap from the dispenser

Level of Cognitive Ability: Application
Client Needs: Safe and Effective Care Environment
Integrated Process: Nursing Process/Implementation
Content Area: Leadership/Management

Answer: 2
Rationale: Proper handwashing procedure involves wetting the hands and wrists and keeping the hands lower than the forearms so that water flows toward the fingertips. The nurse uses 3 to 5 mL of soap and scrubs for 10 to 15 seconds, using rubbing and circular motions. The hands are rinsed and then dried, moving from the fingers to the forearms. The paper towel is then discarded, and a second one is used to turn off the faucet to avoid hand contamination.

Test-Taking Strategy: Note the strategic word "intervene." This strategic word indicates a negative event query and the need to select the option that identifies an incorrect action by the nursing assistant. Use basic principles of medical asepsis and visualize each of the actions in the options to assist in directing you to option 2. Review this fundamental nursing procedure if you had difficulty with this question.

References
Ignatavicius, D., & Workman, M. (2006). *Medical-surgical nursing: Critical thinking for collaborative care* (5th ed., pp. 511-512). Philadelphia: Saunders.
Potter, P., & Perry, A. (2005). *Fundamentals of nursing* (6th ed., pp. 790-793). St. Louis: Mosby.

762. The nurse is developing a plan of care for a client being admitted to the hospital who is immunosuppressed and will be placed on neutropenic precautions. With regard to neutropenic precautions, which intervention is incorrect?
1 Admitting the client to a semiprivate room
2 Placing a precaution sign on the door to the room
3 Placing a mask on the client if the client leaves the room
4 Removing a vase with fresh flowers left by a previous client

Level of Cognitive Ability: Application
Client Needs: Safe and Effective Care Environment
Integrated Process: Nursing Process/Planning
Content Area: Adult Health/Oncology

Answer: 1
Rationale: The client who is on neutropenic precautions is immunosuppressed and is admitted to a single (private) room on the nursing unit. A precaution sign should be placed on the door to the client's room. The client should wear a mask whenever leaving the room to be protected from exposure to microorganisms. Standing water and fresh flowers should be removed to decrease the microorganism count.

Test-Taking Strategy: Use the process of elimination, noting the strategic word "incorrect." This strategic word indicates a negative event query and the need to select the option that identifies an incorrect action. Recalling that neutropenic precautions are instituted when the client is at risk for infection because of impaired immune function will direct you to option 1. Review this type of infection control precaution if you had difficulty with this question.

References
Ignatavicius, D., & Workman, M. (2006). *Medical-surgical nursing: Critical thinking for collaborative care* (5th ed., p. 497). Philadelphia: Saunders.
Lewis, S., Heitkemper, M., Dirksen, S., O'Brien, P., & Bucher, L. (2007). *Medical-surgical nursing: Assessment and management of clinical problems* (7th ed., p. 715). St. Louis: Mosby.

763. The nurse is preparing to change the linens and gown of a client who was incontinent of urine. The client had received an unsealed radiation source earlier in the day for treatment of thyroid cancer. The nurse wears which of the following protective items?
1 Mask and gloves
2 Gown and gloves
3 Mask, gown, and gloves
4 Gown, gloves, and eyewear

Level of Cognitive Ability: Application
Client Needs: Safe and Effective Care Environment
Integrated Process: Nursing Process/Implementation
Content Area: Adult Health/Oncology

Answer: 2
Rationale: In caring for the incontinent client who has received an unsealed radiation source, the nurse should wear gloves and a gown to protect the hands and uniform from contamination with urine. Generally, traces of the radioactive isotope are found in urine, feces, emesis, and wound drainage.

Test-Taking Strategy: Note that the potential source of contamination in this situation is the client's urine. The nurse needs to protect his or her hands, since the radioactive source could be absorbed through the skin if traces exist in the urine. Because urine present on the hospital gown and bedclothes is not likely to splash, eliminate options 1, 3, and 4. Review standard precautions and caring for the client who has received an unsealed radiation source if you had difficulty with this question.

Reference
Potter, P., & Perry, A. (2005). *Fundamentals of nursing* (6th ed., p. 797). St. Louis: Mosby.

764. The nurse receives a telephone call from the hospital admission office and is informed that a client is being admitted who will undergo implantation of a sealed internal radiation source. The nurse asks the admission office clerk if which of the following rooms is selected for the client?

1 A single room near the nurse's station
2 A single room at the distant end of the hall
3 A semiprivate room near the nurse's station
4 A semiprivate room between two isolation rooms

Level of Cognitive Ability: Application
Client Needs: Safe and Effective Care Environment
Integrated Process: Nursing Process/Planning
Content Area: Adult Health/Oncology

Answer: 2
Rationale: The client receiving an implantation of a sealed internal radiation source should be placed in a single room in an area that reduces the risk of exposure to others. For this reason, rooms are often used that are at the end of a hall.

Test-Taking Strategy: Use of the principles of shielding related to radiation therapy will assist to eliminate options 1, 3, and 4 because they do not provide distance to protect other clients or health care personnel. Review the protective measures related to the care of a client with a sealed internal radiation source if you had difficulty with this question.

Reference
Ignatavicius, D., & Workman, M. (2006). *Medical-surgical nursing: Critical thinking for collaborative care* (5th ed., p. 490). Philadelphia: Saunders.

765. The nurse is assessing the corneal reflex on an unconscious client. The nurse would use which of the following as the safest stimulus to touch the client's cornea?

1 Sterile glove
2 Wisp of cotton
3 Sterile tongue depressor
4 Tip of a 1-mL syringe with the needle removed

Level of Cognitive Ability: Application
Client Needs: Safe and Effective Care Environment
Integrated Process: Nursing Process/Assessment
Content Area: Adult Health/Neurological

Answer: 2
Rationale: The corneal reflex is tested in selected situations, such as with the unconscious client. The client who is unconscious is at great risk for corneal abrasion. For this reason, the safest way to test the corneal reflex is by touching the cornea lightly with cotton. Normally, the lids of both eyes blink when the cornea is touched. Use of the items in options 1, 3, and 4 can cause injury to the cornea.

Test-Taking Strategy: Use the process of elimination, noting the strategic words "unconscious" and "safest." Visualize each item in the options and eliminate options 1, 3, and 4 because they are blunt objects. Review care of an unconscious client if you had difficulty with this question.

References
Black, J., & Hawks, J. (2005). *Medical-surgical nursing: Clinical management for positive outcomes* (7th ed., pp. 2028, 2034). Philadelphia: Saunders.
Wilson, S., & Giddens, J. (2005). *Health assessment for nursing practice* (3rd ed., p. 310). St. Louis: Mosby.

766. The nurse prepares to transfer the client from the bed to a chair using a mechanical lift. Which should the nurse implement to move the client safely with this device?

1 Lower the client rapidly onto the chair.
2 Instruct the client to hold onto the sling.
3 Have three people at the bedside to assist.
4 Position the client in the center of the sling.

Answer: 4
Rationale: When using a mechanical lift, the client is positioned in the center of the sling. The client's hands and arms are crossed over the chest, and the client is raised from the bed into a sitting position. The client is lowered slowly once the sling is positioned over the chair to prevent client injury or orthostatic hypotension.

Test-Taking Strategy: Focus on the subject—moving the client safely. Visualize this procedure and each description in the options to direct you to option 4. Review this procedure if you had difficulty with this question.

Level of Cognitive Ability: Application
Client Needs: Safe and Effective Care
   Environment
Integrated Process: Nursing Process/
   Implementation
Content Area: Fundamental Skills

Reference
Potter, P., & Perry, A. (2005). *Fundamentals of nursing* (6th ed., p. 1473). St. Louis:
   Mosby.

---

767. An older client in a long-term care facility has a stable gait and has a nursing diagnosis of Risk for injury related to confusion. Which is the most suitable method of restraint for the nurse to use on this client to prevent injury?
   1 Bed alarm
   2 Vest restraint
   3 Alarm-activating bracelet
   4 Chair with locking lap tray

Level of Cognitive Ability: Analysis
Client Needs: Safe and Effective Care
   Environment
Integrated Process: Nursing Process/
   Implementation
Content Area: Fundamental Skills

Answer: 3
Rationale: For the client who is confused and has a stable gait, the least intrusive method of restraint is the alarm-activating bracelet or "wandering bracelet." This allows the client to move about the residence freely while preventing the client from leaving the premises. Option 1 is indicated for clients who should remain in bed. Options 2 and 4 are restrictive devices and potentially contribute to client injury.

Test-Taking Strategy: Note the strategic words, "most suitable" and "stable gait." Integrate the process of elimination with your knowledge of the ethical and legal ramifications related to restraints to direct you to option 3. Review the guidelines related to the use of restraints if you had difficulty with this question.

References
Perry, A., & Potter, P. (2006). *Clinical nursing skills & techniques* (6th ed., p. 86).
   St. Louis: Mosby.
Potter, P., & Perry, A. (2005). *Fundamentals of nursing* (6th ed., pp. 988, 990).
   St. Louis: Mosby.

---

768. The nurse administers furosemide (Lasix) 80 mg by mouth, but the prescription is written for furosemide 40 mg by mouth. Which should the nurse document on an incident report?
   1 "I gave the wrong dose of the medication."
   2 "Furosemide 80 mg by mouth administered."
   3 "A double dose of furosemide was given to the client."
   4 "Furosemide 80 mg given to the client instead of 40 mg."

Level of Cognitive Ability: Application
Client Needs: Safe and Effective Care
   Environment
Integrated Process: Communication and
   Documentation
Content Area: Fundamental Skills

Answer: 2
Rationale: When completing an incident report, the nurse should state the facts clearly. The nurse avoids documenting subjective data, including assumptions and opinions about what occurred, and avoids assigning blame. Furthermore, the nurse avoids documenting to any wrong doing.

Test-Taking Strategy: Read the occurrence as stated in the question. Use the process of elimination and select the option that clearly and most directly states what occurred. Options 1 and 3 are comparable or alike, provide subjective data or a judgment, and thus are eliminated. Eliminate option 4 because it points out an error. Option 2 clearly and simply states the occurrence. Review the principles associated with incident reports if you had difficulty with this question.

Reference
Potter, P., & Perry, A. (2005). *Fundamentals of nursing* (6th ed., p. 419). St. Louis:
   Mosby.

769. A registered nurse (RN) on the night shift assists a staff member in completing an incident report for a client who was found sitting on the floor. Following completion of the report, the RN intervenes if the staff member prepares to:

1 Notify the nursing supervisor.
2 Ask the unit secretary to telephone the physician.
3 Document in the nurses' notes that an incident report was filed.
4 Forward the incident report to the Continuous Quality Improvement Department.

Level of Cognitive Ability: Application
Client Needs: Safe and Effective Care Environment
Integrated Process: Nursing Process/ Implementation
Content Area: Leadership/Management

Answer: 3
Rationale: Nurses are advised not to document the filing of an incident report in the nurses' notes for legal reasons. Incident reports inform the facility's administration of the incident so that risk management personnel can consider changes that might prevent similar occurrences in the future. Incident reports also alert the facility's insurance company to a potential claim and the need for further investigation. Options 1, 2, and 4 are accurate interventions.

Test-Taking Strategy: Note the strategic word "intervenes." This strategic word indicates a negative event query and the need to select the option that identifies an incorrect action by the staff member. Note that options 1, 2, and 4 all relate to notification of key individuals or departments. Option 3 relates to documentation of filing an incident report. Review the concepts that relate to incident reports if you had difficulty with this question.

References
Huber, D. (2006). *Leadership and nursing care management* (3rd ed., p. 862). Philadelphia: Saunders.
Potter, P., & Perry, A. (2005). *Fundamentals of nursing* (6th ed., p. 419). St. Louis: Mosby.

---

770. A physician visiting a client on the nursing unit is paged and notified that the monthly physician's breakfast meeting is about to start. The physician states to the nurse: "I'm in a hurry. Can you write an order to decrease the atenolol (Tenormin) to 25 mg daily?" Which of the following is the appropriate nursing action?

1 Write the order.
2 Call the nursing supervisor to write the order.
3 Inform the client of the change of medication.
4 Ask the physician to return to the nursing unit to write the order.

Level of Cognitive Ability: Application
Client Needs: Safe and Effective Care Environment
Integrated Process: Nursing Process/ Implementation
Content Area: Leadership/Management

Answer: 4
Rationale: Nurses are encouraged not to accept verbal orders from the physician because of the risks of error. The only exception to this may be in an emergency situation, and then the nurse must follow agency policy and procedure. Although the client will be informed of the change in the treatment plan, this is not the appropriate action at this time. The physician needs to write the new order. It is inappropriate to ask another individual other than the physician to write the order.

Test-Taking Strategy: Use the process of elimination. Recall that verbal orders are not acceptable. Options 1 and 2 are comparable or alike, so eliminate these options. Option 3 is appropriate, but not at this time. Option 4 clearly identifies the nurse's responsibility in this situation. Review these principles if you had difficulty with this question.

Reference
Potter, P., & Perry, A. (2005). *Fundamentals of nursing* (6th ed., pp. 497, 838). St. Louis: Mosby.

771. A nurse is caring for a hospitalized client who has an order for dextroamphetamine sulphate (Dexedrine) 25 mg orally daily. The nurse collaborates with the dietitian to limit the amount of which of the following items on the client's dietary trays?

1 Fat
2 Starch
3 Protein
4 Caffeine

Level of Cognitive Ability: Application
Client Needs: Safe and Effective Care Environment
Integrated Process: Nursing Process/ Implementation
Content Area: Pharmacology

Answer: 4
Rationale: Dextroamphetamine sulfate is a central nervous system (CNS) stimulant. Caffeine is also a stimulant and should be limited in the client taking this medication. The client should be taught to limit caffeine intake as well. Options 1, 2, and 3 are acceptable dietary items.

Test-Taking Strategy: Use the process of elimination. Recalling that this medication is a CNS stimulant will direct you to option 4. Review this medication if you had difficulty with this question.

Reference
Lehne, R. (2007). *Pharmacology for nursing care* (6th ed., p. 388). St. Louis: Saunders.

---

772. The nurse is planning preoperative care for a client scheduled for insertion of an inferior vena cava filter. The nurse questions the physician about withholding which regularly scheduled medication on the day before surgery?

1 Furosemide (Lasix)
2 Docusate sodium (Colace)
3 Potassium chloride (K-Dur)
4 Warfarin sodium (Coumadin)

Level of Cognitive Ability: Application
Client Needs: Safe and Effective Care Environment
Integrated Process: Nursing Process/ Implementation
Content Area: Adult Health/Cardiovascular

Answer: 4
Rationale: In the preoperative period, the nurse consults with the physician about withholding warfarin sodium to avoid the occurrence of hemorrhage. Docusate sodium is a stool softener, furosemide is a diuretic, and potassium chloride is a supplement.

Test-Taking Strategy: Note the subject—withholding a medication. Use the process of elimination, evaluating each medication in terms of its potential harm to the preoperative client. This will direct you to option 4. Review these medications if you had difficulty with this question.

Reference
Ignatavicius, D., & Workman, M. (2006). *Medical-surgical nursing: Critical thinking for collaborative care* (5th ed., p. 815). Philadelphia: Saunders.

---

773. A hospitalized client with hypertension has been started on captopril (Capoten). The nurse ensures that the client does which of the following specific to this medication?

1 Drinks plenty of water
2 Eats foods that are high in potassium
3 Takes in sufficient amounts of high-fiber foods
4 Moves from a sitting to a standing position slowly

Answer: 4
Rationale: Orthostatic hypotension is a concern for clients taking antihypertensive medications. Clients are advised to avoid standing in one position for lengthy amounts of time, to change positions slowly, and to avoid extreme warmth (showers, bath, and weather). Clients are also taught to recognize the symptoms of orthostatic hypotension, including dizziness, light-headedness, weakness, and syncope. Options 1, 2, and 3 are not specific to this medication.

Test-Taking Strategy: Use the process of elimination. Recalling that captopril is an antihypertensive will direct you to option 4. Remember that the risk of orthostatic hypotension is present with all types of antihypertensives. Review the effects of this medication if you had difficulty with this question.

Level of Cognitive Ability: Application
Client Needs: Safe and Effective Care
  Environment
Integrated Process: Nursing Process/
  Implementation
Content Area: Adult Health/Cardiovascular

References
Hodgson, B., & Kizior, R. (2007). *Saunders nursing drug handbook 2007* (p. 182).
  Philadelphia: Saunders.
Kee, J., Hayes, E., & McCuistion, L. (2006). *Pharmacology: A nursing process approach*
  (5th ed., pp. 650-651). Philadelphia: Saunders.
Lewis, S., Heitkemper, M., Dirksen, S., O'Brien, P., & Bucher, L. (2007). *Medical-surgical nursing: Assessment and management of clinical problems* (7th ed., p. 778).
  St. Louis: Mosby.

---

774. The nurse prepares to ambulate a client with left-side weakness. Which is the best and safest position for the nurse in assisting a client to stand?
  1 Behind the client
  2 In front of the client
  3 On the affected side of the client
  4 On the unaffected side of the client

Level of Cognitive Ability: Application
Client Needs: Safe and Effective Care
  Environment
Integrated Process: Nursing Process/
  Implementation
Content Area: Fundamental Skills

Answer: 3
Rationale: When walking with clients, the nurse stands on the affected side and grasps the security belt in the back of the client. The nurse positions the free hand at the shoulder area so that the client can be pulled toward the nurse in the event the client falls forward. The nurse instructs the client to look up and outward rather than at the feet. Options 1, 2, and 4 are incorrect positions.

Test-Taking Strategy: Use the process of elimination. Recalling that support is needed on the affected side will assist in directing you to option 3. Review this procedure if you had difficulty with this question.

Reference
Potter, P., & Perry, A. (2005). *Fundamentals of nursing* (6th ed., pp. 947-948).
  St. Louis: Mosby.

---

775. A client receiving lisinopril (Prinivil) has a white blood cell (WBC) count of 3800/mm³. The nurse plans to do which of the following in the care of this client?
  1 Follow strict aseptic technique.
  2 Place the client on respiratory isolation.
  3 Use antibacterial soap when bathing the client.
  4 Request prophylactic antibiotics from the physician.

Level of Cognitive Ability: Application
Client Needs: Safe and Effective Care
  Environment
Integrated Process: Nursing Process/Planning
Content Area: Pharmacology

Answer: 1
Rationale: The client taking angiotensin-converting enzyme (ACE) inhibitors, such as lisinopril, may be at risk of developing neutropenia. These clients require the use of strict aseptic technique by all who care for the client. The client should also be taught to report signs and symptoms of infection, such as sore throat and fever, to the physician. The WBC count with differential may be monitored monthly for up to 6 months in clients deemed at risk. Options 2, 3, and 4 are not appropriate interventions. No data in the question indicate the need for antibiotics, respiratory isolation, or the use of antibacterial soap.

Test-Taking Strategy: Use the process of elimination. This question can be correctly answered even without knowing that ACE inhibitors cause neutropenia, as long as you can recognize abnormally low WBC values. Recognizing that a WBC count of 3800 mm³ is a low count and that a low count places the client at risk for infection directs you to option 1. Review this medication if you had difficulty with this question.

References
Hodgson, B., & Kizior, R. (2007). *Saunders nursing drug handbook 2007* (p. 697).
  Philadelphia: Saunders.
Ignatavicius, D., & Workman, M. (2006). *Medical-surgical nursing: Critical thinking for collaborative care* (5th ed., p. 497). Philadelphia: Saunders.

776. A nurse is called to a client's room by another nurse. When the nurse arrives at the room, she discovers that a fire has occurred in the client's wastebasket. The first nurse has removed the client from the room. What is the second nurse's next action?

1 Confine the fire.
2 Evacuate the unit.
3 Extinguish the fire.
4 Activate the fire alarm.

Level of Cognitive Ability: Application
Client Needs: Safe and Effective Care Environment
Integrated Process: Nursing Process/ Implementation
Content Area: Delegating/Prioritizing

Answer: 4
Rationale: Remember the acronym RACE (i.e., rescue, alarm, confine, extinguish) to set priorities if a fire occurs. In this situation, the client has been rescued from the immediate vicinity of the fire. The next action is to activate the fire alarm.

Test-Taking Strategy: Use the RACE acronym to set priorities and answer the question. This will direct you to option 4. Review fire safety if you had difficulty with this question.

Reference
Potter, P., & Perry, A. (2005). *Fundamentals of nursing* (6th ed., p. 991). St. Louis: Mosby.

---

777. The nurse is caring for a client with cervical cancer who is receiving brachytherapy. Which is the best radiation safety equipment for the nurse to keep at the client's bedside to prevent unnecessary radiation contamination?

1 A face mask and gown
2 A radiation safety dosimeter badge
3 A bedside commode for urine collection
4 Long-handled forceps and a lead container

Level of Cognitive Ability: Analysis
Client Needs: Safe and Effective Care Environment
Integrated Process: Nursing Process/ Implementation
Content Area: Fundamental Skills

Answer: 4
Rationale: When an internal radiation implant becomes dislodged, the nurse avoids touching the radioactive source with the bare hands. The nurse uses a long-handled forceps and places the radioactive implant into the lead container kept in the client's room. A film badge measures radiation exposure but does not prevent exposure. A bedside commode is used for client convenience; the urine is disposed of properly in the bathroom commode. A face mask and gown would not protect the nurse from radiation.

Test-Taking Strategy: Note the strategic word "best." Eliminate option 1 because it provides no protection. Eliminate option 2 because the dosimeter measures radiation. Eliminate option 3 because the nurse would be exposed to radioactive urine until it is disposed of. Keep in mind suitable methods for containing radiation to direct you to option 4. Review these principles if you had difficulty with this question.

References
Black, J., & Hawks, J. (2005). *Medical-surgical nursing: Clinical management for positive outcomes* (7th ed., p. 363). Philadelphia: Saunders.
Monahan, F., Sands, J., Neighbors, M., Marek, J., & Green, C. (2007). *Phipps', medical-surgical nursing: Health and illness perspectives* (8th ed., pp. 1700-1701). St. Louis: Mosby.

---

778. The nurse understands that incident reports allow the agency to analyze adverse client events by:

1 Evaluating quality care and potential risks for injury to the client
2 Supplying supervisors with objective information for performance reviews
3 Providing a method of reporting injuries to local, state, and federal agencies
4 Determining the effectiveness of nursing interventions in relation to outcomes

Answer: 1
Rationale: Proper documentation of unusual occurrences, incidents, and accidents, as well as the follow-up nursing actions, allow the nursing department and the agency administration to review the quality of care and determine potential risks. Supervisors document the nurse's performance on evaluation documents. Because incident reports are internal documents, they are not used to notify government or regulatory agencies. Quality surveys and nursing research are used to determine the effectiveness of nursing interventions.

Level of Cognitive Ability: Analysis
Client Needs: Safe and Effective Care
  Environment
Integrated Process: Nursing Process/Analysis
Content Area: Fundamental Skills

Test-Taking Strategy: Use the process of elimination and knowledge regarding the purpose of incident reports. Eliminate option 2 because incident reports are not used in performance reviews of nurses. Eliminate option 3 because incident reports are internal documents. Eliminate option 4 because it is unrelated to the purpose of an incident report. Review the purpose of incident reports if you had difficulty with this question.

References
Huber, D. (2006). *Leadership and nursing care management* (3rd ed., p. 862). Philadelphia: Saunders.
Potter, P., & Perry, A. (2005). *Fundamentals of nursing* (6th ed., p. 419). St. Louis: Mosby.

---

779. A registered nurse suspects that a colleague is substance impaired and notes signs of alcohol intoxication in the colleague. The Nurse Practice Act requires that the registered nurse do which of the following?
  1 Talk with the colleague.
  2 Call the impaired nurse organization.
  3 Report the information to a nursing supervisor.
  4 Ask the colleague to go to the nurses' lounge to sleep for awhile.

Level of Cognitive Ability: Application
Client Needs: Safe and Effective Care
  Environment
Integrated Process: Nursing Process/
  Implementation
Content Area: Leadership/Management

Answer: 3
Rationale: Nurse Practice Acts require reporting the suspicion of impaired nurses. The Board of Nursing has jurisdiction over the practice of nursing and may develop plans for treatment and supervision. This suspicion needs to be reported to the nursing supervisor, who will then report to the Board of Nursing. Confronting the colleague may cause conflict. Asking the colleague to go to the nurses' lounge to sleep for awhile does not safeguard clients.

Test-Taking Strategy: Use the process of elimination and knowledge regarding the agency channels of communication when reporting an incident. Remember to report suspicions of substance abuse to the nursing supervisor. Review nursing responsibilities related to suspicion of an impaired nurse if you had difficulty with this question.

Reference
Ignatavicius, D., & Workman, M. (2006). *Medical-surgical nursing: Critical thinking for collaborative care* (5th ed., p. 93). Philadelphia: Saunders.

---

780. A nurse lawyer provides an educational session to the nursing staff regarding client rights. Which of the following actions demonstrates a violation of the client's right to privacy?
  1 Threatening to put a client in restraints
  2 Photographing a client without consent
  3 Performing a surgical procedure without consent
  4 Telling a client that he or she cannot leave the hospital

Level of Cognitive Ability: Analysis
Client Needs: Safe and Effective Care
  Environment
Integrated Process: Nursing Process/Analysis
Content Area: Leadership/Management

Answer: 2
Rationale: Invasion of privacy takes place when an individual's private affairs are unreasonably revealed to the public. Telling the client that he or she cannot leave the hospital constitutes false imprisonment. Threatening to place a client in restraints constitutes assault. Performing a surgical procedure without consent is an example of battery.

Test-Taking Strategy: Use the process of elimination, noting the strategic words "violation of the client's right to privacy." Note the relation of these strategic words to option 2. Review those situations that include invasion of privacy if you had difficulty with this question.

Reference
Potter, P., & Perry, A. (2005). *Fundamentals of nursing* (6th ed., pp. 413-414). St. Louis: Mosby.

781. The nurse accepts compensation from the family for caring for a child at the scene of an accident. The family files suit against the nurse after the child dies. Which is an accurate interpretation of the Good Samaritan law regarding the nurse's liability in this lawsuit?

1 Protects the nurse in civil and criminal court
2 Protects the nurse if the care given was not negligent
3 Provides no immunity if the nurse accepts compensation
4 Protects laypersons but not professional health care providers

Level of Cognitive Ability: Analysis
Client Needs: Safe and Effective Care Environment
Integrated Process: Nursing Process/Analysis
Content Area: Fundamental Skills

Answer: 3
Rationale: A Good Samaritan law is intended to encourage nurses and other health care providers to deliver care to a person when an accident, emergency, or injury occurs. The law provides immunity from prosecution, as long as the health care professional does not accept compensation for the care and the care is not willfully and wantonly negligent.

Test-Taking Strategy: Note the strategic words "accepts compensation" in the question. Note the relation of these words to option 3. Review the Good Samaritan law if you had difficulty with this question.

Reference
Potter, P., & Perry, A. (2005). *Fundamentals of nursing* (6th ed., pp. 411-412). St. Louis: Mosby.

---

782. A client arrives in the emergency department after a serious accident. The client is unconscious, bleeding profusely, and requires life-saving emergency surgery. Which is the best intervention for the nurse to implement before the procedure related to informed consent?

1 Try to call a family member on the telephone.
2 Initiate a court order for the surgical procedure.
3 Ask the client's friend to sign the consent form.
4 Transport the client to the operating room at once.

Level of Cognitive Ability: Analysis
Client Needs: Safe and Effective Care Environment
Integrated Process: Nursing Process/Implementation
Content Area: Fundamental Skills

Answer: 4
Rationale: Generally, the informed consent of an adult client is not needed when an emergency occurs and delay of treatment to obtain informed consent would most likely result in injury or death to the client. The client can also waive the right to give informed consent. Options 1 and 2 potentially delay treatment. The nurse avoids obtaining informed consent from a nonfamily members of the client.

Test-Taking Strategy: Note the strategic words "requires life-saving emergency surgery" and use the process of elimination. Eliminate option 1 and 2 because they would delay treatment; efforts to contact a family member by telephone can be futile, and the court order potentially takes hours to obtain. Eliminate option 3 because a nonfamily member is an unsuitable legal representative of the client. Review the issues surrounding informed consent if you had difficulty with this question.

References
Ignatavicius, D., & Workman, M. (2006). *Medical-surgical nursing: Critical thinking for collaborative care* (5th ed., pp. 304, 306, 857). Philadelphia: Saunders.
Potter, P., & Perry, A. (2005). *Fundamentals of nursing* (6th ed., pp. 416-417). St. Louis: Mosby.

783. A nurse is caring for a 9-month-old child following cleft palate repair who has elbow restraints (security devices) applied. The mother visits the child and asks the nurse to remove the restraints. The nurse takes which appropriate action?

1 Removes both restraints
2 Removes a restraint from one extremity
3 Tells the mother that the restraints cannot be removed
4 Loosens the restraints but tells the mother that they cannot be removed

Level of Cognitive Ability: Application
Client Needs: Safe and Effective Care Environment
Integrated Process: Nursing Process/ Implementation
Content Area: Child Health

Answer: 2
Rationale: Elbow restraints are used following cleft palate repair to prevent the child from touching the repair site, which could cause accidental rupture and tearing of the sutures. The restraints can be removed one at a time only if a parent or nurse is in constant attendance. Options 1, 3, and 4 are inaccurate nursing actions.

Test-Taking Strategy: Use the process of elimination. Eliminate options 3 and 4 first because they are comparable or alike. From the remaining options, recall the purpose of the restraints following this surgical procedure. This will assist in directing you to option 2, the safest nursing action. Review postoperative nursing interventions following cleft palate repair if you had difficulty with this question.

Reference
Hockenberry, M., Wilson, D., & Winkelstein, M. (2005). *Wong's essentials of pediatric nursing* (7th ed., p. 874). St. Louis: Mosby.

---

784. A cooling blanket is prescribed for a child with a fever. A nurse caring for the child has never used this type of equipment, and the charge nurse provides instructions and observes the nurse using the cooling blanket. The charge nurse intervenes if the nurse:

1 Keeps the child uncovered to assist in reducing the fever
2 Places the cooling blanket on the bed and covers the blanket with a sheet
3 Keeps the child dry while on the cooling blanket to reduce the risk of frostbite
4 Checks the skin condition of the child before, during, and after the use of the cooling blanket

Level of Cognitive Ability: Analysis
Client Needs: Safe and Effective Care Environment
Integrated Process: Teaching and Learning
Content Area: Leadership/Management

Answer: 1
Rationale: While on a cooling blanket, the child should be covered lightly to maintain privacy and reduce shivering. Options 2, 3, and 4 are important interventions to prevent shivering, frostbite, and skin breakdown.

Test-Taking Strategy: Note the strategic word "intervenes." This word indicates a negative event query and the need to select the option that identifies an incorrect nursing action. Recalling the physiological response associated with fever and noting the word "uncovered" in option 1 will direct you to this option. Review the procedure associated with the use of a cooling blanket if you had difficulty with this question.

References
Hockenberry, M., & Wilson, D. (2007). *Nursing care of infants and children* (8th ed., p. 1105). St. Louis: Mosby.
McKinney, E., James, S., Murray, S., & Ashwill, J. (2005). *Maternal-child nursing* (2nd ed., pp. 945-946). St. Louis: Saunders.

---

785. A child with respiratory syncytial virus (RSV) who is in an oxygen tent is receiving ribavirin (Virazole). Which precaution will the nurse specifically take while caring for the child?

1 Wear a gown.
2 Wear a head covering.
3 Wear a gown and mask.
4 Wear goggles and a mask.

Answer: 4
Rationale: Some caregivers experience headaches, burning nasal passages and eyes, and crystallization of soft contact lenses as a result of contact with ribavirin (Virazole). Therefore, goggles and a mask should be worn. A gown or head covering is not necessary.

Level of Cognitive Ability: Application
Client Needs: Safe and Effective Care
Environment
Integrated Process: Nursing Process/
Implementation
Content Area: Child Health

Test-Taking Strategy: Note the strategic words "specifically take" in the question. Recalling the effects of this medication on contact with it will direct you to option 4. Review the procedures related to the administration of this medication if you had difficulty with this question.

References

Hockenberry, M., & Wilson, D. (2007). *Nursing care of infants and children* (8th ed., pp. 1106, 1338). St. Louis: Mosby.

McKinney, E., James, S., Murray, S., & Ashwill, J. (2005). *Maternal-child nursing* (2nd ed., p. 1214). St. Louis: Saunders.

ALTERNATE ITEM FORMATS

786. A home care nurse visits a client who has been recently discharged from the hospital following an acute myocardial infarction. The client tells the nurse that a living will was prepared and asks the nurse where a copy of the will can be kept. In which areas will a copy of the client's living will be kept?
Select all that apply.
☐ **1** Lawyer's office
☐ **2** Physician's office
☐ **3** The client's home
☐ **4** The Social Security office
☐ **5** Medical record at the hospital
☐ **6** Hospital emergency department files

Level of Cognitive Ability: Application
Client Needs: Safe and Effective Care
Environment
Integrated Process: Nursing Process/
Implementation
Content Area: Fundamental Skills

Answers: 1, 2, 3, 5
Rationale: Copies of a living will should be kept with the medical record, at the physician's office, and in the client's home. A copy should also be maintained in the lawyer's office. The emergency department does not maintain these documents in its files. A copy of a client's living will is not sent to the Social Security office.

Test-Taking Strategy: Recall that a living will is a legal document, and recall the subjects surrounding confidentiality. Note that the question addresses a home care nurse. Therefore, it seems reasonable that the client should have a copy in the home because this document identifies the client's wishes. It would also seem reasonable that both a physician and lawyer would hold a copy of this document and that a copy would be maintained in the client's medical record to provide guidance to care providers if a situation arose during hospitalization requiring referral to this document. It is not realistic for an emergency department to maintain such documents in its files, especially if the client's medical record will contain this document, anyway. Review the concepts related to living wills if you had difficulty with this question.

References

Ignatavicius, D., & Workman, M. (2006). *Medical-surgical nursing: Critical thinking for collaborative care* (5th ed., p. 64). Philadelphia: Saunders.

Lewis, S., Heitkemper, M., Dirksen, S., O'Brien, P., & Bucher, L. (2007). *Medical-surgical nursing: Assessment and management of clinical problems* (7th ed., pp. 155-156). St. Louis: Mosby.

787. A nurse is providing an educational session to a group of students who are enrolled in a nursing assistant program and prepares an instructional list for the students regarding the correct procedure for handwashing. Select in order of priority the correct procedure for performing handwashing. (Number 1 is the first step in the procedure.)

___Rinse the hands.

___Turn on the water.

___Dry the hands using a paper towel.

___Allow the warm water to wet the hands.

___Turn the water faucet off with a clean and dry paper towel.

___Apply soap to the hands, keep the hands pointed downward, and rub them vigorously.

Level of Cognitive Ability: Application
Client Needs: Safe and Effective Care Environment
Integrated Process: Nursing Process/ Implementation
Content Area: Delegating/Prioritizing

Answers: 4, 1, 5, 2, 6, 3
Rationale: The nurse turns the water on first and then allows the warm water to wet the hands, applies soap to the hands, keeps the hands pointed downward, and rubs them vigorously. Warm water is used for handwashing because it increases the sudsing action of the soap. Hands should be kept downward to enable the unsanitary material to fall off the skin. The nurse then rinses the hands, dries the hands using a paper towel, and turns the water faucet off with a clean and dry paper towel. The faucet is turned off by using a paper towel to prevent the hands from getting recontaminated.

Test-Taking Strategy: Visualize the procedure to answer the question. Recall that care must be taken to avoid recontamination of the hands during and after this procedure. This will assist in determining the order of action. Review the procedure for handwashing if you had difficulty with this question.

References
Ignatavicius, D., & Workman, M. (2006). *Medical-surgical nursing: Critical thinking for collaborative care* (5th ed., pp. 511-512). Philadelphia: Saunders.
Lewis, S., Heitkemper, M., Dirksen, S., O'Brien, P., & Bucher, L. (2007). *Medical-surgical nursing: Assessment and management of clinical problems* (7th ed., p. 248). St. Louis: Mosby.

---

788. A nurse is taking care of a client on contact isolation. After nursing care has been performed and upon leaving the room, the nurse removes protective items in which order of priority? (Number 1 is the first action.)

___Removes the gloves

___Performs handwashing

___Unties the gown at the waist

___Removes the mask and eyewear (goggles)

___Discards the gown in the appropriate receptacle

___Unties the gown at the neck, allows it to fall forward toward the shoulders, and removes it

Level of Cognitive Ability: Application
Client Needs: Safe and Effective Care Environment
Integrated Process: Nursing Process/ Implementation
Content Area: Delegating/Prioritizing

Answers: 2, 6, 1, 5, 4, 3
Rationale: At the door of the room and next to an appropriate receptacle, the nurse unties the gown at the waist but does not remove it yet. The nurse then removes the gloves. The gown is then untied at the neck, allowed to fall forward from the shoulders, and removed. The gown is then discarded in the appropriate receptacle. The nurse then removes the mask and goggles and discards them. The hands are then washed.

Test-Taking Strategy: Use the principles of standard precautions and the methods of preventing contamination to answer the question. Visualize the correct process of removing contaminated clothing and items after caring for a client. Review this procedure if you had difficulty with this question.

References
Monahan, F., Sands, J., Neighbors, M., Marek, J., & Green, C. (2007). *Phipps' medical-surgical nursing: Health and illness perspectives* (8th ed., p. 115). St. Louis: Mosby.
Potter, P., & Perry, A. (2005). *Fundamentals of nursing* (6th ed., pp. 794-795). St. Louis: Mosby.

789. The physician's order reads heparin sodium 25,000 units in 250 mL 5% dextrose in water to infuse intravenously continuously at a rate of 800 units per hour. To ensure that the solution infuses safely at the rate prescribed, the nurse sets the intravenous pump to how many mL per hr?

Answer: _____ mL

Level of Cognitive Ability: Application
Client Needs: Safe and Effective Care Environment
Integrated Process: Nursing Process/ Implementation
Content Area: Fundamental Skills

Answer: 8
Rationale: Use the formula for calculating mL per hour with the use of an infusion pump.
Desired: 800 units per hour
Available: 25,000 units in 250 mL 5% dextrose in water
First, divide the 25,000 units by the 250 mL to yield a concentration of 100 units per mL. Next, 800 units per hour (desired) is divided by 100 units per mL. The nurse would set the pump at 8 mL per hour.

Test-Taking Strategy: Think about what the question is asking. Determine units per mL and then use the standard "desired over available" formula. This will assist in determining that the pump should be set at 8 mL per hour. Review this formula if you had difficulty with this question.

Reference
Kee, J., & Marshall, S. (2004). *Clinical calculations: With applications to general and specialty areas* (5th ed., p. 212). Philadelphia: Saunders.

---

790. The nurse is planning postoperative care for the client who has undergone esophagogastrostomy. To provide a safe environment, which of the following should be included in the plan of care?
Select all that apply.

☐ **1** Place the bed in semi-Fowler's or Fowler's position.

☐ **2** Reposition the nasogastric (NG) tube if drainage stops.

☐ **3** Irrigate the nasogastric tube as needed to promote drainage.

☐ **4** Provide oral hygiene every 2 hours while the NG tube is in place.

☐ **5** Instruct the client to take extra fluids with meals once diet is resumed.

☐ **6** Encourage deep breathing exercises and use of the incentive spirometer.

Level of Cognitive Ability: Application
Client Needs: Safe and Effective Care Environment
Integrated Process: Nursing Process/Planning
Content Area: Adult Health/Gastrointestinal

Answers: 1, 4, 6
Rationale: During esophagogastrostomy the diseased portion of the esophagus and stomach (if involved) is removed and remaining portions of the esophagus and stomach are anastomosed. Measures that could disturb the suture line of anastomosed sites, such as repositioning and irrigation of the NG tube, should be avoided. Absence of drainage from the NG tube warrants a call to the physician. Since the client has an NG tube, frequent and meticulous oral hygiene is essential. Semi-Fowler's or Fowler's position allows for better ventilation and prevention of reflux. When the diet is resumed, the client should ingest fluids between meals rather than during meals to prevent diarrhea. Depending upon the surgical approach, in the client may have an abdominal or thoracic incision but, in either case, will need frequent pulmonary hygiene measures.

Test-Taking Strategy: Think about the anatomy of the esophagus and stomach and the specific surgical procedure to direct you to the appropriate nursing care options. From the selections, immediately eliminate options 2 and 3 because the NG tube of a client after esophagogastrostomy should never be independently manipulated in any way. Knowing that the gastrointestinal tract has been shortened by surgery will guide you in eliminating option 5, because fluids during meals will increase the possibility of diarrhea. Review the postoperative care of the client who has undergone esophageal surgery if you had difficulty with this question.

References
Ignatavicius, D., & Workman, M. (2006). *Medical-surgical nursing: Critical thinking for collaborative care* (5th ed., pp. 1278-1279). Philadelphia: Saunders.
Lewis, S., Heitkemper, M., Dirksen, S., O'Brien, P., & Bucher, L. (2007). *Medical-surgical nursing: Assessment and management of clinical problems* (7th ed., pp. 1010-1011). St. Louis: Mosby.
Monahan, F., Sands, J., Neighbors, M., Marek, J., & Green, C. (2007). *Phipps' medical-surgical nursing: Health and illness perspectives* (8th ed., pp. 1201-1202). St. Louis: Mosby.

791. The medical-surgical nurse who has no experience in critical care and is unfamiliar with the technology of the intensive care unit (ICU) receives an assignment from the supervisor to report to the ICU. Which should the nurse implement? Select all that apply.

- ☐ **1** Refuse to report to the ICU.
- ☐ **2** Ask for the ICU job description.
- ☐ **3** Use one of the accrued sick days.
- ☐ **4** Call the hospital lawyer for advice.
- ☐ **5** Go to the ICU and find the charge nurse.
- ☐ **6** Tell the ICU charge nurse about her nursing experience.

Level of Cognitive Ability: Application
Client Needs: Safe and Effective Care Environment
Integrated Process: Nursing Process/ Implementation
Content Area: Fundamental Skills

Answers: 2, 5, 6
Rationale: Legally, a nurse cannot refuse to float unless it is specified in a contract or the nurse can prove a lack of knowledge for performing nursing tasks related to the assignment. When floated to another unit, the nurse should document the personnel involved in assigning and explaining the new nursing duties, identify potential areas of client injury and the related plan of care, and note all pertinent facts related to client care and safety issues. In addition, the nurse should set priorities and determine areas for collaboration with other, more experienced nurses, because the nurse is legally responsible for implementation of nursing interventions. The float nurse should ask for the job description of the new assignment to identify areas beyond her experience and training. The nurse explains her knowledge and experience to the ICU charge nurse. The charge nurse determines if the float nurse is suitable for the specific assignment in the ICU; if not, the charge nurse notifies the supervisor immediately and avoids assigning the float nurse to clients. The nurse avoids using a sick day because the supervisor knows that the nurse is not ill. This can be construed as client abandonment, and that is unethical. Calling the hospital attorney is unnecessary.

Test-Taking Strategy: Use the process of elimination. Eliminate options 1 and 3, because, if a nurse refuses to care for a client, the nurse can be charged with abandonment. Eliminate option 4 because it is unnecessary. From the remaining options, focus on the subject—the legalities surrounding floating—to direct you to options 2, 5, and 6. Review the issues related to floating and abandonment of the client if you had difficulty with this question.

Reference
Potter, P., & Perry, A. (2005). *Fundamentals of nursing* (6th ed., pp. 418-419). St. Louis: Mosby.

REFERENCES

Black, J., & Hawks, J. (2005). *Medical-surgical nursing: Clinical management for positive outcomes* (7th ed.). Philadelphia: Saunders.

Chernecky, C., & Berger, B. (2008). *Laboratory tests and diagnostic procedures* (5th ed.). Philadelphia: Saunders.

Cohen, E., & Cesta, T. (2005). *Nursing case management: From essentials to advanced practice applications* (4th ed.). St. Louis: Mosby.

Fultz, J., & Sturt, P. (2005). *Emergency nursing reference* (3rd ed.). St. Louis: Mosby.

Gahart, B., & Nazareno, A. (2006). *2006 Intravenous medications* (22nd ed.). St. Louis: Mosby.

Hockenberry, M., & Wilson, D. (2007). *Nursing care of infants and children* (8th ed.). St. Louis: Mosby.

Hockenberry, M., Wilson, D., & Winkelstein, M. (2005). *Wong's essentials of pediatric nursing* (7th ed.). St. Louis: Mosby.

Hodgson, B., & Kizior, R. (2007). *Saunders nursing drug handbook 2007.* Philadelphia: Saunders.

Huber, D. (2006). *Leadership and nursing care management* (3rd ed.). Philadelphia: Saunders.

Ignatavicius, D., & Workman, M. (2006). *Medical-surgical nursing: Critical thinking for collaborative care* (5th ed.). Philadelphia: Saunders.

Kee, J., Hayes, E., & McCuistion, L. (2006). *Pharmacology: A nursing process approach* (5th ed.). Philadelphia: Saunders.

Kee, J., & Marshall, S. (2004). *Clinical calculations: With applications to general and specialty areas* (5th ed.). Philadelphia: Saunders.

Lehne, R. (2007). *Pharmacology for nursing care* (6th ed.). St. Louis: Saunders.

Lewis, S., Heitkemper, M., Dirksen, S., O'Brien, P., & Bucher, L. (2007). *Medical-surgical nursing: Assessment and management of clinical problems* (7th ed.). St. Louis: Mosby.

Lowdermilk, D., & Perry, A. (2006). *Maternity nursing* (7th ed.). St. Louis: Mosby.

McKenry, L., Tressier, E., & Hogan, M. (2006). *Mosby's pharmacology in nursing* (22nd ed.). St. Louis: Mosby.

McKinney, E., James, S., Murray, S., & Ashwill, J. (2005). *Maternal-child nursing* (2nd ed.). St. Louis: Saunders.

Meiner, S., & Leuckenotte, A. (2006). *Gerontologic nursing* (3rd ed.). St. Louis: Mosby.

Monahan, F., Sands, J., Marek, J., Neighbars, M., & Green, C. (2007). *Phipps' medical-surgical nursing: Health and illness pesspectives* (8th ed.). St. Louis, Mosby.

Murray, S., & McKinney, E. (2006). *Foundations of maternal-newborn nursing* (4th ed.). Philadelphia: Saunders.

Pagana, K., & Pagana, T. (2005). *Mosby's diagnostic and laboratory test reference* (7th ed.). St. Louis: Mosby.

Perry, A., & Potter, P. (2006). *Clinical nursing skills & techniques* (6th ed.). St. Louis: Mosby.

Potter, P., & Perry, A. (2005). *Fundamentals of nursing* (6th ed.). St. Louis: Mosby.

Skidmore-Roth, L. (2008). *Mosby's nursing drug reference* (21st ed.). St. Louis: Mosby.

Stuart, G., & Laraia, M. (2005). *Principles and practice of psychiatric nursing* (8th ed.). St. Louis: Mosby.

Varcarolis, E., Carson, V., & Shoemaker, N. (2006). *Foundations of psychiatric mental health nursing* (5th ed., p. 304). Philadelphia: Saunders.

Wilson, S., & Giddens, J. (2005). *Health assessment for nursing practice* (3rd ed.). St. Louis: Mosby.

Wong, D., Hockenberry, M., Perry, S., Lowdermilk, D., & Wilson, D. (2006). *Maternal-child nursing care* (3rd ed.). St. Louis: Mosby.

Health Promotion and Maintenance

792. The nurse is conducting a health screening clinic for osteoporosis. The nurse determines that which client seen in the clinic is at the greatest risk of developing this disorder?

1 A 25-year-old female who jogs
2 A 36-year-old male who has asthma
3 A 70-year-old male who consumes excess alcohol
4 A sedentary 65-year-old female who smokes cigarettes

Level of Cognitive Ability: Analysis
Client Needs: Health Promotion and Maintenance
Integrated Process: Nursing Process/Assessment
Content Area: Adult Health/Musculoskeletal

Answer: 4
Rationale: Risk factors for osteoporosis include being female, postmenopausal status, advanced age, low-calcium diet, excessive alcohol intake, sedentary lifestyle, and cigarette smoking. The long-term use of corticosteroids, anticonvulsants, and furosemide (Lasix) also increase the risk.

Test-Taking Strategy: Use the process of elimination, thinking about the risk factors associated with osteoporosis. Option 1 is eliminated first. The 25-year-old female who jogs (exercise using the long bones) has negligible risk. The 36-year-old male with asthma (option 2) is eliminated next, because the only risk factor may be the long-term use of corticosteroids for asthma. From the remaining options, the 65-year-old female is at higher risk (age, gender, postmenopausal, sedentary, smoking) than the 70-year-old male (age, alcohol consumption). Review the risk factors associated with osteoporosis if you had difficulty with this question.

Reference
Ignatavicius, D., & Workman, M. (2006). *Medical-surgical nursing: Critical thinking for collaborative care* (5th ed., p. 1158). Philadelphia. Saunders.

---

793. A client has been taught to use a walker to aid with mobility after the internal fixation of a hip fracture. The nurse determines that the client is using the walker incorrectly if the client:

1 Holds the walker using the hand grips
2 Advances the walker with reciprocal motion
3 Leans forward slightly when advancing the walker
4 Supports the body weight on the hands while advancing the weaker leg

Answer: 2
Rationale: The client should use the walker by placing the hands on the hand grips for stability. The client lifts the walker to advance it and leans forward slightly while moving it. The client walks into the walker, supporting the body weight on the hands while moving the weaker leg. A disadvantage of the walker is that it does not allow for reciprocal walking motion. If the client were to try to use reciprocal motion with a walker, the walker would advance forward one side at a time as the client walks; thus the client would not be supporting the weaker leg with the walker during ambulation.

Level of Cognitive Ability: Analysis
Client Needs: Health Promotion and
Maintenance
Integrated Process: Nursing Process/Evaluation
Content Area: Adult Health/Musculoskeletal

Test-Taking Strategy: Note the strategic word "incorrectly." Use the process of elimination and visualize this procedure; this will direct you to option 2. Review the client teaching points related to the use of a cane if you had difficulty with this question.

References
Ignatavicius, D., & Workman, M. (2006). *Medical-surgical nursing: Critical thinking for collaborative care* (5th ed., pp. 125-126). Philadelphia: Saunders.
Potter, P., & Perry, A. (2005). *Fundamentals of nursing* (6th ed., pp. 948-949). St. Louis: Mosby.

---

794. The nurse has taught a client with a below-the-knee amputation about prosthesis and residual limb care. The nurse determines that the client has understood the instructions if the client stated that he should:

1 Wear a clean nylon sock over the residual limb every day.
2 Use a mirror to inspect all areas of the residual limb each day.
3 Toughen the skin of the residual limb by rubbing it with alcohol.
4 Prevent cracking of the skin of the residual limb by applying lotion daily.

Level of Cognitive Ability: Analysis
Client Needs: Health Promotion and
Maintenance
Integrated Process: Nursing Process/Evaluation
Content Area: Adult Health/Musculoskeletal

Answer: 2
Rationale: The client should inspect all surfaces of the residual limb daily for irritation, blisters, and breakdown. The client should wear a clean woolen (not nylon) sock each day. The residual limb is cleansed daily with a gentle soap and water and dried carefully. Alcohol is avoided, because it could cause drying or cracking of the skin. Oils and creams are also avoided, because they are too softening to the skin for safe prosthesis use.

Test-Taking Strategy: Use the process of elimination. Recall that nylon is a synthetic material that does not allow for the best air circulation and that holds in moisture. For this reason, option 1 is incorrect. Either alcohol or lotion can interfere with the natural condition of the skin, thus increasing the likelihood of breakdown either from drying or from excess moisture. For these reasons, eliminate options 3 and 4. Review the client teaching points related to residual limb care after amputation if you had difficulty with this question.

Reference
Black, J., & Hawks, J. (2005). *Medical-surgical nursing: Clinical management for positive outcomes* (7th ed., pp. 1524-1525, 1527). Philadelphia: Saunders.

---

795. The nurse is ambulating a client with a right-leg fracture who has an order for partial weight-bearing status. The nurse determines that the client demonstrates compliance with this restriction if the client:

1 Does not bear weight on the right leg
2 Allows the right leg to touch the floor only
3 Puts 30% to 50% of the weight on the right leg
4 Puts 60% to 80% of the weight on the right leg

Level of Cognitive Ability: Analysis
Client Needs: Health Promotion and
Maintenance
Integrated Process: Nursing Process/Evaluation
Content Area: Adult Health/Musculoskeletal

Answer: 3
Rationale: The client who has partial weight-bearing status places 30% to 50% of the body weight on the affected limb. Full weight-bearing status involves placing full weight on the limb. Non–weight-bearing status does not allow the client to let the limb touch the floor. Touchdown weight-bearing allows the client to let the limb touch the floor but not to bear weight. There is no classification for 60% to 80% weight-bearing status.

Test-Taking Strategy: Use the process of elimination, focusing on the strategic words "partial weight-bearing status." Option 3 is the only option that fits the description of partial weight-bearing status. Review the categories related to weight-bearing if you had difficulty with this question.

References
Black, J., & Hawks, J. (2005). *Medical-surgical nursing: Clinical management for positive outcomes* (7th ed., p. 643). Philadelphia: Saunders.
Monahan, F., Sands, J., Neighbors, M., Marek, J., & Green, C. (2007). *Phipps' medical-surgical nursing: Health and illness perspectives* (8th ed., p. 1537). St. Louis: Mosby.

796. The nurse is planning to teach a client in skeletal leg traction about measures to increase bed mobility. Which item would be most helpful for this client?
  1 Television
  2 Fracture bedpan
  3 Overhead trapeze
  4 Reading materials

Level of Cognitive Ability: Analysis
Client Needs: Health Promotion and Maintenance
Integrated Process: Nursing Process/Planning
Content Area: Adult Health/Musculoskeletal

Answer: 3
Rationale: The use of an overhead trapeze is extremely helpful for assisting a client with moving about in bed and getting on and off the bedpan. This device has the greatest value for increasing overall bed mobility. Television and reading materials are helpful to reduce boredom and provide distraction. A fracture bedpan is useful for reducing discomfort with elimination.

Test-Taking Strategy: Note the strategic words "most helpful," and focus on the subject—increased bed mobility. Although all of these options are useful to the client in skeletal traction, the only one that helps with bed mobility is the trapeze. Review the care of the client in traction if you had difficulty with this question.

References
Black, J., & Hawks, J. (2005). *Medical-surgical nursing: Clinical management for positive outcomes* (7th ed., p. 636). Philadelphia: Saunders.
Monahan, F., Sands, J., Neighbors, M., Marek, J., & Green, C. (2007). *Phipps' medical-surgical nursing: Health and illness perspectives* (8th ed., pp. 1528-1529, 1535). St. Louis: Mosby.
Potter, P., & Perry, A. (2005). *Fundamentals of nursing* (6th ed., pp. 1455-1456). St. Louis: Mosby.

---

797. A nurse has given medication instructions to the client who is starting anticonvulsant therapy with carbamazepine (Tegretol). The nurse determines that the client understands the use of the medication if the client stated which of the following?
  1 "I can drive as long as it is not at night."
  2 "I will use sunscreen when out of doors."
  3 "I will keep tissues handy because of excess salivation."
  4 "I will discontinue the medication if fever or a sore throat occurs."

Level of Cognitive Ability: Analysis
Client Needs: Health Promotion and Maintenance
Integrated Process: Teaching and Learning
Content Area: Pharmacology

Answer: 2
Rationale: Carbamazepine acts by depressing synaptic transmission in the central nervous system (CNS). Because of this, the client should avoid driving or doing other activities that require mental alertness until the effect on the client is known. The client should use protective clothing and sunscreen to avoid photosensitivity reactions. The medication may cause dry mouth, and the client should be instructed to provide good oral hygiene and to use sugarless candy or gum as needed. The medication should not be abruptly discontinued, because it could cause the return of seizures. Fever and sore throat should be reported to the physician because they may indicate leukopenia.

Test-Taking Strategy: Use the process of elimination. Recalling that this is an anticonvulsant medication with CNS depressant properties will assist with the elimination of option 1 first. Option 4 is eliminated next, because an anticonvulsant is not discontinued just because side effects or infection occur; rather, the physician should be called. From the remaining options, remembering that carbamazepine causes dry mouth will assist you with eliminating option 3. Review the client teaching points related to this medication if you had difficulty with this question.

Reference
Lehne, R. (2007). *Pharmacology for nursing care* (6th ed., p. 224). Philadelphia: Saunders.

798. The nurse provides discharge instructions to a client with rheumatoid arthritis. The instructions focus on measures to lessen discomfort and to provide joint protection, and the nurse tells the client to:

1 Change positions every hour.
2 Lift items rather than sliding them.
3 Avoid stooping, bending, or overreaching.
4 Perform prescribed exercises even if the joints are inflamed.

Level of Cognitive Ability: Application
Client Needs: Health Promotion and Maintenance
Integrated Process: Nursing Process/ Implementation
Content Area: Adult Health/Musculoskeletal

Answer: 3

Rationale: The client with rheumatoid arthritis is instructed to avoid stooping, bending, or overreaching. The client should avoid remaining in one position and should change positions or stretch every 20 minutes. To reduce efforts by joints, the client should slide objects rather than lift them. The client should avoid exercises and activities other than gentle range-of-motion movements when the joints are inflamed.

Test-Taking Strategy: Use the process of elimination. Eliminate option 1 because, with rheumatoid arthritis, remaining in one position for 1 hour is rather lengthy. Eliminate option 4 on the basis of the basic principle that joints should be rested if they are inflamed. From the remaining options, use the principles related to body mechanics to direct you to option 3. Review the principles for joint protection in rheumatoid arthritis if you had difficulty with this question.

References

Black, J., & Hawks, J. (2005). *Medical-surgical nursing: Clinical management for positive outcomes* (7th ed., p. 2344). Philadelphia: Saunders.

Monahan, F., Sands, J., Neighbors, M., Marek, J., & Green, C. (2007). *Phipps' medical-surgical nursing: Health and illness perspectives* (8th ed., pp. 1651-1653). St. Louis: Mosby.

---

799. The home-care nurse visits an older client with arthritis. The client complains of difficulty instilling glaucoma eye drops because of shaking hands caused by the arthritis. Which instruction should the nurse plan to provide to the client to alleviate this problem?

1 Tilt the head back to instill the eye drops.
2 Lie down on a bed or sofa to instill the eye drops.
3 A family member will have to instill the eye drops.
4 Keep the eye drops in the refrigerator so that they will thicken and be easier to instill.

Level of Cognitive Ability: Application
Client Needs: Health Promotion and Maintenance
Integrated Process: Teaching and Learning
Content Area: Adult Health/Eye

Answer: 2

Rationale: Older clients with arthritis or shaking hands have difficulty instilling their own eye drops. The older client is instructed to lie down on a bed or sofa to instill the eye drops. Tilting the head back can lead to a loss of balance. Eye drop regimens for glaucoma require accurate timing, and it is unreasonable to expect a family member to instill the eye drops. Additionally, this discourages client independence. Placing the eye drops in the refrigerator should not be done unless specifically prescribed.

Test-Taking Strategy: Use the process of elimination. Eliminate option 4 first, because eye medication should not be refrigerated unless specifically prescribed. Considering the subject of promoting client independence and the fact that the question does not provide data regarding the client's family, eliminate option 3. From the remaining options, select option 2, because it provides greater safety for the older client. Review the procedures for instilling eye drops if you had difficulty with this question.

References

Black, J., & Hawks, J. (2005). *Medical-surgical nursing: Clinical management for positive outcomes* (7th ed., p. 1948). Philadelphia: Saunders.

Monahan, F., Sands, J., Neighbors, M., Marek, J., & Green, C. (2007). *Phipp's medical-surgical nursing: Health and illness perspectives* (8th ed., p. 1823). St. Louis: Mosby.

800. A scleral buckling procedure is performed on a client with retinal detachment, and the nurse provides home-care instructions to the client. Which statement by the client indicates a need for further instructions?

1 "I need to avoid heavy lifting."
2 "I need to avoid vigorous activity."
3 "I need to wear an eye shield during naps and at night."
4 "I need to clean the eye daily with sterile water and a clean washcloth."

Level of Cognitive Ability: Analysis
Client Needs: Health Promotion and Maintenance
Integrated Process: Teaching and Learning
Content Area: Adult Health/Eye

Answer: 4
Rationale: In a scleral buckling procedure, the sclera is compressed from the outside by Silastic sponges or silicone bands that are sutured in place permanently. In addition, an intraocular injection of air, a gas bubble, or both may be used to apply pressure on the retina from the inside of the eye to hold the retina in place. If an air or gas bubble has been injected, it may take several weeks to be absorbed. Vigorous activities and heavy lifting are avoided. An eye shield or glasses should be worn during the day, and a shield should be worn during naps and at night. The client is instructed to clean the eye with warm tap water using a clean washcloth.

Test-Taking Strategy: Use the process of elimination, noting the strategic words "need for further instructions." These words indicate a negative event query and ask you to select an option that is an incorrect statement. It is not necessary to use sterile water to clean the eye. In fact, it does not make sense to use a sterile solution with a clean washcloth. Review the client teaching points for care after scleral buckling if you had difficulty with this question.

References
Black, J., & Hawks, J. (2005). *Medical-surgical nursing: Clinical management for positive outcomes* (7th ed., p. 1953). Philadelphia: Saunders.
Ignatavicius, D., & Workman, M. (2006). *Medical-surgical nursing: Critical thinking for collaborative care* (5th ed., pp. 1102-1103). Philadelphia: Saunders.

801. A nurse provides dietary instruction to the parents of a child with a diagnosis of cystic fibrosis. The nurse tells the parents that the diet should be:

1 Fat free
2 Low in protein
3 Low in sodium
4 High in calories

Level of Cognitive Ability: Application
Client Needs: Health Promotion and Maintenance
Integrated Process: Teaching and Learning
Content Area: Child Health

Answer: 4
Rationale: Children with cystic fibrosis are managed with a high-calorie, high-protein diet, pancreatic enzyme replacement therapy, fat-soluble vitamin supplements, and, if nutritional problems are severe, nighttime gastrostomy feedings or parental nutrition. Fats are not restricted unless steatorrhea cannot be controlled by increased pancreatic enzymes. Sodium intake is unrelated to this disorder.

Test-Taking Strategy: Think about the pathophysiology associated with cystic fibrosis, and use the process of elimination. Select option 4 because children require calories for growth and development and because this option is the umbrella one. Review the dietary measures for the child with cystic fibrosis if you had difficulty with this question.

Reference
Hockenberry, M., Wilson, D., & Winkelstein, M. (2005). *Wong's essentials of pediatric nursing* (7th ed., p. 827). St. Louis: Mosby.

802. A clinic nurse instructs an adolescent with iron deficiency anemia about the administration of oral iron preparations. The nurse tells the adolescent that it is best to take the iron with:
1 Cola
2 Soda
3 Water
4 Tomato juice

Level of Cognitive Ability: Application
Client Needs: Health Promotion and Maintenance
Integrated Process: Teaching and Learning
Content Area: Child Health

Answer: 4
Rationale: Iron should be administered with vitamin-C–rich fluids, because vitamin C enhances the absorption of the iron preparation. Tomato juice has a high ascorbic acid (vitamin C) content, whereas water, soda, and cola do not contain vitamin C.

Test-Taking Strategy: Use the process of elimination. Eliminate options 1 and 2 first because they are comparable or alike. From the remaining options, recall that vitamin C increases the absorption of iron to direct you to option 4. Review the administration of oral iron if you had difficulty with this question.

References
Hockenberry, M., Wilson, D., & Winkelstein, M. (2005). *Wong's essentials of pediatric nursing* (7th ed., p. 1519). St. Louis: Mosby.
McKinney, E., James, S., Murray, S., & Ashwill, J. (2005). *Maternal-child nursing* (2nd ed., p. 657). St. Louis: Saunders.

---

803. A nurse is conducting a home visit for the client who started taking a sustained-release preparation of procainamide hydrochloride (Pronestyl SR). The nurse plans to teach the client which of the following items about this medication?
1 A double dose may be taken if the first daily dose is missed.
2 Do not crush, chew, or break the sustained-release preparations.
3 Monitoring the pulse rate is not necessary after this medication is begun.
4 The presence of a tablet wax matrix in the stool indicates poor medication absorption.

Level of Cognitive Ability: Application
Client Needs: Health Promotion and Maintenance
Integrated Process: Teaching and Learning
Content Area: Pharmacology

Answer: 2
Rationale: Procainamide (Pronestyl) is an antidysrhythmic that is available in a sustained-release (SR) form. The SR preparations should not be broken, chewed, or crushed. The SR form has a wax matrix that may be noted in the stool, but, if this occurs, it is not significant. If a dose is missed, an SR tablet may be taken if remembered within 4 hours (2 hours for regular-acting form); otherwise, the dose should be omitted. The client or a family member should be taught to monitor the client's pulse and to report any changes in rate or rhythm.

Test-Taking Strategy: Use the process of elimination. Note the relationship between the medication (Pronestyl SR) and option 2. Remember, SR preparations should not be broken, chewed, or crushed. Review the administration of this type of medication if you had difficulty with this question.

References
Hodgson, B., & Kizior, R. (2007). *Saunders nursing drug handbook 2007* (p. 965). Philadelphia: Saunders.
Skidmore-Roth, L. (2008). *Mosby's nursing drug reference* (21st ed., p. 850). St. Louis: Mosby.

---

804. The nurse has given the client with a nephrostomy tube instructions to follow after hospital discharge. The nurse determines that the client understands the instructions if the client verbalizes the need to drink at least how many glasses of water per day?
1 2 to 4
2 6 to 8
3 10 to 12
4 14 to 16

Answer: 2
Rationale: The client with a nephrostomy tube needs to have adequate fluid intake to dilute urinary particles that could cause calculus and to provide good mechanical flushing of the kidney and the tube. The nurse encourages the client to take in at least 2000 mL of fluid per day, which is roughly equivalent to 6 to 8 glasses of water. Option 1 is an inadequate amount. Options 3 and 4 are amounts that could distend the renal pelvis.

Level of Cognitive Ability: Analysis
Client Needs: Health Promotion and
 Maintenance
Integrated Process: Nursing Process/Evaluation
Content Area: Adult Health/Renal

Test-Taking Strategy: Use the process of elimination, noting that the client has a nephrostomy tube. Recall that the client needs at least 2 L of fluid per day. This will direct you to option 2. Also, avoid options in the much higher range, because these are unnecessary and could possibly place undue distention on the renal pelvis. Review the care of the client with a nephrostomy tube if you had difficulty with this question.

References

Ignatavicius, D., & Workman, M. (2006). *Medical-surgical nursing: Critical thinking for collaborative care* (5th ed., p. 1715). Philadelphia: Saunders.

Monahan, F., Sands, J., Neighbors, M., Marek, J., & Green, C. (2007). *Phipps' medical-surgical nursing: Health and illness perspectives* (8th ed., p. 992). St. Louis: Mosby.

---

805. The primary care nurse provides home-care instructions to a female client who has chronic trichomoniasis, and she then has the client explain the plan of care. Which explanation by the client requires follow-up nursing interventions?

1 Avoid sexual intercourse.
2 Perform good perineal hygiene.
3 Apply an antifungal agent for 7 days.
4 Discontinue treatment during menstruation.

Level of Cognitive Ability: Analysis
Client Needs: Health Promotion and
 Maintenance
Integrated Process: Teaching and Learning
Content Area: Fundamental Skills

Answer: 4
Rationale: Treatment for a recurrent vaginal trichomoniasis (yeast) infection continues through the menstrual period; because the vagina is more alkaline during menses, a flare-up is more likely to occur. While the infection remains active, the client should refrain from sexual intercourse or instruct her partner to wear a condom. To help break the chain of infection, the nurse directs the client to perform perineal hygiene after each voiding and each bowel movement. Antifungal therapy is more effective if it is administered for a continuous, 7-day period.

Test-Taking Strategy: Note the strategic words "requires follow-up nursing interventions." This indicates that the answer will be a client misunderstanding about self-care while treating the yeast infection. Recall the basic principles related to infection control for vaginal fungal infections and medication administration to direct you to option 4. Review the treatment for this infection if you had difficulty with this question.

Reference

Ignatavicius, D., & Workman, M. (2006). *Medical-surgical nursing: Critical thinking for collaborative care* (5th ed., pp. 1832, 1902). Philadelphia: Saunders.

---

806. The nurse has provided home-care instructions to a client recovering from a radical vulvectomy. Which statement by the client indicates the need for further instructions?

1 "I need to take showers rather than tub baths."
2 "I need to monitor for foul-smelling perineal discharge."
3 "I need to wipe from front to back after a bowel movement."
4 "I need to notify the physician if swelling of the groin or genital area persists for longer than 1 week."

Answer: 4
Rationale: The physician needs to be notified if any swelling of the groin or genital area occurs, and the client should not wait 1 week before notifying the physician. Options 1, 2, and 3 are accurate instructions. Additionally, the client should monitor for pain, redness, or tenderness in the calves and for any signs of infection.

Test-Taking Strategy: Use the process of elimination, noting the strategic words "need for further instructions." These words indicate a negative event query and ask you to select an option that is an incorrect statement. Basic hygiene principles will assist you with eliminating options 1 and 3. From the remaining options, select option 4, noting the timeframe given in this option. Review the client teaching points related to a radical vulvectomy if you had difficulty with this question.

Level of Cognitive Ability: Analysis
Client Needs: Health Promotion and
    Maintenance
Integrated Process: Teaching and Learning
Content Area: Adult Health/Oncology

References
Black, J., & Hawks, J. (2005). *Medical-surgical nursing: Clinical management for positive outcomes* (7th ed., pp. 1086-1087). Philadelphia: Saunders.
Ignatavicius, D., & Workman, M. (2006). *Medical-surgical nursing: Critical thinking for collaborative care* (5th ed., pp. 1851-1852). Philadelphia: Saunders.

---

807. A client with a history of depression will be participating in cognitive therapy for health maintenance. The client asks the nurse, "How does this treatment work?" The nurse should make which statement to the client?

1 "This treatment will help you relax and develop new coping skills."

2 "This treatment helps you confront your fears by gradually exposing you to them."

3 "This treatment helps you examine how your past life has contributed to your problems."

4 "This treatment helps examine how your thoughts and feelings contribute to your difficulties."

Level of Cognitive Ability: Application
Client Needs: Health Promotion and
    Maintenance
Integrated Process: Nursing Process/
    Implementation
Content Area: Mental Health

Answer: 4

Rationale: Cognitive therapy is frequently used with clients who have depression. This type of therapy is based on exploring the client's subjective experience. It includes examining the client's thoughts and feelings about situations as well as how these thoughts and feelings contribute to and perpetuate the client's difficulties and mood. Options 1, 2, and 3 are not characteristics of cognitive therapy.

Test-Taking Strategy: Note the strategic word "cognitive," and note the relationship between this word and option 4. Option 4 uses the word "thoughts" when describing the treatment. Review this form of therapy if you had difficulty with this question.

References
Stuart, G., & Laraia, M. (2005). *Principles and practice of psychiatric nursing* (8th ed., p. 793). St. Louis: Mosby.
Varcarolis, E., Carson, V., & Shoemaker, N. (2006). *Foundations of psychiatric mental health nursing* (5th ed., p. 333). Philadelphia: Saunders.

---

808. A client with acquired immunodeficiency syndrome has a nursing diagnosis of Imbalanced Nutrition: Less Than Body Requirements. The nurse has instructed the client regarding methods of maintaining and increasing weight. The nurse determines that the client would benefit from further instruction if the client stated the need to:

1 Eat low-calorie snacks between meals.

2 Eat small, frequent meals throughout the day.

3 Consume nutrient-dense foods and beverages.

4 Keep easy-to-prepare foods available in the home.

Level of Cognitive Ability: Analysis
Client Needs: Health Promotion and
    Maintenance
Integrated Process: Teaching and Learning
Content Area: Adult Health/Immune

Answer: 1

Rationale: The client should eat small, frequent meals throughout the day. The client also should take in nutrient-dense and high-calorie meals and snacks. The client is encouraged to eat favorite foods to keep intake up and to plan meals that are easy to prepare. The client can also avoid taking fluids with meals to increase food intake before satiety occurs.

Test-Taking Strategy: Note the strategic words "would benefit from further instruction." These words indicate a negative event query and ask you to select an option that is an incorrect statement. Also note the nursing diagnosis: Imbalanced Nutrition: Less Than Body Requirements. Recalling that the client should choose snacks that are high in calories (rather than low in calories) will direct you to option 1. Review the care of the client with imbalanced nutrition if you had difficulty with this question.

References
Black, J., & Hawks, J. (2005). *Medical-surgical nursing: Clinical management for positive outcomes* (7th ed., p. 2396). Philadelphia: Saunders.
Monahan, F., Sands, J., Neighbors, M., Marek, J., & Green, C. (2007). *Phipps' medical-surgical nursing: Health and illness perspectives* (8th ed., p. 454). St. Louis: Mosby.

809. The nurse has given a postoperative thoracotomy client instructions about how to perform arm and shoulder exercises after discharge from the hospital. The nurse determines that the client needs further instructions about effective techniques if the client is observed doing which movement on the affected side?
1 Making circles with the wrist
2 Moving the arm up over the head and back down
3 Holding the hands crossed in front and raising them over the head
4 Holding the upper arm straight out while moving the forearm up and down

Level of Cognitive Ability: Analysis
Client Needs: Health Promotion and Maintenance
Integrated Process: Teaching and Learning
Content Area: Adult Health/Respiratory

Answer: 1
Rationale: Exercises that move only the wrist joint are of no use after this surgery. A variety of exercises that involve moving the shoulder and elbow joints are indicated after thoracotomy. These include shrugging the shoulders and moving them back and forth; moving the arms up, down, forward, and backward; holding the hands crossed in front of the waist and then raising them over the head; and holding the upper arm straight out while moving the lower arm up and down.

Test-Taking Strategy: Use the process of elimination, noting the strategic words "needs further instructions about effective techniques." These words indicate a negative event query and ask you to select an option that is an incorrect technique. Also focus on the subject—arm and shoulder exercises. Note that options 2 and 3 involve movement of the shoulder joint. Option 4 involves the movement of the shoulder and elbow joints, and option 1 involves movement of only the wrist joint. Review arm and shoulder exercises after thoracotomy if you had difficulty with this question.

Reference
Black, J., & Hawks, J. (2005). *Medical-surgical nursing: Clinical management for positive outcomes* (7th ed., pp. 306, 1822). Philadelphia: Saunders.

810. The nurse is teaching a client with histoplasmosis infection about the prevention of future exposure to infectious sources. The nurse determines that the client needs further instruction if the client states that potential infectious sources include:
1 Grape arbors
2 Bird droppings
3 Mushroom cellars
4 Floors of chicken houses

Level of Cognitive Ability: Analysis
Client Needs: Health Promotion and Maintenance
Integrated Process: Teaching and Learning
Content Area: Adult Health/Respiratory

Answer: 1
Rationale: The client with histoplasmosis is taught to avoid exposure to potential sources of the fungus, including bird droppings (especially those of starlings and blackbirds), the floors of chicken houses and bat caves, and mushroom cellars.

Test-Taking Strategy: Note the strategic words "needs further instruction." These words indicate a negative event query and ask you to select an option that is an incorrect statement. Eliminate options 2 and 4 first, because they are comparable or alike. Because histoplasmosis is a fungus, recall that there is increased exposure to areas where the fungus thrives. Therefore, the least likely option is the grape arbor, which is above ground and is not in a dark and damp area. Review the sources and causes of histoplasmosis infection if you had difficulty with this question.

References
Black, J., & Hawks, J. (2005). *Medical-surgical nursing: Clinical management for positive outcomes* (7th ed., pp. 420, 2391). Philadelphia: Saunders.
Lewis, S., Heitkemper, M., Dirksen, S., O'Brien, P., & Bucher, L. (2007). *Medical-surgical nursing: Assessment and management of clinical problems* (7th ed., p. 576). St. Louis: Mosby.

811. The nurse is teaching a client with pulmonary sarcoidosis about long-term ongoing management. The nurse plans to include which of the following in the instructions?
1 The usefulness of home oxygen
2 The need for daily corticosteroids
3 The importance of using incentive spirometry daily
4 The need for follow-up chest X-rays every 6 months

Level of Cognitive Ability: Application
Client Needs: Health Promotion and Maintenance
Integrated Process: Nursing Process/Planning
Content Area: Adult Health/Respiratory

Answer: 4
Rationale: The client with pulmonary sarcoidosis needs to have follow-up chest X-rays every 6 months to monitor disease progression. If an exacerbation occurs, treatment is initiated with systemic corticosteroids, but corticosteroids are not a part of long-term ongoing management. Home oxygen and the ongoing use of incentive spirometry are not indicated.

Test-Taking Strategy: Note the strategic words "long-term ongoing management," and focus on the client's diagnosis. Eliminate option 1 first, because there is no specific information in the question to indicate a need for the use of home oxygen. Recalling that corticosteroids are used for exacerbation helps you to eliminate option 2 as well. From the remaining options, it is necessary to know that serial monitoring with x-ray examination is needed to track the progression of the disease. Review the treatment of pulmonary sarcoidosis if you had difficulty with this question.

Reference
Black, J., & Hawks, J. (2005). *Medical-surgical nursing: Clinical management for positive outcomes* (7th ed., pp. 1871-1872). Philadelphia: Saunders.

---

812. The nurse has taught a client with silicosis about situations to avoid to prevent self-exposure to silica dust. The nurse determines that the client understands the instructions if the client verbalizes the need to give up or wear a mask during which of the following hobbies?
1 Painting
2 Gardening
3 Woodworking
4 Pottery making

Level of Cognitive Ability: Analysis
Client Needs: Health Promotion and Maintenance
Integrated Process: Nursing Process/Evaluation
Content Area: Adult Health/Respiratory

Answer: 4
Rationale: Exposure to silica dust occurs with activities such as pottery making and stone masonry. Exposure to the finely ground silica, such as that used in soaps, polishes, and filters, is also dangerous. Silica is not a pesticide and is not found in average soil. Silica is not inhaled in fumes, such as those involved with painting or woodworking.

Test-Taking Strategy: Use the process of elimination, focusing on the subject—silica dust. Think about the materials that could give off silica dust. Recalling that pottery is made from clay, which is dug from the earth, will direct you to option 4. Review the sources of silica dust if you had difficulty with this question.

Reference
Lewis, S., Heitkemper, M., Dirksen, S., O'Brien, P., & Bucher, L. (2007). *Medical-surgical nursing: Assessment and management of clinical problems* (7th ed., p. 578). St. Louis: Mosby.

---

813. The nurse is teaching a client who is hypocalcemic about dietary sources of calcium. Which food should the nurse encourage the client to consume to increase calcium intake?
1 Apples
2 Cheese
3 Cooked pasta
4 Chicken breast

Answer: 2
Rationale: Products that are naturally high in calcium are dairy products, including milk, cheese, ice cream, and yogurt. High-calcium foods generally have more than 100 mg of calcium per serving. The other options are foods that are low in calcium, which means that they have less than 25 mg of calcium per serving.

Test-Taking Strategy: Use the process of elimination, focusing on the client's diagnosis. Recalling that dairy products are naturally high in calcium will direct you to option 2. Review the foods that are high in calcium if you had difficulty with this question.

Level of Cognitive Ability: Application
Client Needs: Health Promotion and
  Maintenance
Integrated Process: Teaching and Learning
Content Area: Fundamental Skills

References
Black, J., & Hawks, J. (2005). *Medical-surgical nursing: Clinical management for positive outcomes* (7th ed., pp. 238-239). Philadelphia: Saunders.
Ignatavicius, D., & Workman, M. (2006). *Medical-surgical nursing: Critical thinking for collaborative care* (5th ed., p. 206). Philadelphia: Saunders.

---

814. A client has hyperphosphatemia. Which food does the nurse instruct the client to avoid to prevent aggravating the condition?
  1 Coffee
  2 Grapes
  3 Bananas
  4 Carbonated beverages

Level of Cognitive Ability: Application
Client Needs: Health Promotion and
  Maintenance
Integrated Process: Teaching and Learning
Content Area: Fundamental Skills

Answer: 4
Rationale: Food items and liquids that are naturally high in phosphates include fish, eggs, milk products, vegetables, whole grains, and carbonated beverages, and they should be avoided by the client with hyperphosphatemia. The food items in options 1, 2, and 3 are acceptable for this client to consume.

Test-Taking Strategy: Focus on the client's diagnosis and the subject—the item to limit because it will aggravate the condition. Recalling the phosphate content of foods and fluids will direct you to option 4. Review the dietary measures for the client with hyperphosphatemia if you had difficulty with this question.

References
Black, J., & Hawks, J. (2005). *Medical-surgical nursing: Clinical management for positive outcomes* (7th ed., p. 242). Philadelphia: Saunders.
Lewis, S., Heitkemper, M., Dirksen, S., O'Brien, P., & Bucher, L. (2007). *Medical-surgical nursing: Assessment and management of clinical problems* (7th ed., p. 331). St. Louis: Mosby.

---

815. The community health nurse provides an educational session regarding the risk factors for cervical cancer to women in the local community. The nurse determines that further teaching is needed if a woman attending the session identifies which of the following as a risk factor for this type of cancer?
  1 White race
  2 Smoking tobacco
  3 Low socioeconomic class
  4 Early age of first intercourse

Level of Cognitive Ability: Analysis
Client Needs: Health Promotion and
  Maintenance
Integrated Process: Teaching and Learning
Content Area: Adult Health/Oncology

Answer: 1
Rationale: Risk factors for cervical cancer include being black or Native American, smoking tobacco, having a low socioeconomic status, an early age of first intercourse, having multiple sexual partners or a partner who had multiple sexual partners, untreated chronic cervicitis, sexually transmitted diseases, and having a partner with a history of penile or prostate cancer.

Test-Taking Strategy: Note the strategic words "further teaching is needed." These words indicate a negative event query and ask you to select an option that is an incorrect risk factor. Recalling the risk factors for cervical cancer will direct you to option 1. Review these risk factors if you had difficulty with this question.

References
Black, J., & Hawks, J. (2005). *Medical-surgical nursing: Clinical management for positive outcomes* (7th ed., p. 1072). Philadelphia: Saunders.
Monahan, F., Sands, J., Neighbors, M., Marek, J., & Green, C. (2007). *Phipps' medical-surgical nursing: Health and illness perspectives* (8th ed., p. 1697). St. Louis: Mosby.

816. A high-school nurse teaches the female students how to prevent pelvic inflammatory disease. The nurse tells the students:
1 To douche monthly
2 To avoid single sexual partners
3 To avoid unprotected intercourse
4 To consult with a gynecologist regarding the placement of an intrauterine device (IUD)

Level of Cognitive Ability: Application
Client Needs: Health Promotion and Maintenance
Integrated Process: Teaching and Learning
Content Area: Fundamental Skills

Answer: 3
Rationale: The primary prevention of pelvic inflammatory disease includes avoiding unprotected intercourse, multiple sexual partners, the use of an IUD, and douching.

Test-Taking Strategy: Use the process of elimination and the principle of the exposure of the pelvic area to factors that cause infection. With this concept in mind, eliminate options 1, 2, and 4. Review the preventive measures for pelvic inflammatory disease if you had difficulty with this question.

References
Black, J., & Hawks, J. (2005). *Medical-surgical nursing: Clinical management for positive outcomes* (7th ed., p. 1063). Philadelphia: Saunders.
Monahan, F., Sands, J., Neighbors, M., Marek, J., & Green, C. (2007). *Phipps' medical-surgical nursing: Health and illness perspectives* (8th ed., p. 1688). St. Louis: Mosby.

---

817. A nurse provides discharge teaching to a client after a vasectomy. Which statement by the client would indicate the need for further teaching?
1 "I can use a scrotal support if I need to."
2 "I don't need to practice birth control any longer."
3 "I can resume sexual intercourse whenever I want."
4 "If I have pain or swelling, I can use an ice bag and take Tylenol."

Level of Cognitive Ability: Analysis
Client Needs: Health Promotion and Maintenance
Integrated Process: Teaching and Learning
Content Area: Fundamental Skills

Answer: 2
Rationale: After vasectomy, the client must continue to practice a method of birth control until the follow-up semen analysis shows azoospermia. Live sperm may be present in the vas deferens after this procedure. Options 1, 3, and 4 are appropriate client statements.

Test-Taking Strategy: Note the strategic words "need for further teaching." These words indicate a negative event query and ask you to select an option that is an incorrect statement. Options 1 and 4 can be eliminated, because these measures assist with alleviating discomfort and swelling after the procedure. Option 3 can be eliminated, because there would be no reason to avoid sexual intercourse unless the client was experiencing discomfort. Thinking about the purpose of a vasectomy will direct you to option 2. Review the client teaching points after a vasectomy if you had difficulty with this question.

References
Black, J., & Hawks, J. (2005). *Medical-surgical nursing: Clinical management for positive outcomes* (7th ed., p. 1040). Philadelphia: Saunders.
Monahan, F., Sands, J., Neighbors, M., Marek, J., & Green, C. (2007). *Phipps' medical-surgical nursing: Health and illness perspectives* (8th ed., p. 1748). St. Louis: Mosby.

818. A nursing instructor asks a student to identify the risk factors for and the methods of preventing prostate cancer. Which statement by the student indicates the need to review this information?
  1 A high-fat diet will assist with preventing this type of cancer.
  2 Men more than 50 years old should be monitored with a yearly digital rectal exam.
  3 Men more than 50 years old should be monitored with a prostate-specific antigen assay.
  4 Employment in the fertilizer, textile, or rubber industries increases the risk of prostate cancer.

Level of Cognitive Ability: Analysis
Client Needs: Health Promotion and Maintenance
Integrated Process: Teaching and Learning
Content Area: Fundamental Skills

Answer: 1
Rationale: A high intake of dietary fat is a risk factor for prostate cancer. Options 2, 3, and 4 are accurate statements regarding the risks and prevention measures related to this type of cancer.

Test-Taking Strategy: Note the strategic words "the need to review this information." These words indicate a negative event query and ask you to select an option that is an incorrect statement. Recalling the general principles related to cancer prevention will direct you to option 1. Review these measures if you had difficulty with this question.

References
Black, J., & Hawks, J. (2005). *Medical-surgical nursing: Clinical management for positive outcomes* (7th ed., p. 1028). Philadelphia: Saunders.
Monahan, F., Sands, J., Neighbors, M., Marek, J., & Green, C. (2007). *Phipps' medical-surgical nursing: Health and illness perspectives* (8th ed., p. 1738). St. Louis: Mosby.

---

819. A clinic nurse provides information to a married couple regarding measures to prevent infertility. Which statement made by the husband indicates the need to provide further information?
  1 "We need to eat a nutritious diet."
  2 "We need to avoid the excessive intake of alcohol."
  3 "We need to decrease exposure to environmental hazards."
  4 "I need to maintain warmth to my scrotum by taking hot baths frequently."

Level of Cognitive Ability: Analysis
Client Needs: Health Promotion and Maintenance
Integrated Process: Teaching and Learning
Content Area: Fundamental Skills

Answer: 4
Rationale: Keeping the testes cool by avoiding hot baths and tight clothing appears to improve the sperm count. Avoiding factors that depress spermatogenesis (such as the use of drugs, alcohol, and marijuana), limiting exposure to occupational and environmental hazards, and maintaining good nutrition are key components of preventing infertility.

Test-Taking Strategy: Note the strategic words "need to provide further information." These words indicate a negative event query and ask you to select an option that is an incorrect statement. Eliminate option 1 first, because the maintenance of a nutritious diet is important in all situations. From the remaining options, recalling that heat decreases the motility of sperm will assist with directing you to the correct option. Review the measures that prevent infertility if you have difficulty with this question.

Reference
Black, J., & Hawks, J. (2005). *Medical-surgical nursing: Clinical management for positive outcomes* (7th ed., p. 1043). Philadelphia: Saunders.

820. The nurse is teaching a client who is preparing for discharge from the hospital after a total hip replacement. Which statement by the client would indicate the need for further instructions?
1 "I cannot drive a car for probably 6 weeks."
2 "I should not sit in one position for more than 4 hours."
3 "I need to wear a support stocking on the unaffected leg."
4 "I need to place a pillow between my knees when I lie down."

Level of Cognitive Ability: Analysis
Client Needs: Health Promotion and Maintenance
Integrated Process: Teaching and Learning
Content Area: Adult Health/Musculoskeletal

Answer: 2
Rationale: The client needs to be instructed to not sit continuously for more than 1 hour. The client should be instructed to stand, stretch, and take a few steps periodically. The client cannot drive a car for 6 weeks after surgery unless allowed to do so by a physician. A support stocking should be worn on the unaffected leg, and an Ace bandage usually is prescribed to be placed on the affected leg until there is no swelling in the legs and feet and until full activities are resumed. The legs are abducted by placing a pillow between them when the client lies down.

Test-Taking Strategy: Note the strategic words "need for further instructions." These words indicate a negative event query and ask you to select an option that is an incorrect statement. Recalling standard measures related to the postoperative period will assist you with eliminating option 1. Knowing that leg abduction is maintained postoperatively during hospitalization will assist you with eliminating option 4. From the remaining options, note the timeframe of 4 hours given in option 2. This is a lengthy time period for the client to remain in one position. Review the client teaching points after total hip replacement if you had difficulty with this question.

References
Black, J., & Hawks, J. (2005). *Medical-surgical nursing: Clinical management for positive outcomes* (7th ed., p. 593). Philadelphia: Saunders.
Monahan, F., Sands, J., Neighbors, M., Marek, J., & Green, C. (2007). *Phipps' medical-surgical nursing: Health and illness perspectives* (8th ed., p. 1634). St. Louis: Mosby.

821. A client is diagnosed with hypothyroidism and is scheduled to begin taking thyroid supplements. The nurse instructs the client about the medication. Which statement by the client would indicate the need for further instructions?
1 "I need to take my daily dose every night at bedtime."
2 "I need to notify my physician if I develop any chest pain."
3 "I may experience some gastrointestinal problems, such as diarrhea."
4 "I need to speak to my physician when I begin to plan for parenthood."

Level of Cognitive Ability: Analysis
Client Needs: Health Promotion and Maintenance
Integrated Process: Teaching and Learning
Content Area: Adult Health/Endocrine

Answer: 1
Rationale: The client is instructed to take the medication in the morning to prevent insomnia. If the client experiences any chest pain, it may indicate an overdose, and the physician needs to be notified. Gastrointestinal complaints from thyroid supplements include increased appetite, nausea, and diarrhea. The dose needs to be adjusted if the client is pregnant or plans to get pregnant.

Test-Taking Strategy: Use the process of elimination, noting the strategic words "need for further instructions." These words indicate a negative event query and ask you to select an option that is an incorrect statement. Eliminate options 2 and 4 on the basis of general principles related to medication therapy. Chest pain warrants follow-up, and pregnancy would require a review of the medication dosage. From the remaining options, think about the disorder—hypothyroidism. You would expect that thyroid hormone would have an effect on increasing body metabolism. This will assist with directing you to option 1. Review the client teaching points related to thyroid supplements if you had difficulty with this question.

Reference
Kee, J., Hayes, E., & McCuistion, L. (2006). *Pharmacology: A nursing process approach.* (5th ed., p. 765). Philadelphia: Saunders.

822. The clinic nurse instructs a client with diabetes mellitus about how to prevent diabetic ketoacidosis on days when the client is feeling ill. Which statement by the client indicates the need for further instructions?

1 "I need to stop my insulin if I am vomiting."

2 "I need to eat 10 to 15 g of carbohydrates every 1 to 2 hours."

3 "I need to call my physician if I am ill for more than 24 hours."

4 "I need to drink small quantities of fluid every 15 to 30 minutes."

Level of Cognitive Ability: Analysis
Client Needs: Health Promotion and Maintenance
Integrated Process: Teaching and Learning
Content Area: Adult Health/Endocrine

Answer: 1
Rationale: The client needs to be instructed to take insulin, even if he or she is vomiting and unable to eat. It is important to self-monitor blood glucose more frequently during illness (every 2 to 4 hours). If the premeal blood glucose is more than 250 mg/dL, the client should test for urine ketones and contact the physician. Options 2, 3, and 4 are accurate interventions.

Test-Taking Strategy: Note the strategic words "need for further instructions." These words indicate a negative event query and ask you to select an option that is an incorrect statement. Recalling that insulin needs to be taken every day will assist with directing you to option 1. Review the sick-day rules for the client with diabetes mellitus if you had difficulty with this question.

Reference
Black, J., & Hawks, J. (2005). *Medical-surgical nursing: Clinical management for positive outcomes* (7th ed., p. 1286). Philadelphia: Saunders.

---

823. The nurse is instructing a client with diabetes mellitus regarding hypoglycemia. Which statement by the client indicates the need for further instructions?

1 "Hypoglycemia can occur at any time of the day or night."

2 "I can drink 6 to 8 ounces of milk if hypoglycemia occurs."

3 "If I feel sweaty or shaky, I might be experiencing hypoglycemia."

4 "If hypoglycemia occurs, I need to take my regular insulin as prescribed."

Level of Cognitive Ability: Analysis
Client Needs: Health Promotion and Maintenance
Integrated Process: Teaching and Learning
Content Area: Adult Health/Endocrine

Answer: 4
Rationale: Insulin is not taken as a treatment for hypoglycemia, because the insulin will lower the blood glucose level. Hypoglycemic reactions can occur at any time of the day or night. If a hypoglycemic reaction occurs, the client will need to consume 10 to 15 g of carbohydrate; 6 to 8 ounces of milk contains this amount of carbohydrate. Tremors and diaphoresis are signs of mild hypoglycemia.

Test-Taking Strategy: Note the strategic words "need for further instructions." These words indicate a negative event query and ask you to select an option that is an incorrect statement. Remember that, in clients with hypoglycemia, the blood glucose level is lowered. Insulin also lowers blood glucose; therefore, it would seem reasonable that insulin is not a treatment for this condition. Review the signs of hypoglycemia and the appropriate interventions if you had difficulty with this question.

Reference
Ignatavicius, D., & Workman, M. (2006). *Medical-surgical nursing: Critical thinking for collaborative care* (5th ed., pp. 1539-1540). Philadelphia: Saunders.

---

824. A client with nephrolithiasis arrives at the clinic for a follow-up visit. The laboratory analysis of the stone that the client passed 1 week ago indicates that the stone is composed of calcium oxalate. On the basis of this analysis, the nurse tells the client to avoid which of the following foods?

1 Pasta

2 Lentils

3 Lettuce

4 Spinach

Answer: 4
Rationale: Many kidney stones are composed of calcium oxalate. Foods that raise urinary oxalate excretion include spinach, rhubarb, strawberries, chocolate, wheat bran, nuts, beets, and tea.

Test-Taking Strategy: Note the strategic word "avoid," and focus on the type of stone. Recalling the foods, such as spinach, that raise urinary oxalate excretion will direct you to option 4. Review the foods that raise urinary oxalate excretion if you had difficulty with this question.

Level of Cognitive Ability: Application
Client Needs: Health Promotion and
Maintenance
Integrated Process: Nursing Process/
Implementation
Content Area: Adult Health/Renal

References
Black, J., & Hawks, J. (2005). *Medical-surgical nursing: Clinical management for
positive outcomes* (7th ed., p. 885). Philadelphia: Saunders.
Monahan, F., Sands, J., Neighbors, M., Marek, J., & Green, C. (2007). *Phipps'
medical-surgical nursing: Health and illness perspectives* (8th ed., p. 979). St. Louis:
Mosby.

---

825. A nurse provides instructions to a new
mother who is about to breast-feed her
newborn infant. The nurse observes the
new mother as she breast-feeds for the first
time and intervenes if the new mother:
1 Turns the newborn infant on his side,
facing the mother
2 Tilts up the nipple or squeezes the
areola, pushing it into the newborn's
mouth
3 Draws the newborn the rest of the way
onto the breast when the newborn
opens his mouth
4 Places a clean finger in the side of the
newborn's mouth to break the suction
before removing the newborn from the
breast

Level of Cognitive Ability: Analysis
Client Needs: Health Promotion and
Maintenance
Integrated Process: Teaching and Learning
Content Area: Maternity/Postpartum

Answer: 2
Rationale: The mother is instructed to avoid tilting up the nipple
or squeezing the areola and pushing it into the newborn's mouth;
doing so does not facilitate the breast-feeding process or the
flow of milk. Options 1, 3, and 4 are correct procedures for breast-
feeding.

Test-Taking Strategy: Note the strategic word "intervenes."
Visualize the descriptions in each of the options. This will eliminate options 1, 3, and 4. Also, carefully reading option 2 and
noting the word "pushing," which suggests force or resistance,
should assist with directing you to this option. Review the procedure for breast-feeding if you had difficulty with this question.

Reference
Murray, S., & McKinney, E. (2006). *Foundations of maternal-newborn nursing*
(4th ed., pp. 546-547). Philadelphia: Saunders.

---

826. A clinic nurse provides instructions to a
mother regarding the care of her child
who is diagnosed with croup. Which
statement by the mother indicates the
need for further instructions?
1 "I will give Tylenol for the fever."
2 "I will give cough syrup every night at
bedtime."
3 "Sips of warm fluids during a croup
attack will help."
4 "I will place a cool-mist humidifier
next to my child's bed."

Level of Cognitive Ability: Analysis
Client Needs: Health Promotion and
Maintenance
Integrated Process: Teaching and Learning
Content Area: Child Health

Answer: 2
Rationale: The mother needs to be instructed that cough syrup
and cold medicines are not to be administered, because they may
dry and thicken secretions. Sips of warm fluid will relax the vocal
cords and thin the mucus. A cool-mist humidifier rather than
a steam vaporizer is recommended because of the danger of the
child pulling the machine over and causing a burn. Acetaminophen
(Tylenol) will reduce the fever.

Test-Taking Strategy: Note the strategic words "need for further
instructions." These words indicate a negative event query and
ask you to select an option that is an incorrect statement.
Option 1 can be eliminated first, recalling that acetaminophen
(Tylenol) is normally prescribed to reduce a fever. Recalling
that warm fluids will thin secretions will assist you with eliminating option 3. From the remaining options, recalling that
cough syrup will dry secretions will assist with directing you to
option 2. Review the home-care instructions for the child with
croup if you had difficulty with this question.

Reference
Hockenberry, M., Wilson, D., & Winkelstein, M. (2005). *Wong's essentials of pediatric
nursing* (7th ed., pp. 800-802). St. Louis: Mosby.

827. A client with anxiety disorder is taking buspirone (BuSpar) orally. The client tells the nurse that it is difficult to swallow the tablets. The nurse provides which instruction to the client?

1 Crush the tablets before taking them.
2 Mix the tablet uncrushed in applesauce.
3 Call the physician for a change in medication.
4 Purchase the liquid preparation with the next refill.

Level of Cognitive Ability: Application
Client Needs: Health Promotion and Maintenance
Integrated Process: Nursing Process/ Implementation
Content Area: Pharmacology

Answer: 1

Rationale: Buspirone (BuSpar) may be administered without regard to meals, and the tablets may be crushed. This medication is not available in liquid form. It is premature to advise the client to call the physician for a change in medication without first trying alternative interventions. Mixing the tablet uncrushed in applesauce will not ensure ease of swallowing.

Test-Taking Strategy: Use the process of elimination. Eliminate option 3 first, because, in most situations, a nursing intervention can be instituted before calling the physician. Next, eliminate option 2, because this instruction will not ensure ease of swallowing. From the remaining options, it is necessary to know that this medication is not available in liquid form. Additionally, many tablets can be crushed. Review the client instructions for administering this medication if you had difficulty with this question.

References
Hodgson, B., & Kizior, R. (2007). *Saunders nursing drug handbook 2007* (p. 164). Philadelphia: Saunders.
Skidmore-Roth, L. (2008). *Mosby's nursing drug reference* (21st ed., p. 213). St. Louis: Mosby.

---

828. A nurse caring for a child with congestive heart failure provides instructions to the parents regarding the administration of digoxin (Lanoxin). Which statement by the mother indicates a need for further instructions?

1 "I will mix the medication with food."
2 "I will check my child's pulse before giving the medication."
3 "If my child vomits after I give the medication, I will not repeat the dose."
4 "I will check the dose of medication with my husband before I give the medication."

Level of Cognitive Ability: Analysis
Client Needs: Health Promotion and Maintenance
Integrated Process: Teaching and Learning
Content Area: Pharmacology

Answer: 1

Rationale: The medication should not be mixed with food or formula, because this method would not ensure that the child receives the entire dose of medication. Options 2, 3, and 4 are correct. Additionally, if a dosage is missed and this is not identified until 4 or more hours later, the dose is not administered. If more than one consecutive dose is missed, the physician needs to be notified.

Test-Taking Strategy: Note the strategic words "need for further instructions." These words indicate a negative event query and ask you to select an option that is an incorrect statement. General principles regarding medication administration to children should assist with directing you to the correct option. Mixing medications with formula or food may alter the effectiveness of the medication. More important, if the child does not consume all of the formula or food, the total dosage may not be administered. Review the parental instructions regarding the administration of digoxin if you had difficulty with this question.

References
Hockenberry, M., Wilson, D., & Winkelstein, M. (2005). *Wong's essentials of pediatric nursing* (7th ed., p. 910). St. Louis: Mosby.
Skidmore-Roth, L. (2007). *2007 Mosby's nursing drug reference* (20th ed., p. 361). St. Louis: Mosby.

829. A nurse provides discharge instructions to the mother of a child who was hospitalized for heart surgery. The nurse tells the mother that:

1 The child can play outside for short periods of time.
2 After bathing, rub lotion and sprinkle powder on the incision.
3 The child may return to school 1 week after hospital discharge.
4 The physician is to be notified if the child develops a fever of more than 100.5° F.

Level of Cognitive Ability: Application
Client Needs: Health Promotion and Maintenance
Integrated Process: Teaching and Learning
Content Area: Child Health

Answer: 4
Rationale: After heart surgery, the child should not return to school until 3 weeks after hospital discharge, at which time the child should go to school for half days for the first few days. No creams, lotions, or powders should be placed on the incision until it is completely healed and without scabs. The mother is instructed to not allow the child to play outside for several weeks. The physician needs to be notified if the child develops a fever of more than 100.5° F.

Test-Taking Strategy: Use the process of elimination, bearing in mind the potential for infection in this child. Eliminate option 3 because of the timeframe of 1 week. Eliminate option 1, because outside play can expose the child to infection and the risk of injury. Basic principles related to incision care should assist you with eliminating option 2. Review the home-care instructions for the child after heart surgery if you had difficulty with this question.

References
Hockenberry, M., & Wilson, D. (2007). *Nursing care of infants and children* (8th ed., pp. 1476-1477). St. Louis: Mosby.
McKinney, E., James, S., Murray, S., & Ashwill, J. (2005). *Maternal-child nursing* (2nd ed., p. 1283). St. Louis: Saunders.

---

830. A clinic nurse provides instructions to a client who will begin taking oral contraceptives. Which statement by the client indicates the need for further instructions?

1 "I will take one pill daily at the same time every day."
2 "If I miss a pill, I need to take it as soon as I remember."
3 "I will not need to use an additional birth-control method after I start these pills."
4 "If I miss two pills, I will take them both as soon as I remember, and I will take two pills the next day, also."

Level of Cognitive Ability: Analysis
Client Needs: Health Promotion and Maintenance
Integrated Process: Teaching and Learning
Content Area: Pharmacology

Answer: 3
Rationale: The client needs to be instructed to use a second birth-control method during the first pill cycle. Options 1, 2, and 4 are correct. Additionally, the client needs to be instructed that, if she misses three pills, she will need to discontinue pill use for that cycle and use another birth-control method.

Test-Taking Strategy: Note the strategic words "need for further instructions." These words indicate a negative event query and ask you to select an option that is an incorrect statement. It would seem reasonable that, during the first pill cycle, a second birth-control method would need to be used to prevent conception. Review these guidelines if you had difficulty with this question.

Reference
Kee, J., Hayes, E., & McCuistion, L. (2006). *Pharmacology: A nursing process approach.* (5th ed., p. 865). Philadelphia: Saunders.

---

831. The nurse is providing dietary instructions to a client who has been hospitalized for pancreatitis. Which of the following foods would the nurse instruct the client to avoid?

1 Chili
2 Bagels
3 Lentil soup
4 Watermelon

Answer: 1
Rationale: The client needs to avoid alcohol, coffee, tea, spicy foods, and heavy meals, which stimulate pancreatic secretions and produce attacks of pancreatitis. The client is instructed regarding the benefit of eating small, frequent meals that are high in protein, low in fat, and moderate to high in carbohydrates.

Level of Cognitive Ability: Application
Client Needs: Health Promotion and Maintenance
Integrated Process: Nursing Process/ Implementation
Content Area: Adult Health/Gastrointestinal

Test-Taking Strategy: Use the process of elimination, noting that options 2, 3, and 4 are foods that are moderately bland. Option 1 is different in that chili is a spicy food. Review the dietary measures for the client with pancreatitis if you had difficulty with this question.

References

Black, J., & Hawks, J. (2005). *Medical-surgical nursing: Clinical management for positive outcomes* (7th ed., p. 1297). Philadelphia: Saunders.

Monahan, F., Sands, J., Neighbors, M., Marek, J., & Green, C. (2007). *Phipps' medical-surgical nursing: Health and illness perspectives* (8th ed., p. 1295). St. Louis: Mosby.

---

832. The home-care nurse visits a client who was recently diagnosed with cirrhosis and provides home-care management instructions to the client. Which statement by the client indicates the need for further instructions?

1 "I will obtain adequate rest."
2 "I should monitor my weight regularly."
3 "I should include sufficient carbohydrates in my diet."
4 "I will take acetaminophen (Tylenol) if I get a headache."

Level of Cognitive Ability: Analysis
Client Needs: Health Promotion and Maintenance
Integrated Process: Teaching and Learning
Content Area: Adult Health/Gastrointestinal

Answer: 4

Rationale: Acetaminophen (Tylenol) is avoided, because it can cause fatal liver damage in the client with cirrhosis. Adequate rest and nutrition are important. The diet should supply sufficient carbohydrates with a total daily intake of 2000 to 3000 calories. The client's weight should be monitored regularly.

Test-Taking Strategy: Note the strategic words "need for further instructions." These words indicate a negative event query and ask you to select an option that is an incorrect statement. Recalling that acetaminophen (Tylenol) is a hepatotoxic agent will assist with directing you to option 4. Review the medications that are restricted or avoided in clients with cirrhosis if you had difficulty with this question.

References

Black, J., & Hawks, J. (2005). *Medical-surgical nursing: Clinical management for positive outcomes* (7th ed., p. 1339). Philadelphia: Saunders.

Canobbio, M. (2006). *Mosby's handbook of patient teaching* (3rd ed., pp. 244-245) St. Louis: Mosby.

---

833. A client has a history of urolithiasis related to hyperuricemia. To prevent the formation of future stones, the nurse instructs the client to avoid certain foods, including:

1 Liver
2 Carrots
3 White rice
4 Skim milk

Level of Cognitive Ability: Application
Client Needs: Health Promotion and Maintenance
Integrated Process: Teaching and Learning
Content Area: Fundamental Skills

Answer: 1

Rationale: Because the client has a high level of uric acid in the blood and a history of kidney stones from crystallized uric acid in the renal pelvis, the nurse instructs the client to avoid foods that contain high amounts of purines, because these foods contain a high concentration of uric acid. This includes limiting or avoiding organ meats, such as liver, brain, heart, and kidney. Other foods to avoid include sweetbreads, herring, sardines, anchovies, meat extracts, consommés, and gravies. Foods that are low in purines include all fruits, many vegetables, milk, cheese, eggs, refined cereals, coffee, tea, chocolate, and carbonated beverages.

Test-Taking Strategy: Use the process of elimination, focusing on the client's diagnosis and noting the strategic word "avoid." Because purines are end products of protein metabolism, eliminate options 2 and 3 first. From the remaining options, recall that organ meats such as liver provide a greater quantity of protein than milk does. Review the dietary instructions for the client with uric acid stones if you had difficulty with this question.

References

Black, J., & Hawks, J. (2005). *Medical-surgical nursing: Clinical management for positive outcomes* (7th ed., pp. 885-886). Philadelphia: Saunders.

Monahan, F., Sands, J., Neighbors, M., Marek, J., & Green, C. (2007). *Phipps' medical-surgical nursing: Health and illness perspectives* (8th ed., pp. 978-979, 1561). St. Louis: Mosby.

---

834. A client tells the nurse that he gets dizzy and lightheaded with each use of the incentive spirometer. The nurse asks the client to demonstrate the use of the device, expecting that the client is:

1 Inhaling too slowly
2 Exhaling too slowly
3 Not resting adequately between breaths
4 Not forming a tight seal around the mouthpiece

Level of Cognitive Ability: Analysis
Client Needs: Health Promotion and Maintenance
Integrated Process: Nursing Process/Evaluation
Content Area: Adult Health/Respiratory

Answer: 3

Rationale: If the client does not breathe normally between incentive spirometer breaths, hyperventilation and fatigue can result. Hyperventilation is the most common cause of respiratory alkalosis, which is characterized by lightheadedness and dizziness.

Test-Taking Strategy: Focus on the subject—the cause of the lightheadedness and dizziness. Think about each of the actions described in the options to direct you to option 3. Options 1, 2, and 4 would result in ineffective use but would not cause dizziness and lightheadedness. Review the procedure for the use of the incentive spirometer if you had difficulty with this question.

Reference

Ignatavicius, D., & Workman, M. (2006). *Medical-surgical nursing: Critical thinking for collaborative care* (5th ed., pp. 309, 637). Philadelphia: Saunders.

---

835. The nurse is conducting a health screening clinic. The nurse interprets that which client participating in the screening has the greatest need for instruction to lower the risk of developing respiratory disease?

1 A 36-year-old who works with pesticides
2 A 40-year-old smoker who works in a hospital
3 A 25-year-old who does woodworking as a hobby
4 A 50-year-old smoker who has cracked asbestos lining on the basement pipes in her home

Level of Cognitive Ability: Analysis
Client Needs: Health Promotion and Maintenance
Integrated Process: Nursing Process/Assessment
Content Area: Adult Health/Respiratory

Answer: 4

Rationale: Smoking greatly enhances the client's risk of developing some form of respiratory disease. Other risk factors include exposure to harmful chemicals, airborne toxins, and dust or fumes. The client who is at the greatest risk has two identified risk factors, one of which is smoking.

Test-Taking Strategy: Use the process of elimination. Eliminate options 1 and 3 first, because the most harmful risk factor for the respiratory system is smoking. From the remaining options, select option 4, because asbestos is toxic to the lungs if its particles are inhaled. In addition, two risk factors are identified in option 4, which makes this client at greater risk than the others, who have only one factor identified. Review the risk factors associated with respiratory disease if you had difficulty with this question.

References

Black, J., & Hawks, J. (2005). *Medical-surgical nursing: Clinical management for positive outcomes* (7th ed., p. 1732). Philadelphia: Saunders.

Ignatavicius, D., & Workman, M. (2006). *Medical-surgical nursing: Critical thinking for collaborative care* (5th ed., p. 650). Philadelphia: Saunders.

836. The nurse has conducted teaching with a client who experienced pulmonary embolism about methods to prevent recurrence after discharge from the hospital. Evaluation of learning is evident if the client states the intention to do which of the following?
1 Limit the intake of fluids.
2 Sit down whenever possible.
3 Continue to wear supportive hose.
4 Cross the legs only at the ankle and not at the knees.

Level of Cognitive Ability: Analysis
Client Needs: Health Promotion and Maintenance
Integrated Process: Nursing Process/Evaluation
Content Area: Adult Health/Respiratory

Answer: 3
Rationale: The recurrence of pulmonary embolism can be minimized with the wearing of elastic or supportive hose, because these hose enhance venous return. The client also enhances venous return by avoiding crossing the legs at the knees or ankles, interspersing periods of sitting with walking, and doing active foot and ankle exercises. The client should also take in sufficient fluids to prevent hemoconcentration and hypercoagulability.

Test-Taking Strategy: Use the process of elimination, noting the strategic words "learning is evident." Recalling that promoting venous return will prevent pulmonary embolism will direct you to option 3. Review the measures that will prevent the recurrence of pulmonary embolism if you had difficulty with this question.

References
Black, J., & Hawks, J. (2005). *Medical-surgical nursing: Clinical management for positive outcomes* (7th ed., pp. 1539-1540). Philadelphia: Saunders.
Canobbio, M. (2006). *Mosby's handbook of patient teaching* (3rd ed., p. 652). St. Louis: Mosby.

---

837. A female client is being discharged from the hospital to home with an indwelling urinary catheter after the surgical repair of the bladder after trauma. The nurse determines that the client understands the principles of catheter management if the client states to:
1 Keep the drainage bag lower than the level of the bladder.
2 Cleanse the perineal area with soap and water once a day.
3 Limit fluid intake so that the bag will not become full so quickly.
4 Coil the tubing and place it under the thigh when sitting to avoid tugging on the bladder.

Level of Cognitive Ability: Analysis
Client Needs: Health Promotion and Maintenance
Integrated Process: Nursing Process/Evaluation
Content Area: Adult Health/Renal

Answer: 1
Rationale: The perineal area should be cleansed twice daily and after each bowel movement with soap and water. The drainage bag should be lower than the level of the bladder, and the tubing should be free of kinks and compression. Coiling the tubing and placing it under the thigh can compress the tube. Adequate fluid intake is necessary to prevent infection and to provide natural irrigation of the catheter from increased urine flow.

Test-Taking Strategy: Note the strategic words "understands the principles." Option 4 is eliminated first, because sitting on coiled tubing could cause compression and obstruct drainage. Option 3 is eliminated next, because increased fluids are important. From the remaining options, noting the words "once a day" in option 2 will assist you with eliminating this option. Review the principles related to catheter care if you had difficulty with this question.

Reference
Black, J., & Hawks, J. (2005). *Medical-surgical nursing: Clinical management for positive outcomes* (7th ed., p. 906). Philadelphia: Saunders.

---

838. A 24-year-old female with a family history of heart disease presents to the physician's office asking to begin oral contraceptive therapy for birth control. The nurse would next inquire whether the client:
1 Exercises regularly
2 Is currently a smoker
3 Eats a low-cholesterol diet
4 Has taken oral contraceptives before

Answer: 2
Rationale: Oral contraceptive use is a risk factor for heart disease, particularly when it is combined with cigarette smoking. Regular exercise and keeping total cholesterol levels less than 200 mg/dL are general measures to decrease cardiovascular risk.

Level of Cognitive Ability: Analysis
Client Needs: Health Promotion and
   Maintenance
Integrated Process: Nursing Process/Assessment
Content Area: Adult Health/Cardiovascular

Test-Taking Strategy: Use the process of elimination, noting the strategic words "family history of heart disease." Remember that smoking is the item that is linked to oral contraceptive use to make it a risk factor for cardiovascular disease. This will direct you to option 2. Review the risks associated with the use of oral contraceptives if you had difficulty with this question.

References
Lewis, S., Heitkemper, M., Dirksen, S., O'Brien, P., & Bucher, L. (2007). *Medical-surgical nursing: Assessment and management of clinical problems* (7th ed., p. 1267). St. Louis: Mosby.
Skidmore-Roth, L. (2007). *Mosby's drug guide for nurses* (7th ed., p. 267). St. Louis: Mosby.

---

839. The nurse is teaching a client with atrial fibrillation about the need to begin long-term anticoagulant therapy. Which explanation would the nurse use to best describe the reasoning for this therapy?
   1 "Because of this dysrhythmia, blood backs up in the legs and puts you at risk for blood clots."
   2 "The antidysrhythmic medications you are taking cause blood clots as a side effect, so you need this medication to prevent them."
   3 "This dysrhythmia decreases the volume of blood flowing from the heart, which can lead to blood clots forming in the brain."
   4 "Because the atria are quivering, blood flows sluggishly through them, and clots can form along the heart wall, which could then loosen and travel to the lungs or brain."

Level of Cognitive Ability: Application
Client Needs: Health Promotion and
   Maintenance
Integrated Process: Nursing Process/
   Implementation
Content Area: Adult Health/Cardiovascular

Answer: 4
Rationale: A severe complication of atrial fibrillation is the development of mural thrombi. The blood stagnates in the "quivering" atria because of the loss of organized atrial muscle contraction and "atrial kick." The blood that pools in the atria can then clot, which increases the risk of pulmonary and cerebral emboli.

Test-Taking Strategy: Use the process of elimination. Note the relationship between the client's diagnosis of atrial fibrillation and the words "atria are quivering" in option 4. Review the pathophysiology of atrial fibrillation if you had difficulty with this question.

Reference
Black, J., & Hawks, J. (2005). *Medical-surgical nursing: Clinical management for positive outcomes* (7th ed., p. 1602). Philadelphia: Saunders.

---

840. A clinic nurse is providing instructions to a client in the third trimester of pregnancy regarding relief measures for heartburn. Which instruction should the nurse provide to the client?
   1 Sip on milk or hot tea.
   2 Use antacids that contain sodium.
   3 Eat fatty foods once a day in the morning only.
   4 Eat three large meals a day rather than small, frequent meals.

Answer: 1
Rationale: Measures to provide relief of heartburn include eating small, frequent meals and avoiding fatty and fried foods, coffee, and cigarettes. Mild antacids can be used if they do not contain aspirin or sodium. Frequent sips of milk or hot tea are helpful.

Level of Cognitive Ability: Application
Client Needs: Health Promotion and
Maintenance
Integrated Process: Nursing Process/
Implementation
Content Area: Maternity/Antepartum

Test-Taking Strategy: Use the process of elimination. Eliminate option 2 first, because sodium will lead to edema, and edema should be avoided. Eliminate option 3 next on the basis of basic nutritional principles that fatty and fried foods should be avoided. From the remaining options, recalling that milk and hot tea can be soothing to the gastrointestinal tract will assist you with eliminating option 4. Review the measures that relieve heartburn if you had difficulty with this question.

References
McKinney, E., James, S., Murray, S., & Ashwill, J. (2005). *Maternal-child nursing* (2nd ed., p. 275). St. Louis: Saunders.
Murray, S., & McKinney, E. (2006). *Foundations of maternal-newborn nursing* (4th ed., pp. 137-138). Philadelphia: Saunders.

---

841. A nurse provides instructions regarding home care to a parent of a 3-year-old child who has been hospitalized with hemophilia. Which statement by the parent indicates the need for further instructions?
   1 "I should not leave my child unattended."
   2 "I need to pad table corners in my home."
   3 "My child should not have any immunizations."
   4 "I need to remove household items that can tip over."

Level of Cognitive Ability: Analysis
Client Needs: Health Promotion and
Maintenance
Integrated Process: Teaching and Learning
Content Area: Child Health

Answer: 3
Rationale: The nurse needs to stress the importance of immunizations, dental hygiene, and routine well-child care. Options 1, 2, and 4 are appropriate. The parent should also be instructed regarding measures to implement if blunt trauma occurs (especially trauma involving the joints) and how to apply prolonged pressure to superficial wounds until the bleeding has stopped.

Test-Taking Strategy: Note the strategic words "need for further instructions." These words indicate a negative event query and ask you to select an option that is an incorrect statement. Recalling that bleeding is a concern in clients with this disorder will assist you with eliminating options 1, 2, and 4, which include measures of protection and safety for the child. Recalling the importance of immunizations will direct you to option 3. Review the care of the child with hemophilia if you had difficulty with this question.

Reference
Hockenberry, M., Wilson, D., & Winkelstein, M. (2005). *Wong's essentials of pediatric nursing* (7th ed., p. 954). St. Louis: Mosby.

---

842. A nurse provides instructions to the client taking clorazepate (Tranxene) for the management of an anxiety disorder. The nurse tell the client that:
   1 Dizziness is a side effect.
   2 If drowsiness occurs, call the physician.
   3 Smoking increases the effectiveness of the medication.
   4 If gastrointestinal disturbances occur, discontinue the medication.

Level of Cognitive Ability: Application
Client Needs: Health Promotion and
Maintenance
Integrated Process: Teaching and Learning
Content Area: Mental Health

Answer: 1
Rationale: Dizziness is a side effect of this medication. The client should be instructed that, if dizziness occurs, he or she should change positions slowly from lying to sitting to standing. Drowsiness is also a side effect that diminishes with continued therapy and that does not warrant the need to contact the physician. Smoking reduces medication effectiveness. Gastrointestinal disturbance is an occasional side effect, and the medication can be given with food if this occurs.

Test-Taking Strategy: Use the process of elimination. Eliminate option 4 first, because the client should not be instructed to discontinue the medication. Eliminate option 2, because episodes of drowsiness commonly occur with antianxiety medications. Eliminate option 3 next, because smoking reduces medication effectiveness. Review the client teaching points related to this medication if you had difficulty with this question.

References
Hodgson, B., & Kizior, R. (2007). *Saunders nursing drug handbook 2007* (p. 276). Philadelphia: Saunders.
Stuart, G., & Laraia, M. (2005). *Principles and practice of psychiatric nursing* (8th ed., pp. 574-575). St. Louis: Mosby.

---

843. The client with prostatitis asks the nurse, "Why do I need to take a stool softener? The problem is with my urine, not my bowels!" The nurse makes which response to the client?
1 "This is a standard medication order for anyone with an abdominal problem."
2 "This will keep the bowel free of feces, which helps decrease the swelling inside."
3 "Being constipated puts you at more risk for developing complications of prostatitis."
4 "This will help you prevent constipation, because straining is painful with prostatitis."

Level of Cognitive Ability: Application
Client Needs: Health Promotion and Maintenance
Integrated Process: Nursing Process/ Implementation
Content Area: Adult Health/Renal

Answer: 4
Rationale: Stool softeners are ordered for the client with prostatitis to prevent constipation, which can be painful. It has no direct effect on decreasing swelling. Constipation does not cause complications of prostatitis. Stool softeners are not a standard prescription for "anyone with an abdominal problem."

Test-Taking Strategy: Use the process of elimination. Recalling the purpose and use of stool softeners to prevent constipation will direct you to option 4. Review the care of the client with prostatitis if you had difficulty with this question.

Reference
Ignatavicius, D., & Workman, M. (2006). *Medical-surgical nursing: Critical thinking for collaborative care* (5th ed., p. 1880). Philadelphia: Saunders.

---

844. A client with Parkinson's disease has begun therapy with levodopa. The nurse determines that the client understands the action of the medication if the client verbalizes that results may not be apparent for:
1 1 week
2 24 hours
3 5 to 7 days
4 2 to 3 weeks

Level of Cognitive Ability: Analysis
Client Needs: Health Promotion and Maintenance
Integrated Process: Nursing Process/Evaluation
Content Area: Pharmacology

Answer: 4
Rationale: Signs and symptoms of Parkinson's disease usually begin to resolve within 2 to 3 weeks of starting therapy, although in some clients marked improvement may not be seen for up to 6 months. Clients need to understand this concept to aid in their compliance with medication therapy.

Test-Taking Strategy: Use the process of elimination and knowledge regarding this medication. Eliminate options 1 and 3, because they involve similar timeframes. From the remaining options, eliminate option 2, because it is unlikely that results would be noted in 24 hours. Review this medication if you had difficulty with this question.

References
Hodgson, B., & Kizior, R. (2007). *Saunders nursing drug handbook 2007* (p. 186). Philadelphia: Saunders.
McKenry, L., Tressier, E., & Hogan, M. (2006). *Mosby's pharmacology in nursing* (22nd ed., pp. 495-496). St. Louis: Mosby.

845. The nurse is conducting a prostate screening clinic and discussing prevention and risk factors for prostate cancer. The nurse determines that a client understands the educational information that was shared if the nurse overhears the client tell another participant that:

1 A low-fiber diet helps to prevent prostate cancer.
2 Eating foods high in fat is not a risk factor for prostate cancer.
3 Green and yellow vegetables should be limited in the diet to prevent prostate cancer.
4 An annual prostate exam and a prostate-specific antigen (PSA) test should be performed beginning at the age of 50 years.

Level of Cognitive Ability: Analysis
Client Needs: Health Promotion and Maintenance
Integrated Process: Nursing Process/Evaluation
Content Area: Adult Health/Renal

Answer: 4
Rationale: An annual prostate exam and a PSA test should be performed beginning at the age of 50 years or at the age of 45 years if the client is at high risk for this type of cancer. A low-fat, high-fiber diet diminishes prostate cancer risk. The increased intake of green or yellow vegetables or of the lycopenes contained in tomatoes may be helpful to reduce risk.

Test-Taking Strategy: Use the process of elimination, and focus on the subject—prostate screening and prevention and the risk factors for prostate cancer. Using general health principles will direct you to option 4. Review the screening measures for prostate cancer if you had difficulty with this question.

References
Black, J., & Hawks, J. (2005). *Medical-surgical nursing: Clinical management for positive outcomes* (7th ed., p. 1027). Philadelphia: Saunders.
Lewis, S., Heitkemper, M., Dirksen, S., O'Brien, P., & Bucher, L. (2007). *Medical-surgical nursing: Assessment and management of clinical problems* (7th ed., p. 282). St. Louis: Mosby.

---

846. A client is being discharged to home without an indwelling urinary catheter after prostatectomy. The nurse plans to teach the client which of the following points as part of the discharge teaching?

1 Mowing the lawn is allowed after 1 week.
2 Avoid lifting more than 50 pounds for 4 to 6 weeks after surgery.
3 Drink at least 15 glasses of water a day to minimize clot formation.
4 Notify the physician if fever, increased pain, or an inability to void occurs.

Level of Cognitive Ability: Application
Client Needs: Health Promotion and Maintenance
Integrated Process: Nursing Process/Planning
Content Area: Adult Health/Renal

Answer: 4
Rationale: The client should notify the physician if there are any signs of infection, bleeding, increased pain, or urinary obstruction. Strenuous activities that could increase intra-abdominal tension are restricted, such as mowing the lawn. Lifting more than 20 pounds is prohibited for 4 to 6 weeks after surgery. The client should take in 6 to 8 glasses of water or nonalcoholic beverages per day to minimize the risk of clot formation.

Test-Taking Strategy: Use the process of elimination, and focus on the client's diagnosis. Eliminate option 3 first as an excessive fluid intake. Noting that the activities identified in options 1 and 2 are also excessive will assist you with eliminating these options. Review the home-care measures after prostatectomy if you had difficulty with this question.

References
Black, J., & Hawks, J. (2005). *Medical-surgical nursing: Clinical management for positive outcomes* (7th ed., p. 1024). Philadelphia: Saunders.
Ignatavicius, D., & Workman, M. (2006). *Medical-surgical nursing: Critical thinking for collaborative care* (5th ed., pp. 1867-1868). Philadelphia: Saunders.

---

847. The nurse is teaching a client with acute renal failure to include proteins in the diet that are considered high quality. Which food item should the nurse discourage because it is a low-quality protein source?

1 Fish
2 Eggs
3 Chicken
4 Broccoli

Answer: 4
Rationale: High-quality proteins come from animal sources and include such foods as eggs, chicken, meat, and fish. Low-quality proteins are derived from plant sources and include vegetables and foods made from grains. Because the renal diet is limited in protein, it is important that the proteins ingested are of high quality.

Level of Cognitive Ability: Application
Client Needs: Health Promotion and
  Maintenance
Integrated Process: Nursing Process/
  Implementation
Content Area: Adult Health/Renal

Test-Taking Strategy: Use the process of elimination, noting the strategic words "low-quality protein source." When comparing the options, note that option 4 is the only item that does not derive from an animal source. Chicken, eggs, and fish derive from animal sources, whereas broccoli is a plant. Review the food items that are high- and low-quality proteins if you had difficulty with this question.

References
Black, J., & Hawks, J. (2005). *Medical-surgical nursing: Clinical management for positive outcomes* (7th ed., pp. 946-948). Philadelphia: Saunders.
Grodner, M., Long, S., & DeYoung, S. (2004). *Foundations and clinical applications of nutrition: A nursing approach.* (3rd ed., pp. 150-151, 614). St. Louis: Mosby.

---

848. The home-care nurse visits a client who had a brain attack (stroke) with resultant unilateral neglect who was recently discharged from the hospital. The nurse provides instructions to the family regarding care and tells the family to:
  1 Assist the client from the affected side.
  2 Place personal items directly in front of the client.
  3 Discourage the client from scanning the environment.
  4 Assist the client with grooming the unaffected side first.

Level of Cognitive Ability: Application
Client Needs: Health Promotion and
  Maintenance
Integrated Process: Teaching and Learning
Content Area: Adult Health/Neurological

Answer: 1
Rationale: Unilateral neglect is a pattern of a lack of awareness of body parts such as paralyzed arms or legs. Initially the environment is adapted to the deficit by focusing on the client's unaffected side, and the client's personal items are placed on the unaffected side; gradually the client's attention is focused to the affected side. The client is assisted from the affected side, and the client grooms the affected side first. The client needs to scan the entire environment.

Test-Taking Strategy: Note the client's diagnosis of unilateral neglect and the subject of home-care instructions. Recalling the physiological alteration that occurs with unilateral neglect and that it involves a pattern of a lack of awareness of body parts will direct you to option 1. Review the interventions associated with unilateral neglect if you had difficulty with this question.

Reference
Black, J., & Hawks, J. (2005). *Medical-surgical nursing: Clinical management for positive outcomes* (7th ed., p. 2131). Philadelphia: Saunders.

---

849. The nurse has completed discharge teaching with a client who has had surgery for lung cancer. The nurse determines that the client has misunderstood essential elements of home management if the client verbalizes the need to:
  1 Avoid exposure to crowds.
  2 Deal with any increases in pain independently.
  3 Sit up and lean forward to breathe more easily.
  4 Call the physician in case of increased temperature or shortness of breath.

Level of Cognitive Ability: Analysis
Client Needs: Health Promotion and
  Maintenance
Integrated Process: Teaching and Learning
Content Area: Adult Health/Oncology

Answer: 2
Rationale: Health teaching for this condition includes using positions that facilitate respiration, such as sitting up and leaning forward. It also includes avoiding exposure to crowds or persons with respiratory infections and reporting signs and symptoms of respiratory infection or increases in pain. The client should not be expected to deal with increases in pain independently.

Test-Taking Strategy: Note the strategic words "has misunderstood." These words indicate a negative event query and ask you to select an option that is an incorrect statement. Focusing on the client's diagnosis of lung cancer will direct you to option 2. Review the home-care measures for the client who has had surgery for lung cancer if you had difficulty with this question.

References
Black, J., & Hawks, J. (2005). *Medical-surgical nursing: Clinical management for positive outcomes* (7th ed., p. 1862). Philadelphia: Saunders.
Ignatavicius, D., & Workman, M. (2006). *Medical-surgical nursing: Critical thinking for collaborative care* (5th ed., p. 625). Philadelphia: Saunders.

850. A client weighed 165 pounds at admission. After a surgical procedure, the nurse determines that the client is maintaining adequate nutritional status if the client's weight is between baseline and:
1 160 pounds
2 157 pounds
3 155 pounds
4 153 pounds

Level of Cognitive Ability: Analysis
Client Needs: Health Promotion and Maintenance
Integrated Process: Nursing Process/Evaluation
Content Area: Fundamental Skills

Answer: 1
Rationale: The nurse determines that the client has maintained adequate nutritional status if the client maintains the baseline body weight or loses less than 5 pounds. The client's baseline weight is 165 pounds, so the acceptable range for the client's postoperative weight is 160 to 165 pounds.

Test-Taking Strategy: Focus on the subject—maintaining adequate nutritional status. In this situation, it is best to select the option that identifies the least amount of weight loss; this will direct you to option 1. Review nutritional principles if you had difficulty with this question.

Reference
Black, J., & Hawks, J. (2005). *Medical-surgical nursing: Clinical management for positive outcomes* (7th ed., p. 1791). Philadelphia: Saunders.

---

851. The nurse has given the client with a non-plaster (fiberglass) leg cast instructions regarding cast care at home. The nurse determines that the client needs further instructions if the client makes which statement?
1 "I should avoid walking on wet, slippery floors."
2 "I'm not supposed to scratch the skin underneath the cast."
3 "It's all right to wipe dirt off of the top of the cast with a damp cloth."
4 "If the cast gets wet, I can dry it with a hair dryer turned to the hot setting."

Level of Cognitive Ability: Analysis
Client Needs: Health Promotion and Maintenance
Integrated Process: Teaching and Learning
Content Area: Adult Health/Musculoskeletal

Answer: 4
Rationale: If the cast gets wet, it can be dried with a hair dryer set to a cool setting. The client is instructed to avoid walking on wet, slippery floors to prevent falls. If the skin under the cast itches, cool air from a hair dryer may be used to relieve it. The client should never scratch under the cast because of the risk of skin breakdown and infection. Surface soil on a cast may be removed with a damp cloth.

Test-Taking Strategy: Note the strategic words "needs further instructions." These words indicate a negative event query and ask you to select an option that is an incorrect statement. Noting the word "hot" in option 4 will direct you to this option. Review the home-care instructions for a client with a cast if you had difficulty with this question.

References
Black, J., & Hawks, J. (2005). *Medical-surgical nursing: Clinical management for positive outcomes* (7th ed., pp. 631-632). Philadelphia: Saunders.
Ignatavicius, D., & Workman, M. (2006). *Medical-surgical nursing: Critical thinking for collaborative care* (5th ed., p. 1198). Philadelphia: Saunders.

---

852. A child is seen in the health care clinic, and initial testing for human immunodeficiency virus (HIV) is performed because of the child's exposure to HIV infection. Which home-care instruction would the nurse provide to the parents of the child?
1 Avoid sharing toothbrushes.
2 Avoid all immunizations until the diagnosis is established.
3 Wipe up any blood spills with soap and water, and allow them to air dry.
4 Wash your hands with half-strength bleach if they come in contact with the child's blood.

Answer: 1
Rationale: Immunizations must be kept up to date. Blood spills are wiped up with a paper towel; the area is then washed with soap and water, rinsed with bleach and water, and allowed to air dry. Hands are washed with soap and water if they come in contact with blood. Parents are instructed that toothbrushes are not to be shared.

Test-Taking Strategy: Use the process of elimination. Eliminate option 2 first because of the close-ended word "all." Eliminate option 3 next on the basis of the knowledge that blood spills need to be cleaned with a bleach solution. Eliminate option 4, because bleach would be irritating and caustic to the skin. Review the home-care instructions for the child exposed to HIV infection if you had difficulty with this question.

Level of Cognitive Ability: Application
Client Needs: Health Promotion and
Maintenance
Integrated Process: Teaching and Learning
Content Area: Child Health

References
Hockenberry, M., Wilson, D., & Winkelstein, M. (2005). *Wong's essentials of pediatric nursing* (7th ed., p. 1550). St. Louis: Mosby.
McKinney, E., James, S., Murray, S., & Ashwill, J. (2005). *Maternal-child nursing* (2nd ed., p. 1058). St. Louis: Saunders.

---

853. The nurse prepares a client who is ready for discharge for care at home. The client needs to receive continued intravenous (IV) therapy, so the nurse provides the client with instructions on caring for the IV site. Which is the best method of evaluating the client's ability to care for the IV site?
  1 Have the client role-play an IV dressing change.
  2 Direct the client to explain IV site care completely.
  3 Invite the client to change the IV dressing unaided.
  4 Ask the client to provide self-care before being discharged.

Level of Cognitive Ability: Application
Client Needs: Health Promotion and
Maintenance
Integrated Process: Teaching and Learning
Content Area: Fundamental Skills

Answer: 3
Rationale: The best method for the nurse to use to evaluate the client's acquisition of psychomotor skills is to observe the client performing the skill; in this case, it is an IV dressing change. This is the best method, because the client cannot perform the skill correctly without understanding the directions and having the fine motor skills to perform the skill. Role playing is a suitable method of rehearsing a skill. Explanations are suitable to evaluate client knowledge of a skill, but they will not draw attention to the client's physical inability to perform the psychomotor function. If the nurse was evaluating client self-care, having the client function independently before discharge is suitable; however, the question is asking about IV site care.

Test-Taking Strategy: Use teaching and learning principles to answer the question, and note the strategic word "best." This means that all options are correct and so you must choose the option that is the best choice. The correct option needs to identify some type of active client participation. This concept will direct you to option 3. Review teaching and learning principles if you had difficulty with this question.

Reference
Potter, P., & Perry, A. (2005). *Fundamentals of nursing* (6th ed., pp. 451-454, 1194). St. Louis: Mosby.

---

854. A nurse provides home-care instructions to a client with an implanted vascular access port. Which statement by the client indicates the need for further instructions?
  1 "I should keep the site clean and dry."
  2 "I should pump the port daily to maintain patency."
  3 "If the site becomes red, I will notify my physician."
  4 "The port will need to be flushed with saline to maintain patency."

Level of Cognitive Ability: Analysis
Client Needs: Health Promotion and
Maintenance
Integrated Process: Teaching and Learning
Content Area: Fundamental Skills

Answer: 2
Rationale: An implanted vascular access port does not need to be pumped to maintain patency. The site will need to be kept clean and dry, and the physician would need to be notified about signs and symptoms of infection. Saline is used to flush the site to maintain patency.

Test-Taking Strategy: Note the strategic words "need for further instructions." These words indicate a negative event query and ask you to select an option that is an incorrect statement. Using the principles related to vascular access ports and care of an intravenous line will direct you to option 2. Review these principles if you had difficulty with this question.

Reference
Perry, A., & Potter, P. (2006). *Clinical nursing skills & techniques* (6th ed., pp. 924-925). St. Louis: Mosby.

855. The nurse is planning to teach a client with a below-the-knee amputation about skin care to prevent breakdown. Which of the following points should the nurse include in the teaching plan?
1 A stump sock must be worn at all times and changed twice a week.
2 The socket of the prosthesis must be dried carefully before it is used.
3 The residual limb (stump) is washed gently and dried every other day.
4 The socket of the prosthesis needs to be washed with a strong bactericidal agent daily.

Level of Cognitive Ability: Application
Client Needs: Health Promotion and Maintenance
Integrated Process: Nursing Process/Planning
Content Area: Adult Health/Musculoskeletal

Answer: 2
Rationale: The socket of the prosthesis is cleansed with a mild detergent, rinsed, and dried carefully each day. A strong bactericidal agent would not be used. A stump sock must be worn at all times to absorb perspiration, and it is changed daily. The residual limb (stump) is washed, dried, and inspected for breakdown twice each day.

Test-Taking Strategy: Use the process of elimination. Recalling that the residual limb is cared for twice a day will assist you with eliminating options 1 and 3. From the remaining options, noting the strategic word "strong" in option 4 will assist you with eliminating this option. Review the home-care instructions for the client with an amputation if you had difficulty with this question.

Reference
Black, J., & Hawks, J. (2005). *Medical-surgical nursing: Clinical management for positive outcomes* (7th ed., p. 1527). Philadelphia: Saunders.

---

856. The nurse has completed instructions regarding diet and fluid restriction for the client with chronic renal failure. The nurse determines that the client understands the information presented if the client selected which dessert from the dietary menu?
1 Jell-O
2 Sherbet
3 Ice cream
4 Angel food cake

Level of Cognitive Ability: Analysis
Client Needs: Health Promotion and Maintenance
Integrated Process: Nursing Process/Evaluation
Content Area: Adult Health/Renal

Answer: 4
Rationale: Dietary fluid includes anything that is liquid at room temperature. This includes items such as Jell-O, sherbet, and ice cream. For clients on a fluid-restricted diet, it is helpful to avoid "hidden" fluids to whatever extent possible. This allows the client to take in more fluid by drinking, which can help alleviate thirst.

Test-Taking Strategy: Use the process of elimination, noting the strategic words "fluid restriction." Recalling that dietary fluid includes anything that is liquid at room temperature will direct you to option 4. Review this type of dietary restriction if you had difficulty with this question.

Reference
Ignatavicius, D., & Workman, M. (2006). *Medical-surgical nursing: Critical thinking for collaborative care* (5th ed., p. 1736). Philadelphia: Saunders.

---

857. The nurse has given instructions to the client with chronic renal failure about reducing pruritus from uremia. The nurse determines that the client needs further instructions if the client states to use which item for skin care?
1 Mild soap
2 Oil in the bathwater
3 Lanolin-based lotion
4 Alcohol cleansing pads

Answer: 4
Rationale: The client with chronic renal failure often has dry skin that is accompanied by itching (pruritus) from uremia. Products that contain perfumes or alcohol increase dryness and pruritus and should be avoided. The client should use mild soaps, lotions, and bath oils to reduce dryness without increasing skin irritation.

Level of Cognitive Ability: Analysis
Client Needs: Health Promotion and
  Maintenance
Integrated Process: Teaching and Learning
Content Area: Adult Health/Renal

Test-Taking Strategy: Focus on the subject of reducing pruritus, and note the strategic words "needs further instructions." These words indicate a negative event query and ask you to select an incorrect statement. Eliminate options 2 and 3 first, because they are comparable or alike. From the remaining options, eliminate option 1, knowing that the client should avoid putting irritating products on the skin. Review the mea-sures for the treatment of pruritus if you had difficulty with this question.

References

Black, J., & Hawks, J. (2005). *Medical-surgical nursing: Clinical management for positive outcomes* (7th ed., pp. 965; 966). Philadelphia: Saunders.

Ignatavicius, D., & Workman, M. (2006). *Medical-surgical nursing: Critical thinking for collaborative care* (5th ed., p. 1744). Philadelphia: Saunders.

---

858. A physician in a community clinic diagnoses a client with prostatitis, and a nurse provides home-care instructions to the client. Which statement by the client would indicate a need for further instructions?
  1 "There are no restrictions to my diet."
  2 "I need to avoid sexual activity for 2 weeks."
  3 "The warm sitz baths will help my condition."
  4 "I need to take the anti-inflammatory medications as prescribed."

Level of Cognitive Ability: Analysis
Client Needs: Health Promotion and
  Maintenance
Integrated Process: Teaching and Learning
Content Area: Fundamental Skills

Answer: 2

Rationale: Interventions for prostatitis include anti-inflammatory agents or short-term antimicrobial medication. Warm sitz baths and normal sexual activity are recommended. Dietary restrictions are not necessary unless the person finds that certain foods are associated with manifestations.

Test-Taking Strategy: Note the strategic words "need for further instructions." These words indicate a negative event query and ask you to select an option that is an incorrect statement. Eliminate option 4 first, using the general principles associated with medication prescriptions. Option 1 can be eliminated next, because there is no specific relationship of diet with this disorder. From the remaining options, eliminate option 3, because it would seem reasonable that sitz baths would provide comfort. Review the home-care instructions for the client with prostatitis if you had difficulty with this question.

References

Black, J., & Hawks, J. (2005). *Medical-surgical nursing: Clinical management for positive outcomes* (7th ed., p. 1036). Philadelphia: Saunders.

Monahan, F., Sands, J., Neighbors, M., Marek, J., & Green, C. (2007). *Phipps' medical-surgical nursing: Health and illness perspectives* (8th ed., p. 1727). St. Louis: Mosby.

---

859. The nurse provides information to a client who is scheduled for the implantation of an implantable cardioverter defibrillator (ICD) regarding care after implantation. The nurse tells the client that there is a need to keep a diary and that its primary purpose is to:
  1 Analyze which activities to avoid.
  2 Document events that precipitate a countershock.
  3 Provide a count of the number of shocks delivered.
  4 Record a variety of data that are useful for the physician during medical management.

Answer: 4

Rationale: The client with an ICD maintains a log or diary of a variety of data. This includes recording the date and time of the shock, any activity that took place before the shock, any symptoms experienced, the number of shocks delivered, and how the client felt after the shock. The information is used by the physician to adjust the medical regimen and especially the medication therapy, which must be maintained after ICD insertion.

Test-Taking Strategy: Use the process of elimination. Each of the incorrect options lists one of the items that should be logged in the diary, but the correct option is the only one that could be considered a "primary" purpose. Option 4 is the umbrella option. Review the home-care instructions for the client with an ICD if you had difficulty with this question.

Level of Cognitive Ability: Application
Client Needs: Health Promotion and
  Maintenance
Integrated Process: Teaching and Learning
Content Area: Adult Health/Cardiovascular

References
Black, J., & Hawks, J. (2005). *Medical-surgical nursing: Clinical management for positive outcomes* (7th ed., p. 1698). Philadelphia: Saunders.
Canobbio, M. (2006). *Mosby's handbook of patient teaching* (3rd ed., pp. 479-481). St. Louis: Mosby.

---

860. The nurse is evaluating a hypertensive client's understanding of dietary modifications to control the disease process. The nurse determines that the client's understanding is satisfactory if the client made which of the following meal selections?
1 Corned beef, fresh carrots, boiled potato
2 Hot dog on a bun, sauerkraut, baked beans
3 Turkey, baked potato, salad with oil and vinegar
4 Scallops, French fries, salad with bleu cheese dressing

Level of Cognitive Ability: Analysis
Client Needs: Health Promotion and
  Maintenance
Integrated Process: Nursing Process/Evaluation
Content Area: Adult Health/Cardiovascular

Answer: 3
Rationale: The client with hypertension should avoid foods that are high in sodium. Foods from the meat group that are higher in sodium include bacon, hot dogs, luncheon meat, chipped or corned beef, Kosher meat, smoked or salted meat or fish, peanut butter, and a variety of shellfish.

Test-Taking Strategy: Use the process of elimination, and focus on the client's diagnosis. Eliminate options 1 and 2, because they are highly processed meats that would be high in sodium. From the remaining options, recalling that shellfish and commercial salad dressing are high in sodium will assist you with eliminating option 4. Review foods that are high in sodium if you had difficulty with this question.

References
Black, J., & Hawks, J. (2005). *Medical-surgical nursing: Clinical management for positive outcomes* (7th ed., pp. 1499, 1501, 1503, 1707). Philadelphia: Saunders.
Canobbio, M. (2006). *Mosby's handbook of patient teaching* (3rd ed., p. 928). St. Louis: Mosby.
Grodner, M., Long, S., & DeYoung, S. (2004). *Foundations and clinical applications of nutrition: A nursing approach* (3rd ed., pp. 592, 609). St. Louis: Mosby.

---

861. A nurse has taught a client who will be taking warfarin sodium (Coumadin) indefinitely. Which statement by the client indicates the need for further teaching?
1 "I need to use a soft toothbrush."
2 "I need to use a straight razor for shaving."
3 "I need to avoid drinking alcohol while taking this medication."
4 "I need to carry identification regarding the medication being taken."

Level of Cognitive Ability: Analysis
Client Needs: Health Promotion and
  Maintenance
Integrated Process: Teaching and Learning
Content Area: Pharmacology

Answer: 2
Rationale: Client instructions for oral anticoagulant therapy include taking the medication only as prescribed and at the same time each day; avoiding other medications (including over-the-counter medications) without physician approval; avoiding alcohol; notifying all caregivers about the medication; carrying a Medic-Alert bracelet or card; reporting any signs of bleeding and implementing measures to prevent bleeding; and adhering to the schedule for follow-up blood work.

Test-Taking Strategy: Note the strategic words "need for further teaching." These words indicate a negative event query and ask you to select an option that is an incorrect statement. Recalling that warfarin sodium is an anticoagulant and that the client is at risk for bleeding will direct you to option 2. Review the home-care instructions for the client taking an anticoagulant if you had difficulty with this question.

References
Hodgson, B., & Kizior, R. (2007). *Saunders nursing drug handbook 2007* (p. 1222). Philadelphia: Saunders.
Skidmore-Roth, L. (2008). *Mosby's nursing drug reference* (21st ed., p. 1069). St. Louis: Mosby.

862. The home-care nurse has given instructions to a client who was recently discharged from the hospital regarding the care of an arterial ischemic leg ulcer. The nurse determines that further instruction is needed if the client makes which of the following statements?

1 "I should inspect my feet daily."
2 "I should wear shoes and socks."
3 "I should cut my toenails straight across."
4 "I should raise my legs above the level of my heart periodically."

Level of Cognitive Ability: Analysis
Client Needs: Health Promotion and Maintenance
Integrated Process: Teaching and Learning
Content Area: Adult Health/Cardiovascular

Answer: 4

Rationale: Foot-care instructions for the client with peripheral arterial ischemia are the same instructions given to the client with diabetic mellitus. The client with arterial disease, however, should avoid raising the legs above heart level unless instructed to do so as part of an exercise program (such as Buerger's postural exercises) or unless venous stasis is also present. Options 1, 2, and 3 are accurate client statements.

Test-Taking Strategy: Note the strategic words "further instruction is needed." These words indicate a negative event query and ask you to select an option that is an incorrect statement. Note that the client has an arterial disorder. Recalling the anatomy of the blood vessels and the pattern of blood flow in the arteries will direct you to option 4. Review the home-care instructions for the client with an arterial disorder if you had difficulty with this question.

Reference

Ignatavicius, D., & Workman, M. (2006). *Medical-surgical nursing: Critical thinking for collaborative care* (5th ed., p. 796). Philadelphia: Saunders.

---

863. A client with chronic renal failure is about to begin hemodialysis therapy. The client asks the nurse about the frequency and scheduling of hemodialysis treatments. The nurse tells the client that the typical schedule is:

1 2 hours of treatment 6 days per week
2 5 hours of treatment 2 days per week
3 2 to 3 hours of treatment 5 days per week
4 3 to 4 hours of treatment 3 days per week

Level of Cognitive Ability: Application
Client Needs: Health Promotion and Maintenance
Integrated Process: Nursing Process/ Implementation
Content Area: Adult Health/Renal

Answer: 4

Rationale: The typical schedule for hemodialysis is 3 to 4 hours of treatment 3 days per week. Individual adjustments may be made according to certain variables, such as the size of the client, the type of dialyzer, the rate of blood flow, and personal client preferences.

Test-Taking Strategy: Focus on the subject—the "typical" dialysis schedule. Recalling that the client receives dialysis 3 days per week will direct you to option 4. Review the typical dialysis schedule if you had difficulty with this question.

References

Black, J., & Hawks, J. (2005). *Medical-surgical nursing: Clinical management for positive outcomes* (7th ed., p. 957). Philadelphia: Saunders.

Lewis, S., Heitkemper, M., Dirksen, S., O'Brien, P., & Bucher, L. (2007). *Medical-surgical nursing: Assessment and management of clinical problems* (7th ed., p. 1223). St. Louis: Mosby.

---

864. The nurse prepares a client for discharge from the hospital with a peripheral intravenous (IV) site for home IV therapy. Which should the nurse teach the client to help prevent phlebitis and infiltration?

1 Massage the IV site daily.
2 Immobilize the extremity.
3 Stabilize the cannula with tape.
4 Cleanse the site daily with alcohol.

Answer: 3

Rationale: Providing IV therapy at home involves the same principles as are used in the hospital. Protecting the IV site and securing it with tape are extremely important to ensure that the IV site remains immobile to reduce the risk of phlebitis and infiltration; however, the extremity does not need to be immobilized. Massaging the site potentially contributes to catheter movement and tissue damage. Alcohol skin preparation is used during the catheter insertion; because of the potential for excessive drying and client discomfort, alcohol is not used in IV site care. Immobilization devices such as arm boards are used if a site is near a joint and the IV flow rate is affected by joint movement.

Level of Cognitive Ability: Application
Client Needs: Health Promotion and
Maintenance
Integrated Process: Teaching and Learning
Content Area: Fundamental Skills

Test-Taking Strategy: Use the process of elimination, focusing on the subject—preventing phlebitis and infiltration. Eliminate options 1, 2, and 4 because of the words "massage," "immobilize," and "alcohol," respectively. Review the interventions related to the prevention of phlebitis and infiltration if you had difficulty with this question.

Reference
Potter, P., & Perry, A. (2005). *Fundamentals of nursing* (6th ed., pp. 1189, 1194). St. Louis: Mosby.

---

865. The nurse is teaching a client how to stand on crutches. The nurse tells the client to place the crutches:
1 3 inches to the front and side of the toes
2 8 inches to the front and side of the toes
3 15 inches to the front and side of the toes
4 20 inches to the front and side of the toes

Level of Cognitive Ability: Application
Client Needs: Health Promotion and
Maintenance
Integrated Process: Nursing Process/
Implementation
Content Area: Adult Health/Musculoskeletal

Answer: 2
Rationale: The classic tripod position is taught to the client before instructions regarding gait are given. The crutches are placed anywhere from 6 to 10 inches in front of and to the side of the client's toes, depending on the client's body size. This provides a wide enough base of support for the client and improves balance.

Test-Taking Strategy: Use the process of elimination. Three inches (option 1) and 20 inches (option 4) seem excessively short and long, respectively, and these options should be eliminated first. From the remaining options, visualize this procedure. Eight inches seems more in keeping with the normal length of a stride than 15 inches. Review this procedure if you had difficulty with this question.

Reference
Ignatavicius, D., & Workman, M. (2006). *Medical-surgical nursing: Critical thinking for collaborative care* (5th ed., p. 1204). Philadelphia: Saunders.

---

866. A nurse is giving instructions to a client who is beginning therapy with digoxin (Lanoxin). The nurse teaches the client to:
1 Take the pulse daily.
2 Have electrolyte levels drawn weekly.
3 Monitor the blood pressure once a week.
4 Measure the weight each morning before breakfast.

Level of Cognitive Ability: Application
Client Needs: Health Promotion and
Maintenance
Integrated Process: Teaching and Learning
Content Area: Pharmacology

Answer: 1
Rationale: Clients taking digoxin should take the pulse each day and notify the physician if the heart rate is less than 60 beats/min or more than 100 beats/min. Options 2, 3, and 4 are not necessary interventions for the client taking digoxin.

Test-Taking Strategy: Use the process of elimination, focusing on the medication identified in the question. Recalling that digoxin is a cardiac medication will direct you to option 1. Review the client instructions regarding digoxin if you had difficulty with this question.

Reference
Skidmore-Roth, L. (2008). *Mosby's nursing drug reference* (21st ed., p. 364). St. Louis: Mosby.

867. The nurse has completed client teaching with a hemodialysis client regarding the self-monitoring of the fluid status between hemodialysis treatments. The nurse determines that the client understands the information given if the client states the need to record which of the following on a daily basis?

1 Activity
2 Pulse and respiratory rate
3 Intake, output, and weight
4 Blood urea nitrogen and creatinine levels

Level of Cognitive Ability: Analysis
Client Needs: Health Promotion and Maintenance
Integrated Process: Nursing Process/Evaluation
Content Area: Adult Health/Renal

Answer: 3
Rationale: The client receiving hemodialysis should monitor his or her fluid status between hemodialysis treatments. This can be done by recording intake and output and measuring weight on a daily basis. Ideally the hemodialysis client should not gain more than 0.5 kg of weight per day. Options 1, 2, and 4 are not necessary.

Test-Taking Strategy: Use the process of elimination. Immediately eliminate option 4, because it would not be the client's responsibility to obtain or record this information. Note the strategic words "daily basis." Focusing on these strategic words and the subject of fluid status will direct you to option 3. Review the self-care instructions for the hemodialysis client if you had difficulty with this question.

References
Black, J., & Hawks, J. (2005). *Medical-surgical nursing: Clinical management for positive outcomes* (7th ed., p. 964). Philadelphia: Saunders.
Ignatavicius, D., & Workman, M. (2006). *Medical-surgical nursing: Critical thinking for collaborative care* (5th ed., p. 1756). Philadelphia: Saunders.

---

868. Diltiazem hydrochloride (Cardizem) is prescribed for the client with Prinzmetal angina. A nurse provides instructions to the client regarding this medication. Which statement by the client indicates the need for further instructions?

1 "I will take the medication after meals."
2 "I will call the physician if shortness of breath occurs."
3 "I will rise slowly when getting out of bed in the morning."
4 "I will avoid activities that require alertness until my body gets used to the medication."

Level of Cognitive Ability: Analysis
Client Needs: Health Promotion and Maintenance
Integrated Process: Teaching and Learning
Content Area: Pharmacology

Answer: 1
Rationale: Diltiazem hydrochloride (Cardizem) is a calcium-channel blocker. It is administered before meals and at bedtime, as prescribed. Hypotension can occur, and the client is instructed to rise slowly. The client should avoid tasks that require alertness until a response to the medication is established. The client should call the physician if an irregular heartbeat, shortness of breath, pronounced dizziness, nausea, or constipation occurs.

Test-Taking Strategy: Note the strategic words "need for further instructions." These words indicate a negative event query and ask you to select an option that is an incorrect statement. Focusing on the client's diagnosis will assist you with eliminating options 2, 3, and 4. Review the home-care instructions regarding diltiazem hydrochloride if you had difficulty with this question.

Reference
Skidmore-Roth, L. (2008). *Mosby's nursing drug reference* (21st ed., p. 369). St. Louis: Mosby.

---

869. The nurse has provided instructions to a client being discharged from the hospital to home after an abdominal aortic aneurysm (AAA) resection. The nurse determines that the client understands the instructions if the client stated that an appropriate activity would be to:

1 Mow the lawn.
2 Play a game of 18-hole golf.
3 Lift objects up to 30 pounds.
4 Walk as tolerated, including up and down stairs and outdoors.

Answer: 4
Rationale: The client can walk as tolerated after the repair or resection of an AAA, including climbing stairs and walking outdoors. The client should not lift objects that weigh more than 15 to 20 pounds for 6 to 12 weeks or engage in any activities that involve pushing, pulling, or straining. Driving is also prohibited for several weeks.

Level of Cognitive Ability: Analysis
Client Needs: Health Promotion and
  Maintenance
Integrated Process: Nursing Process/Evaluation
Content Area: Adult Health/Cardiovascular

Test-Taking Strategy: Use the process of elimination, noting the strategic words "understands the instructions." Evaluate each option in terms of the strain that it could put on the sutured graft. This will direct you to option 4. Review the discharge instructions after AAA if you had difficulty with this question.

Reference
Black, J., & Hawks, J. (2005). *Medical-surgical nursing: Clinical management for positive outcomes* (7th ed., pp. 1531-1532). Philadelphia: Saunders.

870. A nurse is planning dietary counseling for the client taking triamterene (Dyrenium). The nurse plans to include which of the following in a list of foods that are acceptable?
  1 Bananas
  2 Oranges
  3 Baked potato
  4 Canned pears

Level of Cognitive Ability: Application
Client Needs: Health Promotion and
  Maintenance
Integrated Process: Teaching and Learning
Content Area: Pharmacology

Answer: 4
Rationale: Triamterene is a potassium-sparing diuretic, and clients taking this medication should be cautioned against eating foods that are high in potassium, including many vegetables, fruits, and fresh meats. Because potassium is very soluble in water, foods that are prepared in cans are often lower in potassium.

Test-Taking Strategy: Focus on the medication, noting the strategic words "foods that are acceptable." Recall that triamterene is a potassium-sparing diuretic. Next, review the options, identifying the food item that is lowest in potassium. Review high-potassium foods and triamterene if you had difficulty with this question.

References
Hodgson, B., & Kizior, R. (2007). *Saunders nursing drug handbook 2007* (p. 1175). Philadelphia: Saunders.
Kee, J., Hayes, E., & McCuistion, L. (2006). *Pharmacology: A nursing process approach.* (5th ed., p. 638). Philadelphia: Saunders.
McKenry, L., Tessier, E., & Hogan, M. (2006). *Mosby's pharmacology in nursing* (22nd ed., p. 678). St. Louis: Mosby.

871. Cyclophosphamide (Cytoxan) is prescribed for the client with breast cancer, and the nurse provides instructions to the client regarding the medication. Which statement by the client indicates the need for further instructions?
  1 "If I lose my hair, it will grow back."
  2 "If I develop a sore throat, I should notify the physician."
  3 "I need to limit my fluid intake while taking this medication."
  4 "I need to avoid contact with anyone who recently received a live virus vaccine."

Level of Cognitive Ability: Analysis
Client Needs: Health Promotion and
  Maintenance
Integrated Process: Teaching and Learning
Content Area: Pharmacology

Answer: 3
Rationale: Hemorrhagic cystitis is an adverse reaction associated with cyclophosphamide. The client needs to be instructed to consume copious amounts of fluid during therapy. Avoiding contact with anyone who recently received a live virus vaccine is important, because cyclophosphamide produces immunosuppression, thus placing the client at risk for infection. The client's hair will grow back, although it may have a different color and texture. A sore throat may be an indication of an infection, and it needs to be reported to the physician.

Test-Taking Strategy: Note the strategic words "need for further instructions." These words indicate a negative event query and ask you to select an option that is an incorrect statement. Eliminate options 2 and 4, because they are comparable or alike in that they both relate to the risk of infection. From the remaining options, recalling that hemorrhagic cystitis is an adverse effect of cyclophosphamide will direct you to option 3. Review the adverse effects of cyclophosphamide if you had difficulty with this question.

References
Hodgson, B., & Kizior, R. (2007). *Saunders nursing drug handbook 2007* (p. 300). Philadelphia: Saunders.
Skidmore-Roth, L. (2008). *Mosby's nursing drug reference* (21st ed., p. 315). St. Louis: Mosby.

---

872. The community health nurse has reviewed information about the population of a local community and has determined that there are groups in the population that are at high risk for infection with tuberculosis (TB). The nurse targets which high-risk group for screening?
1 French Canadians
2 White, Anglo-Saxon Americans
3 Older clients in long-term care facilities
4 Adolescents between the ages of 13 and 17 years

Level of Cognitive Ability: Analysis
Client Needs: Health Promotion and Maintenance
Integrated Process: Nursing Process/Assessment
Content Area: Adult Health/Respiratory

Answer: 3
Rationale: Older clients, particularly those in long-term care facilities, are at high risk for infection with TB. Other people at risk include children who are 5 years old and younger, the malnourished, the immunosuppressed, the economically disadvantaged, foreign-born persons, and persons of a minority race who formerly lived in a place where TB is common, such as Asia or the Pacific islands.

Test-Taking Strategy: Recalling the risk factors associated with TB will direct you to option 3. Remember that the very young and the very old often fall into high-risk categories. Review the risk factors associated with TB if you had difficulty with this question.

Reference
Black, J., & Hawks, J. (2005). *Medical-surgical nursing: Clinical management for positive outcomes* (7th ed., p. 1844). Philadelphia: Saunders.

---

873. The nurse prepares a discharge plan of care for a postoperative client who had a cystectomy and a urinary diversion (vesicostomy) created to treat bladder cancer. The nurse identifies which nursing diagnosis as a priority?
1 Risk for infection related to a direct opening into the bladder
2 Risk for disturbed body image related to the presence of a pouch
3 Risk for a toileting self-care deficit related to poor hand-eye coordination
4 Impaired urinary elimination related to urinary diversion and the loss of the ability to void normally

Level of Cognitive Ability: Analysis
Client Needs: Health Promotion and Maintenance
Integrated Process: Nursing Process/Planning
Content Area: Adult Health/Renal

Answer: 4
Rationale: A urinary diversion is a surgical diversion of urinary flow from its usual path through the urinary tract. As a result, the client has impaired urinary elimination. The nursing diagnosis of impaired urinary elimination is the first priority, because it is identified as an actual problem and directly relates to the client's surgical procedure. The client is also at risk for infection as a result of the direct opening into the bladder. Because infection can be life-threatening if it occurs, the nursing diagnosis of risk for infection is the second priority. Because the risk for a toileting self-care deficit is a physiological need, it takes priority over the risk for a disturbed body image, which is a psychosocial need. Therefore, the risk for a toileting self-care deficit is the third priority, followed by the risk for a disturbed body image.

Test-Taking Strategy: When presented with nursing diagnoses and asked to prioritize them, remember that, in most situations, an actual nursing diagnosis is the priority. This guideline assists you with selecting option 4, impaired urinary elimination, as the first priority. Review the care of the client with a urinary diversion if you had difficulty with this question.

References
Black, J., & Hawks, J. (2005). *Medical-surgical nursing: Clinical management for positive outcomes* (7th ed., pp. 875, 877). Philadelphia: Saunders.
Gulanick, M., & Myers, J. (2007). *Nursing care plans: Nursing diagnosis and intervention* (6th ed., pp. 960-972). St. Louis: Mosby.

874. The mother of a teenage client with an anxiety disorder is concerned about her daughter's progress after discharge. She states that her daughter "stashes food, eats all the wrong things that make her hyperactive," and "hangs out with the wrong crowd." To promote optimal health and to assist the mother with preparing for her daughter's discharge, the nurse advises the mother to:

1 Restrict the daughter's socializing time with her school friends.
2 Consider taking time off to help her daughter readjust to the home environment.
3 Limit the amount of chocolate and caffeine products that are available in the home.
4 Keep her daughter out of school until she proves that she can adjust to the school environment.

Level of Cognitive Ability: Application
Client Needs: Health Promotion and Maintenance
Integrated Process: Teaching and Learning
Content Area: Mental Health

Answer: 3
Rationale: Clients with anxiety disorders are advised to limit their intake of caffeine, chocolate, and alcohol, because these products have the potential to increase anxiety. Options 1 and 4 are unreasonable and involve unhealthy approaches. In addition, it may not be realistic for a family member to take time off from work.

Test-Taking Strategy: Note the daughter's diagnosis, and focus on the subject—to promote health. Options 1, 2, and 4 are comparable or alike, and they are concerned with monitoring or curtailing the daughter's physical activities, whereas option 3 focuses on the subject. Review the health promotion measures for the client with an anxiety disorder if you had difficulty with this question.

References
Stuart, G., & Laraia, M. (2005). *Principles and practice of psychiatric nursing* (8th ed., p. 266). St. Louis: Mosby.
Varcarolis, E., Carson, V., & Shoemaker, N. (2006). *Foundations of psychiatric mental health nursing* (5th ed., p. 757). Philadelphia: Saunders.

875. The nurse assesses a client with hepatic encephalopathy for the presence of asterixis. To appropriately test for asterixis, the nurse:

1 Examines the client's handwriting movements
2 Checks the stool for clay-colored pigmentation
3 Asks the client to extend the wrist and the fingers
4 Checks the serum bilirubin and liver enzyme levels

Level of Cognitive Ability: Application
Client Needs: Health Promotion and Maintenance
Integrated Process: Nursing Process/Assessment
Content Area: Fundamental Skills

Answer: 3
Rationale: Asterixis is a nonrhythmic, abnormal muscle tremor of the wrists and fingers that is commonly associated with hepatic encephalopathy and referred to as "liver flap." Clients with hepatic encephalopathy can experience changes in bowel habits and flatulence. Handwriting is a nonspecific and insensitive test of motor function, so the nurse avoids using this to assess for asterixis. The nurse expects the liver function studies of a client with hepatic encephalopathy to have above-normal results.

Test-Taking Strategy: Recalling the signs and symptoms of hepatic encephalopathy will direct you to option 3. Focus on the definition of asterixis to answer correctly. Review this technique if you are unfamiliar with assessment for asterixis.

Reference
Ignatavicius, D., & Workman, M. (2006). *Medical-surgical nursing: Critical thinking for collaborative care* (5th ed., pp. 1369, 1373). Philadelphia: Saunders.

876. The nurse assesses the cranial nerve XII in the client who sustained a brain attack (stroke). To assess this cranial nerve, the nurse asks the client to perform which of the following?
1 Extend the arms.
2 Extend the tongue.
3 Turn the head toward the nurse's arm.
4 Focus the eyes on an object held by the nurse.

Level of Cognitive Ability: Application
Client Needs: Health Promotion and Maintenance
Integrated Process: Nursing Process/Assessment
Content Area: Adult Health/Neurological

Answer: 2
Rationale: To assess the function of cranial nerve XII (hypoglossal), the nurse would assess the client's ability to extend the tongue. Impairment of cranial nerve XII can occur with a stroke. Options 1, 3, and 4 do not test the function of the 12th cranial nerve.

Test-Taking Strategy: Recalling that cranial nerve XII is the hypoglossal nerve will direct you to option 2. Review the cranial nerves and the methods of testing these nerves if you had difficulty with this question.

References
Black, J., & Hawks, J. (2005). *Medical-surgical nursing: Clinical management for positive outcomes* (7th ed., p. 2029). Philadelphia: Saunders.
Ignatavicius, D., & Workman, M. (2006). *Medical-surgical nursing: Critical thinking for collaborative care* (5th ed., p. 931). Philadelphia: Saunders.

---

877. A client with type 2 diabetes mellitus is being discharged from the hospital after an occurrence of hyperglycemic hyperosmolar nonketotic syndrome (HHNS). The nurse develops a discharge teaching plan for the client and identifies which of the following as a priority?
1 Exercise routines
2 Controlling dietary intake
3 Keeping follow-up appointments
4 Monitoring for signs of dehydration

Level of Cognitive Ability: Application
Client Needs: Health Promotion and Maintenance
Integrated Process: Teaching and Learning
Content Area: Delegating/Prioritizing

Answer: 4
Rationale: Clients at risk for HHNS should immediately report signs and symptoms of dehydration to health care providers. Dehydration can be severe, and it may progress rapidly. Although options 1, 2, and 3 are components of the teaching plan, for the client with HHNS, dehydration is the priority.

Test-Taking Strategy: Use the process of elimination, noting the strategic word "priority." Look at each option in terms of its seriousness, and recall that dehydration can rapidly progress to HHNS. Review HHNS if you had difficulty with this question.

References
Black, J., & Hawks, J. (2005). *Medical-surgical nursing: Clinical management for positive outcomes* (7th ed., p. 1273). Philadelphia: Saunders.
Ignatavicius, D., & Workman, M. (2006). *Medical-surgical nursing: Critical thinking for collaborative care* (5th ed., p. 1546). Philadelphia: Saunders.

---

878. The nurse develops a plan of care for an older client with diabetes mellitus. The nurse plans to first:
1 Structure menus for adherence to diet.
2 Teach with videotapes showing insulin administration to ensure competence.
3 Encourage dependence on others to prepare the client for the chronicity of the disease.
4 Assess the client's ability to read label markings on syringes and blood glucose monitoring equipment.

Answer: 4
Rationale: The nurse first assesses the client's ability for self-care. Structuring menus for the client promotes dependence. Allowing the client to have hands-on experience rather than teaching with videos is more effective. Independence should be encouraged.

Test-Taking Strategy: Use the steps of the nursing process. Option 4 reflects assessment, which is the first step of the nursing process. Review teaching and learning principles and the teaching and learning needs of the older client if you had difficulty with this question.

Level of Cognitive Ability: Application
Client Needs: Health Promotion and
  Maintenance
Integrated Process: Teaching and Learning
Content Area: Adult Health/Endocrine

References
Black, J., & Hawks, J. (2005). *Medical-surgical nursing: Clinical management for positive outcomes* (7th ed., pp. 154, 1265-1266). Philadelphia: Saunders.
Meiner, S., & Leuckenotte, A. (2006). *Gerontologic nursing* (3rd ed., pp. 544-545). St. Louis: Mosby.

---

879. The nurse is conducting a health screening on a client with a family history of hypertension. Which assessment finding would alert the nurse to the need for teaching related to brain attack (stroke) prevention?

  1 Eats two bowls of high-fiber grain cereal with skim milk for breakfast
  2 Has a blood pressure of 136/86 mm Hg and has lost 10 pounds recently
  3 Uses oral contraceptives and condoms for pregnancy and disease prevention
  4 Works as the manager of a busy medical-surgical unit and jogs 2 miles daily

Level of Cognitive Ability: Analysis
Client Needs: Health Promotion and
  Maintenance
Integrated Process: Nursing Process/Assessment
Content Area: Adult Health/Neurological

Answer: 3
Rationale: Obesity, hypertension, hypercholesterolemia, smoking, and the use of oral contraceptives are all modifiable risk factors for stroke. Oral contraceptive use is discouraged in some clients because of the side effect of clot formation. Low-fat diet and stress-reduction methods are encouraged and identified in options 1 and 4. Although option 2 identifies an elevated blood pressure, the client has made a change in eating habits as noted by the weight loss that is also mentioned in this option.

Test-Taking Strategy: Note the strategic words "need for teaching." These words indicate a negative event query and ask you to select the option that is a risk factor for stroke. Noting the words "oral contraceptives" in option 3 will direct you to this option. Review the risk factors related to stroke if you had difficulty with this question.

References
Ignatavicius, D., & Workman, M. (2006). *Medical-surgical nursing: Critical thinking for collaborative care* (5th ed., p. 1031). Philadelphia: Saunders.
Lewis, S., Heitkemper, M., Dirksen, S., O'Brien, P., & Bucher, L. (2007). *Medical-surgical nursing: Assessment and management of clinical problems* (7th ed., pp. 768, 770). St. Louis: Mosby.

---

880. The nurse is reviewing the assessment data of a clinic client. Which finding would be most important for the client to modify to lessen the risk for coronary artery disease (CAD)?

  1 Elevated triglyceride levels
  2 Elevated serum lipase levels
  3 Elevated low-density lipoprotein (LDL) levels
  4 Elevated high-density lipoprotein (HDL) levels

Level of Cognitive Ability: Analysis
Client Needs: Health Promotion and
  Maintenance
Integrated Process: Nursing Process/Assessment
Content Area: Adult Health/Cardiovascular

Answer: 3
Rationale: LDLs are more directly associated with CAD than are other lipoproteins. LDL levels, along with levels of cholesterol, have a higher predictive association with CAD than levels of triglycerides. Additionally, HDL is inversely associated with the risk of CAD. Lipase is a digestive enzyme that breaks down ingested fats in the gastrointestinal tract.

Test-Taking Strategy: Focus on the subject—the risk factor related to CAD. Recalling that LDL is the "bad" cholesterol will direct you to option 3. Review this content if you are unfamiliar with these risk factors.

References
Ignatavicius, D., & Workman, M. (2006). *Medical-surgical nursing: Critical thinking for collaborative care* (5th ed., pp. 695, 842-843). Philadelphia: Saunders.
Lewis, S., Heitkemper, M., Dirksen, S., O'Brien, P., & Bucher, L. (2007). *Medical-surgical nursing: Assessment and management of clinical problems* (7th ed., p. 793). St. Louis: Mosby.

881. The nurse is taking a history from a client who is suspected of having testicular cancer. Which of the following data will be most helpful for determining the client's risk factors for this type of cancer?
1 Age and race
2 Marital status
3 Number of children
4 Number of sexual partners

Level of Cognitive Ability: Analysis
Client Needs: Health Promotion and Maintenance
Integrated Process: Nursing Process/Assessment
Content Area: Adult Health/Oncology

Answer: 1
Rationale: Two basic but important risk factors for testicular cancer are age and race. The incidence of testicular cancer is four times higher among white males than black males. It is the most common type of cancer to occur in males between the ages of 15 and 34 years. Other risk factors include a history of an undescended testis and a family history of testicular cancer. Marital status and the number of children are not resk factors for testicular cancer.

Test-Taking Strategy: Use your knowledge of the risk factors associated with this type of cancer to answer the question. Recalling that testicular cancer most often occurs in males between the ages of 15 and 34 years will direct you to option 1. Review the risk factors related to testicular cancer if you had difficulty with this question.

References
Black, J., & Hawks, J. (2005). *Medical-surgical nursing: Clinical management for positive outcomes* (7th ed., p. 1036). Philadelphia: Saunders.
Ignatavicius, D., & Workman, M. (2006). *Medical-surgical nursing: Critical thinking for collaborative care* (5th ed., p. 1866). Philadelphia: Saunders.
Lewis, S., Heitkemper, M., Dirksen, S., O'Brien, P., & Bucher, L. (2007). *Medical-surgical nursing: Assessment and management of clinical problems* (7th ed., p. 1432). St. Louis: Mosby.

882. A nurse instructs a perinatal client about measures to prevent urinary tract infections. Which statement by the client would indicate an understanding of these measures?
1 "I can wear my tight-fitting jeans."
2 "I should always use scented toilet paper."
3 "I should choose underwear with a cotton panel liner."
4 "I can take a bubble bath as long as the soap doesn't contain any oils."

Level of Cognitive Ability: Analysis
Client Need: Health Promotion and Maintenance
Integrated Process: Nursing Process/Evaluation
Content Area: Maternity/Antepartum

Answer: 3
Rationale: Wearing items with a cotton panel liner allows for air movement in and around the genital area. Bubble bath or other bath oils should be avoided, because these may be irritating to the urethra. Harsh, scented, or printed toilet paper may cause irritation. Wearing tight clothes irritates the genital area and does not allow for air circulation.

Test-Taking Strategy: Use the process of elimination, and note the strategic words "indicate an understanding." Eliminate option 2 because of the close-ended word "always" and option 1 because of the words "tight-fitting." From the remaining options, recall that bubble baths need to be avoided. Review the measures to prevent urinary tract infections if you had difficulty with this question.

Reference
Wong, D., Hockenberry, M., Perry, S., Lowdermilk, D., & Wilson, D. (2006). *Maternal-child nursing care* (3rd ed., pp. 275-277). St. Louis: Mosby.

883. A nurse instructs a client with mild preeclampsia about home-care measures. The nurse determines that the teaching has been effective concerning the assessment of complications when the client states:
1 "I need to check my weight every day at different times during the day."
2 "I need to take my blood pressure each morning and alternate arms each time."
3 "As long as the home-care nurse is visiting me daily, I do not have to keep my next physician's appointment."
4 "I need to check my urine with a dipstick every day for protein and call the physician if it is 2+ or more."

Level of Cognitive Ability: Analysis
Client Needs: Health Promotion and Maintenance
Integrated Process: Nursing Process/Evaluation
Content Area: Maternity/Antepartum

Answer: 4
Rationale: The client needs to be instructed to report any increases in blood pressure, 2+ proteinuria, weight gain of more than 1 pound per week, the presence of edema, and decreased fetal activity to the physician or health care provider immediately to prevent worsening of the preeclamptic condition. It is important to keep physician appointments even if the client is receiving visits from a home-care nurse. Blood pressure measurements need to be taken in the same arm everyday in a sitting position to obtain consistent and accurate readings. The weight needs to be checked at the same time each day, after voiding, before breakfast, with the client wearing the same clothes, to obtain reliable weight readings.

Test-Taking Strategy: Use the process of elimination, noting the strategic words "teaching has been effective." Basic principles related to health care teaching and focusing on the specific subject of the question—mild preeclampsia—will assist with directing you to option 4. Review the home-care teaching points for the client with preeclampsia if you had difficulty with this question.

Reference
Wong, D., Hockenberry, M., Perry, S., Lowdermilk, D., & Wilson, D. (2006). *Maternal-child nursing care* (3rd ed., p. 379). St. Louis: Mosby.

884. The nurse is providing instructions to a client and family regarding home care after left-eye cataract removal. The nurse tells the client and family which of the following about positioning during the postoperative period?
1 Sleep only on the left side.
2 Sleep on the right side or the back.
3 Bend below the waist as often as you are able.
4 Lower the head between the knees three times a day.

Level of Cognitive Ability: Application
Client Needs: Health Promotion and Maintenance
Integrated Process: Teaching and Learning
Content Area: Adult Health/Eye

Answer: 2
Rationale: After cataract surgery, the client should not sleep on the operative side. The client should also avoid bending below the level of the waist or lowering the head, because these actions will increase intraocular pressure.

Test-Taking Strategy: Use the process of elimination. Eliminate options 3 and 4 first, because they are comparable or alike and indicate that lowering the head below waist level is acceptable. From the remaining options, remembering that the client needs to be instructed to remain off of the operative side will direct you to option 2. Review the postoperative instructions for the client after cataract surgery if you had difficulty with this question.

References
Black, J., & Hawks, J. (2005). *Medical-surgical nursing: Clinical management for positive outcomes* (7th ed., p. 1951). Philadelphia: Saunders.
Ignatavicius, D., & Workman, M. (2006). *Medical-surgical nursing: Critical thinking for collaborative care* (5th ed., p. 1096). Philadelphia: Saunders.
Lewis, S., Heitkemper, M., Dirksen, S., O'Brien, P., & Bucher, L. (2007). *Medical-surgical nursing: Assessment and management of clinical problems* (7th ed., p. 428). St. Louis: Mosby.

885. A nurse has provided instructions to a new mother with a urinary tract infection regarding foods and fluids to consume that will acidify the urine. The nurse determines that further instructions are needed if the mother indicates that which fluid will acidify the urine?
1 Prune juice
2 Apricot juice
3 Cranberry juice
4 Carbonated drinks

Level of Cognitive Ability: Analysis
Client Needs: Health Promotion and Maintenance
Integrated Process: Teaching and Learning
Content Area: Maternity/Postpartum

Answer: 4
Rationale: Acidification of the urine inhibits the multiplication of bacteria. Fluids that acidify the urine include apricot, prune, and cranberry juice. Carbonated drinks should be avoided, because they increase urine alkalinity.

Test-Taking Strategy: Use the process of elimination, noting the strategic words "further instructions are needed." These words indicate a negative event query and ask you to select the fluid item that will not acidify the urine. Note the similarity between options 1, 2, and 3 in that these items are fruit juices. This will assist with directing you to option 4. Review the foods and fluids that cause urine acidification if you had difficulty with this question.

References
Ignatavicius, D., & Workman, M. (2006). *Medical-surgical nursing: Critical thinking for collaborative care* (5th ed., pp. 1684-1685). Philadelphia: Saunders.
Wong, D., Hockenberry, M., Perry, S., Lowdermilk, D., & Wilson, D. (2006). *Maternal-child nursing care* (3rd ed., pp. 276-277). St. Louis: Mosby.

886. A postpartum nurse has instructed a new mother regarding how to bathe her newborn infant. The nurse demonstrates the procedure to the mother and, on the following day, asks the mother to perform the procedure. Which observation by the nurse indicates that the mother is performing the procedure correctly?
1 The mother cleans the ears and then moves to the eyes and the face.
2 The mother begins to wash the newborn infant by starting with the eyes and face.
3 The mother washes the arms, chest, and back followed by the neck, arms, and face.
4 The mother washes the entire newborn infant's body and then washes the eyes, face, and scalp.

Level of Cognitive Ability: Analysis
Client Needs: Health Promotion and Maintenance
Integrated Process: Nursing Process/Evaluation
Content Area: Maternity/Postpartum

Answer: 2
Rationale: Bathing should start at the eyes and face and with the cleanest area first. Next, the external ears and behind the ears are cleaned. The newborn infant's neck should be washed, because formula, lint, and breast milk will often accumulate in the folds of the neck. The hands and arms are then washed. The newborn infant's legs are washed next, with the diaper area being washed last.

Test-Taking Strategy: Use the process of elimination, and use the basic techniques and principles of bathing a client to answer this question. Remember to always start with the cleanest area of the body and proceed to the dirtiest area. This principle will direct you to option 2. Review the home-care measures related to the care of the newborn infant if you had difficulty with this question.

Reference
Wong, D., Hockenberry, M., Perry, S., Lowdermilk, D., & Wilson, D. (2006). *Maternal-child nursing care* (3rd ed., p. 763). St. Louis: Mosby.

887. A nurse is teaching umbilical cord care to a new mother. The nurse tells the mother that:

1 Alcohol is the only agent to use to clean the cord.
2 Cord care is done only at birth to control bleeding.
3 It takes at least 21 days for the cord to dry up and fall off.
4 The process of keeping the cord clean and dry will decrease bacterial growth.

Level of Cognitive Ability: Application
Client Needs: Health Promotion and Maintenance
Integrated Process: Teaching and Learning
Content Area: Maternity/Postpartum

Answer: 4

Rationale: The cord should be kept clean and dry to decrease bacterial growth. It should be cleansed two to three times a day using alcohol or other agents. Cord care is required until the cord dries up and falls off between 7 and 14 days after birth. Additionally, the diaper should be folded below the cord to keep urine away from the cord.

Test-Taking Strategy: Use the process of elimination. Eliminate options 1 and 2 first because of the close-ended word "only." From the remaining options, recalling the purpose of cord care will direct you to option 4. Review the concepts related to cord care if you had difficulty with this question.

Reference
Wong, D., Hockenberry, M., Perry, S., Lowdermilk, D., & Wilson, D. (2006). *Maternal-child nursing care* (3rd ed., pp. 733-734). St. Louis: Mosby.

---

888. The parents of a male newborn infant who is uncircumcised request information about how to clean the newborn's penis. The nurse tells the parents to:

1 "Retract the foreskin and cleanse with every diaper change."
2 "Retract the foreskin and cleanse the glans when bathing the infant."
3 "Avoid the retraction of the foreskin to clean the penis, because this may cause adhesions."
4 "Retract the foreskin no farther than it will easily go, and replace it over the glans after cleaning."

Level of Cognitive Ability: Application
Client Needs: Health Promotion and Maintenance
Integrated Process: Teaching and Learning
Content Area: Maternity/Postpartum

Answer: 3

Rationale: In male newborn infants, the prepuce is continuous with the epidermis of the gland, and it is not retractable. If retraction is forced, this may cause adhesions to develop. The mother should be told to allow separation to occur naturally, which usually occurs between the ages of 3 years and puberty. Most foreskins are retractable by the time the child is 3 years old and should be pushed back gently at this time for cleaning once a week. Options 1, 2, and 4 identify an action that includes the retraction of the foreskin.

Test-Taking Strategy: Use the process of elimination. Note that options 1, 2, and 4 are comparable or alike in that they all identify retracting the foreskin. Option 3 is the option that is different. Review the teaching points related to cleaning the penis of an uncircumcised newborn infant if you had difficulty with this question.

Reference
McKinney, E., James, S., Murray, S., & Ashwill, J. (2005). *Maternal-child nursing* (2nd ed., pp. 562-563). St. Louis: Saunders.

---

889. The nurse prepares a teaching plan regarding the administration of eardrops for the parents of a 6-year-old child. The nurse tells the parents that, when administering the drops, they should:

1 Wear gloves.
2 Pull the ear up and back.
3 Hold the child in a sitting position.
4 Position the child so that the affected ear is facing downward.

Answer: 2

Rationale: To administer eardrops in a child who is more than 3 years old, the ear is pulled upward and back. The ear is pulled down and back in children less than 3 years old. Gloves do not need to be worn by the parents, but handwashing before and after the procedure needs to be performed. The child needs to be in a side-lying position with the affected ear facing upward to facilitate the flow of medication down the ear canal with the help of gravity.

Test-Taking Strategy: Visualizing this procedure will assist you with eliminating options 1, 3, and 4. Recalling the anatomy of the child's ear canal and noting the age of the child will direct you to option 2. Review this procedure if you had difficulty with this question.

Level of Cognitive Ability: Application
Client Needs: Health Promotion and
  Maintenance
Integrated Process: Teaching and Learning
Content Area: Child Health

Reference
Wong, D., Hockenberry, M., Perry, S., Lowdermilk, D., & Wilson, D. (2006). *Maternal-child nursing care* (3rd ed., pp. 1402-1403). St. Louis: Mosby.

---

890. A nurse is providing discharge instructions to the mother of an 8-year-old child who had a tonsillectomy. The mother tells the nurse that the child loves tacos and asks when the child can safely eat one. The appropriate response to the mother is:
  1 "In 1 week."
  2 "In 3 weeks."
  3 "Six days after surgery."
  4 "When the physician says it's okay."

Level of Cognitive Ability: Application
Client Needs: Health Promotion and
  Maintenance
Integrated Process: Teaching and Learning
Content Area: Child Health

Answer: 2
Rationale: Rough or scratchy foods as well as spicy foods are to be avoided for 3 weeks after a tonsillectomy. Citrus juices that irritate the throat need to be avoided for 10 days. Red liquids are avoided, because they will give the appearance of blood if the child vomits. The mother is instructed to add full liquids on the second day and soft foods as the child tolerates them.

Test-Taking Strategy: Use the process of elimination. Eliminate options 1 and 3 first, because they identify similar timeframes. From the remaining options, focus on the strategic word "appropriate." Eliminate option 4, because it places the mother's question on hold. Review the dietary instructions after tonsillectomy if you had difficulty with this question.

References
Hockenberry, M., & Wilson, D. (2007). *Nursing care of infants and children* (8th ed., p. 1322). St. Louis: Mosby.
McKinney, E., James, S., Murray, S., & Ashwill, J. (2005). *Maternal-child nursing* (2nd ed., p. 1203). St. Louis: Saunders.

---

891. After a cleft lip repair, the nurse instructs the parents about the cleaning of the lip repair site. The nurse uses which solution when demonstrating this procedure to the parents?
  1 Tap water
  2 Sterile water
  3 Full-strength hydrogen peroxide
  4 Half-strength hydrogen peroxide

Level of Cognitive Ability: Application
Client Needs: Health Promotion and
  Maintenance
Integrated Process: Teaching and Learning
Content Area: Child Health

Answer: 2
Rationale: Th e lip repair site is cleansed with sterile water using a cotton swab after feeding and as prescribed. The parents should be instructed to use a rolling motion starting at the suture line and rolling out. Tap water is not a sterile solution. Hydrogen peroxide may disrupt the integrity of the site.

Test-Taking Strategy: Use the process of elimination. Eliminate options 3 and 4 first, because they are comparable or alike. From the remaining options, recall the importance of asepsis when treating a surgical site to direct you to option 2. Review this procedure if you had difficulty with this question.

References
McKinney, E., James, S., Murray, S., & Ashwill, J. (2005). *Maternal-child nursing* (2nd ed., p. 1110). St. Louis: Saunders.
Wong, D., Hockenberry, M., Perry, S., Lowdermilk, D., & Wilson, D. (2006). *Maternal-child nursing care* (3rd ed., p. 1527). St. Louis: Mosby.

892. A child with a diagnosis of umbilical hernia has been scheduled for surgical repair in 2 weeks. The clinic nurse instructs the parents about the signs of possible hernial strangulation. The nurse tells the parents that which sign would require physician notification?

1 Fever
2 Diarrhea
3 Vomiting
4 Constipation

Level of Cognitive Ability: Application
Client Needs: Health Promotion and Maintenance
Integrated Process: Teaching and Learning
Content Area: Child Health

Answer: 3
Rationale: The parents of a child with an umbilical hernia need to be instructed regarding the signs of strangulation, which include vomiting, pain, and an irreducible mass at the umbilicus. The parents should be instructed to contact the physician immediately if strangulation is suspected.

Test-Taking Strategy: Use the process of elimination and the definition of the word "strangulation" to assist you with eliminating options 1 and 2. From the remaining options, think about the anatomy of the body and the expected occurrence if strangulation developed to direct you to option 3. Review the signs of strangulation if you had difficulty with this question.

Reference
Wong, D., Hockenberry, M., Perry, S., Lowdermilk, D., & Wilson, D. (2006). *Maternal-child nursing care* (3rd ed., p. 1532). St. Louis: Mosby.

---

893. A client with a compound (open) fracture of the radius has a plaster cast applied in the emergency department. The nurse provides home-care instructions and tells the client to seek medical attention if which of the following occurs?

1 Numbness and tingling are felt in the fingers.
2 The cast feels heavy and damp after 24 hours of application.
3 The entire cast feels warm during the first 24 hours after application.
4 Bloody drainage is noted on the cast during the first 6 hours after application.

Level of Cognitive Ability: Application
Client Needs: Health Promotion and Maintenance
Integrated Process: Teaching and Learning
Content Area: Adult Health/Musculoskeletal

Answer: 1
Rationale: A limb encased in a cast is at risk for nerve damage and diminished circulation from increased pressure caused by edema. Signs of increased pressure from the cast include numbness, tingling, and increased pain. A cast can take up to 48 hours to dry and generates heat while drying. Some drainage may occur initially with a compound (open) fracture.

Test-Taking Strategy: Note the strategic words "compound (open)" in the question. These strategic words and the use of the ABCs—airway, breathing, and circulation—will direct you to option 1. Review the teaching points for the client with a plaster cast if you had difficulty with this question.

Reference
Monahan, F., Sands, J., Neighbors, M., Marek, J., & Green, C. (2007). *Phipps' medical-surgical nursing: Health and illness perspectives* (8th ed., p. 1536). St. Louis: Mosby.

---

894. The mother of a child with celiac disease asks the nurse how long a special diet is necessary. The nurse tells the mother that:

1 A gluten-free diet will need to be followed for life.
2 A lactose-free diet will need to be followed temporarily.
3 Adequate nutritional status will help prevent celiac crisis.
4 Supplemental vitamins, iron, and folate will prevent complications.

Answer: 1
Rationale: The main nursing consideration with celiac disease is helping the child adhere to dietary management. The treatment of celiac disease consists primarily of dietary management with a gluten-free diet. Options 2, 3, and 4 are all true statements, but they do not answer the question that the client is asking. Children with untreated celiac disease may have lactose intolerance, which usually improves with gluten withdrawal. Nutritional deficiencies resulting from malabsorption are treated with appropriate supplements.

Level of Cognitive Ability: Application
Client Needs: Health Promotion and
  Maintenance
Integrated Process: Teaching and Learning
Content Area: Child Health

References
Hockenberry, M., Wilson, D., & Winkelstein, M. (2005). *Wong's essentials of pediatric nursing* (7th ed., p. 886). St. Louis: Mosby.
McKinney, E., James, S., Murray, S., & Ashwill, J. (2005). *Maternal-child nursing* (2nd ed., p. 1145). St. Louis: Saunders.

Test-Taking Strategy: Focus on the subject of the question—the length of time that a special diet is necessary. Option 1 relates directly to this subject. Review the dietary requirements for celiac disease if you had difficulty with this question.

---

895. A nurse teaches the mother of a newly circumcised infant about postcircumcision care. Which statement by the mother indicates an understanding of the care required?

  1 "I need to clean the penis every hour with baby wipes."
  2 "I need to check for bleeding every hour for the first 12 hours."
  3 "My baby will not urinate for the next 24 hours because of swelling."
  4 "I need to wrap the penis completely in dry sterile gauze, making sure that it is dry when I change his diaper."

Level of Cognitive Ability: Analysis
Client Needs: Health Promotion and
  Maintenance
Integrated Process: Nursing Process/Evaluation
Content Area: Maternity/Postpartum

Answer: 2
Rationale: The mother needs to be taught to observe for bleeding and to assess the site hourly for 8 to 12 hours after the circumcision. Voiding needs to be assessed. The mother should call the physician if the baby has not urinated within 24 hours, because swelling or damage may obstruct urine output. When the diaper is changed, Vaseline gauze should be reapplied. Frequent diaper changing prevents contamination of the site. Water is used for cleaning, because soap or baby wipes may irritate the area and cause discomfort.

Test-Taking Strategy: Use the process of elimination. Eliminate option 1, because baby wipes will cause stinging of the newly circumcised penis. Eliminate option 3, because penile swelling that prevents voiding needs to be reported to the physician. Eliminate option 4, because gauze will stick to the penis if it is completely dry. Review postcircumcision care if you had difficulty answering the question.

Reference
Wong, D., Hockenberry, M., Perry, S., Lowdermilk, D., & Wilson, D. (2006). *Maternal-child nursing care* (3rd ed., p. 755). St. Louis: Mosby.

---

896. A nurse is developing a teaching plan for a client who will be receiving phenelzine sulfate (Nardil). The nurse plans to tell the client to avoid:

  1 Vasodilators
  2 Aged cheeses
  3 Digitalis preparations
  4 Cherries and blueberries

Level of Cognitive Ability: Application
Client Needs: Health Promotion and
  Maintenance
Integrated Process: Teaching and Learning
Content Area: Pharmacology

Answer: 2
Rationale: Phenelzine sulfate is in the monoamine oxidase inhibitor (MAOI) class of antidepressant medications. An individual taking an MAOI must avoid aged cheeses, alcoholic beverages, avocados, bananas, and caffeine drinks. There are also other food items to avoid, including chocolate, meat tenderizers, pickled herring, raisins, sour cream, yogurt, and soy sauce. Medications that should be avoided include amphetamines, antiasthmatics, and certain antidepressants. The client should also avoid antihistamines, antihypertensive medications, levodopa (L-dopa), and

Test-Taking Strategy: Note the strategic word "avoid." This word indicates a negative event query and asks you to select the food item that the client is not allowed to consume. Recalling that phenelzine sulfate is an MAOI and recalling the foods that need to be avoided will direct you to option 2. Review phenelzine sulfate if you had difficulty with this question.

References
Hodgson, B., & Kizior, R. (2007). *Saunders nursing drug handbook 2007* (p. 921). Philadelphia: Saunders.
Skidmore-Roth, L. (2008). *Mosby's nursing drug reference* (21st ed., p. 811). St. Louis: Mosby.

---

897. A nurse is providing home-care instructions to the parents of an infant who had surgical repair of an inguinal hernia. The nurse instructs the parents to do which of the following to prevent infection at the surgical site?

1 Report a fever immediately.
2 Restrict the infant's physical activity.
3 Change the diapers as soon as they become damp.
4 Soak the infant in a tub bath twice a day for the next 5 days.

Level of Cognitive Ability: Application
Client Needs: Health Promotion and Maintenance
Integrated Process: Teaching and Learning
Content Area: Child Health

Answer: 3

Rationale: Changing diapers as soon as they become damp helps prevent infection at the surgical site. Parents are instructed to change diapers more frequently than usual during the day and once or twice during the night. Parents are also instructed to give the infant sponge baths rather than tub baths for 2 to 5 days postoperatively. There are no restrictions placed on the infant's activity. A fever could indicate the presence of an infection.

Test-Taking Strategy: Focus on the subject—preventing infection. This will assist you with eliminating options 1 and 4. From the remaining options, thinking about the anatomical location of an inguinal hernia will direct you to option 3. Review the measures to prevent infection after inguinal hernia repair if you had difficulty with this question.

Reference

Wong, D., Hockenberry, M., Perry, S., Lowdermilk, D., & Wilson, D. (2006). *Maternal-child nursing care* (3rd ed., pp. 1653, 1775). St. Louis: Mosby.

---

898. The nurse determines the need for further instruction regarding the use of the incentive spirometer if the client does which of the following?

1 Inhales slowly
2 Breathes through the nose
3 Removes the mouthpiece to exhale
4 Forms a tight seal around the mouthpiece with the lips

Level of Cognitive Ability: Application
Client Needs: Health Promotion and Maintenance
Integrated Process: Teaching and Learning
Content Area: Adult Health/Respiratory

Answer: 2

Rationale: Incentive spirometry is ineffective if the client breathes through the nose. The client should exhale, form a tight seal around the mouthpiece, inhale slowly, hold to the count of 3, and remove the mouthpiece to exhale. The client should repeat the exercise approximately 10 times every hour for best results.

Test-Taking Strategy: Note the strategic words "need for further instruction." These words indicate a negative event query and ask you to select the option that identifies an incorrect client action. Visualizing the use of this device will direct you to option 2. Review the procedure for the use of the incentive spirometer if you had difficulty with this question.

References

Black, J., & Hawks, J. (2005). *Medical-surgical nursing: Clinical management for positive outcomes* (7th ed., p. 306). Philadelphia: Saunders.
Ignatavicius, D., & Workman, M. (2006). *Medical-surgical nursing: Critical thinking for collaborative care* (5th ed., pp. 309-310). Philadelphia: Saunders.

899. A client with chronic obstructive pulmonary disease has a knowledge deficit related to the positions used to breathe more easily. The nurse teaches the client to assume which of the following positions?

1 Sit bolt upright in bed with the arms crossed over the chest.
2 Lie on the side with the head of the bed at a 45-degree angle.
3 Sit in a reclining chair tilted slightly back with the feet elevated.
4 Sit on the edge of the bed with the arms leaning on an over-bed table.

Level of Cognitive Ability: Application
Client Needs: Health Promotion and Maintenance
Integrated Process: Teaching and Learning
Content Area: Adult Health/Respiratory

Answer: 4
Rationale: Proper positioning can decrease episodes of dyspnea in a client. Appropriate positions include sitting upright while leaning on an over-bed table, sitting upright in a chair with the arms resting on the knees, and leaning against a wall while standing. Option 1 restricts the movement of the anterior and posterior walls of the lung, and option 2 restricts the expansion of the lateral wall of the lung. Option 3 restricts posterior lung expansion.

Test-Taking Strategy: Use the process of elimination. Visualize each of the positions described in the options, and think about how each position affects lung expansion to direct you to option 4. Review the positions that relieve dyspnea in the client with chronic obstructive pulmonary disease if you had difficulty with this question.

Reference
Ignatavicius, D., & Workman, M. (2006). *Medical-surgical nursing: Critical thinking for collaborative care* (5th ed., pp. 602-605). Philadelphia: Saunders.

---

900. The nurse has taught the client with pleurisy about measures to promote comfort during recuperation. The nurse determines that the client has understood the instructions if the client states the need to:

1 Try to take only small, shallow breaths.
2 Take as much pain medication as possible.
3 Lie as much as possible on the unaffected side.
4 Splint the chest wall during coughing and deep breathing.

Level of Cognitive Ability: Analysis
Client Needs: Health Promotion and Maintenance
Integrated Process: Nursing Process/Evaluation
Content Area: Adult Health/Respiratory

Answer: 4
Rationale: The client with pleurisy should splint the chest wall during coughing and deep breathing. The client may also lie on the affected side to minimize the movement of the affected chest wall. Taking small, shallow breaths promotes atelectasis. The client should take medication cautiously so that adequate coughing and deep breathing are performed and an adequate level of comfort is maintained.

Test-Taking Strategy: Focus on the subject—to promote comfort. Eliminate option 1 because of the close-ended word "only." From the remaining options, noting the word "splint" in option 4 will direct you to this option. Review the measures that will promote comfort in a client with pleurisy if you had difficulty with this question.

Reference
Lewis, S., Heitkemper, M., Dirksen, S., O'Brien, P., & Bucher, L. (2007). *Medical-surgical nursing: Assessment and management of clinical problems* (7th ed., p. 597). St. Louis: Mosby.

901. A client with a diagnosis of trigeminal neuralgia is started on a regimen of carbamazepine (Tegretol). The nurse provides instructions to the client about the medication and determines that the client understands the instructions if the client states:

1 "I will report a fever or sore throat to my doctor."

2 "Some joint pain is expected and is nothing to worry about."

3 "I must brush my teeth frequently to avoid damage to my gums."

4 "My urine may turn red in color, but this is nothing to be concerned about."

Level of Cognitive Ability: Analysis
Client Needs: Health Promotion and Maintenance
Integrated Process: Nursing Process/Evaluation
Content Area: Pharmacology

Answer: 1
Rationale: Agranulocytosis is an adverse effect of carbamazepine, and it places the client at risk for infection. If the client develops a fever or a sore throat, the physician should be notified. Unusual bruising and bleeding are also adverse effects of the medication, and they need to be reported to the physician if they occur.

Test-Taking Strategy: Use the process of elimination. Eliminate option 3 because of the close-ended word "must." Next, eliminate options 2 and 4, because both indicate that the development of an adverse effect is "nothing to be concerned about." Recalling that agranulocytosis is an adverse effect will direct you to option 1. Review the adverse effects of carbamazepine and the laboratory tests that need monitoring if you had difficulty with this question.

Reference
Hodgson, B., & Kizior, R. (2007). *Saunders nursing drug handbook 2007* (p. 184). Philadelphia: Saunders.

---

902. The nurse teaches a preoperative client about the nasogastric (NG) tube that will be inserted in preparation for surgery. The nurse determines that the client understands when the tube will be removed during the postoperative period when the client states that it will come out:

1 "When the doctor says so."

2 "When I can tolerate food without vomiting."

3 "When my gastrointestinal (GI) system is healed."

4 "When my bowels begin to function again and I begin to pass gas."

Level of Cognitive Ability: Analysis
Client Needs: Health Promotion and Maintenance
Integrated Process: Nursing Process/Evaluation
Content Area: Adult Health/Gastrointestinal

Answer: 4
Rationale: NG tubes are discontinued when normal function returns to the GI tract. The tube will be removed before GI healing. Food would not be administered unless bowel function returns. Although the physician determines when the NG tube will be removed, option 1 does not determine the effectiveness of teaching.

Test-Taking Strategy: Use the process of elimination. Option 1 can be easily eliminated first. Eliminate option 3 next, considering the time factor associated with the healing of the GI tract. From the remaining options, recalling that food would not be administered unless bowel function returns will assist you with eliminating option 2. Review the use and care of the NG tube if you had difficulty with this question.

References
Ignatavicius, D., & Workman, M. (2006). *Medical-surgical nursing: Critical thinking for collaborative care* (5th ed., p. 345). Philadelphia: Saunders.
Potter, P., & Perry, A. (2005). *Fundamentals of nursing* (6th ed., p. 1408). St. Louis: Mosby.

903. A client is receiving intralipids (fat emulsion) intravenously at home, and the client's spouse manages the infusion. The health care nurse makes a visit and discusses potential adverse reactions and the side effects of the therapy with the client and the spouse. After the discussion, the nurse expects the spouse to verbalize that, in case of a suspected adverse reaction, the priority action is to:

1 Stop the infusion.
2 Contact the nurse.
3 Take the client's blood pressure.
4 Contact the local area emergency response team.

Level of Cognitive Ability: Analysis
Client Needs: Health Promotion and Maintenance
Integrated Process: Teaching and Learning
Content Area: Delegating/Prioritizing

Answer: 1
Rationale: Fat-emulsion therapy can cause overloading syndrome (i.e., focal seizures, fever, and shock) and adverse effects, including chest pain, chills, and shock. The priority action is to stop the infusion to limit the adverse response. Although options 2, 3, and 4 are correct interventions, the priority is to stop the infusion.

Test-Taking Strategy: Note the strategic words "suspected adverse reaction" and "priority." Remembering that the priority action when an adverse reaction occurs is to stop the infusion will direct you to the correct option. Review the adverse reactions of fat-emulsion therapy and the priority actions to take if an adverse reaction occurs if you had difficulty with this question.

References
Back, J., & Hawks, J. (2005). *Medical-surgical nursing: Clinical management for positive outcomes* (7th ed., p. 708). Philadelphia: Saunders.
Gahart, B., & Nazareno, A. (2008). 2008 *Intravenous medications* (24th ed., p. 566). St. Louis: Mosby.

---

904. The home-care nurse suspects that a client's spouse is experiencing caregiver strain. The nurse assesses for this condition by:

1 Referring the family to a social services agency
2 Waiting for the caregiver to talk about the stress
3 Obtaining feedback from the client about the caregiver
4 Gathering assessment data from the caregiver and the client

Level of Cognitive Ability: Application
Client Needs: Health Promotion and Maintenance
Integrated Process: Nursing Process/Assessment
Content Area: Fundamental Skills

Answer: 4
Rationale: Caregiver strain can occur when a client is significantly dependent on the caregiver for personal and health care needs. The nurse gathers data from the client and the caregiver to determine the caregiver's stressors and coping abilities and withholds making any referrals until the assessment is complete and the plan of care is in place. Because the nurse suspects caregiver strain, the nurse fulfills the duty to the client and family by approaching the family with the concern, gathering assessment data, and planning care. The nurse does not expect the client to assess the coping abilities of the caregiver, because assessment is part of the nursing process and should not be delegated.

Test-Taking Strategy: Use the steps of the nursing process to eliminate options 1 and 3. From the remaining options, eliminate option 2, because it breaches the duty that the nurse owes to the family; however, the nurse begins to fulfill that duty by performing a comprehensive assessment that addresses both the client and the caregiver. Review the concepts of caregiver strain if you had difficulty with this question.

References
Ignatavicius, D., & Workman, M. (2006). *Medical-surgical nursing: Critical thinking for collaborative care* (5th ed., pp. 7, 971). Philadelphia: Saunders.
Potter, P., & Perry, A. (2005). *Fundamentals of nursing* (6th ed., pp. 609-610). St. Louis: Mosby.

905. A client being discharged from the hospital will be taking warfarin sodium (Coumadin) at home on a daily basis. The nurse has provided instructions to the client about the medication and determines that further teaching is needed if the client states:

1 "I need to have a prothrombin time checked in 2 weeks."
2 "This medicine thins my blood and allows me to clot more slowly."
3 "I need to increase the intake of foods high in vitamin K in my diet."
4 "If I notice any increased bleeding or bruising, I need to call my doctor."

Level of Cognitive Ability: Analysis
Client Needs: Health Promotion and Maintenance
Integrated Process: Teaching and Learning
Content Area: Pharmacology

Answer: 3
Rationale: Warfarin sodium (Coumadin) is an oral anticoagulant that is used mainly to prevent thrombotic events, such as thrombophlebitis, pulmonary embolism, and embolism formation caused by atrial fibrillation or other disorders. Oral anticoagulants prolong the clotting time and are monitored by the prothrombin time and the international normalized ratio. Client education should include signs and symptoms of adverse effects and dietary restrictions such as limiting foods high in vitamin K (e.g., leafy green vegetables, liver, cheese, egg yolks), because these increase clotting times.

Test-Taking Strategy: Note the strategic words "further teaching is needed." These words indicate a negative event query and ask you to select an option that is an incorrect statement. Recalling that warfarin sodium is an anticoagulant will assist you with eliminating options 1, 2, and 4. Also, remembering the role that vitamin K plays in the clotting mechanism will direct you to option 3. Review the client teaching points related to warfarin sodium if you had difficulty with this question.

Reference
Hodgson, B., & Kizior, R. (2007). *Saunders nursing drug handbook 2007* (p. 1221). Philadelphia: Saunders.

906. A teenager returns to the gynecological clinic for a follow-up visit for a sexually transmitted infection (STI). Which statement by the teenager indicates the need for further teaching?

1 "I know you won't tell my parents I'm sick."
2 "I finished all of the antibiotics, just like you said."
3 "I always make sure that my boyfriend uses a condom."
4 "My boyfriend doesn't have to come in for treatment, does he?"

Level of Cognitive Ability: Analysis
Client Needs: Health Promotion and Maintenance
Integrated Process: Teaching and Learning
Content Area: Child Health

Answer: 4
Rationale: When treating STIs, all sexual contacts must be contacted and treated with medication. Clients should always use a condom with any sexual contact. The treatment of a teenager at a gynecological clinic is confidential, and parents will not be contacted, even if the client is less than 18 years old. Clients should always finish the course of antibiotics prescribed by the health care provider.

Test-Taking Strategy: Note the strategic words "need for further teaching." These words indicate a negative event query and ask you to select an option that is an incorrect statement. Recalling the concepts related to safe sex, the treatment of STIs in the teenager, and the principles related to antibiotic therapy will direct you to option 4. Review these concepts if you had difficulty with this question.

References
Hockenberry, M., & Wilson, D. (2007). *Nursing care of infants and children* (8th ed., p. 839). St. Louis: Mosby.
McKinney, E., James, S., Murray, S., & Ashwill, J. (2005). *Maternal-child nursing* (2nd ed., p. 791). St. Louis: Saunders.

907. A nurse is teaching a client who had been newly diagnosed with diabetes mellitus about blood glucose monitoring. The nurse teaches the client to report glucose levels that consistently exceed:

1 150 mg/dL
2 200 mg/dL
3 250 mg/dL
4 350 mg/dL

Level of Cognitive Ability: Application
Client Needs: Health Promotion and Maintenance
Integrated Process: Teaching and Learning
Content Area: Adult Health/Endocrine

Answer: 3
Rationale: The client should be taught to report blood glucose levels that exceed 250 mg/dL, unless otherwise instructed by the physician. Options 1 and 2 are low levels that do not require physician notification. Option 4 is a high value.

Test-Taking Strategy: Use the process of elimination. Recalling the basic principles related to diabetic home-care instructions will direct you to option 3. Review the principles related to blood glucose monitoring for clients with diabetes mellitus if you had difficulty with this question.

References
Black, J., & Hawks, J. (2005). *Medical-surgical nursing: Clinical management for positive outcomes* (7th ed., p. 1249). Philadelphia: Saunders.
Ignatavicius, D., & Workman, M. (2006). *Medical-surgical nursing: Critical thinking for collaborative care* (5th ed., p. 1525). Philadelphia: Saunders.

---

908. A client with gastritis asks the nurse at a screening clinic about analgesics that will not cause epigastric distress. The nurse tells the client to take which of the following medications?

1 Ecotrin
2 Tylenol
3 Bufferin
4 Ascriptin

Level of Cognitive Ability: Application
Client Needs: Health Promotion and Maintenance
Integrated Process: Teaching and Learning
Content Area: Pharmacology

Answer: 2
Rationale: Aspirin is irritating to the gastrointestinal tract of the client with a history of gastritis. The client should be advised to take analgesics that do not contain aspirin, such as acetaminophen (Tylenol). The other medications listed have aspirin in them. Other medications that are irritating to the gastrointestinal tract are the nonsteroidal anti-inflammatory drugs.

Test-Taking Strategy: Use the process of elimination. Note that options 1, 3, and 4 are comparable or alike and that they are aspirin-containing medications. Review these medications if you had difficulty with this question.

Reference
Kee, J., Hayes, E., & McCuistion, L. (2006). *Pharmacology: A nursing process approach.* (5th ed., p. 324). Philadelphia: Saunders.

---

909. A client is diagnosed with thromboangiitis obliterans (Buerger disease). The nurse places highest priority on teaching the client about modifications of which risk factor related to this disorder?

1 Exposure to heat
2 Cigarette smoking
3 Diet low in vitamin C
4 Excessive water intake

Level of Cognitive Ability: Application
Client Needs: Health Promotion and Maintenance
Integrated Process: Teaching and Learning
Content Area: Adult Health/Cardiovascular

Answer: 2
Rationale: Buerger disease occurs predominantly among men who are more than 40 years old who smoke cigarettes. A familial tendency is noted, but cigarette smoking is consistently a risk factor. Symptoms of the disease improve with smoking cessation. Options 1, 3, and 4 are not risk factors.

Test-Taking Strategy: Note the strategic words "highest priority" and "risk factor." Recalling the pathophysiology related to this disorder will direct you to option 2. Review the risk factors for Buerger disease if you had difficulty with this question.

Reference
Ignatavicius, D., & Workman, M. (2006). *Medical-surgical nursing: Critical thinking for collaborative care* (5th ed., p. 810). Philadelphia: Saunders.

910. A client has a new prescription for timolol (Betimol). The nurse determines that the client has misunderstood instructions given about the medication if the client states the need to:

1 Change positions slowly.
2 Report shortness of breath to the physician.
3 Taper or discontinue the medication when the client feels well.
4 Have enough medication on hand to last through weekends and vacations.

Level of Cognitive Ability: Analysis
Client Needs: Health Promotion and Maintenance
Integrated Process: Teaching and Learning
Content Area: Pharmacology

Answer: 3
Rationale: Common client teaching points about β-adrenergic blocking agents include taking the pulse daily and holding it to for a rate of less than 60 beats/min (and notifying the physician) and reporting shortness of breath. The client should not discontinue or change the medication dose. The client is also instructed to keep enough medication on hand, to change positions slowly, to not take over-the-counter medications (especially decongestants, cough, and cold preparations) without consulting the physician, and to carry medical identification that states that a β-blocker is being taken.

Test-Taking Strategy: Use the process of elimination, and note the strategic words "has misunderstood." These words indicate a negative event query and ask you to select an option that is an incorrect statement. Noting the word "discontinue" in option 3 will direct you to this option. Review client teaching points related to timolol if you had difficulty with this question.

References
Hodgson, B., & Kizior, R. (2007). *Saunders nursing drug handbook 2007* (p. 1135). Philadelphia: Saunders.
Skidmore-Roth, L. (2007). *2007 Mosby's nursing drug reference* (20th ed., p. 978). St. Louis: Mosby.

---

911. A nurse has completed giving medication instructions to a client receiving benazepril (Lotensin) to treat hypertension. The nurse determines that the client needs further instruction if the client states the need to:

1 Change positions slowly.
2 Monitor the blood pressure every week.
3 Use salt moderately in cooking and on foods.
4 Report signs and symptoms of infection to the physician.

Level of Cognitive Ability: Analysis
Client Needs: Health Promotion and Maintenance
Integrated Process: Teaching and Learning
Content Area: Pharmacology

Answer: 3
Rationale: The client taking an angiotensin-converting enzyme inhibitor is instructed to take the medication exactly as prescribed, monitor the blood pressure weekly, and continue with other lifestyle changes to control hypertension. The client should change positions slowly to avoid orthostatic hypotension; report fever, mouth sores, and sore throats to the physician (neutropenia); and avoid the use of salt.

Test-Taking Strategy: Use the process of elimination, and note the strategic words "needs further instruction." These words indicate a negative event query and ask you to select an option that is an incorrect statement. Noting that the medication is prescribed to treat hypertension will assist you with eliminating options 1, 2, and 4. Review benazepril if you had difficulty with this question.

References
Hodgson, B., & Kizior, R. (2007). *Saunders nursing drug handbook 2007* (pp. 126-127). Philadelphia: Saunders.
Kee, J., Hayes, E., & McCuistion, L. (2006). *Pharmacology: A nursing process approach.* (5th ed., p. 652). Philadelphia: Saunders.

912. A nurse has given medication instructions to a client receiving lovastatin (Mevacor). The nurse determines that the client understands the effects of the medication if the client stated the need to adhere to the periodic evaluation of serum:

1 Bleeding times
2 Creatinine levels
3 Blood glucose levels
4 Liver function studies

Level of Cognitive Ability: Analysis
Client Needs: Health Promotion and Maintenance
Integrated Process: Nursing Process/Evaluation
Content Area: Pharmacology

Answer: 4
Rationale: Lovastatin is a reductase inhibitor. It results in an increase in high-density lipoprotein cholesterol and a decrease in triglycerides and low-density lipoprotein cholesterol. This medication is converted by the liver to active metabolites and therefore not used in clients with active hepatic disease or elevated transaminase levels. For this reason, it is recommended that clients have periodic liver function studies. Periodic cholesterol levels are also needed to monitor the effectiveness of therapy.

Test-Taking Strategy: Focus on the name of the medication. Recalling that medication names that end with *-statin* are cholesterol-lowering medications and that cholesterol is synthesized in the liver will direct you to option 4. Review lovastatin if you had difficulty with this question.

Reference
Hodgson, B., & Kizior, R. (2007). *Saunders nursing drug handbook 2007* (p. 714). Philadelphia: Saunders.

---

913. A home-care nurse visits a client. Clonazepam (Klonopin) has been prescribed for the client, and the nurse teaches the client about the medication. Which statement by the client indicates that further teaching is necessary?

1 "If I experience slurred speech, it will disappear in about 8 weeks."
2 "My drowsiness will decrease over time with continued treatment."
3 "I should take my medicine with food to decrease stomach problems."
4 "I can take my medicine at bedtime if it tends to make me feel drowsy."

Level of Cognitive Ability: Analysis
Client Needs: Health Promotion and Maintenance
Integrated Process: Teaching and Learning
Content Area: Pharmacology

Answer: 1
Rationale: Clients who experience signs and symptoms of toxicity with the administration of clonazepam exhibit slurred speech, sedation, confusion, respiratory depression, hypotension, and eventually coma. Some drowsiness may occur, but it will decrease with continued use. The medication may be taken with food to decrease gastrointestinal irritation. Options 2, 3, and 4 are correct and show an accurate understanding of the medication.

Test-Taking Strategy: Use the process of elimination, and note the strategic words "further teaching is necessary." These words indicate a negative event query and ask you to select an incorrect statement. Recalling the toxic effects that can occur with the use of this medication will direct you to option 1. Review clonazepam if you had difficulty with this question.

References
Hodgson, B., & Kizior, R. (2007). *Saunders nursing drug handbook 2007* (pp. 271-272). Philadelphia: Saunders.
Kee, J., Hayes, E., & McCuistion, L. (2006). *Pharmacology: A nursing process approach.* (5th ed., p. 348). Philadelphia: Saunders.

---

914. Dipyridamole (Persantine) has been prescribed for the client, and the nurse has provided teaching to the client about the medication. Which statement indicates that the client understands the medication instructions?

1 "This medication will prevent a stroke."
2 "This medication will prevent a heart attack."
3 "This medicine will protect my artificial heart valve."
4 "This medication will help me keep my blood pressure down."

Answer: 3
Rationale: Dipyridamole combined with warfarin sodium is prescribed to protect the client's artificial heart valves. Dipyridamole does not prevent heart attacks or strokes. It is an antiplatelet medication rather than an antihypertensive.

Test-Taking Strategy: Use the process of elimination. Recalling that this medication is an antiplatelet medication rather than an antihypertensive will assist you with eliminating option 4. Noting the word "prevent" in options 1 and 2 will assist you with eliminating these options. Review the use of dipyridamole Persantine if you had difficulty with this question.

Level of Cognitive Ability: Analysis
Client Needs: Health Promotion and
Maintenance
Integrated Process: Nursing Process/Evaluation
Content Area: Pharmacology

References
Hodgson, B., & Kizior, R. (2007). *Saunders nursing drug handbook 2007* (p. 369). Philadelphia: Saunders.
McKenry, L., Tressier, E., & Hogan, M. (2006). *Mosby's pharmacology in nursing* (22nd ed., p. 601). St. Louis: Mosby.

---

915. A nurse is preparing to care for the mother of a preterm infant. The nurse plans to begin discharge planning:
  1 When the mother is in labor
  2 When the discharge date is set
  3 After stabilization of the infant during the early stages of hospitalization
  4 When the parents feel comfortable with and can demonstrate adequate care of the infant

Level of Cognitive Ability: Application
Client Needs: Health Promotion and
Maintenance
Integrated Process: Nursing Process/Planning
Content Area: Maternity/Postpartum

Answer: 3
Rationale: Discharge planning begins at admission. The determination of the services, needs, supplies, and equipment requirements should not be made on the day of discharge. Options 2 and 4 are incorrect, because these times are much too late to make the plans that need to be made. Option 1 is incorrect, because, during labor, the outcome of the delivery is not known.

Test-Taking Strategy: Use the process of elimination, remembering that discharge planning always begins at admission to the hospital. Noting the strategic words "early stages of hospitalization" will direct you to option 3. Review the guidelines related to discharge planning if you had difficulty with this question.

References
Murray, S., & McKinney, E. (2006). *Foundations of maternal-newborn nursing* (4th ed., pp. 570, 572). Philadelphia: Saunders.
Wong, D., Hockenberry, M., Perry, S., Lowdermilk, D., & Wilson, D. (2006). *Maternal-child nursing care* (3rd ed., p. 824). St. Louis: Mosby.

---

916. The nurse is providing home-care instructions to a client recovering from an acute inferior myocardial infarction (MI) with recurrent angina. The nurse teaches the client to:
  1 Avoid sexual intercourse for at least 4 months.
  2 Replace sublingual nitroglycerin tablets yearly.
  3 Participate in an exercise program that includes overhead lifting and reaching.
  4 Recognize the adverse effects of acetylsalicylic acid (aspirin), which include tinnitus and hearing loss.

Level of Cognitive Ability: Application
Client Needs: Health Promotion and
Maintenance
Integrated Process: Teaching and Learning
Content Area: Adult Health/Cardiovascular

Answer: 4
Rationale: After an acute MI, many clients are instructed to take an aspirin daily. Adverse effects include tinnitus, hearing loss, epigastric distress, gastrointestinal bleeding, and nausea. Sexual intercourse usually can be resumed in 4 to 8 weeks after an acute MI if the physician agrees and if the client has been able to achieve traditional parameters such as climbing two flights of steps without chest pain or dyspnea. Clients should be advised to purchase a new supply of nitroglycerin tablets every 6 months. Expiration dates on the medication bottle should also be checked. Activities that include lifting and reaching over the head should be avoided, because they reduce cardiac output.

Test-Taking Strategy: Use the process of elimination, and focus on the client's diagnosis. Noting the time limits in options 1 and 2 ("4 months" and "yearly," respectively) will assist you with eliminating these options. From the remaining options, "overhead lifting and reaching" in option 3 should indicate that this is incorrect. Review the client teaching points after an MI if you had difficulty with this question.

References
Black, J., & Hawks, J. (2005). *Medical-surgical nursing: Clinical management for positive outcomes* (7th ed., p. 1637). Philadelphia: Saunders.
Ignatavicius, D., & Workman, M. (2006). *Medical-surgical nursing: Critical thinking for collaborative care* (5th ed., pp. 851-852). Philadelphia: Saunders.

917. The nurse is reviewing home-care instructions with an older client who has type 1 diabetes mellitus and a history of diabetic ketoacidosis (DKA). The client's spouse is present when the instructions are given. Which statement by the spouse indicates that further teaching is necessary?
1 "If he is vomiting, I shouldn't give him any insulin."
2 "I should bring him to the physician's office if he develops a fever."
3 "If the grandchildren are sick, they probably shouldn't come to visit."
4 "I should call the doctor if he has nausea or abdominal pain lasting for more than 1 or 2 days."

Level of Cognitive Ability: Analysis
Client Needs: Health Promotion and Maintenance
Integrated Process: Teaching and Learning
Content Area: Adult Health/Endocrine

Answer: 1
Rationale: Infection and the stopping of insulin are precipitating factors for DKA. Nausea and abdominal pain that last more than 1 or 2 days need to be reported to the physician, because these signs may be indicative of DKA.

Test-Taking Strategy: Note the strategic words "further teaching is necessary." These words indicate a negative event query and ask you to select an option that is an incorrect statement. Eliminate options 2 and 3 first, because both relate to infection. From the remaining options, recalling the causes of DKA will direct you to option 1. Review the precipitating factors associated with DKA if you had difficulty with this question.

Reference
Black, J., & Hawks, J. (2005). *Medical-surgical nursing: Clinical management for positive outcomes* (7th ed., pp. 1269, 1271). Philadelphia: Saunders.

---

918. The home-care nurse provides self-care instructions to a client with chronic venous insufficiency caused by deep vein thrombosis. Which statement by the client indicates the need for further instructions?
1 "I need to avoid prolonged standing or sitting."
2 "I need to elevate the foot of the bed during sleep."
3 "I can cross my legs at the knee but not at the ankle."
4 "I should continue to wear elastic hose for at least 6 to 8 weeks."

Level of Cognitive Ability: Analysis
Client Needs: Health Promotion and Maintenance
Integrated Process: Teaching and Learning
Content Area: Adult Health/Cardiovascular

Answer: 3
Rationale: Clients with chronic venous insufficiency are advised to avoid crossing their legs, sitting in chairs where their feet do not touch the floor, and wearing garters or sources of pressure above the legs (such as girdles). The client should sleep with the foot of the bed elevated to promote venous return during sleep. The client should wear elastic hose for 6 to 8 weeks or, in some situations, for life. Venous problems are characterized by the insufficient drainage of blood from the legs returning to the heart. Because of this, interventions need to be aimed at promoting the flow of blood out of the legs and back to the heart.

Test-Taking Strategy: Note the strategic words "need for further instructions." These words indicate a negative event query and ask you to select an option that is an incorrect statement. Use the concept of gravity when answering questions that relate to peripheral vascular problems. Option 3 is the only action that does not promote venous drainage. Review the home-care instructions for the client with chronic venous insufficiency if you had difficulty with this question.

Reference
Lewis, S., Heitkemper, M., Dirksen, S., O'Brien, P., & Bucher, L. (2007). *Medical-surgical nursing: Assessment and management of clinical problems* (7th ed., pp. 919-920). St. Louis: Mosby.

919. The nurse is providing home-care instructions to a client who had varicose vein stripping and ligation and who is being discharged from the ambulatory care unit. The nurse tells the client to:

1 Remove elastic hose after 24 hours.
2 Maintain bedrest for the first 3 days.
3 Elevate the foot of the bed while in bed.
4 Ambulate for 5 to 10 minutes twice a day beginning the day after surgery.

Level of Cognitive Ability: Application
Client Needs: Health Promotion and Maintenance
Integrated Process: Teaching and Learning
Content Area: Adult Health/Cardiovascular

Answer: 3
Rationale: The foot of the bed should be elevated 15 degrees to promote venous drainage. Standard postoperative care after vein ligation and stripping consists of bedrest for 24 hours with ambulation for 5 to 10 minutes every 2 hours thereafter. The continuous elastic compression of the leg is maintained usually for 1 week after the procedure, and this is followed by the long-term use of elastic hose.

Test-Taking Strategy: Use your knowledge of the concepts related to blood flow and immobility to answer this question. Options 1 and 2 will promote venous stasis, so they are eliminated first. From the remaining options, noting the words "twice a day" in option 4 will eliminate this option. Review postoperative teaching points after varicose vein stripping and ligation if you had difficulty with this question.

Reference
Ignatavicius, D., & Workman, M. (2006). *Medical-surgical nursing: Critical thinking for collaborative care* (5th ed., pp. 817-818). Philadelphia: Saunders.

---

920. The nurse is developing a teaching plan for the client with Raynaud disease. Which of the following instructions should the nurse include?

1 Daily cool baths will provide an analgesic effect.
2 A high-protein diet will minimize tissue malnutrition.
3 Vitamin K administration will prevent tendencies toward bleeding.
4 Keeping the hands and feet warm and dry will prevent vasoconstriction.

Level of Cognitive Ability: Application
Client Needs: Health Promotion and Maintenance
Integrated Process: Teaching and Learning
Content Area: Adult Health/Cardiovascular

Answer: 4
Rationale: The use of measures to prevent vasoconstriction are helpful for the management of Raynaud disease. The hands and feet should be kept dry. Gloves and warm fabrics should be worn in cold weather, and the client should avoid exposure to nicotine and caffeine. The avoidance of situations that trigger stress is also helpful. Options 1, 2, and 3 are not components of the treatment for this disorder.

Test-Taking Strategy: Use the process of elimination. Recalling the pathophysiology of the disorder and the need to promote vasodilation will direct you to option 4. Review the teaching points related to Raynaud disease if you had difficulty with this question.

References
Ignatavicius, D., & Workman, M. (2006). *Medical-surgical nursing: Critical thinking for collaborative care* (5th ed., p. 811). Philadelphia: Saunders.
Lewis, S., Heitkemper, M., Dirksen, S., O'Brien, P., & Bucher, I. (2007). *Medical-surgical nursing: Assessment and management of clinical problems* (7th ed., pp. 908-909). St. Louis: Mosby.

921. A client with peripheral arterial disease has received instructions from the nurse about how to limit the progression of the disease. The nurse determines that the client needs further instructions if which statement was made by the client?

1 "I need to eat a balanced diet."
2 "A heating pad on my leg will help soothe the leg pain."
3 "I need to take special care of my feet to prevent injury."
4 "I should walk daily to increase the circulation to my legs."

Level of Cognitive Ability: Analysis
Client Needs: Health Promotion and Maintenance
Integrated Process: Teaching and Learning
Content Area: Adult Health/Cardiovascular

Answer: 2
Rationale: The long-term management of peripheral arterial disease consists of measures that increase peripheral circulation (exercise), promote vasodilation (warmth), relieve pain, and maintain tissue integrity (foot care and nutrition). The application of heat directly to the extremity is contraindicated. The limb may have decreased sensitivity and be more at risk for burns. Additionally, the direct application of heat raises the oxygen and nutritional requirements of the tissue even further.

Test-Taking Strategy: Focus on the client's diagnosis, and note the strategic words "needs further instructions." These words indicate a negative event query and ask you to select an option that is an incorrect statement. Noting the strategic word "heating" in option 2 will direct you to the correct option. Review the teaching points related to peripheral arterial disease if you had difficulty with this question.

References
Black, J., & Hawks, J. (2005). *Medical-surgical nursing: Clinical management for positive outcomes* (7th ed., pp. 1515-1516). Philadelphia: Saunders.
Ignatavicius, D., & Workman, M. (2006). *Medical-surgical nursing: Critical thinking for collaborative care* (5th ed., pp. 796, 804). Philadelphia: Saunders.

922. The nurse is teaching a client with hypertension about items that contain sodium and reviews a written list of items sent from the cardiac rehabilitation department. The nurse tells the client that which of the following items is lowest in sodium content?

1 Antacids
2 Laxatives
3 Toothpaste
4 Demineralized water

Level of Cognitive Ability: Application
Client Needs: Health Promotion and Maintenance
Integrated Process: Teaching and Learning
Content Area: Adult Health/Cardiovascular

Answer: 4
Rationale: Sodium intake can be increased with the use of several types of products, including toothpaste and mouthwashes; over-the-counter medications such as analgesics, antacids, cough remedies, laxatives, and sedatives; and softened water as well as some mineral waters. Water that is bottled, distilled, deionized, or demineralized may be used for drinking and cooking. Clients are advised to read labels for sodium content.

Test-Taking Strategy: Focus on the subject—the item that is lowest in sodium. Noting the word "demineralized," which means having the minerals taken out of, will direct you to option 4. Review items that are low and high in sodium content if you had difficulty with this question.

References
Grodner, M., Long, S., & DeYoung, S. (2004). *Foundations and clinical applications of nutrition: A nursing approach.* (3rd ed., pp. 201, 597, 609). St. Louis: Mosby.
Nix, S. (2005). *Williams' basic nutrition & diet therapy* (12th ed., p. 356). St. Louis: Mosby.

923. The school nurse provides teaching about the hazards of smoking to a group of high school students. Which comment by a student indicates the need for additional teaching?
1 "Chewing tobacco is much safer than is smoking tobacco."
2 "Smoking during pregnancy increases the risk of stillbirth."
3 "My health is at risk when my family smokes in the house."
4 "Inhaling smoke from other people is a public health issue."

Level of Cognitive Ability: Analysis
Client Needs: Health Promotion and Maintenance
Integrated Process: Teaching and Learning
Content Area: Fundamental Skills

Answer: 1
Rationale: All forms of tobacco use are health hazards. Options 2, 3, and 4 are accurate regarding the health hazards of tobacco use.

Test-Taking Strategy: Note the strategic words "need for additional teaching." These words indicate a negative event query and ask you to select an option that is an incorrect statement. This should direct you to option 1. Review the hazards of tobacco use if you had difficulty with this question.

References
Black, J., & Hawks, J. (2005). *Medical-surgical nursing: Clinical management for positive outcomes* (7th ed., pp. 39-40, 337). Philadelphia: Saunders.
Monahan, F., Sands, J., Neighbors, M., Marek, J., & Green, C. (2007). *Phipps' medical-surgical nursing: Health and illness perspectives* (8th ed., p. 37). St. Louis: Mosby.

---

924. A nurse is developing goals for the postpartum client who is at risk for uterine infection. Which goal would be most appropriate for this client?
1 The client will verbalize a reduction of pain.
2 The client will report how to treat an infection.
3 The client will no longer have a positive Homan sign.
4 The client will be able to identify measures to prevent infection.

Level of Cognitive Ability: Analysis
Client Needs: Health Promotion and Maintenance
Integrated Process: Nursing Process/Planning
Content Area: Maternity/Postpartum

Answer: 4
Rationale: The uterus is theoretically sterile during pregnancy until the membranes rupture. However, it is capable of being invaded by pathogens after membrane rupture. Options 1 and 3 are unrelated to the subject of infection. Option 2 indicates that an infection is present. Option 4 is a goal for the client who is at risk for infection.

Test-Taking Strategy: Focus on the strategic words "at risk for uterine infection." Noting the word "prevent" in option 4 will direct you to this option. Options 1 and 3 are unrelated to the subject of the question. Option 2 implies that an infection has been diagnosed. Review the goals for a client who is at risk for infection if you had difficulty with this question.

Reference
Murray, S., & McKinney, E. (2006). *Foundations of maternal-newborn nursing* (4th ed., pp. 406-407). Philadelphia: Saunders.

---

925. A neonatal intensive care unit (NICU) nurse teaches handwashing techniques to the parents of an infant who is receiving antibiotic treatment for a neonatal infection. The nurse determines that the parents understand the purpose of handwashing if they state that this is primarily done to:
1 Reduce their fears.
2 Minimize the spread of infection to other siblings.
3 Allow them an opportunity to communicate with each other and staff.
4 Reduce the possibility of transmitting an environmental infection to the infant

Answer: 4
Rationale: Appropriate handwashing by staff and parents has been effective for the prevention of nosocomial infections in nursery units. This action also promotes parents taking an active part in the care of their infant. Options 1 and 3 are not the primary reason to perform handwashing. Because the infant has the infection and is in the NICU, option 2 is incorrect.

Test-Taking Strategy: Note the strategic word "primarily" to assist you with eliminating options 1 and 3. Noting that the infant is in the NICU will assist you with eliminating option 2. Review the purposes of handwashing if you had difficulty with this question.

Level of Cognitive Ability: Analysis
Client Needs: Health Promotion and
    Maintenance
Integrated Process: Nursing Process/Evaluation
Content Area: Maternity/Postpartum

Reference
Murray, S., & McKinney, E. (2006). *Foundations of maternal-newborn nursing* (4th ed., pp. 420, 771). Philadelphia: Saunders.

---

926. The nurse monitors a client for brachial plexus compromise after shoulder arthroplasty and is checking the status of the ulnar nerve. Which technique should the nurse use to assess the status of this nerve?
1 Ask the client to raise the forearm above the head.
2 Have the client spread all of the fingers wide and resist pressure.
3 Ask the client to move the thumb toward the palm and then back to the neutral position.
4 Have the client grasp the nurse's hand, and note the strength of the client's first and second fingers.

Level of Cognitive Ability: Application
Client Needs: Health Promotion and
    Maintenance
Integrated Process: Nursing Process/Assessment
Content Area: Adult Health/Musculoskeletal

Answer: 2
Rationale: So that the nurse may assess the ulnar nerve status, the client is asked to spread all of the fingers wide and resist pressure. Weakness against pressure may indicate compromise of the ulnar nerve. Option 1 assesses the flexion of the biceps and determines the status of the cutaneous nerve. Option 3 describes the assessment of the status of the radial nerve. Option 4 describes the assessment of the status of the medial nerve.

Test-Taking Strategy: Focus on the subject—the status of the ulnar nerve. Recalling the location and function of this nerve will direct you to option 2. Review this assessment technique if you are unfamiliar with this procedure.

Reference
Black, J., & Hawks, J. (2005). *Medical-surgical nursing: Clinical management for positive outcomes* (7th ed., pp. 1482-1483, 2010). Philadelphia: Saunders.

---

927. A hospitalized client with active pulmonary tuberculosis has been receiving multidrug therapy for the past month and is being prepared for discharge. The nurse determines that respiratory isolation is no longer required and that medication therapy has been effective when:
1 Stools are clay colored.
2 The Mantoux test is negative.
3 Sputum cultures are negative.
4 Nausea and vomiting have stopped.

Level of Cognitive Ability: Analysis
Client Needs: Health Promotion and
    Maintenance
Integrated Process: Nursing Process/Evaluation
Content Area: Adult Health/Respiratory

Answer: 3
Rationale: The primary diagnostic tool for pulmonary tuberculosis is a sputum culture. A negative culture indicates the effectiveness of treatment. Nausea, vomiting, and clay-colored stools are side effects of the medication that is used to treat tuberculosis; their presence or absence does not measure the therapeutic effectiveness of the medication. The Mantoux test is a screening tool rather than a diagnostic test for tuberculosis. Because the Mantoux test indicates exposure to the organism but not active disease, the test results will remain positive.

Test-Taking Strategy: Use the process of elimination, and note the strategic words "therapy has been effective." Remember that the absence of infectious organisms is a desired outcome in clients with communicable diseases. The sputum is the only diagnostic test that will determine the absence of infectious organisms. Review the measures that prevent the spread of pulmonary tuberculosis if you had difficulty with this question.

Reference
Ignatavicius, D., & Workman, M. (2006). *Medical-surgical nursing: Critical thinking for collaborative care* (5th ed., p. 644). Philadelphia: Saunders.

928. A nurse has conducted a class for pregnant clients with diabetes mellitus about the signs and symptoms of potential complications. The nurse determines that the teaching was effective if a client makes which of the following statements?

1 "I should not have ultrasounds done because I am diabetic."
2 "I'm glad I don't have to worry about developing hypoglycemia while I am pregnant."
3 "I need to watch my weight for any sudden gains because I am prone to gestational hypertension."
4 "My insulin needs should decrease during the last 2 months because I will be using some of the baby's insulin supply."

Level of Cognitive Ability: Analysis
Client Needs: Health Promotion and Maintenance
Integrated Process: Nursing Process/Evaluation
Content Area: Maternity/Antepartum

Answer: 3
Rationale: Hypoglycemia is a problem during pregnancy and needs to be assessed. A diabetic pregnant client has a higher incidence of developing gestational hypertension than the nondiabetic pregnant client does. Insulin needs will increase during the last trimester because of increased placenta degradation. Ultrasounds are done frequently during a diabetic pregnancy to check for congenital anomalies and to determine appropriate growth patterns.

Test-Taking Strategy: Use the process of elimination, and focus on the subject—a pregnant client with diabetes mellitus. Options 1 and 2 can be easily eliminated by recalling that hypoglycemia is a concern and that ultrasounds need to be performed. From the remaining options, remember that insulin needs will increase during the last trimester of pregnancy. This will assist you with eliminating option 4. Review the complications associated with diabetes and pregnancy if you had difficulty with this question.

Reference
Murray, S., & McKinney, E. (2006). *Foundations of maternal-newborn nursing* (4th ed., pp. 666-667). Philadelphia: Saunders.

929. A postpartum client recovering from disseminated intravascular coagulopathy is to be discharged on low dosages of an anticoagulant medication. The nurse provides home-care instructions and tells the client to avoid which of the following?

1 Brushing her teeth
2 Taking acetylsalicylic acid (aspirin)
3 Walking long distances and climbing stairs
4 All activities, because bruising injuries can occur

Level of Cognitive Ability: Application
Client Needs: Health Promotion and Maintenance
Integrated Process: Teaching and Learning
Content Area: Pharmacology

Answer: 2
Rationale: Aspirin can interact with the anticoagulant medication and increase the clotting time beyond therapeutic ranges, so avoiding aspirin is a priority. However, not all activities need to be avoided. Walking and climbing stairs are acceptable activities. The client does not need to avoid brushing the teeth, but he or she should be instructed to use a soft toothbrush.

Test-Taking Strategy: Note the strategic word "avoid" in the question. Recalling that bleeding is an adverse effect of anticoagulants will direct you to the correct option. Review the teaching points related to anticoagulants if you had difficulty with this question.

References
Kee, J., Hayes, E., & McCuistion, L. (2006). *Pharmacology: A nursing process approach.* (5th ed., p. 411). Philadelphia: Saunders.
McKenry, L., Tressier, E., & Hogan, M. (2006). *Mosby's pharmacology in nursing* (21st ed., p. 211). St. Louis: Mosby.

930. A client with a diagnosis of depression admits that one reason for her depression is that too many demands drain her energy. The client also admits that one reason the situation is bad is because the word "no" is not part of her vocabulary when it comes to the requests and needs of others. After 7 days of hospitalization, another client asks for assistance with cleaning the unit immediately. The client with depression says, "No, I can't help you now. I am enjoying watching this movie." The nurse interprets this response as:

1 Withdrawal from peers
2 A shirking of responsibility
3 Increased control over decisions
4 Decreased cooperation with others

Level of Cognitive Ability: Analysis
Client Needs: Health Promotion and Maintenance
Integrated Process: Nursing Process/Analysis
Content Area: Mental Health

Answer: 3
Rationale: The client has been unable to refuse requests in the past. Saying "no" now indicates that the client is trying to meet her own needs. The word is being said now without guilt and apology. During the treatment process, the client has learned how to meet her own needs, and this can help her to maintain her health after discharge. Options 1, 2, and 4 are incorrect interpretations.

Test-Taking Strategy: Use the process of elimination. Focusing on the data in the question will direct you to option 3. Review the measures that assist with increasing control in the client with depression if you had difficulty with this question.

Reference
Varcarolis, E., Carson, V., & Shoemaker, N. (2006). *Foundations of psychiatric mental health nursing* (5th ed., pp. 338, 340). Philadelphia: Saunders.

---

931. A client with depression who was admitted to the mental health unit approximately 7 days ago is preparing for discharge, and the nurse is evaluating the client's understanding of depression and of the coping strategies learned during hospitalization. The nurse determines that further teaching needs to occur if the client makes which of the following statements?

1 "I now know that I can't be all things to all people all of the time."
2 "I know that I probably won't have depression again in the future."
3 "I know I must continue to take my medications just as prescribed."
4 "This hospital experience has been a positive experience in my life."

Level of Cognitive Ability: Analysis
Client Needs: Health Promotion and Maintenance
Integrated Process: Teaching and Learning
Content Area: Mental Health

Answer: 2
Rationale: Depression may be a recurring illness for some people. The client needs to understand the symptoms of depression and to recognize when or if treatment needs to begin again. The other statements indicate that the client has learned some coping skills, such as setting limits, taking medications, and reframing a potentially unpleasant experience into a more positive one.

Test-Taking Strategy: Note the strategic words "further teaching needs to occur." These words indicate a negative event query and ask you to select the option that indicates a lack of client understanding about depression. Recalling that depression may recur will direct you to option 2. Review the characteristics of depression if you had difficulty with this question.

Reference
Stuart, G., & Laraia, M. (2005). *Principles and practice of psychiatric nursing* (8th ed., pp. 358-359). St. Louis: Mosby.

932. A nurse demonstrates to a mother how to correctly take an axillary temperature using a nonelectronic device to determine if the child has a fever. Which action by the mother would indicate the need for further teaching?

1 She selects a thermometer with a slender tip.
2 She holds the thermometer in the axilla for 1 minute.
3 She records the actual temperature reading and route.
4 She places the thermometer in the center of the axilla.

Level of Cognitive Ability: Analysis
Client Needs: Health Promotion and Maintenance
Integrated Process: Teaching and Learning
Content Area: Child Health

Answer: 2
Rationale: Taking an axillary temperature for at least 5 minutes is most accurate. Options 1, 3, and 4 are correct steps for taking the axillary temperature.

Test-Taking Strategy: Note the strategic words "need for further teaching." These words indicate a negative event query and ask you to select the option that identifies an incorrect action by the mother. Visualizing the procedure and noting the words "1 minute" in option 2 will direct you to this option. Review the procedure for obtaining an axillary temperature if you had difficulty with this question.

References
Hockenberry, M., Wilson, D., & Winkelstein, M. (2005). *Wong's essentials of pediatric nursing* (7th ed., p. 183). St. Louis: Mosby.
Wong, D., Hockenberry, M., Perry, S., Lowdermilk, D., & Wilson, D. (2006). *Maternal-child nursing care.* (3rd ed., pp. 991-993). St. Louis: Mosby.

---

933. The school nurse teaches an athletic coach how to prevent dehydration among athletes practicing in the hot weather. What is the best advice for the nurse to give to the coach?

1 Drink plenty of fluids before and after practice.
2 Have the athletes take a salt tablet before practice.
3 Reschedule practice for before school and after sunset.
4 Provide a fluid break every 30 minutes during practice.

Level of Cognitive Ability: Application
Client Needs: Health Promotion and Maintenance
Integrated Process: Teaching and Learning
Content Area: Fundamental Skills

Answer: 4
Rationale: Hot weather accelerates the body's loss of fluid and electrolytes during strenuous physical activity, so the nurse encourages the coach to schedule fluid breaks at 30-minute intervals so that the athletes can periodically rest and restore body fluids. Drinking fluid before and after practice is a reasonable suggestion; however, because the hot weather accelerates fluid and electrolyte losses, body fluids must be periodically replenished to maintain the fluid and electrolyte balance. Although a sodium load increases fluid retention, the nurse avoids suggesting salt tablets for the athletes, because the nurse needs approval from each athlete's health care provider before recommending the salt. Rescheduling practice times is unrealistic.

Test-Taking Strategy: Note the strategic words "prevent dehydration." The presence of the word "best" in the question indicates that each option is a reasonable response for preventing dehydration. However, you must choose the option that is a better choice than the other three. Recall the principles of fluid and electrolyte balance and the causes of dehydration. Option 4 is the best answer, because it is the most effective response that addresses fluid and electrolyte balance directly, and it is also the most practical choice. Review the measures used to prevent dehydration if you had difficulty with this question.

References
Black, J., & Hawks, J. (2005). Medical-surgical nursing: *Clinical management for positive outcomes* (7th ed., pp. 208-209). Philadelphia: Saunders.
Ignatavicius, D., & Workman, M. (2006). *Medical-surgical nursing: Critical thinking for collaborative care* (5th ed., pp. 215-216). Philadelphia: Saunders.

934. The nurse instructs a client who is hospitalized and on a low-fat diet. Which menu does the nurse provide for the client?

1 Shrimp, avocado, and tomato salad
2 Calf's liver, potato salad, and sherbet
3 Lean steak, mashed potatoes, and gravy
4 Turkey breast, boiled rice, and strawberries

Level of Cognitive Ability: Application
Client Needs: Health Promotion and Maintenance
Integrated Process: Teaching and Learning
Content Area: Fundamental Skills

Answer: 4
Rationale: Turkey breast without the skin, boiled rice, and strawberries offer the client nourishing foods that are low in fat. Some sources of fat include meats, avocado, salad dressing, mayonnaise, butter, cheese, and bacon. Options 1, 2, and 3 contain high-fat foods.

Test-Taking Strategy: Use the process of elimination. Eliminate options 1 and 2 first, because avocado and liver have a very high fat content. Potato salad usually contains mayonnaise, which is high in fat. Next, eliminate option 3, because meat is high in fat and mashed potatoes are not very palatable without butter or gravy, and both are high in fat. Option 4 does not contain high-fat foods. Review the foods that contain fat if you had difficulty with this question.

References
Grodner, M., Long, S., & DeYoung, S. (2004). *Foundations and clinical applications of nutrition: A nursing approach* (3rd ed., pp. 123-124). St. Louis: Mosby.
Nix, S. (2005). *Williams' basic nutrition & diet therapy* (12th ed., pp. 39-40). St. Louis: Mosby.

---

935. The nurse has provided discharge instructions regarding nitroglycerin therapy to the client with angina. Which statement by the client indicates an understanding of the home use of the nitroglycerin?

1 "If I use the nitroglycerin and the pain does not subside in 15 minutes, I should go to the hospital."
2 "When I have pain, I should lie down and place a tablet under my tongue. If unrelieved in 5 minutes, I should take another tablet."
3 "When I have chest pain, I should put a tablet under my tongue. If I have a burning sensation, I should call my doctor immediately."
4 "When I experience chest pain, I can continue what I'm doing. If it doesn't go away in 10 minutes, I should use a nitroglycerin tablet."

Level of Cognitive Ability: Analysis
Client Needs: Health Promotion and Maintenance
Integrated Process: Nursing Process/Evaluation
Content Area: Adult Health/Cardiovascular

Answer: 2
Rationale: The client taking sublingual nitroglycerin should lie down when taking the medication, because lightheadedness and dizziness may occur as a result of postural hypotension. The client should use up to three tablets at 5-minute intervals before seeking medical attention. Options 1, 3, and 4 are incorrect regarding the use of nitroglycerin. A burning sensation is a common side effect of nitroglycerin. Nitroglycerin should be taken with the onset of anginal pain. The client should take another dose of nitroglycerin if relief is not obtained with the first or second dose.

Test-Taking Strategy: Use the process of elimination. Recalling that nitroglycerin may be taken three times at 5-minute intervals will direct you to option 2. Review the client teaching related to nitroglycerin if you had difficulty with this question.

References
Hodgson, B., & Kizior, R. (2008). *Saunders nursing drug handbook 2008* (p. 847). St. Louis: Saunders.
Lehne, R. (2007). *Pharmacology for nursing care* (6th ed., p. 583). St. Louis: Saunders.

936. A client has urinary calculi that are composed of uric acid, and the nurse teaches the client dietary measures to prevent the further development of the calculi. The nurse determines that the client understands the dietary measures if the client states that it is necessary to avoid consuming:

1 Milk
2 Dairy products
3 Foods such as spinach, chocolate, and tea
4 Foods such as fish with fine bones and organ meats

Level of Cognitive Ability: Analysis
Client Needs: Health Promotion and Maintenance
Integrated Process: Nursing Process/Evaluation
Content Area: Adult Health/Renal

Answer: 4
Rationale: The client with a uric acid stone should limit the intake of foods that are high in purines. Organ meats, sardines, herring, and other high-purine foods are eliminated from the diet. Foods with moderate levels of purines, such as red and white meats and some seafood, are also limited. Options 1, 2, and 3 are recommended dietary changes to prevent calculi that are composed of calcium phosphate or calcium oxalate.

Test-Taking Strategy: Note the strategic words "uric acid." Remembering that organ meats are high in purines will direct you to the correct option. Also note that options 1, 2, and 3 are comparable or alike in that they are foods that are avoided if the client has calcium phosphate or calcium oxalate calculi. Review the foods to avoid with uric acid calculi if you had difficulty with this question.

Reference
Ignatavicius, D., & Workman, M. (2006). *Medical-surgical nursing: Critical thinking for collaborative care* (5th ed., p. 1701). Philadelphia: Saunders.

---

937. A nurse is teaching a mother with diabetes mellitus who delivered a large-for-gestational-age (LGA) male infant about the care of the infant. The nurse tells the mother that LGA infants appear to be more mature because of their large size, but that, in reality, these infants frequently need to be aroused to facilitate nutritional intake and attachment. Which statement by the mother indicates the need for additional information about the care of the infant?

1 "I will talk to my baby when he is in a quiet, alert state."
2 "I will allow my baby to sleep through the night, because he needs his rest."
3 "I will breast-feed my baby every 2½ to 3 hours and will use arousal techniques."
4 "I will watch my baby closely, because I know that he may not be as mature in his motor development."

Level of Cognitive Ability: Analysis
Client Needs: Health Promotion and Maintenance
Integrated Process: Teaching and Learning
Content Area: Maternity/Postpartum

Answer: 2
Rationale: LGA infants tend to be more difficult to arouse and therefore will need to be aroused to facilitate nutritional intake and attachment opportunities. These infants also have problems maintaining a quiet, alert state. It is beneficial for the mother to interact with the infant during this time to enhance and lengthen the quiet, alert state. Although the infant is large, motor function is not usually as mature as it is in the term infant. LGA infants need to be aroused for feedings, usually every 2½ to 3 hours for breast-feeding.

Test-Taking Strategy: Note the strategic words "need for additional information." These words indicate a negative event query and ask you to select an option that is an incorrect statement. Focusing on the words "frequently need to be aroused" in the question will direct you to option 2. Options 1, 3, and 4 address observation and arousal, whereas option 2 does not. Review the care of the LGA infant if you had difficulty with this question.

Reference
Wong, D., Hockenberry, M., Perry, S., Lowdermilk, D., & Wilson, D. (2006). *Maternal-child nursing care* (3rd ed., pp. 797-798, 821). St. Louis: Mosby.

938. A client has been experiencing muscle weakness for a period of several months. The physician suspects polymyositis, and the client asks the nurse about the disorder. The nurse tells the client that in this disorder:
1 Muscle fibers are inflamed.
2 Muscle fibers are thickened.
3 There is a decrease in elastic tissue.
4 There are increased fibers and tissue.

Level of Cognitive Ability: Application
Client Needs: Health Promotion and Maintenance
Integrated Process: Teaching and Learning
Content Area: Adult Health/Musculoskeletal

Answer: 1
Rationale: Polymyositis is a diffuse inflammatory disorder of skeletal (striated) muscle that is characterized by symmetric weakness and atrophy. Option 2 describes the opposite of what is noted with this disorder. Option 3 is incorrect, but decreased elastic tissue in the aorta would be noted in a client with Marfan syndrome. Option 4 refers to the increased fibrous tissue seen in clients with ankylosis.

Test-Taking Strategy: Note the subject of the question: polymyositis. The ending *-itis* indicates inflammation. The only option that addresses inflammation is option 1. Review the description of polymyositis if you had difficulty with this question.

Reference
Ignatavicius, D., & Workman, M. (2006). *Medical-surgical nursing: Critical thinking for collaborative care* (5th ed., p. 416). Philadelphia: Saunders.

---

939. The nurse in an ambulatory clinic administers a Mantoux skin test to a client on a Monday. The nurse tells the client to return to the clinic to have the results read on:
1 Thursday or Friday
2 The following Monday
3 Tuesday or Wednesday
4 Wednesday or Thursday

Level of Cognitive Ability: Application
Client Needs: Health Promotion and Maintenance
Integrated Process: Nursing Process/Implementation
Content Area: Adult Health/Respiratory

Answer: 4
Rationale: The Mantoux skin test for tuberculosis is read in 48 to 72 hours. The client should return to the clinic on Wednesday or Thursday.

Test-Taking Strategy: Use the process of elimination. Recalling that this test is read within 48 to 72 hours will direct you to option 4. Review the procedure for the Mantoux test if you had difficulty with this question.

References
Chernecky, C., & Berger, B. (2008). *Laboratory tests and diagnostic procedures* (5th ed., pp. 758-759). Philadelphia: Saunders.
Lewis, S., Heitkemper, M., Dirksen, S., O'Brien, P., & Bucher, L. (2007). *Medical-surgical nursing: Assessment and management of clinical problems* (7th ed., p. 571). St. Louis: Mosby.

---

940. A client with chronic airflow limitation is admitted to the hospital with an exacerbation and has a nursing diagnosis of Ineffective Airway Clearance. The nurse assesses the client and determines that which factor contributed most to this nursing diagnosis?
1 Fat intake
2 Fluid intake
3 Anxiety level
4 Amount of sleep

Level of Cognitive Ability: Analysis
Client Needs: Health Promotion and Maintenance
Integrated Process: Nursing Process/Assessment
Content Area: Adult Health/Respiratory

Answer: 2
Rationale: The client with Ineffective Airway Clearance has ineffective coughing and excess sputum in the airways. The nurse assesses the client for contributing factors such as dehydration and a lack of knowledge of proper coughing techniques. The reduction of these factors helps to limit exacerbations of the disease. Options 1, 3, and 4 are not directly associated with this nursing diagnosis.

Test-Taking Strategy: Note the nursing diagnosis: Ineffective Airway Clearance. This calls to mind the concept of sputum production and clearance. Evaluate each of the options in terms of their potential ability to inhibit sputum production or clearance. The fluid intake is the only factor that could affect the viscosity of secretions, thus affecting airway clearance. Review the defining characteristics of Ineffective Airway Clearance if you had difficulty with this question.

References
Gulanick, M., & Myers, J. (2007). *Nursing care plans: Nursing diagnosis and intervention* (6th ed., p. 442). St. Louis: Mosby.
Ignatavicius, D., & Workman, M. (2006). *Medical-surgical nursing: Critical thinking for collaborative care* (5th ed., pp. 584-585). Philadelphia: Saunders.

---

941. A client with acquired immunodeficiency syndrome gets recurrent *Candida* infections of the mouth (thrush). The nurse has given the client instructions to minimize the occurrence of thrush and determines that the client understands the instructions if which statement is made by the client?
  1 "I should use warm saline or water to rinse my mouth."
  2 "I should use a strong mouthwash at least once a week."
  3 "I should brush my teeth and rinse my mouth once a day."
  4 "Increasing the amount of red meat in my diet will keep this from recurring."

Level of Cognitive Ability: Analysis
Client Needs: Health Promotion and Maintenance
Integrated Process: Nursing Process/Evaluation
Content Area: Adult Health/Immune

Answer: 1
Rationale: When a client is in a state of immunosuppression or has decreased levels of some normal oral flora, an overgrowth of the normal flora *Candida* can occur. Careful routine mouth care is helpful to prevent the recurrence of *Candida* infections. The client should use a mouthwash that consists of warm saline or water. Red meat will not prevent thrush. The timeframes given for oral hygiene in options 2 and 3 are too infrequent.

Test-Taking Strategy: Use the process of elimination. Eliminate options 2 and 3, because they are comparable or alike and the timeframes are too infrequent. From the remaining options, recalling that red meat is not likely to minimize the occurrence of thrush will direct you to option 1. Review the teaching points related to the prevention of *Candida* infections if you had difficulty with this question.

References
Black, J., & Hawks, J. (2005). *Medical-surgical nursing: Clinical management for positive outcomes* (7th ed., p. 2391). Philadelphia: Saunders.
Ignatavicius, D., & Workman, M. (2006). *Medical-surgical nursing: Critical thinking for collaborative care* (5th ed., pp. 1249-1250). Philadelphia: Saunders.

---

942. The nurse is teaching a client with acquired immunodeficiency syndrome (AIDS) how to avoid foodborne illnesses. The nurse instructs the client to prevent acquiring infection from food by avoiding which of the following items?
  1 Raw oysters
  2 Bottled water
  3 Pasteurized milk
  4 Products with sorbitol

Level of Cognitive Ability: Application
Client Needs: Health Promotion and Maintenance
Integrated Process: Teaching and Learning
Content Area: Adult Health/Immune

Answer: 1
Rationale: The client is taught to avoid raw or undercooked seafood, meat, poultry, and eggs. The client should also avoid unpasteurized milk and dairy products. Fruits that can be peeled, as well as bottled beverages, are safe. The client may be taught to avoid sorbitol, but this is to diminish diarrhea and has nothing to do with foodborne infections.

Test-Taking Strategy: Use the process of elimination, and focus on the subject—foodborne illness. Sorbitol can cause diarrhea, but it is unrelated to foodborne illness, so option 4 is eliminated first. Eliminate option 3 next, because products that are pasteurized are free of microbes. From the remaining options, noting the strategic word "raw" in option 1 will direct you to this option. Review dietary teaching for the client with AIDS if you had difficulty with this question.

References
Black, J., & Hawks, J. (2005). *Medical-surgical nursing: Clinical management for positive outcomes* (7th ed., p. 2396). Philadelphia: Saunders.
Ignatavicius, D., & Workman, M. (2006). *Medical-surgical nursing: Critical thinking for collaborative care* (5th ed., p. 443). Philadelphia: Saunders.

943. A client with histoplasmosis has an order for ketoconazole (Nizoral). The nurse teaches the client to do which of the following while taking this medication?
1 Avoid exposure to sunlight.
2 Limit alcohol to 2 ounces per day.
3 Take the medication with an antacid.
4 Take the medication on an empty stomach.

Level of Cognitive Ability: Application
Client Needs: Health Promotion and Maintenance
Integrated Process: Teaching and Learning
Content Area: Pharmacology

Answer: 1
Rationale: The client should be taught that ketoconazole is an antifungal medication. It should be taken with food or milk. Antacids should be avoided for 2 hours after it is taken, because gastric acid is needed to activate the medication. The client should avoid the concurrent use of alcohol, because the medication is hepatotoxic. The client should also avoid exposure to sunlight, because the medication increases photosensitivity.

Test-Taking Strategy: Use the process of elimination and general guidelines related to medication administration to eliminate options 2 and 3. From the remaining options, it is necessary to know that the medication causes photosensitivity reaction and should be taken with food or milk. Review ketoconazole if you had difficulty with this question.

Reference
McKenry, L., Tressier, E., & Hogan, M. (2006). *Mosby's pharmacology in nursing* (22nd ed., p. 1059). St. Louis: Mosby.

---

944. A nurse is planning to teach a teenage client about sexuality. The nurse would begin the instruction by:
1 Informing the teenager about the dangers of pregnancy
2 Establishing a relationship and determining prior knowledge
3 Providing written information about sexually transmitted diseases
4 Advising the teenager to maintain sexual abstinence until marriage

Level of Cognitive Ability: Application
Client Needs: Health Promotion and Maintenance
Integrated Process: Teaching and Learning
Content Area: Child Health

Answer: 2
Rationale: The first step in effective communication is establishing a relationship. By exploring the client's interest and prior knowledge, rapport is established, and learning needs are assessed. The other options may or may not be later steps, depending on the data obtained.

Test-Taking Strategy: Use the steps of the nursing process, and select an assessment option. This will direct you to option 2. When teaching, assessing motivation, interest, and level of knowledge is done before providing information. Review the principles of teaching and learning if you had difficulty with this question.

Reference
Hockenberry, M., Wilson, D., & Winkelstein, M. (2005). *Wong's essentials of pediatric nursing* (7th ed., pp. 510-511). St. Louis: Mosby.

---

945. The nurse provides home-care instructions to a client with Cushing's syndrome. The nurse determines that the client understands the hospital discharge instructions if the client makes which statement?
1 "I need to eat foods low in potassium."
2 "I need to check the color of my stools."
3 "I need to check the temperature of my legs twice a day."
4 "I need to take aspirin rather than Tylenol for a headache."

Answer: 2
Rationale: Cushing's syndrome results in an increased secretion of cortisol. Cortisol stimulates the secretion of gastric acid, and this can result in the development of peptic ulcers and gastrointestinal bleeding. The client should be encouraged to eat potassium-rich foods to correct the hypokalemia that occurs with this disorder. Cushing's syndrome does not affect temperature changes in the lower extremities. Aspirin can increase the risk for gastric bleeding and skin bruising.

Test-Taking Strategy: Note the strategic words "understands the hospital discharge instructions." Recalling the pathophysiology of this disorder and that cortisol stimulates the secretion of gastric acid will direct you to option 2. Review Cushing's syndrome if you had difficulty with this question.

Level of Cognitive Ability: Analysis
Client Needs: Health Promotion and
 Maintenance
Integrated Process: Nursing Process/Evaluation
Content Area: Adult Health/Endocrine

References
Black, J., & Hawks, J. (2005). *Medical-surgical nursing: Clinical management for positive outcomes* (7th ed., p. 1156). Philadelphia: Saunders.
Ignatavicius, D., & Workman, M. (2006). *Medical-surgical nursing: Critical thinking for collaborative care* (5th ed., p. 1471). Philadelphia: Saunders.

---

946. A client with congestive heart failure and secondary hyperaldosteronism is started on spironolactone (Aldactone) to manage this disorder. The nurse informs the client that the need for dosage adjustment may be necessary if which of the following medications is also being taken?
1 Potassium chloride
2 Alprazolam (Xanax)
3 Warfarin sodium (Coumadin)
4 Verapamil hydrochloride (Calan)

Level of Cognitive Ability: Analysis
Client Needs: Health Promotion and
 Maintenance
Integrated Process: Nursing Process/
 Implementation
Content Area: Adult Health/Cardiovascular

Answer: 1
Rationale: Spironolactone (Aldactone) is a potassium-sparing diuretic. If the client is also taking potassium chloride or another potassium supplement, the risk for hyperkalemia exists. Potassium doses would need to be adjusted while the client is taking this medication. A dosage adjustment would not be necessary if the client was taking the medications identified in options 2, 3, or 4.

Test-Taking Strategy: Focus on the subject—dosage adjustment. Recalling that spironolactone is a potassium-sparing diuretic will direct you to option 1. Review potassium-sparing diuretics if you had difficulty with this question.

Reference
Hodgson, B., & Kizior, R. (2008). *Saunders nursing drug handbook 2008.* (p. 1083). St. Louis: Saunders.

---

947. A nurse is teaching health education classes to a group of expectant parents, and the topic is preventing mental retardation caused by congenital hypothyroidism. The nurse tells the parents that the most effective means of preventing this disorder is by:
1 Vitamin intake
2 Neonatal screening
3 Adequate protein intake
4 Limiting alcohol consumption

Level of Cognitive Ability: Application
Client Needs: Health Promotion and
 Maintenance
Integrated Process: Teaching and Learning
Content Area: Maternity/Antepartum

Answer: 2
Rationale: Congenital hypothyroidism is the most common preventable cause of mental retardation. Neonatal screening is the only means of early diagnosis and the subsequent prevention of mental retardation. Newborn infants are screened for congenital hypothyroidism before discharge from the nursery and before 7 days of life. Treatment is begun immediately, if necessary. Adequate protein and vitamin intake will not specifically prevent this disorder. Alcohol consumption during pregnancy needs to be restricted rather than just limited.

Test-Taking Strategy: Focus on the subject—preventing the mental retardation caused by congenital hypothyroidism. Options 1, 3, and 4 are measures to prevent all birth defects. In addition, note that neonatal screening is the umbrella option. Review congenital hypothyroidism and its complications if you had difficulty with this question.

References
Murray, S., & McKinney, E. (2006). *Foundations of maternal-newborn nursing* (4th ed., p. 533). Philadelphia: Saunders.
Wong, D., Hockenberry, M., Perry, S., Lowdermilk, D., & Wilson, D. (2006). *Maternal-child nursing care* (3rd ed., p. 742). St. Louis: Mosby.

948. The nurse in an outpatient diabetes clinic is monitoring a client with type 1 diabetes mellitus. Today's blood work reveals a glycosylated hemoglobin level of 10%. The nurse creates a teaching plan on the basis of the understanding that this result indicates which of the following?

1 A normal value that indicates that the client is managing blood glucose control well

2 A low value that indicates that the client is not managing blood glucose control very well

3 A value that does not offer information regarding the client's management of the disease

4 A high value that indicates that the client is not managing blood glucose control very well

Level of Cognitive Ability: Analysis
Client Needs: Health Promotion and Maintenance
Integrated Process: Teaching and Learning
Content Area: Adult Health/Endocrine

Answer: 4
Rationale: Glycosylated hemoglobin is a measure of glucose control during the 6 to 8 weeks before the test. It is a reliable measure for determining the degree of glucose control in diabetic clients over a period of time, and it is not influenced by dietary management a day or two before the test is done. The glycosylated hemoglobin level should be 7.0% or less, with elevated levels indicating poor glucose control.

Test-Taking Strategy: Specific knowledge regarding the normal values for this test will direct you to option 4. Remember that the level should be 7.0% or less. Review glycosylated hemoglobin testing if you had difficulty with this question.

References
Chernecky, C., & Berger, B. (2008). *Laboratory tests and diagnostic procedures* (5th ed., pp. 594-595). Philadelphia: Saunders.
Lewis, S., Heitkemper, M., Dirksen, S., O'Brien, P., & Bucher, L. (2007). *Medical-surgical nursing: Assessment and management of clinical problems* (7th ed., pp. 1251, 1258). St. Louis: Mosby.

949. The nurse is instructing a client with type 1 diabetes mellitus about the management of hypoglycemic reactions. The nurse instructs the client that hypoglycemia most likely occurs during what time interval after insulin administration?

1 Peak

2 Onset

3 Duration

4 Anytime

Level of Cognitive Ability: Application
Client Needs: Health Promotion and Maintenance
Integrated Process: Teaching and Learning
Content Area: Adult Health/Endocrine

Answer: 1
Rationale: Insulin reactions are most likely to occur during the peak time after insulin administration, when the medication is at its maximum action. Peak action depends on the type of insulin, the amount administered, the injection site, and other factors.

Test-Taking Strategy: Remember that insulin is a hypoglycemic agent. The word "peak" means the highest point. Remembering this should assist with directing you to option 1. Review the occurrence of hypoglycemia when a client is taking insulin if you had difficulty with this question.

References
Black, J., & Hawks, J. (2005). *Medical-surgical nursing: Clinical management for positive outcomes* (7th ed., pp. 1273-1274). Philadelphia: Saunders.
Ignatavicius, D., & Workman, M. (2006). *Medical-surgical nursing: Critical thinking for collaborative care* (5th ed., pp. 1519, 1539). Philadelphia: Saunders.

950. The nurse is caring for a client who is scheduled to have a thyroidectomy and provides instructions to the client about the surgical procedure. Which statement by the client would indicate an understanding of the nurse's instructions?

1 "I expect to experience some tingling of my toes, fingers, and lips after surgery."
2 "I will definitely have to continue taking antithyroid medication after this surgery."
3 "I need to place my hands behind my neck when I have to cough or change positions."
4 "I need to turn my head and neck front, back, and side to side every hour for the first 12 hours after surgery."

Level of Cognitive Ability: Analysis
Client Needs: Health Promotion and Maintenance
Integrated Process: Nursing Process/Evaluation
Content Area: Adult Health/Endocrine

Answer: 3
Rationale: The client is taught that tension needs to be avoided on the suture line, because hemorrhage may develop. One way of reducing incisional tension is to teach the client how to support the neck when coughing or being repositioned. Likewise, during the postoperative period, the client should avoid any unnecessary movement of the neck; that is why sandbags and pillows are frequently used to support the head and neck. If a client experiences tingling in the fingers, toes, and lips, it is probably a result of injury to the parathyroid gland during surgery, resulting in hypocalcemia. These signs and symptoms need to be reported immediately. The removal of the thyroid does not mean that the client will be taking antithyroid medications postoperatively.

Test-Taking Strategy: Use the process of elimination. Focusing on the type of surgery and the anatomical location of the surgical procedure will assist you with eliminating options 1, 2, and 4. Review postoperative care after thyroidectomy if you had difficulty with this question.

Reference
Ignatavicius, D., & Workman, M. (2006). *Medical-surgical nursing: Critical thinking for collaborative care* (5th ed., p. 1487). Philadelphia: Saunders.

---

951. The nurse has been preparing a client with chronic obstructive pulmonary disease for discharge. Which statement by the client indicates the need for further teaching about nutrition?

1 "I will rest a few minutes before I eat."
2 "I will not eat as much cabbage as I once did."
3 "I will certainly try to drink 3 L of fluid every day."
4 "It's best to eat three large meals a day so that I will get all my nutrients."

Level of Cognitive Ability: Analysis
Client Needs: Health Promotion and Maintenance
Integrated Process: Teaching and Learning
Content Area: Adult Health/Respiratory

Answer: 4
Rationale: Large meals distend the abdomen and elevate the diaphragm, which may interfere with breathing. Resting before eating may decrease the fatigue that is often associated with chronic obstructive pulmonary disease. Gas-forming foods may cause bloating, which interferes with normal diaphragmatic breathing. Adequate fluid intake helps to liquefy pulmonary secretions.

Test-Taking Strategy: Use the process of elimination, and note the strategic words "need for further teaching." These words indicate a negative event query and ask you to select an option that is an incorrect statement. Focusing on the client's diagnosis and recalling the activities that produce dyspnea will direct you to option 4. Review nutrition and the client with a chronic respiratory disorder if you had difficulty with this question.

References
Black, J., & Hawks, J. (2005). *Medical-surgical nursing: Clinical management for positive outcomes* (7th ed., p. 1829). Philadelphia: Saunders.
Ignatavicius, D., & Workman, M. (2006). *Medical-surgical nursing: Critical thinking for collaborative care* (5th ed., pp. 604, 606). Philadelphia: Saunders.

952. The nurse is preparing a client with pneumonia for discharge. Which statement by the client would alert the nurse to the fact that the client is in need of further discharge teaching?

1 "I will take all of my antibiotics, even if I do feel 100% better."
2 "You can toss out that incentive spirometer as soon as I leave for home."
3 "I realize that it may be weeks before my usual sense of well-being returns."
4 "It is a good idea for me to take a nap every afternoon for the next couple of weeks."

Level of Cognitive Ability: Analysis
Client Needs: Health Promotion and Maintenance
Integrated Process: Teaching and Learning
Content Area: Adult Health/Respiratory

Answer: 2
Rationale: Deep breathing and coughing exercises and the use of incentive spirometry should be practiced for 6 to 8 weeks after the client is discharged from the hospital to keep the alveoli expanded and to promote the removal of lung secretions. If the entire regimen of antibiotics is not taken, the client may suffer a relapse. Adequate rest is needed to maintain progress toward recovery. The period of convalescence with pneumonia is often lengthy, and it may be weeks before the client feels a sense of well-being.

Test-Taking Strategy: Note the strategic words "in need of further discharge teaching." These words indicate a negative event query and ask you to select an option that is an incorrect statement. Focusing on the client's diagnosis and recalling the need to promote the removal of lung secretions will direct you to option 2. Review the teaching points for the client with pneumonia if you had difficulty with this question.

References
Ignatavicius, D., & Workman, M. (2006). *Medical-surgical nursing: Critical thinking for collaborative care* (5th ed., pp. 638-639). Philadelphia: Saunders.
Lewis, S., Heitkemper, M., Dirksen, S., O'Brien, P., & Bucher, L. (2007). *Medical-surgical nursing: Assessment and management of clinical problems* (7th ed., p. 569). St. Louis: Mosby.

---

953. The community health nurse provides an educational session to members of the local community regarding breast self-examination (BSE). Which statement by a member indicates the need for further education?

1 "I need to perform a BSE every month."
2 "I should perform a BSE when I have my period."
3 "It is easiest to perform a BSE when I am in the shower when my hands are soapy."
4 "I'll use the finger pads of my three middle fingers to feel for lumps and thickening."

Level of Cognitive Ability: Analysis
Client Needs: Health Promotion and Maintenance
Integrated Process: Teaching and Learning
Content Area: Adult Health/Oncology

Answer: 2
Rationale: The best time to perform a BSE is after (not during) the monthly period, when the breasts are not tender and swollen. Options 1, 3, and 4 identify accurate information regarding the BSE.

Test-Taking Strategy: Note the strategic words "need for further education." These words indicate a negative event query and ask you to select an option that is an incorrect statement. Focusing on the subject of BSE and visualizing this procedure will direct you to option 2. Review the BSE procedure if you had difficulty with this question.

References
Ignatavicius, D., & Workman, M. (2006). *Medical-surgical nursing: Critical thinking for collaborative care* (5th ed., pp. 1796-1798). Philadelphia: Saunders.
Potter, P., & Perry, A. (2005). *Fundamentals of nursing* (6th ed., pp. 736-737). St. Louis: Mosby.

954. The nurse makes a home-care visit to a client with Bell's palsy. Which statement by the client requires clarification by the nurse?
1 "I wear an eye patch at night."
2 "I am staying on a liquid diet."
3 "I wear dark glasses when I go out."
4 "I have been gently massaging my face."

Level of Cognitive Ability: Analysis
Client Needs: Health Promotion and Maintenance
Integrated Process: Teaching and Learning
Content Area: Adult Health/Neurological

Answer: 2
Rationale: It is not necessary for a client with Bell's palsy to stay on a liquid diet. The client should be encouraged to chew on the unaffected side. Options 1, 3, and 4 identify accurate statements related to the management of Bell's palsy.

Test-Taking Strategy: Note the strategic words "requires clarification by the nurse." These words indicate a negative event query and ask you to select an option that is an incorrect statement. Recalling that Bell's palsy relates to the face will assist you with eliminating options 1, 3, and 4. Review interventions associated with Bell's palsy if you had difficulty with this question.

References
Lewis, S., Heitkemper, M., Dirksen, S., O'Brien, P., & Bucher, L. (2007). *Medical-surgical nursing: Assessment and management of clinical problems* (7th ed., p. 1585). St. Louis: Mosby.
Monahan, F., Sands, J., Neighbors, M., Marek, J., & Green, C. (2007). *Phipps' medical-surgical nursing: Health and illness perspectives* (8th ed., p. 1486). St. Louis: Mosby.

---

955. The home-care nurse is evaluating a client's understanding of the self-management of trigeminal neuralgia. Which client statement indicates that teaching is necessary?
1 "I should chew on my good side."
2 "An analgesic will relieve my pain."
3 "I should use warm mouthwash for oral hygiene."
4 "Taking my carbamazepine (Tegretol) will help control my pain."

Level of Cognitive Ability: Analysis
Client Needs: Health Promotion and Maintenance
Integrated Process: Teaching and Learning
Content Area: Adult Health/Neurological

Answer: 2
Rationale: Chronic irritation of cranial nerve V results in trigeminal neuralgia, and it is characterized by intermittent episodes of intense pain of sudden onset on the affected side of the face. The pain is rarely relieved by analgesics. It is recommended that clients chew on the unaffected side and use warm mouthwash for oral hygiene. Medications such as carbamazepine (Tegretol) help control the pain of trigeminal neuralgia.

Test-Taking Strategy: Use the process of elimination, and note the strategic words "indicates that teaching is necessary." These words indicate a negative event query and ask you to select an option that is an incorrect statement. Recalling that trigeminal neuralgia is characterized by intense pain will direct you to option 2. Review trigeminal neuralgia if you had difficulty with this question.

Reference
Black, J., & Hawks, J. (2005). *Medical-surgical nursing: Clinical management for positive outcomes* (7th ed., pp. 2153-2154). Philadelphia: Saunders.

---

956. The nurse is caring for a client with type 1 diabetes mellitus. Because the client is at risk for hypoglycemia, the nurse teaches the client to:
1 Monitor the urine for acetone.
2 Report any feelings of drowsiness.
3 Keep glucose tablets and subcutaneous glucagon available.
4 Omit the evening dose of NPH insulin if the client has been exercising.

Answer: 3
Rationale: Glucose tablets are taken if a hypoglycemic reaction occurs. Glucagon is administered subcutaneously or intramuscularly if the client loses consciousness and is unable to take glucose by mouth. Glucagon releases glycogen stores and raises the blood glucose levels of hypoglycemic clients. Family members can be taught to administer this medication and possibly to prevent an emergency department visit. Acetone in the urine may indicate hyperglycemia. Although signs of hypoglycemia need to be taught to the client, drowsiness and coma are not the initial and key signs of this complication. The nurse would not instruct a client to omit insulin.

Level of Cognitive Ability: Application
Client Needs: Health Promotion and
  Maintenance
Integrated Process: Teaching and Learning
Content Area: Adult Health/Endocrine

Test-Taking Strategy: Use the process of elimination. Eliminate option 4 first, because the nurse would not instruct a client to omit insulin doses. Options 1 and 2 can be eliminated next, because they are not related to the subject of hypoglycemia. Review the signs of hypoglycemia and the appropriate interventions if you had difficulty with this question.

References

Black, J., & Hawks, J. (2005). *Medical-surgical nursing: Clinical management for positive outcomes* (7th ed., pp. 1274-1275). Philadelphia: Saunders.
Hodgson, B., & Kizior, R. (2008). *Saunders nursing drug handbook 2008* (p. 554). St. Louis: Saunders.

---

957. A nurse is caring for a client with a precipitate labor. The nurse tells the client that in this type of labor:
  1 Induction may be necessary.
  2 The onset of contractions is gradual.
  3 The labor may last less than 3 hours.
  4 A lengthy period of pushing may be necessary.

Level of Cognitive Ability: Application
Client Needs: Health Promotion and
  Maintenance
Integrated Process: Nursing Process/
  Implementation
Content Area: Maternity/Intrapartum

Answer: 3
Rationale: Precipitate labor is defined as labor that lasts 3 hours or less for the entire labor and delivery. It usually has an abrupt rather than a gradual onset. Induction, particularly with an oxytocic agent, is contraindicated because of the enhanced stimulatory effects on the uterine muscle and an increased risk for fetal hypoxia.

Test-Taking Strategy: The word "precipitate" should assist you with defining this condition. Note the relationship between this word and "less than 3 hours" in option 3. Review the information related to precipitate labor if you had difficulty with this question.

Reference

Murray, S., & McKinney, E. (2006). *Foundations of maternal-newborn nursing* (4th ed., p. 706). Philadelphia: Saunders.

---

958. A nurse is instructing a pregnant client regarding measures to prevent a recurrent episode of preterm labor. Which statement by the client indicates the need for further teaching?
  1 "I will report any feeling of pelvic pressure."
  2 "I will not engage in sexual intercourse at this time."
  3 "I will adhere to the limitations in activity and stay off my feet."
  4 "I will limit my fluid intake to three 8-ounce glasses of fluid per day."

Level of Cognitive Ability: Analysis
Client Needs: Health Promotion and
  Maintenance
Integrated Process: Teaching and Learning
Content Area: Maternity/Antepartum

Answer: 4
Rationale: Risks for preterm labor include dehydration. A client should not restrict fluids (except for those containing alcohol and caffeine). A sign of preterm labor may be pelvic pressure without the perception of a contraction. A decrease in activity and bedrest are often prescribed in an attempt to decrease pressure on the cervix and to increase uterine blood flow. Mechanical stimulation of the cervix during intercourse can stimulate contractions.

Test-Taking Strategy: Note the strategic words "need for further teaching." These words indicate a negative event query and ask you to select an option that is an incorrect statement. Focusing on the subject of the prevention of preterm labor will direct you to option 4. Remember that it is generally not a good practice for the client to limit fluid intake to three 8-ounce glasses of fluid per day. Review the measures to prevent preterm labor if you had difficulty with this question.

Reference

Murray, S., & McKinney, E. (2006). *Foundations of maternal-newborn nursing* (4th ed., pp. 712-714). Philadelphia: Saunders.

959. The nurse has completed discharge teaching with the parents of a child with glomerulonephritis. Which statement by the parents indicates that further teaching is necessary?
1 "We'll check our child's blood pressure every day."
2 "We'll test our child's urine for albumin every week."
3 "It'll be so good to have our child back in tap-dancing classes next week."
4 "We'll be sure that our child eats a lot of vegetables and does not add extra salt to food."

Level of Cognitive Ability: Analysis
Client Needs: Health Promotion and Maintenance
Integrated Process: Teaching and Learning
Content Area: Child Health

Answer: 3
Rationale: After discharge, parents should allow the child to return to his or her normal routine and activities, with adequate periods allowed for rest. Tap-dancing classes 1 week after discharge would be unrealistic and involve a too-rapid increase in activity. Options 1, 2, and 4 are appropriate home-care measures.

Test-Taking Strategy: Use the process of elimination, and note the strategic words "further teaching is necessary." These words indicate a negative event query and ask you to select an option that is an incorrect statement. Select option 3, because tap dancing is an aggressive exercise. Review the home-care measures for glomerulonephritis if you had difficulty with this question.

Reference
Hockenberry, M., Wilson, D., & Winkelstein, M. (2005). *Wong's essentials of pediatric nursing* (7th ed., p. 999). St. Louis: Mosby.

---

960. A nurse is planning discharge teaching for the parents of a child who sustained a head injury and who is now receiving tapering doses of dexamethasone sodium phosphate (Decadron). The nurse plans to make which statement to the parents?
1 "This medication decreases the chance of infection."
2 "This medication will be discontinued after two doses."
3 "If your child's face becomes puffy, the medication dose needs to be increased."
4 "This medication is tapered to decrease the chance of recurring swelling in the brain."

Level of Cognitive Ability: Application
Client Needs: Health Promotion and Maintenance
Integrated Process: Teaching and Learning
Content Area: Pharmacology

Answer: 4
Rationale: The rebounding of cerebral edema is a side effect of dexamethasone sodium phosphate (Decadron) withdrawal if it is done abruptly. Dexamethasone sodium phosphate decreases inflammation rather than infection. Facial edema is a common side effect that disappears when the medication is discontinued.

Test-Taking Strategy: Focus on the name of the medication, and recall that it is a corticosteroid. Remember that tapering is required with corticosteroids to prevent a rebound effect as a result of adrenal insufficiency. Review dexamethasone sodium phosphate if you had difficulty with this question.

Reference
McKenry, L., Tessier, E., & Hogan, M. (2006). *Mosby's pharmacology in nursing* (22nd ed., p. 852). St. Louis: Mosby.

---

961. The nurse has implemented a plan of care for a client with a C5 spinal cord injury to promote health maintenance. Which client outcome would indicate the effectiveness of the interventions?
1 Maintenance of intact skin
2 Regaining of bladder and bowel control
3 Performance of activities of daily living independently
4 Independent transfer of self to and from the wheelchair

Answer: 1
Rationale: A C5 spinal cord injury results in quadriplegia with no sensation below the clavicle, including most of the arms and hands. The client maintains the partial movement of the shoulders and elbows. Maintaining intact skin is an outcome for spinal cord injury clients. The remaining options are inappropriate for this client.

Level of Cognitive Ability: Analysis
Client Needs: Health Promotion and
  Maintenance
Integrated Process: Nursing Process/Evaluation
Content Area: Adult Health/Neurological

Test-Taking Strategy: Focus on the strategic words "C5 spinal cord injury." Eliminate options 3 and 4 first, because they are comparable or alike. From the remaining options, recalling the effects of a C5 spinal cord injury will assist you with eliminating option 2, because it is unrealistic. Review C5 spinal cord injuries if you had difficulty with this question.

Reference
Ignatavicius, D., & Workman, M. (2006). *Medical-surgical nursing: Critical thinking for collaborative care* (5th ed., pp. 987, 992, 994). Philadelphia: Saunders.

---

962. A home-care nurse visits a child who is being treated with penicillin G potassium (Pfizerpen) for scarlet fever. The mother tells the nurse that the child has only voided a small amount of tea-colored urine since the previous day. The mother also reports that the child's appetite has decreased and that the child's face was swollen this morning. The nurse interprets that these new symptoms are:

1 Nothing to be concerned about
2 Symptoms of acute glomerulonephritis
3 Signs of the normal progression of scarlet fever
4 Symptoms of an allergic reaction to penicillin G potassium

Level of Cognitive Ability: Analysis
Client Needs: Health Promotion and
  Maintenance
Integrated Process: Nursing Process/Analysis
Content Area: Child Health

Answer: 2
Rationale: The symptoms identified in the question indicate acute glomerulonephritis. Although the child is recieving penicillin G potassium, these are not symptoms of an allergic reaction. These symptoms are not normal and should not be ignored.

Test-Taking Strategy: Use the process of elimination. Eliminate options 1 and 3, because they are comparable or alike. From the remaining options, recalling the complications of scarlet fever and the symptoms of a medication reaction will direct you to option 2. Review the complications of scarlet fever and the symptoms of acute glomerulonephritis if you had difficulty with this question.

Reference
Hockenberry, M., Wilson, D., & Winkelstein, M. (2005). *Wong's essentials of pediatric nursing* (7th ed., pp. 997-998). St. Louis: Mosby.

---

963. A client who sustained a thoracic cord injury a year ago returns to the clinic for a follow-up visit, and the nurse notes a small reddened area on the coccyx. The client is not aware of the reddened area. After counseling the client to relieve pressure on the area according to a turning schedule, which action by the nurse is appropriate?

1 Teaching the client to feel for reddened areas
2 Asking a family member to assess the skin daily
3 Teaching the client to use a mirror for skin assessment
4 Scheduling the client to return to the clinic daily for a skin check

Answer: 3
Rationale: The client should be encouraged to be as independent as possible. The most effective means of skin self-assessment for this client is with the use of a mirror. Asking a family member to assess the skin daily does not promote independence. It is unnecessary and unrealistic for the client to return to the clinic daily for a skin check, and redness cannot be felt.

Test-Taking Strategy: Use the process of elimination, and recall that independence is key to the rehabilitation of clients. Options 2 and 4 involve others in performing a task that the client can do independently. Option 1 is an inaccurate assessment technique, because redness cannot be felt. Option 3 is the only option that addresses client self-assessment. Review the home-care measures for the client with a thoracic cord injury if you had difficulty with this question.

Level of Cognitive Ability: Application
Client Needs: Health Promotion and
Maintenance
Integrated Process: Nursing Process/
Implementation
Content Area: Adult Health/Neurological

Reference
Black, J., & Hawks, J. (2005). *Medical-surgical nursing: Clinical management for positive outcomes* (7th ed., pp. 2228, 2234). Philadelphia: Saunders.

---

964. The nurse has given instructions to a client who is returning home after an arthroscopy of the knee. The nurse determines that the client understands the home-care instructions if the client states the need to:
  1 Resume strenuous exercise the following day.
  2 Stay off the leg entirely for the rest of the day.
  3 Report fever or site inflammation to the physician.
  4 Refrain from eating food for the remainder of the day.

Level of Cognitive Ability: Analysis
Client Needs: Health Promotion and
Maintenance
Integrated Process: Nursing Process/Evaluation
Content Area: Adult Health/Musculoskeletal

Answer: 3
Rationale: After arthroscopy, the client can usually walk carefully on the leg after sensation has returned. The client is instructed to avoid strenuous exercise for at least a few days. The client may resume the usual diet. Signs and symptoms of infection should be reported to the physician.

Test-Taking Strategy: Use the process of elimination, and focus on the procedure—arthroscopy. Recalling that the procedure is invasive will direct you to option 3. Additionally, the client is always taught which signs and symptoms of infection to report to the physician. Review the home-care instructions for the client after arthroscopy if you had difficulty with this question.

References
Black, J., & Hawks, J. (2005). *Medical-surgical nursing: Clinical management for positive outcomes* (7th ed., p. 577). Philadelphia: Saunders.
Monahan, F., Sands, J., Neighbors, M., Marek, J., & Green, C. (2007). *Phipps' medical-surgical nursing: Health and illness perspectives* (8th ed., p. 1521). St. Louis: Mosby.

---

965. Allopurinol (Zyloprim) has been prescribed for a client to treat gouty arthritis. The nurse teaches the client to anticipate which of the following prescriptions if an acute attack occurs?
  1 Doubling the dose of the allopurinol
  2 Stopping the allopurinol and taking acetylsalicylic acid (aspirin)
  3 Stopping the allopurinol and taking a nonsteroidal anti-inflammatory drug
  4 Adding colchicine or a nonsteroidal anti-inflammatory drug to the treatment plan

Level of Cognitive Ability: Application
Client Needs: Health Promotion and
Maintenance
Integrated Process: Teaching and Learning
Content Area: Pharmacology

Answer: 4
Rationale: Allopurinol helps prevent an attack of gouty arthritis, but it does not relieve the pain. Therefore, another medication such as colchicine or a nonsteroidal anti-inflammatory drug must be added if an acute attack occurs. Because acute attacks may occur more frequently early during the course of therapy with allopurinol, some physicians recommend taking the two products concurrently during the first 3 to 6 months.

Test-Taking Strategy: Use the process of elimination. Eliminate options 2 and 3 first, because it is unlikely that medication will be stopped. From the remaining options, recalling that an acute attack of gouty arthritis is painful will assist you with selecting option 4 because of the anti-inflammatory action of the nonsteroidal anti-inflammatory drug. Review the interventions for an acute attack of gouty arthritis if you had difficulty with this question.

References
Ignatavicius, D., & Workman, M. (2006). *Medical-surgical nursing: Critical thinking for collaborative care* (5th ed., p. 416). Philadelphia: Saunders.
Lehne, R. (2007). *Pharmacology for nursing care* (6th ed., p. 844). Philadelphia: Saunders.

966. A nursing instructor asks a nursing student to describe live or attenuated vaccines. The student tells the instructor that these types of vaccines are:
1 Bacterial toxins that have been made inactive by either chemicals or heat
2 Vaccines that contain pathogens made inactive by either chemicals or heat
3 Vaccines that have their virulence (potency) diminished so as to not produce a full-blown clinical illness
4 Vaccines that have been obtained from the pooled blood of many people and provide antibodies to a variety of diseases

Level of Cognitive Ability: Comprehension
Client Needs: Health Promotion and Maintenance
Integrated Process: Teaching and Learning
Content Area: Child Health

Answer: 3
Rationale: Live or attenuated vaccines have their virulence (potency) diminished so as to not produce a full-blown clinical illness. In response to vaccination, the body produces antibodies and causes immunity to be established. Option 1 identifies toxoids. Option 2 identifies killed or inactivated vaccines. Option 4 identifies human immune globulin.

Test-Taking Strategy: Use the process of elimination, and focus on the subject of the question: live or attenuated vaccines. Noting the strategic word "live" in the question will assist you with eliminating options 1, 2, and 4. Review the different types of vaccines if you had difficulty with this question.

Reference
McKinney, E., James, S., Murray, S., & Ashwill, J. (2005). *Maternal-child nursing* (2nd ed., p. 69). St. Louis: Saunders.

---

967. A client has received a prescription for lisinopril (Prinivil). The nurse teaches the client that which of the following frequent side effects may occur?
1 Cough
2 Polyuria
3 Hypothermia
4 Hypertension

Level of Cognitive Ability: Application
Client Needs: Health Promotion and Maintenance
Integrated Process: Teaching and Learning
Content Area: Pharmacology

Answer: 1
Rationale: Cough is a frequent side effect of therapy with any of the angiotensin-converting enzyme (ACE) inhibitors. Fever is an occasional side effect. Proteinuria is another common side effect, but polyuria is not. Hypertension is the reason to administer the medication rather than a side effect.

Test-Taking Strategy: Note the name of the medication. Recalling that most ACE inhibitor medication names end in *-pril* and that ACE inhibitors are used to treat hypertension will assist you with eliminating option 4. From the remaining options, it is necessary to know that cough is a frequent side effect of these medications. Review the side effects of lisinopril if you had difficulty with this question.

Reference
McKenry, L., Tressier, E., & Hogan, M. (2006). *Mosby's pharmacology in nursing* (22nd ed., p. 556). St. Louis: Mosby.

---

968. A nurse has provided home-care instructions to a client who is taking lithium carbonate (Eskalith). Which client statement indicates that the client understands the prescribed regimen?
1 "I will restrict my water intake."
2 "I will make sure that my diet contains salt."
3 "I will keep my medication in the refrigerator."
4 "I will be careful to avoid eating foods high in potassium."

Answer: 2
Rationale: Lithium replaces sodium ions in the cells and induces the excretion of sodium and potassium from the body. Client teaching includes the maintenance of sodium intake in the daily diet and increased fluid intake (at least 1 to 1½ L per day) during maintenance therapy. Lithium is stored at room temperature and protected from light and moisture.

Test-Taking Strategy: Note the strategic words "understands the prescribed regimen." Recalling that lithium is a salt that replaces sodium ions and that induces the excretion of sodium and potassium will direct you to the correct option. Review lithium carbonate if you had difficulty with this question.

Level of Cognitive Ability: Analysis
Client Needs: Health Promotion and
   Maintenance
Integrated Process: Nursing Process/Evaluation
Content Area: Pharmacology

Reference
Lehne, R. (2007). *Pharmacology for nursing care* (6th ed., p. 357). Philadelphia: Saunders.

---

969. An older client is given a prescription for haloperidol (Haldol). The nurse instructs the client and family to report any signs of pseudoparkinsonism and tells the family to monitor for:

1 Tremors and hyperpyrexia
2 Motor restlessness and aphasia
3 Stooped posture and a shuffling gait
4 Muscle weakness and decreased salivation

Level of Cognitive Ability: Application
Client Needs: Health Promotion and
   Maintenance
Integrated Process: Teaching and Learning
Content Area: Pharmacology

Answer: 3
Rationale: Pseudoparkinsonism is a common extrapyramidal side effect of antipsychotic medications. This condition is characterized by a stooped posture, a shuffling gait, a mask-like facial appearance, drooling, tremors, and pill-rolling motions of the fingers. Hyperpyrexia is characteristic of the extrapyramidal side effect of neuroleptic malignant syndrome. Motor restlessness, asphasia, muscle weakness, and decreased salivation are not characteristic of pseudoparkinsonism.

Test-Taking Strategy: Focus on the word "pseudoparkinsonism." Recalling the characteristics of Parkinson disease will direct you to option 3. Review the characteristics and side effects of antipsychotic medications if you had difficulty with this question.

Reference
McKenry, L., Tressier, E., & Hogan, M. (2006). *Mosby's pharmacology in nursing* (22nd ed., p. 386). St. Louis: Mosby.

---

970. A client who is taking tranylcypromine sulfate (Parnate) requests information about foods that are acceptable to eat while taking the medication. The nurse tells the client that it is safe to eat:

1 Yogurt
2 Raisins
3 Oranges
4 Smoked fish

Level of Cognitive Ability: Application
Client Needs: Health Promotion and
   Maintenance
Integrated Process: Teaching and Learning
Content Area: Pharmacology

Answer: 3
Rationale: Tranylcypromine sulfate is classified as a monoamine oxidase inhibitor (MAOI); as such, tyramine-containing food should be avoided. Types of food to be avoided include—but are not limited to—those items identified in options 1, 2, and 4. Additionally, beer, wine, caffeinated beverages, pickled meats, yeast preparations, avocados, bananas, and plums are to be avoided. Oranges are permissible.

Test-Taking Strategy: Note the similarity in the food items in options 1, 2, and 4. These are food items that are either processed or that contain some type of additive. The only natural food is option 3. Remember that, although bananas, avocados, and plums are natural foods, they are not permitted while taking an MAOI. Review foods that are high in tyramine if you had difficulty with this question.

Reference
Lehne, R. (2007). *Pharmacology for nursing care* (6th ed., p. 346). Philadelphia: Saunders.

971. A nurse is performing an assessment on a 3-year-old child with chickenpox. The child's mother tells the nurse that the child keeps scratching at night, and the nurse teaches the mother about measures that will prevent an alteration in skin integrity. Which statement by the mother indicates that teaching was effective?

1 "I need to place white gloves on my child's hands at night."
2 "I will apply generous amounts of a cortisone cream to prevent itching."
3 "I will give my child a glass of warm milk at bedtime to help my child sleep."
4 "I need to keep my child in a warm room at night so that the covers will not cause my child to scratch."

Level of Cognitive Ability: Analysis
Client Needs: Health Promotion and Maintenance
Integrated Process: Nursing Process/Evaluation
Content Area: Child Health

Answer: 1
Rationale: Gloves will keep the child from causing an alteration in skin integrity from scratching. Generous amounts of any topical cream can lead to medication toxicity. A warm room will increase the child's skin temperature and make the itching worse. Warm milk will have no effect on itching.

Test-Taking Strategy: Use the process of elimination. Note the strategic words "prevent an alteration in skin integrity." Eliminate option 4 first, because this action will promote itching. Option 3 is eliminated next, because it is unrelated to skin integrity. From the remaining options, the words "generous amounts" in option 2 should provide you with a clue that this option is incorrect. Review the measures related to the child with chickenpox if you had difficulty with this question.

Reference
Hockenberry, M., Wilson, D., & Winkelstein, M. (2005). *Wong's essentials of pediatric nursing* (7th ed., p. 437). St. Louis: Mosby.

---

972. The nurse is providing instructions to a client with peptic ulcer disease about symptom management. Client learning is evident if the client makes which of the following statements?

1 "I should eat a snack at bedtime."
2 "I can take aspirin to relieve gastric pain."
3 "It is important that I eat slowly and chew my food thoroughly."
4 "I should take my antacid and famotidine (Pepcid) at the same time."

Level of Cognitive Ability: Analysis
Client Needs: Health Promotion and Maintenance
Integrated Process: Nursing Process/Evaluation
Content Area: Adult Health/Gastrointestinal

Answer: 3
Rationale: Eating slowly and chewing thoroughly helps to prevent overdistention and reflux. Bedtime snacks are avoided, because they can promote nighttime acid secretion. Acetaminophen (Tylenol) is administered for routine pain relief during treatment. All nonsteroidal anti-inflammatory drugs, and aspirin are avoided. Antacids will interfere with the absorption of the famotidine (Pepcid), so they should not be taken at the same time.

Test-Taking Strategy: Focus on the words "learning is evident" and the concepts related to digestion to direct you to option 3. Review the teaching points related to the client with peptic ulcer disease if you had difficulty with this question.

References
Grodner, M., Long, S., & DeYoung, S. (2004). *Foundations and clinical applications of nutrition: A nursing approach* (3rd ed., pp. 508, 510). St. Louis: Mosby.
Ignatavicius, D., & Workman, M. (2006). *Medical-surgical nursing: Critical thinking for collaborative care* (5th ed., pp. 1294, 1301). Philadelphia: Saunders.

---

973. A client with a hiatal hernia asks the nurse about fluids that are safe to drink and that will not irritate the gastric mucosa. The nurse tells the client to drink:

1 Apple juice
2 Orange juice
3 Tomato juice
4 Grapefruit juice

Answer: 1
Rationale: Substances that are irritating to the client with hiatal hernia include tomato products and citrus fruits, which should be avoided. Because caffeine stimulates gastric acid secretion, beverages that contain caffeine, such as coffee, tea, cola, and cocoa, are also eliminated from the diet.

Level of Cognitive Ability: Application
Client Needs: Health Promotion and
Maintenance
Integrated Process: Nursing Process/
Implementation
Content Area: Adult Health/Gastrointestinal

Test-Taking Strategy: Use the process of elimination. Eliminate options 2, 3, and 4, because they are comparable or alike and are all citrus products. Additionally, option 1 is the least irritating to the stomach. Review the dietary measures for the client with hiatal hernia if you had difficulty with this question.

References

Black, J., & Hawks, J. (2005). *Medical-surgical nursing: Clinical management for positive outcomes* (7th ed., pp. 732-733). Philadelphia: Saunders.
Grodner, M., Long, S., & DeYoung, S. (2004). *Foundations and clinical applications of nutrition: A nursing approach* (3rd ed., p. 508). St. Louis: Mosby.

---

974. The nurse determines that the client with gastroesophageal reflux disease (GERD) needs further dietary teaching if which of the following statements is made?
 1 "I must avoid coffee, tea, and chocolate."
 2 "I should eat four to six small meals a day."
 3 "It is important that I drink extra fluids during meals."
 4 "I need to avoid snacking for 2 to 3 hours before bedtime."

Level of Cognitive Ability: Application
Client Needs: Health Promotion and
Maintenance
Integrated Process: Teaching and Learning
Content Area: Adult Health/Gastrointestinal

Answer: 3
Rationale: Fluids need to be taken between meals rather than with meals to prevent the overdistention that leads to reflux. Coffee, tea, cola, and chocolate are also eliminated from the diet, because they decrease lower esophageal sphincter pressure and can potentiate reflux. Four to six smaller meals per day will help to prevent gastric overdistention. One of the primary factors in GERD is an incompetent lower esophageal sphincter. Adequate time needs to pass before the client assumes the supine position to decrease the risk for the reflux of gastric contents.

Test-Taking Strategy: Focus on the words "needs further dietary teaching." Eliminate options 1, 2, and 4, because they indicate that the client has a proper understanding of the dietary management of GERD. Review the dietary measures for the client with GERD if you had difficulty with this question.

Reference

Lewis, S., Heitkemper, M., Dirksen, S., O'Brien, P., & Bucher, L. (2007). *Medical-surgical nursing: Assessment and management of clinical problems* (7th ed., pp. 1004-1005). St. Louis: Mosby.

---

975. When preparing the client with a spinal cord injury who is experiencing bladder spasms and reflex incontinence for discharge to home, the nurse instructs the client to institute which of the following measures to deal with the issue?
 1 "Avoid caffeine in your diet."
 2 "Take your temperature every day."
 3 "Limit your fluid intake to 1000 mL per 24 hours."
 4 "Catheterize yourself every 2 hours as needed to prevent spasm."

Level of Cognitive Ability: Application
Client Needs: Health Promotion and
Maintenance
Integrated Process: Teaching and Learning
Content Area: Adult Health/Neurological

Answer: 1
Rationale: Caffeine in the diet can contribute to bladder spasms and reflex incontinence; thus it should be eliminated in the diet of the client with a spinal cord injury. The self-monitoring of the temperature would be useful to detect infection, but it does nothing to alleviate bladder spasms. Limiting fluid intake does not prevent spasm, and it could place the client at further risk for urinary tract infection. Self-catheterization every 2 hours is too frequent and serves no useful purpose.

Test-Taking Strategy: Focus on the subject—preventive measures for bladder spasms and reflex incontinence. Eliminate options 3 and 4 first, because they place the client at increased risk for urinary tract infection and are therefore not appropriate. From the remaining options, eliminate option 2, because this action would detect infection but does not deal with spasms and incontinence. Review the measures to prevent bladder spasms and reflex incontinence if you had difficulty with this question.

References

Black, J., & Hawks, J. (2005). *Medical-surgical nursing: Clinical management for positive outcomes* (7th ed., p. 2227). Philadelphia: Saunders.

Lewis, S., Heitkemper, M., Dirksen, S., O'Brien, P., & Bucher, L. (2007). *Medical-surgical nursing: Assessment and management of clinical problems* (7th ed., p. 1180). St. Louis: Mosby.

---

976. A client seeks treatment in an ambulatory care center for symptoms of Raynaud's disease. The nurse instructs the client to:

1 Decrease cigarette smoking by one half.
2 Alternate exposures to both heat and cold.
3 Continue activity during vasospasm for quicker relief of symptoms.
4 Wear protective items, such as gloves and warm socks, as necessary.

Level of Cognitive Ability: Application
Client Needs: Health Promotion and Maintenance
Integrated Process: Teaching and Learning
Content Area: Adult Health/Cardiovascular

Answer: 4

Rationale: Treatment for Raynaud's disease includes the avoidance of precipitating factors such as cold or damp weather, stress, and cigarettes. The client should get sufficient rest and sleep, protect the extremities by wearing protective clothing, and stop activity during vasospasm.

Test-Taking Strategy: Use the process of elimination. Recall that the symptoms of Raynaud's disease are caused by vasospasm. Eliminate options 1, 2, and 3, because they will all cause vasospasm. Review the client teaching points related to Raynaud's disease if you had difficulty with this question.

References

Ignatavicius, D., & Workman, M. (2006). *Medical-surgical nursing: Critical thinking for collaborative care* (5th ed., p. 811). Philadelphia: Saunders.

Monahan, F., Sands, J., Neighbors, M., Marek, J., & Green, C. (2007). *Phipps' medical-surgical nursing: Health and illness perspectives* (8th ed., p. 875). St. Louis: Mosby.

---

977. The nurse determines that the client with atherosclerosis understands dietary modifications to lower the risk of heart disease if which of the following food selections is made?

1 Roast beef
2 Fresh cantaloupe
3 Broiled cheeseburger
4 Mashed potato with gravy

Level of Cognitive Ability: Analysis
Client Needs: Health Promotion and Maintenance
Integrated Process: Nursing Process/Evaluation
Content Area: Adult Health/Cardiovascular

Answer: 2

Rationale: To lower the risk of heart disease, the diet should be low in saturated fat with the appropriate number of total calories. The diet should include less red meat and more white meat with the skin removed. Dairy products used should be low in fat, and foods with high amounts of empty calories should be avoided.

Test-Taking Strategy: Focus on the subject—lowering the risk of heart disease. Use the fat content of the foods in the options as a guide to answering this question. Eliminate options 1 and 3 first because of the fat content of the described meats. From the remaining options, eliminate option 4, because fresh fruits and vegetables are naturally low in fat. Review the dietary measures that will lower the risk of heart disease if you had difficulty with this question.

References

Grodner, M., Long, S., & DeYoung, S. (2004). *Foundations and clinical applications of nutrition: A nursing approach* (3rd ed., pp. 601-602). St. Louis: Mosby.

Ignatavicius, D., & Workman, M. (2006). *Medical-surgical nursing: Critical thinking for collaborative care* (5th ed., pp. 20, 757, 1676). Philadelphia: Saunders.

978. A client being discharged to home after angioplasty via the right femoral groin as the catheter insertion site has received discharge instructions from the nurse. Client learning is evident if which of the following statements is made?
1 "Coolness or discoloration of the right foot is expected."
2 "I should expect a large area of bruising at the right groin."
3 "Temperature as high as 101° F is not unusual a few days after the procedure."
4 "Mild discomfort in the right groin may occur, and Tylenol should relieve the pain."

Level of Cognitive Ability: Analysis
Client Needs: Health Promotion and Maintenance
Integrated Process: Nursing Process/Evaluation
Content Area: Adult Health/Cardiovascular

Answer: 4
Rationale: The client may feel some mild discomfort at the catheter insertion site after angioplasty. This is usually relieved by analgesics such as acetaminophen (Tylenol). The client is taught to report to the physician any neurovascular changes to the affected leg, bleeding or bruising at the insertion site, and signs of local infection, such as drainage at the site or increased temperature.

Test-Taking Strategy: Use the process of elimination, and note the strategic words "learning is evident." Knowing that bleeding and infection are complications of the procedure guides you to eliminate options 2 and 3. From the remaining options, eliminate option 1 knowing that neurovascular status should not be impaired by the procedure or by knowing that the area may be mildly uncomfortable. Review the complications associated with angioplasty if you had difficulty with this question.

References
Ignatavicius, D., & Workman, M. (2006). *Medical-surgical nursing: Critical thinking for collaborative care* (5th ed., p. 698). Philadelphia: Saunders.
Pagana, K., & Pagana, T. (2005). *Mosby's diagnostic and laboratory test reference* (7th ed., pp. 236-237). St. Louis: Mosby.

979. The nurse is teaching dietary modifications to the client with hypertension. The nurse instructs the client to eat which of the following snack foods?
1 Raw carrots
2 Frozen pizza
3 Cheese and crackers
4 Canned tomato soup

Level of Cognitive Ability: Application
Client Needs: Health Promotion and Maintenance
Integrated Process: Teaching and Learning
Content Area: Adult Health/Cardiovascular

Answer: 1
Rationale: Sodium should be avoided by the client with hypertension. Fresh fruits and vegetables are naturally low in sodium. Hypertensive clients are also advised to keep fat intake to less than 30% of their total calories as part of prudent heart living. Each of the incorrect options contain high amounts of sodium, and options 2 and 3 are also likely to be higher in fat.

Test-Taking Strategy: Focus on the subject—the dietary modifications needed with hypertension. Eliminate options 2, 3, and 4, because they are comparable or alike and because they are all processed food items. Review the dietary measures for the client with hypertension if you had difficulty with this question.

References
Grodner, M., Long, S., & DeYoung, S. (2004). *Foundations and clinical applications of nutrition: A nursing approach* (3rd ed., p. 592). St. Louis: Mosby.
Ignatavicius, D., & Workman, M. (2006). *Medical-surgical nursing: Critical thinking for collaborative care* (5th ed., p. 757). Philadelphia: Saunders.

980. The nurse teaches a client with hypertension to recognize the signs and symptoms that may occur during periods of elevated blood pressure. The nurse determines that the client needs additional teaching if the client states that which sign or symptom is associated with this condition?
1 Epistaxis
2 Dizziness
3 Blurred vision
4 A feeling of fullness in the head

Answer: 4
Rationale: Cerebrovascular symptoms of hypertension include early morning headaches, occipital headaches, blurred vision, lightheadedness, vertigo, dizziness, and epistaxis. The client should be aware of these symptoms and report them if they occur. The client should also be taught to self-monitor the blood pressure. A feeling of fullness in the head is more likely associated with a sinus condition.

Level of Cognitive Ability: Analysis
Client Needs: Health Promotion and
    Maintenance
Integrated Process: Teaching and Learning
Content Area: Adult Health/Cardiovascular

Test-Taking Strategy: Note the strategic words "needs additional teaching." These words indicate a negative event query and ask you to select an option that is an incorrect sign or symptom. Focus on the subject—signs of an elevated blood pressure. Option 4 is the vague option, whereas options 1, 2, and 3 are specific and related to hypertension. Review the signs and symptoms of hypertension if you had difficulty with this question.

References

Black, J., & Hawks, J. (2005). *Medical-surgical nursing: Clinical management for positive outcomes* (7th ed., p. 1495). Philadelphia: Saunders.
Ignatavicius, D., & Workman, M. (2006). *Medical-surgical nursing: Critical thinking for collaborative care* (5th ed., p. 691). Philadelphia: Saunders.

---

981. Which of the following instructions should the nurse include in the teaching plan for a client taking iron supplements to correct iron deficiency anemia?
1 Eat a low-fiber diet.
2 Limit the intake of fluids.
3 Limit the intake of meat, fish, and poultry.
4 Avoid taking the iron supplements with milk or antacids.

Level of Cognitive Ability: Application
Client Needs: Health Promotion and
    Maintenance
Integrated Process: Teaching and Learning
Content Area: Pharmacology

Answer: 4
Rationale: The client should avoid taking the iron supplements with milk or antacids, because these items decrease the absorption of iron. The client should also avoid taking the iron with food, if possible. The client should increase the intake of natural sources of iron, such as meats, fish, and poultry. Finally, the client should take in sufficient fiber and fluids to prevent constipation as a side effect of iron therapy.

Test-Taking Strategy: Use the process of elimination. Eliminate options 1 and 2, because constipation is a common side effect of iron therapy. Recalling that meat products contain iron helps you to eliminate option 3 next. Remember that several medications have impaired absorption with milk products or antacids. Review the home-care measures for the client with iron deficiency anemia if you had difficulty with this question.

Reference

McKenry, L., Tressier, E., & Hogan, M. (2006). *Mosby's pharmacology in nursing* (22nd ed., p. 1225). St. Louis: Mosby.

---

982. A client with a colostomy complains to the nurse of appliance odor. The nurse recommends that the client take in which of the following deodorizing foods?
1 Eggs
2 Yogurt
3 Cucumbers
4 Mushrooms

Level of Cognitive Ability: Application
Client Needs: Health Promotion and
    Maintenance
Integrated Process: Teaching and Learning
Content Area: Adult Health/Gastrointestinal

Answer: 2
Rationale: Foods that help eliminate odor with a colostomy include yogurt, buttermilk, cranberry juice, and parsley. Foods that cause odor are many and include alcohol, beans, turnips, radishes, asparagus, onions, cucumbers, mushrooms, cabbage, eggs, and fish.

Test-Taking Strategy: Use the process of elimination. Remember that foods that cause gas in the client with normal gastrointestinal function also form gas in the gastrointestinal tract of the client with a colostomy. Use basic nutritional knowledge to eliminate options 1, 3, and 4. Review the foods that cause gas formation if you had difficulty with this question.

References
Ignatavicius, D., & Workman, M. (2006). *Medical-surgical nursing: Critical thinking for collaborative care* (5th ed., p. 1325). Philadelphia: Saunders.
Lewis, S., Heitkemper, M., Dirksen, S., O'Brien, P., & Bucher, L. (2007). *Medical-surgical nursing: Assessment and management of clinical problems* (7th ed., pp. 1073, 1075). St. Louis: Mosby.

---

983. The nurse is demonstrating colostomy care to a client with a newly created colostomy. The nurse demonstrates the correct cutting of the appliance by making the circle how much larger than the client's stoma?

1 ½ inch
2 ⅛ inch
3 ¼ inch
4 1⁄16 inch

Level of Cognitive Ability: Application
Client Needs: Health Promotion and Maintenance
Integrated Process: Teaching and Learning
Content Area: Adult Health/Gastrointestinal

Answer: 2

Rationale: The size of the opening for the appliance is generally cut ⅛ inch larger than the size of the client's stoma. This minimizes the amount of exposed skin but does not put pressure on the stoma. Option 4 is an extremely small size that would cause irritation to the stoma. Options 1 and 3 leave too much skin area exposed for possible irritation by gastrointestinal contents.

Test-Taking Strategy: Use the process of elimination, and remember that the goal is to prevent stoma and skin irritation. Visualizing each of the appliance sizes in the options will direct you to option 2. Review the home-care instructions for the client with a colostomy if you had difficulty with this question.

Reference
Ignatavicius, D., & Workman, M. (2006). *Medical-surgical nursing: Critical thinking for collaborative care* (5th ed., p. 1325). Philadelphia: Saunders.

---

984. The nurse teaches a client with a spinal cord injury about measures to prevent autonomic hyperreflexia. Which statement by the client would indicate the need for additional teaching?

1 "It is best if I avoid tight clothing and lumpy bedclothes."
2 "I should watch for headache, congestion, and flushed skin."
3 "Symptoms I should watch for include fever and chest pain."
4 "I need to pay close attention to how frequently my bowels move."

Level of Cognitive Ability: Analysis
Client Needs: Health Promotion and Maintenance
Integrated Process: Teaching and Learning
Content Area: Adult Health/Neurological

Answer: 3

Rationale: Symptoms of autonomic hyperreflexia include headache, congestion, flushed skin above the level of injury and cold skin below it, diaphoresis, nausea, and anxiety. Fever and chest pain are not associated with this condition.

Test-Taking Strategy: Use the process of elimination, and note the strategic words "need for additional teaching." These words indicate a negative event query and ask you to select an option that is an incorrect statement. Recalling the signs, symptoms, and causes of autonomic hyperreflexia will direct you to option 3. Review this content if you are unfamiliar with this syndrome.

Reference
Ignatavicius, D., & Workman, M. (2006). *Medical-surgical nursing: Critical thinking for collaborative care* (5th ed., p. 987). Philadelphia: Saunders.

985. The nurse is discharging a female client from the hospital who has a diagnosis of a T11 fracture with cord transection. The nurse has provided home-care instructions to the client. Which of the following would indicate the need for further discharge teaching?

  1 The client jokes about no longer needing to worry about birth control.

  2 The client states that she will be careful to not eat as many dairy products.

  3 The client verbalizes the need to eat her meals at the same time every day.

  4 The client states that she will wash her hands, her perineum, and the catheter with soap and water before performing self-catheterization.

Level of Cognitive Ability: Analysis
Client Needs: Health Promotion and Maintenance
Integrated Process: Teaching and Learning
Content Area: Adult Health/Neurological

Answer: 1

Rationale: Female spinal cord trauma clients remain fertile during their reproductive years, and contraception is necessary for those who are sexually active. However, oral contraceptives may increase the risk for thrombophlebitis. Clients with paralysis should avoid dairy products to control the formation of urinary calculi. Meals should be eaten at the same time everyday, and they should include fiber and warm solid and liquid foods to promote and maintain the regular evacuation of the bowel. Clients who lack bladder control are taught to self-catheterize using clean technique.

Test-Taking Strategy: Note the strategic words "need for further discharge teaching." These words indicate a negative event query and ask you to select an option that is an incorrect statement. Remember that the key aspects of dealing with a spinal cord injury client are nutrition and elimination. Options 2, 3, and 4 address these key areas. Review the teaching points for a client with a transection of the spinalcord if you had difficulty with this question.

References
Ignatavicius, D., & Workman, M. (2006). *Medical-surgical nursing: Critical thinking for collaborative care* (5th ed., p. 994). Philadelphia: Saunders.
Lewis, S., Heitkemper, M., Dirksen, S., O'Brien, P., & Bucher, L. (2007). *Medical-surgical nursing: Assessment and management of clinical problems* (7th ed., pp. 1597, 1608). St. Louis: Mosby.

---

986. A client has been started on a monoamine oxidase inhibitor (MAOI). Which of the following should the nurse include when teaching the client about the medication?

  1 This medication can cause severe drowsiness.

  2 The client must avoid foods that contain tyramine.

  3 The medication is associated with a high rate of abuse.

  4 The medication will begin to alleviate symptoms of depression almost immediately.

Level of Cognitive Ability: Application
Client Needs: Health Promotion and Maintenance
Integrated Process: Teaching/Learning
Content Area: Pharmacology

Answer: 2

Rationale: Although MAOIs usually produce hypotension as a side effect, potentially lethal hypertension can occur if the client eats foods that contain tyramine. Such foods include aged cheeses, hot dogs, and beer, among others. Options 1, 3, and 4 are incorrect statements.

Test-Taking Strategy: Note the strategic words "monoamine oxidase inhibitor (MAOI)." Recalling that MAOIs are associated with a food-medication interaction will direct you to option 2. Review these food–medication interactions if you had difficulty with this question.

References
Kee, J., Hayes, E., & McCuistion, L. (2006). *Pharmacology: A nursing process approach.* (5th ed., p. 395). Philadelphia: Saunders.
Lehne, R. (2007). *Pharmacology for nursing care* (6th ed., p. 344). Philadelphia: Saunders.

987. A nurse is developing a plan of care for an older client with dementia and formulates a nursing diagnosis of a self-care deficit. The nurse develops which realistic outcome for the client?

1 The client will function at the highest level of independence possible.
2 The client will be admitted to a nursing home to have the needs of activities of daily living met.
3 The nursing staff will attend to all of the client's activities of daily living needs during the hospital stay.
4 The client will complete all activities of daily living independently within a 1- to 1½-hour timeframe.

Level of Cognitive Ability: Analysis
Client Needs: Health Promotion and Maintenance
Integrated Process: Nursing Process/Planning
Content Area: Mental Health

Answer: 1
Rationale: All clients, regardless of age, need to be encouraged to perform at the highest level of independence possible. This contributes to the client's sense of control and well-being. Options 2 and 3 are not client-centered goals, and a 1- to 1½-hour timeframe may not be realistic for an older client with dementia.

Test-Taking Strategy: Use the process of elimination, and focus on the strategic words "realistic outcome for the client." Eliminate options 2 and 3 first, because they are not client-centered. From the remaining options, eliminate option 4 because of the unrealistic timeframe. Review the care of the client with dementia if you had difficulty with this question.

Reference
Stuart, G., & Laraia, M. (2005). *Principles and practice of psychiatric nursing* (8th ed., p. 461). St. Louis: Mosby.

---

988. A client who is receiving haloperidol (Haldol) at bedtime is prescribed to receive benztropine mesylate (Cogentin) at the same time. The nurse explains to the client that the benztropine mesylate is given to:

1 Enhance sleep.
2 Enhance the effects of haloperidol.
3 Combat extrapyramidal syndrome (EPS).
4 Enhance the anticholinergic effects of the medications.

Level of Cognitive Ability: Application
Client Needs: Health Promotion and Maintenance
Integrated Process: Teaching and Learning
Content Area: Pharmacology

Answer: 3
Rationale: Haloperidol is a neuroleptic medication that may cause the client to experience EPS. Antiparkinsonian medications such as benztropine mesylate may be administered concurrently to decrease the symptoms of EPS. Options 1, 2, and 4 are incorrect.

Test-Taking Strategy: Focus on the name of the medication, and recall that haloperidol is a neuroleptic medication. Recalling that EPS is a concern with the use of neuroleptic medications will direct you to option 3. Review the purposes of these medications if you had difficulty with this question.

References
Kee, J., Hayes, E., & McCuistion, L. (2006). *Pharmacology: A nursing process approach.* (5th ed., p. 379). Philadelphia: Saunders.
Lehne, R. (2007). *Pharmacology for nursing care* (6th ed., p. 320) Philadelphia: Saunders.

---

989. A client is newly diagnosed with chronic obstructive pulmonary disease (COPD). The client returns home after a short hospitalization. The home-care nurse visits the client and most importantly plans teaching strategies that are designed to:

1 Promote membership in support groups.
2 Encourage the client to become a more active person.
3 Identify irritants in the home that interfere with breathing.
4 Improve oxygenation and minimize carbon dioxide retention.

Answer: 4
Rationale: Improving oxygenation and minimizing carbon dioxide retention are the primary goals. The other options are interventions that will help with the achievement of this primary goal.

Test-Taking Strategy: Note the strategic words "most importantly." Use the ABCs—airway, breathing, and circulation—to direct you to option 4. Review care of the client with COPD if you had difficulty with this question.

Level of Cognitive Ability: Application
Client Needs: Health Promotion and
    Maintenance
Integrated Process: Teaching and Learning
Content Area: Adult Health/Respiratory

Reference
Ignatavicius, D., & Workman, M. (2006). *Medical-surgical nursing: Critical thinking for collaborative care* (5th ed., p. 606). Philadelphia: Saunders.

---

990. A client is being discharged from the hospital after a bronchoscopy that was performed a day prior. After the discharge teaching, the client makes all of the following statements to the nurse. Which statement would the nurse identify as indicating a need for further teaching?
  1 "I will stop smoking my cigarettes."
  2 "I can expect to cough up bright red blood."
  3 "I will get help immediately if I start having trouble breathing."
  4 "I will use the throat lozenges as directed by the physician until my sore throat goes away."

Level of Cognitive Ability: Analysis
Client Needs: Health Promotion and
    Maintenance
Integrated Process: Teaching and Learning
Content Area: Adult Health/Respiratory

Answer: 2
Rationale: After the procedure, the client should be observed for signs of respiratory distress, including dyspnea, changes in respiratory rate, the use of accessory muscles, and changes in or absent lung sounds. Expectorated secretions are inspected for hemoptysis, and, if the client expectorates bright red blood, the physician is to be notified. The client needs to avoid smoking. A sore throat is common, and lozenges would be helpful to alleviate it.

Test-Taking Strategy: Note the strategic words "need for further teaching." These words indicate a negative event query and ask you to select an option that is an incorrect statement. Note the words "bright red" in option 2. Remember that bright red blood indicates active bleeding and that this needs to be reported to the physician. Review the care of the client after bronchoscopy if you had difficulty with this question.

References
Black, J., & Hawks, J. (2005). *Medical-surgical nursing: Clinical management for positive outcomes* (7th ed., pp. 1768-1769). Philadelphia: Saunders.
Pagana, K., & Pagana, T. (2005). *Mosby's diagnostic and laboratory test reference* (7th ed., p. 209). St. Louis: Mosby.

---

991. A client who is taking chlorpromazine (Thorazine) is preparing for discharge. When developing a health promotion plan for the client, the nurse instructs the client to:
  1 Avoid prolonged exposure to the sun.
  2 Adhere to a strict tyramine-restricted diet.
  3 Recognize the signs and symptoms of a relapse of depression.
  4 Have therapeutic blood levels drawn, because the medication has a narrow therapeutic range.

Level of Cognitive Ability: Application
Client Needs: Health Promotion and
    Maintenance
Integrated Process: Teaching and Learning
Content Area: Pharmacology

Answer: 1
Rationale: Chlorpromazine is an antipsychotic medication that is often used for the treatment of psychosis. Photosensitivity is sometimes a side effect of the phenothiazine class of antipsychotic medications to which chlorpromazine (Thorazine) belongs. Options 2, 3, and 4 are unrelated to the administration of this medication.

Test-Taking Strategy: Focus on the name of the medication. Because chlorpromazine is an antipsychotic medication, option 3 can be eliminated. Eliminate option 2, because this option relates to medications that are monoamine oxidase inhibitors. There is not a narrow range between therapeutic and toxic levels such as there is with lithium carbonate (Eskalith); therefore, option 4 can be eliminated. Review chlorpromazine if you had difficulty with this question.

Reference
Lehne, R. (2007). *Pharmacology for nursing care* (6th ed., p. 318). Philadelphia: Saunders.

992. The nurse instructs a client with hepatitis about measures to use to control fatigue. The nurse determines that the client needs additional instructions if the client states the need to:

1 Rest between activities.
2 Plan rest periods after meals.
3 Perform personal hygiene if not fatigued.
4 Complete all daily activities in the morning when the client is most rested.

Level of Cognitive Ability: Analysis
Client Needs: Health Promotion and Maintenance
Integrated Process: Teaching and Learning
Content Area: Adult Health/Gastrointestinal

Answer: 4
Rationale: A client with hepatitis has tremendous metabolic demands that lead to fatigue and that interfere with activities of daily living. The nurse encourages activities of daily living, unless they cause excessive fatigue. The client is advised to plan rest periods after activities such as meals. Activities should be spaced throughout the day with frequent planned rest periods. Clients who engage in excessive activity too early during the recovery stage may experience a relapse.

Test-Taking Strategy: Note the strategic word "needs additional instructions." These words indicate a negative event query and ask you to select an option that is an incorrect statement. Use the basic principles associated with a balance of rest and activities to answer the question. By the process of elimination, the only option that does not provide this balance is option 4. Review the measures to use to alleviate fatigue in the client with hepatitis if you had difficulty with this question.

Reference
Black, J., & Hawks, J. (2005). *Medical-surgical nursing: Clinical management for positive outcomes* (7th ed., p. 1329). Philadelphia: Saunders.

993. The nurse provides home care instructions to a client with multiple sclerosis. The nurse teaches the client to:

1 Maintain a low-fiber diet.
2 Avoid becoming pregnant.
3 Avoid taking hot baths or showers.
4 Restrict fluid intake to 1000 mL daily.

Level of Cognitive Ability: Application
Client Needs: Health Promotion and Maintenance
Integrated Process: Teaching and Learning
Content Area: Adult Health/Musculoskeletal

Answer: 3
Rationale: Because fatigue can be precipitated by warm temperatures, the client is instructed to take cool baths and to maintain a cool environmental temperature. The client should not be told to avoid pregnancy, but the nurse should assist the client with the making of informed decisions regarding pregnancy. A high-fiber diet and an adequate fluid intake of 2000 mL daily are encouraged to prevent alterations in elimination and bowel patterns.

Test-Taking Strategy: Use the process of elimination and your knowledge regarding the effects of multiple sclerosis when answering the question. Eliminate option 2 first, because it is inappropriate to tell a client to avoid pregnancy. Eliminate options 1 and 4 next, because these measures are unhealthy for this client and would promote alterations in elimination patterns. Review the teaching points related to the client with multiple sclerosis if you had difficulty with this question.

References
Black, J., & Hawks, J. (2005). *Medical-surgical nursing: Clinical management for positive outcomes* (7th ed., p. 2180). Philadelphia: Saunders.
Monahan, F., Sands, J., Neighbors, M., Marek, J., & Green, C. (2007). *Phipps' medical-surgical nursing: Health and illness perspectives* (8th ed., p. 1444). St. Louis: Mosby.

994. The home-care nurse provides instructions to the client with a halo vest. The nurse tells the client to:
1 Loosen the bolts once a day for bathing.
2 Have the spouse use the metal frame to assist the client to sit up.
3 Carry the correct-size wrench to loosen the bolts during an emergency.
4 Perform pin care three times a week using hydrogen peroxide or alcohol.

Level of Cognitive Ability: Application
Client Needs: Health Promotion and Maintenance
Integrated Process: Teaching and Learning
Content Area: Adult Health/Neurological

Answer: 3
Rationale: The bolts should never be loosened except in an emergency. In fact, the physician should be notified if the bolts loosen. The client is instructed to carry the correct-size wrench in case of an emergency requiring cardiopulmonary resuscitation (CPR). In such a situation, the anterior portion of the vest, including the anterior bolts, will need to be loosened, and the posterior portion should remain in place to provide stability for the spine during CPR. The metal frame is never used or pulled on for turning or lifting. Pin care should be performed at least once a day using soap and water with cotton-tipped or alcohol swabs.

Test-Taking Strategy: Try to visualize the appearance of a halo vest. Recall that the purpose of this vest is to stabilize a cervical fracture. Eliminate option 4 first, because pin care should be done at least once a day. Eliminate option 2, because pulling on the frame will disrupt the stabilization of the fracture and possibly lead to serious complications. Remember that bolts should never be loosened except in an emergency situation. Review the home-care instructions for a client with a halo vest if you had difficulty with this question.

References
Ignatavicius, D., & Workman, M. (2006). *Medical-surgical nursing: Critical thinking for collaborative care* (5th ed., p. 990). Philadelphia: Saunders.
Lewis, S., Heitkemper, M., Dirksen, S., O'Brien, P., & Bucher, L. (2007). *Medical-surgical nursing: Assessment and management of clinical problems* (7th ed., p. 1606). St. Louis: Mosby.

995. Haloperidol (Haldol) has been prescribed for a client with Tourette syndrome, and the nurse instructs the client about the medication. Which statement by the client indicates the need for further instructions?
1 "It may take 6 weeks before the medication works."
2 "I need to avoid alcohol while taking this medication."
3 "The drowsiness will probably go away as I continue the medication."
4 "I should stop the medication immediately if my vision becomes blurred."

Level of Cognitive Ability: Analysis
Client Needs: Health Promotion and Maintenance
Integrated Process: Teaching and Learning
Content Area: Pharmacology

Answer: 4
Rationale: The client needs to be instructed to not abruptly stop taking the medication. The client is informed that, if visual disturbances occur, the physician should be notified. Options 1, 2, and 3 are accurate statements regarding the medication.

Test-Taking Strategy: Use the process of elimination, and focus on the strategic words "need for further instructions." These words indicate a negative event query and ask you to select an option that is an incorrect statement. Eliminate option 2 first, because this is a general principle with most medications. Knowledge that this medication is an antipsychotic will assist you with eliminating options 1 and 3. Additionally, knowing that the medication should not be abruptly stopped will assist with directing you to option 4. Review haloperidol if you had difficulty with this question.

References
Hodgson, B., & Kizior, R. (2007). *Saunders nursing drug handbook 2007* (p. 570). Philadelphia: Saunders.
Skidmore-Roth, L. (2008). *Mosby's nursing drug reference* (21st ed., p. 523). St. Louis: Mosby.

996. A client with diabetes mellitus has received instructions about foot care. Which statement by the client would indicate that the client needs further instructions?

1 "I'll trim my nails straight across after my bath."
2 "My feet should be inspected daily using a mirror."
3 "The cuticles of my nails must be cut to prevent overgrowth."
4 "Cotton stockings should be worn to absorb excess moisture."

Level of Cognitive Ability: Analysis
Client Needs: Health Promotion and Maintenance
Integrated Process: Teaching and Learning
Content Area: Adult Health/Endocrine

Answer: 3
Rationale: Trimming or cutting the cuticles of the nails can lead to injury to the foot by scratching the skin. Even small injuries can be dangerous to the client with diabetes mellitus who has decreased peripheral vascular circulation. A manicure stick can be used to gently push the cuticle back under the nail. Nails can be cut straight across; after a bath is the best time, because the nails are softest then. White cotton stockings are best, and the client needs to inspect the feet daily. The client can use a mirror for those areas that are difficult to inspect.

Test-Taking Strategy: Use the process of elimination, noting the strategic words "needs further instructions." These words indicate a negative event query and ask you to select an option that is an incorrect statement. Look for the option that could result in altered skin integrity. Using this principle, eliminate options 1, 2, and 4. Review diabetic foot care if you had difficulty with this question.

Reference
Ignatavicius, D., & Workman, M. (2006). *Medical-surgical nursing: Critical thinking for collaborative care* (5th ed., pp. 1535-1537). Philadelphia: Saunders.

---

997. The nurse has taught a client about the signs and symptoms and treatment of hyperglycemia. Which statement by the client reflects an accurate understanding?

1 "I may become diaphoretic and faint."
2 "I may notice that I have dry skin and increased urination and thirst."
3 "I should restrict my fluid intake if my blood glucose level is more than 250 mg/dL."
4 "I need to take an extra diabetic pill if my blood glucose level is more than 300 mg/dL."

Level of Cognitive Ability: Analysis
Client Needs: Health Promotion and Maintenance
Integrated Process: Nursing Process/Evaluation
Content Area: Adult Health/Endocrine

Answer: 2
Rationale: Dry skin, polyuria (excess urination), and polydipsia (excess thirst) are classic symptoms of hyperglycemia. Dry skin occurs as a result of dehydration related to the polyuria. Polydipsia occurs as a result of fluid loss. Diaphoresis is associated with hypoglycemia. Clients should not take extra oral hypoglycemic agents to reduce an elevated blood glucose level. A client with hyperglycemia becomes dehydrated as a result of the osmotic effect of elevated glucose; therefore, the client must increase fluid intake.

Test-Taking Strategy: Note the strategic words "reflects an accurate understanding," and focus on the subject—hyperglycemia. Recalling that polyuria and polydipsia are signs of hyperglycemia will direct you to option 2. Review these signs if you had difficulty with this question.

Reference
Ignatavicius, D., & Workman, M. (2006). *Medical-surgical nursing: Critical thinking for collaborative care* (5th ed., p. 1541). Philadelphia: Saunders.

---

998. A client taking famotidine (Pepcid) asks the home-care nurse what would be the best medication to take for a headache. The nurse tells the client that it would be best to take:

1 Ibuprofen (Motrin)
2 Naproxen (Naprosyn)
3 Acetaminophen (Tylenol)
4 Aspirin (acetylsalicylic acid)

Answer: 3
Rationale: The client is taking famotidine, which is a histamine receptor antagonist. This implies that the client has a disorder characterized by gastrointestinal (GI) irritation. The only medication of the ones listed in the options that is not irritating to the GI tract is acetaminophen. The other medications could aggravate an already existing GI problem.

Level of Cognitive Ability: Application
Client Needs: Health Promotion and Maintenance
Integrated Process: Teaching and Learning
Content Area: Pharmacology

Test-Taking Strategy: Note the medication that the client is taking. Recalling that this medication is used for GI irritation will direct you to option 3. Also, note that options 1, 2, and 4 are comparable or alike and that they are anti-inflammatory medications. Review the listed medications if you had difficulty with this question.

References
Hodgson, B., & Kizior, R. (2007). *Saunders nursing drug handbook 2007* (p. 463). Philadelphia: Saunders.
Lehne, R. (2007). *Pharmacology for nursing care* (6th ed., pp. 893, 902). Philadelphia: Saunders.

---

999. A nurse is teaching the client who is taking cyclosporine (Sandimmune) after renal transplant about the medication. The nurse tells the client to be especially alert for:

1 Hair loss
2 Weight loss
3 Hypotension
4 Signs of infection

Level of Cognitive Ability: Application
Client Needs: Health Promotion and Maintenance
Integrated Process: Teaching and Learning
Content Area: Pharmacology

Answer: 4
Rationale: Cyclosporine is an immunosuppressant medication that is used to prevent transplant rejection. The client should be especially alert for signs and symptoms of infection while taking this medication and report them to the physician if they occur. The client is also taught about other side effects of the medication, including hypertension, increased facial hair, tremors, gingival hyperplasia, and gastrointestinal complaints.

Test-Taking Strategy: Recalling that cyclosporine is an immunosuppressant and that the client is at risk for infection while taking this medication will direct you to option 4. Review the client teaching points related to cyclosporine if you had difficulty with this question.

Reference
Skidmore-Roth, L. (2008). *Mosby's nursing drug reference* (21st ed., p. 317). St. Louis: Mosby.

1000. A client has undergone surgery for glaucoma. The nurse provides which discharge instructions to the client?

1 The sutures are removed after 1 week.
2 Wound healing usually takes 12 weeks.
3 Expect that vision will be permanently impaired.
4 A shield or eye patch should be worn to protect the eye.

Level of Cognitive Ability: Application
Client Needs: Health Promotion and Maintenance
Integrated Process: Teaching and Learning
Content Area: Adult Health/Eye

Answer: 4
Rationale: After ocular surgery, the client should wear an eye patch or eyeglasses for the protection of the eye. Healing takes place in about 6 weeks. When the postoperative inflammation subsides, the client's vision should return to the preoperative level of acuity. Sutures are usually absorbable.

Test-Taking Strategy: Use the process of elimination, and focus on the subject—ocular surgery. Recalling that the eye requires protection after surgery will direct you to option 4. Review postoperative teaching points after eye surgery if you had difficulty with this question.

References
Black, J., & Hawks, J. (2005). *Medical-surgical nursing: Clinical management for positive outcomes* (7th ed., p. 1951). Philadelphia: Saunders.
Ignatavicius, D., & Workman, M. (2006). *Medical-surgical nursing: Critical thinking for collaborative care* (5th ed., pp. 1096-1097). Philadelphia: Saunders.

1001. A client has undergone surgery for cataracts. The nurse instructs the client to call the physician for which of the following complaints?
1 A sudden decrease in vision
2 A gradual resolution of eye redness
3 Eye pain relieved by acetaminophen (Tylenol)
4 Small amounts of dried matter on the eyelashes after sleep

Level of Cognitive Ability: Application
Client Needs: Health Promotion and Maintenance
Integrated Process: Teaching and Learning
Content Area: Adult Health/Eye

Answer: 1
Rationale: The client should report a noticeable or sudden decrease in vision to the physician. The eye may be slightly reddened postoperatively, but this should gradually resolve. The client is taught to take acetaminophen, which is usually effective for relieving discomfort. Small amounts of dried material may be present on the lashes after sleep; this is expected and should be removed with a warm facecloth.

Test-Taking Strategy: Use the process of elimination, and note the strategic words "call the physician." Noting the words "sudden decrease" in option 1 will direct you to this option. Review the home-care instructions after eye surgery if you had difficulty with this question.

Reference
Black, J., & Hawks, J. (2005). *Medical-surgical nursing: Clinical management for positive outcomes* (7th ed., p. 1951). Philadelphia: Saunders.

1002. The home-care nurse visits a client with a diagnosis of cirrhosis and ascites. The nurse provides dietary instructions and tells the client to:
1 Restrict sodium intake.
2 Maintain a low-calorie diet.
3 Decrease carbohydrate intake.
4 Restrict calories to 1500 daily.

Level of Cognitive Ability: Application
Client Needs: Health Promotion and Maintenance
Integrated Process: Nursing Process/ Implementation
Content Area: Adult Health/Gastrointestinal

Answer: 1
Rationale: If the client has ascites, sodium and possibly fluids should be restricted in the diet. The client should follow a high-caloric, high-carbohydrate diet to maintain the weight and spare protein. The diet should provide ample protein to rebuild tissue but not enough protein to precipitate hepatic encephalopathy.

Test-Taking Strategy: Focus on the client's diagnosis—cirrhosis and ascites. Recalling that ascites indicates the accumulation of fluid will direct you to option 1. Review the dietary measures for the client with cirrhosis and ascites if you had difficulty with this question.

Reference
Ignatavicius, D., & Workman, M. (2006). *Medical-surgical nursing: Critical thinking for collaborative care* (5th ed., p. 1375). Philadelphia: Saunders.

1003. The nurse is preparing a client with a diagnosis of multiple myeloma for discharge. The nurse tells the client to:
1 Maintain bedrest.
2 Restrict fluid intake to 1000 mL daily.
3 Maintain a high-calorie, low-fiber diet.
4 Notify the physician if anorexia and nausea occur and persist.

Level of Cognitive Ability: Application
Client Needs: Health Promotion and Maintenance
Integrated Process: Teaching and Learning
Content Area: Adult Health/Oncology

Answer: 4
Rationale: Clients with multiple myeloma need to be taught to monitor for signs of hypercalcemia and to report them immediately to the physician. Anorexia, nausea, vomiting, polyuria, weakness, fatigue, constipation, and signs of dehydration are signs of moderate hypercalcemia. Activity is encouraged. A fluid intake of 3000 mL daily is required to dilute the calcium overload and to prevent protein from precipitating in the renal tubules. Although a high-calorie diet is encouraged, a low-fiber diet can lead to constipation.

Test-Taking Strategy: Recall that hypercalcemia is a concern for clients with multiple myeloma. Eliminate option 1, because bedrest will promote hypercalcemia. Next, eliminate option 2, because this amount of fluid is rather low. Finally, eliminate option 3, because a low-fiber diet can lead to constipation. Review the signs of hypercalcemia if you had difficulty with this question.

Reference
Ignatavicius, D., & Workman, M. (2006). *Medical-surgical nursing: Critical thinking for collaborative care* (5th ed., p. 241). Philadelphia: Saunders.

1004. The nurse provides discharge instructions to the client who had a mastectomy and axillary lymph node dissection. The nurse teaches the client to:
1 Avoid the use of insect repellent.
2 Wear protective gloves when doing the dishes.
3 Avoid the use of lanolin hand cream on the affected arm.
4 Cut the cuticles on the nails carefully using clean cuticle scissors.

Level of Cognitive Ability: Application
Client Needs: Health Promotion and Maintenance
Integrated Process: Teaching and Learning
Content Area: Adult Health/Oncology

Answer: 2
Rationale: After axillary lymph node dissection, the affected arm may swell and be at risk for infection. The client needs to be instructed regarding the several measures required to prevent complications. Protective gloves should be worn while doing dishes and cleaning. The client should use insect repellent to avoid bites and stings. Lanolin hand cream should be applied a few times daily. Picking at or cutting the cuticles should not be done, because this could cause an alteration in skin integrity and result in infection.

Test-Taking Strategy: Note the client's diagnosis, and focus on the subject—preventing altered skin integrity and thus infection. Keeping this in mind will assist you with eliminating options 1, 3, and 4, all of which could potentially lead to a skin alteration. Review the client teaching points related to mastectomy and lymph node dissection if you had difficulty with this question.

References
Black, J., & Hawks, J. (2005). *Medical-surgical nursing: Clinical management for positive outcomes* (7th ed., p. 1108). Philadelphia: Saunders.
Monahan, F., Sands, J., Neighbors, M., Marek, J., & Green, C. (2007). *Phipps' medical-surgical nursing: Health and illness perspectives* (8th ed., p. 1771). St. Louis: Mosby.

1005. A client is receiving a course of chemotherapy on an outpatient basis for the diagnosis of lung cancer. Which home-care instruction should the nurse provide to the client?
1 A bathroom can be shared with any member of the family.
2 Urinary and bowel excreta are not considered contaminated.
3 Disposable plates and plastic utensils must be used during the entire course of chemotherapy.
4 Contaminated linens should be washed separately and then washed a second time, if necessary.

Level of Cognitive Ability: Application
Client Needs: Health Promotion and Maintenance
Integrated Process: Teaching and Learning
Content Area: Adult Health/Oncology

Answer: 4
Rationale: The client may excrete the chemotherapeutic agent for 48 hours or more after administration, depending on the medication administered. Blood, emesis, and excreta may be considered contaminated during this time, and the client should not share a bathroom with children or pregnant women during this time. Any contaminated linens or clothing should be washed separately and then washed a second time, if necessary. All contaminated disposable items should be sealed in plastic bags and disposed of as hazardous waste. Option 3 is unnecessary.

Test-Taking Strategy: Use the process of elimination. Eliminate options 1 and 2 first, because they are comparable or alike. Eliminate option 3 next, because it would seem unreasonable to have to use disposable utensils for the "entire" course of therapy. Also note the close-ended word "must" in option 3. Review the client teaching points related to chemotherapy if you had difficulty with this question.

References
Black, J., & Hawks, J. (2005). *Medical-surgical nursing: Clinical management for positive outcomes* (7th ed., pp. 374-375). Philadelphia: Saunders.
Monahan, F., Sands, J., Neighbors, M., Marek, J., & Green, C. (2007). *Phipps' medical-surgical nursing: Health and illness perspectives* (8th ed., p. 553). St. Louis: Mosby.

1006. The home-care nurse visits a client with bowel cancer who recently received a course of chemotherapy. The client has developed stomatitis, and the nurse provides instructions to the client about the care of the mouth. The nurse determines that the client needs further instructions if the client states the need to:

1 Eat foods without spices.
2 Maintain a diet of soft foods.
3 Drink juices that are not citrus.
4 Drink foods and liquids that are hot.

Level of Cognitive Ability: Analysis
Client Needs: Health Promotion and Maintenance
Integrated Process: Teaching and Learning
Content Area: Adult Health/Oncology

Answer: 4
Rationale: *Stomatitis* is a term that is used to describe the inflammation and ulceration of the mucosal lining of the mouth. Dietary modifications for this condition include avoiding extremely hot foods, spices, and citrus fruits and juices. The client should be instructed to eat soft foods and to take nutritional supplements as prescribed. Food and fluid should be lukewarm or cold.

Test-Taking Strategy: Note the words "needs further instructions." These words indicate a negative event query and ask you to select an option that is an incorrect statement. Recalling that stomatitis is an inflammation of the mucosal lining of the mouth will assist you with eliminating options 1, 2, and 3, because these measures will alleviate further irritation and prevent discomfort. Review the client teaching points for stomatitis if you had difficulty with this question.

References
Black, J., & Hawks, J. (2005). *Medical-surgical nursing: Clinical management for positive outcomes* (7th ed., p. 386). Philadelphia: Saunders.
Lewis, S., Heitkemper, M., Dirksen, S., O'Brien, P., & Bucher, L. (2007). *Medical-surgical nursing: Assessment and management of clinical problems* (7th ed., pp. 295, 1000). St. Louis: Mosby.

1007. A home-care nurse provides instructions to a breast-feeding postpartum client who has developed breast engorgement. The nurse tells the client to:

1 Avoid the use of a bra during engorgement.
2 Apply cool packs to both breasts 20 minutes before a feeding.
3 Gently massage the breast from the outer areas to the nipple during feeding.
4 Feed the infant less frequently, every 4 to 6 hours, and use bottle-feeding in between.

Level of Cognitive Ability: Application
Client Needs: Health Promotion and Maintenance
Integrated Process: Teaching and Learning
Content Area: Maternity/Postpartum

Answer: 3
Rationale: The client with breast engorgement should be advised to breast-feed frequently: at least every 2½ hours for 15 to 20 minutes per side. Moist heat should be applied to both breasts for about 20 minutes before a feeding. Between feedings, the mother should wear a supportive bra. During a feeding, it is helpful to gently massage the breast from the outer areas to the nipple to stimulate the let-down and flow of milk.

Test-Taking Strategy: Note the client's diagnosis: breast engorgement. Think about the manifestations that occur with engorgement, and recall that measures are initiated to facilitate the flow of milk. With this concept in mind, eliminate options 1, 2, and 4, because they will not facilitate the flow of milk. Review the measures that are used for breast engorgement if you had difficulty with this question.

References
Murray, S., & McKinney, E. (2006). *Foundations of maternal-newborn nursing* (4th ed., pp. 555-557). Philadelphia: Saunders.
Wong, D., Hockenberry, M., Perry, S., Lowdermilk, D., & Wilson, D. (2006). *Maternal-child nursing care* (3rd ed., pp. 783-784). St. Louis: Mosby.

1008. A client in the third trimester of pregnancy arrives at the clinic and tells the nurse that she frequently has a backache. Which instructions would the nurse provide to the client to alleviate the backache?
1 Eat small meals frequently.
2 Elevate the legs when sitting.
3 Perform pelvic rock exercises.
4 Sleep in a supine position and on a firm mattress.

Level of Cognitive Ability: Application
Client Needs: Health Promotion and Maintenance
Integrated Process: Teaching and Learning
Content Area: Maternity/Antepartum

Answer: 3
Rationale: To provide relief from backache, the nurse would advise the client to use good posture and body mechanics, to perform pelvic rock exercises, and to wear flat, supportive shoes. The client may also be advised to wear a maternity girdle, to avoid overexertion, and to sleep in the lateral position on a firm mattress. Back massage is also helpful. Eating small meals would more specifically assist with the relief of dyspnea. Leg elevation assists the client with varicosities.

Test-Taking Strategy: Use the process of elimination, keeping in mind that the subject of the question is backache. This should assist you with eliminating options 1 and 2, because they are unrelated to the relief of backache. From the remaining options, recalling that the lateral position is most appropriate for the pregnant client will assist with directing you to option 3. Review the relief measures for backache if you had difficulty with this question.

Reference
Murray, S., & McKinney, E. (2006). *Foundations of maternal-newborn nursing* (4th ed., pp. 137, 140). Philadelphia: Saunders.

1009. A nurse provides dietary instructions to the client receiving spironolactone (Aldactone). Which food item would the nurse instruct the client to avoid while taking this medication?
1 Shrimp
2 Apricots
3 Popcorn
4 Crackers

Level of Cognitive Ability: Application
Client Needs: Health Promotion and Maintenance
Integrated Process: Teaching and Learning
Content Area: Pharmacology

Answer: 2
Rationale: Spironolactone is a potassium-sparing diuretic, and the client needs to avoid foods that are high in potassium, such as whole-grain cereals, legumes, meat, bananas, apricots, orange juice, potatoes, and raisins. Option 2 provides the highest source of potassium and should be avoided.

Test-Taking Strategy: Use the process of elimination, and note the strategic word "avoid." Recall that this medication is a potassium-sparing diuretic. Eliminate options 3 and 4, because they are food items that are comparable or alike. Remembering that fruits, vegetables, and fresh meats are high in potassium will direct you to option 2 as the food to avoid. Review spironolactone if you had difficulty with this question.

References
Lehne, R. (2007). *Pharmacology for nursing care* (6th ed., p. 446). Philadelphia: Saunders.
Skidmore-Roth, L. (2007). *2007 Mosby's nursing drug reference* (20th ed., p. 922). St. Louis: Mosby.

1010. Oral lactulose (Chronulac) is prescribed for a client with a hepatic disorder, and the home-care nurse provides instructions to the client regarding the medication. The nurse determines that the client needs additional instructions if the client states the need to:

1 Increase fluid intake.
2 Increase fiber in the diet.
3 Take the medication with water.
4 Notify the physician immediately if nausea occurs.

Level of Cognitive Ability: Analysis
Client Needs: Health Promotion and Maintenance
Integrated Process: Teaching and Learning
Content Area: Pharmacology

Answer: 4

Rationale: Lactulose retains ammonia in the colon and promotes increased peristalsis and bowel evacuation to expel ammonia from the colon. It should be taken with water or juice to aid in the softening of the stool. An increased fluid intake and a high-fiber diet will promote defecation. If nausea occurs, the client should be instructed to drink cola or to eat unsalted crackers or dry toast. Notifying the physician immediately is not necessary.

Test-Taking Strategy: Use the process of elimination, and note the strategic words "needs additional instructions." These words indicate a negative event query and ask you to select an option that is an incorrect statement. Eliminate options 1, 2, and 3, because they are comparable or alike in that they will promote defecation. Also, recall that measures can be provided to the client to relieve nausea before the physician needs to be notified. Review the client teaching points related to oral lactulose if you had difficulty with this question.

References

Lehne, R. (2007). *Pharmacology for nursing care* (6th ed., p. 908). Philadelphia: Saunders.

Skidmore-Roth, L. (2007). *2007 Mosby's nursing drug reference* (20th ed., p. 587). St. Louis: Mosby.

1011. A client with leukemia receives a course of chemotherapy. The home-care nurse who is scheduled to visit the client receives a telephone call from the client's physician. The physician informs the nurse that the client's neutrophil count is 600/mm³. On the basis of this laboratory value, the home-care nurse tells the client to avoid doing which of the following?

1 Straining at bowel movements
2 Using a straight razor for shaving
3 Eating any raw fruits or vegetables
4 Taking aspirin or medications that contain aspirin

Level of Cognitive Ability: Application
Client Needs: Health Promotion and Maintenance
Integrated Process: Teaching and Learning
Content Area: Adult Health/Oncology

Answer: 3

Rationale: Neutrophil counts should range between 3000 and 5800/mm³. A low neutrophil count places the client at risk for infection. When the client is at risk for infection, he or she should avoid exposure to individuals with colds or infections. All live plants, flowers, and objects that may harbor bacteria should be removed from the client's environment. The client should be on a low-bacteria diet and avoid eating any raw fruits and vegetables. Options 1, 2, and 4 are measures that would be implemented if the client was at risk for bleeding.

Test-Taking Strategy: Use the process of elimination. Recalling that a low neutrophil count places the client at risk for infection will direct you to option 3. Also, bearing in mind that the subject of the question relates to infection will assist you with eliminating options 1, 2, and 4, because these options identify measures that reduce the risk of bleeding. Review the care of the client with a low neutrophil count if you had difficulty with this question.

References

Ignatavicius, D., & Workman, M. (2006). *Medical-surgical nursing: Critical thinking for collaborative care* (5th ed., p. 497). Philadelphia: Saunders.

Monahan, F., Sands, J., Neighbors, M., Marek, J., & Green, C. (2007). *Phipps' medical-surgical nursing: Health and illness perspectives* (8th ed., p. 556). St. Louis: Mosby.

1012. The nurse provides instructions to the client who received cryosurgery for a local stage 0 cervical tumor. The nurse tells the client:

1 To avoid tub baths
2 To call the physician if a watery discharge occurs
3 That pain indicates a complication of the procedure
4 To call the physician if the discharge remains odorous after 1 week

Level of Cognitive Ability: Application
Client Needs: Health Promotion and Maintenance
Integrated Process: Nursing Process/ Implementation
Content Area: Adult Health/Oncology

Answer: 1
Rationale: Healing takes about 10 weeks. Showers or sponge baths should be taken during this time; tub baths and sitz baths need to be avoided. Mild pain may occur and continue for several days after this procedure. A clear, watery discharge is expected. For about 14 days, this is followed by discharge that contains debris, which may be odorous. If the discharge continues for more than 8 weeks, an infection is suspected.

Test-Taking Strategy: Use the process of elimination. Think about the anatomical area of the body in terms of where this procedure is performed. It would seem likely that the client would be instructed to avoid tub baths after this procedure. Review the teaching points related to cryosurgery if you had difficulty with this question.

Reference
Black, J., & Hawks, J. (2005). *Medical-surgical nursing: Clinical management for positive outcomes* (7th ed., p. 1076). Philadelphia: Saunders.

1013. A home-care nurse provides instructions to the client taking 0.25 mg of digoxin (Lanoxin) daily. Which client statement would indicate the need for further instructions?

1 "I will check my pulse before I take my medication."
2 "I will carry a medication identification card with me."
3 "I will take my prescribed antacid if I become nauseated."
4 "It is important to have my blood drawn when prescribed."

Level of Cognitive Ability: Analysis
Client Needs: Health Promotion and Maintenance
Integrated Process: Teaching and Learning
Content Area: Pharmacology

Answer: 3
Rationale: Digoxin is an antidysrhythmic. The most common early manifestations of toxicity are gastrointestinal (GI) disturbances such as anorexia, nausea, and vomiting. Digoxin blood levels need to be obtained as prescribed to monitor for therapeutic plasma levels (0.5 to 2.0 ng/mL). The client is instructed to take the pulse, to hold the medication if the pulse is less than 60 beats/ minute, and to notify the physician. The client is instructed to wear or carry an identification bracelet or card.

Test-Taking Strategy: Use the process of elimination, and recall that toxicity can occur with the use of this medication. Also, note the strategic words "the need for further instructions." These words indicate a negative event query and ask you to select an option that is an incorrect statement. Remembering that GI disturbances are the earliest signs of digoxin toxicity will assist with directing you to option 3. Review digoxin if you had difficulty with this question.

Reference
Skidmore-Roth, L. (2008). *Mosby's nursing drug reference* (21st ed., p. 364). St. Louis: Mosby.

1014. The nurse is providing immediate post-procedure care to a client who had a thoracentesis to relieve a tension pneumothorax that resulted from rib fractures. The goal is to have the client exhibit normal respiratory functioning. The nurse provides instructions to assist the client with achieving this goal. Which statement by the client indicates that further instructions are needed?

1 "I will lie on the affected side for an hour."
2 "I can expect a chest x-ray to be done shortly."
3 "I will let you know at once if I have trouble breathing."
4 "I will notify you if I feel a crackling sensation on my chest."

Level of Cognitive Ability: Analysis
Client Needs: Health Promotion and Maintenance
Integrated Process: Teaching and Learning
Content Area: Adult Health/Respiratory

Answer: 1
Rationale: After the procedure, the client is usually turned onto the unaffected side for 1 hour to facilitate lung expansion. A chest x-ray examination may be performed to evaluate the degree of lung reexpansion or pneumothorax. Tachypnea, dyspnea, cyanosis, retractions, or diminished breath sounds, which may indicate pneumothorax, should be reported to the physician. Subcutaneous emphysema may occur after this procedure, because air in the pleural cavity leaks into the subcutaneous tissues. The tissues feel like lumpy paper and crackle when palpated (crepitus). Usually subcutaneous emphysema causes no problems unless it is increasing and constricting vital organs such as the trachea.

Test-Taking Strategy: Note the strategic words "further instructions are needed." These words indicate a negative event query and ask you to select an option that is an incorrect statement. Focus on the subject of postprocedure care after thoracentesis, and recall that facilitating lung expansion is important. Noting the words "affected side" in option 1 will direct you to this option. Review the postprocedure care for a thoracentesis if you had difficulty with this question.

References
Black, J., & Hawks, J. (2005). *Medical-surgical nursing: Clinical management for positive outcomes* (7th ed., p. 1772). Philadelphia: Saunders.
Pagana, K., & Pagana, T. (2005). *Mosby's diagnostic and laboratory test reference* (7th ed., p. 902). St. Louis: Mosby.

1015. As the nurse prepares an older female client for discharge, she states "I don't know how I'll be able to remember all these instructions and take care of myself at home." The nurse plans which of the following actions to assist the client?

1 Delay the discharge until the client can provide effective self-care.
2 Ask an out-of-town relative to stay with the client for several days.
3 Ask the social worker to follow up with telephone calls to the client.
4 Collaborate for a home health care referral for nursing care and support.

Level of Cognitive Ability: Application
Client Needs: Health Promotion and Maintenance
Integrated Process: Nursing Process/Planning
Content Area: Fundamental Skills

Answer: 4
Rationale: Following hospital discharge, a client can require support from a home health nurse until he or she can perform self-care independently. Discharge should not be delayed as a result of a client's need for additional teaching, because teaching can be provided in the home. Finding an out-of-town relative is likely to delay the discharge until the relative arrives, and it does not ensure that the client will receive the proper care at home. A social worker cannot provide nursing care, but a referral to social services can be helpful for other client-related issues. Option 4 ensures that the client has necessary assistance for as long as is required.

Test-Taking Strategy: Use the process of elimination, and focus on the client's need to perform self-care. Note that option 4 is the umbrella option and that it ensures client assistance at home. Review the home-care resources after hospital discharge if you had difficulty with this question.

References
Black, J., & Hawks, J. (2005). *Medical-surgical nursing: Clinical management for positive outcomes* (7th ed., pp. 170, 173). Philadelphia: Saunders.
Potter, P., & Perry, A. (2005). *Fundamentals of nursing* (6th ed., p. 36). St. Louis: Mosby.

1016. A client who has been newly diagnosed with angina pectoris asks the nurse how to prevent future angina attacks. The nurse plans to incorporate which instruction in a teaching session?

1 Eat fewer, larger meals for more efficient digestion.
2 Dress appropriately in very cold or very hot weather.
3 Adjust medication doses freely until your symptoms do not recur.
4 Plan all activities for early in the morning, when you are the most rested.

Level of Cognitive Ability: Application
Client Needs: Health Promotion and Maintenance
Integrated Process: Teaching and Learning
Content Area: Adult Health/Cardiovascular

Answer: 2
Rationale: Anginal episodes are triggered by events such as eating heavy meals, straining during bowel movements, smoking, over-exertion, and experiencing emotional upset or temperature extremes. Medication therapy is monitored and regulated by the physician.

Test-Taking Strategy: Use the process of elimination, and focus on the subject—preventing angina attacks. Recalling the causes of chest pain and the principles of medication therapy will direct you to option 2. Review the teaching points for the client with angina if you had difficulty with this question.

References
Black, J., & Hawks, J. (2005). *Medical-surgical nursing: Clinical management for positive outcomes* (7th ed., p. 1706). Philadelphia: Saunders.
Lewis, S., Heitkemper, M., Dirksen, S., O'Brien, P., & Bucher, L. (2007). *Medical-surgical nursing: Assessment and management of clinical problems* (7th ed., p. 797). St. Louis: Mosby.

1017. The nurse has performed a nutritional assessment for a client with cystitis. The nurse tells the client to consume which of the following beverages to minimize the recurrence of cystitis?

1 Tea
2 Water
3 Coffee
4 White wine

Level of Cognitive Ability: Application
Client Needs: Health Promotion and Maintenance
Integrated Process: Nursing Process/ Implementation
Content Area: Adult Health/Renal

Answer: 2
Rationale: Water helps flush bacteria out of the bladder, and an intake of 6 to 8 glasses per day is encouraged. Caffeine and alcohol can irritate the bladder. Therefore, alcohol and caffeine-containing beverages such as coffee, tea, and wine are avoided to minimize risk.

Test-Taking Strategy: Use the process of elimination. Option 4 is eliminated first, because alcohol intake is not encouraged for any disorder. Options 1 and 3 are comparable or alike in that they both contain caffeine. Thus, it is unlikely that either of these are the correct options. Review the client teaching points related to the prevention of cystitis if you had difficulty with this question.

References
Black, J., & Hawks, J. (2005). *Medical-surgical nursing: Clinical management for positive outcomes* (7th ed., p. 860). Philadelphia: Saunders.
Lewis, S., Heitkemper, M., Dirksen, S., O'Brien, P., & Bucher, L. (2007). *Medical-surgical nursing: Assessment and management of clinical problems* (7th ed., pp. 1159, 1161). St. Louis: Mosby.

1018. The home-care nurse has given instructions to a female client with cystitis about measures to help prevent recurrence. Which statement made by the client indicates the need for further instructions?

1 "I will avoid wearing pantyhose while wearing slacks."
2 "I should take bubble baths for more effective hygiene."
3 "I should drink a glass of water and void after intercourse."
4 "I will wear underwear made of cotton or with cotton panels."

Answer: 2
Rationale: Measures to prevent cystitis include increasing fluid intake to 3 L per day; eating an acid–ash diet; wiping front to back after urination; taking showers instead of tub baths; drinking water and voiding after intercourse; avoiding bubble baths, feminine hygiene sprays, and perfumed toilet tissue or sanitary pads; and wearing clothes that "breathe" (cotton pants, no tight jeans, no pantyhose under slacks). Other measures include teaching pregnant women to void every 2 hours and teaching menopausal women to use estrogen vaginal creams to restore the vaginal pH.

Level of Cognitive Ability: Analysis
Client Needs: Health Promotion and
   Maintenance
Integrated Process: Teaching and Learning
Content Area: Adult Health/Renal

Test-Taking Strategy: Note the strategic words "need for further instructions." These words indicate a negative event query and ask you to select an option that is an incorrect statement. Eliminate option 3 first, because drinking water is a basic measure for preventing cystitis. Next, eliminate options 1 and 4, because they are comparable or alike. Review the teaching measures to prevent cystitis if you had difficulty with this question.

References

Ignatavicius, D., & Workman, M. (2006). *Medical-surgical nursing: Critical thinking for collaborative care* (5th ed., p. 1684). Philadelphia: Saunders.

Lewis, S., Heitkemper, M., Dirksen, S., O'Brien, P., & Bucher, L. (2007). *Medical-surgical nursing: Assessment and management of clinical problems* (7th ed., p. 1161). St. Louis: Mosby.

1019. A client with pyelonephritis is being discharged from the hospital, and the nurse provides the client with discharge instructions to prevent recurrence. The nurse determines that the client understands the information that was given if the client states an intention to:

1 Take the prescribed antibiotics until all symptoms subside.
2 Modify fluid intake for the day on the basis of the previous day's output.
3 Return to the physician's office for the scheduled follow-up urine cultures.
4 Report any signs and symptoms of urinary tract infection (UTI) if they persist for more than 1 week.

Level of Cognitive Ability: Analysis
Client Needs: Health Promotion and
   Maintenance
Integrated Process: Nursing Process/Evaluation
Content Area: Adult Health/Renal

Answer: 3

Rationale: The client with pyelonephritis should take the full course of antibiotic therapy that has been prescribed and return to the physician's office for follow-up urine cultures if so instructed. The client should learn the signs and symptoms of UTI and report them immediately if they occur. The client should use all measures that are used to prevent cystitis, including consuming up to 3 L of fluid per day.

Test-Taking Strategy: Use the process of elimination. Eliminate option 4 first, because UTI symptoms should never go unreported for a week. Option 1 is eliminated next, because antibiotics should be taken for the full course of treatment for the adequate elimination of the infection. From the remaining options, recalling the importance of increased fluids will direct you to option 3. Review the client teaching points related to pyelonephritis if you had difficulty with this question.

Reference

Black, J., & Hawks, J. (2005). *Medical-surgical nursing: Clinical management for positive outcomes* (7th ed., p. 920). Philadelphia: Saunders.

1020. A client with nephrotic syndrome needs dietary teaching about how the diet can help counteract the effects of altered renal function. The nurse plans to include which of the following statements in instructions to the client?

1 "Increase your intake of fish, meat, and eggs."
2 "Plan to drink at least 12 glasses of water a day."
3 "Increase your intake of fatty foods to prevent protein loss."
4 "Add salt during cooking to replace sodium lost in the urine."

Answer: 1

Rationale: Protein is increased unless the glomerular filtration rate is impaired. This helps to replace the protein lost in the urine, and it ultimately helps to control edema. The diet for clients with nephrotic syndrome is limited in sodium. This is also done to help control edema, which is a predominant part of the clinical picture. Fluids are not limited unless hyponatremia is present. Alternatively, the client is not encouraged to force fluids. A part of the clinical picture in nephrotic syndrome is hyperlipidemia, which results from the liver's synthesis of lipoproteins in response to hypoalbuminemia. Increasing the intake of fatty foods would not be helpful in this circumstance.

Level of Cognitive Ability: Application
Client Needs: Health Promotion and
   Maintenance
Integrated Process: Nursing Process/Planning
Content Area: Adult Health/Renal

Test-Taking Strategy: Use the process of elimination. Recalling that nephrotic syndrome is characterized by fluid retention and hypoalbuminemia will help you to eliminate options 2 and 4. From the remaining options, knowing that hyperlipidemia (option 3) accompanies this disorder will direct you to option 1. Review the home-care instructions for the client with nephrotic syndrome if you had difficulty with this question.

References
Black, J., & Hawks, J. (2005). *Medical-surgical nursing: Clinical management for positive outcomes* (7th ed., p. 926). Philadelphia: Saunders.
Monahan, F., Sands, J., Neighbors, M., Marek, J., & Green, C. (2007). *Phipps' medical-surgical nursing: Health and illness perspectives* (8th ed., p. 972). St. Louis: Mosby.

1021. The nurse is giving the client with polycystic kidney disease instructions for replacing the elements that are lost in the urine as a result of impaired kidney function. The nurse instructs the client to increase the intake of which of the following in the diet?
   1 Sodium and water
   2 Water and phosphorus
   3 Sodium and potassium
   4 Calcium and phosphorus

Level of Cognitive Ability: Application
Client Needs: Health Promotion and
   Maintenance
Integrated Process: Teaching and Learning
Content Area: Adult Health/Renal

Answer: 1
Rationale: Clients with polycystic kidney disease waste sodium rather than retain it and therefore require an increase in sodium and water in the diet. Potassium, calcium, and phosphorus need no special attention.

Test-Taking Strategy: Use the process of elimination. Recalling that this disorder causes sodium (not phosphorus) to be wasted will assist you with eliminating options 2 and 4. From the remaining options, recall that, when the kidney excretes sodium, water is carried with it. This will direct you to option 1. Review the care of the client with polycystic kidney disease if you had difficulty with this question.

Reference
Black, J., & Hawks, J. (2005). *Medical-surgical nursing: Clinical management for positive outcomes* (7th ed., p. 938). Philadelphia: Saunders.

1022. A client with acquired immunodeficiency syndrome is being treated for tuberculosis with isoniazid (INH). The nurse plans to teach the client which of the following regarding the administration of the medication?
   1 Administer it with food to prevent the rapid absorption of INH.
   2 Administer it with an antacid to prevent gastrointestinal distress.
   3 Administer it with a corticosteroid to potentiate the effects of INH.
   4 Administer it at least 1 hour before administering an aluminum-containing antacid to prevent a medication interaction.

Answer: 4
Rationale: Aluminum hydroxide, which is a common ingredient in antacids, significantly decreases INH absorption. INH should be administered at least 1 hour before aluminum-containing antacids. Food affects the rate of absorption of rifampin (Rifadin) rather than INH. INH administration with a corticosteroid decreases INH's effects and increases the effects of the corticosteroid.

Test-Taking Strategy: Recall the general principles related to medication administration. In general, you would not usually administer a medication with an antacid, because the antacid would decrease the absorption of the medication. Remembering this principle will direct you to option 4. Review INH for the treatment of tuberculosis if you had difficulty with this question.

Level of Cognitive Ability: Application
Client Needs: Health Promotion and
  Maintenance
Integrated Process: Nursing Process/Planning
Content Area: Adult Health/Immune

References
Hodgson, B., & Kizior, R. (2007). *Saunders nursing drug handbook 2007* (pp. 46, 643). Philadelphia: Saunders.
Monahan, F., Sands, J., Neighbors, M., Marek, J., & Green, C. (2007). *Phipps' medical-surgical nursing: Health and illness perspectives* (8th ed., pp. 1212-1213). St. Louis: Mosby.

1023. The nurse has provided dietary instructions to a client to minimize the risk of osteoporosis. The nurse determines that the client understands the recommended changes if the client verbalizes the need to increase the intake of which food?

  1 Rice
  2 Yogurt
  3 Chicken
  4 Sardines

Level of Cognitive Ability: Analysis
Client Needs: Health Promotion and
  Maintenance
Integrated Process: Nursing Process/Evaluation
Content Area: Adult Health/Musculoskeletal

Answer: 2

Rationale: Calcium intake is encouraged to minimize the risk of osteoporosis. The major dietary source of calcium is from dairy foods, including milk, yogurt, and a variety of cheeses. Calcium may also be added to certain products, such as orange juice, which are then advertised as being fortified with calcium. Calcium supplements are available and recommended for those with typically low calcium intake. Rice, sardines, and chicken are not high-calcium foods.

Test-Taking Strategy: Note the client's diagnosis, and recall that calcium intake is encouraged to minimize the risk of osteoporosis. Recalling that dairy products are high in calcium and that yogurt is a dairy product will direct you to option 2. Review osteoporosis and foods high in calcium if you had difficulty with this question.

References
Black, J., & Hawks, J. (2005). *Medical-surgical nursing: Clinical management for positive outcomes* (7th ed., p. 601). Philadelphia: Saunders.
Ignatavicius, D., & Workman, M. (2006). *Medical-surgical nursing: Critical thinking for collaborative care* (5th ed., pp. 206, 1167, 1170). Philadelphia: Saunders.

1024. A client with a history of ear problems is going on vacation by aircraft. The nurse advises the client to avoid which of the following to prevent barotrauma during the ascent and descent of the airplane?

  1 Yawning
  2 Swallowing
  3 Sucking hard candy
  4 Keeping the mouth motionless

Level of Cognitive Ability: Application
Client Needs: Health Promotion and
  Maintenance
Integrated Process: Nursing Process/
  Implementation
Content Area: Adult Health/Ear

Answer: 4

Rationale: Clients who are prone to barotrauma should perform any of a variety of mouth movements to equalize pressure in the ear, particularly during the ascent and descent of an aircraft. These can include yawning, swallowing, drinking, chewing, or sucking on hard candy. The Valsalva maneuver may also be helpful. The client should avoid sitting with the mouth motionless during this time, because this aggravates pressure buildup behind the tympanic membrane.

Test-Taking Strategy: Use the process of elimination, and note the strategic word "avoid." This word indicates a negative event query and asks you to select the option that identifies an incorrect client action. Eliminate options 1, 2, and 3, because they are comparable or alike and involve the movement of the mouth. Review the measures that will prevent barotrauma of the ear if you had difficulty with this question.

References
Black, J., & Hawks, J. (2005). *Medical-surgical nursing: Clinical management for positive outcomes* (7th ed., pp. 1981-1982). Philadelphia: Saunders.
Ignatavicius, D., & Workman, M. (2006). *Medical-surgical nursing: Critical thinking for collaborative care* (5th ed., p. 1131). Philadelphia: Saunders.

1025. The community health nurse is planning a school dietary program to help prevent nutritional deficiencies through healthy dietary practices. Which should the nurse use as primary prevention in the program?
1 Community-wide dietary screenings
2 Identifying individual dietary practices
3 Screening programs for poor eating habits
4 Educational programs about healthy eating

Level of Cognitive Ability: Application
Client Needs: Health Promotion and Maintenance
Integrated Process: Nursing Process/ Implementation
Content Area: Fundamental Skills

Answer: 4
Rationale: Primary prevention includes interventions that help with the avoidance of illness, injury, or potential problems; thus, for the nurse's program to prevent nutritional deficiencies, the nurse plans educational programs to teach healthy dietary practices. Options 1, 2, and 3 are secondary prevention measures that seek to detect existing health problems or trends.

Test-Taking Strategy: Note the subject of the question—primary prevention intervention. Knowledge that primary prevention interventions are those measures that keep illness from occurring will direct you to option 4. Review the levels of prevention if you had difficulty with this question.

References
Black, J., & Hawks, J. (2005). *Medical-surgical nursing: Clinical management for positive outcomes* (7th ed., pp. 22, 668-669). Philadelphia: Saunders.
Ignatavicius, D., & Workman, M. (2006). *Medical-surgical nursing: Critical thinking for collaborative care* (5th ed., p. 6). Philadelphia: Saunders.

1026. A nursing instructor asks a nursing student to identify situations that indicate a secondary level of prevention in health care. Which situation, if identified by the student, would indicate the need for further study of the levels of prevention?
1 Teaching a stroke client how to use a walker
2 Screening for hypertension in a community group
3 Screening for hyperlipidemia in a community group
4 Encouraging a woman who is more than 40 years old to obtain periodic mammograms

Level of Cognitive Ability: Analysis
Client Needs: Health Promotion and Maintenance
Integrated Process: Teaching and Learning
Content Area: Leadership/Management

Answer: 1
Rationale: Secondary prevention focuses on the early diagnosis and prompt treatment of disease. Tertiary prevention is represented by rehabilitation services. Options 2, 3, and 4 identify screening procedures. Option 1 identifies a rehabilitative service.

Test-Taking Strategy: Note the strategic words "indicate the need for further study." These words indicate a negative event query and ask you to select the option that does not represent a secondary level of prevention. Recalling that secondary prevention focuses on the early diagnosis and prompt treatment of disease will direct you to option 1. Review the levels of prevention if you had difficulty with this question.

References
Ignatavicius, D., & Workman, M. (2006). *Medical-surgical nursing: Critical thinking for collaborative care* (5th ed., p. 6). Philadelphia: Saunders.
Potter, P., & Perry, A. (2005). *Fundamentals of nursing* (6th ed., p. 97). St. Louis: Mosby.

1027. Which food does the nurse suggest to the client to increase the dietary intake of thiamine?
1 Milk
2 Pork
3 Chicken
4 Broccoli

Answer: 2
Rationale: Thiamine is present in a variety of foods of plant and animal origin. Pork, nuts, whole-grain cereals, and legumes are especially rich in this vitamin. Chicken is a good source of protein, broccoli is high in iron and vitamin K, and milk is a good source of calcium.

Level of Cognitive Ability: Comprehension
Client Needs: Health Promotion and Maintenance
Integrated Process: Teaching and Learning
Content Area: Fundamental Skills

Test-Taking Strategy: Focus on the subject—the food items that are high in thiamine. Remember that pork is high in thiamine. Review the foods that contain thiamine if you had difficulty with this question.

Reference
Grodner, M., Long, S., & DeYoung, S. (2004). *Foundations and clinical applications of nutrition: A nursing approach* (3rd ed., p. 170). St. Louis: Mosby.

1028. A nurse provides home-care instructions to the mother of an infant with a diagnosis of hydrocephalus. Which statement by the mother indicates an understanding of the care of the infant?
1 "I need to support my infant's neck and head."
2 "I need to feed my infant in a flat, side-lying position."
3 "I need to keep my infant's head in a pushed-back position during sleep."
4 "I need to place my infant on its stomach with a towel under the neck for sleep."

Level of Cognitive Ability: Analysis
Client Needs: Health Promotion and Maintenance
Integrated Process: Nursing Process/Evaluation
Content Area: Child Health

Answer: 1
Rationale: Hydrocephalus is a condition that is characterized by the enlargement of the cranium caused by an abnormal accumulation of cerebrospinal fluid within the cerebral ventricular system. This characteristic causes an increase in the weight of the infant's head, which causes the infant's head to become top heavy. Supporting the infant's head and neck when picking the infant up will prevent the hyperextension of the neck area and keep the infant from falling backward. The hyperextension of the infant's head can put pressure on the neck vertebrae, which can cause injury. Options 3 and 4 will cause hyperextension. The infant should be fed with the head elevated for the proper motility of food processing.

Test-Taking Strategy: Note the strategic words "indicates an understanding." Use the process of elimination, and eliminate option 2 first, because feeding any infant in this position is unsafe. Eliminate options 3 and 4 next, because they are comparable or alike. Both of these positions will cause hyperextension of the infant's neck. Review the care of the infant with hydrocephalus if you had difficulty with this question.

Reference
Hockenberry, M., Wilson, D., & Winkelstein, M. (2005). *Wong's essentials of pediatric nursing* (7th ed., p. 1059). St. Louis: Mosby.

1029. A nurse is preparing a teaching plan for the parents of an infant with a ventricular peritoneal shunt who will be discharged from the hospital. The nurse includes which instructions in the plan of care?
1 Call the physician if the infant is fussy.
2 Expect an increased urine output from the shunt.
3 Call the physician if the infant has a high-pitched cry.
4 Position the infant on the side of the shunt when the infant is put to bed.

Level of Cognitive Ability: Application
Client Needs: Health Promotion and Maintenance
Integrated Process: Teaching and Learning
Content Area: Child Health

Answer: 3
Rationale: If the shunt is broken or malfunctioning, the fluid from the ventricular part of the brain will not be diverted to the peritoneal cavity, and the cerebrospinal fluid will build up in the cranial area. The result is intracranial pressure, which then causes a high-pitched cry in the infant. The infant should not be positioned on the side of the shunt, because this will cause pressure on the shunt as well as skin breakdown. This type of shunt affects the gastrointestinal system rather than the genitourinary system, and an increased urinary output is not expected. Option 1 is only a concern if other signs that are indicative of a complication are occurring.

Test-Taking Strategy: Use the process of elimination. Remember that a high-pitched cry in an infant indicates a concern or problem. Review significant assessment findings and home-care instructions for the parents of an infant with a ventricular peritoneal shunt if you had difficulty with this question.

References
McKinney, E., James, S., Murray, S., & Ashwill, J. (2005). *Maternal-child nursing* (2nd ed., p. 1506). St. Louis: Saunders.
Wong, D., Hockenberry, M., Perry, S., Lowdermilk, D., & Wilson, D. (2006). *Maternal-child nursing care* (3rd ed., p. 1715). St. Louis: Mosby.

1030. A home-care nurse visits a child with Reye syndrome and plans to provide instructions to the mother regarding care of the child. The nurse instructs the mother to:

1 Increase the stimuli in the environment.
2 Avoid daytime naps so the child will sleep at night.
3 Give the child frequent, small meals if vomiting occurs.
4 Check the child's skin and eyes every-day for a yellow discoloration.

Level of Cognitive Ability: Application
Client Needs: Health Promotion and Maintenance
Integrated Process: Teaching and Learning
Content Area: Child Health

Answer: 4
Rationale: Checking for jaundice will assist with the identification of the presence of the liver complications that are characteristic of Reye syndrome. If vomiting occurs in a client with Reye syndrome, it is caused by cerebral edema, and it is a sign of increased intra-cranial pressure, so it needs to be reported. Decreasing stimuli and providing rest decrease stress on the brain tissue. Options 1 and 2 do not promote a restful environment for the child.

Test-Taking Strategy: Read each option carefully, and think about the manifestations and complications associated with Reye syndrome. Recalling that increased intracranial pressure is a concern will assist you with eliminating option 3. Eliminate options 1 and 2 next, because they are comparable or alike in that they do not promote a restful environment for the child. Review the care of the child with Reye syndrome if you had difficulty with this question.

References
Hockenberry, M., & Wilson, D. (2007). *Nursing care of infants and children* (8th ed., p. 1651). St. Louis: Mosby.
Hockenberry, M., Wilson, D., & Winkelstein, M. (2005). *Wong's essentials of pediatric nursing* (7th ed., p. 1045). St. Louis: Mosby.

1031. A nurse in the well-baby clinic has pro-vided instructions regarding dental care to the mother of a 10-month-old child. Which statement by the mother indi-cates the need for further instructions?

1 "I need to limit the amount of con-centrated sweets."
2 "I need to start dental hygiene as soon as the primary teeth erupt."
3 "I need to use fluoride supplements if the water is not fluoridated."
4 "I can coat a pacifier with honey during the day as long as I do not give my child a bottle during a nap or at bedtime."

Level of Cognitive Ability: Analysis
Client Needs: Health Promotion and Maintenance
Integrated Process: Teaching and Learning
Content Area: Child Health

Answer: 4
Rationale: The practice of coating pacifiers with honey or using commercially available hard-candy pacifiers is discouraged. In addition to being cariogenic, honey may also cause botulism. Also, a bottle at nap or bedtime that contains sweet milk or other fluids such as juice bathes the teeth, thus producing caries. Fluoride, which is an essential mineral for building caries-resist-ant teeth, is needed beginning when the child is 6 months old or as directed by the physician if the infant does not receive adequate fluoride content. A diet that is low in sweets and high in nutritious food promotes dental health. Dental hygiene should start as soon as primary teeth erupt.

Test-Taking Strategy: Note the strategic words "indicates the need for further instructions." These words indicate a negative event query and ask you to select an option that is an incorrect statement. Focus on the subject as it relates to the prevention of dental caries, and recall that honey is cariogenic and that it may also cause botulism. This will direct you to option 4. Review dental care measures if you had difficulty with this question.

Reference
Hockenberry, M., Wilson, D., & Winkelstein, M. (2005). *Wong's essentials of pediatric nursing* (7th ed., p. 405). St. Louis: Mosby.

1032. A 7-year-old child is hospitalized with a fracture of the femur and placed in traction. To help meet the growth and development needs of the child, the nurse selects which appropriate play activity for the child?
  1 A board game
  2 A large puzzle
  3 A finger-painting set
  4 A coloring book with crayons

Level of Cognitive Ability: Application
Client Needs: Health Promotion and Maintenance
Integrated Process: Nursing Process/ Implementation
Content Area: Child Health

Answer: 1
Rationale: The school-age child becomes organized with more direction with play activities. Such activities include collections, drawing, construction, dolls, pets, guessing games, board games, riddles, hobbies, competitive games, and listening to the radio or television. Options 3 and 4 are most appropriate for a preschooler, and option 2 is most appropriate for a toddler.

Test-Taking Strategy: Note the age and the diagnosis of the child to answer this question. Recalling the specific types of age-related play activities that are appropriate for the school-age child will direct you to option 1. Review the age-appropriate activities for the school-age child if you had difficulty with this question.

Reference
Hockenberry, M., Wilson, D., & Winkelstein, M. (2005). *Wong's essentials of pediatric nursing* (7th ed., p. 486). St. Louis: Mosby.

1033. The nurse is providing medication instructions to a client about diclofenac sodium (Voltaren). The nurse teaches the client to immediately report which of the following symptoms to the health care provider?
  1 Hiccups
  2 Constipation
  3 Jaundice, fatigue, and nausea
  4 An increase in muscle and joint pain

Level of Cognitive Ability: Application
Client Needs: Health Promotion and Maintenance
Integrated Process: Teaching and Learning
Content Area: Pharmacology

Answer: 3
Rationale: The risk of liver dysfunction is present with the use of diclofenac sodium. Accordingly, the client should receive periodic tests of liver function and should be instructed to report any manifestations of liver injury (jaundice, fatigue, and nausea). Options 1 and 2 are not of concern. Some clients may experience muscle and joint pain; although this should be reported, it is not as critical as the risk of liver dysfunction.

Test-Taking Strategy: Noting the strategic word "immediately" will help you to eliminate options 1 and 2. From the remaining options, recalling that liver dysfunction is a concern with the use of this medication will direct you to option 3. Review the adverse effects of diclofenac sodium if you had difficulty with this question.

Reference
Lehne, R. A. (2007). *Pharmacology for nursing care* (6th ed., p. 818). Philadelphia: Saunders.

1034. A clinic nurse has provided information to the mother of a toddler regarding toilet training. Which statement by the mother would indicate the need for further instruction?
  1 "I should have my child sit on the potty until she urinates."
  2 "I should wait until my child is between 18 and 24 months old."
  3 "I know my child is ready to begin toilet training if my child is walking."
  4 "I know that my child will develop bowel control before bladder control."

Answer: 1
Rationale: The child should not be forced to sit on the potty for long periods of time. The physical ability to control the anal and urethral sphincters is achieved some time after the child is walking, probably between ages of 18 and 24 months. Bowel control is usually achieved before bladder control.

Test-Taking Strategy: Note the strategic words "the need for further instruction." These words indicate a negative event query and ask you to select an option that is an incorrect statement. Recall that forcing a child to develop this behavior will result in a negative response. This will direct you to option 1. Review the task of toilet training if you had difficulty with this question.

Level of Cognitive Ability: Analysis
Client Needs: Health Promotion and
    Maintenance
Integrated Process: Teaching and Learning
Content Area: Child Health

Reference
Hockenberry, M., Wilson, D., & Winkelstein, M. (2005). *Wong's essentials of pediatric nursing* (7th ed., pp. 396-397). St. Louis: Mosby.

1035. A clinic nurse is performing an assessment on a 12-month-old infant. The nurse determines that the infant is demonstrating the highest level of developmental achievement if the 12-month-old infant is able to:

1 Produce cooing sounds.
2 Obey simple commands.
3 Produce babbling sounds.
4 Begin to use simple words.

Level of Cognitive Ability: Analysis
Client Needs: Health Promotion and
    Maintenance
Integrated Process: Nursing Process/Assessment
Content Area: Child Health

Answer: 4
Rationale: Simple words such as "mama" and the use of gestures to communicate begins when the infant is between 9 and 12 months old. A 1- to 3-month-old infant will produce cooing sounds. Babbling is common in a 3- to 4-month-old infant. Between the ages of 8 and 9 months, the infant begins to understand and obey simple commands such as "wave bye-bye." The use of single-consonant babbling occurs between the ages of 6 and 8 months.

Test-Taking Strategy: Note that the infant is 12 months old, and note the strategic words "highest level." Use the process of elimination and your knowledge of language and communication developmental milestones to answer the question. Review these milestones if you had difficulty with this question.

Reference
Hockenberry, M., Wilson, D., & Winkelstein, M. (2005). *Wong's essentials of pediatric nursing* (7th ed., p. 325). St. Louis: Mosby.

1036. A nurse is assisting with conducting a session about relaxation techniques for a group of pregnant women attending a childbirth class. The nurse informs the group that active relaxation techniques will assist them with coping with the discomfort of contractions. The nurse determines that teaching has been effective when a client says that active relaxation includes:

1 Relaxing uninvolved muscles while the uterus contracts
2 Remembering that the contractions will be over after delivery
3 Assuming a state of mind that is open to suggestions from a coach
4 Understanding that the causes of contraction discomfort are more psychological than physical

Level of Cognitive Ability: Analysis
Client Needs: Health Promotion and
    Maintenance
Integrated Process: Nursing Process/Evaluation
Content Area: Maternity/Antepartum

Answer: 1
Rationale: Active relaxation includes specific relaxation exercises and conditioned responses such as distraction from the discomfort of labor. The woman is an active participant in the use of the technique, which focuses on relaxing the uninvolved muscles while the uterus contracts. Options 2, 3, and 4 are incorrect.

Test-Taking Strategy: Use the process of elimination, and note the strategic words "active relaxation." Option 1 contains an active verb and is different from the other options. Options 2, 3, and 4 are all comparable or alike in that the verb is passive. Review the purpose of active relaxation techniques during labor if you had difficulty with this question.

Reference
Wong, D., Hockenberry, M., Perry, S., Lowdermilk, D., & Wilson, D. (2006). *Maternal-child nursing care* (3rd ed., pp. 442-443). St. Louis: Mosby.

1037. The nurse is performing an assessment of a prenatal client who is being seen in the clinic for the first time. After the assessment, the nurse determines that which piece of data places the client in a high-risk category for contracting human immunodeficiency virus (HIV)?

1 A history of one sexual partner within the past 10 years
2 A history of intravenous drug use during the past year
3 Living in an area where the population rate of HIV infection is low
4 A spouse who is heterosexual and who has had only one sexual partner during the past 10 years

Level of Cognitive Ability: Analysis
Client Needs: Health Promotion and Maintenance
Integrated Process: Nursing Process/Assessment
Content Area: Adult Health/Immune

Answer: 2
Rationale: HIV is transmitted by intimate sexual contact and the exchange of body fluids, exposure to infected blood, and transmission from an infected woman to her fetus. Women who fall into the high-risk category for HIV infection include those with persistent and recurrent sexually transmitted diseases, those with a history of multiple sexual partners, and those who have used intravenous drugs. A heterosexual partner, particularly a partner who has had only one sexual partner in 10 years, is not a high-risk factor for the development of HIV.

Test-Taking Strategy: Use the process of elimination, recalling that the exchange of blood and body fluids places the client at high risk for HIV infection. This will assist with directing you to the correct option. Review the risk factors for HIV if you had difficulty with this question.

References
McKinney, E., James, S., Murray, S., & Ashwill, J. (2005). *Maternal-child nursing* (2nd ed., pp. 665-666). St. Louis: Saunders.
Wong, D., Hockenberry, M., Perry, S., Lowdermilk, D., & Wilson, D. (2006). *Maternal-child nursing care* (3rd ed., p. 271). St. Louis: Mosby.

ALTERNATE ITEM FORMATS

1038. The nurse working at a health screening clinic gathers data from a client to identify the client's risk factors associated with coronary artery disease. The nurse is specifically interested in modifiable risk factors so that a health promotion and maintenance plan of care can be developed for the client. Which risk factors are modifiable? Select all that apply.

☐ 1 Is black
☐ 2 Is a cigarette smoker
☐ 3 Is physically inactive
☐ 4 Is a 45-year-old female
☐ 5 Has a family history of heart disease
☐ 6 Has a personal history of diabetes mellitus

Level of Cognitive Ability: Analysis
Client Needs: Health Promotion and Maintenance
Integrated Process: Nursing Process/Assessment
Content Area: Adult Health/Cardiovascular

Answers: 2, 3, 6
Rationale: Modifiable risk factors for coronary artery disease are those that can be modified or reduced with treatment. These include physical inactivity, cigarette smoking, hypertension, an elevated serum cholesterol level, diabetes mellitus, and obesity. Nonmodifiable risk factors are those that cannot be modified or reduced by treatment and include such factors as heredity, race, age, and gender. Those clients whose parents had coronary heart disease are at higher risk. Increasing age influences both the risk and severity of the disease. Although men are at higher risk for heart attacks at a younger age, the risk for women increases significantly at menopause. The incidence of coronary artery disease is more prevalent among black women.

Test-Taking Strategy: Focus on the subject—modifiable risk factors. Recalling that modifiable risk factors are those that can be modified or reduced by treatment will assist you with answering this question. Look at each risk factor listed, and select the risk factors that can be changed. Review the modifiable and nonmodifiable risk factors for coronary artery disease if you had difficulty with this question.

References
Black, J., & Hawks, J. (2005). *Medical-surgical nursing: Clinical management for positive outcomes* (7th ed., p. 1628). Philadelphia: Saunders.
Lewis, S., Heitkemper, M., Dirksen, S., O'Brien, P., & Bucher, L. (2007). *Medical-surgical nursing: Assessment and management of clinical problems* (7th ed., pp. 787, 792). St. Louis: Mosby.

1039. The nurse instructs a client who is at risk for urinary tract infections to drink 3000 mL of fluid daily to decrease the risk. How many 10-ounce glasses of fluid per day should the nurse instruct the client to drink to consume 3000 mL?

Answer: _____ glasses

Level of Cognitive Ability: Application
Client Needs: Health Promotion and Maintenance
Integrated Process: Teaching and Learning
Content Area: Fundamental Skills

Answer: 10
Rationale: Each 10-ounce glass of fluid contains 300 mL (1 oz = 30 mL, so 10 oz = 300 mL). Therefore, the client will need to drink ten 10-ounce glasses of fluid daily (3000 mL divided by 300 mL = 10).

Test-Taking Strategy: Focus on the subject—the number of 10-ounce glasses of fluid that will equal 3000 mL. First, change ounces to mL to determine the number of mL in each 10-ounce glass of fluid. Next, divide the amount of fluid prescribed by the number of mL in each 10-ounce glass of fluid. Review the formula for converting ounces to mL if you had difficulty with this question.

References
Lewis, S., Heitkemper, M., Dirksen, S., O'Brien, P., & Bucher, L. (2007). *Medical-surgical nursing: Assessment and management of clinical problems* (7th ed., p. 1159). St. Louis: Mosby.
Monahan, F., Sands, J., Neighbors, M., Marek, J., & Green, C. (2007). *Phipps' medical-surgical nursing: Health and illness perspectives* (8th ed., p. 964). St. Louis: Mosby.

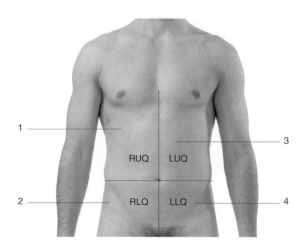

From Wilson, S., & Giddens, J. (2005). *Health assessment for nursing practice* (3rd ed.). St. Louis: Mosby.

1040. The nurse is performing a physical assessment on an adult client and is preparing to palpate the liver to assess for the location of the liver's lower border. The nurse plans to palpate in which abdominal quadrant?

Answer: _____

Level of Cognitive Ability: Application
Client Needs: Health Promotion and Maintenance
Integrated Process: Nursing Process/Assessment
Content Area: Adult Health/Gastrointestinal

Answer: 1
Rationale: The liver is the largest organ in the body, weighing about 3.5 pounds (1.6 kg). It lies under the right diaphragm, and it spans the upper quadrant of the abdomen from the fifth intercostal space to slightly below the costal margin. The rib cage covers a substantial portion of the liver; only the lower margin is exposed beneath it.

Test-Taking Strategy: Use your knowledge of the anatomy of the body. Recalling that the liver is located on the right side of the body in the upper quadrant will direct you to the correct answer. Review the anatomical location of the liver and the technique for palpation if you had difficulty with this question.

Reference
Wilson, S., & Giddens, J. (2005). *Health assessment for nursing practice* (3rd ed., pp. 432, 443). St. Louis: Mosby.

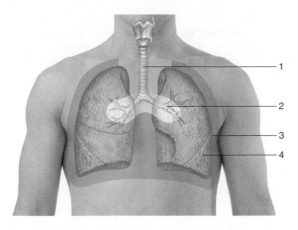

From Wilson, S., & Giddens, J. (2005). *Health assessment for nursing practice* (3rd ed.). St. Louis: Mosby.

1041. The nurse is performing a physical assessment on a client and is preparing to auscultate the breath sounds. The nurse places the stethoscope in which area to assess the bronchovesicular sounds?

Answer: _____

Level of Cognitive Ability: Application
Client Needs: Health Promotion and Maintenance
Integrated Process: Nursing Process/Assessment
Content Area: Adult Health/Respiratory

Answer: 2
Rationale: Bronchovesicular breath sounds are heard over the main bronchi. Specifically, their normal location is between the first and second intercostal spaces at the sternal border anteriorly and posteriorly at T4 medial to the scapula. These sounds are moderate in pitch and medium in intensity, and the durations of inspiration and expiration are equal. Bronchial breath sounds are heard over the trachea. Vesicular breath sounds are heard over the lesser bronchi, the bronchioles, and the lobes.

Test-Taking Strategy: Focus on the locations identified. Eliminate options 3 and 4, because they identify similar locations (peripheral lung fields). From the remaining options, recall that bronchial breath sounds are heard over the trachea. Review respiratory assessment techniques if you had difficulty with this question.

Reference
Wilson, S., & Giddens, J. (2005). *Health assessment for nursing practice* (3rd ed., pp. 347-348). St. Louis: Mosby.

1042. The nurse is developing a discharge teaching plan for a client with chronic arterial insufficiency. Which of the following should the nurse plan to include during the instruction? Select all that apply.

☐ **1** Cross the legs at the ankles only.

☐ **2** Avoid the use of tobacco products.

☐ **3** Wear rounded-toe shoes with soft insoles.

☐ **4** Wash the feet daily with warm water and mild soap, and dry well.

☐ **5** Use a mirror to visualize the hard-to-access places of the feet weekly.

☐ **6** Seek assistance from a podiatrist for the removal of corns, calluses, and ingrown toenails.

Answers: 2, 3, 4, 6
Rationale: Foot care for the client with vascular disease includes the daily inspection and cleansing of the feet with warm water and a mild soap; drying well, especially between the toes; and wearing shoes that fit well without pressure areas. The client is also instructed to avoid crossing the legs at the knees or ankles and to avoid the use of tobacco products to prevent vasoconstriction. Conditions such as ingrown toenails, corns, and calluses should be treated by a podiatrist to avoid further complications.

Test-Taking Strategy: Recall that vascular disease can result in the impairment of the tissues of the feet. Eliminate option 1, because crossing the legs at either the knees or the ankles restricts circulation. Next, eliminate option 5 because of the word "weekly," knowing that this practice should be incorporated daily. The remaining options are all appropriate to incorporate in the teaching plan. Review the foot care for the client with vascular disease if you had difficulty with this question.

Level of Cognitive Ability: Application
Client Needs: Health Promotion and
  Maintenance
Integrated Process: Teaching and Learning
Content Area: Adult Health/Cardiovascular

References
Ignatavicius, D., & Workman, M. (2006). *Medical-surgical nursing: Critical thinking for collaborative care* (5th ed., pp. 795, 804). Philadelphia: Saunders.
Lewis, S., Heitkemper, M., Dirksen, S., O'Brien, P., & Bucher, L. (2007). *Medical-surgical nursing: Assessment and management of clinical problems* (7th ed., p. 907). St. Louis: Mosby.

1043. The camp nurse provides instructions for families about protecting the skin from the harmful ultraviolet (UV) rays of the sun. Which would the nurse recommend as effective skin protection measures for preventing these effects? Select all that apply.

☐ **1** Bring long-sleeved shirts and long pants.

☐ **2** Wear a wide-brimmed hat and sunglasses.

☐ **3** Use sunscreen mixed with insect repellent.

☐ **4** Select tightly woven materials for better sun protection.

☐ **5** Avoid using sunscreen on cloudy days and in the shade.

☐ **6** Purchase sunscreen with a sun protection factor (SPF) of 15 or higher.

Level of Cognitive Ability: Application
Client Needs: Health Promotion and
  Maintenance
Integrated Process: Teaching and Learning
Content Area: Fundamental Skills

Answers: 1, 2, 4, 6
Rationale: Effective measures to block UV rays include tightly woven clothing, hats, and sunglasses. To be effective, liberal amounts of sunscreen with an SPF of 15 or higher should be applied 30 minutes before exposure to UV rays, every 2 hours throughout the day, and after exposure to water. A hat, a long-sleeved shirt, and long pants should be worn when out in the sun, and tightly woven materials provide greater protection from the sun's rays. The nurse recommends that families provide protection from some insects with insect-repellent–impregnated clothing or a product that contains insect repellent only. This is to prevent overexposure to the chemicals in the insect repellent when combination products are reapplied throughout the day. Most commercial insect repellents should not be used on young children. The sun's rays are as damaging to the skin on cloudy, hazy days as they are on sunny days, and they can also cause damage when an individual is in the shade as a result of reflection.

Test-Taking Strategy: Note the strategic words "effective skin protection measures." Recall the concepts that UV rays are damaging with both direct and indirect exposure to the sun, that sunscreen must be used properly to be effective, and that the reapplication of combination products that include insect repellent can be harmful. Therefore, eliminate option 3 first, because it mentions a combination product. Next, eliminate option 5 because of the sun's potential to damage the skin with direct and indirect exposure. The remaining options should provide effective protection from the UV rays of the sun. Review the guidelines that protect the skin from the damaging rays of the sun if you had difficulty with this question.

Reference
Lewis, S., Heitkemper, M., Dirksen, S., O'Brien, P., & Bucher, L. (2007). *Medical-surgical nursing: Assessment and management of clinical problems* (7th ed., pp. 460-461). St. Louis: Mosby.

1044. A client with a chlamydia infection receives instructions regarding self-care and methods to prevent reinfection. Which instructions does the nurse provide to the client? Select all that apply.

- ☐ **1** Use antibiotics prophylactically.
- ☐ **2** Inform sexual partners of infection.
- ☐ **3** Douche with antibacterial solution.
- ☐ **4** Limit the number of sexual partners.
- ☐ **5** Use latex condoms during intercourse.
- ☐ **6** Return to the clinic for a follow-up culture.

Level of Cognitive Ability: Application
Client Needs: Health Promotion and Maintenance
Integrated Process: Teaching and Learning
Content Area: Fundamental Skills

Answers: 2, 4, 5, 6
Rationale: The nurse instructs the client to reduce the risk of reinfection and decrease the risk of transmission by limiting the number of sexual partners, using condoms, and informing sexual partners so that they can seek screening and treatment as necessary. Returning for the follow-up culture helps to confirm a cure, because, if the chlamydia is not resolved with the initial treatment, the client will continue to be infected and capable of spreading the infection. Antibiotic therapy and douching will not prevent a chlamydia infection.

Test-Taking Strategy: Note the strategic words "self-care and methods to prevent reinfection," and note that the client has a sexually transmitted disease. Recall the basic principles of the chain of infection, and use the process of elimination. Eliminate options 1 and 3, because these instructions are ineffective for preventing reinfection or the transmission of microorganisms. Review the treatment measures for chlamydia infection if you had difficulty with this question.

Reference
Black, J., & Hawks, J. (2005). *Medical-surgical nursing: Clinical management for positive outcomes* (7th ed., p. 1132). Philadelphia: Saunders.

1045. Instructions for the self-care for a client with preterm premature rupture of membranes (PPROM) should include which of the following? Select all that apply.

- ☐ **1** Take daily tub baths.
- ☐ **2** Sexual activity is allowed.
- ☐ **3** Remain on modified bedrest.
- ☐ **4** Douche daily with a vinegar solution.
- ☐ **5** Report a temperature of more than 38° C.
- ☐ **6** Watch for foul-smelling vaginal discharge.

Level of Cognitive Ability: Application
Client Needs: Health Promotion and Maintenance
Integrated Process: Teaching and Learning
Content Area: Maternity/Antepartum

Answers: 3, 5, 6
Rationale: Vigilance for signs of infection is a major part of the nursing care and client education after PPROM. The client should be taught to remain on modified bedrest, to report a temperature of more than 38° C, and to watch for foul-smelling vaginal discharge. Other instructions should include taking the temperature and the pulse every 4 hours when awake, inserting nothing into the vagina, avoiding sexual activity, assessing for uterine contractions, counting fetal movements daily, avoiding tub baths, wiping from front to back after urinating or having a bowel movement, taking antibiotics (if prescribed), and making visits to the primary health care provider as scheduled. Daily tub baths, douching with a vinegar solution, and engaging in sexual activity would be contraindicated.

Test-Taking Strategy: Focus on the data in the question, and remember that, after the membranes have ruptured, the risk is infection. Eliminate the options that could introduce any infection (options 1, 2, and 4). Options that would prevent or monitor for infection are options 3, 5, and 6. Review the care of the client after PPROM if you had difficulty with this question.

Reference
Lowdermilk, D., & Perry, S. (2006). *Maternity nursing* (7th ed., p. 782). St. Louis: Mosby.

1046. A nurse is discussing contraceptive methods with a postpartum client. The nurse tells the client that combined oral contraceptives (COCs) are contraindicated if the client has a medical history of which of the following? Select all that apply.

☐ **1** Acne

☐ **2** Infertility

☐ **3** Breast cancer

☐ **4** Dysmenorrhea

☐ **5** Coronary artery disease

☐ **6** Thromboembolic disorders

Level of Cognitive Ability: Analysis
Client Needs: Health Promotion and Maintenance
Integrated Process: Nursing Process/Implementation
Content Area: Maternity/Postpartum

Answers: 3, 5, 6
Rationale: Contraindications for COC use include a history of thromboembolic disorders, coronary artery disease, and breast cancer. The use of oral contraceptives is also contraindicated in a client with impaired liver function, liver tumor, smoking (if the client is more than 35 years old and smokes more than 15 cigarettes a day), headaches with focal neurological symptoms, surgery with prolonged immobilization or any surgery on the legs, hypertension, and diabetes mellitus (of more than 20 years' duration) with vascular disease. COC is not contraindicated with dysmenorrhea, although dysmenorrhea may be a side effect of therapy. COC is sometimes used to treat acne. COC is not contraindicated for a client who has a history of infertility.

Test-Taking Strategy: Focus on the subject—contraindications to the use of COC. Recall the contraindications, uses, and side effects of COC to direct you to the correct options. Remember that options 3, 5, and 6 are disorders that would contraindicate the use of COC. Option 4 is a side effect but not a contraindication. COC is sometimes used to treat acne, and it is not contraindicated for clients with infertility. Review the contraindications for the use of COC if you had difficulty with this question.

References
Lowdermilk, D., & Perry, S. (2006). *Maternity nursing* (7th ed., p. 149). St. Louis: Mosby.
Skidmore-Roth, L. (2008). *Mosby's nursing drug reference* (21st ed., p. 307). St. Louis: Mosby.

REFERENCES

Black, J., & Hawks, J. (2005). *Medical-surgical nursing: Clinical management for positive outcomes* (7th ed.). Philadelphia: Saunders.

Canobbio, M. (2006). *Mosby's handbook of patient teaching* (3rd ed.). St. Louis: Mosby.

Chernecky, C., & Berger, B. (2008). *Laboratory tests and diagnostic procedures* (5th ed.). Philadelphia: Saunders.

Gahart, B., & Nazareno, A. (2008). *2008 Intravenous medications* (22nd ed.). St. Louis: Mosby.

Grodner, M., Long, S., & DeYoung, S. (2004). *Foundations and clinical applications of nutrition: A nursing approach* (3rd ed.). St. Louis: Mosby.

Gulanick, M., & Myers, J. (2007). *Nursing care plans: Nursing diagnosis and intervention* (6th ed.). St. Louis: Mosby.

Hockenberry, M., & Wilson, D. (2007). *Nursing care of infants and children* (8th ed.). St. Louis: Mosby.

Hockenberry, M., Wilson, D., & Winkelstein, M. (2005). *Wong's essentials of pediatric nursing* (7th ed.). St. Louis: Mosby.

Hodgson, B., & Kizior, R. (2007). *Saunders nursing drug handbook 2007*. Philadelphia: Saunders.

Hodgson, B., & Kizior, R. (2008). *Saunders nursing drug handbook 2008*. Philadelphia: Saunders.

Ignatavicius, D., & Workman, M. (2006). *Medical-surgical nursing: Critical thinking for collaborative care* (5th ed.). Philadelphia: Saunders.

Kee, J., Hayes, E., & McCuistion, L. (2006). *Pharmacology: A nursing process approach* (5th ed.). Philadelphia: Saunders.

Lehne, R. (2007). *Pharmacology for nursing care* (6th ed.). Philadelphia: Saunders.

Lewis, S., Heitkemper, M., Dirksen, S., O'Brien, P., & Bucher, L. (2007). *Medical-surgical nursing: Assessment and management of clinical problems* (7th ed.). St. Louis: Mosby.

Lowdermilk, D., & Perry, S. (2006). *Maternity nursing* (7th ed.). St. Louis: Mosby.

McKenry, L., Tressier, E., & Hogan, M. (2006). *Mosby's pharmacology in nursing* (22nd ed.). St. Louis: Mosby.

McKinney, E., James, S., Murray, S., & Ashwill, J. (2005). *Maternal-child nursing* (2nd ed.). St. Louis: Saunders.

Meiner, S., & Leuckenotte, A. (2006). *Gerontologic nursing* (3rd ed.). St. Louis: Mosby.

Monahan, F., Sands, J., Neighbors, M., Marek, J., & Green, C. (2007). *Phipps' medical-surgical nursing: Health and illness perspectives* (8th ed.). St. Louis: Mosby.

Murray, S., & McKinney, E. (2006). *Foundations of maternal-newborn nursing* (4th ed.). Philadelphia: Saunders.

National Council of State Boards of Nursing (Eds.). (2007). *2007 NCLEX-RN® detailed test plan*. Chicago: Author.

Nix, S. (2005). *Williams' basic nutrition & diet therapy* (12th ed.). St. Louis: Mosby.

Pagana, K., & Pagana, T. (2005). *Mosby's diagnostic and laboratory test reference* (7th ed.). St. Louis: Mosby.

Perry, A., & Potter, P. (2006). *Clinical nursing skills & techniques* (6th ed.). St. Louis: Mosby.

Potter, P., & Perry, A. (2005). *Fundamentals of nursing* (6th ed.). St. Louis: Mosby.

Skidmore-Roth, L. (2005). *Mosby's drug guide for nurses* (6th ed.). St. Louis: Mosby.

Skidmore-Roth, L. (2007). *2007 Mosby's nursing drug reference* (20th ed.). St. Louis: Mosby.

Skidmore-Roth, L. (2008). *Mosby's nursing drug reference* (21st ed.). St. Louis: Mosby.

Stuart, G., & Laraia, M. (2005). *Principles and practice of psychiatric nursing* (8th ed.). St. Louis: Mosby.

Varcarolis, E., Carson, V., & Shoemaker, N. (2006). *Foundations of psychiatric mental health nursing* (5th ed.). Philadelphia: Saunders.

Wilson, S., & Giddens, J. (2005). *Health assessment for nursing practice* (3rd ed.). St. Louis: Mosby.

Wong, D., Hockenberry, M., Perry, S., Lowdermilk, D., & Wilson, D. (2006). *Maternal-child nursing care* (3rd ed.). St. Louis: Mosby.

Psychosocial Integrity

1047. A toddler with suspected conjunctivitis is crying and refuses to sit still during the eye examination. Which of the following is the most appropriate statement for the nurse to make to the child?
1 "Would you like to see my flashlight?"
2 "Don't be scared, the light won't hurt you."
3 "If you will sit still, the exam will be over soon."
4 "I know you are upset. We can do this exam later."

Level of Cognitive Ability: Application
Client Needs: Psychosocial Integrity
Integrated Process: Communication and Documentation
Content Area: Child Health

Answer: 1
Rationale: Fears in this age group can be decreased by getting the child actively involved in the examination. Option 2 tells the toddler how to feel. Option 3 ignores the toddler's feelings. Although option 4 acknowledges the toddler's feelings, it falsely puts off the inevitable.

Test-Taking Strategy: Use knowledge regarding the stages of growth and development, noting that the child is a toddler. The use of therapeutic communication techniques will direct you to option 1. Review the growth and development related to the toddler if you had difficulty with this question.

Reference
Hockenberry, M., Wilson, D., & Winkelstein, M. (2005). *Wong's essentials of pediatric nursing* (7th ed., pp. 133-134, 444-445). St. Louis: Mosby.

1048. A client with acute pyelonephritis is scheduled for a voiding cystourethrogram. The client is very shy and modest. The nurse determines that this client would benefit from increased support and teaching about the procedure because:
1 Radioactive material is inserted into the bladder.
2 Radiopaque contrast is injected into the bloodstream.
3 The client must void while the voiding process is filmed.
4 The client must lie on an X-ray table in a cold, barren room.

Answer: 3
Rationale: Having to void in the presence of others can be very embarrassing for clients, and it may actually interfere with the client's ability to void. The nurse teaches the client about the procedure to try to minimize stress from a lack of preparation and gives the client encouragement and emotional support. Screens may be used in the radiology department to try to provide an element of privacy during this procedure. Options 1, 2, and 4 are incorrect and do not address the subject of support.

Test-Taking Strategy: Use the process of elimination and your knowledge regarding this procedure. Noting the strategic words "shy" and "modest" will direct you to option 3. Review the procedure for a voiding cystourethrogram if you had difficulty with this question.

Level of Cognitive Ability: Analysis
Client Needs: Psychosocial Integrity
Integrated Process: Nursing Process/Analysis
Content Area: Adult Health/Renal

References
Chernecky, C., & Berger, B. (2008). *Laboratory tests and diagnostic procedures* (5th ed., pp. 420-421). Philadelphia: Saunders.
Pagana, K., & Pagana, T. (2005). *Mosby's diagnostic and laboratory test reference* (7th ed., pp. 334-335). St. Louis: Mosby.

1049. A female client who is in a manic state emerges from her room topless while making sexual remarks and lewd gestures toward the staff and her peers. The nurse should initiate which intervention first?

1 Quietly approach the client, escort her to her room, and help her to get dressed.
2 Confront the client on the inappropriateness of her behavior and offer her a time out.
3 Approach the client in the hallway and insist that she go to her own room immediately.
4 Ask the other clients to ignore her behavior; eventually she will return to her own room.

Level of Cognitive Ability: Application
Client Needs: Psychosocial Integrity
Integrated Process: Nursing Process/ Implementation
Content Area: Mental Health

Answer: 1
Rationale: A person who is experiencing mania lacks insight and judgment, has poor impulse control, and is highly excitable. The nurse must take control without creating increased stress or anxiety for the client. Insisting that the client go to her room may cause the nurse to be met with a great deal of resistance. Confronting the client and offering her a consequence of time out may be meaningless to her. Asking other clients to ignore her is inappropriate. A quiet but firm approach while distracting the client (walking her to her room and helping her get dressed) achieves the goal of having the client dressed appropriately and preserving her psychosocial integrity.

Test-Taking Strategy: Use the process of elimination, and note that the client is in a manic state. Recalling that the nurse must take control to protect the client will direct you to option 1. Review the care of the client with mania if you had difficulty with this question.

References
Stuart, G., & Laraia, M. (2005). *Principles and practice of psychiatric nursing* (8th ed., p. 336). St. Louis: Mosby.
Varcarolis, E., Carson, V., & Shoemaker, N. (2006). *Foundations of psychiatric mental health nursing* (5th ed., p. 367). Philadelphia: Saunders.

1050. Both the client who had cardiac surgery and the client's family express anxiety regarding how to cope with the recuperative process when they are home alone after discharge. The nurse plans to tell the client and family about which available resource?

1 The United Way
2 The local library
3 The American Cancer Society Reach for Recovery
4 The American Heart Association Mended Hearts Club

Answer: 4
Rationale: Most clients and families benefit from knowing that there are available resources to help them cope with the stress of self-care management at home. These can include telephone contact with the surgeon, the cardiologist, and the nurse; cardiac rehabilitation programs; and community support groups such as the American Heart Association Mended Hearts Club, which is a nationwide program with local chapters. The United Way provides a wide variety of services to people who may not otherwise be able to afford them. The library normally does not provide resources for coping with the recuperative process. The American Cancer Society Reach for Recovery helps women recover after mastectomy.

Test-Taking Strategy: Use the process of elimination. Note that the options identify three organizations and a library. Eliminate the library first, because the client and family need resources to cope, which implies the need for an interactive process. From the remaining options, noting that the client had cardiac surgery will direct you to option 4. Review the support services for clients who have had cardiac surgery if you had difficulty with this question.

Level of Cognitive Ability: Application
Client Needs: Psychosocial Integrity
Integrated Process: Nursing Process/Planning
Content Area: Adult Health/Cardiovascular

References
Black, J., & Hawks, J. (2005). *Medical-surgical nursing: Clinical management for positive outcomes* (7th ed., pp. 1644, 1699). Philadelphia: Saunders.
Lewis, S., Heitkemper, M., Dirksen, S., O'Brien, P., & Bucher, L. (2007). *Medical-surgical nursing: Assessment and management of clinical problems* (7th ed., pp. 811-812). St. Louis: Mosby.

1051. An older client who has never been hospitalized before is to have a 12-lead electrocardiogram (ECG). The nurse would alleviate the client's anxiety about the test by giving which of the following explanations?
  1 "It's important to lie still during the procedure."
  2 "It should only take about 20 minutes to complete the ECG tracing."
  3 "The ECG electrodes are painless and will record the electrical activity of the heart."
  4 "The ECG can give the doctor information about what might be wrong with your heart."

Level of Cognitive Ability: Application
Client Needs: Psychosocial Integrity
Integrated Process: Communication and Documentation
Content Area: Adult Health/Cardiovascular

Answer: 3
Rationale: The ECG uses painless electrodes that are applied to the chest and limbs. The procedure takes less than 5 minutes to complete, and it requires the client to lie still. The ECG measures the heart's electrical activity to determine rate, rhythm, and a variety of abnormalities. Options 1 and 4 are factual statements, but they are not stated to reduce anxiety.

Test-Taking Strategy: Use the process of elimination, and focus on the subject: alleviating the client's anxiety. Eliminate option 2, because it is inaccurate. Next, eliminate options 1 and 4, because they will not alleviate anxiety. Review the ECG and measures to alleviate anxiety if you had difficulty with this question.

References
Black, J., & Hawks, J. (2005). *Medical-surgical nursing: Clinical management for positive outcomes* (7th ed., pp. 1582-1583). Philadelphia: Saunders.
Pagana, K., & Pagana, T. (2005). *Mosby's diagnostic and laboratory test reference* (7th ed., p. 371). St. Louis: Mosby.

1052. A spouse of a client who is scheduled for the insertion of an implantable cardioverter-defibrillator (ICD) expresses anxiety about what would happen if the device discharges during physical contact. The nurse tells the spouse that:
  1 Physical contact should be avoided whenever possible.
  2 The spouse would not feel or be harmed by the countershock.
  3 The shock would be felt, but it would not cause the spouse any harm.
  4 A warning device sounds before countershock, so there is time to move away.

Level of Cognitive Ability: Application
Client Needs: Psychosocial Integrity
Integrated Process: Nursing Process/ Implementation
Content Area: Adult Health/Cardiovascular

Answer: 3
Rationale: Clients and families are often fearful about the activation of the ICD. Their fears are about the device itself and also about the occurrence of life-threatening dysrhythmias that trigger its function. Family members need reassurance that, even if the device activates while they are touching the client, the level of the charge is not high enough to harm the family member, although it will be felt. The ICD emits a warning beep when the client is near magnetic fields, which could possibly deactivate it, but it does not beep before countershock.

Test-Taking Strategy: Focus on the subject of anxiety, and use your knowledge of the function of the ICD to answer this question. This will direct you to option 3. Review the concepts related to the ICD if you had difficulty with this question.

Reference
Ignatavicius, D., & Workman, M. (2006). *Medical-surgical nursing: Critical thinking for collaborative care* (5th ed., pp. 745-746). Philadelphia: Saunders.

1053. A client who is scheduled for permanent transvenous pacemaker insertion says to the nurse, "I know I need it, but I'm not sure this surgery is the best idea." Which nursing response will best help the nurse assess the client's preoperative concerns?

1 "How does your family feel about the surgery?"

2 "Has anyone taught you about the procedure yet?"

3 "You sound uncertain about the procedure. Can you tell me more about what has you concerned?"

4 "You sound unnecessarily worried. Has anyone told you that the technology is quite advanced now?"

Level of Cognitive Ability: Application
Client Needs: Psychosocial Integrity
Integrated Process: Communication and Documentation
Content Area: Adult Health/Cardiovascular

Answer: 3

Rationale: Anxiety is common in the client with the need for pacemaker insertion. This can be related to a fear of life-threatening dysrhythmias or of the surgical procedure. Option 1 is not indicated, because it asks about the family and deflects attention away from the client's concerns. Options 2 and 4 are close-ended and not exploratory. Option 3 is open-ended and uses clarification as a communication technique to explore the client's concerns.

Test-Taking Strategy: Use therapeutic communication techniques, focusing on the subject: addressing the client's preoperative concerns. Option 1 can be eliminated first, because it addresses the family rather than the client. From the remaining options, the only option that addresses the client's concerns is option 3. Review therapeutic communication techniques if you had difficulty with this question.

References

Ignatavicius, D., & Workman, M. (2006). *Medical-surgical nursing: Critical thinking for collaborative care* (5th ed., p. 793). Philadelphia: Saunders.

Potter, P., & Perry, A. (2005). *Fundamentals of nursing* (6th ed., p. 437). St. Louis: Mosby.

1054. A client with superficial varicose veins says to the nurse, "I hate these things. They're so ugly. I wish I could get them to go away." The nurse makes which therapeutic response to the client?

1 "You should try sclerotherapy. It's great."

2 "There's not much you can do once you get them."

3 "What have you been told about varicose veins and their management?"

4 "I understand how you feel, but you know, they really don't look too bad."

Level of Cognitive Ability: Application
Client Needs: Psychosocial Integrity
Integrated Process: Communication and Documentation
Content Area: Adult Health/Cardiovascular

Answer: 3

Rationale: The client expressing distress about the physical appearance has a risk for a nursing diagnosis of Disturbed Body Image. The nurse assesses the client's knowledge and self-management of the condition as a means of empowering the client and helping him or her adapt to the body change. Options 1, 2, and 4 are nontherapeutic.

Test-Taking Strategy: Use the process of elimination. With questions that deal with client's feelings, select the option that facilitates the sharing of information and concerns by the client. Options 1, 2, and 4 cut off or limit further comments by the client. Additionally, option 3 addresses assessment, which is the first step of the nursing process. Review therapeutic communication techniques if you had difficulty with this question.

References

Black, J., & Hawks, J. (2005). *Medical-surgical nursing: Clinical management for positive outcomes* (7th ed., p. 1539). Philadelphia: Saunders.

Potter, P., & Perry, A. (2005). *Fundamentals of nursing* (6th ed., p. 437). St. Louis: Mosby.

1055. A client who has been diagnosed with chronic renal failure has been told that hemodialysis will be required. The client becomes angry and states, "I'll never be the same now." The nurse formulates which nursing diagnosis for the client?

1 Anxiety
2 Noncompliance
3 Disturbed body image
4 Disturbed thought processes

Level of Cognitive Ability: Analysis
Client Needs: Psychosocial Integrity
Integrated Process: Nursing Process/Analysis
Content Area: Adult Health/Renal

Answer: 3
Rationale: A client with a renal disorder such as renal failure may become angry in response to the permanence of the condition. Because of the physical changes and the change in lifestyle that may be required to manage a severe renal condition, the client may experience Disturbed body image. Anxiety is not appropriate, because the client is able to identify the cause of concern. The client is not stating a refusal to undergo therapy (option 2) and is not cognitively impaired (option 4).

Test-Taking Strategy: Use the process of elimination, and focus on the client's statement. Note that the client's statement focuses on the self, which is consistent with Disturbed body image. Review the defining characteristics of Disturbed body image if you had difficulty with this question.

Reference
Black, J., & Hawks, J. (2005). *Medical-surgical nursing: Clinical management for positive outcomes* (7th ed., p. 1423). Philadelphia: Saunders.

1056. A client with the diagnosis of hyperparathyroidism says to the nurse, "I can't stay on this diet. It is too difficult for me." When intervening in this situation, how should the nurse respond?

1 "Why do you think you find this diet plan difficult to adhere to?"
2 "It really isn't difficult to stick to this diet. Just avoid milk products."
3 "You are having a difficult time staying on this plan. Let's discuss this."
4 "It is very important that you stay on this diet to avoid forming renal calculi."

Level of Cognitive Ability: Application
Client Needs: Psychosocial Integrity
Integrated Process: Communication and Documentation
Content Area: Adult Health/Endocrine

Answer: 3
Rationale: By paraphrasing the client's statement, the nurse can encourage the client to verbalize emotions. The nurse also sends feedback to the client that the message was understood. An open-ended statement or question such as this prompts a lengthy response from the client. Option 1 requests information that the client may not be able to express. Option 2 devalues the client's feelings. Option 4 gives advice, which blocks communication.

Test-Taking Strategy: Use therapeutic communication techniques, and focus on the client's statement. Note that option 3 paraphrases the client's statement. Review therapeutic communication techniques if you had difficulty with this question.

References
Black, J., & Hawks, J. (2005). *Medical-surgical nursing: Clinical management for positive outcomes* (7th ed., p. 1201). Philadelphia: Saunders.
Potter, P., & Perry, A. (2005). *Fundamentals of nursing* (6th ed., p. 437). St. Louis: Mosby.

1057. The nurse is caring for a client with newly diagnosed type 1 diabetes mellitus. To develop an effective teaching plan, it would be most important for the nurse to assess the client for:

1 Knowledge of the diabetic diet
2 Expressions of denial of having diabetes
3 Fear of performing insulin administration
4 Feelings of depression about lifestyle changes

Answer: 2
Rationale: When diabetes mellitus is first diagnosed, the client may go through the phases of grief: denial, fear, anger, bargaining, depression, and acceptance. Denial is the phase that is the most detrimental to the teaching and learning process. If the client is denying the fact that he or she has diabetes, then he or she probably will not listen to discussions about the disease or how to manage it. Denial must be identified before the nurse can develop a teaching plan.

Level of Cognitive Ability: Application
Client Needs: Psychosocial Integrity
Integrated Process: Teaching and Learning
Content Area: Adult Health/Endocrine

Test-Taking Strategy: Use the process of elimination, and note the strategic words "most important." All of the options may be appropriate to assess, but note that options 1, 3, and 4 relate to specific components of the teaching. Option 2 is the umbrella option, and, considering the principles of teaching and learning, this aspect needs to be assessed before the implementation of teaching. Review the principles of teaching and learning if you had difficulty with this question.

Reference

Black, J., & Hawks, J. (2005). *Medical-surgical nursing: Clinical management for positive outcomes* (7th ed., pp. 525-526). Philadelphia: Saunders.

1058. A client with newly diagnosed type 1 diabetes mellitus has been seen for 3 consecutive days in the emergency department with hyperglycemia. During the assessment, the client says to the nurse, "I'm sorry to keep bothering you every day, but I just can't give myself those awful shots." The nurse makes which therapeutic response?

1 "I couldn't give myself a shot either."
2 "You must learn to give yourself the shots."
3 "Let me see if the doctor can change your medication."
4 "I'm sorry that you are having trouble with your injections. Has someone given you instructions about how to perform them?"

Level of Cognitive Ability: Application
Client Needs: Psychosocial Integrity
Integrated Process: Communication and Documentation
Content Area: Adult Health/Endocrine

Answer: 4
Rationale: It is important to determine and deal with a client's underlying fear of self-injection. The nurse should determine whether a knowledge deficit exists. Positive reinforcement should occur rather than focusing on negative behaviors (option 1). Demanding that the client perform a behavior or skill is inappropriate (option 2). The nurse should not offer a change in regimen that cannot be accomplished (option 3).

Test-Taking Strategy: Use therapeutic communication techniques. Options 1, 2, and 3 are nontherapeutic. In addition, option 3 may provide false reassurance regarding a potential change in medications. Review therapeutic communication techniques if you had difficulty with this question.

References

Black, J., & Hawks, J. (2005). *Medical-surgical nursing: Clinical management for positive outcomes* (7th ed., pp. 1262-1263). Philadelphia: Saunders.
Ignatavicius, D., & Workman, M. (2006). *Medical-surgical nursing: Critical thinking for collaborative care* (5th ed., pp. 1548-1549). Philadelphia: Saunders.
Potter, P., & Perry, A. (2005). *Fundamentals of nursing* (6th ed., p. 437). St. Louis: Mosby.

1059. The nurse requests that a client with diabetes mellitus ask his or her significant other(s) to attend an educational conference about the self-administration of insulin. The client questions why significant others need to be included. The nurse's best response would be:

1 "Family members can take you to the doctor."
2 "Family members are at risk of developing diabetes."
3 "Nurses need someone to call and check on a client's progress."
4 "Clients and families often work together to develop strategies for the management of diabetes."

Answer: 4
Rationale: Families and significant others may be included in diabetes education to assist with adjustments of the diabetic regimen. Although options 1 and 2 may be accurate, they are not the most appropriate responses. Option 3 devalues the client, disregards the issue of independence, and promotes powerlessness.

Test-Taking Strategy: Use the process of elimination and therapeutic communication techniques. Eliminate option 3 first, because it devalues the client. From the remaining options, note that option 4 is the umbrella option. Review therapeutic communication techniques if you had difficulty with this question.

Level of Cognitive Ability: Application
Client Needs: Psychosocial Integrity
Integrated Process: Communication and
Documentation
Content Area: Adult Health/Endocrine

References
Black, J., & Hawks, J. (2005). *Medical-surgical nursing: Clinical management for positive outcomes* (7th ed., p. 1265). Philadelphia: Saunders.
Ignatavicius, D., & Workman, M. (2006). *Medical-surgical nursing: Critical thinking for collaborative care* (5th ed., pp. 1546-1547). Philadelphia: Saunders.
Potter, P., & Perry, A. (2005). *Fundamentals of nursing* (6th ed., p. 437). St. Louis: Mosby.

1060. A 22-year-old female client has recently been diagnosed with polycystic kidney disease. The nurse has a series of discussions with the client that are intended to help the client adjust to the disorder. The nurse plans to include which item as part of one of these discussions?

1 Ongoing fluid restriction
2 The need for genetic counseling
3 The risk of hypotensive episodes
4 Depression regarding massive edema

Level of Cognitive Ability: Application
Client Needs: Psychosocial Integrity
Integrated Process: Nursing Process/Planning
Content Area: Adult Health/Renal

Answer: 2

Rationale: Adult polycystic kidney disease is a hereditary disorder that is inherited as an autosomal-dominant trait. Because of this, the client and his or her extended family should have genetic counseling. Ongoing fluid restriction is unnecessary. The client is likely to have hypertension rather than hypotension. Massive edema is not part of the clinical picture of this disorder.

Test-Taking Strategy: Use the process of elimination. Because massive edema and the need for fluid restriction are not part of the clinical picture of the client with polycystic kidney disease, eliminate options 1 and 4. From the remaining options, recalling either that this disorder is hereditary in nature or that the client would exhibit hypertension rather than hypotension will direct you to option 2. Review the psychosocial aspects related to polycystic kidney disease if you had difficulty with this question.

Reference
Black, J., & Hawks, J. (2005). *Medical-surgical nursing: Clinical management for positive outcomes* (7th ed., p. 937). Philadelphia: Saunders.

1061. The nurse is admitting a client to the hospital who is to undergo ureterolithotomy for urinary calculi removal. The nurse understands that it is unnecessary to assess which of the following to determine the client's readiness for surgery?

1 The need for a visit from a support group
2 The knowledge of postoperative activities
3 An understanding of the surgical procedure
4 Feelings or anxieties about the surgical procedure

Level of Cognitive Ability: Application
Client Needs: Psychosocial Integrity
Integrated Process: Nursing Process/Assessment
Content Area: Adult Health/Renal

Answer: 1

Rationale: Ureterolithotomy is the removal of a calculus from the ureter using either a flank or abdominal incision. Because no urinary diversion is created during this procedure, the client has no need for a visit from a member of a support group. The client should have an understanding of the same items as are required for any surgery, including a knowledge of the procedures, the expected outcome, the postoperative routines, and any expected discomfort. The client should also be assessed for any concerns or anxieties before surgery.

Test-Taking Strategy: Use the process of elimination, and note the strategic word "unnecessary." Eliminate options 2, 3, and 4, because they are assessments that should be performed before surgery. Recalling that a urinary diversion is not needed for this type of surgery will direct you to option 1. Review preoperative assessments if you had difficulty with this question.

References
Black, J., & Hawks, J. (2005). *Medical-surgical nursing: Clinical management for positive outcomes* (7th ed., pp. 889-890). Philadelphia: Saunders.
Stuart, G., & Laraia, M. (2005). *Principles and practice of psychiatric nursing* (8th ed., p. 678). St. Louis: Mosby.
Varcarolis, E., Carson, V., & Shoemaker, N. (2006). *Foundations of psychiatric mental health nursing* (5th ed., p. 597). Philadelphia: Saunders.

1062. The spouse of a dying client says to the nurse, "I don't think I can come anymore and watch her die. It's chewing me up too much!" The nurse should make which therapeutic response to the spouse?

1 "Focus on your wife's pain rather than yours. I know it's hard, but this isn't about what's happening to you, you know."

2 "I know it's hard for you, but she would know if you're not there, and you would feel so very guilty all of the rest of your days."

3 "It's hard to watch someone you love die. You've been here with your wife every day. Are you taking any time for yourself?"

4 "I think you're making the right decision. Your wife knows you love her. You don't have to come everyday. I'll take care of her."

Level of Cognitive Ability: Application
Client Needs: Psychosocial Integrity
Integrated Process: Communication and Documentation
Content Area: Mental Health

Answer: 3
Rationale: The most therapeutic response is the one that is empathic and that reflects the nurse's understanding of the client's (in this case, the husband) stress and emotional pain. In the correct option, the nurse suggests that the client take time for himself. Option 1 is an example of a nontherapeutic and judgmental attitude that places blame. Option 2 makes statements that the nurse cannot know are true (the client's wife may not in fact know if the husband visits) and that predicts feelings of guilt, which is inappropriate. Option 4 fosters dependency and gives advice, which is nontherapeutic.

Test-Taking Strategy: Use therapeutic communication techniques to answer the question. Note that the client of the question is the husband. Option 3 is the only option that is therapeutic and that addresses the husband's feelings. Review therapeutic communication techniques if you had difficulty with this question.

References
Stuart, G., & Laraia, M. (2005). *Principles and practice of psychiatric nursing* (8th ed., pp. 30-34). St. Louis: Mosby.
Varcarolis, E., Carson, V., & Shoemaker, N. (2006). *Foundations of psychiatric mental health nursing* (5th ed., pp. 617-618). Philadelphia: Saunders.

1063. An older adult client at the retirement center spits her food out and throws it on the floor. She yells, "This turkey is dry and cold! I can't stand the food here!" How should the nurse respond to the client?

1 "Now look what you've done! You're ruining this meal for the whole community. Aren't you ashamed of yourself?"

2 "I think you had better return to your apartment now. I'll make arrangements for a new meal to be served to you there."

3 "Let me get you another serving that is more to your liking. Would you like to come visit the chef and select your own serving?"

4 "One of the things that was agreed upon was that anyone who did not use appropriate behavior would be asked to leave the dining room. Please leave now."

Level of Cognitive Ability: Application
Client Needs: Psychosocial Integrity
Integrated Process: Communication and Documentation
Content Area: Mental Health

Answer: 3
Rationale: Asking the client to accompany the nurse to the kitchen respects the client's need for control, removes the angry client from the dining room, and may offer the nurse an opportunity to assess what is happening to the client. Option 2 could provoke a regressive struggle between the nurse and the client and cause more anger in the client. Option 1 is angry, aggressive, and nontherapeutic. In option 4, the nurse is authoritative, and it would not be appropriate to ask the client to leave. This action may set up an aggressive struggle between the nurse and the client.

Test-Taking Strategy: Use therapeutic communication techniques and your knowledge about the care of an angry client. Option 3 is the only option that addresses the client's angry feelings, and it also provides the nurse with an opportunity to further assess the client. Review therapeutic communication techniques if you had difficulty with this question.

References
Stuart, G., & Laraia, M. (2005). *Principles and practice of psychiatric nursing* (8th ed., pp. 30-34). St. Louis: Mosby.
Varcarolis, E., Carson, V., & Shoemaker, N. (2006). *Foundations of psychiatric mental health nursing* (5th ed., pp. 490, 500). Philadelphia: Saunders.

1064. A physician orders a follow-up home-care visit for an older adult client with emphysema. When the home-care nurse arrives, the client is smoking. Which statement by the nurse would be therapeutic?

  1 "Well, I can see you never got to the stop-smoking clinic!"

  2 "I'm glad I caught you smoking! Now that your secret is out, let's decide what you are going to do."

  3 "I notice that you are smoking. Did you explore the stop-smoking program at the senior citizens center?"

  4 "I wonder if you realize that you are slowly killing yourself. Why prolong the agony? You can just jump off the bridge!"

Level of Cognitive Ability: Application
Client Needs: Psychosocial Integrity
Integrated Process: Communication and Documentation
Content Area: Adult Health/Respiratory

Answer: 3

Rationale: Emphysema clients need to avoid smoking and all airborne irritants. The nurse who observes a maladaptive behavior in a client should not make judgmental comments and should instead explore an adaptive strategy with the client without being overly controlling. This will place the decision making in the client's hands and provide an avenue for the client to share what may be expressions of frustration about an inability to stop what is essentially a physiological addiction. Option 1 is an intrusive use of sarcastic humor that is degrading to the client. Option 2 is a disciplinary remark and places a barrier between the nurse and the client within the therapeutic relationship. In Option 4, the nurse preaches and is judgmental.

Test-Taking Strategy: Use therapeutic communication techniques. Option 3 recognizes and addresses the client's behavior and explores an avenue for dealing with the behavior. Review therapeutic communication techniques if you had difficulty with this question.

References

Black, J., & Hawks, J. (2005). *Medical-surgical nursing: Clinical management for positive outcomes* (7th ed., pp. 1818, 1828). Philadelphia: Saunders.

Potter, P., & Perry, A. (2005). *Fundamentals of nursing* (6th ed., p. 437). St. Louis: Mosby.

1065. A client is to have arterial blood gases drawn. While the nurse is performing Allen's test, the client says to the nurse, "What are you doing? No one else has done that!" The nurse makes which therapeutic response to the client?

  1 "I assure you that I am doing the correct procedure. I cannot account for what others do."

  2 "This step is crucial to safe blood withdrawal. I would not let anyone take my blood until they did this."

  3 "Oh? You have questions about this? You should insist that they all do this procedure before drawing up your blood."

  4 "This is a routine precautionary step that simply makes certain your circulation is intact before a blood sample is obtained."

Level of Cognitive Ability: Application
Client Needs: Psychosocial Integrity
Integrated Process: Communication and Documentation
Content Area: Adult Health/Cardiovascular

Answer: 4

Rationale: Allen's test is performed to assess collateral circulation in the hand before drawing a radial artery blood specimen. The therapeutic response provides information to the client. Option 1 is defensive and nontherapeutic in that it offers false reassurance. Option 2 identifies client advocacy, but it is overly controlling and aggressive, and it undermines treatment. Option 3 is aggressive, controlling, and nontherapeutic in its disapproving stance.

Test-Taking Strategy: Use therapeutic communication techniques and the process of elimination. Option 4 addresses the subject of the question and provides information to the client. Review therapeutic communication techniques if you had difficulty with this question.

References

Black, J., & Hawks, J. (2005). *Medical-surgical nursing: Clinical management for positive outcomes* (7th ed., pp. 258, 1764). Philadelphia: Saunders.

Potter, P., & Perry, A. (2005). *Fundamentals of nursing* (6th ed., p. 437). St. Louis: Mosby.

1066. A client reports having difficulty concentrating and outbursts of anger as well as feeling "keyed up" all the time. The nurse obtaining the client's history discovers that the symptoms started about 6 months ago. The client reveals that, around that same time, a best friend was killed in a drive-by shooting while they were talking together. The nurse suspects that the client is experiencing:
  1 Social phobia
  2 Panic disorder
  3 Post-traumatic stress disorder (PTSD)
  4 Obsessive-compulsive disorder (OCD)

Level of Cognitive Ability: Analysis
Client Needs: Psychosocial Integrity
Integrated Process: Nursing Process/Analysis
Content Area: Mental Health

Answer: 3
Rationale: PTSD is a response to an event that would be markedly distressing to almost anyone. Characteristic symptoms include a sustained level of anxiety, difficulty sleeping, irritability, difficulty concentrating, and outbursts of anger. OCD involves some repetitive thoughts or behaviors. Panic disorders and social phobia are characterized by a specific fear of an object or situation.

Test-Taking Strategy: Focus on the data in the question, and use the process of elimination. Eliminate options 1 and 2 first, because they are comparable or alike. From the remaining options, recalling that OCD relates to a repetitive thought or behavior will direct you to option 3. Review PTSD if you had difficulty with this question.

Reference
Stuart, G., & Laraia, M. (2005). *Principles and practice of psychiatric nursing* (8th ed., p. 273). St. Louis: Mosby.

1067. A client says to the nurse, "I can't get any help with my care! I call and call but the nurses never answer my light. Last night one of them told me she had other clients besides me! I'm very sick, but the nurses don't care!" Which of the following statements from the nurse is therapeutic?
  1 "I think you are being very impatient. The nurses come as quickly as they can."
  2 "I can hear your anger. That nurse had no right to speak to you that way. I will report her."
  3 "It's hard to be in bed and to have to ask for help. You feel that the nurses do not seem to care?"
  4 "You poor thing! I'm so sorry this happened to you. That nurse should be fired immediately."

Level of Cognitive Ability: Application
Client Needs: Psychosocial Integrity
Integrated Process: Communication and Documentation
Content Area: Mental Health

Answer: 3
Rationale: Empathy is a term that describes the nurse's capacity to enter into the life of another person and to perceive how the client is feeling and what meaning this has for the client. In option 3, the nurse displays empathy and shares perceptions. The sharing of perceptions asks the client to validate the nurse's understanding of what the client is feeling and thinking. It opens the door for the client to share concerns, fears, and anxieties. In option 1, the nurse is assertive and also defends the nursing staff. In option 2, the nurse expresses the client's frustration by labeling the client's feelings as "angry" and disapproving of the nursing staff. This is splitting, and it is nontherapeutic. Option 4 is a social response, and it is demeaning to the client.

Test-Taking Strategy: Use therapeutic communication techniques and the process of elimination. Focus on the client's statement in the question. Note the relationship between the client's statement and option 3. In addition, in this option, the nurse validates the client's feelings. Review therapeutic communication techniques if you had difficulty with this question.

References
Stuart, G., & Laraia, M. (2005). *Principles and practice of psychiatric nursing* (8th ed., pp. 30-34). St. Louis: Mosby.
Varcarolis, E., Carson, V., & Shoemaker, N. (2006). *Foundations of psychiatric mental health nursing* (5th ed., p. 157). Philadelphia: Saunders.

1068. An English-speaking Hispanic male with a newly applied long leg cast has a right proximal fractured tibia. During rounds at night, the nurse finds the client restless, withdrawn, and quiet. Which initial nursing statement would be appropriate?

1 "Are you uncomfortable?"
2 "Tell me what you are feeling."
3 "You'll feel better in the morning."
4 "I'll get you pain medication right away."

Level of Cognitive Ability: Application
Client Needs: Psychosocial Integrity
Integrated Process: Communication and Documentation
Content Area: Adult Health/Musculoskeletal

Answer: 2
Rationale: Option 2 is open-ended and makes no assumptions about the client's psychological or emotional state. Option 1 is incorrect, because males in traditional standard Hispanic cultures practice "machismo" in which stoicism is valued, so this client may deny any pain when asked. False reassurance is never therapeutic, which makes option 3 incorrect. Option 4 is incorrect, because an assessment is necessary before administering medication for pain.

Test-Taking Strategy: Use therapeutic communication techniques. Recalling that the client's feelings are the priority will direct you to option 2. Review therapeutic communication techniques if you had difficulty with this question.

References

Giger, J., & Davidhizar, R. (2004). *Transcultural nursing* (5th ed, p. 224). St. Louis: Mosby.
Potter, P , & Perry, A. (2005). *Fundamentals of nursing* (6th ed., p. 437). St. Louis: Mosby.

1069. A client was started on oral anticoagulant therapy while hospitalized. The client is now being discharged to home and is intermittently confused. The nurse determines that the client has the best support system for successful anticoagulant therapy monitoring if the client:

1 Has a home health aide coming to the house for 9 weeks
2 Was going to stay with a daughter in the daughter's home indefinitely
3 Was going to have blood work drawn in the home by a local laboratory
4 Has a good friend living next door who would take the client to the doctor

Level of Cognitive Ability: Analysis
Client Needs: Psychosocial Integrity
Integrated Process: Nursing Process/Evaluation
Content Area: Adult Health/Cardiovascular

Answer: 2
Rationale: The client taking anticoagulant therapy should be informed about the medication, its purpose, and the necessity of taking the proper dose at the specified times. If the client is unwilling or unable to comply with the medication regimen, the continuance of the regimen should be questioned. Clients may need support systems in place to enhance compliance with therapy. Option 1 facilitates reminding the client to take the medication, option 3 facilitates blood work only, and option 4 facilitates medical care. Option 2 provides a direct support system.

Test-Taking Strategy: Use the process of elimination, and note the subject: the best support system. Note that option 2 is the only option that indicates direct support for the client. Review the concepts surrounding support systems for the client if you had difficulty with this question.

References

Black, J., & Hawks, J. (2005). *Medical-surgical nursing: Clinical management for positive outcomes* (7th ed., p. 489). Philadelphia: Saunders.
Ignatavicius, D., & Workman, M. (2006). *Medical-surgical nursing: Critical thinking for collaborative care* (5th ed., pp. 654-655). Philadelphia: Saunders.

1070. A client who has undergone successful femoral-popliteal bypass grafting of the leg says to the nurse, "I hope everything goes well after this and that I don't lose my leg. I'm so afraid that I'll have gone through this for nothing." The nurse makes which therapeutic response to the client?

1 "I can understand what you mean. I'd be nervous too, if I were in your shoes."

2 "This surgery is so successful that I wouldn't be concerned at all if I were you."

3 "Complications are possible, but you have a good deal of control if you make the lifestyle adjustments we talked about."

4 "Stress isn't helpful for you. You should probably just try to relax. You shouldn't worry unless something actually happens."

Level of Cognitive Ability: Application
Client Needs: Psychosocial Integrity
Integrated Process: Communication and Documentation
Content Area: Adult Health/Cardiovascular

Answer: 3

Rationale: Clients frequently fear that they will ultimately lose a limb or become debilitated in some other way. Option 1 feeds into the client's anxiety and is not therapeutic. Option 2 gives false reassurance. Option 4 is meant to be reassuring, but it offers no suggestions to empower the client. Option 3 acknowledges the client's concerns and empowers the client to improve his or her health, which will ultimately reduce concern about the risk of complications.

Test-Taking Strategy: Use the process of elimination and therapeutic communication techniques. Option 3 is the only option that acknowledges the client's concerns and addresses the client's control over the situation. Review therapeutic communication techniques if you had difficulty with this question.

References

Black, J., & Hawks, J. (2005). *Medical-surgical nursing: Clinical management for positive outcomes* (7th ed., pp. 1517-1518). Philadelphia: Saunders.

Ignatavicius, D., & Workman, M. (2006). *Medical-surgical nursing: Critical thinking for collaborative care* (5th ed., p. 857). Philadelphia: Saunders.

Potter, P., & Perry, A. (2005). *Fundamentals of nursing* (6th ed., p. 437). St. Louis: Mosby.

1071. A client in the coronary care unit is about to have a pericardiocentesis done for a rapidly accumulating pericardial effusion. The nurse's best plan to alleviate the apprehension of the client is by:

1 Telling the client to watch television during the procedure as a distraction

2 Talking to the client from the foot of the bed and being available to get needed supplies

3 Staying beside the client and giving information and encouragement during the procedure

4 Telling the client that she (the nurse) will take care of another assigned client at this time so that she will be available when the procedure is complete

Level of Cognitive Ability: Application
Client Needs: Psychosocial Integrity
Integrated Process: Caring
Content Area: Adult Health/Cardiovascular

Answer: 3

Rationale: Clients who develop sudden complications are in situational crisis and need therapeutic intervention. Staying with the client and giving information and encouragement is part of building and maintaining trust in the nurse–client relationship. Options 1 and 4 distance the nurse from the client in a psychosocial as well as physical sense. The nurse should ask another caregiver to be available to get extra supplies if they are needed.

Test-Taking Strategy: Use the process of elimination and therapeutic communication techniques. Option 3 is the only option that provides direct contact with and assistance to the client. Review therapeutic communication techniques if you had difficulty with this question.

References

Black, J., & Hawks, J. (2005). *Medical-surgical nursing: Clinical management for positive outcomes* (7th ed., p. 1622). Philadelphia: Saunders.

Ignatavicius, D., & Workman, M. (2006). *Medical-surgical nursing: Critical thinking for collaborative care* (5th ed., p. 694). Philadelphia: Saunders.

1072. A nurse has formulated a nursing diagnosis of Disturbed body image for the male client taking spironolactone (Aldactone). The nurse based this diagnosis on the assessment of which of the following side effects of the medication?

1 Edema
2 Hair loss
3 Alopecia
4 Decreased libido

Level of Cognitive Ability: Analysis
Client Needs: Psychosocial Integrity
Integrated Process: Nursing Process/Analysis
Content Area: Pharmacology

Answer: 4

Rationale: The nurse should be aware of the fact that the client taking spironolactone may experience body image changes that result from a threatened sexual identity. These are related to decreased libido, gynecomastia in males, and hirsutism in females. Edema and hair loss are not specifically associated with the use of this medication.

Test-Taking Strategy: Use the process of elimination and your knowledge regarding the side effects of spironolactone. Eliminate options 2 and 3, because they are comparable or alike. From the remaining options, focusing on the nursing diagnosis in the question will direct you to option 4. Review the side effects of spironolactone if you had difficulty with this question.

Reference
Skidmore-Roth, L. (2008). *Mosby's nursing drug reference* (21st ed., p. 940). St. Louis: Mosby.

1073. The nurse is caring for a client who is recovering from the signs and symptoms of autonomic hyperreflexia. The nurse makes which therapeutic statement to the client?

1 "How could your home-care nurse let this happen?"
2 "Now that this problem is taken care of, I'm sure you'll be fine."
3 "I have some time if you would like to talk about what happened to you."
4 "I'm sure you now understand the importance of preventing this from occurring."

Level of Cognitive Ability: Application
Client Needs: Psychosocial Integrity
Integrated Process: Communication and Documentation
Content Area: Adult Health/Neurological

Answer: 3

Rationale: Option 3 encourages the client to discuss his or her feelings. Options 1 and 4 show disapproval, and option 2 provides false reassurance; these are nontherapeutic techniques.

Test-Taking Strategy: Use the process of elimination and therapeutic communication techniques. Remembering to always address the client's concerns and feelings first will direct you to option 3. Review therapeutic communication techniques if you had difficulty with this question.

References
Black, J., & Hawks, J. (2005). *Medical-surgical nursing: Clinical management for positive outcomes* (7th ed., p. 2229). Philadelphia: Saunders.
Potter, P., & Perry, A. (2005). *Fundamentals of nursing* (6th ed., p. 437). St. Louis: Mosby.

1074. While assisting a client with a spinal cord injury with activities of daily living, the client states, "I can't do this. I wish I were dead." The nurse makes which therapeutic response to the client?

1 "Why do you say that?"
2 "You wish you were dead?"
3 "Let's wash your back now."
4 "I'm sure you are frustrated, but things will work out just fine for you."

Answer: 2

Rationale: Clarifying is a therapeutic technique that involves restating what was said to obtain additional information. By asking "why" (option 1), the nurse puts the client on the defensive. Option 3 changes the subject. In option 4, false reassurance is offered. Options 1, 3, and 4 are nontherapeutic and block communication.

Level of Cognitive Ability: Application
Client Needs: Psychosocial Integrity
Integrated Process: Communication and
Documentation
Content Area: Adult Health/Neurological

Test-Taking Strategy: Use the process of elimination and therapeutic communication techniques. Remember to focus on the client's feelings. Option 2 involves clarifying and restating, and it is the only option that will encourage the client to verbalize feelings and concerns. Review therapeutic communication techniques if you had difficulty with this question.

References

Black, J., & Hawks, J. (2005). *Medical-surgical nursing: Clinical management for positive outcomes* (7th ed., p. 2224). Philadelphia: Saunders.

Potter, P., & Perry, A. (2005). *Fundamentals of nursing* (6th ed., p. 437). St. Louis: Mosby.

1075. Family members of a client who attempted suicide are tearful. Which statement by the nurse would be therapeutic?
1 "I'll check on when you will be able to see your loved one."
2 "Believe me when I say that everything possible is being done."
3 "Don't worry, you have absolutely nothing to feel guilty about."
4 "I certainly can see that you are terribly worried about your loved one."

Level of Cognitive Ability: Application
Client Needs: Psychosocial Integrity
Integrated Process: Caring
Content Area: Mental Health

Answer: 4

Rationale: Options 1, 2, and 3 are communication blocks. Option 1 focuses on an important issue at an inappropriate time. Option 2 uses clichés and false reassurance. Option 3 labels the family's behavior without their validation. Option 4 addresses the family's feelings and displays empathy.

Test-Taking Strategy: Use the process of elimination and therapeutic communication techniques. Option 4 involves clarifying, and it is the only option that will encourage the family to verbalize feelings and concerns. Review therapeutic communication techniques if you had difficulty with this question.

Reference

Stuart, G., & Laraia, M. (2005). *Principles and practice of psychiatric nursing* (8th ed., pp. 30-34, 367). St. Louis: Mosby.

1076. A nurse is caring for an 11-year-old child who has been abused. The nurse includes which therapeutic action in the plan of care?
1 Encourage the child to fear the abuser.
2 Provide a care environment that allows for the development of trust.
3 Teach the child to make wise choices when confronted with an abusive situation.
4 Have the child point out the abuser if he or she should visit while the child is hospitalized.

Level of Cognitive Ability: Application
Client Needs: Psychosocial Integrity
Integrated Process: Caring
Content Area: Child Health

Answer: 2

Rationale: The abused child usually requires long-term therapeutic support. The environment provided during the child's healing must include one in which trust and empathy are modeled and provided for the child. Option 1 reinforces fear, which should not be encouraged. Options 3 and 4 ask the child to behave with a maturity beyond that which would be expected for an 11-year-old child. Option 2 is therapeutic, because it provides the child with a nurturing and supportive environment in which to begin the healing process.

Test-Taking Strategy: Use the process of elimination and therapeutic techniques. Option 2 is the only option that provides support to the child. Review therapeutic interventions for a child who has been abused if you had difficulty with this question.

Reference

Hockenberry, M., Wilson, D., & Winkelstein, M. (2005). *Wong's essentials of pediatric nursing* (7th ed., p. 468). St. Louis: Mosby.

1077. Which of the following psychosocial factors obtained during an assessment of an older client places the client at risk for abuse?

 1 The client resides in an apartment in a low-income neighborhood.
 2 The client shows several signs and symptoms of clinical depression.
 3 The client is completely dependent on family members for both food and medicine.
 4 The client has been diagnosed with and is receiving treatment for several chronic illnesses.

Level of Cognitive Ability: Analysis
Client Needs: Psychosocial Integrity
Integrated Process: Nursing Process/Assessment
Content Area: Mental Health

Answer: 3
Rationale: Elder abuse is sometimes the result of frustrated adult children who find themselves caring for dependent parents. Increasing demands by parents for care and financial support can cause resentment and a feeling of being burdened. Option 2 relates to depression rather than the risk for abuse. Option 4 relates to a physical factor rather than a psychosocial factor. The issues of abuse are not bound to socioeconomic status (option 1).

Test-Taking Strategy: Note the strategic words "psychosocial factors," and focus on the subject: the risk for abuse. Noting the strategic words "completely dependent" in option 3 will direct you to this option. Review the risk factors associated with elder abuse if you had difficulty with this question.

References
Stuart, G., & Laraia, M. (2005). *Principles and practice of psychiatric nursing* (8th ed., pp. 810-811). St. Louis: Mosby.
Varcarolis, E., Carson, V., & Shoemaker, N. (2006). *Foundations of psychiatric mental health nursing* (5th ed., p. 508). Philadelphia: Saunders.

1078. The nurse is caring for a dying male client who says, "Will you be the executor of my will?" How should the nurse respond to this client?

 1 "Tell me more so that I can understand your thinking."
 2 "I must decline your offer, because I am your nurse."
 3 "I will carry out your will according to your wishes."
 4 "It is an honor to be named the executor of your will."

Level of Cognitive Ability: Application
Client Needs: Psychosocial Integrity
Integrated Process: Communication and Documentation
Content Area: Fundamental Skills

Answer: 1
Rationale: The client's question reflects his thoughts about the will and how to obtain an executor, but the question does not reveal why the client is asking the nurse to be executor, and it also does not address other important information. In option 1, the nurse seeks clarification while acknowledging the client's statement. Most agencies do not allow a nurse to be the executor of a client's will (option 2) or to witness other legal documents, to avoid conflict-of-interest charges. In addition, option 3 is an unsuitable response. In option 4, the nurse, who is responding with social communication, fails to regard the potential consequences, think critically, or explore the client's motivation and needs.

Test-Taking Strategy: Use therapeutic communication techniques and the process of elimination. Option 1 is the only option that addresses the client's thoughts and feelings. Review therapeutic communication techniques if you had difficulty with this question.

References
Black, J., & Hawks, J. (2005). *Medical-surgical nursing: Clinical management for positive outcomes* (7th ed., pp. 63-64). Philadelphia: Saunders.
Ignatavicius, D., & Workman, M. (2006). *Medical-surgical nursing: Critical thinking for collaborative care* (5th ed., p. 106). Philadelphia: Saunders.
Potter, P., & Perry, A. (2005). *Fundamentals of nursing* (6th ed., p. 437). St. Louis: Mosby.

1079. A client who is suffering from urticaria (hives) and pruritus says to the nurse, "What am I going to do? I'm getting married next week, and I'll probably be covered in this rash and itching like crazy." Which of the following statements made by the nurse is the most therapeutic?
  1 "You're troubled that this will extend into your wedding?"
  2 "It's probably just due to prewedding jitters. You'll be fine."
  3 "The antihistamine will help a great deal, just you wait and see."
  4 "I hope your husband-to-be has a sense of humor and can laugh about this."

Level of Cognitive Ability: Application
Client Needs: Psychosocial Integrity
Integrated Process: Communication and Documentation
Content Area: Mental Health

Answer: 1
Rationale: The therapeutic communication technique that the nurse uses in option 1 is reflection. In option 2, the nurse minimizes the client's anxiety and fears. In option 3, the nurse talks about antihistamines and asks the client to "wait and see." This is nontherapeutic, because the nurse is making promises that may not be kept. In addition, the response is close-ended and shuts off the client's expression of feelings. In option 4, the nurse uses humor inappropriately and without sensitivity.

Test-Taking Strategy: Use the process of elimination and therapeutic communication techniques. Options 2, 3, and 4 are nontherapeutic responses. Option 1 addresses the client's feelings. Review therapeutic communication techniques if you had difficulty with this question.

References
Ignatavicius, D., & Workman, M. (2006). *Medical-surgical nursing: Critical thinking for collaborative care* (5th ed., p. 1577). Philadelphia: Saunders.
Stuart, G., & Laraia, M. (2005). *Principles and practice of psychiatric nursing* (8th ed., pp. 30-34). St. Louis: Mosby.

1080. A client with a spinal cord injury makes the following comments. Which comment warrants additional intervention by the nurse?
  1 "I'm so angry that this happened to me."
  2 "I'm really looking forward to going home."
  3 "I know I will have to make major adjustments in my life."
  4 "I would like my family members to be here for my teaching sessions."

Level of Cognitive Ability: Analysis
Client Needs: Psychosocial Integrity
Integrated Process: Nursing Process/Analysis
Content Area: Adult Health/Neurological

Answer: 1
Rationale: It is important to allow the client with a spinal cord injury to verbalize his or her feelings. If the client indicates a desire to discuss his or her feelings, the nurse should respond therapeutically. Options 3 and 4 indicate that the client understands that changes will be occurring and that family involvement is best. No data in the question indicate that the client will not be going home; therefore, this comment does not require further intervention.

Test-Taking Strategy: Use the process of elimination, noting the strategic words "warrants additional intervention." Noting the word "angry" in option 1 will direct you to this option. Review psychosocial issues related to the care of a client with a spinal cord injury if you had difficulty with this question.

Reference
Black, J., & Hawks, J. (2005). *Medical-surgical nursing: Clinical management for positive outcomes* (7th ed., p. 2224). Philadelphia: Saunders.

1081. The nurse is caring for a client with a grade II (mild) cerebral aneurysm rupture. The client becomes restless and anxious before visiting hours. The nurse determines that the client's behavior is likely related to:
  1 Spiritual distress
  2 Disturbed body image
  3 Disabled family coping
  4 The severity of the aneurysm rupture

Answer: 2
Rationale: A grade II cerebral aneurysm rupture is a mild bleed in which the client remains alert but has nuchal rigidity with possible neurological deficits, depending on the area of the bleed. Because these clients remain alert, they are acutely aware of the neurological deficits and frequently have some degree of body image disturbance. No data in the question indicate that the client's behavior is related to options 1, 3, or 4.

Level of Cognitive Ability: Analysis
Client Needs: Psychosocial Integrity
Integrated Process: Nursing Process/Analysis
Content Area: Adult Health/Neurological

Test-Taking Strategy: Focus on the client's behavior, and note the strategic words "before visiting hours." Using your knowledge of the effects of this disorder and focusing on the client's behavior will direct you to option 2. Review the effects of a grade II cerebral aneurysm rupture if you had difficulty with this question.

References

Black, J., & Hawks, J. (2005). *Medical-surgical nursing: Clinical management for positive outcomes* (7th ed., p. 2089). Philadelphia: Saunders.
Ignatavicius, D., & Workman, M. (2006). *Medical-surgical nursing: Critical thinking for collaborative care* (5th ed., p. 1037). Philadelphia: Saunders.

1082. When planning the care of the client with thromboangiitis obliterans (Buerger's disease), the nurse incorporates measures to help the client cope with the lifestyle changes that are needed to control the disease process. The nurse can accomplish this by recommending a:

1 Consult with a dietician
2 Pain management clinic
3 Smoking cessation program
4 Referral to a medical social worker

Level of Cognitive Ability: Application
Client Needs: Psychosocial Integrity
Integrated Process: Nursing Process/ Implementation
Content Area: Adult Health/Cardiovascular

Answer: 3
Rationale: Smoking is highly detrimental to the client with Buerger's disease, and clients are recommended to stop completely. Because smoking is a form of chemical dependency, referral to a smoking cessation program may be helpful for many clients. For many clients, symptoms are relieved or alleviated when smoking stops. Options 1, 2, and 4 are not directly related to the physiology associated with this condition.

Test-Taking Strategy: Use the process of elimination, and focus on the client's diagnosis. Recalling that the treatment goals are the same as for peripheral vascular disease will direct you to option 3. Review the treatment goals for Buerger's disease if you had difficulty with this question.

Reference

Black, J., & Hawks, J. (2005). *Medical-surgical nursing: Clinical management for positive outcomes* (7th ed., p. 1534). Philadelphia: Saunders.

1083. While assessing a 14-year-old child, the nurse notes bruises and cigarette burns on the child's chest and rope burns on the buttocks. The child states, "I'm afraid to go home because my stepfather will be angry for telling on him!" The nurse should respond by saying:

1 "You can't go back there with that man. How do you think your mother will react?"
2 "You must know that your presence in the house will only tease your stepfather more."
3 "I am sorry that this has happened to you, but you will be safe here until plans can be made."
4 "Let's keep this between you, me, and the physician until we formulate further plans to assist you."

Answer: 3
Rationale: A child who has been physically and sexually abused should be admitted to the hospital. This will provide time for a more comprehensive evaluation while protecting the child from further abuse. The correct option also provides an empathic statement that supports the child to appropriately perceive himself or herself as the victim while assuring the child of protection from abuse. In option 1, the nurse does not respond with a calm and reassuring communication style or maintain a professional attitude. Option 2, which holds an innuendo, appears to accuse the victim of teasing the stepfather and is thus incorrect; it is also judgmental, controlling, and demeaning. The nurse's suggestion in option 4 is not only incorrect but also passive in its stance.

Test-Taking Strategy: Use the process of elimination, therapeutic communication techniques, and your knowledge of the care of the child who has been physically abused. Recalling that the priority is the safety of the victim will direct you to option 3. Review the care of the child who has been abused if you had difficulty with this question.

Level of Cognitive Ability: Application
Client Needs: Psychosocial Integrity
Integrated Process: Caring
Content Area: Mental Health

Reference
Stuart, G., & Laraia, M. (2005). *Principles and practice of psychiatric nursing* (8th ed., p. 808). St. Louis: Mosby.

1084. A nurse is caring for a 12-year-old female client who has been physically and sexually abused by her father. The father angrily approaches the nurse and says, "I'm taking my daughter home. She's told me what you people are up to, and we're out of here!" The nurse makes which therapeutic response?

1. "Your daughter will remain here until the doctor discharges her. I'll call hospital security and the police if you attempt to take her."
2. "Try to listen to me, please. If you are insistent and do take your daughter from this unit, the police will most certainly order you to bring her back again."
3. "Your daughter is ill and needs to be here. I know you want to help her to recover and that you will work to help everyone straighten out the circumstances that caused this."
4. "You seem very upset. Let's talk at the nurse's station. I know you're very concerned and that you want to help your daughter. It will be best if you agree to let your daughter stay here for now."

Level of Cognitive Ability: Application
Client Needs: Psychosocial Integrity
Integrated Process: Communication and Documentation
Content Area: Mental Health

Answer: 4
Rationale: When a suspected abused child is admitted to the hospital for further evaluation and protection, the physician will usually work with the parents so that they will agree to the admission. If the parents refuse to do this, the hospital can request an immediate court order to retain the child for a specific length of time. In option 1, the nurse is angry and verbally abusive. It is clear that the nurse has decided that the father is guilty of child abuse. In addition, the nurse is aggressive and challenging; this may antagonize the father and cause the nurse to become a victim of violence, as well. In option 2, the command to listen is somewhat demanding. Option 3 seems somewhat pompous and lecturing.

Test-Taking Strategy: Use the process of elimination and therapeutic communication techniques. Note that the client of the question is the child's father. Note that option 4 addresses the father's behavior yet protects the child. Review the psychosocial issues related to child abuse if you had difficulty with this question.

References
Stuart, G., & Laraia, M. (2005). *Principles and practice of psychiatric nursing* (8th ed., p. 808). St. Louis: Mosby.
Varcarolis, E., Carson, V., & Shoemaker, N. (2006). *Foundations of psychiatric mental health nursing* (5th ed., p. 508). Philadelphia: Saunders.

1085. A client with chronic arterial leg ulcers complains of pain and tells the nurse, "I'm so discouraged. I have had this pain for more than a year now. The pain never seems to go away. I can't do anything, and I feel as though I'll never get better." The nurse formulates which nursing diagnosis for this client?

1. Ineffective coping, related to chronic illness
2. Acute pain, related to the effects of leg ischemia
3. Fatigue, related to lack of sleep and frustration with illness
4. Chronic pain, related to the nonhealing arterial ulcerations

Answer: 4
Rationale: The major focus of the client's complaint is the experience of pain. Pain that has a duration of more than 6 months is defined as chronic pain rather than acute pain. NANDA International defines Fatigue as "a sense of exhaustion and decreased capacity for physical and mental work." NANDA International defines Ineffective coping as the "impairment of adaptive behaviors and abilities of a person in meeting life's demands and roles."

Level of Cognitive Ability: Analysis
Client Needs: Psychosocial Integrity
Integrated Process: Nursing Process/Analysis
Content Area: Adult Health/Cardiovascular

Test-Taking Strategy: Use the process of elimination. Focus on the client's statement, "I have had this pain for more than a year now." This statement and noting the word "chronic" in the question and in option 4 will direct you to this option. Review the defining characteristics for the nursing diagnosis of Chronic Pain if you had difficulty with this question.

Reference
Black, J., & Hawks, J. (2005). *Medical-surgical nursing: Clinical management for positive outcomes* (7th ed., p. 446). Philadelphia: Saunders.

1086. A client with valvular heart disease is being considered for mechanical valve replacement. Which item is essential to assess before the surgery is performed?
1 The physical demands of the client's lifestyle
2 The ability to comply with anticoagulant therapy for life
3 The ability to participate in a cardiac rehabilitation program
4 The likelihood of the client experiencing body image problems

Level of Cognitive Ability: Application
Client Needs: Psychosocial Integrity
Integrated Process: Nursing Process/Assessment
Content Area: Adult Health/Cardiovascular

Answer: 2
Rationale: Mechanical valves carry the associated risk of thromboemboli, which require long-term anticoagulation with warfarin sodium (Coumadin). No data in the question indicate that physical demands exist in the client's lifestyle. Body image problems are important but not critical. Not all clients who undergo cardiac surgery require cardiac rehabilitation.

Test-Taking Strategy: Use the process of elimination, and focus on the strategic word "essential." Recalling that mechanical valves are thrombogenic will direct you to option 2. Review the care of the client undergoing a mechanical valve replacement if you had difficulty with this question.

Reference
Black, J., & Hawks, J. (2005). *Medical-surgical nursing: Clinical management for positive outcomes* (7th ed., p. 1605). Philadelphia: Saunders.

1087. A client who has a history of depression has been prescribed nadolol (Corgard) for the management of angina pectoris. Which item is most important when the nurse plans to counsel this client about the effects of this medication?
1 Risk of tachycardia
2 Probability of fatigue
3 High incidence of hypoglycemia
4 Possible exacerbation of depression

Level of Cognitive Ability: Application
Client Needs: Psychosocial Integrity
Integrated Process: Teaching and Learning
Content Area: Pharmacology

Answer: 4
Rationale: Clients with depression or a history of depression have experienced an exacerbation of depression after beginning therapy with β-adrenergic blocking agents. These clients should be monitored carefully if these agents are prescribed. The medication would cause bradycardia rather than tachycardia. Fatigue is a possible side effect, but it is not the most important item. Hypoglycemia is a sign that is masked with β-blockers.

Test-Taking Strategy: Use the process of elimination. Noting the relationship between the client's history and option 4 will direct you to this option. Review nadolol if you had difficulty with this question.

References
Lehne, R. (2007). *Pharmacology for nursing care* (6th ed., p. 173). Philadelphia: Saunders.
Skidmore-Roth, L. (2008). *Mosby's nursing drug reference* (21st ed., p. 712). St. Louis: Mosby.

1088. The nurse is caring for a client with terminal cancer of the throat. The family approaches the nurse and tells the nurse that they have spoken to the physician regarding taking their loved one home. The nurse plans to coordinate discharge planning. Which of the following services would be most supportive to the client and the family?

1 Hospice care
2 The American Cancer Society
3 The American Lung Association
4 Local religious and social organizations

Level of Cognitive Ability: Analysis
Client Needs: Psychosocial Integrity
Integrated Process: Caring
Content Area: Adult Health/Oncology

Answer: 1
Rationale: Hospice care provides an environment that emphasizes caring rather than curing; the emphasis is on palliative care. One of the major goals of hospice care is that clients be free of pain and other symptoms that do not allow them to maintain a quality life. An interdisciplinary approach is used. Options 2, 3, and 4 would be helpful, but they are not the most supportive of the options provided.

Test-Taking Strategy: Note the strategic words "most supportive." Knowledge regarding the goals and services provided by hospice care will assist you with answering the question. Think about what each support service presented in the options will provide for meeting this client's needs. This will assist with directing you to option 1. Review the goals of these different support systems and hospice care if you had difficulty with this question.

References
Black, J., & Hawks, J. (2005). *Medical-surgical nursing: Clinical management for positive outcomes* (7th ed., p. 187). Philadelphia: Saunders.
Lewis, S., Heitkemper, M., Dirksen, S., O'Brien, P., & Bucher, L. (2007). *Medical-surgical nursing: Assessment and management of clinical problems* (7th ed., pp. 92, 156-157). St. Louis: Mosby.

1089. The home-care nurse is caring for a client with acute cancer pain. The most appropriate assessment of the client's pain should include which of the following?

1 The client's pain rating
2 The nurse's impression of the client's pain
3 Verbal and nonverbal clues from the client
4 Pain relief after appropriate nursing intervention

Level of Cognitive Ability: Application
Client Needs: Psychosocial Integrity
Integrated Process: Caring
Content Area: Adult Health/Oncology

Answer: 1
Rationale: The client's perception of pain is the hallmark of pain assessment. Usually noted by the client's rating on a scale of 1 to 10, the assessment is documented and followed with appropriate medical and nursing interventions. The nurse's impression and the verbal and nonverbal clues are subjective data. Pain relief after intervention is appropriate but relates to evaluation.

Test-Taking Strategy: Use the process of elimination. Eliminate option 4 first, because it relates to evaluation. Next, eliminate options 2 and 3, because they relate to subjective data. In addition, note that option 1 is client focused. Review the techniques of pain assessment if you had difficulty with this question.

Reference
Ignatavicius, D., & Workman, M. (2006). *Medical-surgical nursing: Critical thinking for collaborative care* (5th ed., pp. 65, 68). Philadelphia: Saunders.

1090. A prenatal client has been told during a physician office visit that she is positive for human immunodeficiency virus (HIV). The client cried and was significantly distressed regarding this news. Which nursing diagnosis would these data best support?

1 Acute pain
2 Noncompliance
3 Anticipatory grieving
4 High risk for infection

Answer: 3
Rationale: A life-threatening diagnosis such as HIV will stimulate the anticipatory grief response. Anticipatory grief occurs when the client, family, and loved ones know that the client will die. The prenatal HIV client is forced to make important changes in her life, frequently resulting in grief related to lost future dreams and diminished self-esteem as a result of an inability to achieve life goals. Although options 1, 2, and 4 may be appropriate nursing diagnoses at some point, they do not address the information given in the question.

Level of Cognitive Ability: Analysis
Client Needs: Psychosocial Integrity
Integrated Process: Caring
Content Area: Adult Health/Immune

Test-Taking Strategy: Note the strategic words "best support." Use the process of elimination, and focus on the data in the question. A client who is distressed and crying is supporting data for the nursing diagnosis of Anticipatory grieving. Review this nursing diagnosis if you had difficulty with this question.

References

Lewis, S., Heitkemper, M., Dirksen, S., O'Brien, P., & Bucher, L. (2007). *Medical-surgical nursing: Assessment and management of clinical problems* (7th ed., p. 264). St. Louis: Mosby.

Murray, S., & McKinney, E. (2006). *Foundations of maternal-newborn nursing* (4th ed., pp. 608-609). Philadelphia: Saunders.

1091. A nurse is assessing a client's suicide potential. The nurse asks the client which most important question?

1 "Why do you want to hurt yourself?"
2 "Do you have a plan to commit suicide?"
3 "Has anyone in your family committed suicide?"
4 "Can you describe how you are feeling right now?"

Level of Cognitive Ability: Application
Client Needs: Psychosocial Integrity
Integrated Process: Nursing Process/Assessment
Content Area: Mental Health

Answer: 2

Rationale: When assessing for suicide risk, the nurse must evaluate whether the client has a suicide plan. Clients who have a definitive plan pose a greater risk for suicide. Options 3 and 4 may also be questions that the nurse would ask, but they are not the most important. The nurse avoids the use of the word "why" when communicating with a client. The use of this word may place the client on the defensive; additionally, the client may not even know the reason that he or she wants to hurt himself or herself.

Test-Taking Strategy: Use the process of elimination, and note the strategic words "most important." Recalling the importance of assessing for a suicide plan will direct you to option 2. Review the assessment of suicide potential if you had difficulty with this question.

Reference

Stuart, G., & Laraia, M. (2005). *Principles and practice of psychiatric nursing* (8th ed., pp. 367-368). St. Louis: Mosby.

1092. A nurse is caring for a client who is receiving electroconvulsive therapy (ECT) for a major depressive disorder. Which assessment finding would the nurse identify as an unexpected side effect of ECT that requires notifying the physician?

1 Confusion
2 Memory loss
3 Hypertension
4 Disorientation

Level of Cognitive Ability: Analysis
Client Needs: Psychosocial Integrity
Integrated Process: Nursing Process/Assessment
Content Area: Mental Health

Answer: 3

Rationale: The major side effects of ECT are confusion, disorientation, and memory loss. A change in blood pressure would not be an anticipated side effect, and it would be a cause for concern. If hypertension occurred after ECT, the physician should be notified.

Test-Taking Strategy: Use the process of elimination, and focus on the subject: an unexpected side effect. Recall the side effects of ECT, and note that options 1, 2, and 4 are comparable or alike. Review the expected and unexpected side effects of ECT if you had difficulty with this question.

Reference

Stuart, G., & Laraia, M. (2005). *Principles and practice of psychiatric nursing* (8th ed., p. 608). St. Louis: Mosby.

1093. During the admission assessment of a client admitted to the hospital for ruptured esophageal varices, the client says, "I deserve this. I brought it on myself." The nurse makes which therapeutic response to the client?
1 "Would you like to talk to the chaplain?"
2 "Is there some reason you feel you deserve this?"
3 "Not all esophageal varices are caused by alcohol."
4 "That is something to think about when you leave the hospital."

Level of Cognitive Ability: Application
Client Needs: Psychosocial Integrity
Integrated Process: Communication and Documentation
Content Area: Adult Health/Gastrointestinal

Answer: 2
Rationale: Ruptured esophageal varices are often a complication of cirrhosis of the liver, and the most common type of cirrhosis is caused by chronic alcohol abuse. It is important to obtain an accurate history regarding the client's alcohol intake. If the client is ashamed or embarrassed, he or she may not respond accurately. Option 2 is open-ended and allows the client to discuss his or her feelings about drinking. Option 1 blocks the nurse–client communication process. Options 3 and 4 are somewhat judgmental.

Test-Taking Strategy: Use the process of elimination and therapeutic communication techniques to direct you to option 2. Remember that the client's feelings should be addressed first. Review therapeutic communication techniques if you had difficulty with this question.

References
Ignatavicius, D., & Workman, M. (2006). *Medical-surgical nursing: Critical thinking for collaborative care* (5th ed., p. 1369). Philadelphia: Saunders.
Potter, P., & Perry, A. (2005). *Fundamentals of nursing* (6th ed., p. 437). St. Louis: Mosby.

1094. A nurse is performing a neurological assessment on a client with dementia and assessing the function of the frontal lobe of the brain. The assessment of which of the following items by the nurse would yield the best information about this area of functioning?
1 Eye movements
2 Feelings or emotions
3 Level of consciousness
4 Insight, judgment, and planning

Level of Cognitive Ability: Application
Client Needs: Psychosocial Integrity
Integrated Process: Nursing Process/Assessment
Content Area: Adult Health/Neurological

Answer: 4
Rationale: Insight, judgment, and planning are part of the function of the frontal lobe. The level of consciousness is controlled by the reticular activating system. Feelings and emotions are part of the role of the limbic system. Eye movements are under the control of cranial nerves III, IV, and VI.

Test-Taking Strategy: A specific understanding of the function of the frontal lobe of the brain will direct you to option 4. Review the function of the frontal lobe if you had difficulty with this question.

Reference
Ignatavicius, D., & Workman, M. (2006). *Medical-surgical nursing: Critical thinking for collaborative care* (5th ed., p. 925). Philadelphia: Saunders.

1095. The nurse caring for a client who is dying formulates a nursing diagnosis of Fear and identifies appropriate nursing interventions. From the following list of nursing interventions, which intervention should the nurse implement first?
1 Help the client express fears.
2 Assess the nature of the client's fears.
3 Help the client identify coping mechanisms that were successful in the past.
4 Document verbal and nonverbal expressions of fear and other significant data.

Answer: 2
Rationale: Fear can range from a paralyzing, overwhelming feeling to a mild concern. Therefore, the nurse would first assess the nature of the client's fears to know how best to help the client. Next, the nurse would help the client express his or her fears. The client's fear may not be limited to the fear of dying, and the nurse needs this information to help the client. After the nurse is aware of the client's fears, the methods that the client used to cope with fear in the past are identified. From the interventions listed, the nurse would document verbal and nonverbal expressions of fear and any other significant data as a final intervention.

Level of Cognitive Ability: Application
Client Needs: Psychosocial Integrity
Integrated Process: Nursing Process/
Implementation
Content Area: Delegating/Prioritizing

Test-Taking Strategy: Use the steps of the nursing process to assist you with determining the order of priority of the nursing interventions. An assessment of the client's fear would be the first intervention. Review the care of the dying client who is experiencing fear if you had difficulty with this question.

Reference
Ackley, B., & Ladwig, G. (2006). *Nursing diagnosis handbook: A guide for planning care* (7th ed., p. 523). St. Louis: Mosby.

1096. Fluoxetine hydrochloride (Prozac) is prescribed for a client with depression. The nurse provides instructions to the client regarding the administration of the medication. Which statement by the client indicates an understanding about administration of the medication?

1 "I should take the medication with my evening meal."
2 "I should take the medication at noon with an antacid."
3 "I should take the medication in the morning when I first arise."
4 "I should take the medication right before bedtime with a snack."

Level of Cognitive Ability: Analysis
Client Needs: Psychosocial Integrity
Integrated Process: Nursing Process/Evaluation
Content Area: Pharmacology

Answer: 3
Rationale: Fluoxetine hydrochloride is administered in the early morning without consideration to meals. Options 1, 2, and 4 are incorrect.

Test-Taking Strategy: Use the process of elimination. Eliminate options 1, 2, and 4 because they are comparable or alike and indicate taking the medication with an antacid or food. If you are unfamiliar with the use of this medication and the client teaching points, review this content.

Reference
Lehne, R. (2007). *Pharmacology for nursing care* (6the ed., p. 351). Philadelphia: Saunders.

1097. A mother comes to the pediatric clinic because her previously continent 6-year-old son has resumed bedwetting. After discovering that there is a new baby in the home, the nurse explains to the mother that the son is most likely using the defense mechanism of:

1 Regression
2 Repression
3 Identification
4 Rationalization

Level of Cognitive Ability: Application
Client Needs: Psychosocial Integrity
Integrated Process: Nursing Process/
Implementation
Content Area: Child Health

Answer: 1
Rationale: The defense mechanism of regression is characterized by returning to an earlier form of expressing an impulse. Option 2 is characterized by blocking a wish or desire from conscious expression. Option 3 occurs when a person models behavior after someone else. Option 4 occurs when a person unconsciously falsifies an experience by giving a "rational" explanation.

Test-Taking Strategy: Focus on the data in the question. Noting the strategic words "resumed bedwetting" will direct you to option 1. Review defense mechanisms if you had difficulty with this question.

Reference
Hockenberry, M., Wilson, D., & Winkelstein, M. (2005). *Wong's essentials of pediatric nursing* (7th ed., pp. 538-539). St. Louis: Mosby.

1098. A nurse is obtaining a health history from an adolescent. Which statement by the adolescent indicates a need for follow-up assessment and intervention?
1 "When I get stressed out about school, I just like to be alone."
2 "I find myself very moody. I'm happy one minute and crying the next."
3 "I can't seem to wake up in the morning. I would sleep until noon if I could."
4 "I don't eat anything with any fat in it, and I've lost 8 pounds in 2 weeks."

Level of Cognitive Ability: Analysis
Client Needs: Psychosocial Integrity
Integrated Process: Nursing Process/Analysis
Content Area: Child Health

Answer: 4
Rationale: During the adolescent period, there is a heightened awareness of body image and peer pressure to go on excessively restrictive diets. The extreme limitation of omitting all fat in the diet and losing weight during a time of growth suggests inadequate nutrition and a possible eating disorder. Options 1, 2, and 3 are common and normal behaviors or feelings that occur during adolescence.

Test-Taking Strategy: Note the strategic words "need for follow-up." These words indicate a negative event query and ask you to select the option that identifies a statement made by the adolescent that is of concern. Options 1, 2, and 3 are common and normal behaviors or feelings during adolescence. Option 4 indicates a problem or abnormality. Review the developmental stage of adolescence if you had difficulty with this question.

References
Hockenberry, M., & Wilson, D. (2007). *Nursing care of infants and children* (8th ed., p. 837). St. Louis: Mosby.
Hockenberry, M., Wilson, D., & Winkelstein, M. (2005). *Wong's essentials of pediatric nursing* (7th ed., pp. 532-534). St. Louis: Mosby.

1099. A nurse is caring for a client who has bipolar disorder and is in a manic state. The nurse determines that which menu choice would be best for this client?
1 Beef stew, fruit salad, tea
2 Cheeseburger, banana, milk
3 Macaroni and cheese, apple, milk
4 Scrambled eggs, orange juice, coffee with cream and sugar

Level of Cognitive Ability: Application
Client Needs: Psychosocial Integrity
Integrated Process: Nursing Process/Planning
Content Area: Mental Health

Answer: 2
Rationale: The client in a manic state often has inadequate food and fluid intake as a result of physical agitation. Foods that the client can eat "on the run" are best, because the client is too active to sit at meals and use utensils. Additionally, clients in a manic state should not have any products that contain caffeine.

Test-Taking Strategy: Use the process of elimination, and focus on the strategic words "manic state." Note that options 1, 3, and 4 are comparable or alike in that the client needs to sit to eat some of these food items. Remember the concept of "finger foods" with regard to the client with mania. Review the care of the client with mania if you had difficulty with this question.

References
Stuart, G., & Laraia, M. (2005). *Principles and practice of psychiatric nursing* (8th ed., pp. 266, 351). St. Louis: Mosby.
Varcarolis, E., Carson, V., & Shoemaker, N. (2006). *Foundations of psychiatric mental health nursing* (5th ed., p. 370). Philadelphia: Saunders.

1100. A nurse is caring for a child who is a victim of child abuse and has determined that the child uses repression to cope with past life experiences. The nurse implements a plan of care that includes:

1 Having the child talk about the abuse in detail during the first therapy session
2 Telling the child to let the past go and to concentrate on the present and future
3 Placing the child on medications that will help the child forget the incidents
4 Encouraging the child to use therapeutic play to act out past experiences

Level of Cognitive Ability: Application
Client Needs: Psychosocial Integrity
Integrated Process: Nursing Process/ Implementation
Content Area: Child Health

Answer: 4
Rationale: Therapeutic play is used to reduce the trauma of illness and hospitalizations. It is a nonthreatening avenue through which the child can use artwork, dolls, or puppets to act out frightening life experiences. Option 1 would be extremely threatening to the child and nontherapeutic. Options 2 and 3 devalue the child and force the child to further repress harmful past experiences rather than facing them and moving on.

Test-Taking Strategy: Use therapeutic communication techniques to eliminate options 2 and 3. From the remaining options, note the relationship of the words "past life experiences" in the question and "past experiences" in the correct option. Review the care of the child who is a victim of abuse if you had difficulty with this question.

References
Hockenberry, M., Wilson, D., & Winkelstein, M. (2005). *Wong's essentials of pediatric nursing* (7th ed., p. 468). St. Louis: Mosby.
Wong, D., Hockenberry, M., Perry, S., Lowdermilk, D., & Wilson, D. (2006). *Maternal-child nursing care* (3rd ed., p. 1147). St. Louis: Mosby.

1101. An older female client is brought to the emergency department by a family member with whom she lives. The nurse notes that the client has poor hygiene, contractures, and pressure ulcers on the sacrum, the scapula, and the heels. The client is suspected of which form of victimization?

1 Sexual abuse
2 Physical abuse
3 Emotional abuse
4 Psychological abuse

Level of Cognitive Ability: Analysis
Client Needs: Psychosocial Integrity
Integrated Process: Nursing Process/Analysis
Content Area: Mental Health

Answer: 2
Rationale: Victimization in a family can take many forms. When analyzing a specific client situation, it is important to understand which form of abuse is being considered. Physical abuse can take the form of battering (hitting, slapping, striking), or it can be more subtle, such as neglect (the failure to meet basic needs). Emotional and psychological abuse can involve inflicting verbal statements that cause mental anguish or alienation of the victim. Sexual abuse can involve unwanted sexual remarks, sexual advances, and physical sexual acts.

Test-Taking Strategy: Focus on the data in the question. This question identifies only the physical signs of victimization. Option 2 is the only option that fits the description in the question. Review the signs of physical abuse in the older client if you had difficulty with this question.

References
Stuart, G., & Laraia, M. (2005). *Principles and practice of psychiatric nursing* (8th ed., p. 811). St. Louis: Mosby.
Varcarolis, E., Carson, V., & Shoemaker, N. (2006). *Foundations of psychiatric mental health nursing* (5th ed., pp. 508, 516). Philadelphia: Saunders.

1102. A female client is admitted to the inpatient mental health unit. When asked her name, she responds, "I am Elizabeth, the Queen of England." The nurse recognizes this response as a(n):

1 Visual illusion
2 Loose association
3 Grandiose delusion
4 Auditory hallucination

Answer: 3
Rationale: A delusion is an important personal belief that is almost certainly not true and that resists modification. An illusion is a misperception or misinterpretation of externally real stimuli. Loose association is thinking that is characterized by speech in which ideas that are unrelated shift from one subject to another. A hallucination is a false perception.

Level of Cognitive Ability: Analysis
Client Needs: Psychosocial Integrity
Integrated Process: Nursing Process/Assessment
Content Area: Mental Health

Test-Taking Strategy: Use the process of elimination, and focus on the information in the question. Eliminate options 1 and 4, because the client is not having any visual or auditory disturbances. Option 2 is eliminated next, because there is no indication that the client is shifting from one subject to another. Making a reference to being a queen is a grandiose assumption. Review the description of grandiose delusions if you had difficulty with this question.

References
Stuart, G., & Laraia, M. (2005). *Principles and practice of psychiatric nursing* (8th ed., p. 112). St. Louis: Mosby.
Varcarolis, E., Carson, V., & Shoemaker, N. (2006). *Foundations of psychiatric mental health nursing* (5th ed., pp. 401-402). Philadelphia: Saunders.

1103. A client who has been newly admitted to the mental health unit with a diagnosis of bipolar disorder is trying to organize a dance with the other clients on the unit and is planning an on-unit supper. To decrease stimulation, the nurse should encourage the client to:

1 Seek assistance from other staff members.
2 Postpone the dance and engage in a writing activity.
3 Engage the help of other clients on the unit to accomplish the task.
4 Stop the planning and firmly tell the client that this task is inappropriate.

Level of Cognitive Ability: Application
Client Needs: Psychosocial Integrity
Integrated Process: Nursing Process/ Implementation
Content Area: Mental Health

Answer: 2
Rationale: Because the client with bipolar disorder is easily stimulated by the environment, sedentary activities are the best outlets for energy release. Most bipolar clients enjoy writing, so the writing task is appropriate. An activity such as planning a dance or supper may be appropriate at some point, but not for the newly admitted client who is likely to have impaired judgment and a short attention span. Options 1 and 3 encourage planning the activity and therefore increase client stimulation. Option 4 could result in an angry outburst by the client.

Test-Taking Strategy: Use the process of elimination. Note the strategic words "to decrease stimulation." Options 1 and 3 encourage activity and should be eliminated. Option 4 tells the client that the activity is inappropriate, and this could result in an angry outburst by the client. Option 2 is the only option that limits activity. Review the appropriate activities for the bipolar client if you had difficulty with this question.

References
Stuart, G., & Laraia, M. (2005). *Principles and practice of psychiatric nursing* (8th ed., pp. 355-356). St. Louis: Mosby.
Varcarolis, E., Carson, V., & Shoemaker, N. (2006). *Foundations of psychiatric mental health nursing* (5th ed., p. 375). Philadelphia: Saunders.

1104. A client with obsessive-compulsive disorder spends many hours during the day and night washing her hands. When initially planning for a safe environment, the nurse allows the client to continue this behavior because it:

1 Relieves the client's anxiety
2 Decreases the chance of infection
3 Gives the client a feeling of self-control
4 Increases the client's sense of self-esteem

Answer: 1
Rationale: The compulsive act provides immediate relief from anxiety and is used to cope with stress, conflict, or pain. Although the client may feel the need to increase self-esteem, that is not the primary goal of this behavior. Options 2 and 3 are also incorrect interpretations of the client's need to perform this behavior.

Level of Cognitive Ability: Application
Client Needs: Psychosocial Integrity
Integrated Process: Nursing Process/
   Implementation
Content Area: Mental Health

Test-Taking Strategy: Use the process of elimination. Focusing on the strategic word "initially" and recalling the effect of compulsive acts will direct you to option 1. Review this disorder if you are unfamiliar with this content.

References

Stuart, G., & Laraia, M. (2005). *Principles and practice of psychiatric nursing* (8th ed., p. 273). St. Louis: Mosby.
Varcarolis, E., Carson, V., & Shoemaker, N. (2006). *Foundations of psychiatric mental health nursing* (5th ed., p. 234). Philadelphia: Saunders.

1105. An adolescent is preparing to return home after psychiatric hospitalization for a suicide attempt. Which of the following would be the least effective for preparing the client to return home?
1 Identify the family's strengths and weaknesses.
2 Ask that the mother's boyfriend move out of the home.
3 Provide and offer the family appropriate options and resources.
4 Encourage communication and the sharing of feelings among the family members.

Level of Cognitive Ability: Application
Client Needs: Psychosocial Integrity
Integrated Process: Nursing Process/
   Implementation
Content Area: Mental Health

Answer: 2
Rationale: Option 2 is clearly the least effective option, because there is no information in the question that indicates that the boyfriend's involvement has anything to do with the suicide attempt. Options 1, 3, and 4 offer helpful ways to enhance the family processes.

Test-Taking Strategy: Note the strategic words "least effective." These words indicate a negative event query and ask you to select the option that would be the least helpful. Focus on the data in the question, and note that options 1, 3, and 4 are comparable or alike and that they identify positive measures. Review the psychosocial issues related to preparing a client for discharge if you had difficulty with this question.

References

Stuart, G., & Laraia, M. (2005). *Principles and practice of psychiatric nursing* (8th ed., p. 773). St. Louis: Mosby.
Varcarolis, E., Carson, V., & Shoemaker, N. (2006). *Foundations of psychiatric mental health nursing* (5th ed., pp. 481, 485). Philadelphia: Saunders.

1106. An 11-year-old child scheduled for a diagnostic procedure will have an intravenous line inserted and will receive an intramuscular injection. The nurse appropriately prepares the child for the procedure by:
1 Reassuring the child that he or she will not feel any pain
2 Teaching the parents so that they can explain everything to the child
3 Telling the child not to worry, because the doctors take care of everything
4 Using pictures, concrete words, and demonstrations to describe what will happen

Level of Cognitive Ability: Application
Client Needs: Psychosocial Integrity
Integrated Process: Nursing Process/
   Implementation
Content Area: Child Health

Answer: 4
Rationale: The school-age child understands best with visual aids and concrete language. Option 1 is inaccurate information, because the injection will cause some discomfort. Option 2 inappropriately delegates the responsibility for teaching to the parents. Option 3 is not therapeutic.

Test-Taking Strategy: Use the process of elimination and therapeutic communication techniques. Option 1 presents inaccurate information. In option 2, a nursing responsibility is inappropriately delegated to parents, and option 3 is nontherapeutic. Review the care of the school-age child if you had difficulty with this question.

Reference

Hockenberry, M., Wilson, D., & Winkelstein, M. (2005). *Wong's essentials of pediatric nursing* (7th ed., p. 691). St. Louis: Mosby.

1107. A nurse observes an anxious client blocking the hallway, walking three steps forward and then two steps backward. Other clients are agitated and trying to get past the client. The nurse intervenes by:
1 Standing alongside the client and saying, "You're very anxious today."
2 Attempting to stop the behavior and saying, "You're going to get exhausted."
3 Taking the client to the lounge and saying, "Relax and watch television now."
4 Walking alongside the client and saying, "You're not going anywhere very fast doing this."

Level of Cognitive Ability: Application
Client Needs: Psychosocial Integrity
Integrated Process: Nursing Process/ Implementation
Content Area: Mental Health

Answer: 1
Rationale: An important consideration when alleviating anxiety is to assist the client with recognizing the behavior. Options 2 and 3 do not address the increased anxiety and the need to control the underlying behavior, and they may even escalate the behavior. Option 4 does not raise the client to a functioning level.

Test-Taking Strategy: Use the process of elimination. Note the relationship between the word "anxious" in the question and in the correct option. Remember, it is important to assist the client with recognizing his or her behavior. Review the measures related to the care of an anxious client if you had difficulty with this question.

References
Stuart, G., & Laraia, M. (2005). *Principles and practice of psychiatric nursing* (8th ed., p. 268). St. Louis: Mosby.
Varcarolis, E., Carson, V., & Shoemaker, N. (2006). *Foundations of psychiatric mental health nursing* (5th ed., p. 244). Philadelphia: Saunders.

1108. A nurse is assisting with providing a form of psychotherapy in which the client acts out situations that are of emotional significance. The nurse understands that this form of therapy is known as:
1 Psychodrama
2 Reality therapy
3 Psychoanalytic therapy
4 Short-term dynamic psychotherapy

Level of Cognitive Ability: Analysis
Client Needs: Psychosocial Integrity
Integrated Process: Nursing Process/Analysis
Content Area: Mental Health

Answer: 1
Rationale: Psychodrama involves the enactment of emotionally charged situations. Reality therapy is used for individuals with cognitive impairment. Both short-term dynamic psychotherapy and psychoanalytic therapy depend on techniques that are drawn from psychoanalysis.

Test-Taking Strategy: Note the strategic words "the client acts out situations." These words will assist you by providing you with the definition of psychodrama. Review the different types of psychotherapy listed if you had difficulty with this question.

Reference
Varcarolis, E., Carson, V., & Shoemaker, N. (2006). *Foundations of psychiatric mental health nursing* (5th ed., p. 652). Philadelphia: Saunders.

1109. A manic client is placed in a seclusion room after an outburst of violent behavior that involved a physical assault on another client. As the client is secluded, the nurse:
1 Asks the client if she understands why the seclusion is necessary
2 Remains silent, because verbal interaction would be too stimulating
3 Tells the client that she will be allowed to come out when she can behave
4 Informs the client that she is being secluded to help her to regain her self-control

Answer: 4
Rationale: The client is removed to a nonstimulating environment as a result of her behavior. Options 1, 2, and 3 are nontherapeutic actions. Additionally, option 2 implies punishment. It is best to directly inform the client of the purpose of the seclusion.

Test-Taking Strategy: Use therapeutic communication techniques. Select the option that presents reality most clearly to the client. Option 4 is the only option that provides a clear and direct purpose of the seclusion. Review the care of the client who requires seclusion if you had difficulty with this question.

Level of Cognitive Ability: Application
Client Needs: Psychosocial Integrity
Integrated Process: Nursing Process/
   Implementation
Content Area: Mental Health

References
Stuart, G., & Laraia, M. (2005). *Principles and practice of psychiatric nursing* (8th ed., p. 646). St. Louis: Mosby.
Varcarolis, E., Carson, V., & Shoemaker, N. (2006). *Foundations of psychiatric mental health nursing* (5th ed., pp. 496-497). Philadelphia: Saunders.

1110. A client with angina pectoris is extremely anxious after being hospitalized for the first time. The nurse plans to do which of the following to minimize the client's anxiety?
   1 Provide care choices to the client.
   2 Keep the door open and the hallway lights on at night.
   3 Encourage the client to limit visitors to as few as possible.
   4 Admit the client to a room as far as possible from the nursing station.

Level of Cognitive Ability: Application
Client Needs: Psychosocial Integrity
Integrated Process: Nursing Process/Planning
Content Area: Adult Health/Cardiovascular

Answer: 1
Rationale: General interventions to minimize anxiety in the hospitalized client include providing information, social support, and control over choices related to care as well as acknowledging the client's feelings. Leaving the door open with the hallway lights on may keep the client oriented, but these actions may interfere with sleep and increase anxiety. Limiting visitors reduces social support. Being far from the nursing station is unlikely to reduce anxiety for this client.

Test-Taking Strategy: Use the process of elimination, and focus on the subject: minimizing anxiety. Thinking about each option and how it may either increase or minimize anxiety will direct you to option 1. Review the interventions used to minimize anxiety in the hospitalized client if you had difficulty with this question.

References
Ignatavicius, D., & Workman, M. (2006). *Medical-surgical nursing: Critical thinking for collaborative care* (5th ed., p. 687). Philadelphia: Saunders.
Lewis, S., Heitkemper, M., Dirksen, S., O'Brien, P., & Bucher, L. (2007). *Medical-surgical nursing: Assessment and management of clinical problems* (7th ed., pp. 813-814, 829). St. Louis: Mosby.

1111. A male client diagnosed with catatonic stupor demonstrates severe withdrawal by lying on the bed with his body pulled into a fetal position. The nurse plans to:
   1 Ask the client direct questions to encourage talking.
   2 Leave the client alone and intermittently check on him.
   3 Sit beside the client in silence and occasionally ask open-ended questions.
   4 Take the client into the dayroom with the other clients so that they can help watch him.

Level of Cognitive Ability: Application
Client Needs: Psychosocial Integrity
Integrated Process: Nursing Process/Planning
Content Area: Mental Health

Answer: 3
Rationale: Clients who are withdrawn may be immobile and mute, and they require consistent, repeated approaches. Intervention includes the establishment of interpersonal contact. The nurse facilitates communication with the client by sitting in silence, asking open-ended questions, and pausing to provide opportunities for the client to respond. The client is not to be left alone. Asking this client direct questions is not therapeutic.

Test-Taking Strategy: Use the process of elimination. Eliminate option 2, because the nurse would not leave the client alone. Option 4 relies on other clients to care for this client; this is inappropriate, and it should be eliminated next. From the remaining options, recall that asking direct questions to this client would not be therapeutic. Review the care of the client with catatonic stupor if you had difficulty with this question.

References
Stuart, G., & Laraia, M. (2005). *Principles and practice of psychiatric nursing* (8th ed., p. 404). St. Louis: Mosby.
Varcarolis, E., Carson, V., & Shoemaker, N. (2006). *Foundations of psychiatric mental health nursing* (5th ed., pp. 413-414). Philadelphia: Saunders.

1112. A nurse is interviewing a client being admitted to the mental health inpatient unit who was involved in a fire 2 months ago. The client is complaining of insomnia, difficulty concentrating, nervousness, hypervigilance, and frequently thinking about fires. The nurse assesses these symptoms to be indicative of:

1 Phobia
2 Dissociative disorder
3 Obsessive-compulsive disorder
4 Post-traumatic stress disorder (PTSD)

Level of Cognitive Ability: Analysis
Client Needs: Psychosocial Integrity
Integrated Process: Nursing Process/Assessment
Content Area: Mental Health

Answer: 4
Rationale: PTSD is precipitated by events that are overwhelming, unpredictable, and sometimes life-threatening. Typical symptoms of PTSD include difficulty concentrating, sleep disturbances, intrusive recollections of the traumatic event, hypervigilance, and anxiety. These symptoms are not characteristic of the disorders noted in options 1, 2, and 3.

Test-Taking Strategy: Focus on the data in the question regarding the client's complaints. Recalling that having flashbacks of traumatic events is a common symptom of PTSD will direct you to option 4. Review the clinical manifestations of PTSD if you had difficulty with this question.

Reference
Stuart, G., & Laraia, M. (2005). *Principles and practice of psychiatric nursing* (8th ed., pp. 271, 273). St. Louis: Mosby.

1113. A 16-year-old client is hospitalized. Which statement by the client would alert the nurse to a potential developmental problem?

1 "I'd like my hair washed before my friends get here."
2 "Is it okay if I have a couple of friends in to visit me this evening?"
3 "Please tell my friends not to visit since I'll see them back at school next week."
4 "When my friends get here, I would like to play some computer games with them."

Level of Cognitive Ability: Analysis
Client Needs: Psychosocial Integrity
Integrated Process: Nursing Process/Assessment
Content Area: Child Health

Answer: 3
Rationale: Adolescents who withdraw from peers into isolation struggle with developing identity, so option 3 should cause the nurse to be concerned. Option 2 indicates that the client is eager for companionship. Adolescents often develop special interests within their groups that may help them to maximize certain skills, such as with computers. It is appropriate for the client to ask for hygiene measures to be attended to before the peer group arrives.

Test-Taking Strategy: Use the process of elimination. Options 1, 2, and 4 indicate that the client is anticipating the arrival of a peer group, which is appropriate. Option 3 indicates that the client may be withdrawing from appropriate relationships. Review the concepts of growth and development related to an adolescent if you had difficulty with this question.

Reference
Hockenberry, M., Wilson, D., & Winkelstein, M. (2005). *Wong's essentials of pediatric nursing* (7th ed., p. 541). St. Louis: Mosby.

1114. The nurse obtains an electrocardiogram (ECG) rhythm strip for an adult client who is anxious about the result. The ECG shows that the rate is 90 beats per minute. To relieve anxiety, the nurse tells the client that:

1 The rate is normal.
2 There is no need to worry.
3 A slower heart rate is preferred.
4 Medication specific to the problem will be prescribed.

Answer: 1
Rationale: A normal adult resting pulse rate ranges between 60 and 100 beats per minute; therefore, the rate is normal. The nurse would not tell a client not to worry. Options 3 and 4 indicate that the ECG is abnormal.

Test-Taking Strategy: Use the process of elimination and your knowledge of the basic range of pulse rates for an adult. Eliminate option 2, because telling the client not to worry is an inappropriate action. Eliminate options 3 and 4, because they are comparable or alike and indicate that a problem exists. Review the normal adult vital signs if you had difficulty with this question.

Level of Cognitive Ability: Application
Client Needs: Psychosocial Integrity
Integrated Process: Nursing Process/
  Implementation
Content Area: Adult Health/Cardiovascular

References
Chernecky, C., & Berger, B. (2008). *Laboratory tests and diagnostic procedures* (5th ed., pp. 461-462). Philadelphia: Saunders.
Lewis, S., Heitkemper, M., Dirksen, S., O'Brien, P., & Bucher, L. (2007). *Medical-surgical nursing: Assessment and management of clinical problems* (7th ed., pp. 743-744). St. Louis: Mosby.

1115. The nurse determines that a client recovering from a myocardial infarction is exhibiting signs of depression when the client:

  1 Reports insomnia at night
  2 Consumes 25% of meals and shows little interest when doing client teaching
  3 Ignores activity restrictions and does not report the experience of chest pain with activity
  4 Expresses apprehension about leaving the hospital and requests that someone stay in the room at night

Level of Cognitive Ability: Analysis
Client Needs: Psychosocial Integrity
Integrated Process: Nursing Process/Analysis
Content Area: Adult Health/Cardiovascular

Answer: 2
Rationale: Signs of depression include withdrawal, lack of interest, crying, anorexia, and apathy. Insomnia may be a sign of anxiety or fear. Ignoring symptoms and activity restrictions are signs of denial. Apprehension is a sign of anxiety.

Test-Taking Strategy: Use the process of elimination, and focus on the subject: signs of depression. Recalling that anorexia and a lack of interest are associated with depression will direct you to option 2. Review the signs of depression if you had difficulty with this question.

References
Black, J., & Hawks, J. (2005). *Medical-surgical nursing: Clinical management for positive outcomes* (7th ed., p. 532). Philadelphia: Saunders.
Ignatavicius, D., & Workman, M. (2006). *Medical-surgical nursing: Critical thinking for collaborative care* (5th ed., p. 852). Philadelphia: Saunders.
Lewis, S., Heitkemper, M., Dirksen, S., O'Brien, P., & Bucher, L. (2007). *Medical-surgical nursing: Assessment and management of clinical problems* (7th ed., p. 814). St. Louis: Mosby.

1116. A client who recently had a gastrostomy feeding tube inserted refuses to participate in the plan of care, will not make eye contact, and does not speak to family or visitors. The nurse assesses that the client is using which type of coping mechanism?

  1 Distancing
  2 Self-control
  3 Problem solving
  4 Accepting responsibility

Level of Cognitive Ability: Analysis
Client Needs: Psychosocial Integrity
Integrated Process: Nursing Process/Assessment
Content Area: Adult Health/Gastrointestinal

Answer: 1
Rationale: Distancing is an unwillingness or inability to discuss events. Self-control is demonstrated by stoicism and hiding feelings. Problem solving involves making plans and verbalizing what will be done. Accepting responsibility places the responsibility for a situation on oneself.

Test-Taking Strategy: Focus on the data in the question. Noting the client's behavior will direct you to option 1, which is the least effective coping strategy. Review coping mechanisms if you had difficulty with this question.

References
Black, J., & Hawks, J. (2005). *Medical-surgical nursing: Clinical management for positive outcomes* (7th ed., pp. 24-25, 820). Philadelphia: Saunders.
Stuart, G., & Laraia, M. (2005). *Principles and practice of psychiatric nursing* (8th ed., pp. 68, 226). St. Louis: Mosby.
Varcarolis, E., Carson, V., & Shoemaker, N. (2006). *Foundations of psychiatric mental health nursing* (5th ed., p. 243). Philadelphia: Saunders.

1117. A nurse reviews the preoperative teaching plan for a client scheduled for a radical neck dissection. When implementing the plan, the nurse initially focuses on:
1 The financial status of the client
2 Postoperative communication techniques
3 Information given to the client by the surgeon
4 The client's support systems and coping behaviors

Level of Cognitive Ability: Application
Client Needs: Psychosocial Integrity
Integrated Process: Teaching and Learning
Content Area: Delegating/Prioritizing

Answer: 3
Rationale: The first step in client teaching is establishing what the client already knows. This allows the nurse not only to correct any misinformation but also to determine the starting point for teaching and to implement the education at the client's level. Although options 1, 2, and 4 may be components of the plan, they are not the initial focus.

Test-Taking Strategy: Note the strategic word "initially." Remember that determining what the client already knows provides a starting point for teaching. Review the teaching and learning process if you had difficulty with this question.

References
Ignatavicius, D., & Workman, M. (2006). *Medical-surgical nursing: Critical thinking for collaborative care* (5th ed., p. 312). Philadelphia: Saunders.
Potter, P., & Perry, A. (2005). *Fundamentals of nursing* (6th ed., pp. 451-454). St. Louis: Mosby.

1118. A nurse is monitoring a client for signs of alcohol withdrawal. Which assessment data indicate early signs of withdrawal?
1 Anxiety, tremor, and irritability
2 Dizziness, vomiting, and headache
3 Disorientation, nausea, and sleepiness
4 Clouding of the consciousness, tiredness, and fatigue

Level of Cognitive Ability: Analysis
Client Needs: Psychosocial Integrity
Integrated Process: Nursing Process/Assessment
Content Area: Mental Health

Answer: 1
Rationale: The signs of alcohol withdrawal develop within a few hours after the cessation or reduction of alcohol, and they peak after 24 to 48 hours. Early signs include anxiety, anorexia, insomnia, tremor, irritability, an elevation in pulse and blood pressure, nausea, vomiting, and poorly formed hallucinations or illusions.

Test-Taking Strategy: Use the process of elimination, and eliminate options 3 and 4 first, because they are comparable or alike. From the remaining options, focus on the strategic word "early," and remember that the client will become irritable and anxious. Review the signs and symptoms of alcohol withdrawal if you had difficulty with this question.

References
Stuart, G., & Laraia, M. (2005). *Principles and practice of psychiatric nursing* (8th ed., p. 491). St. Louis: Mosby.
Varcarolis, E., Carson, V., & Shoemaker, N. (2006). *Foundations of psychiatric mental health nursing* (5th ed., pp. 550, 554). Philadelphia: Saunders.

1119. A preschool child is placed in traction for the treatment of a femur fracture. The child, who has reportedly been toilet trained for at least 1 year, begins bedwetting. The nurse recognizes this as:
1 A body image disturbance
2 A loss of developmental milestones caused by prolonged immobilization
3 Attention-seeking behavior requiring intervention by the child psychologist
4 Regressing to earlier developmental behavior, which is a normal psychological effect of immobilization

Answer: 4
Rationale: The monotony of immobilization can lead to sluggish intellectual and psychomotor responses. Regressive behaviors are not uncommon in immobilized children, and they usually do not require professional intervention. Although the "loss of developmental milestones" may seem like an appropriate option, "regressing to earlier developmental behavior" is a more accurate description of the psychological effects of immobilization. Body image may or may not be affected by long-term immobilization, but it does not relate to the information presented in the question.

Level of Cognitive Ability: Analysis
Client Needs: Psychosocial Integrity
Integrated Process: Nursing Process/Assessment
Content Area: Child Health

Test-Taking Strategy: Use the process of elimination. Eliminate option 1 first, because it is unrelated to the question. Eliminate option 3, because bedwetting by an immobilized child is not unusual, and a child psychologist is not needed. From the remaining options, recalling that regression is a normal psychological response to immobilization will direct you to option 4. Review the psychological effects of immobilization if you had difficulty with this question.

Reference
Hockenberry, M., Wilson, D., & Winkelstein, M. (2005). *Wong's essentials of pediatric nursing* (7th ed., pp. 1148-1150). St. Louis: Mosby.

1120. The nurse is assessing a client to determine the client's adjustment to presbycusis. Which of the following indicates successful adaptation to this problem?
  1 Proper use of a hearing aid
  2 Denial of a hearing impairment
  3 Withdrawal from social activities
  4 Reluctance to answer the telephone

Level of Cognitive Ability: Analysis
Client Needs: Psychosocial Integrity
Integrated Process: Nursing Process/Evaluation
Content Area: Adult Health/Ear

Answer: 1
Rationale: Presbycusis occurs as part of the aging process; it is a progressive sensorineural hearing loss. Some clients may not adapt well to the impairment, denying its presence. Others withdraw from social interactions and contact with others, embarrassed by the problem and the need to wear a hearing aid. Clients show adequate adaptation by obtaining and regularly using a hearing aid.

Test-Taking Strategy: The strategic words in the question are "successful adaptation." A review of each of the options shows that the only option with positive wording is option 1. The incorrect options indicate a need for further adaptation. Review the psychosocial issues related to the care of the client with a hearing aid if you had difficulty with this question.

References
Ignatavicius, D., & Workman, M. (2006). *Medical-surgical nursing: Critical thinking for collaborative care* (5th ed., pp. 1134-1135, 1137). Philadelphia: Saunders.
Lewis, S., Heitkemper, M., Dirksen, S., O'Brien, P., & Bucher, L. (2007). *Medical-surgical nursing: Assessment and management of clinical problems* (7th ed., pp. 109, 446). St. Louis: Mosby.

1121. A nurse is performing an admission assessment on a child and notes the presence of old and new bruises on the child's back and legs. The nurse suspects physical abuse and would:
  1 Report the case to legal authorities.
  2 File charges against the mother and father of the child.
  3 Ask the mother to identify the individual who is physically abusing the child.
  4 Tell the child that she will need to go to a foster home until the situation is straightened out.

Answer: 1
Rationale: The primary legal nursing responsibility when child abuse is suspected is to report the case. All 50 states require health care professionals to report all cases of suspected abuse. It is not appropriate for the nurse to file charges against the father or mother. It is also inappropriate to ask the mother to identify the abuser, because the abuser may in fact be the mother. If so, the possibility exists that the mother may become defensive and leave the emergency department with the child. Option 4 is clearly inappropriate and will produce fear in the child.

Level of Cognitive Ability: Application
Client Needs: Psychosocial Integrity
Integrated Process: Nursing Process/
  Implementation
Content Area: Child Health

Test-Taking Strategy: Use the process of elimination. In addition to the many implications associated with child abuse, abuse is a crime. With this in mind, option 1 describes the primary responsibility of the nurse. Review the responsibilities of the nurse when child abuse is suspected if you had difficulty with this question.

References

Hockenberry, M., & Wilson, D. (2007). *Nursing care of infants and children* (8th ed., pp. 705-706). St. Louis: Mosby.
Hockenberry, M., Wilson, D., & Winkelstein, M. (2005). *Wong's essentials of pediatric nursing* (7th ed., pp. 467-468). St. Louis: Mosby.

1122. The emergency department nurse is performing an assessment on a 7-year-old child with a fractured arm. The child is hesitant to answer questions that the nurse is asking and consistently looks at the parents in a fearful manner. The nurse suspects physical abuse and continues with the assessment procedures. Which assessment finding would most likely assist the nurse with verifying the suspicion?
1 Poor hygiene
2 Bald spots on the scalp
3 Swelling of the genitals
4 Lacerations in the anal area

Level of Cognitive Ability: Analysis
Client Needs: Psychosocial Integrity
Integrated Process: Nursing Process/Assessment
Content Area: Child Health

Answer: 2
Rationale: Bald spots on the scalp are most likely associated with physical abuse. The most likely assessment findings of sexual abuse include difficulty walking or sitting; torn, stained, or bloody underclothing; pain, swelling, or itching of the genitals; and bruises, bleeding, or lacerations in the genital or anal area. Poor hygiene may be indicative of physical neglect.

Test-Taking Strategy: Read the question carefully, and note the strategic words "physical abuse." The only option that specifically addresses an assessment finding related to physical abuse is option 2. Review the assessment findings of suspected physical abuse of a child if you had difficulty with this question.

Reference

Hockenberry, M., Wilson, D., & Winkelstein, M. (2005). *Wong's essentials of pediatric nursing* (7th ed., p. 465). St. Louis: Mosby.

1123. A 4-year-old child who was recently hospitalized is brought to the clinic by his mother for a follow-up visit. The mother tells the nurse that the child has begun to wet the bed ever since he was brought home from the hospital. The mother is concerned and asks the nurse what to do. Which of the following is the appropriate nursing response?
1 "You need to discipline the child."
2 "This is a normal occurrence after hospitalization."
3 "We will need to discuss this behavior with the physician."
4 "The child probably has developed a urinary tract infection."

Answer: 2
Rationale: Regression can occur in a preschooler, and it is most often a result of the stress of the hospitalization. It is best to accept the regression if it occurs. Parents may be overly concerned about the regressive behavior, and they should be told that regression is normal after hospitalization. It is premature to discuss the situation with the physician. Options 1 and 4 are inappropriate responses to the mother.

Test-Taking Strategy: Note the strategic word "appropriate," and use the process of elimination. Eliminate option 4 first, because there are no data in the question to support this statement. Knowledge regarding the behavior patterns of a preschooler after hospitalization and the use of therapeutic communication techniques will assist you with eliminating options 1 and 3. Review the psychosocial issues related to the hospitalized preschool child if you had difficulty with this question.

Level of Cognitive Ability: Application
Client Needs: Psychosocial Integrity
Integrated Process: Communication and
    Documentation
Content Area: Child Health

Reference
Hockenberry, M., Wilson, D., & Winkelstein, M. (2005). *Wong's essentials of pediatric nursing* (7th ed., pp. 401, 646). St. Louis: Mosby.

1124. During an office visit, a prenatal client with mitral stenosis states that she has been under a lot of stress lately. During the examination, the client questions the nurse and behaves anxiously. The appropriate nursing action at this time should be to:

1 Tell the client not to worry.
2 Refer the client to a counselor.
3 Ignore the client's unfounded concerns and continue with the assessment.
4 Explain the purpose of the nurse's actions and answer all of the client's questions.

Answer: 4
Rationale: In the prenatal cardiac client, stress should be reduced as much as possible. The client should be provided with honest and informed answers to questions to help alleviate unnecessary fears and emotional stress. Explaining the purpose of nursing actions will assist with decreasing the stress level of the client. Options 1, 2, and 3 are nontherapeutic methods of communication at this time.

Test-Taking Strategy: Use the process of elimination and therapeutic communication techniques to answer the question. The client's concerns and feelings should always be addressed, and option 4 is the only option that does this. Review therapeutic communication techniques if you had difficulty with this question.

Level of Cognitive Ability: Application
Client Needs: Psychosocial Integrity
Integrated Process: Nursing Process/
    Implementation
Content Area: Maternity/Antepartum

Reference
Murray, S., & McKinney, E. (2006). *Foundations of maternal-newborn nursing* (4th ed., pp. 24-26). Philadelphia: Saunders.

1125. A postpartum client with gestational diabetes is scheduled for discharge. During the discharge teaching, the client asks the nurse, "Do I have to worry about this diabetes anymore?" Which of the following is the appropriate response by the nurse?

1 "Your blood glucose level is within normal limits now, so you will be all right."
2 "You will only have to worry about the diabetes if you become pregnant again."
3 "You will be at risk for developing gestational diabetes with your next pregnancy and also for developing diabetes mellitus."
4 "When you have gestational diabetes, you have diabetes forever, and you must be treated with medication for the rest of your life."

Answer: 3
Rationale: The client is at risk for developing gestational diabetes with each pregnancy. The client also has an increased risk for developing diabetes mellitus and needs to comply with follow-up assessments. She also needs to be taught techniques to lower her risk for developing diabetes mellitus, such as weight control. The diagnosis of gestational diabetes mellitus indicates that this client has an increased risk for developing diabetes mellitus; however, with proper care, it may not develop.

Test-Taking Strategy: Identify the subject of the question, which is the long-term effect of gestational diabetes. In addition, use therapeutic communication techniques to answer the question and to direct you to option 3. Review the long-term effects of gestational diabetes if you had difficulty with this question.

Reference
Murray, S., & McKinney, E. (2006). *Foundations of maternal-newborn nursing* (4th ed., pp. 665, 667). Philadelphia: Saunders.

Level of Cognitive Ability: Application
Client Needs: Psychosocial Integrity
Integrated Process: Communication and
    Documentation
Content Area: Maternity/Postpartum

1126. A nurse is performing an assessment on a 16-year-old female client who has been diagnosed with anorexia nervosa. Which statement by the client would the nurse identify as a priority requiring further assessment?

1 "I check my weight every day without fail."
2 "I exercise 3 to 4 hours every day to keep my slim figure."
3 "I've been told that I am 10% below my ideal body weight."
4 "My best friend was in the hospital with this disorder a year ago."

Level of Cognitive Ability: Analysis
Client Needs: Psychosocial Integrity
Integrated Process: Nursing Process/Analysis
Content Area: Mental Health

Answer: 2
Rationale: Exercising 3 to 4 hours every day is excessive physical activity and unrealistic for a 16-year-old girl. The nurse needs to further assess this statement immediately to find out why the client feels the need to exercise this much to maintain her figure. Although it is unfortunate that the client's best friend had this disorder, this is not considered a major threat to this client's physical well-being. A weight that exceeds 15% below the ideal weight is significant for clients with anorexia nervosa. It is not considered abnormal to check the weight every day; many clients with anorexia nervosa check their weight close to 20 times a day.

Test-Taking Strategy: Note the strategic words "requiring further assessment." These words indicate a negative event query and ask you to select the option that identifies a concern. Eliminate options 3 and 4 first, because these client statements are not significant or abnormal. From the remaining options, knowledge regarding the manifestations associated with anorexia nervosa will direct you to option 2. Review the significant manifestations of anorexia nervosa if you had difficulty with this question.

References
Stuart, G., & Laraia, M. (2005). *Principles and practice of psychiatric nursing* (8th ed., pp. 527, 530). St. Louis: Mosby.
Varcarolis, E., Carson, V., & Shoemaker, N. (2006). *Foundations of psychiatric mental health nursing* (5th ed., p. 314). Philadelphia: Saunders.

1127. A client who has confusion as a result of bedrest and a prolonged length of hospital stay receives a prescription for progressive ambulation as tolerated. Which is the best nursing intervention to use to implement the prescription?

1 Ambulate in the room for short distances frequently.
2 Ambulate in the hall progressively three times a day.
3 Ambulate to the client's bathroom three times a day.
4 Assist with range-of-motion exercises three times a day.

Level of Cognitive Ability: Analysis
Client Needs: Psychosocial Integrity
Integrated Process: Nursing Process/Planning
Content Area: Fundamental Skills

Answer: 2
Rationale: The cause of the client's confusion is bedrest and decreased sensory stimulation from a prolonged length of stay; therefore, the best intervention is to ambulate the client in the hall to increase sensory stimulation. Hopefully the stimulation can help to decrease the confusion. Options 1 and 3 do not address the client's need for sensory stimulation. The nurse performs option 4 in preparation for ambulation while the client is on bedrest.

Test-Taking Strategy: Focus on the subject of "confusion as a result of bedrest and a prolonged length of hospital stay." Eliminate option 4 first, because this action should have been performed in preparation for ambulation. Next, eliminate options 1 and 3, because they are comparable or alike in that they both address ambulating the client in the hospital room. Review the interventions related to promoting sensory stimulation if you had difficulty with this question.

References
Ignatavicius, D., & Workman, M. (2006). *Medical-surgical nursing: Critical thinking for collaborative care* (5th ed., pp. 311-312). Philadelphia: Saunders.
Potter, P., & Perry, A. (2005). *Fundamentals of nursing* (6th ed., p. 1477). St. Louis: Mosby.

1128. The nurse is caring for an older client who has been placed in Buck's extension traction after a hip fracture. During the assessment of the client, the nurse notes that the client is disoriented. What is the appropriate nursing intervention?
1 Apply restraints to the client.
2 Ask the family to stay with the client.
3 Ask the laboratory to perform electrolyte studies.
4 Reorient the client frequently and place a clock and a calendar in the client's room.

Level of Cognitive Ability: Application
Client Needs: Psychosocial Integrity
Integrated Process: Nursing Process/
  Implementation
Content Area: Adult Health/Musculoskeletal

Answer: 4
Rationale: An inactive older person may become disoriented as a result of a lack of sensory stimulation. The appropriate nursing intervention would be to frequently reorient the client and to place objects such as a clock and a calendar in the client's room to maintain orientation. Restraints may cause further disorientation and should not be applied unless specifically prescribed. Agency policies and procedures should be followed before the application of restraints. The family can assist with the orientation of the client, but it is not appropriate to ask the family to stay with the client. It is not within the scope of nursing practice to prescribe laboratory studies.

Test-Taking Strategy: Note the strategic word "appropriate." Eliminate option 3 first, because it is not within the realm of nursing practice to prescribe laboratory studies. Next, eliminate option 1, because restraints may add to the disorientation that the client is experiencing. It is not appropriate to place the responsibility of the client on the family, so option 2 should be eliminated. In addition, note the relationship between the words "disoriented" in the question and "reorient" in option 4. Review the measures related to caring for a client who is disoriented if you had difficulty with this question.

References
Black, J., & Hawks, J. (2005). *Medical-surgical nursing: Clinical management for positive outcomes* (7th ed., pp. 641, 2169). Philadelphia: Saunders.
Monahan, F., Sands, J., Neighbors, M., Marek, J., & Green, C. (2007). *Phipps' medical-surgical nursing: Health and illness perspectives* (8th ed., p. 1547). St. Louis: Mosby.

1129. An 8-year-old boy is admitted to the hospital. He was sexually abused by an adult family member, and he is withdrawn and appears frightened. Which of the following describes the best plan for the initial nursing encounter to convey concern and support?
1 Introduce self and explain to the child that he is safe now that he is in the hospital.
2 Introduce self and tell the child that the nurse would like to sit with him for a little while.
3 Introduce self and then ask the child to express how he feels about the events leading up to this hospital admission.
4 Introduce self, explain your role, and ask the child to act out the sexual encounter with the abuser with the use of art therapy.

Level of Cognitive Ability: Application
Client Needs: Psychosocial Integrity
Integrated Process: Caring
Content Area: Child Health

Answer: 2
Rationale: Victims of sexual abuse may exhibit fear and anxiety regarding what has just occurred. In addition, they may fear that the abuse could be repeated. When initiating contact with a child victim of sexual abuse who demonstrates a fear of others, it is best to convey a willingness to spend time and to move slowly to initiate activities that may be perceived as threatening. After a rapport is established, the nurse may explore the child's feelings or use various therapeutic modalities to encourage the recounting of the sexual encounter. Option 2 conveys a plan for an initial encounter that establishes trust by sitting with the child in a nonthreatening atmosphere. Option 1 does not convey concern and support by the nurse. Options 3 and 4 may be implemented after trust and rapport are established.

Test-Taking Strategy: Use the process of elimination, and focus on the child's experience and the fact that the child is frightened. This will assist you with eliminating options 3 and 4. From the remaining options, recalling that rapport needs to be established first will direct you to option 2. Review the care of the abused child if you had difficulty with this question.

References
Hockenberry, M., Wilson, D., & Winkelstein, M. (2005). *Wong's essentials of pediatric nursing* (7th ed., pp. 463, 465). St. Louis: Mosby.
Wong, D., Hockenberry, M., Perry, S., Lowdermilk, D., & Wilson, D. (2006). *Maternal-child nursing care* (3rd ed., p. 1144). St. Louis: Mosby.

1130. A female victim of a sexual assault is being seen in the crisis center for a third visit. She states that, although the rape occurred nearly 2 months ago, she still feels "as though the rape just happened yesterday." The nurse would respond by stating:

1 "In reality, the rape did not just occur. It has been over 2 months now."

2 "What can you do to alleviate some of your fears about being assaulted again?"

3 "In time, our goal will be to help you move on from these strong feelings about your rape."

4 "Tell me more about those aspects of the rape that cause you to feel like the rape just occurred."

Level of Cognitive Ability: Application
Client Needs: Psychosocial Integrity
Integrated Process: Communication and Documentation
Content Area: Mental Health

Answer: 4
Rationale: Option 4 allows for the client to express her ideas and feelings more fully and portrays a nonhurried, nonjudgmental, supportive attitude. Clients need to be reassured that their feelings are normal and that they may freely express their concerns in a safe care environment. Although option 1 is true, it immediately blocks communication. Option 2 places the problem solving totally on the client. Option 3 places the client's feelings on hold.

Test-Taking Strategy: Use therapeutic communication techniques. Option 4 specifically addresses the client's feelings and concerns. Remember to always address the client's feelings first. Review therapeutic communication techniques if you had difficulty with this question.

Reference
Stuart, G., & Laraia, M. (2005). *Principles and practice of psychiatric nursing* (8th ed., pp. 30-34, 235). St. Louis: Mosby.

1131. When formulating the plan of care for a client with a nursing diagnosis of Disturbed thought processes as a result of paranoia, the nurse instructs the staff to do which of the following?

1 Avoid laughing or whispering in front of the client.

2 Have the client sign a release of information form.

3 Increase the socialization of the client with unit peers.

4 Begin educating the client about available social supports.

Level of Cognitive Ability: Application
Client Needs: Psychosocial Integrity
Integrated Process: Nursing Process/ Implementation
Content Area: Mental Health

Answer: 1
Rationale: A client experiencing paranoia is distrustful and suspicious of others. The health care team needs to establish rapport and trust with the client. Laughing or whispering in front of the client would increase the client's paranoia. Options 2, 3, and 4 ask the client to trust on a multitude of levels. These options are too intrusive for a client who is paranoid.

Test-Taking Strategy: Focus on the client's problem: paranoia. Recalling that the client with paranoia is distrustful and suspicious of others will direct you to option 1. Review paranoia if you had difficulty with this question.

Reference
Stuart, G., & Laraia, M. (2005). *Principles and practice of psychiatric nursing* (8th ed., p. 786). St. Louis: Mosby.

1132. A nurse is assessing a client who has a nursing diagnosis of Risk for self-directed violence. The client says, "You won't have to worry about me much longer." The nurse interprets this statement as:

1 An intention of suicide

2 An expression of depression

3 An intention of self-mutilation

4 An expression of hopelessness

Answer: 1
Rationale: A client with a Risk for self-directed violence who says, "You won't have to worry about me much longer," is making an expression of a suicidal intent. Although hopelessness, depression, and self-mutilation may relate to self-directed violence, the statement that he or she will not be around is a direct comment about the act of suicide.

Level of Cognitive Ability: Analysis
Client Needs: Psychosocial Integrity
Integrated Process: Nursing Process/Analysis
Content Area: Mental Health

Test-Taking Strategy: Use the process of elimination. Focus on the client's statement to direct you to option 1. Review the characteristics related to risk for self-directed violence if you had difficulty with this question.

Reference
Stuart, G., & Laraia, M. (2005). *Principles and practice of psychiatric nursing* (8th ed., pp. 308-309). St. Louis: Mosby.

1133. The nurse notes that an assigned client is lying tense in bed and staring at the cardiac monitor. The client states, "There sure are a lot of wires around there. I sure hope we don't get hit by lightning." Which of the following is the appropriate nursing response?
1 "Your family can stay tonight if they wish."
2 "Would you like a mild sedative to help you relax?"
3 "Oh, don't worry, the weather is supposed to be sunny and clear today."
4 "Yes, all of those wires must be a little scary. Did someone explain to you what the cardiac monitor is for?"

Level of Cognitive Ability: Application
Client Needs: Psychosocial Integrity
Integrated Process: Nursing Process/Implementation
Content Area: Adult Health/Cardiovascular

Answer: 4
Rationale: The nurse should initially validate the client's concern and then assess the client's knowledge regarding the cardiac monitor. This gives the nurse an opportunity to provide client education, if necessary. Options 1, 2, and 3 do not address the client's concern. In addition, pharmacological interventions should be considered only if necessary.

Test-Taking Strategy: Use therapeutic communication techniques. Remember to address the client's feelings first. Option 4 is the only option that addresses the client's feelings. Review therapeutic communication techniques if you had difficulty with this question.

References
Ignatavicius, D., & Workman, M. (2006). *Medical-surgical nursing: Critical thinking for collaborative care* (5th ed., p. 343). Philadelphia: Saunders.
Potter, P., & Perry, A. (2005). *Fundamentals of nursing* (6th ed., p. 437). St. Louis: Mosby.

1134. A young adult male client with a spinal cord injury tells the nurse, "It's so depressing that I'll never get to have sex again." The nurse replies in a realistic way by making which of the following statements to the client?
1 "It must feel horrible to know you can never have sex again."
2 "It's still possible to have a sexual relationship, but it will be different."
3 "You're young, so you'll adapt to this more easily than if you were older."
4 "Because of body reflexes, sexual functioning will be no different than before."

Answer: 2
Rationale: It is possible to have a sexual relationship after a spinal cord injury, but it is different than what the client will have experienced before the injury. Males may experience reflex erections, although they may not ejaculate. Females can have adductor spasm. Sexual counseling may help the client adapt to changes in sexuality after a spinal cord injury.

Test-Taking Strategy: Use the process of elimination, your knowledge regarding the effects of a spinal cord injury, and therapeutic communication techniques. Option 2 addresses the subject, is accurate, and is a therapeutic response. Review the effects of a spinal cord injury if you had difficulty with this question.

Level of Cognitive Ability: Application
Client Needs: Psychosocial Integrity
Integrated Process: Communication and
     Documentation
Content Area: Adult Health/Neurological

References
Black, J., & Hawks, J. (2005). *Medical-surgical nursing: Clinical management for positive outcomes* (7th ed., p. 2224). Philadelphia: Saunders.
Ignatavicius, D., & Workman, M. (2006). *Medical-surgical nursing: Critical thinking for collaborative care* (5th ed., p. 994). Philadelphia: Saunders.
Potter, P., & Perry, A. (2005). *Fundamentals of nursing* (6th ed., p. 437). St. Louis: Mosby.

1135. A family member of a client with a brain tumor states that he is feeling distraught and guilty for not encouraging the client to seek medical evaluation earlier. The nurse should incorporate which of the following items when formulating a response to the family member's statement?

1 There are no symptoms of a brain tumor.

2 It is true that brain tumors are easily recognizable.

3 Brain tumors are never detected until very late in their course.

4 The symptoms of a brain tumor may be easily attributed to another cause.

Level of Cognitive Ability: Application
Client Needs: Psychosocial Integrity
Integrated Process: Caring
Content Area: Adult Health/Neurological

Answer: 4

Rationale: Signs and symptoms of a brain tumor vary depending on location, and they may easily be attributed to another cause. Symptoms include headache, vomiting, visual disturbances, and changes in intellectual abilities or personality. Seizures occur in some clients. These symptoms can be easily attributed to other causes. The family requires support to assist them during the normal grieving process. Options 1, 2, and 3 are inaccurate.

Test-Taking Strategy: Use the process of elimination. Eliminate options 1 and 3 first, because they contain the close-ended words "no" and "never," respectively. From the remaining options, recall that the symptoms of a brain tumor may be easily attributed to another cause. Also, note the word "may" in the correct option. Review the symptoms of a brain tumor if you had difficulty with this question.

References
Ignatavicius, D., & Workman, M. (2006). *Medical-surgical nursing: Critical thinking for collaborative care* (5th ed., p. 1057). Philadelphia: Saunders.
Potter, P., & Perry, A. (2005). *Fundamentals of nursing* (6th ed., p. 437). St. Louis: Mosby.

1136. A male client is in a hip spica cast as a result of a hip fracture. On the day after the cast has been applied, the nurse finds the client surrounded by papers from his briefcase and planning a phone meeting. The nurse's interaction with the client about the client's activities should be based on the knowledge that:

1 Rest is an essential component of bone healing.

2 Setting limits on a client's behavior is a mandated nursing role.

3 Not keeping up with his job will increase the client's stress level.

4 Immediate involvement in his job will keep the client from becoming bored while on bedrest.

Level of Cognitive Ability: Analysis
Client Needs: Psychosocial Integrity
Integrated Process: Caring
Content Area: Adult Health/Musculoskeletal

Answer: 1

Rationale: Rest is an essential component of bone healing. Nurses can help clients understand the importance of rest and find ways to balance work demands to promote healing. Stress should be kept to a minimum to promote bone healing. Nurses cannot demand these changes, but they need to encourage clients to choose them. It may relieve stress to do work; however, during the immediate period after the cast is applied, it may not be therapeutic. Setting limits on a client's behavior is not a mandated nursing role.

Test-Taking Strategy: Use the process of elimination. Eliminate options 3 and 4, because they are comparable or alike. From the remaining options, note that option 1 is the umbrella option and that it addresses the subject of rest. Review the physiological and psychosocial needs of the client in a hip spica cast if you had difficulty with this question.

Reference
Black, J., & Hawks, J. (2005). *Medical-surgical nursing: Clinical management for positive outcomes* (7th ed., p. 636). Philadelphia: Saunders.

1137. A charge nurse observes a nursing assistant talking in an unusually loud voice to a client with delirium. The charge nurse takes which action?

1 The nurse enters the room and informs the client that everything is all right.

2 The nurse speaks to the nursing assistant immediately while in the client's room to solve the problem.

3 The nurse ensures the client's safety, calmly asks the nursing assistant to step outside the room, and informs the nursing assistant that her voice was unusually loud.

4 The nurse explains to the nursing assistant that yelling in the client's room is tolerated only if the client is talking loudly and the nursing assistant needs to get the client's attention.

Level of Cognitive Ability: Application
Client Needs: Psychosocial Integrity
Integrated Process: Nursing Process/
  Implementation
Content Area: Leadership/Management

Answer: 3
Rationale: The nurse must ascertain that the client is safe and then discuss the matter with the nursing assistant in an area away from the hearing of the client. If the client hears the conversation, the client may become more confused or agitated. Options 1, 2, and 4 are incorrect actions.

Test-Taking Strategy: Use Maslow's Hierarchy of Needs theory. Remember that, when a physiological need is not present, safety needs are the priority. Review appropriate and therapeutic communication techniques and the care of the client with delirium if you had difficulty with this question.

References
Huber, D. (2006). *Leadership and nursing care management* (3rd ed., pp. 125-127). Philadelphia: Saunders.
Stuart, G., & Laraia, M. (2005). *Principles and practice of psychiatric nursing* (8th ed., pp. 464, 467). St. Louis: Mosby.

1138. A teenager who has celiac disease arrives at the emergency department complaining of profuse, watery diarrhea after a pizza party the night before. The client states, "I don't want to be different from my friends." Which nursing diagnosis is most appropriate for this client?

1 Celiac crisis

2 Deficient knowledge

3 Deficient fluid volume

4 Risk for situational low self-esteem

Level of Cognitive Ability: Analysis
Client Needs: Psychosocial Integrity
Integrated Process: Nursing Process/Analysis
Content Area: Child Health

Answer: 4
Rationale: The client expresses concern about being different from friends. Although the question states that the client has profuse, watery diarrhea, no data identify an actual deficient fluid volume. In addition, the assessment data provided do not support a diagnosis of Deficient knowledge. Celiac crisis is a medical diagnosis.

Test-Taking Strategy: Use the process of elimination, and focus on the data in the question. Eliminate option 1, because it is a medical diagnosis. Next, focus on the client's feelings of "being different." This will direct you to option 4. Review the defining characteristics of the Risk for situational low self-esteem if you had difficulty with this question.

References
Hockenberry, M., Wilson, D., & Winkelstein, M. (2005). *Wong's essentials of pediatric nursing* (7th ed., pp. 91, 504). St. Louis: Mosby.
Wong, D., Hockenberry, M., Perry, S., Lowdermilk, D., & Wilson, D. (2006). *Maternal-child nursing care* (3rd ed., p. 1192). St. Louis: Mosby.

1139. A nurse develops a plan of care for a 1-month-old infant hospitalized for intussusception. Which nursing measure would be most effective to provide psychosocial support for the parent–child relationship?

1 Provide educational materials.
2 Encourage the parents to room-in with their infant.
3 Initiate home nutritional support as early as possible.
4 Encourage the parents to go home and get some sleep.

Level of Cognitive Ability: Application
Client Needs: Psychosocial Integrity
Integrated Process: Caring
Content Area: Child Health

Answer: 2
Rationale: Rooming-in is effective for reducing separation anxiety and preserving the parent–child relationship. Parents are under stress when a child is ill and hospitalized, and telling a parent to go home and sleep will not relieve this stress. Educational materials may be beneficial, but they will not provide psychosocial support for the parent–child relationship. Home nutritional support is not usually necessary in the situation described.

Test-Taking Strategy: Focus on the strategic words "parent–child relationship." Use the process of elimination, and focus on this concept. The only option that addresses the parent–child relationship is option 2. Review the measures that promote the parent–child relationship in a hospitalized infant if you had difficulty with this question.

Reference
Hockenberry, M., Wilson, D., & Winkelstein, M. (2005). *Wong's essentials of pediatric nursing* (7th ed., pp. 652-653). St. Louis: Mosby.

1140. The parents of a male infant who will have a surgical repair of a hernia make the following comments. Which comment would require follow-up assessment by a nurse?

1 "I understand that surgery will repair the hernia."
2 "I don't know if he will be able to father a child when he grows up."
3 "The day nurse told me to give him sponge baths for a few days after surgery."
4 "I'll need to buy extra diapers, because we need to change them more frequently now."

Level of Cognitive Ability: Analysis
Client Needs: Psychosocial Integrity
Integrated Process: Nursing Process/Analysis
Content Area: Child Health

Answer: 2
Rationale: The anatomical location of a hernia frequently causes more psychological concern to the parents than does the actual condition or treatment. Options 1, 3, and 4 all indicate accurate understanding. Option 2 is an incorrect comment.

Test-Taking Strategy: Focus on the strategic words "would require follow-up assessment." Options 1, 3, and 4 do not require follow-up, whereas option 2 reflects parental fear and identifies a need for further assessment. Review parental instructions regarding the effects of a hernia repair if you had difficulty with this question.

Reference
Wong, D., Hockenberry, M., Perry, S., Lowdermilk, D., & Wilson, D. (2006). *Maternal-child nursing care* (3rd ed., p. 1534). St. Louis: Mosby.

1141. A nurse is leading a crisis intervention group comprised of high school students who have experienced the recent death of a classmate who committed suicide. The students are experiencing disbelief as they review the details of finding the classmate dead in a bathroom. Initially, the nurse would:

1 Ask how the students recovered from a death event in the past.
2 Reinforce the students' ability to work through this death event.
3 Reinforce the students' sense of growth through this death experience.
4 Inquire about the students' perception of their classmate's suicide.

Level of Cognitive Ability: Analysis
Client Needs: Psychosocial Integrity
Integrated Process: Nursing Process/Assessment
Content Area: Mental Health

Answer: 4

Rationale: It is essential to determine the students' views. Inquiring about the students' perception of the suicide will specifically identify the appraisal of the suicide and the meaning of the perception. Options 2 and 3 are comparable or alike in that they are attempts to foster students' self-esteem. Such an approach is premature at this point. Although option 1 is exploratory, it does not address the "here and now" appraisal in terms of the classmate's suicide. Although the nurse is interested in how students' have coped in the past, this inquiry should not be the most immediate assessment.

Test-Taking Strategy: Use the steps of the nursing process to eliminate options 2 and 3. From the remaining options, consider the subject of the question and select the option that deals with the here and now. The nurse must first determine the students' perception and appraisal of the stressful event. Review the phases of crisis if you had difficulty with this question.

Reference
Stuart, G., & Laraia, M. (2005). *Principles and practice of psychiatric nursing* (8th ed., pp. 227-229). St. Louis: Mosby.

1142. A hospitalized client has participated in substance abuse therapy group sessions. The nurse is monitoring the client's response to these sessions. Which statement by the client would best indicate that the client has assimilated session topics, understood coping response styles, and processed information effectively for self-use?

1 "I'll keep all my appointments, and I'll do everything I'm supposed to. I just know nothing will go wrong that way."
2 "I know I'm ready to be discharged. I feel like I'll have no problem saying no and leaving a group of friends if they are drinking."
3 "This group has really helped a lot. I know it will be different when I go home. But I'm sure that my family and friends will all help me, like the people in this group have. They'll all help me, I know they will. They won't let me go back to old ways."
4 "I'm looking forward to leaving here, but I know that I will miss all of you. So, I'm happy, and I'm sad. I'm excited, and I'm scared. I know that I have to work hard to be strong and that everyone isn't going to be as helpful as you all have been. I know it isn't going to be easy, but I'm going to try as hard as I can."

Answer: 4

Rationale: With the defense mechanism of denial, the person denies reality. There can be varying degrees of this denial. In option 4, the client is expressing real concern and ambivalence about discharge from the hospital. The client demonstrates an ability to perceive reality in the appraisal regarding the lifestyle changes that will have to be initiated as well as the fact that the client will have to work hard and develop new friends and meeting places. In option 1, the client is concrete and procedure oriented; again, the client verbalizes denial. Option 2 identifies denial. In option 3, the client is relying heavily on others, and the client's locus of control is external.

Test-Taking Strategy: Note the strategic words "processed information effectively." Select the option that identifies the most realistic client verbalization. Recalling that a person in denial is unable to face reality will assist you with eliminating options 1, 2, and 3. Review the defense mechanism of denial if you had difficulty with this question.

Level of Cognitive Ability: Analysis
Client Needs: Psychosocial Integrity
Integrated Process: Nursing Process/Analysis
Content Area: Mental Health

References
Stuart, G., & Laraia, M. (2005). *Principles and practice of psychiatric nursing* (8th ed., p. 492). St. Louis: Mosby.
Varcarolis, E., Carson, V., & Shoemaker, N. (2006). *Foundations of psychiatric mental health nursing* (5th ed., p. 220). Philadelphia: Saunders.

1143. A client recovering from a head injury becomes agitated at times. Which action should the nurse incorporate to calm this client?
  1 Assign the client a new task to master.
  2 Turn on the television to a musical program.
  3 Make the client aware that the behavior is undesirable.
  4 Talk to the client about the familiar objects, such as family pictures, that are kept in the client's room.

Level of Cognitive Ability: Application
Client Needs: Psychosocial Integrity
Integrated Process: Caring
Content Area: Adult Health/Neurological

Answer: 4
Rationale: Decreasing environmental stimuli aids in reducing agitation for the head-injured client. Option 1 does not simplify the environment, because a new task may be frustrating. Option 2 increases stimuli. In option 3, the nurse uses negative reinforcement to help the client adjust. Providing familiar objects will decrease anxiety.

Test-Taking Strategy: Use the process of elimination, and identify those options that may increase stimuli, agitation, and frustration. This will assist you with eliminating options 1, 2, and 3. Review the measures that will relieve agitation if you had difficulty with this question.

References
Black, J., & Hawks, J. (2005). *Medical-surgical nursing: Clinical management for positive outcomes* (7th ed., pp. 528-530). Philadelphia: Saunders.
Ignatavicius, D., & Workman, M. (2006). *Medical-surgical nursing: Critical thinking for collaborative care* (5th ed., p. 1050). Philadelphia: Saunders.

1144. A client recovering from a brain attack (stroke) has become irritable and angry regarding limitations. Which of the following is the best nursing approach to help the client regain motivation to succeed?
  1 Ignore the behavior, knowing that the client is grieving.
  2 Allow longer and more frequent visitation by the spouse.
  3 Use supportive statements to correct the client's behavior.
  4 Tell the client that the nurses are experienced and know how the client feels.

Level of Cognitive Ability: Application
Client Needs: Psychosocial Integrity
Integrated Process: Caring
Content Area: Adult Health/Neurological

Answer: 3
Rationale: Clients who have experienced a stroke have many and varied needs. It is also important to support and praise the client for accomplishments. The client may need his or her behavior pointed out so that correction can take place, and the client's behavior should not be ignored. Spouses of a stroke client are often grieving; therefore, more visitation may not be helpful. Additionally, short visits are often encouraged. Stating that the nurse knows how the client feels is inappropriate.

Test-Taking Strategy: Use therapeutic communication techniques to eliminate options 1 and 4. From the remaining options, option 3 is the only option that addresses the client's behavior described in the question. Review the psychosocial aspects related to a stroke if you had difficulty with this question.

Reference
Ignatavicius, D., & Workman, M. (2006). *Medical-surgical nursing: Critical thinking for collaborative care* (5th ed., p. 1035). Philadelphia: Saunders.

1145. A client is admitted to the hospital with a fractured hip and is experiencing periods of confusion. The nurse formulates a nursing diagnosis of Disturbed thought processes and identifies which psychosocial outcome as a priority?

1 Improved sleep patterns
2 Reduced family fears and anxiety
3 Meeting self-care needs independently
4 Increased ability to concentrate and make decisions

Level of Cognitive Ability: Analysis
Client Needs: Psychosocial Integrity
Integrated Process: Nursing Process/Planning
Content Area: Adult Health/Musculoskeletal

Answer: 4

Rationale: The client needs to be able to concentrate and make decisions. When the client is able to do that, the nurse can work with the client to achieve the other outcomes. The client is the center of the nurse's concern. Options 1 and 3 address physiological needs rather than psychosocial outcomes. Option 2 is a secondary need and does not address the client.

Test-Taking Strategy: Use the process of elimination, and note the strategic words "psychosocial outcome." Select the option that will have the greatest impact on the client's ability to function psychosocially. Option 2 can be eliminated, because it does not address the client described in the question. Options 1 and 3 address physiological rather than psychosocial needs. Review the expected outcomes for the client with Disturbed thought processes if you had difficulty with this question.

References

Black, J., & Hawks, J. (2005). *Medical-surgical nursing: Clinical management for positive outcomes* (7th ed., p. 641). Philadelphia: Saunders.

Stuart, G., & Laraia, M. (2005). *Principles and practice of psychiatric nursing* (8th ed., pp. 785-786). St. Louis: Mosby.

1146. The nurse is caring for a young woman who is dying from breast cancer. The nurse determines that a defining characteristic of anticipatory grieving is present when the woman:

1 Discusses thoughts and feelings related to loss
2 Verbalizes unrealistic goals and plans for the future
3 Has prolonged emotional reactions and outbursts
4 Ignores untreated medical conditions that require treatment

Level of Cognitive Ability: Analysis
Client Needs: Psychosocial Integrity
Integrated Process: Nursing Process/Analysis
Content Area: Adult Health/Neurological

Answer: 1

Rationale: The nurse can determine the client's stage of grief by observing the client's behavior. This is extremely important, because the appropriate nursing diagnoses need to be developed so that the plan of care is appropriate. Options 2, 3, and 4 are examples of dysfunctional grieving.

Test-Taking Strategy: Focus on the subject: anticipatory grieving. Note the similarity of options 2, 3, and 4 in that they indicate dysfunctional grieving. Also noting the words "prolonged," "unrealistic," and "ignores" in these options will assist you with eliminating them. Review the stages of grief and anticipatory grieving if you had difficulty with this question.

Reference

Ignatavicius, D., & Workman, M. (2006). *Medical-surgical nursing: Critical thinking for collaborative care* (5th ed., p. 113). Philadelphia: Saunders.

1147. A nurse determines that a client is beginning to experience shock and hemorrhage as a result of a partial inversion of the uterus. The nurse pages the obstetrician to come immediately and calls for assistance. The client asks in an apprehensive voice, "What is happening to me? I feel so funny, and I know I'm bleeding. Am I dying?" The nurse responds to the client, knowing that the client is feeling:

1 Panic as a result of shock
2 Anticipatory grieving related to the fear of dying
3 Depression related to postpartum hormonal changes
4 Fear and anxiety related to unexpected and ambiguous sensations

Level of Cognitive Ability: Analysis
Client Needs: Psychosocial Integrity
Integrated Process: Nursing Process/Analysis
Content Area: Maternity/Postpartum

Answer: 4
Rationale: Feelings of loss of control are common causes of anxiety, and the unknown is the most common cause of fear. Apprehension and feelings of impending doom are also associated with shock, but the information in the question does not suggest panic at this point. Anticipatory grieving occurs when there is knowledge of the impending loss, but it is not associated with a sudden situational crisis such as this one. It is far too early for the onset of postpartum depression.

Test-Taking Strategy: Focus on the data and the client's statement. Note the relationship between "I feel so funny" in the question and "unexpected and ambiguous sensations" in option 4. Review client responses when a sudden situational crisis occurs if you had difficulty with this question.

Reference
Murray, S., & McKinney, E. (2006). *Foundations of maternal-newborn nursing* (4th ed., pp. 340-341). Philadelphia: Saunders.

1148. A perinatal home-care nurse has just assessed the fetal status of a client with a diagnosis of partial placental abruption of 20 weeks' gestation. The client is experiencing new bleeding and reports less fetal movement. The nurse informs the client that the physician will be contacted for possible hospital admission. The client begins to cry quietly while holding her abdomen with her hands. She murmurs, "No, no, you can't go, my little man." The nurse recognizes the client's behavior as an indication of:

1 Pain related to abdominal tetany
2 Cognitive confusion as a result of shock
3 Situational crisis related to fear, loss, and the death of the fetus
4 Anticipatory grieving related to the perceived potential loss of the fetus

Level of Cognitive Ability: Analysis
Client Needs: Psychosocial Integrity
Integrated Process: Nursing Process/Analysis
Content Area: Maternity/Antepartum

Answer: 4
Rationale: Anticipatory grieving occurs when a client has knowledge of an impending loss, such as when signs of fetal distress accelerate. The first stages of anticipatory grieving may be characterized by shock, emotional numbness, disbelief, and strong emotions such as tears, screaming, or anger. There are no data that indicate the presence of pain, confusion, or fetal death.

Test-Taking Strategy: Use the process of elimination, and focus on the data in the question. Options 1 and 2 can be eliminated, because there is no indication of pain or confusion. Note that, in this situation, there is a situational crisis with feelings of grief, but no fetal loss has occurred at this point. Therefore, eliminate option 3. Review the defining characteristics of anticipatory grieving if you had difficulty with this question.

References
Murray, S., & McKinney, E. (2006). *Foundations of maternal-newborn nursing* (4th ed., p. 608). Philadelphia: Saunders.
Wong, D., Hockenberry, M., Perry, S., Lowdermilk, D., & Wilson, D. (2006). *Maternal-child nursing care* (3rd ed., p. 800). St. Louis: Mosby.

1149. A postoperative client has been vomiting and has absent bowel sounds, and paralytic ileus has been diagnosed. The physician orders the insertion of a nasogastric tube. The nurse explains the purpose of the tube and the insertion procedure to the client. The client says to the nurse, "I'm not sure I can take any more of this treatment." The nurse makes which response to the client?

1 "Let's just put the tube down so that you can get well."

2 "It is your right to refuse any treatment. I'll notify the physician."

3 "If you don't have this tube put down, you will just continue to vomit."

4 "You are feeling tired and frustrated with your recovery from surgery?"

Level of Cognitive Ability: Application
Client Needs: Psychosocial Integrity
Integrated Process: Communication and Documentation
Content Area: Adult Health/Gastrointestinal

Answer: 4
Rationale: In option 4, the nurse uses empathy. Empathy, comprehending, and sharing a client's frame of reference are important components of the nurse–client relationship. They assist clients with expressing and exploring feelings, which can lead to problem solving. The other options are examples of barriers to effective communication, including stereotyping (option 1), defensiveness (option 2), and showing disapproval (option 3).

Test-Taking Strategy: Use therapeutic communication techniques. Option 4 is an open-ended question and a communication tool; it also focuses on the client's feelings. Review therapeutic communication techniques if you had difficulty with this question.

References
Ignatavicius, D., & Workman, M. (2006). *Medical-surgical nursing: Critical thinking for collaborative care* (5th ed., p. 1327). Philadelphia: Saunders.
Potter, P., & Perry, A. (2005). *Fundamentals of nursing* (6th ed., p. 437). St. Louis: Mosby.

1150. A client is admitted to the hospital with a bowel obstruction as a result of a recurrent malignancy, and the physician inserts a Miller-Abbott tube. After the procedure, the client asks the nurse, "Do you think this is worth all this trouble?" What is the appropriate action or response by the nurse?

1 "Let's give this tube a chance."

2 To stay with the client and be silent

3 "Are you wondering whether you are going to get better?"

4 "I remember a case similar to yours, and the tube relieved the obstruction."

Level of Cognitive Ability: Application
Client Needs: Psychosocial Integrity
Integrated Process: Communication and Documentation
Content Area: Adult Health/Oncology

Answer: 3
Rationale: The nurse uses therapeutic communication tools to assist a client with a chronic terminal illness to express feelings. The nurse listens attentively to the client and uses clarifying and focusing to assist the client with expressing feelings. Changing the subject (option 1), responding with inappropriate silence (option 2), and offering false reassurance (option 4) are not therapeutic communication techniques.

Test-Taking Strategy: Use therapeutic communications techniques. Option 3 encourages the client to verbalize. Review therapeutic communication techniques if you had difficulty with this question.

References
Ignatavicius, D., & Workman, M. (2006). *Medical-surgical nursing: Critical thinking for collaborative care* (5th ed., p. 1329). Philadelphia: Saunders.
Potter, P., & Perry, A. (2005). *Fundamentals of nursing* (6th ed., p. 437). St. Louis: Mosby.

1151. A client who is receiving parenteral nutrition (PN) tells the nurse, "I'm not sure that I want to receive an infusion of intralipids because it could make me obese." Which of the following should the nurse include in the initial response to the client?

1 Inquire how illness affects the client's self-concept.
2 Ask the provider to discuss the benefits of intralipids.
3 State that intralipids supply essential fatty acids for life.
4 Explain how intralipids replace dietary sources of lipids.

Level of Cognitive Ability: Analysis
Client Needs: Psychosocial Integrity
Integrated Process: Communication and Documentation
Content Area: Fundamental Skills

Answer: 1
Rationale: A client who receives PN is at risk for developing an essential fatty acid deficiency; however, this client's comment requires more than a simple informational response initially. Thus, the nurse responds with option 1 to assist the client with self-expression and to deal with aspects of illness and treatment. Option 2 delays client self-expression and devalues the client's feelings. Options 3 and 4 provide information only.

Test-Taking Strategy: Note the strategic words "initial response." This should cue you to use therapeutic communication techniques to focus on the client's feelings, because, before the nurse can provide comprehensive information, the client's feelings must be assessed, and the nurse adapts the information accordingly. Option 1 is the only option that addresses the client's feelings. Review therapeutic communication techniques if you had difficulty with this question.

References
Ignatavicius, D., & Workman, M. (2006). *Medical-surgical nursing: Critical thinking for collaborative care* (5th ed., pp. 1430-1431). Philadelphia: Saunders.
Potter, P., & Perry, A. (2005). *Fundamentals of nursing* (6th ed., p. 437). St. Louis: Mosby.

1152. A client has terminal cancer and is using opioid analgesics for pain relief. The client is concerned about becoming addicted to the pain medication. The home-care nurse allays the client's anxiety by:

1 Encouraging the client to hold off as long as possible between doses of pain medication
2 Telling the client to take lower doses of medications even though the pain is not well controlled
3 Explaining to the client that the fears are justified but should be of no concern during the final stages of care
4 Explaining to the client that addiction rarely occurs in individuals who are taking medication to relieve pain

Level of Cognitive Ability: Application
Client Needs: Psychosocial Integrity
Integrated Process: Caring
Content Area: Adult Health/Oncology

Answer: 4
Rationale: Clients who are on opioid analgesics often have well-founded fears about addiction, even in the face of pain. The nurse has the responsibility to provide correct information about the likelihood of addiction while still maintaining adequate pain control. Addiction is rare for individuals who are taking medication to relieve pain. Allowing the client to be in pain, as in options 1 and 2, is not acceptable nursing practice. Option 3 is only partially correct in that it acknowledges the client's fear.

Test-Taking Strategy: Use the process of elimination. Eliminate options 1 and 2, because these are not acceptable nursing practices. From the remaining options, eliminate option 3, because it is only partially correct. Review pain management if you had difficulty with this question.

Reference
Black, J., & Hawks, J. (2005). *Medical-surgical nursing: Clinical management for positive outcomes* (7th ed., p. 450). Philadelphia: Saunders.

1153. A client is very anxious about receiving chest physical therapy (CPT) for the first time at home. When planning for the client's care, the home-care nurse reassures the client that:

1 There are no risks associated with this procedure.

2 CPT will help the client cough more effectively.

3 CPT will resolve all of the client's respiratory symptoms.

4 CPT will assist with mobilizing secretions to enhance more effective breathing.

Level of Cognitive Ability: Application
Client Needs: Psychosocial Integrity
Integrated Process: Teaching and Learning
Content Area: Adult Health/Respiratory

Answer: 4

Rationale: There are risks associated with CPT, including cardiac, gastrointestinal, neurological, and pulmonary effects. CPT is an intervention to assist with mobilizing and clearing secretions to enhance more effective breathing. It will not resolve all of the client's respiratory symptoms. CPT will assist the client with coughing if the secretions have been mobilized and the cough stimulus is present.

Test-Taking Strategy: Use the process of elimination. Eliminate options 1 and 3 because they contain the close-ended words "no" and "all." From the remaining options, focus on the purpose of CPT, and recall that coughing will be effective after secretions are mobilized. Review the purpose of CPT if you had difficulty with this question.

References

Ignatavicius, D., & Workman, M. (2006). *Medical-surgical nursing: Critical thinking for collaborative care* (5th ed., pp. 634-637). Philadelphia: Saunders.

Lewis, S., Heitkemper, M., Dirksen, S., O'Brien, P., & Bucher, L. (2007). *Medical-surgical nursing: Assessment and management of clinical problems* (7th ed., pp. 646-647). St. Louis: Mosby.

1154. A client with cardiomyopathy stops eating, takes long naps, and turns away from the nurse when the nurse talks to the client. The nurse interprets that this client is most likely experiencing:

1 Depression

2 Intractable pain

3 Noncompliance

4 Activity intolerance

Level of Cognitive Ability: Analysis
Client Needs: Psychosocial Integrity
Integrated Process: Nursing Process/Analysis
Content Area: Adult Health/Cardiovascular

Answer: 1

Rationale: Depression is a common problem related to clients who have long-term and debilitating illnesses. Options 2, 3, and 4 are not related to the symptoms present in the question and therefore are not appropriate interpretations.

Test-Taking Strategy: When a question asks for an interpretation of a client's symptoms, focus on the information in the question. On the basis of the data presented, the only appropriate interpretation is depression. Review the characteristics of depression if you had difficulty with this question.

References

Black, J., & Hawks, J. (2005). *Medical-surgical nursing: Clinical management for positive outcomes* (7th ed., pp. 532, 1607). Philadelphia: Saunders.

Lewis, S., Heitkemper, M., Dirksen, S., O'Brien, P., & Bucher, L. (2007). *Medical-surgical nursing: Assessment and management of clinical problems* (7th ed., p. 814). St. Louis: Mosby.

1155. A nurse is caring for a pregnant client who has been hospitalized for the stabilization of diabetes mellitus. The client tells the nurse that her husband is caring for their 2-year-old daughter. The nurse develops which short-term psychosocial outcome for the client?

1 Be alert to the risks of early labor and birth.

2 Protect the client from injuries that can result from seizures.

3 Teach the client and family about diabetes and its implications.

4 Provide emotional support and education about interrupted family processes related to the pregnant woman's hospitalization.

Level of Cognitive Ability: Analysis
Client Needs: Psychosocial Integrity
Integrated Process: Nursing Process/Planning
Content Area: Maternity/Antepartum

Answer: 4

Rationale: The short-term psychosocial well-being of the family is at risk as a result of the hospitalization of the client. Teaching about diabetes mellitus is a long-term goal related to diabetes. Options 1 and 2 are unrelated to diabetes mellitus and are more related to gestational hypertension.

Test-Taking Strategy: Use the process of elimination. Eliminate options 1 and 2, because they are unrelated to diabetes mellitus. From the remaining options, note the words "short-term psychosocial outcome" and focus on the data in the question to direct you to option 4. Review the outcomes for interrupted family processes if you had difficulty with this question.

Reference
McKinney, E., James, S., Murray, S., & Ashwill, J. (2005). *Maternal-child nursing* (2nd ed., pp. 43, 654). St. Louis: Saunders.

1156. A new mother is trying to decide whether to have her baby boy circumcised. The nurse makes which statement to assist the client with making the decision?

1 "I had my son circumcised, and I am so glad."

2 "Circumcision is a difficult decision, but your physician is the best, and you know it's better to get it done now than later."

3 "You know they say it prevents cancer and sexually transmitted infections, so I would definitely have my son circumcised."

4 "Circumcision is a difficult decision. There are various controversies surrounding circumcision. Here, read this pamphlet that discusses the pros and cons, and we will talk about any questions that you have after you read it."

Level of Cognitive Ability: Application
Client Needs: Psychosocial Integrity
Integrated Process: Communication and Documentation
Content Area: Maternity/Postpartum

Answer: 4

Rationale: Informed decision making is the strategic point when answering this question. The nurse should provide educational materials and answer questions pertaining to the education of the mother. Providing written information to the mother will give her the information she needs to make an educated and informed decision. The nurse's personal thoughts and feelings should not be part of the educational process.

Test-Taking Strategy: Use therapeutic communication techniques and the process of elimination. Options 1, 2, and 3 are communication blocks, because the nurse is providing a personal opinion to the client. Review therapeutic communication techniques if you had difficulty with this question.

Reference
Murray, S., & McKinney, E. (2006). *Foundations of maternal-newborn nursing* (4th ed., pp. 24-25, 526-527). Philadelphia: Saunders.

1157. The nurse is planning care for a client who is experiencing anxiety after a myocardial infarction. Which prioritized nursing intervention should be included in the plan of care?

1 Answer questions with factual information.
2 Provide detailed explanations of all procedures.
3 Limit family involvement during the acute phase.
4 Administer an antianxiety medication to promote relaxation.

Level of Cognitive Ability: Application
Client Needs: Psychosocial Integrity
Integrated Process: Nursing Process/ Implementation
Content Area: Adult Health/Cardiovascular

Answer: 1
Rationale: Accurate information reduces fear, strengthens the nurse–client relationship, and assists the client with dealing realistically with the situation. Providing detailed information may increase the client's anxiety. The client's family may be a source of support for the client. Information should be provided simply and clearly. Medication should not be used unless necessary. Limiting family involvement may or may not be helpful.

Test-Taking Strategy: Note that the client is experiencing anxiety. Eliminate option 2 first because of the word "detailed." Eliminate option 4 next, because medication should not be the first intervention to alleviate anxiety; however, it may be necessary if other strategies are not effective. From the remaining options, eliminate option 3, because limiting family involvement does not reduce anxiety in all situations. Review the measures to reduce anxiety if you had difficulty with this question.

Reference
Black, J., & Hawks, J. (2005). *Medical-surgical nursing: Clinical management for positive outcomes* (7th ed., p. 1723). Philadelphia: Saunders.

1158. A client recovering from an acute myocardial infarction will be discharged in 1 day. Which client action on the evening before discharge suggests that the client is in the denial phase?

1 Requests a sedative for sleep at 10:00 PM
2 Expresses a hesitancy to leave the hospital
3 Consumes 25% of foods and fluids given for supper
4 Walks up and down three flights of stairs unsupervised

Level of Cognitive Ability: Analysis
Client Needs: Psychosocial Integrity
Integrated Process: Nursing Process/Analysis
Content Area: Adult Health/Cardiovascular

Answer: 4
Rationale: Ignoring activity limitations and avoiding lifestyle changes are signs of the denial stage. Walking three flights of stairs should be a supervised activity during this phase of the recovery process. Option 1 is an appropriate client action on the evening before discharge. Option 2 may be a manifestation of anxiety or fear rather than of denial. Option 3 is a manifestation of depression rather than denial.

Test-Taking Strategy: Focus on the strategic word "denial," and use the process of elimination. Option 1 is an appropriate client request. Option 2 identifies anxiety or fear. Option 3 identifies depression. Option 4 is the only option that identifies denial. Review the manifestations associated with denial if you had difficulty with this question.

Reference
Black, J., & Hawks, J. (2005). *Medical-surgical nursing: Clinical management for positive outcomes* (7th ed., pp. 525-526, 1723, 1729). Philadelphia: Saunders.

1159. The nurse is caring for a client with Hodgkin's disease who will be receiving radiation and chemotherapy. Which statement by the client indicates a positive coping mechanism to be used during these treatments?

1 "I won't leave the house bald."
2 "Losing my hair won't bother me."
3 "I will be one of the few who doesn't lose my hair."
4 "I have selected a wig even though I will miss my own hair."

Answer: 4
Rationale: A combination of radiation and chemotherapy often causes alopecia. To make use of positive coping mechanisms, the client must identify personal feelings and positive interventions to deal with side effects. Options 1, 2, and 3 are not positive coping mechanisms.

Test-Taking Strategy: Focus on the subject: a positive coping mechanism. Options 1, 2, and 3 involve avoidance and denial. Option 4 is the only option that addresses a positive coping mechanism. Review coping mechanisms if you had difficulty with this question.

Level of Cognitive Ability: Analysis
Client Needs: Psychosocial Integrity
Integrated Process: Nursing Process/Analysis
Content Area: Adult Health/Oncology

Reference
Black, J., & Hawks, J. (2005). *Medical-surgical nursing: Clinical management for positive outcomes* (7th ed., pp. 391, 2411-2413). Philadelphia: Saunders.

1160. A male client is admitted to the hospital with diabetic ketoacidosis (DKA). The client's daughter says to the nurse, "My mother died last month, and now this. I've been trying to follow all of the instructions from the doctor, but what have I done wrong?" The nurse makes which response to the client's daughter?

1 "Tell me what you think you did wrong."

2 "Maybe we can keep your father in the hospital for a while longer to give you a rest."

3 "You should talk to the social worker about getting you someone at home who is more capable with managing a diabetic's care."

4 "An emotional stress such as your mother's death can trigger DKA in a diabetic client, even though the prescribed regimen is being followed."

Level of Cognitive Ability: Application
Client Needs: Psychosocial Integrity
Integrated Process: Caring
Content Area: Adult Health/Endocrine

Answer: 4

Rationale: Environment, infection, or an emotional stressor can initiate the physiological mechanism of DKA. Options 1 and 3 substantiate the daughters' feelings of guilt and incompetence. Option 2 is not a cost-effective intervention.

Test-Taking Strategy: Use the process of elimination. Eliminate option 2 first, because this option is not cost effective. Options 1 and 3 devalue the client (the daughter) and block therapeutic communication, so they are eliminated next. Review therapeutic communication techniques if you had difficulty with this question.

References
Black, J., & Hawks, J. (2005). *Medical-surgical nursing: Clinical management for positive outcomes* (7th ed., p. 1269). Philadelphia: Saunders.
Potter, P., & Perry, A. (2005). *Fundamentals of nursing* (6th ed., p. 437). St. Louis: Mosby.

1161. A nurse has been working with a victim of rape in an outpatient setting for the past 4 weeks. The nurse identifies which client objective as an unrealistic short-term goal?

1 The client will verbalize feelings about the rape event.

2 The client will resolve feelings of fear and anxiety related to the rape trauma.

3 The client will experience physical healing of the wounds that were incurred during the rape.

4 The client will participate in the treatment plan by following through with treatment options.

Level of Cognitive Ability: Analysis
Client Needs: Psychosocial Integrity
Integrated Process: Nursing Process/Analysis
Content Area: Mental Health

Answer: 2

Rationale: Short-term goals include the beginning stages of dealing with the rape trauma. Clients will initially be expected to keep appointments, participate in care, start to explore feelings, and begin to heal the physical wounds that were inflicted at the time of the rape. The resolution of feelings of anxiety and fear is a long-term goal.

Test-Taking Strategy: Focus on the subject: an unrealistic short-term goal. Use the process of elimination, considering each option and the reality of it being achieved in the short term. Note the word "resolve" in option 2. This word should provide you with the clue that this option is a long-term goal. Review the appropriate goals for the client who is a victim of rape if you had difficulty with this question.

References
Stuart, G., & Laraia, M. (2005). *Principles and practice of psychiatric nursing* (8th ed., p. 235). St. Louis: Mosby.
Varcarolis, E., Carson, V., & Shoemaker, N. (2006). *Foundations of psychiatric mental health nursing* (5th ed., p. 538). Philadelphia: Saunders.

1162. A client is admitted to a surgical unit with a diagnosis of cancer. The client is scheduled for surgery in the morning. When the nurse enters the room and begins the surgical preparation, the client states, "I'm not having surgery. You must have the wrong person! My test results were negative. I'll be going home tomorrow." The nurse recognizes that the ego defense mechanism that may be operating here is:

1 Denial
2 Psychosis
3 Delusions
4 Displacement

Level of Cognitive Ability: Analysis
Client Needs: Psychosocial Integrity
Integrated Process: Nursing Process/Analysis
Content Area: Adult Health/Oncology

Answer: 1

Rationale: By definition, ego defense mechanisms are operations outside of a person's awareness that the ego calls into play to protect against anxiety. Denial is the defense mechanism that blocks out painful or anxiety-inducing events or feelings. In this case, the client cannot deal with the upcoming surgery for cancer and therefore denies the illness. Psychosis and delusions are not defense mechanisms. Displacement is the discharging of pent-up feelings on people who are less dangerous than those who initially aroused the feelings.

Test-Taking Strategy: Focus on the subject: ego defense mechanisms. Options 2 and 3 are eliminated first, because these are not ego defense mechanisms. From the remaining options, focus on the client's statement to direct you to option 1. Review ego defense mechanisms if you had difficulty with this question.

References
Stuart, G., & Laraia, M. (2005). *Principles and practice of psychiatric nursing* (8th ed., pp. 279, 296). St. Louis: Mosby.
Varcarolis, E., Carson, V., & Shoemaker, N. (2006). *Foundations of psychiatric mental health nursing* (5th ed., p. 220). Philadelphia: Saunders.

1163. A community health nurse working in an industrial setting has received a memo indicating that a large number of employees will be laid off during the next 2 weeks. An analysis of previous layoffs suggested that workers experienced role crises, indecision, and depression. Using this data, the nurse should begin to:

1 Help the workers acquire unemployment benefits to avoid a gap in income.
2 Reduce the staff in the occupational health department of the industrial setting.
3 Notify insurance carriers of the upcoming event to assist with potential health care alterations.
4 Identify referral, counseling, and vocational rehabilitative services for the employees being laid off.

Level of Cognitive Ability: Analysis
Client Needs: Psychosocial Integrity
Integrated Process: Nursing Process/Planning
Content Area: Mental Health

Answer: 4

Rationale: In preparation for this crisis, the nurse should identify the services that are available to the employees. These resources will provide immediate avenues for assistance when the layoff occurs. Additional information about the industrial setting is needed to determine whether options 1, 2, and 3 are necessary or possible.

Test-Taking Strategy: Use the steps of the nursing process to direct you to option 4. This option refers to the assessment of resources and services for employees. Review crisis intervention if you had difficulty with this question.

References
Stuart, G., & Laraia, M. (2005). *Principles and practice of psychiatric nursing* (8th ed., pp. 228-229). St. Louis: Mosby.
Varcarolis, E., Carson, V., & Shoemaker, N. (2006). *Foundations of psychiatric mental health nursing* (5th ed., pp. 458-459). Philadelphia: Saunders.

1164. A primigravid client comes to the clinic and has been diagnosed with a urinary tract infection. She has repeatedly verbalized concern regarding the safety of the fetus. Which of the following nursing diagnoses is appropriate at this time?
1 Fear
2 Acute pain
3 Urinary tract infection
4 Impaired tissue integrity

Level of Cognitive Ability: Analysis
Client Needs: Psychosocial Integrity
Integrated Process: Nursing Process/Analysis
Content Area: Maternity/Antepartum

Answer: 1
Rationale: The primary concern of this client is the safety of her fetus rather than of herself. The priority nursing diagnosis at this time is Fear. Option 3 is a medical diagnosis and outside of the scope of nursing practice. Acute pain and Impaired tissue integrity are commonly seen among clients experiencing urinary tract infections, but the question includes no data to support either of these options.

Test-Taking Strategy: Focus on the data in the question, and note the strategic words "verbalized concern." Eliminate option 3, because it is a medical diagnosis. In addition, note that options 2, 3, and 4 are comparable or alike in that they are all physiological. Option 1 addresses the psychosocial issue. Review the defining characteristics of Fear if you had difficulty with this question.

References
Black, J., & Hawks, J. (2005). *Medical-surgical nursing: Clinical management for positive outcomes* (7th ed., p. 278). Philadelphia: Saunders.
Murray, S., & McKinney, E. (2006). *Foundations of maternal-newborn nursing* (4th ed., p. 685). Philadelphia: Saunders.

1165. A nurse is planning interventions for counseling a maternal client who has been newly diagnosed with sickle cell anemia. Which of the following would be the most important psychosocial intervention at this time?
1 Provide emotional support.
2 Avoid the topic of the disease at all costs.
3 Allow the client to be alone if she is crying.
4 Provide the client with all of the information regarding the disease.

Level of Cognitive Ability: Application
Client Needs: Psychosocial Integrity
Integrated Process: Caring
Content Area: Maternity/Antepartum

Answer: 1
Rationale: One of the most important nursing roles is providing emotional support to the client and family during the counseling process. Option 4 overwhelms the client with information while she is trying to cope with the news of the disease. Option 3 is only appropriate if the client requests to be alone; if this is not requested, the nurse is abandoning the client in a time of need. Option 2, like option 4, is nontherapeutic.

Test-Taking Strategy: Use the process of elimination. Eliminate options 2 and 4 because of the close-ended words "avoid" and "all." Additionally, these actions are nontherapeutic. From the remaining options, remember that the client's feelings are the priority, and an extremely important role of the nurse is to provide emotional support. Review the interventions related to providing emotional support if you had difficulty with this question.

Reference
Murray, S., & McKinney, E. (2006). *Foundations of maternal-newborn nursing* (4th ed., pp. 678-679). Philadelphia: Saunders.

1166. A neonatal intensive care nurse is caring for a newborn infant immediately after delivery. The infant has a suspected diagnosis of erythroblastosis fetalis. The nurse should make which of the following statements to the parents at this time?

1 "Your infant is very sick. The next 24 hours are the most crucial."

2 "This is a common neonatal problem, so you shouldn't be concerned."

3 "There is no need to worry. We have the most updated equipment in this hospital."

4 "You must have many concerns. Please ask me any questions that you have so that I can explain your infant's care."

Level of Cognitive Ability: Application
Client Needs: Psychosocial Integrity
Integrated Process: Caring
Content Area: Maternity/Postpartum

Answer: 4

Rationale: Parental anxiety is expected in relation to the care of the infant with erythroblastosis fetalis. This anxiety is caused by a lack of knowledge regarding the disease process, treatments, and expected outcomes. Parents need to be encouraged to verbalize concerns and to participate in the care as appropriate. The nurse would not tell the parents to be or to not be concerned. Option 1 will produce anxiety in the parents.

Test-Taking Strategy: Use therapeutic communication techniques. Eliminate options 2 and 3, because they are comparable or alike, and they are blocks to communication. Eliminate option 1, because it will produce anxiety in the parents. Remember to address the clients' feelings and concerns. Option 4 is the only option that encourages communication. Review therapeutic communication techniques if you had difficulty with this question.

References

Hockenberry, M., Wilson, D., & Winkelstein, M. (2005). *Wong's essentials of pediatric nursing* (7th ed., p. 269). St. Louis: Mosby.

Murray, S., & McKinney, F. (2006). *Foundations of maternal-newborn nursing* (4th ed., pp. 24-25). Philadelphia: Saunders.

1167. A school nurse is weighing all of the high school students. One of the teenagers who has type 1 diabetes mellitus has gained 15 pounds during the last year with no gain in height. The nurse also notices this student eating alone in the cafeteria at lunch time and avoiding any interaction with her peers. On the basis of these data, the nurse is most concerned that the student may have:

1 Bulimia nervosa

2 A drug abuse problem

3 Self-destructive thoughts

4 An alcohol abuse problem

Level of Cognitive Ability: Analysis
Client Needs: Psychosocial Integrity
Integrated Process: Nursing Process/Analysis
Content Area: Child Health

Answer: 3

Rationale: Diabetic teenagers are at risk for depression and suicide (self-destructive thoughts), and this is frequently manifested by changing insulin and eating patterns. Social isolation is another indicator. Bulimics may be of normal weight, but they may control weight gain by purging. Alcohol and drug abuse are more likely to be related to weight loss.

Test-Taking Strategy: Focus on the data in the question, and use the process of elimination. Eliminate options 2 and 4 first, because they are comparable or alike. From the remaining options, noting the social isolation issue and the age of the client should direct you to option 3. Review the manifestations associated with depression and self-destructive thoughts if you had difficulty with this question.

References

Black, J., & Hawks, J. (2005). *Medical-surgical nursing: Clinical management for positive outcomes* (7th ed., pp. 532, 534). Philadelphia: Saunders.

Hockenberry, M., & Wilson, D. (2007). *Nursing care of infants and children* (8th ed., pp. 1726-1727). St. Louis: Mosby.

1168. A nurse is planning care for a client with an intrauterine fetal demise. Which of the following is an inappropriate goal for this client?
1 The woman and her family will discuss plans for going home without the infant.
2 The woman and her family will express their grief about the loss of their desired infant.
3 The woman will recognize that thoughts of worthlessness and suicide are normal after a loss.
4 The woman and her family will contact their pastor or grief counselor for support after discharge.

Level of Cognitive Ability: Analysis
Client Needs: Psychosocial Integrity
Integrated Process: Caring
Content Area: Maternity/Postpartum

Answer: 3
Rationale: It is important for the nurse to assess whether the client is undergoing the normal grieving process. Signs that are a cause for concern and that are not part of the normal grieving process include thoughts of worthlessness and suicide. Options 1, 2, and 4 are appropriate goals.

Test-Taking Strategy: Use the process of elimination, and note the strategic words "inappropriate goal." These words should direct you to option 3, because thoughts of worthlessness and suicide are cause for concern. Review the care of the client who has experienced intrauterine fetal demise if you had difficulty with this question.

Reference
Wong, D., Hockenberry, M., Perry, S., Lowdermilk, D., & Wilson, D. (2006). *Maternal-child nursing care* (3rd ed., pp. 679-680). St. Louis: Mosby.

1169. A client with severe preeclampsia is admitted to the hospital. The client is a student at a local college and insists on continuing her studies while in the hospital, despite being instructed to rest. The client studies approximately 10 hours a day and has numerous visits from fellow students, family, and friends. The nurse plans to:
1 Ask her why she is not complying with the order of bedrest.
2 Develop a routine with the client to balance her studies and her rest needs.
3 Include a significant other in helping the client understand the need for bedrest.
4 Instruct the client that the health of the baby is more important than her studies at this time.

Level of Cognitive Ability: Application
Client Needs: Psychosocial Integrity
Integrated Process: Nursing Process/ Implementation
Content Area: Maternity/Antepartum

Answer: 2
Rationale: In options 1 and 4, the nurse is judging the client's choices and asking probing questions; this will cause a breakdown in communication. Option 3 persuades the client's significant other to disagree with the client's actions. This could cause problems with the relationship between the client and the significant other, and it could also cause conflict in the client's communication with the health care workers. Option 2 involves the client in the decision-making process.

Test-Taking Strategy: Use the process of elimination. Eliminate options 1, 3, and 4, because these are blocks to both communication and a therapeutic nurse–client relationship. Option 2 is the most thorough nursing action, because it addresses both rest and studies, and it involves the client in the decision-making process. Review the care of the client with preeclampsia if you had difficulty with this question.

References
Murray, S., & McKinney, E. (2006). *Foundations of maternal-newborn nursing* (4th ed., p. 645). Philadelphia: Saunders.
Potter, P., & Perry, A. (2005). *Fundamentals of nursing* (6th ed., p. 437). St. Louis: Mosby.

1170. A pregnant client is newly diagnosed with gestational diabetes. The client cries when receiving this information and keeps repeating, "What have I done to cause this? If I could only live my life over." Which nursing diagnosis should direct nursing care at this time?

1 Risk for injury to the fetus related to maternal distress

2 Disturbed body image related to complications of pregnancy

3 Situational low self-esteem related to complications of pregnancy

4 Deficient knowledge related to diabetic self-care during pregnancy

Level of Cognitive Ability: Analysis
Client Needs: Psychosocial Integrity
Integrated Process: Nursing Process/Analysis
Content Area: Maternity/Antepartum

Answer: 3
Rationale: The client is putting the blame for the diabetes on herself, thus lowering her self-esteem. She is expressing fear and grief. Deficient knowledge is an important nursing diagnosis for this client, but not at this time, because the client will not be able to comprehend information at this time. There are no data in the question to support the nursing diagnoses in options 1 and 2.

Test-Taking Strategy: Use the data presented in the question to direct you to the correct option. The words "what have I done" should assist you with eliminating options 1, 2, and 4. Review the defining characteristics of the nursing diagnosis of Situational low self-esteem if you had difficulty with this question.

References
McKinney, E., James, S., Murray, S., & Ashwill, J. (2005). *Maternal-child nursing* (2nd ed., p. 647). St. Louis: Saunders.
Murray, S., & McKinney, E. (2006) *Foundations of maternal-newborn nursing* (4th ed., p. 672). Philadelphia: Saunders.

1171. A client says to the nurse, "I'm going to die, and I wish my family would stop hoping for a cure! I get so angry when they carry on like this! After all, I'm the one who's dying." The nurse makes which therapeutic response to the client?

1 "Have you shared your feelings with your family?"

2 "I think we should talk more about your anger at your family."

3 "You're feeling angry that your family continues to hope for you to be cured?"

4 "Well, it sounds like you're being pretty pessimistic. After all, years ago people died of pneumonia."

Level of Cognitive Ability: Application
Client Needs: Psychosocial Integrity
Integrated Process: Caring
Content Area: Mental Health

Answer: 3
Rationale: Reflection is the therapeutic communication technique that redirects the client's feelings back at the client to validate what the client is saying. Option 3 uses the therapeutic technique of reflection. In option 1, the nurse is attempting to assess the client's ability to openly discuss feelings with family members. In option 2, the nurse attempts to use focusing, but the attempt to discuss central issues seems premature. In option 4, the nurse makes a judgment, and this is not therapeutic in the one-to-one relationship. Although this is an appropriate assessment for this client, the timing is somewhat premature, and it closes off the facilitation of the client's feelings.

Test-Taking Strategy: Use therapeutic communication techniques to answer the question. Option 3 is the only option that uses a therapeutic technique. Also, note the word "angry" in the question and in the correct option. Review the technique of reflection if you had difficulty with this question.

Reference
Stuart, G., & Laraia, M. (2005). *Principles and practice of psychiatric nursing* (8th ed., pp. 31-32, 34, 43). St. Louis: Mosby.

1172. The nurse is caring for a client who says, "I don't want to talk with you, because you're only the nurse. I'll wait for my doctor." What should the nurse say in response to the client?

1 "I'm angry with the way you dismissed me."

2 "You would prefer to speak with your doctor?"

3 "I understand. So should I call your doctor?"

4 "Your doctor directs me in your nursing care."

Level of Cognitive Ability: Application
Client Needs: Psychosocial Integrity
Integrated Process: Communication and Documentation
Content Area: Fundamental Skills

Answer: 2

Rationale: The nurse uses techniques of therapeutic communication to reflect the client's statement (option 2), to redirect feelings back to the client for validation, and to focus on the client's desire to talk with the doctor. Option 1 is a nontherapeutic response. Option 3 reinforces the client's behavior. Option 4 is a defensive response, although it does provide information.

Test-Taking Strategy: Use therapeutic communication techniques. Option 2 is the only therapeutic response. Review therapeutic communication techniques if you had difficulty with this question.

Reference
Potter, P., & Perry, A. (2005). *Fundamentals of nursing* (6th ed., p. 437). St. Louis: Mosby.

1173. A client is awaiting surgery for the removal of a pancreatic mass, and she tells the nurse that she is scared that she will not wake up after receiving the anesthesia. The nurse should make which therapeutic response to the client?

1 "This is a very common concern."

2 "Tell me what makes you feel concerned about the anesthesia."

3 "I had surgery a year ago and was afraid of the same thing. I did just fine."

4 "You have the best anesthesiologist in this hospital. There is no need to be scared."

Level of Cognitive Ability: Application
Client Needs: Psychosocial Integrity
Integrated Process: Communication and Documentation
Content Area: Fundamental Skills

Answer: 2

Rationale: This client is concerned about surgery and is expressing fear about the anesthesia. The therapeutic response to the client is the one that encourages the client to express her concerns. Option 1 is a stereotypical response. Option 3 avoids the client's concern and focuses on the nurse's personal experience. Option 4 also avoids the client's concern.

Test-Taking Strategy: Use therapeutic communication techniques, and focus on the client's feelings. The only response that addresses the client's feelings is option 2. Review therapeutic communication techniques if you had difficulty with this question.

References
Potter, P., & Perry, A. (2005). *Fundamentals of nursing* (6th ed., p. 437). St. Louis: Mosby.
Stuart, G., & Laraia, M. (2005). *Principles and practice of psychiatric nursing* (8th ed., pp. 228-229). St. Louis: Mosby.

1174. A community health nurse visits a recently widowed retired military man. He is estranged from his only child because his son was discharged from the service for being "gay." When the nurse visits, the ordinarily immaculate house is in chaos and the client is disheveled and has an alcohol type of odor on his breath. The nurse makes which therapeutic statement to the client?
  1 "I can see this isn't a good time to visit."
  2 "You seem to be having a very troubling time."
  3 "Do you think your wife would want you to behave like this?"
  4 "What are you doing? How much are you drinking and for how long?"

Level of Cognitive Ability: Application
Client Needs: Psychosocial Integrity
Integrated Process: Communication and Documentation
Content Area: Mental Health

Answer: 2
Rationale: The therapeutic statement is the one that helps the client to explore his situation and to express his feelings. Reflection, by telling to the client that the nurse feels that he is experiencing a troubled or difficult time, is empathic, and it will assist the client with beginning to ventilate his feelings. As the client begins to ventilate, the nurse can assist the client with discussing the reasons behind his alienation from his only child. Option 1 uses humor to avoid therapeutic intimacy and effective problem solving. Option 3 uses admonishment and tries to shame the client, which is not therapeutic or professional. This social communication belittles the client, will likely cause anger, and may evoke "acting out" by the client. Option 4 uses social communication.

Test-Taking Strategy: Use therapeutic communication techniques. Remember to focus on the client's behavior and feelings. This will direct you to option 2. Review therapeutic communication techniques if you had difficulty with this question.

Reference
Stuart, G., & Laraia, M. (2005). *Principles and practice of psychiatric nursing* (8th ed., pp. 30-34). St. Louis. Mosby.

1175. A client says to the nurse, "I don't do anything right. I'm such a loser." The nurse makes which therapeutic statement to the client?
  1 "Everything will get better."
  2 "You don't do anything right?"
  3 "You do things right all the time."
  4 "You are not a loser, you are sick."

Level of Cognitive Ability: Application
Client Needs: Psychosocial Integrity
Integrated Process: Communication and Documentation
Content Area: Mental Health

Answer: 2
Rationale: Option 2 provides the client with the opportunity to verbalize. With this statement, the nurse can learn more about what the client really means by the statement. Options 1, 3, and 4 are closed statements and do not encourage the client to explore further.

Test-Taking Strategy: Use the process of elimination and therapeutic communication techniques. Option 2 repeats the client's statement and encourages further communication. Review therapeutic communication techniques if you had difficulty with this question.

Reference
Stuart, G., & Laraia, M. (2005). *Principles and practice of psychiatric nursing* (8th ed., pp. 30-34). St. Louis: Mosby.

1176. A client who is experiencing suicidal thoughts greets the nurse with the following statement, "It just doesn't seem worth it anymore. Why not just end it all?" The nurse would further assess the client by making which of the following responses?
  1 "Did you sleep at all last night?"
  2 "Tell me what you mean by that."
  3 "I know you have had a stressful night."
  4 "I'm sure that your family is worried about you."

Answer: 2
Rationale: Option 2 allows the client the opportunity to tell the nurse more about what his or her current thoughts are. Option 1 changes the subject and may block communication. Although option 3 offers empathy to the client, it does not further assess the client. Option 4 is false reassurance and may block communication.

Level of Cognitive Ability: Application
Client Needs: Psychosocial Integrity
Integrated Process: Communication and
   Documentation
Content Area: Mental Health

Test-Taking Strategy: Note the strategic words "further assess." Use the nursing process and therapeutic communication techniques to select the correct option. Options 3 and 4 can be eliminated first, because they do not reflect assessment. Both options 1 and 2 relate to assessment, but option 2 is directly related to the subject of the question and is the most therapeutic. Review therapeutic communication techniques if you had difficulty with this question.

Reference

Stuart, G., & Laraia, M. (2005). *Principles and practice of psychiatric nursing* (8th ed., pp. 30-34, 111). St. Louis: Mosby.

1177. A mother says to the nurse, "I am afraid that my child might have another febrile seizure." The nurse makes which therapeutic statement to the mother?
   1 "Tell me what frightens you the most about seizures."
   2 "Tylenol can prevent another seizure from occurring."
   3 "Most children will never experience a second seizure."
   4 "Why worry about something that you cannot control?"

Level of Cognitive Ability: Application
Client Needs: Psychosocial Integrity
Integrated Process: Communication and
   Documentation
Content Area: Child Health

Answer: 1
Rationale: Option 1 is the only response that is an open-ended statement and that provides the mother with an opportunity to express her feelings. Options 2 and 3 are incorrect, because the nurse is giving false reassurance that a seizure will not recur or that it can be prevented in this child. Option 4 is incorrect, because it blocks communication by giving a flippant response to an expressed fear.

Test-Taking Strategy: Note the strategic word "therapeutic." Use the process of elimination, and seek the option that is an example of a therapeutic communication technique. Options 2, 3, and 4 violate the principles of therapeutic communication and actually block communication. Review therapeutic communication techniques if you had difficulty with this question.

References

Hockenberry, M., Wilson, D., & Winkelstein, M. (2005). *Wong's essentials of pediatric nursing* (7th ed., pp. 107, 1053). St. Louis: Mosby.
Murray, S., & McKinney, E. (2006). *Foundations of maternal-newborn nursing* (4th ed., pp. 24-25). Philadelphia: Saunders.

1178. A client has just given birth to a newborn who has a cleft lip and palate. When planning to talk to the client, the nurse recognizes that the client needs to work through which emotion before maternal bonding can occur?
   1 Guilt
   2 Grief
   3 Anger
   4 Depression

Level of Cognitive Ability: Analysis
Client Needs: Psychosocial Integrity
Integrated Process: Nursing Process/Planning
Content Area: Maternity/Postpartum

Answer: 2
Rationale: The mother must first be assisted to grieve for the anticipated perfect child that she did not have. After this is accomplished, the mother can begin to focus on bonding with the infant to whom she did give birth. Options 1, 3, and 4 are incorrect, because they are each only one component of the grief process.

Test-Taking Strategy: Use the process of elimination and your knowledge of the grief process. Options 1, 3, and 4 are incorrect, because they are each only one component of the grief process. Review the grief process if you had difficulty with this question.

Reference

Hockenberry, M., Wilson, D., & Winkelstein, M. (2005). *Wong's essentials of pediatric nursing* (7th ed., pp. 691, 876). St. Louis: Mosby.

1179. An infant who has been diagnosed with acute chalasia is admitted to the hospital. During the nursing history, the mother tells the nurse, "I am concerned that I am somehow causing my infant to vomit after feeding her." Considering this statement, which nursing diagnosis is most appropriate?

1 Anxiety related to hospitalization of the infant for chalasia

2 Impaired parenting related to an unrealistic expectation of self

3 Noncompliance related to denial that chalasia is a physiological defect

4 Deficient knowledge related to a lack of exposure to feeding an infant with chalasia

Level of Cognitive Ability: Analysis
Client Needs: Psychosocial Integrity
Integrated Process: Nursing Process/Analysis
Content Area: Child Health

Answer: 2
Rationale: The infant is vomiting because of a physiological problem that is not caused by the parent. The misconception that the mother is responsible for the problem is an unrealistic expectation of self and may result in the mother having a decreased perception of her ability to adequately parent the child. The nurse should assist the mother with understanding that she is not responsible for the child's condition. The mother's statement does not reflect symptoms of Anxiety regarding the child's hospitalization. The mother states a concern regarding her own behavior. There are no data in the question to support that the mother is experiencing denial that chalasia is a physiological defect. Again, there are insufficient data to support that the mother has not been instructed on feeding techniques for a child with chalasia.

Test-Taking Strategy: Use the process of elimination. Note that the mother is blaming herself for the child's health problem. As a result, the mother is at risk for Impaired parenting. Review the defining characteristics of Impaired parenting if you had difficulty with this question.

References
Hockenberry, M., Wilson, D., & Winkelstein, M. (2005). *Wong's essentials of pediatric nursing* (7th ed., pp. 712-713). St. Louis: Mosby.
McKinney, E., James, S., Murray, S., & Ashwill, J. (2005). *Maternal child nursing* (2nd ed., pp. 1096-1097). St. Louis: Saunders.

1180. A client who experienced a myocardial infarction (MI) 4 days ago refuses to dangle at the bedside, saying, "If my doctor tells me to do it, I will. Otherwise, I won't." The nurse determines that the client is likely displaying:

1 Anger
2 Denial
3 Depression
4 Dependency

Level of Cognitive Ability: Analysis
Client Needs: Psychosocial Integrity
Integrated Process: Nursing Process/Assessment
Content Area: Adult Health/Cardiovascular

Answer: 4
Rationale: Clients may experience numerous emotional and behavioral responses after an MI. Dependency is one response that may be manifested by the client's refusal to perform any tasks or activities unless specifically approved by the physician. There are no data in the question to support denial or depression. Although the client's statement may express anger to some degree, it most specifically addresses dependency.

Test-Taking Strategy: Focus on the data in the question to determine the correct option. Begin by eliminating options 2 and 3, because the client is not exhibiting signs of denial or depression. From the remaining options, focus on the client's statement to direct you to option 4. Review the characteristics of dependency if you had difficulty with this question.

References
Black, J., & Hawks, J. (2005). *Medical-surgical nursing: Clinical management for positive outcomes* (7th ed., p. 1701). Philadelphia: Saunders.
Ignatavicius, D., & Workman, M. (2006). *Medical-surgical nursing: Critical thinking for collaborative care* (5th ed., p. 845). Philadelphia: Saunders.

1181. A nurse is assessing a 45-year-old client who was admitted to the hospital for urinary calculi. The client received 4 mg of morphine sulfate approximately 2 hours previously. The client states to the nurse, "I'm scared to death that it'll come back. That was the worst pain I ever had. Like a knife going from my right side to my groin." Which nursing diagnosis would be appropriate for the nurse to make regarding this statement?

1 Anxiety related to the anticipation of recurrent severe pain
2 Acute pain related to the presence of the calculus in right ureter
3 Urinary retention related to the obstruction of the urinary tract by calculi
4 Deficient knowledge related to a lack of information about the disease process

Level of Cognitive Ability: Analysis
Client Needs: Psychosocial Integrity
Integrated Process: Nursing Process/Analysis
Content Area: Mental Health

Answer: 1
Rationale: The client stated, "I'm scared to death that it'll come back." The anticipation of the recurring pain produces Anxiety and threatens the client's psychological integrity. There is no evidence that the client has a calculus in the right ureter. There is also no evidence that either Urinary retention or Deficient knowledge exists.

Test-Taking Strategy: Use the data presented in the question to assist you with answering the question. Note the strategic words "I'm scared to death that it'll come back," and notice the relationship of these words to option 1. Review the defining characteristics of Anxiety if you had difficulty with this question.

References
Stuart, G., & Laraia, M. (2005). *Principles and practice of psychiatric nursing* (8th ed., pp. 260, 267). St. Louis: Mosby.
Varcarolis, E., Carson, V., & Shoemaker, N. (2006). *Foundations of psychiatric mental health nursing* (5th ed., pp. 238-239). Philadelphia: Saunders.

1182. A nurse is observing the parents at the bedside of their small for gestational age (SGA) female infant, who was born at 27 weeks' gestation. The infant's mother states, "She is so tiny and fragile. I'll never be able to hold her with all those tubes." The nurse interprets the mother's statement to indicate which of the following nursing diagnoses?

1 Impaired adjustment
2 Risk for impaired parenting
3 Compromised family coping
4 Risk for caregiver role strain

Level of Cognitive Ability: Analysis
Client Needs: Psychosocial Integrity
Integrated Process: Nursing Process/Analysis
Content Area: Maternity/Postpartum

Answer: 2
Rationale: One of the nursing diagnoses for the parents of a high-risk neonate, such as a preterm SGA infant, is a Risk for impaired parenting. Parent–infant bonding is affected if the infant does not exhibit normal newborn characteristics. Option 1 involves the nonacceptance of a health status change or an inability to solve a problem or set a goal. Option 3 involves the identification of compromised coping. Option 4 addresses the strain of a caregiver, which, during the initial hospitalization, does not yet apply. At this time, there are inadequate data for these diagnoses, although they may become relevant at a later time.

Test-Taking Strategy: Use the data presented in the question to assist you with answering this question. Eliminate options 1 and 3 first, because these are actual—rather than risk for—nursing diagnoses. From the remaining options, note the strategic words, "I'll never be able to hold her." This should assist with directing you to the strategic words "Impaired parenting" in the correct option. Review the defining characteristics of Impaired parenting if you had difficulty with this question.

References
Hockenberry, M., Wilson, D., & Winkelstein, M. (2005). *Wong's essentials of pediatric nursing* (7th ed., pp. 712-713). St. Louis: Mosby.
McKinney, E., James, S., Murray, S., & Ashwill, J. (2005). *Maternal-child nursing* (2nd ed., pp. 909-910). St. Louis: Saunders.

1183. A client has just delivered a large for gestational age (LGA) infant by the vaginal route. The client verbalizes concern regarding the infant's facial bruising. To enhance attachment, the nurse makes which therapeutic statement?

1 "It is a normal finding in large babies and nothing to be concerned about."
2 "The bruising is caused by polycythemia, which usually leads to jaundice."
3 "The bruising is temporary, and it is important to interact with your infant."
4 "Because the bruising is painful, it is advisable that you not touch the baby's face."

Level of Cognitive Ability: Application
Client Needs: Psychosocial Integrity
Integrated Process: Nursing Process/ Implementation
Content Area: Maternity/Postpartum

Answer: 3
Rationale: The mother of an LGA infant with facial bruising may be reluctant to interact with the infant because of concern about causing additional pain to the infant. The bruising is temporary. Option 4 advises the mother not to touch the baby's face because the bruising is painful, but touch is an important component of the attachment process. Touching the infant gently with the fingertips should be encouraged. The LGA infant may have polycythemia, which can contribute to bruising, but the bruising is not actually caused by the polycythemia. Option 1 does not address the mother's verbalized concerns.

Test-Taking Strategy: Use the process of elimination, and note the subject: to enhance attachment. Eliminate options 1 and 2 first, because they do not specifically address the subject of attachment. From the remaining options, note the relationship of the word "attachment" in the question and the word "interact" in the correct option. Review the interventions that promote mother–infant bonding if you had difficulty with this question.

Reference
Murray, S., & McKinney, E. (2006). *Foundations of maternal-newborn nursing* (4th ed., pp. 431, 783). Philadelphia: Saunders.

1184. A client with myasthenia gravis is ready to return home. The client confides that she is concerned that her husband will no longer find her physically attractive. What should the nurse include in the plan of care?

1 Encourage the client to start a support group.
2 Tell the client to stop dwelling on the negative.
3 Insist that the client reach out and face this fear.
4 Encourage the client to share her feelings with her husband.

Level of Cognitive Ability: Application
Client Needs: Psychosocial Integrity
Integrated Process: Caring
Content Area: Adult Health/Neurological

Answer: 4
Rationale: Talking to the client about sharing her feelings with her husband directly addresses the subject of the question. Encouraging the client to start a support group will not address the client's immediate and individual concerns. Options 2 and 3 are blocks to communication and avoid the client's concern.

Test-Taking Strategy: Focus on the subject of the question, and use therapeutic communication techniques. Option 4 is the only option that addresses the client's immediate concern. Remember to address the client's feelings and concerns first. Review therapeutic communication techniques if you had difficulty with this question.

References
Black, J., & Hawks, J. (2005). *Medical-surgical nursing: Clinical management for positive outcomes* (7th ed., p. 2183). Philadelphia: Saunders.
Potter, P., & Perry, A. (2005). *Fundamentals of nursing* (6th ed., p. 437). St. Louis: Mosby.

1185. A 9-year-old child is hospitalized for 2 months after a car accident. The best way to promote the psychosocial development of this child is to plan for:

1 A phone for calling family and friends
2 Tutoring to keep the child up with schoolwork
3 A portable radio and a tape player with headphones
4 Computer games, a television, and videos at the bedside

Level of Cognitive Ability: Application
Client Needs: Psychosocial Integrity
Integrated Process: Nursing Process/Planning
Content Area: Child Health

Answer: 2
Rationale: The developmental task of the school-age child is industry versus inferiority. The child achieves success by mastering skills and knowledge. Maintaining school work provides for accomplishment and prevents feelings of inferiority that may be caused by lagging behind the rest of the class. The other options provide diversion and are of lesser importance for a child of this age.

Test-Taking Strategy: Note the strategic words "psychosocial development" in the query of the question. Note the age of the child, and determine the developmental task for this child. Options 1, 3, and 4 address social and diversional issues, whereas option 2 specifically addresses psychosocial development. Review the growth and development of the school-age child if you had difficulty with this question.

References
Hockenberry, M., Wilson, D., & Winkelstein, M. (2005). *Wong's essentials of pediatric nursing* (7th ed., pp. 482-483, 697). St. Louis: Mosby.
McKinney, E., James, S., Murray, S., & Ashwill, J. (2005). *Maternal-child nursing* (2nd ed., p. 894). St. Louis: Saunders.

1186. A client who is in halo traction says to the visiting nurse, "I can't get used to this contraption. I can't see properly on the side, and I keep misjudging where everything is." The nurse makes which therapeutic response to the client?

1 "If I were you, I would have had the surgery rather than suffer like this."
2 "No one ever gets used to that thing! It's horrible. Many of our sports people who are in it complain vigorously."
3 "Halo traction involves many difficult adjustments. Practice scanning with your eyes after standing up and before you move around."
4 "Why do you feel like this when you could have died from a broken neck? This is the way it is for several months. You need be more accepting, don't you think?"

Level of Cognitive Ability: Application
Client Needs: Psychosocial Integrity
Integrated Process: Nursing Process/ Implementation
Content Area: Adult Health/Neurological

Answer: 3
Rationale: In option 3, the nurse employs empathy and reflection. The nurse then offers a strategy for problem solving, which helps to increase the peripheral vision of the client in halo traction. In option 1, the nurse undermines the client's faith in the medical treatment being employed by giving advice that is insensitive and unprofessional. In option 2, the nurse provides a social response that contains emotionally charged language that could increase the client's anxiety. In option 4, the nurse uses excessive questioning and gives advice, which is nontherapeutic.

Test-Taking Strategy: Use the process of elimination, and seek the option that represents a therapeutic communication technique. Focus on the client's statement, and note that option 3 is the only statement that addresses the client's concern. Review therapeutic communication techniques if you had difficulty with this question.

References
Ignatavicius, D., & Workman, M. (2006). *Medical-surgical nursing: Critical thinking for collaborative care* (5th ed., pp. 989-990). Philadelphia: Saunders.
Potter, P., & Perry, A. (2005). *Fundamentals of nursing* (6th ed., p. 437). St. Louis: Mosby.

1187. An older client has been admitted to the hospital with a hip fracture. The nurse prepares a plan of care for the client and identifies desired outcomes related to surgery and impaired physical mobility. Which statement by the client supports a positive adjustment to the surgery and impairment in mobility?

1 "Hurry up and go away. I want to be alone."

2 "What took you so long? I called for you 30 minutes ago."

3 "I wish you nurses would leave me alone! You are all telling me what to do!"

4 "I find it difficult to concentrate since the doctor talked with me about the surgery tomorrow."

Level of Cognitive Ability: Analysis
Client Needs: Psychosocial Integrity
Integrated Process: Nursing Process/Evaluation
Content Area: Adult Health/Musculoskeletal

Answer: 4
Rationale: Option 1 demonstrates withdrawal behavior. Option 2 is a demanding response. Option 3 demonstrates acting out by the client. Demanding, acting out, and withdrawn clients have not coped with or adjusted to the injury or disease. Option 4 reflects an individual with moderate anxiety caused by a difficulty to concentrate. It most appropriately supports a positive adjustment.

Test-Taking Strategy: Focus on the subject of "positive adjustment," and use the process of elimination. You should easily be able to eliminate options 1, 2, and 3. Remember that age and impaired mobility in combination with medications often contribute to anxiety and difficulty concentrating. Review the psychosocial issues related to an older client with a hip fracture if you had difficulty with this question.

Reference
Black, J., & Hawks, J. (2005). *Medical-surgical nursing: Clinical management for positive outcomes* (7th ed., pp. 641, 645). Philadelphia: Saunders.

1188. A client who is quadriplegic frequently makes lewd sexual suggestions and uses profanity. The nurse interprets that the client is inappropriately using the defense mechanism of displacement and determines that the appropriate nursing diagnosis for this client is:

1 Ineffective coping

2 Disturbed body image

3 Risk for disuse syndrome

4 Impaired environmental interpretation syndrome

Level of Cognitive Ability: Analysis
Client Needs: Psychosocial Integrity
Integrated Process: Nursing Process/Analysis
Content Area: Mental Health

Answer: 1
Rationale: The definition of Ineffective coping is the "state in which an individual demonstrates impaired adaptive behaviors and problem-solving abilities in meeting life's demands and roles." This nursing diagnosis clearly applies in this situation, because the client is displacing feelings onto the environment instead of using them in a constructive fashion. Option 2 may be appropriate, but it has nothing to do with the displacement that the client is currently using. Options 3 and 4 have no relation to this situation.

Test-Taking Strategy: Focus on the data in the question to identify the correct option. Note that the question addresses the defense mechanism of displacement. Remember that the use of displacement indicates ineffective coping abilities. This will direct you to option 1. Review displacement if you had difficulty with this question.

References
Lewis, S., Heitkemper, M., Dirksen, S., O'Brien, P., & Bucher, L. (2007). *Medical-surgical nursing: Assessment and management of clinical problems* (7th ed., p. 121). St. Louis: Mosby.
Stuart, G., & Laraia, M. (2005). *Principles and practice of psychiatric nursing* (8th ed., pp. 296, 314-315). St. Louis: Mosby.

1189. A nurse in the newborn nursery is caring for a premature infant. The best way to assist the parents with developing attachment behaviors is to:
1 Place family pictures within the infant's view.
2 Encourage the parents to touch and speak to their infant.
3 Report only positive qualities and progress to the parents.
4 Provide information regarding infant development and stimulation.

Level of Cognitive Ability: Application
Client Needs: Psychosocial Integrity
Integrated Process: Nursing Process/
   Implementation
Content Area: Maternity/Postpartum

Answer: 2
Rationale: Parents' involvement through touch and voice establishes and initiates the bonding process in the parent–infant relationship. Their active participation builds their confidence and supports the parenting role. Providing information and emphasizing only positives are not incorrect actions, but they do not relate to the attachment process. Family pictures are ineffective for an infant.

Test-Taking Strategy: Use the process of elimination, and focus on the subject: attachment behaviors. The only option that addresses attachment behaviors is option 2. Review the measures that promote parent–infant bonding if you had difficulty with this question.

Reference
Murray, S., & McKinney, E. (2006). *Foundations of maternal-newborn nursing* (4th ed., p. 785). Philadelphia: Saunders.

1190. A 16-year-old child is admitted to the hospital with hyperglycemia as a result of a failure to follow the diet, insulin, and glucose monitoring regimen. The child states, "I'm fed up with having my life ruled by doctors' orders and machines!" Which of the following is a priority nursing diagnosis?
1 Interrupted family processes related to chronic illness
2 Disturbed thought processes related to a personal crisis
3 Imbalanced nutrition that is greater than body requirements related to high blood glucose
4 Ineffective health maintenance of the therapeutic regimen related to feelings of loss of control

Level of Cognitive Ability: Analysis
Client Needs: Psychosocial Integrity
Integrated Process: Nursing Process/Analysis
Content Area: Child Health

Answer: 4
Rationale: Adolescents strive for identity and independence, and the situation describes a common fear of loss of control. The correct nursing diagnosis relates to the subjects of the question, which are not following the prescribed regimen and the feelings of powerlessness. There is no indication of Interrupted family processes or Disturbed thought processes in the question. Imbalanced nutrition is inaccurate and limited.

Test-Taking Strategy: Focus on the information in the question. Eliminate options 1 and 3, because there are no data to support these nursing diagnoses. Eliminate option 2, because, although the client may be experiencing a personal crisis, there is no evidence of Disturbed thought processes. Review the defining characteristics of Ineffective health maintenance if you had difficulty with this question.

References
Hockenberry, M., Wilson, D., & Winkelstein, M. (2005). *Wong's essentials of pediatric nursing* (7th ed., p. 1089). St. Louis: Mosby.
McKinney, E., James, S., Murray, S., & Ashwill, J. (2005). *Maternal-child nursing* (2nd ed., p. 894). St. Louis: Saunders.

1191. A client angrily tells a nurse that the doctor purposefully provided incorrect information. Which of the following responses would hinder therapeutic communication?

1 "I'm certain that the doctor would not lie to you."
2 "I'm not sure what information you are referring to."
3 "Can you describe the information that you are referring to?"
4 "Do you think it would be helpful to talk to your doctor about this?"

Level of Cognitive Ability: Application
Client Needs: Psychosocial Integrity
Integrated Process: Communication and Documentation
Content Area: Mental Health

Answer: 1
Rationale: Option 1 hinders communication by disagreeing with the client. This technique could make the client defensive and block further communication. Options 2 and 3 attempt to clarify the information to which the client is referring. Option 4 attempts to explore whether the client is comfortable talking to the doctor about this issue and encourages direct confrontation.

Test-Taking Strategy: Use the process of elimination and therapeutic communication techniques, noting the strategic word "hinder." This word indicates a negative event query and asks you to select an option that is an incorrect response. Disagreeing or challenging a client's response will hinder or block therapeutic communication. Review therapeutic communication techniques if you had difficulty with this question.

Reference
Stuart, G., & Laraia, M. (2005). *Principles and practice of psychiatric nursing* (8th ed., p. 34). St. Louis: Mosby.

1192. A client with a diagnosis of major depression says to the nurse, "I should have died. I've always been a failure." The nurse makes which therapeutic response to the nurse?

1 "I see a lot of positive things in you."
2 "You still have a great deal to live for."
3 "Feeling like a failure is part of your illness."
4 "You've been feeling like a failure for some time now?"

Level of Cognitive Ability: Application
Client Needs: Psychosocial Integrity
Integrated Process: Communication and Documentation
Content Area: Mental Health

Answer: 4
Rationale: Responding to the feelings expressed by a client is an effective therapeutic communication technique. The correct option is an example of the use of restating. Options 1, 2, and 3 block communication, because they minimize the client's experience and do not facilitate the exploration of the client's expressed feelings.

Test-Taking Strategy: Use the techniques that facilitate therapeutic communication to answer this question. Remember to address the client's feelings and concerns. Option 4 is the only option that is stated in the form of a question and that is open-ended, thus encouraging the verbalization of feelings. Review therapeutic communication techniques if you had difficulty with this question.

Reference
Stuart, G., & Laraia, M. (2005). *Principles and practice of psychiatric nursing* (8th ed., pp. 30-34). St. Louis: Mosby.

1193. Two months after a right mastectomy for breast cancer, a client comes to the office for a follow-up appointment. After being diagnosed with cancer in the right breast, the client was told that the risk for cancer in the left breast existed. When asked about her breast self-examination (BSE) practices since the surgery, the client replied, "I don't need to do that anymore." The nurse interprets that this response may indicate:

1 Denial
2 Grief and mourning
3 Change in body image
4 Change in role pattern

Answer: 1
Rationale: The coping strategy of denying or minimizing a health problem can produce health situations that may be life-threatening. Denial can lead to an avoidance of self-care measures, such as taking medications or performing a BSE. Options 2, 3, and 4 are unrelated to the client's statement.

Test-Taking Strategy: Focus on the data in the question. Note the client's statement "I don't need to do that anymore." Eliminate options 2, 3, and 4, because they are not directly related to the client's statement. Review the indicators of denial if you had difficulty with this question.

Level of Cognitive Ability: Analysis
Client Needs: Psychosocial Integrity
Integrated Process: Nursing Process/Analysis
Content Area: Adult Health/Oncology

References
Black, J., & Hawks, J. (2005). *Medical-surgical nursing: Clinical management for positive outcomes* (7th ed., pp. 525-526). Philadelphia: Saunders.
Ignatavicius, D., & Workman, M. (2006). *Medical-surgical nursing: Critical thinking for collaborative care* (5th ed., pp. 1807-1808). Philadelphia: Saunders.

1194. When planning for the care of the client who is dying of cancer, one of the goals is that the client verbalize his or her acceptance of impending death. Which client statement indicates to the nurse that this goal has been reached?
1 "I just want to live until my 100th birthday."
2 "I would like to have my family here when I die."
3 "I'll be ready to die when my children finish school."
4 "I want to go to my daughter's wedding. Then I'll be ready to die."

Level of Cognitive Ability: Analysis
Client Needs: Psychosocial Integrity
Integrated Process: Nursing Process/Evaluation
Content Area: Adult Health/Oncology

Answer: 2
Rationale: Acceptance is often characterized by plans for death. Often the client wants loved ones nearby. Options 1, 3, and 4 all reflect the bargaining stage of coping during which the client tries to negotiate with his or her higher power or fate.

Test-Taking Strategy: Use the process of elimination. Note that options 1, 3, and 4 are comparable or alike. These options all demonstrate negotiating for something else to happen before death occurs. Option 2 is different, and it is the option that reflects acceptance. Review the stages of death and dying if you had difficulty with this question.

Reference
Black, J., & Hawks, J. (2005). *Medical-surgical nursing: Clinical management for positive outcomes* (7th ed., p. 500). Philadelphia: Saunders.

1195. The nurse is caring for a client with cancer who has a nursing diagnosis of Disturbed body image related to alopecia. The nurse plans to teach the client about which of the following that is related to this nursing diagnosis?
1 The importance of rinsing the mouth after eating
2 The use of cosmetics to hide drug-induced rashes
3 The use of wigs, which are often covered by insurance
4 Proper dental hygiene with the use of a foam toothbrush

Level of Cognitive Ability: Application
Client Needs: Psychosocial Integrity
Integrated Process: Nursing Process/ Implementation
Content Area: Adult Health/Oncology

Answer: 3
Rationale: The temporary or permanent thinning or loss of hair, known as alopecia, is common among clients with cancer who are receiving chemotherapy. This often causes a body image disturbance that can be easily addressed with the use of wigs, hats, or scarves. Options 1, 2, and 4 are all unrelated to alopecia.

Test-Taking Strategy: Focus on the definition of alopecia. Recalling that alopecia refers to hair loss will direct you to option 3. Review the interventions used to treat alopecia if you had difficulty with this question.

References
Black, J., & Hawks, J. (2005). *Medical-surgical nursing: Clinical management for positive outcomes* (7th ed., p. 386). Philadelphia: Saunders.
Ignatavicius, D., & Workman, M. (2006). *Medical-surgical nursing: Critical thinking for collaborative care* (5th ed., pp. 494-495). Philadelphia: Saunders.
Lewis, S., Heitkemper, M., Dirksen, S., O'Brien, P., & Bucher, L. (2007). *Medical-surgical nursing: Assessment and management of clinical problems* (7th ed., p. 1580). St. Louis: Mosby.

1196. A client with hyperaldosteronism has developed renal failure and says to the nurse, "This means that I will die very soon." The nurse makes which appropriate response to the client?

1 "You will do just fine."
2 "What are you thinking about?"
3 "You sound discouraged today."
4 "I read that death is a beautiful experience."

Level of Cognitive Ability: Application
Client Needs: Psychosocial Integrity
Integrated Process: Communication and Documentation
Content Area: Adult Health/Endocrine

Answer: 3
Rationale: Option 3 uses the therapeutic communication technique of reflection, and it both clarifies and encourages the further expression of the client's feelings. Options 1 and 4 deny the client's concerns and provide false reassurance. Option 2 requests an explanation and does not encourage the expression of feelings.

Test-Taking Strategy: Use therapeutic communication techniques. Note that option 3 facilitates the client's expression of feelings. Remember to focus on the client's feelings. Review therapeutic communication techniques if you had difficulty with this question.

References
Ignatavicius, D., & Workman, M. (2006). *Medical-surgical nursing: Critical thinking for collaborative care* (5th ed., p. 1741). Philadelphia: Saunders.
Potter, P., & Perry, A. (2005). *Fundamentals of nursing* (6th ed., p. 437). St. Louis: Mosby.

1197. A client with diabetes mellitus has expressed frustration with learning the diabetic regimen and insulin administration. Which of the following is an initial action by the home care nurse?

1 Attempt to identify the cause of the frustration.
2 Call the physician to discuss the termination of home-care services.
3 Offer to administer the insulin on a daily basis until the client is ready to learn.
4 Continue with diabetic teaching, knowing that the client will overcome any frustrations.

Level of Cognitive Ability: Application
Client Needs: Psychosocial Integrity
Integrated Process: Teaching and Learning
Content Area: Adult Health/Endocrine

Answer: 1
Rationale: The home-care nurse must determine what is causing the client's frustration. Continuing to teach may only further block the learning process. Administering the insulin provides only a short-term solution. Terminating the client from home-care services achieves nothing and is considered abandonment unless other follow-up care is arranged.

Test-Taking Strategy: Use the steps of the nursing process. Assessment is the first step. Of the options presented, options 2, 3, and 4 represent implementation phases of the nursing process. The only assessment option is option 1. Review the teaching and learning principles if you had difficulty with this question.

References
Ignatavicius, D., & Workman, M. (2006). *Medical-surgical nursing: Critical thinking for collaborative care* (5th ed., pp. 1546-1549). Philadelphia: Saunders.
Potter, P., & Perry, A. (2005). *Fundamentals of nursing* (6th ed., pp. 451-454). St. Louis: Mosby.

1198. A client with cancer is placed on permanent parenteral nutrition as a means of providing nutrition. The nurse includes psychosocial support when planning care for this client because:

1 Death is imminent.
2 Parenteral nutrition requires disfiguring surgery for permanent port implantation.
3 The client will need to adjust to the idea of living without eating by the usual route.
4 Nausea and vomiting occur regularly with this type of treatment and will prevent the client from participating in social activity.

Level of Cognitive Ability: Application
Client Needs: Psychosocial Integrity
Integrated Process: Nursing Process/Planning
Content Area: Adult Health/Oncology

Answer: 3
Rationale: Permanent parenteral nutrition is indicated for clients who can no longer absorb nutrients via the enteral route. These clients will no longer take nutrition orally. Options 1, 2, and 4 are inaccurate. There is no indication in the question that death is imminent. Permanent port implantation is not disfiguring. Parenteral nutrition does not cause nausea and vomiting.

Test-Taking Strategy: Note the strategic words "permanent" and "as a means of providing nutrition" in the question, and note the relationship between these words and option 3. Option 3 states "living without eating by the usual route." Also, knowledge regarding parenteral nutrition therapy will assist you with eliminating options 1, 2, and 4. Review the care of the client receiving permanent parenteral nutrition if you had difficulty with this question.

References
Black, J., & Hawks, J. (2005). *Medical-surgical nursing: Clinical management for positive outcomes* (7th ed., p. 709). Philadelphia: Saunders.
Lewis, S., Heitkemper, M., Dirksen, S., O'Brien, P., & Bucher, L. (2007). *Medical-surgical nursing: Assessment and management of clinical problems* (7th ed., p. 968). St. Louis: Mosby.

1199. A client who is to be discharged to home with a temporary colostomy says to the nurse, "I know I've changed this thing once, but I just don't know how I'll do it by myself when I'm home alone. Can't I stay here until the doctor puts it back?" The nurse makes which therapeutic response to the client?

1 "This is only temporary, but you need to hire a nurse companion until your surgery."
2 "So you're saying that, although you've practiced changing your colostomy bag once, you don't feel comfortable on your own yet?"
3 "Well, your insurance will not pay for a longer stay just to practice changing your colostomy, so you'll have to fight it out with them."
4 "Going home to care for yourself still feels pretty overwhelming? I will schedule you for home visits until you're feeling more comfortable."

Level of Cognitive Ability: Application
Client Needs: Psychosocial Integrity
Integrated Process: Nursing Process/Implementation
Content Area: Adult Health/Gastrointestinal

Answer: 4
Rationale: The client is expressing feelings of fear and helplessness. Option 4 assists with meeting this client's needs. Option 1 provides information that the client already knows and then problem solves by using a client-centered action, which would probably overwhelm the client. Option 2 is restating, but this response could cause the client to feel more helpless, because the client's fears are reflected back to the client. Option 3 provides what is probably accurate information, but the words "just to practice" can be interpreted by the client as belittling.

Test-Taking Strategy: Use therapeutic communication techniques, and focus on the subject of the question: fear and helplessness. This will eliminate options 1 and 3. From the remaining options, remember the subject of the question, and address the client's feelings and concerns. Option 2 is restating, but this intervention could cause the client to feel more helpless. Option 4 addresses the client's fear and dependency (helplessness) needs. Review therapeutic communication techniques if you had difficulty with this question.

References
Ignatavicius, D., & Workman, M. (2006). *Medical-surgical nursing: Critical thinking for collaborative care* (5th ed., pp. 1325-1326). Philadelphia: Saunders.
Lewis, S., Heitkemper, M., Dirksen, S., O'Brien, P., & Bucher, L. (2007). *Medical-surgical nursing: Assessment and management of clinical problems* (7th ed., p. 1075). St. Louis: Mosby.
Potter, P., & Perry, A. (2005). *Fundamentals of nursing* (6th ed., p. 437). St. Louis: Mosby.

1200. The parents of a newborn infant with congenital hypothyroidism and Down syndrome tell the nurse how sad they are that their child was born with these problems. They had many plans for a normal child, and now these will need to be adjusted. On the basis of these statements, the nurse plans to address which nursing diagnosis?
1 Impaired adjustment
2 Anticipatory grieving
3 Dysfunctional grieving
4 Disabled family coping

Level of Cognitive Ability: Analysis
Client Needs: Psychosocial Integrity
Integrated Process: Nursing Process/Analysis
Content Area: Maternity/Postpartum

Answer: 2
Rationale: Anticipatory grieving involves the intellectual and emotional responses and behaviors by which individuals and families work through the process of modifying their self-concepts on the basis of the perception of potential loss. Defining characteristics include expressions of sorrow and distress at the potential loss. Dysfunctional grieving and Impaired adjustment are abnormal responses to changes in health status. The nursing diagnosis of Disabled family coping is used when a usually supportive person is providing insufficient, ineffective, or compromised support, comfort, assistance, or encouragement.

Test-Taking Strategy: Focus on the data in the question. Noting the strategic words "how sad they are" should lead you to one of the options related to grieving. Recalling the defining characteristics of Anticipatory grieving will direct you to this option. Review Anticipatory grieving and Dysfunctional grieving if you had difficulty with this question.

References
Hockenberry, M., Wilson, D., & Winkelstein, M. (2005). *Wong's essentials of pediatric nursing* (7th ed., p. 939). St. Louis: Mosby.
McKinney, E., James, S., Murray, S., & Ashwill, J. (2005). *Maternal-child nursing* (2nd ed., pp. 607-608). St. Louis: Saunders.

1201. A nurse is caring for a client who has been diagnosed with schizophrenia. The client is unable to speak, although there is no known pathological dysfunction. The nurse documents that the client is experiencing:
1 Mutism
2 Verbigeration
3 Pressured speech
4 Poverty of speech

Level of Cognitive Ability: Analysis
Client Needs: Psychosocial Integrity
Integrated Process: Communication and Documentation
Content Area: Mental Health

Answer: 1
Rationale: Mutism is the absence of verbal speech. The client does not communicate verbally despite an intact physical and structural ability to speak. Verbigeration is the purposeless repetition of words or phrases. Poverty of speech involves diminished amounts of speech or monotonic replies. Pressured speech refers to a rapidity of speech that reflects the client's racing thoughts.

Test-Taking Strategy: Use the process of elimination, and focus on the subject: an inability to speak. This should assist you with eliminating options 2 and 3. From the remaining options, recalling that poverty of speech indicates a diminished amount of speech will assist you with eliminating option 4. Review altered thought and speech patterns if you had difficulty with this question.

Reference
Varcarolis, E., Carson, V., & Shoemaker, N. (2006). *Foundations of psychiatric mental health nursing* (5th ed., p. 397). Philadelphia: Saunders.

1202. A client tells the nurse, "I am a spy for the FBI. I am an eye, an eye in the sky." The nurse recognizes that this is an example of:

1 Echolalia
2 Word salad
3 Clang associations
4 Loosened associations

Level of Cognitive Ability: Analysis
Client Needs: Psychosocial Integrity
Integrated Process: Nursing Process/Analysis
Content Area: Mental Health

Answer: 3

Rationale: The repetition of words or phrases that are similar in sound and in no other way (rhyming) is one altered thought and language pattern seen in clients with schizophrenia. Clang associations often take the form of rhyming. Echolalia is the involuntary parrot-like repetition of words spoken by others. Word salad is the use of words with no apparent meaning attached to them or to their relationship to one another. Loosened associations occur when the individual speaks with frequent changes of subject and when the content is only obliquely related.

Test-Taking Strategy: Use the process of elimination, and focus on the client's statement. Recalling that clang associations often take the form of rhyming will direct you to option 3. Review altered thought and language patterns if you had difficulty with this question.

Reference

Varcarolis, E., Carson, V., & Shoemaker, N. (2006). *Foundations of psychiatric mental health nursing* (5th ed., p. 397). Philadelphia: Saunders.

1203. The nurse is planning the hospital discharge of a young client who has been newly diagnosed with type 1 diabetes mellitus. The client tells the nurse that she is concerned about self-administering insulin while in school with other students around. Which statement by the nurse best supports the client's need at this time?

1 "Oh, don't worry about that! You'll do fine!"
2 "You could leave school early and take your insulin at home."
3 "You shouldn't be embarrassed by your diabetes. Lots of people have this disease."
4 "You could contact the school nurse, who could provide a private area for you to administer your insulin."

Level of Cognitive Ability: Application
Client Needs: Psychosocial Integrity
Integrated Process: Nursing Process/ Implementation
Content Area: Child Health

Answer: 4

Rationale: When planning this client's role transition, the nurse functions in the role of a problem solver by assisting the client with adapting to his or her illness. In option 4, the nurse offers information that addresses the client's need and that promotes or assists the client with reaching a decision that optimizes a sense of well-being. Options 1 and 3 are inappropriate statements and are comparable or alike in that they are both blocks to communication. Option 2 requires a change in lifestyle.

Test-Taking Strategy: Use therapeutic communication techniques, and focus on the subject: a concern about self-administering insulin while in school. Eliminate options 1 and 3 first, because they are nontherapeutic. From the remaining options, select option 4, because it promotes the client's ability to continue her present lifestyle, whereas option 2 requires her to change her lifestyle. Review the measures that will assist the client with making a role transition if you had difficulty with this question.

References

Black, J., & Hawks, J. (2005). *Medical-surgical nursing: Clinical management for positive outcomes* (7th ed., p. 1265). Philadelphia: Saunders.
Hockenberry, M., Wilson, D., & Winkelstein, M. (2005). *Wong's essentials of pediatric nursing* (7th ed., p. 1093). St. Louis: Mosby.
Ignatavicius, D., & Workman, M. (2006). *Medical-surgical nursing: Critical thinking for collaborative care* (5th ed., pp. 1547-1548). Philadelphia: Saunders.

1204. The nurse prepares a client for a parathyroidectomy when the client states, "I guess I'll have to wear a scarf after this surgery." Which nursing diagnosis should the nurse use to address this client's need?

1 Risk for anxiety
2 Ineffective denial
3 Ineffective coping
4 Disturbed body image

Level of Cognitive Ability: Application
Client Needs: Psychosocial Integrity
Integrated Process: Nursing Process/Planning
Content Area: Fundamental Skills

Answer: 4

Rationale: The client's statement reflects a psychosocial concern regarding his or her appearance after surgery, so Disturbed body image is the correct option. The remaining options identify unsuitable nursing diagnoses that are not supported by the provided client data.

Test-Taking Strategy: Note that the client is expressing a concern. With that in mind, eliminate option 1, because the client is not demonstrating anxious behavior. Next, option 2 can be eliminated, because denial is a way of avoiding concerns. Eliminate option 3, because the client expresses a realistic method of coping with a surgical scar. Review the psychosocial concerns after parathyroidectomy if you had difficulty with this question.

Reference

Ignatavicius, D., & Workman, M. (2006). *Medical-surgical nursing: Critical thinking for collaborative care* (5th ed., p. 1488). Philadelphia: Saunders.

1205. The husband of a client with Graves' disease expresses concern regarding his wife's health, because, during the past 3 months, she has been experiencing bursts of temper, nervousness, and an inability to concentrate on even trivial tasks. On the basis of this information, which nursing diagnosis would be appropriate for the client?

1 Grieving
2 Social isolation
3 Ineffective coping
4 Disturbed sensory perception

Level of Cognitive Ability: Analysis
Client Needs: Psychosocial Integrity
Integrated Process: Nursing Process/Analysis
Content Area: Adult Health/Endocrine

Answer: 3

Rationale: A client with Graves' disease may become irritable, nervous, or depressed. The signs and symptoms in the question support the nursing diagnosis of Ineffective coping. The information in the question does not support options 1, 2, and 4.

Test-Taking Strategy: Use the process of elimination. Focusing on the data in the question will direct you to option 3. Review the defining characteristics of Ineffective coping if you had difficulty with this question.

Reference

Black, J., & Hawks, J. (2005). *Medical-surgical nursing: Clinical management for positive outcomes* (7th ed., p. 1203). Philadelphia: Saunders.

1206. A client who was admitted to the hospital for the treatment of thyroid storm (hyperthyroidism) is preparing for discharge. The client is anxious about his illness and is, at times, emotionally labile. Which intervention should the nurse include in the discharge plan of care for this client?
1 Avoid teaching the client anything about the disease until he is emotionally stable.
2 Assist the client with identifying coping skills, support systems, and potential stressors.
3 Reassure the client that everything will be fine after he returns to his home environment.
4 Confront the client and explain that he must control his behavior if he wants to go home.

Level of Cognitive Ability: Application
Client Needs: Psychosocial Integrity
Integrated Process: Nursing Process/Planning
Content Area: Adult Health/Endocrine

Answer: 2
Rationale: It is normal for clients who experience thyroid storm (hyperthyroidism) to continue to be anxious and emotionally labile at the time of discharge. The confrontation described in option 4 will only heighten his anxiety. In addition, options 1 and 3 block communication by either avoiding the issue or providing false reassurance. The best intervention is to help the client cope with these changes in behavior and to anticipate potential stressors so that symptoms will not be as severe.

Test-Taking Strategy: Use the process of elimination and therapeutic communication techniques. Eliminate options 1 and 3, because they are blocks to communication. From the remaining options, note the strategic words "anxious about his illness." Eliminate option 4, because it will heighten the client's anxiety. When asked about psychosocial issues, always select the option that addresses the client's feelings and concerns. Review therapeutic communication techniques if you had difficulty with this question.

References
Black, J., & Hawks, J. (2005). *Medical-surgical nursing: Clinical management for positive outcomes* (7th ed., p. 1211). Philadelphia: Saunders.
Lewis, S., Heitkemper, M., Dirksen, S., O'Brien, P., & Bucher, L. (2007). *Medical-surgical nursing: Assessment and management of clinical problems* (7th ed., pp. 1299-1300). St. Louis: Mosby.
Potter, P., & Perry, A. (2005). *Fundamentals of nursing* (6th ed., p. 437). St. Louis: Mosby.

1207. The nurse cares for a client who has been admitted to the hospital for the insertion of a subclavian central venous catheter (CVC). Which psychosocial area should the nurse assess with this client?
1 Ineffective health maintenance
2 Risk for body image disturbance
3 Neck range of motion restrictions
4 Uncontrolled pain related to the CVC

Level of Cognitive Ability: Analysis
Client Needs: Psychosocial Integrity
Integrated Process: Nursing Process/Assessment
Content Area: Fundamental Skills

Answer: 2
Rationale: Psychosocial assessment includes client data related to psychological and social issues. Because the CVC can create socially awkward situations and impair the client's self-concept and body image, the nurse assesses the client for body image disturbance. The client data presented do not support assessing the client for ineffective health maintenance. Although pain and neck range of motion are valid issues for this client, options 3 and 4 are physiological issues.

Test-Taking Strategy: Use the process of elimination, and note the strategic words "psychosocial area." The client data presented do not support ineffective health maintenance. Pain and restricted neck movements are physical concerns. Review the psychosocial effects of a subclavian CVC if you had difficulty with this question.

References
Ignatavicius, D., & Workman, M. (2006). *Medical-surgical nursing: Critical thinking for collaborative care* (5th ed., pp. 907-908). Philadelphia: Saunders.
Perry, A., & Potter, P. (2006). *Clinical nursing skills & techniques* (6th ed., p. 1048). St. Louis: Mosby.
Potter, P., & Perry, A. (2005). *Fundamentals of nursing* (6th ed., pp. 506-507). St. Louis: Mosby.

1208. A 12-year-old child is seen in the health care clinic. During the assessment, which finding would suggest to the nurse that the child is experiencing a disruption in the development of self-concept?
1 The child has many friends.
2 The child has a part-time babysitting job.
3 The child has an intimate relationship with a significant other.
4 The child enjoys playing chess and mastering new skills with this game.

Level of Cognitive Ability: Analysis
Client Needs: Psychosocial Integrity
Integrated Process: Nursing Process/Assessment
Content Area: Child Health

Answer: 3
Rationale: A sense of industry is appropriate for this age group, and it may be exhibited by the child having a part-time job. The increase in self-esteem associated with skill mastery is an important part of development for the school-age child. Friends are also important and appropriate for members of this age group. The formation of an intimate relationship would not be expected until young adulthood.

Test-Taking Strategy: Note the strategic words "disruption in the development of self-concept." Use the process of elimination, and focus on normal growth and development. Noting the age of the child in the question will assist you with eliminating options 1, 2, and 4. Review normal growth and development and the developmental tasks associated with this age group if you had difficulty with this question.

Reference
Hockenberry, M., Wilson, D., & Winkelstein, M. (2005). *Wong's essentials of pediatric nursing* (7th ed., p. 505). St. Louis: Mosby.

1209. A client who has been newly diagnosed with tuberculosis (TB) is hospitalized and will be on respiratory isolation for at least 2 weeks. Which of the following would be appropriate to prevent psychosocial distress in the client?
1 Noting whether the client has visitors
2 Instructing all staff members to not touch the client
3 Giving the client a roommate with TB who persistently tries to talk
4 Removing the calendar and clock in the room so that the client will not obsess about time

Level of Cognitive Ability: Application
Client Needs: Psychosocial Integrity
Integrated Process: Nursing Process/ Implementation
Content Area: Adult Health/Respiratory

Answer: 1
Rationale: The nurse should note whether the client has visitors and social contacts, because the presence of others can offer positive stimulation. Touch may be important to help the client feel socially acceptable. A roommate who insists on talking could create sensory overload. In addition, the client on respiratory isolation should be in a private room. The calendar and clock are needed to promote orientation to time.

Test-Taking Strategy: Note the strategic words "prevent psychosocial distress." Eliminate option 3 first, because the client should be in a private room. From the remaining options, noting that the client will be on respiratory isolation for at least 2 weeks and recalling the basic principles related to sensory overload will direct you to option 1. Review the psychosocial concerns related to isolation if you had difficulty with this question.

References
Ignatavicius, D., & Workman, M. (2006). *Medical-surgical nursing: Critical thinking for collaborative care* (5th ed., p. 644). Philadelphia: Saunders.
Potter, P., & Perry, A. (2005). *Fundamentals of nursing* (6th ed., pp. 797-798). St. Louis: Mosby.

1210. The nurse is interviewing a client with chronic obstructive pulmonary disease (COPD) who has a respiratory rate of 35 breaths per minute and who is experiencing extreme dyspnea. On the basis of the nurse's observations, which nursing diagnosis would be appropriate for the client?

1 Deficient knowledge related to COPD
2 Disturbed body image related to a neurological deficit
3 Impaired verbal communication related to a physical barrier
4 Ineffective coping related to an inability to handle a situational crisis

Level of Cognitive Ability: Analysis
Client Needs: Psychosocial Integrity
Integrated Process: Nursing Process/Analysis
Content Area: Adult Health/Respiratory

Answer: 3
Rationale: A client with COPD may suffer physical or psychological alterations that impair communication. To speak spontaneously and clearly, a person must have an intact respiratory system. Extreme dyspnea is a physical alteration that affects speech. There are no data in the question that support options 1, 2, and 4.

Test-Taking Strategy: Use the process of elimination, and focus on the data in the question. Option 3 clearly addresses the problem that the client is experiencing. Option 1 identifies a medical diagnosis. There is nothing to indicate that the client has a neurological deficit. Option 4 is judgmental and inappropriate. Review the defining characteristics associated with Impaired verbal communication if you had difficulty with this question.

References
Black, J., & Hawks, J. (2005). *Medical-surgical nursing: Clinical management for positive outcomes* (7th ed., pp. 74, 2026). Philadelphia: Saunders.
Ignatavicius, D., & Workman, M. (2006). *Medical-surgical nursing: Critical thinking for collaborative care* (5th ed., p. 654). Philadelphia: Saunders.
Potter, P., & Perry, A. (2005). *Fundamentals of nursing* (6th ed., p. 436). St. Louis: Mosby.

1211. While inebriated, a client received a severe full-thickness burn to his left leg, and he has recently signed an informed consent form for the amputation of the limb. The nurse observes that the client appears withdrawn. Which action should the nurse take at this time?

1 Let the client have some time alone to grieve about the future loss of the limb.
2 Teach the client that the injury was a result of alcohol abuse, and suggest counseling.
3 Inform the physician of the client's behavior, and request medication to assist with coping.
4 Communicate with the client in a manner that reflects back to the client that he appears to be upset.

Level of Cognitive Ability: Application
Client Needs: Psychosocial Integrity
Integrated Process: Nursing Process/ Implementation
Content Area: Mental Health

Answer: 4
Rationale: Reflection statements tend to elicit a deeper awareness of feelings. A well-timed reflection can reveal an emotion that has escaped the client's notice. Additionally, option 4 validates the perception that the client is upset. Option 2 is inappropriate and a block to communication. Options 1 and 3 address interventions before assessing the situation.

Test-Taking Strategy: Use therapeutic communication techniques. Focus on the client's feelings, and select the option that encourages the client to express his feelings and to talk more. This will direct you to option 4. Review therapeutic communication techniques if you had difficulty with this question.

References
Stuart, G., & Laraia, M. (2005). *Principles and practice of psychiatric nursing* (8th ed., pp. 30-32). St. Louis: Mosby.
Varcarolis, E., Carson, V., & Shoemaker, N. (2006). *Foundations of psychiatric mental health nursing* (5th ed., p. 721). Philadelphia: Saunders.

1212. The nurse is caring for a client with left-sided Bell's palsy. Which statement by the client requires further exploration by the nurse?

1 "My left eye is tearing a lot."
2 "I have trouble closing my left eyelid."
3 "I can't taste anything on the left side."
4 "I don't know how I'll live with the effects of this stroke for the rest of my life."

Level of Cognitive Ability: Analysis
Client Needs: Psychosocial Integrity
Integrated Process: Nursing Process/Evaluation
Content Area: Adult Health/Neurological

Answer: 4

Rationale: Bell's palsy is an inflammatory condition that involves the facial nerve (cranial nerve VII). Although it results in facial paralysis, it is not the same as a stroke. Many clients fear that they have had a stroke when the symptoms of Bell's palsy appear, and they commonly believe that the paralysis is permanent. Symptoms resolve, although it may take several weeks. Options 1, 2, and 3 are expected assessment findings of the client with Bell's palsy.

Test-Taking Strategy: Note the strategic words "requires further exploration." These strategic words indicate a negative event query and ask you to select an option that is an incorrect statement. Recalling that this disorder is a temporary condition will direct you to option 4, which identifies an inaccurate understanding of the disorder and thus requires further exploration. Review Bell's palsy if you had difficulty with this question.

References

Black, J., & Hawks, J. (2005). *Medical-surgical nursing: Clinical management for positive outcomes* (7th ed., p. 2154). Philadelphia: Saunders.
Potter, P., & Perry, A. (2005). *Fundamentals of nursing* (6th ed., p. 437). St. Louis: Mosby.

1213. A client who has been newly diagnosed with diabetes mellitus has a nursing diagnosis of Ineffective health maintenance related to anxiety regarding the self-administration of insulin. Initially, the nurse should plan to:

1 Teach a family member to give the client the insulin.
2 Use an orange for the client to inject into until the client is less anxious.
3 Insert the needle, and have the client push in the plunger and remove the needle.
4 Give the injection until the client feels confident enough to do so by himself or herself.

Level of Cognitive Ability: Application
Client Needs: Psychosocial Integrity
Integrated Process: Teaching and Learning
Content Area: Adult Health/Endocrine

Answer: 3

Rationale: Some clients find it difficult to insert a needle into their own skin. For these clients, the nurse might assist by selecting the site and inserting the needle. Then, as a first step in self-injection, the client can push in the plunger and remove the needle. Options 1 and 4 place the client in a dependent role. Option 2 is not realistic, considering the subject of the question.

Test-Taking Strategy: Use the process of elimination, and focus on the subject: anxiety regarding the self-administration of insulin. Eliminate options 1 and 4, because they place the client in a dependent position. From the remaining options, select option 3, because it addresses the subject of self-administration. Review the teaching and learning principles related to an anxious client if you had difficulty with this question.

References

Ignatavicius, D., & Workman, M. (2006). *Medical-surgical nursing: Critical thinking for collaborative care* (5th ed., p. 1509). Philadelphia: Saunders.
Potter, P., & Perry, A. (2005). *Fundamentals of nursing* (6th ed., pp 451-454). St. Louis: Mosby.

1214. A client who is in labor has human immunodeficiency virus (HIV) and says to the nurse, "I know I will have a sick-looking baby." The nurse makes which appropriate response?
1 "You are very sick, but your baby may not be."
2 "All babies are beautiful. I am sure your baby will be, too."
3 "You have concerns about how HIV will affect your baby?"
4 "There is no reason to worry. Our neonatal unit offers the latest treatments available."

Level of Cognitive Ability: Analysis
Client Needs: Psychosocial Integrity
Integrated Process: Communication and Documentation
Content Area: Maternity/Intrapartum

Answer: 3
Rationale: Option 3 is the most therapeutic response, and it will elicit the best information. It addresses the therapeutic communication technique of paraphrasing. Parents need to know that their baby will not look sick from HIV at birth and that there may be a period of uncertainty before it is known whether the baby has acquired the infection. The client should not be told that there is no reason to worry. Options 1 and 2 provide false reassurances. Option 3 is an open-ended response that will provide an opportunity for the client to verbalize her concerns.

Test-Taking Strategy: Use therapeutic communication techniques. Remember to address the client's feelings and concerns. This will direct you to option 3. Review therapeutic communication techniques if you had difficulty with this question.

References
Murray, S., & McKinney, E. (2006). *Foundations of maternal-newborn nursing* (4th ed., pp. 24-25, 688). Philadelphia: Saunders.
Potter, P., & Perry, A. (2005). *Fundamentals of nursing* (6th ed., p. 437). St. Louis: Mosby.

1215. A client who is scheduled for an abdominal peritoneoscopy tells the home-care nurse, "The doctor told me to restrict food and liquids for at least 8 hours before this procedure and to use a Fleet enema 4 hours before entering the hospital. Do people ever get into trouble after this procedure?" The nurse makes which appropriate response to the client?
1 "Any invasive procedure brings risk with it. You need to report any shoulder pain immediately."
2 "You seem to understand the preparation very well. Are you having any concerns about the procedure?"
3 "Trouble? There is never any trouble with this procedure. That's why the surgeon will use local anesthesia."
4 "There are relatively few problems, especially if you are having local anesthesia, but vaginal bleeding should be reported immediately."

Level of Cognitive Ability: Application
Client Needs: Psychosocial Integrity
Integrated Process: Communication and Documentation
Content Area: Adult Health/Gastrointestinal

Answer: 2
Rationale: Abdominal peritoneoscopy is performed to directly visualize the liver, gallbladder, spleen, and stomach after the insufflation of nitrous oxide. During the procedure, a rigid laparoscope is inserted through a small incision in the abdomen. A microscope in the endoscope allows for the visualization of the organs and provides a way to collect a specimen for biopsy or to remove small tumors. The appropriate response is the one that facilitates the expression of the client's feelings. Option 1 may increase the client's anxiety. In option 3, the nurse states that no problems are associated with this procedure; this is close-ended and is incorrect. Although option 4 contains accurate information, the word "immediately" can increase the client's anxiety.

Test-Taking Strategy: Use the process of elimination. Remember to focus on the client's feelings and concerns. Option 2 is the appropriate response, because it provides an opportunity for the client to verbalize concerns. Review therapeutic communication techniques if you had difficulty with this question.

References
Black, J., & Hawks, J. (2005). *Medical-surgical nursing: Clinical management for positive outcomes* (7th ed., pp. 1184-1185). Philadelphia: Saunders.
Potter, P., & Perry, A. (2005). *Fundamentals of nursing* (6th ed., p. 437). St. Louis: Mosby.

1216. A nurse is caring for a client during a precipitate labor. When assessing the client's emotional needs, the nurse can anticipate the client having:
   1 Less pain and anxiety than with a normal labor
   2 A sense of satisfaction regarding her quick labor
   3 A need for support in maintaining a sense of control
   4 Fewer fears regarding the effect of labor on the newborn infant

Level of Cognitive Ability: Analysis
Client Needs: Psychosocial Integrity
Integrated Process: Nursing Process/Assessment
Content Area: Maternity/Intrapartum

Answer: 3
Rationale: The client experiencing a precipitate labor may have more difficulty maintaining control because of the abrupt onset and quick progression of the labor. This may be very different from previous labor experiences; therefore, the client needs support from the nurse to understand and adapt to the rapid progression. The contractions often increase in intensity very quickly, which adds to the client's pain, anxiety, and lack of control. The client may also have an increased amount of concern about the effect of the labor on the newborn infant. A lack of control over the situation in combination with increased pain and anxiety can result in a decreased level of satisfaction with the labor and delivery experience.

Test-Taking Strategy: Use the process of elimination, and focus on the client's condition: a precipitate labor. Note the strategic words "emotional needs" in the question and the strategic words "need for support" in the correct option. Review the care of the client with a precipitate labor if you had difficulty with this question.

Reference
Murray, S., & McKinney, E. (2006). *Foundations of maternal-newborn nursing* (4th ed., p. 706). Philadelphia: Saunders.

1217. A nurse is planning care for a client who presents in active labor with a history of a previous cesarean delivery. The client complains of a "tearing" sensation in the lower abdomen. She is upset, and she expresses concern for the safety of her baby. The nurse makes which response to the client?
   1 "Don't worry, you are in good hands."
   2 "You'll have to talk to your doctor about that."
   3 "I don't have time to answer questions now. We'll talk later."
   4 "I can understand that you are fearful. We are doing everything possible for your baby."

Level of Cognitive Ability: Application
Client Needs: Psychosocial Integrity
Integrated Process: Communication and Documentation
Content Area: Maternity/Intrapartum

Answer: 4
Rationale: Clients have a concern for the safety of their baby during labor and delivery, especially when a problem arises. Empathy and a calm attitude with realistic reassurances are important aspects of client care. Dismissing or ignoring the client's concerns can lead to increased fear and a lack of cooperation. Option 1 uses a cliché and provides false reassurance. Options 2 and 3 place the client's feelings on hold.

Test-Taking Strategy: Use therapeutic communication techniques. Eliminate options 2 and 3, because they place the client's feelings on hold. Next, eliminate option 1, because the client should not be told to not worry. Review therapeutic communication techniques if you had difficulty with this question.

Reference
Murray, S., & McKinney, E. (2006). *Foundations of maternal-newborn nursing* (4th ed., pp. 24-25, 337-338). Philadelphia: Saunders.

1218. A newborn male infant is diagnosed with an undescended testicle (cryptorchidism), and these findings are shared with the parents. The parents ask questions about the condition. The nurse responds, knowing that which of the following could have a psychosocial impact if this condition is not corrected?

1 Atrophy
2 Infertility
3 Malignancy
4 Feminization

Level of Cognitive Ability: Analysis
Client Needs: Psychosocial Integrity
Integrated Process: Nursing Process/Analysis
Content Area: Maternity/Postpartum

Answer: 2

Rationale: Infertility can occur males with this condition, because proper function of the testes in producing fertile sperm depends on a temperature of less than 98.6° F. The psychological effects of an "empty scrotum" could affect the client's perception of self and the ability to reproduce. Options 1 and 3 are possible physical consequences of a failure to treat cryptorchidism rather than psychosocial consequences. Because all of the hormones that are responsible for secondary sex characteristics continue to be secreted directly into the bloodstream, option 4 is not correct.

Test-Taking Strategy: Use the process of elimination. Focusing on the subject of psychosocial impact will assist you with eliminating options 1 and 3. From the remaining options, it is necessary to know that infertility can occur if the condition is not corrected. Review cryptorchidism if you had difficulty with this question.

References

Hockenberry, M., Wilson, D., & Winkelstein, M. (2005). *Wong's essentials of pediatric nursing* (7th ed., p. 486). St. Louis: Mosby.

McKinney, E., James, S., Murray, S., & Ashwill, J. (2005). *Maternal-child nursing* (2nd ed., p. 1169). St. Louis: Saunders.

1219. The mother of an infant with hydrocephalus is concerned about the complication of mental retardation. The mother states to the nurse, "I'm not sure if I can care for my baby at home." The nurse makes which therapeutic response to the mother?

1 "All babies have individual needs."
2 "Mothers instinctively know what is best for their babies."
3 "You have concerns about your baby's condition and care?"
4 "There is no reason to worry. You have a good pediatrician."

Level of Cognitive Ability: Application
Client Needs: Psychosocial Integrity
Integrated Process: Communication and Documentation
Content Area: Maternity/Postpartum

Answer: 3

Rationale: Paraphrasing is restating the mother's message in the nurse's own words. Option 3 demonstrates the therapeutic technique of paraphrasing. In options 2 and 4, the nurse is offering false reassurance, and these types of responses will block communication. In option 1, the nurse is minimizing the social needs involved with the baby's diagnosis, which is harmful for the nurse–parent relationship.

Test-Taking Strategy: Use therapeutic communication techniques and the process of elimination to answer the question. Option 3 is the only therapeutic response, and it demonstrates paraphrasing. This is the only option that will provide the client with an opportunity to verbalize her concerns. Review therapeutic communication techniques if you had difficulty with this question.

References

McKinney, E., James, S., Murray, S., & Ashwill, J. (2005). *Maternal-child nursing* (2nd ed., p. 1507). St. Louis: Saunders.

Murray, S., & McKinney, E. (2006). *Foundations of maternal-newborn nursing* (4th ed., pp. 24-25). Philadelphia: Saunders.

Potter, P., & Perry, A. (2005). *Fundamentals of nursing* (6th ed., p. 437). St. Louis: Mosby.

1220. A preschooler has just been diagnosed with impetigo. The child's mother tells the nurse, "But my children take baths every day." The nurse makes which therapeutic response to the mother?
1 "You are concerned about how your child got impetigo?"
2 "There is no need to worry. We will not tell your day care provider why your child is absent."
3 "Not only do you have to do a better job of keeping your children clean, you must also wash your hands more frequently."
4 "You should have seen the doctor before the wound became infected, and then you would not have had to worry about the child having impetigo."

Level of Cognitive Ability: Application
Client Needs: Psychosocial Integrity
Integrated Process: Communication and Documentation
Content Area: Child Health

Answer: 1
Rationale: By paraphrasing what the parent tells the nurse, the nurse is addressing the parent's thoughts. Option 1 demonstrates the therapeutic technique of paraphrasing. Options 2, 3, and 4 are blocks to communication, because they make the parent feel guilty for the child's illness.

Test-Taking Strategy: Use therapeutic communication techniques and the process of elimination to answer the question. Option 1 is the only therapeutic technique, and it demonstrates paraphrasing. This is the only option that will provide the client with an opportunity to verbalize her concerns. Options 2, 3, and 4 are blocks to communication. Review therapeutic communication techniques if you had difficulty with this question.

References
Hockenberry, M., Wilson, D., & Winkelstein, M. (2005). *Wong's essentials of pediatric nursing* (7th ed., pp. 106, 1107). St. Louis: Mosby.
McKinney, E., James, S., Murray, S., & Ashwill, J. (2005). *Maternal-child nursing* (2nd ed., p. 1365). St. Louis: Saunders.
Murray, S., & McKinney, E. (2006). *Foundations of maternal-newborn nursing* (4th ed., pp. 24-25). Philadelphia: Saunders.
Potter, P., & Perry, A. (2005). *Fundamentals of nursing* (6th ed., p. 437). St. Louis: Mosby.

1221. A nurse is preparing to care for a child from a culture that is different from the nurse's. What is the best way to address the cultural needs of the child and family when the child is admitted to the health care facility?
1 Ask questions, and explain to the family why the questions are being asked.
2 Address only those issues that directly affect the nurse's care of the child.
3 Ignore cultural needs, because they are not important to health care professionals.
4 Explain to the family that, while the child is being treated, they need to discontinue their cultural practices, because they may be harmful to the child.

Level of Cognitive Ability: Application
Client Needs: Psychosocial Integrity
Integrated Process: Caring
Content Area: Child Health

Answer: 1
Rationale: When caring for individuals from a different culture, it is important to ask questions about their specific cultural needs and means of treatment. An understanding of the family's beliefs and health practices is essential to successful interventions for that particular family. Options 2, 3, and 4 ignore the cultural beliefs and values of the client.

Test-Taking Strategy: Use the process of elimination, and focus on the subject: cultural needs. Options 2, 3, and 4 are judgmental. In addition, these options are comparable or alike in that they ignore the cultural practices and values of the client. Review the nursing interventions related to cultural diversity if you had difficulty with this question.

Reference
Hockenberry, M., Wilson, D., & Winkelstein, M. (2005). *Wong's essentials of pediatric nursing* (7th ed., pp. 108-109). St. Louis: Mosby.

1222. A client with a T1 spinal cord injury has just learned that the cord was completely severed. The client says, "I'm no good to anyone. I might as well be dead." The nurse makes which appropriate response to the client?
1 "You're not a useless person at all."
2 "I'll ask the psychologist to see you about this."
3 "You are feeling pretty bad about things right now."
4 "It makes me uncomfortable when you talk this way."

Level of Cognitive Ability: Application
Client Needs: Psychosocial Integrity
Integrated Process: Communication and Documentation
Content Area: Adult Health/Neurological

Answer: 3
Rationale: Restating and reflecting keep the lines of communication open and encourage the client to expand on current feelings of unworthiness and loss that require exploration. The nurse can block communication by showing discomfort and disapproval or by postponing the discussion of issues. Grief is a common reaction to a loss of function. The nurse facilitates grieving through open communication.

Test-Taking Strategy: Use therapeutic communication techniques and the process of elimination. Options 1, 2, and 4 block communication. Option 3 identifies the therapeutic communication technique of restating and reflecting. Review therapeutic communication techniques if you had difficulty with this question.

References
Black, J., & Hawks, J. (2005). *Medical-surgical nursing: Clinical management for positive outcomes* (7th ed., pp. 2224-2231). Philadelphia: Saunders.
Potter, P., & Perry, A. (2005). *Fundamentals of nursing* (6th ed., p. 437). St. Louis: Mosby.

1223. The nurse enters the room of a client who has had a myocardial infarction (MI) and finds the client quietly crying. After determining that there is no physiological reason for the client's distress, the nurse replies:
1 "Do you want me to call your daughter?"
2 "Can you tell me a little about what has you so upset?"
3 "Try not to be so upset. Psychological stress is bad for your heart."
4 "I understand how you feel. I'd cry, too, if I had a major heart attack."

Level of Cognitive Ability: Application
Client Needs: Psychosocial Integrity
Integrated Process: Communication and Documentation
Content Area: Adult Health/Cardiovascular

Answer: 2
Rationale: Clients with MI often have a nursing diagnosis of Anxiety or Fear. The nurse allows the client to express concerns by showing genuine interest and concern and by facilitating communication using therapeutic communication techniques. Option 2 provides the client with an opportunity to express concerns. Options 1, 3, and 4 do not address the client's feelings or promote client verbalization.

Test-Taking Strategy: Use the process of elimination. Select the option that has an exploratory approach, because the question does not identify why the client is upset. This technique helps you eliminate each of the incorrect options. Review therapeutic communication techniques if you had difficulty with this question.

References
Black, J., & Hawks, J. (2005). *Medical-surgical nursing: Clinical management for positive outcomes* (7th ed., p. 1723). Philadelphia: Saunders.
Potter, P. & Perry, A. (2005). *Fundamentals of nursing* (6th ed., p. 437). St. Louis: Mosby.

1224. A client with a recent complete T4 spinal cord transection tells the nurse that he will walk again as soon as the spinal shock resolves. Which of the following will provide the most accurate basis for planning a response to the client?

1 The client is projecting by insisting that walking is the rehabilitation goal.

2 To speed acceptance, the client needs reinforcement that he will not walk again.

3 The client needs to move through the grieving process rapidly to benefit from rehabilitation.

4 Denial can be protective while the client deals with the anxiety created by the new disability.

Level of Cognitive Ability: Analysis
Client Needs: Psychosocial Integrity
Integrated Process: Nursing Process/Planning
Content Area: Adult Health/Neurological

Answer: 4

Rationale: During the adjustment period that occurs the first few weeks after spinal cord injury, clients may use denial as a defense mechanism. Denial may decrease anxiety temporarily, and it is a normal part of grieving. After the spinal shock resolves, the prolonged or excessive use of denial may impair rehabilitation. However, rehabilitation programs include psychological counseling to deal with denial and grief.

Test-Taking Strategy: Use the process of elimination and your knowledge of the physiological effects of a T4 spinal cord injury. The words "walking is the rehabilitation goal," "speed acceptance," and "move through the grieving process rapidly," should be indicators that these are incorrect options. Focus on the client's statement, which is an indication of denial, to direct you to option 4. Review the defining characteristics of denial if you had difficulty with this question.

Reference

Black, J., & Hawks, J. (2005). *Medical-surgical nursing: Clinical management for positive outcomes* (7th ed., pp. 525-526). Philadelphia: Saunders.

1225. A nurse is developing a plan of care for a client scheduled for an above-the-knee leg amputation. The nurse should include which action in the plan when addressing the psychosocial needs of the client?

1 Explain to the client that open grieving is abnormal.

2 Encourage the client to express feelings about body changes.

3 Discourage sharing with others who have had similar experiences.

4 Advise the client to seek psychological treatment after surgery.

Level of Cognitive Ability: Application
Client Needs: Psychosocial Integrity
Integrated Process: Caring
Content Area: Mental Health

Answer: 2

Rationale: Surgical incisions or the loss of a body part can alter a client's body image. The onset of problems coping with these changes may occur during the immediate or extended postoperative stage. Nursing interventions primarily involve providing psychological support. The nurse should encourage the client to express how he or she feels about these postoperative changes that will affect his or her life. Option 1 is an incorrect statement, because open grieving is normal. Option 3 indicates disapproval, and, in option 4, the nurse is giving advice.

Test-Taking Strategy: Use therapeutic communication techniques. Remember to always focus on the client's feelings first. This will direct you to option 2. Review therapeutic communication techniques if you had difficulty with this question.

References

Black, J., & Hawks, J. (2005). *Medical-surgical nursing: Clinical management for positive outcomes* (7th ed., pp. 1430-1431). Philadelphia: Saunders.
Stuart, G., & Laraia, M. (2005). *Principles and practice of psychiatric nursing* (8th ed., pp. 30-34). St. Louis: Mosby.

1226. A client with pulmonary edema exhibits severe anxiety. The nurse is preparing to carry out the medically prescribed orders. Which intervention should the nurse use to meet the needs of the client in a holistic manner?

1 Ask a family member to stay with the client.
2 Give the client the call bell, and encourage its use if the client feels worse.
3 Leave the client alone while gathering required equipment and medications.
4 Stay with the client, and ask another nurse to gather equipment and supplies that are not already in the room.

Level of Cognitive Ability: Application
Client Needs: Psychosocial Integrity
Integrated Process: Nursing Process/
  Implementation
Content Area: Adult Health/Respiratory

Answer: 4
Rationale: Pulmonary edema is accompanied by extreme fear and anxiety. Because the client typically experiences a sense of impending doom, the nurse should remain with the client as much as possible. Options 2 and 3 do not provide for the psychological needs of the client in distress. Family members can emotionally support the client, but they are not able to respond to physiological needs and symptoms. In fact, they are typically in psychological distress themselves.

Test-Taking Strategy: Use the process of elimination. The word "holistic" in the query of the question guides you to consider both the physical and emotional well-being of the client. Option 4 is the only option that addresses both needs. Review the psychosocial aspects of care for the client with pulmonary edema if you had difficulty with this question.

Reference
Black, J., & Hawks, J. (2005). *Medical-surgical nursing: Clinical management for positive outcomes* (7th ed., pp. 1890-1891). Philadelphia: Saunders.

1227. The family of a client with a myocardial infarction complicated by cardiogenic shock is visibly anxious and upset about the client's condition. The nurse plans to do which of the following to provide support to the family?

1 Offer them coffee and other beverages on a regular basis.
2 Insist that they go home to sleep at night to keep up their own strength.
3 Ask the hospital chaplain to sit with them until the client's condition stabilizes.
4 Provide flexibility with visiting times according to the client's condition and family needs.

Level of Cognitive Ability: Application
Client Needs: Psychosocial Integrity
Integrated Process: Caring
Content Area: Adult Health/Cardiovascular

Answer: 4
Rationale: The use of flexible visiting hours meets the needs of both the client and family for reducing the anxiety levels of both. Offering the family beverages does not provide support. Insisting that the family go home is nontherapeutic. Although the chaplain may provide support, it is unrealistic for the chaplain to stay until the client stabilizes.

Test-Taking Strategy: Note the subject: the method of providing support. Options 2 and 3 may or may not be helpful, depending on the client and family situation. Coffee and beverages, while probably helpful to many, do not provide support. Review the measures to provide support to the family of a client with a critical disorder if you had difficulty with this question.

References
Ignatavicius, D., & Workman, M. (2006). *Medical-surgical nursing: Critical thinking for collaborative care* (5th ed., p. 845). Philadelphia: Saunders.
Lewis, S., Heitkemper, M., Dirksen, S., O'Brien, P., & Bucher, L. (2007). *Medical-surgical nursing: Assessment and management of clinical problems* (7th ed., p. 1736). St. Louis: Mosby.

1228. A client with premature ventricular contractions says to the nurse, "I'm so afraid that something bad will happen." Which action by the nurse provides the most immediate help to the client?
1 Telephoning the client's family
2 Using a television to distract the client
3 Having a staff member stay with the client
4 Giving reassurance that nothing will happen to the client

Level of Cognitive Ability: Application
Client Needs: Psychosocial Integrity
Integrated Process: Caring
Content Area: Adult Health/Cardiovascular

Answer: 3
Rationale: When a client experiences fear, the nurse can provide a calm, safe environment by offering appropriate reassurance, using therapeutic touch, and having someone remain with the client as much as possible. Options 1 and 2 do not address the client's fear, and option 4 provides false reassurance.

Test-Taking Strategy: Use the process of elimination. Noting the strategic words "most immediate help" will direct you to option 3. Review the measures to reduce a client's fear if you had difficulty with this question.

References
Black, J., & Hawks, J. (2005). *Medical-surgical nursing: Clinical management for positive outcomes* (7th ed., p. 1668). Philadelphia: Saunders.
Lewis, S., Heitkemper, M., Dirksen, S., O'Brien, P., & Bucher, L. (2007). *Medical-surgical nursing: Assessment and management of clinical problems* (7th ed., p. 346). St. Louis: Mosby.
Potter, P., & Perry, A. (2005). *Fundamentals of nursing* (6th ed., pp. 437, 920-921). St. Louis: Mosby.

1229. A client with Raynaud's disease tells the nurse that he has a stressful job and that he does not handle stressful situations well. The nurse appropriately guides the client to:
1 Change jobs.
2 Seek help from a psychologist.
3 Consider a stress management program.
4 Use earplugs to minimize environmental noise.

Level of Cognitive Ability: Application
Client Needs: Psychosocial Integrity
Integrated Process: Nursing Process/ Implementation
Content Area: Adult Health/Cardiovascular

Answer: 3
Rationale: Stress can trigger the vasospasm that occurs with Raynaud's disease, so referral to a stress management program or the use of biofeedback training may be helpful. Option 1 is unrealistic. Option 2 is not necessarily required at this time. Option 4 does not specifically address the subject.

Test-Taking Strategy: Use the process of elimination, and focus on the subject: stress. Note the relationship between this subject and option 3. Review the measures that reduce stress if you had difficulty with this question.

References
Black, J., & Hawks, J. (2005). *Medical-surgical nursing: Clinical management for positive outcomes* (7th ed., pp. 1533-1534). Philadelphia: Saunders.
Lewis, S., Heitkemper, M., Dirksen, S., O'Brien, P., & Bucher, L. (2007). *Medical-surgical nursing: Assessment and management of clinical problems* (7th ed., p. 122). St. Louis: Mosby.
Potter, P., & Perry, A. (2005). *Fundamentals of nursing* (6th ed., pp. 610-611). St. Louis: Mosby.

1230. A client with a history of pulmonary emboli is scheduled for the insertion of an inferior vena cava filter. The nurse checks on the client 1 hour after the physician has explained the procedure and obtained consent from the client. The client is lying in bed, wringing his hands, and says to the nurse, "I'm not sure about this. What if it doesn't work and I'm just as bad off as before?" The nurse formulates which nursing diagnosis for the client?

1 Anxiety related to the fear of death
2 Ineffective coping related to the treatment regimen
3 Deficient knowledge related to the surgical procedure
4 Fear related to the potential risks and outcomes of surgery

Level of Cognitive Ability: Analysis
Client Needs: Psychosocial Integrity
Integrated Process: Nursing Process/Analysis
Content Area: Adult Health/Respiratory

Answer: 4
Rationale: NANDA International defines Fear as "a feeling of dread related to an identifiable source that the person validates." This client has indicated the surgical procedure and its outcome as the object of fear. Anxiety is present when the client cannot identify the source of the uneasy feelings. Ineffective coping is an appropriate diagnosis when the client is not making needed adaptations to deal with daily life. Deficient knowledge is characterized by a lack of appropriate information.

Test-Taking Strategy: Focus on the data in the question and on the client's statement. Note the relationship of the client's statement and option 4. Review the defining characteristics of Fear if you had difficulty with this question.

References
Black, J., & Hawks, J. (2005). *Medical-surgical nursing: Clinical management for positive outcomes* (7th ed., p. 278). Philadelphia: Saunders.
Potter, P., & Perry, A. (2005). *Fundamentals of nursing* (6th ed., p. 1601). St. Louis: Mosby.

1231. A client has an oral endotracheal tube attached to a mechanical ventilator and is about to begin the weaning process. The nurse determines that which of the following items—which were previously used to minimize the client's anxiety—should now be limited?

1 Radio
2 Television
3 Family visitors
4 Antianxiety medications

Level of Cognitive Ability: Analysis
Client Needs: Psychosocial Integrity
Integrated Process: Nursing Process/Analysis
Content Area: Adult Health/Respiratory

Answer: 4
Rationale: Antianxiety medications and opioid analgesics are used cautiously in the client who is being weaned from a mechanical ventilator. These medications may interfere with the weaning process by suppressing the respiratory drive. The client may exhibit anxiety during the weaning process as well as for a variety of reasons; therefore, distractions such as radio, television, and visitors are still very useful.

Test-Taking Strategy: Note the strategic words "should now be limited." Think about the items that could interfere with the client's strength, endurance, and respiratory drive to maintain independent ventilation. Using this as the guideline, the only possible option is option 4. The side effects of these medications could include sedation, which could interfere with optimal respiratory function. Review the care of the client who is being weaned from a mechanical ventilator if you had difficulty with this question.

References
Black, J., & Hawks, J. (2005). *Medical-surgical nursing: Clinical management for positive outcomes* (7th ed., pp. 1893-1894). Philadelphia: Saunders.
Lewis, S., Heitkemper, M., Dirksen, S., O'Brien, P., & Bucher, L. (2007). *Medical-surgical nursing: Assessment and management of clinical problems* (7th ed., p. 1767). St. Louis: Mosby.

1232. A client scheduled for pulmonary angiography is fearful about the procedure and asks the nurse if the procedure involves significant pain and radiation exposure. The nurse provides a response to the client that provides reassurance on the basis of the understanding that:

1 The procedure is somewhat painful, but there is minimal exposure to radiation.
2 Discomfort may occur with needle insertion, and there is minimal exposure to radiation.
3 There is very mild pain throughout the procedure, and the exposure to radiation is negligible.
4 There is absolutely no pain, although a moderate amount of radiation must be used to get accurate results.

Level of Cognitive Ability: Analysis
Client Needs: Psychosocial Integrity
Integrated Process: Nursing Process/Analysis
Content Area: Adult Health/Respiratory

Answer: 2

Rationale: Pulmonary angiography involves minimal exposure to radiation. The procedure is painless, although the client may feel discomfort with insertion of the needle for the catheter that is used for dye injection. Options 1, 3, and 4 are incorrect.

Test-Taking Strategy: Focus on the diagnostic procedure. Eliminate option 4 because of the close-ended word "no." From the remaining options, recalling that discomfort occurs with needle insertion will direct you to option 2. Review pulmonary angiography if you had difficulty with this question.

References

Black, J., & Hawks, J. (2005). *Medical-surgical nursing: Clinical management for positive outcomes* (7th ed., pp. 102-103). Philadelphia: Saunders.
Chernecky, C., & Berger, B. (2008). *Laboratory tests and diagnostic procedures* (5th ed., pp. 936-937). Philadelphia: Saunders.
Pagana, K., & Pagana, T. (2005). *Mosby's diagnostic and laboratory test reference* (7th ed., p. 772). St. Louis: Mosby.

1233. The nurse is caring for an anxious client who has an open pneumothorax and a sucking chest wound. An occlusive dressing has been applied to the site. Which intervention by the nurse would best relieve the client's anxiety?

1 Staying with the client
2 Distracting the client with television
3 Interpreting the arterial blood gas report
4 Encouraging the client to cough and breathe deeply

Level of Cognitive Ability: Application
Client Needs: Psychosocial Integrity
Integrated Process: Nursing Process/ Implementation
Content Area: Adult Health/Respiratory

Answer: 1

Rationale: Staying with the client has a twofold benefit. First, it relieves the anxiety of the dyspneic client. In addition, the nurse must stay with the client to observe respiratory status after the application of the occlusive dressing. It is possible that the dressing could convert the open pneumothorax to a closed (tension) pneumothorax, which would result in a sudden decline in respiratory status and a mediastinal shift. If this occurs, the nurse is present and able to remove the dressing immediately. Interpreting the arterial blood gas report and promoting coughing and deep breathing have no immediate benefits for the client who is in distress. Option 2 is nontherapeutic.

Test-Taking Strategy: Focus on the subject: relieving the client's anxiety. Eliminate option 2 first, because the client is in distress. From the remaining options, use therapeutic nursing measures to direct you to option 1. Review the measures used to relieve anxiety if you had difficulty with this question.

References

Black, J., & Hawks, J. (2005). *Medical-surgical nursing: Clinical management for positive outcomes* (7th ed., pp. 525-526). Philadelphia: Saunders.
Ignatavicius, D., & Workman, M. (2006). *Medical-surgical nursing: Critical thinking for collaborative care* (5th ed., pp. 605-606, 670). Philadelphia: Saunders.

1234. A client with acquired immunodeficiency syndrome (AIDS) shares with the nurse feelings of social isolation since the diagnosis was made. The nurse suggests which of the following strategies as the most useful way to decrease the client's stated loneliness?

1 Reinstituting contact with the client's family, who live in a distant city
2 Contacting a support group for clients with AIDS that is available in the local region
3 Using the Internet or the computer to facilitate communication while maintaining isolation
4 Using the television and newspapers to maintain a feeling of being "in touch" with the world

Level of Cognitive Ability: Application
Client Needs: Psychosocial Integrity
Integrated Process: Nursing Process/ Implementation
Content Area: Adult Health/Immune

Answer: 2
Rationale: The nurse encourages the client to maintain social contact and support and assists the client with reducing barriers to social contact. This can include educating the client's family about the disease and its transmission as well as suggesting the use of community resources and support groups. Option 1, although feasible, is less likely to address the client's current feelings of loneliness. Options 3 and 4 will not decrease the client's loneliness.

Test-Taking Strategy: Use the process of elimination. Eliminate options 3 and 4 first, because they do not actually decrease the client's isolation and loneliness. Rather, these options maintain a measure of distance between the client and others. From the remaining options, note that the wording of option 1 implies that contact has been lost over time, and the logistics of distance make this an unlikely solution to the client's current feelings of isolation. Review the strategies related to reducing social isolation if you had difficulty with this question.

References
Black, J., & Hawks, J. (2005). *Medical-surgical nursing: Clinical management for positive outcomes* (7th ed., pp. 445-447, 2388). Philadelphia: Saunders.
Ignatavicius, D., & Workman, M. (2006). *Medical-surgical nursing: Critical thinking for collaborative care* (5th ed., pp. 435-436). Philadelphia: Saunders.

1235. A client was just told by the primary care physician that she will have an exercise stress test to evaluate the client's status after recent episodes of severe chest pain. As the nurse enters the examining room, the client states, "Maybe I shouldn't bother going. I wonder if I should just take more medication, instead." The nurse makes which therapeutic response to the client?

1 "Can you tell me more about how you're feeling?"
2 "Don't you really want to control your heart disease?"
3 "Most people tolerate the procedure well without any complications."
4 "Don't worry. Emergency equipment is available if it should be needed."

Level of Cognitive Ability: Application
Client Needs: Psychosocial Integrity
Integrated Process: Communication and Documentation
Content Area: Adult Health/Cardiovascular

Answer: 1
Rationale: Anxiety and fear are often present before stress testing. The nurse should explore a client's feelings if concerns are expressed. Options 2, 3, and 4 are inappropriate statements and limit communication. Option 1 is open-ended and is the only option that is phrased to engender trust and the sharing of concerns by the client.

Test-Taking Strategy: Use therapeutic communication techniques and the process of elimination. Remember to focus on the client's feelings. This will direct you to option 1. Review therapeutic communication techniques if you had difficulty with this question.

References
Lewis, S., Heitkemper, M., Dirksen, S., O'Brien, P., & Bucher, L. (2007). *Medical-surgical nursing: Assessment and management of clinical problems* (7th ed., p. 121). St. Louis: Mosby.
Pagana, K., & Pagana, T. (2005). *Mosby's diagnostic and laboratory test reference* (7th ed., pp. 239-242). St. Louis: Mosby.
Potter, P., & Perry, A. (2005). *Fundamentals of nursing* (6th ed., p. 437). St. Louis: Mosby.

1236. The nurse is giving a client with heart failure home-care instructions for use after hospital discharge. The client interrupts, saying, "What's the use? I'll never remember all of this, and I'll probably die, anyway!" The nurse interprets that the client's response is most likely the result of:

1 Anger about the new medical regimen
2 The teaching strategies used by the nurse
3 Insufficient financial resources to pay for the medications
4 Anxiety about the ability to manage the disease process at home

Level of Cognitive Ability: Analysis
Client Needs: Psychosocial Integrity
Integrated Process: Nursing Process/Analysis
Content Area: Adult Health/Cardiovascular

Answer: 4
Rationale: Anxiety and fear often develop after heart failure, and they can further tax the failing heart. The client's statement is made in the middle of receiving self-care instructions. There is no evidence in the question to support options 1, 2, or 3.

Test-Taking Strategy: Use the process of elimination, and focus on the data in the question. Note that the client's comment is made when preparing for self-care at home, which implies anxiety about disease self-management. Review the psychosocial concerns of a client with heart failure if you had difficulty with this question.

Reference
Black, J., & Hawks, J. (2005). *Medical-surgical nursing: Clinical management for positive outcomes* (7th ed., pp. 1648-1649). Philadelphia: Saunders.

1237. Before inserting a peripheral intravenous (IV) catheter, the nurse notes that the female client's muscles are tense and that she is fidgeting with the bedsheet. Which statement should the nurse verbalize to the client?

1 "Inserting the IV does not hurt very much."
2 "The IV adds fluid into your bloodstream."
3 "This will be finished before you know it."
4 "The IV catheter is a 18-gauge angiocatheter."

Level of Cognitive Ability: Application
Client Needs: Psychosocial Integrity
Integrated Process: Communication and Documentation
Content Area: Fundamental Skills

Answer: 2
Rationale: The nurse uses simple terms to clearly inform the client about the IV's purpose (option 2). Avoiding the client's feelings (option 3) blocks client communication regarding justifiable fears and feelings related to the IV insertion. Option 1 is an unethical statement for the nurse to make, because the information is incorrect. Option 4 is an unsuitable statement, because the client potentially would not understand the word "angiocatheter."

Test-Taking Strategy: Note the client's nonverbal signals that potentially indicate anxiety about the pending IV catheter insertion. Use therapeutic communication techniques and the process of elimination to determine that option 2 provides accurate information without using medical jargon and terminology and that it also promotes therapeutic communication. Review IV insertion and therapeutic communication techniques if you had difficulty with this question.

Reference
Potter, P., & Perry, A. (2005). *Fundamentals of nursing* (6th ed., pp. 437, 1162). St. Louis: Mosby.

1238. A male client who received an implanted port for intermittent chemotherapy says, "I'm not sure if I can handle having a tube coming out of me. What will my friends think?" Which of the following should the nurse implement first?

1 Ask the client if his friends are close to him.
2 Notify the provider of the client's concerns.
3 Show the client various central line catheters.
4 Explain that implanted ports are subcutaneous.

Level of Cognitive Ability: Analysis
Client Needs: Psychosocial Integrity
Integrated Process: Nursing Process/ Implementation
Content Area: Fundamental Skills

Answer: 4
Rationale: An implanted port is subcutaneous; it is not visible, and it has no external tubing. Tubing is used when an intravenous line is connected and the port is accessed for therapy. The remaining options do not correct the client's confusion about the implanted port. Notifying the provider is not indicated. Inquiring about the client's friends is a reasonable response, but it can also provide false hope that the friends will be accepting. In addition, the nurse is likely to cause more anxiety and concern by providing information about the catheter's subcutaneous location. Showing various central line catheters is unlikely to be beneficial, because the client will not be using them; in addition, this can heighten client anxiety and concerns.

Test-Taking Strategy: Note the words "implanted port" in the question and in option 4, and note the strategic word "first" in the query of the question. The criteria for the correct option involve the first nursing intervention that the nurse should implement to promote therapeutic communication. Review the concepts related to implanted catheters and to the teaching and learning process if you had difficulty with this question.

References
Ignatavicius, D., & Workman, M. (2006). *Medical-surgical nursing: Critical thinking for collaborative care* (5th ed., p. 81). Philadelphia: Saunders.
Perry, A., & Potter, P. (2006). *Clinical nursing skills & techniques* (6th ed., pp. 927-928). St. Louis: Mosby.

1239. A client displays signs of anxiety when the nurse explains that the intravenous (IV) line will need to be discontinued as a result of an infiltration. The nurse makes which appropriate statement to the client?

1 "This will be a totally painless experience. It is nothing to worry about."
2 "I'm sure it will be a real relief for you just as soon as I discontinue this IV for good."
3 "Just relax and take a deep breath. This procedure will not take long, and it will be over soon."
4 "I can see that you're anxious. Removal of the IV shouldn't be painful, but the IV will need to be restarted in another location."

Level of Cognitive Ability: Application
Client Needs: Psychosocial Integrity
Integrated Process: Communication and Documentation
Content Area: Fundamental Skills

Answer: 4
Rationale: Although discontinuing an IV is a painless experience, it is not therapeutic to tell a client not to worry. Option 2 does not acknowledge the client's feelings, and it does not tell the client that an infiltrated IV may need to be restarted. Option 3 does not address the client's feelings. Option 4 addresses the client's anxiety and honestly informs the client that the IV may need to be restarted. This option uses the therapeutic technique of giving information, and it also acknowledges the client's feelings.

Test-Taking Strategy: Use therapeutic communication techniques, and recall that an infiltrated IV may need to be restarted. This will direct you to option 4. In addition, note that the correct option acknowledges the client's feelings. Review therapeutic communication techniques if you had difficulty with this question.

References
Ignatavicius, D., & Workman, M. (2006). *Medical-surgical nursing: Critical thinking for collaborative care* (5th ed., p. 259). Philadelphia: Saunders.
Potter, P., & Perry, A. (2005). *Fundamentals of nursing* (6th ed., p. 437). St. Louis: Mosby.

1240. A client has an initial positive result of an enzyme-linked immunosorbent assay (ELISA) test for human immunodeficiency virus (HIV). The client begins to cry and asks the nurse what this means. The nurse is able to provide support to the client using the knowledge that:

1 The client is HIV positive, but the client's CD4 cell count is high.
2 The client is HIV positive, but the disease has been detected early.
3 There are occasional false-positive readings with this test, which can be cleared up by repeating it one more time.
4 False-positive results can occur, and more testing is needed before diagnosing the client as being HIV positive.

Level of Cognitive Ability: Analysis
Client Needs: Psychosocial Integrity
Integrated Process: Nursing Process/
Implementation
Content Area: Adult Health/Immune

Answer: 4

Rationale: If the client tests positive for HIV with the ELISA test, the test is repeated because of the potential for a false-positive result (for example, from a recent influenza or hepatitis B vaccine) or a false-negative result if drawn too early after infection. If the test is positive a second time, the Western blot (a more specific test) is done to confirm the finding. The client is not diagnosed as HIV positive unless the Western blot is positive. Some laboratories also run the Western blot a second time with a new specimen before making a final determination.

Test-Taking Strategy: Recall that HIV is not diagnosed with a single laboratory test. With this in mind, eliminate options 1 and 2 first. From the remaining options, knowing that the ELISA would be repeated and then a Western blot would be done to confirm these results will direct you to option 4. Review the methods of diagnosing HIV if you had difficulty with this question.

References

Ignatavicius, D., & Workman, M. (2006). *Medical-surgical nursing: Critical thinking for collaborative care* (5th ed., p. 436). Philadelphia: Saunders.
Pagana, K., & Pagana, T. (2005). *Mosby's diagnostic and laboratory test reference* (7th ed., pp. 26-27). St. Louis: Mosby.

1241. When performing an assessment on a suicidal client, the nurse most appropriately asks the client which of the following?

1 "Do you have a death wish?"
2 "Do you wish your life was over?"
3 "Do you ever think about ending it all?"
4 "Do you have any thoughts of killing yourself?"

Level of Cognitive Ability: Application
Client Needs: Psychosocial Integrity
Integrated Process: Nursing Process/Assessment
Content Area: Mental Health

Answer: 4

Rationale: A lethality assessment requires direct communication between the client and the nurse concerning the client's intent. It is important to provide a question that is directly related to lethality. Euphemisms should be avoided.

Test-Taking Strategy: Use the process of elimination. Note the relationship between the words "suicidal" in the question and "killing" in the correct option. Although options 1, 2, and 3 infer a suicide intent, option 4 is the most direct. Review the assessment for suicide risk if you had difficulty with this question.

References

Stuart, G., & Laraia, M. (2005). *Principles and practice of psychiatric nursing* (8th ed., p. 367). St. Louis: Mosby.
Varcarolis, E., Carson, V., & Shoemaker, N. (2006). *Foundations of psychiatric mental health nursing* (5th ed., pp. 477-478). Philadelphia: Saunders.

1242. A client diagnosed with cancer of the bladder has a nursing diagnosis of Fear related to the uncertain outcome of an upcoming cystectomy and urinary diversion. The nurse assesses that this diagnosis still applies if the client makes which of the following statements?
1 "I wish I'd never gone to the doctor at all."
2 "I'm so afraid that I won't live through all this."
3 "I'll never feel like myself if I can't go to the bathroom normally."
4 "What if I have no help at home after going through this awful surgery?"

Level of Cognitive Ability: Analysis
Client Needs: Psychosocial Integrity
Integrated Process: Nursing Process/Analysis
Content Area: Adult Health/Renal

Answer: 2
Rationale: For Fear to be an actual diagnosis, the client must be able to identify the object of fear. In this question, the client is expressing a fear of an uncertain outcome related to cancer and possibly a fear of death. Option 1 is vague and nonspecific. Option 3 reflects a disturbed body image. The statement in option 4 reflects a risk for impaired home maintenance. Further exploration would be required to associate this statement with a nursing diagnosis.

Test-Taking Strategy: Note that the diagnostic statement includes wording regarding the uncertain outcome of surgery. Because option 1 is a general statement, it should be eliminated first. Options 3 and 4 focus on the self after surgery, but they do not contain statements about an uncertain outcome. In option 2, the client expresses a fear of dying after enduring the ordeal of surgery. Review the defining characteristics of Fear if you had difficulty with this question.

Reference
Black, J., & Hawks, J. (2005). *Medical-surgical nursing: Clinical management for positive outcomes* (7th ed., pp. 278, 870). Philadelphia: Saunders.

1243. A client with nephrotic syndrome asks the nurse, "Why should I even bother trying to control my diet and the edema? It doesn't really matter what I do if I can never get rid of this kidney problem, anyway!" The nurse selects which of the following as the most appropriate nursing diagnosis for this client?
1 Anxiety
2 Powerlessness
3 Ineffective coping
4 Disturbed body image

Level of Cognitive Ability: Analysis
Client Needs: Psychosocial Integrity
Integrated Process: Nursing Process/Analysis
Content Area: Adult Health/Renal

Answer: 2
Rationale: Powerlessness is present when the client believes that personal actions will not affect an outcome in any significant way. Because nephrotic syndrome is progressive, the client may feel that personal actions may not affect the disease process. Anxiety is diagnosed when the client has a feeling of unease with a vague or undefined source. Ineffective Coping occurs when the client has impaired adaptive abilities or behaviors with regard to meeting expected demands or roles. Disturbed body image occurs when there is an alteration in the way that the client perceives his or her body image.

Test-Taking Strategy: Focus on the data in the question and in the client's statement. Note the statement, "It doesn't really matter what I do." This implies that the client feels a lack of control over the situation, and it will direct you to option 2. Review the defining characteristics of powerlessness if you had difficulty with this question.

Reference
Black, J., & Hawks, J. (2005). *Medical-surgical nursing: Clinical management for positive outcomes* (7th ed., pp. 870, 926). Philadelphia: Saunders.

1244. A client with renal cell carcinoma of the left kidney is scheduled for nephrectomy. The right kidney appears to be normal at this time. The client is anxious about whether dialysis will ultimately be a necessity. The nurse should provide which of the following pieces of information to the client?

1 It is very likely that the client will need dialysis within 5 to 10 years.

2 One kidney is adequate to meet the needs of the body, as long as it has normal function.

3 There is absolutely no chance of the client needing dialysis because of the nature of the surgery.

4 Dialysis could become likely, but it depends on how well the client complies with fluid restriction after surgery.

Level of Cognitive Ability: Application
Client Needs: Psychosocial Integrity
Integrated Process: Nursing Process/
  Implementation
Content Area: Adult Health/Oncology

Answer: 2

Rationale: Fears about having only one functioning kidney are common among clients who must undergo nephrectomy for renal cancer. These clients need emotional support and reassurance that the remaining kidney should be able to fully meet the body's metabolic needs as long as it has normal function. Options 1, 3, and 4 are inaccurate.

Test-Taking Strategy: Use the process of elimination. Eliminate option 3 because of the words "absolutely no chance." Knowing that there is no need for fluid restriction with a functioning kidney guides you to eliminate option 4 next. From the remaining options, recalling that an individual can donate a kidney without adverse consequences or the need for dialysis will direct you to option 2. Review the psychosocial aspects related to nephrectomy if you had difficulty with this question.

References

Black, J., & Hawks, J. (2005). *Medical-surgical nursing: Clinical management for positive outcomes* (7th ed., p. 923). Philadelphia: Saunders.

Ignatavicius, D., & Workman, M. (2006). *Medical-surgical nursing: Critical thinking for collaborative care* (5th ed., p. 1724). Philadelphia: Saunders.

1245. A charge nurse is supervising a new registered nurse (RN) who is providing care to a client with end-stage heart failure. The client is withdrawn and reluctant to talk, and she shows little interest in participating in hygienic care or activities. Which statement, if made by the new RN to the client, indicates that the new RN requires further teaching regarding the use of therapeutic communication techniques?

1 "What are your feelings right now?"

2 "Why don't you feel like getting up for your bath?"

3 "These dreams you mentioned, what are they like?"

4 "Many clients with end-stage heart failure fear death."

Level of Cognitive Ability: Analysis
Client Needs: Psychosocial Integrity
Integrated Process: Teaching and Learning
Content Area: Leadership/Management

Answer: 2

Rationale: When the nurse asks a "why" question of the client, the nurse is requesting an explanation for feelings and behaviors when the client may not know the reason. Requesting an explanation is a nontherapeutic communication technique. In option 1, the nurse is encouraging the verbalization of emotions or feelings, which is a therapeutic communication technique. In option 3, the nurse is using the therapeutic communication technique of exploring, which involves asking the client to describe something in more detail or to discuss it more fully. In option 4, the nurse is using the therapeutic communication technique of giving information. Identifying the common fear of death among clients with end-stage heart failure may encourage the client to voice concerns.

Test-Taking Strategy: Note the strategic words "requires further teaching regarding the use of therapeutic communication techniques." These words indicate a negative event query and ask you to select an option that is an incorrect statement made by the new RN. Select the option that is a block to communication. The word "why" in option 2 should guide you to this option. Review therapeutic communication techniques if you had difficulty with this question.

References

Ignatavicius, D., & Workman, M. (2006). *Medical-surgical nursing: Critical thinking for collaborative care* (5th ed., p. 754). Philadelphia: Saunders.

Potter, P., & Perry, A. (2005). *Fundamentals of nursing* (6th ed., p. 437). St. Louis: Mosby.

1246. The nurse is caring for a client with acute pulmonary edema. The nurse should plan to incorporate strategies for which of the following into the care of the client?

1 Reducing anxiety
2 Increasing fluid volume
3 Decreasing cardiac output
4 Promoting a positive body image

Level of Cognitive Ability: Application
Client Needs: Psychosocial Integrity
Integrated Process: Nursing Process/Planning
Content Area: Adult Health/Cardiovascular

Answer: 1
Rationale: When cardiac output falls as a result of acute pulmonary edema, the sympathetic nervous system is stimulated. Stimulation of the sympathetic nervous system results in the fight-or-flight reaction, which further impairs cardiac function. The goals of treatment are to increase cardiac output and to decrease fluid volume. A disturbed body image is not a common problem among clients with acute pulmonary edema.

Test-Taking Strategy: Use the process of elimination. Thinking about the physiological occurrences of this condition will assist you with eliminating options 2, 3, and 4. In addition, recalling that severe dyspnea occurs should assist with directing you to the correct option. Review the care of the client with pulmonary edema if you had difficulty with this question.

Reference
Ignatavicius, D., & Workman, M. (2006). *Medical-surgical nursing: Critical thinking for collaborative care* (5th ed., p. 755). Philadelphia: Saunders.

1247. A client with acute renal failure is having trouble remembering information and instructions as a result of altered laboratory values. The nurse avoids doing which of the following when communicating with this client?

1 Giving simple, clear directions
2 Including the family in discussions related to care
3 Explaining treatments using understandable language
4 Giving thorough and complete explanations of treatment options

Level of Cognitive Ability: Application
Client Needs: Psychosocial Integrity
Integrated Process: Nursing Process/ Implementation
Content Area: Adult Health/Renal

Answer: 4
Rationale: The client with acute renal failure may have difficulty remembering information and instructions because of anxiety and altered laboratory values. Communications should be clear, simple, and understandable. The family is included whenever possible. Information about treatment should be explained using understandable language.

Test-Taking Strategy: Use the process of elimination, and note the strategic word "avoids." This word indicates a negative event query and asks you to select the option that identifies an incorrect nursing action. Recalling the basic principles of effective communication would lead you to recognize that options 1, 2, and 3 are helpful for maintaining effective communication. Review the basic principles of effective communication if you had difficulty with this question.

Reference
Black, J., & Hawks, J. (2005). *Medical-surgical nursing: Clinical management for positive outcomes* (7th ed., p. 948). Philadelphia: Saunders.

1248. The rehabilitation nurse witnessed a postoperative coronary artery bypass graft client and his spouse arguing after a rehabilitation session. An appropriate statement by the nurse to identify the feelings of the client would be which of the following?

1 "You seem upset."
2 "Oh, don't let this get you down."
3 "It will seem better tomorrow. Now, smile."
4 "You shouldn't get upset. It'll affect your heart."

Answer: 1
Rationale: Acknowledging the client's feelings without inserting your own values or judgments is a method of therapeutic communication. Therapeutic communication techniques assist with the flow of communication, and they always focus on the client. Option 1 is an open-ended statement that allows the client to verbalize, which gives the nurse a direction or clarification of the client's true feelings. Options 2, 3, and 4 do not encourage verbalization by the client.

Level of Cognitive Ability: Application
Client Needs: Psychosocial Integrity
Integrated Process: Communication and
  Documentation
Content Area: Adult Health/Cardiovascular

Test-Taking Strategy: Use therapeutic communication techniques. Focusing on the subject of identifying the feelings of the client will direct you to option 1. Review therapeutic communication techniques if you had difficulty with this question.

References
Ignatavicius, D., & Workman, M. (2006). *Medical-surgical nursing: Critical thinking for collaborative care* (5th ed., p. 862). Philadelphia: Saunders.
Potter, P., & Perry, A. (2005). *Fundamentals of nursing* (6th ed., p. 437). St. Louis: Mosby.

1249. A nurse is monitoring the neurological status on a client with dementia and assessing the limbic system. The assessment of which of the following items by the nurse would yield the best information about this area of functioning?
  1 Eye movements
  2 Feelings or emotions
  3 Level of consciousness
  4 Insight, judgment, and planning

Level of Cognitive Ability: Application
Client Needs: Psychosocial Integrity
Integrated Process: Nursing Process/Assessment
Content Area: Adult Health/Neurological

Answer: 2
Rationale: Feelings and emotions are part of the role of the limbic system. Insight, judgment, and planning are part of the function of the frontal lobe. The level of consciousness is controlled by the reticular activating system. Eye movements are under the control of cranial nerves III, IV, and VI.

Test-Taking Strategy: A specific understanding of the function of the limbic system will direct you to option 2. Review the function of the limbic system if you had difficulty with this question.

Reference
Ignatavicius, D., & Workman, M. (2006). *Medical-surgical nursing: Critical thinking for collaborative care* (5th ed., p. 925). Philadelphia: Saunders.

1250. A client is admitted to the mental health unit with a diagnosis of panic disorder. The nurse anticipates that the physician will prescribe a benzodiazepine and checks the physician's order sheet for which medication order?
  1 Alprazolam (Xanax)
  2 Doxepin (Sinequan)
  3 Imipramine (Tofranil)
  4 Bupropion (Wellbutrin)

Level of Cognitive Ability: Analysis
Client Needs: Psychosocial Integrity
Integrated Process: Nursing Process/Analysis
Content Area: Pharmacology

Answer: 1
Rationale: Options 2, 3, and 4 are classified as antidepressants, and they act by stimulating the central nervous system (CNS) to elevate mood. Alprazolam (Xanax), which is a benzodiazepine antianxiety agent, depresses the CNS and induces relaxation in clients with panic disorders.

Test-Taking Strategy: Knowledge regarding panic disorders and the classification of the medications identified in the options is needed to answer this question. Eliminate options 2, 3, and 4, because they are comparable or alike and because they are all antidepressants. Review the listed medications if you had difficulty with this question.

Reference
Skidmore-Roth, L. (2005). *Mosby's drug guide for nurses* (6th ed., p. 29). St. Louis: Mosby.

1251. A client with empyema is to undergo decortication to remove inflamed tissue, pus, and debris. The nurse offers emotional support to the client on the basis of the understanding that:

1 This problem may decrease the client's life expectancy.
2 The client is likely to be in excruciating pain after surgery.
3 The client will probably have chronic dyspnea after the surgery.
4 Chest tubes will be in place after surgery for some time, and the healing process is slow.

Level of Cognitive Ability: Analysis
Client Needs: Psychosocial Integrity
Integrated Process: Caring
Content Area: Adult Health/Respiratory

Answer: 4
Rationale: The client undergoing decortication to treat empyema needs ongoing support from the nurse. This is especially true because the client will have chest tubes in place after surgery, and these must remain until the former pus-filled space is completely obliterated. This may take some time, and it may be discouraging to the client. Progress is monitored by chest x-ray. Options 1, 2, and 3 are not accurate.

Test-Taking Strategy: Use the process of elimination. Option 1 is the least likely response, and it is thus eliminated first. Option 2 is eliminated next, because no client should be in "excruciating pain" postoperatively. From the remaining options, it is necessary to know that the client will require chest tubes and that it may take some time for full healing to occur. Recalling that the client has chest tubes after thoracic surgery may be sufficient to help you select between these last two options. Review the psychosocial aspects of care after decortication if you had difficulty with this question.

References
Black, J., & Hawks, J. (2005). *Medical-surgical nursing: Clinical management for positive outcomes* (7th ed., p. 1873). Philadelphia: Saunders.
Ignatavicius, D., & Workman, M. (2006). *Medical-surgical nursing: Critical thinking for collaborative care* (5th ed., pp. 646-647). Philadelphia: Saunders.

1252. A client who has never been hospitalized before is having trouble initiating the stream of urine. Knowing that there is no pathological reason for this difficulty, the nurse avoids which of the following because it is the least helpful method of assisting the client?

1 Running tap water in the sink
2 Assisting the client to a commode behind a closed curtain
3 Instructing the client to pour warm water over the perineum
4 Closing the bathroom door and instructing the client to pull the call bell when done

Level of Cognitive Ability: Application
Client Needs: Psychosocial Integrity
Integrated Process: Nursing Process/ Implementation
Content Area: Adult Health/Renal

Answer: 2
Rationale: A lack of privacy is a key issue that may inhibit the ability of the client to void in the absence of known pathology. Using a commode behind a curtain may inhibit voiding in some people. The use of a bathroom is preferable, and this may be supplemented with the use of running water or pouring water over the perineum, as needed.

Test-Taking Strategy: Use the process of elimination, and note the strategic words "least helpful." Think about the issue related to decreased privacy and its effects on elimination. Review the measures used to assist with promoting urinary elimination if you had difficulty with this question.

References
Ignatavicius, D., & Workman, M. (2006). *Medical-surgical nursing: Critical thinking for collaborative care* (5th ed., p. 1710). Philadelphia: Saunders.
Potter, P., & Perry, A. (2005). *Fundamentals of nursing* (6th ed., p. 1327). St. Louis: Mosby.

1253. The client tells the nurse, "I'm scheduled for outpatient surgery, but I live alone with my only child 300 miles away. I'm afraid. What happens if something goes wrong after I go home?" Which of the following statements by the nurse is therapeutic?

1 "Don't worry about the details. This procedure is done all the time and generally without any problems. You'll be fine!"

2 "They say managed care is no care! Get an alarm system so that, if you fall, it will alert someone. If necessary, I'll come."

3 "Your concern is well voiced. I advise you to call your son and insist that he come home immediately! You can't be too careful."

4 "You seem very concerned about going home without help. Have you discussed your concerns with both your doctor and your family?"

Level of Cognitive Ability: Application
Client Needs: Psychosocial Integrity
Integrated Process: Communication and Documentation
Content Area: Mental Health

Answer: 4
Rationale: The client has verbalized concerns. In option 4, the nurse uses reflection to direct the client's feelings and concerns. In option 1, the nurse provides false reassurance and then minimizes the client's concerns. In option 2, the nurse is ventilating the nurse's own anger, frustration, and powerlessness. In addition, the nurse is trying to problem solve for the client but is overly controlling and takes the decision making out of the client's hands. In option 3, the nurse is projecting the client's own fears, and the problem solving suggested by the nurse will increase fear and anxiety in the client.

Test-Taking Strategy: Use therapeutic communication techniques. Remember that the priority is to address the client's feelings, and option 4 is the only option that does this. Review therapeutic communication techniques if you had difficulty with this question.

References
Stuart, G., & Laraia, M. (2005). *Principles and practice of psychiatric nursing* (8th ed., pp. 30-31). St. Louis: Mosby.
Varcarolis, E., Carson, V., & Shoemaker, N. (2006). *Foundations of psychiatric mental health nursing* (5th ed., p. 213). Philadelphia: Saunders.

1254. During the nursing assessment, the client says, "My doctor just told me that my cancer has spread and that I have less than 6 months to live." Which of the following nursing responses would be therapeutic?

1 "I am sorry. Would you like to discuss this with me some more?"

2 "I am sorry. There are no easy answers in times like this, are there?"

3 "I hope you'll focus on the fact that your doctor says you have 6 months to live and that you'll think of how you'd like to live."

4 "I know it seems desperate, but there have been a lot of breakthroughs. Something might come along in a month or so to change your status drastically."

Answer: 1
Rationale: The client has received very distressing news and is most likely still experiencing shock and denial. In option 1, the nurse invites the client to ventilate feelings. Option 2 is social and expresses the nurse's feelings rather than the client's feelings. Option 3 is patronizing and stereotypical. Option 4 provides social communication and false hope.

Test-Taking Strategy: Use therapeutic communication techniques. Note that option 1 provides the opportunity for the client to express feelings. Remember to focus on the client's feelings. Review therapeutic communication techniques if you had difficulty with this question.

Level of Cognitive Ability: Application
Client Needs: Psychosocial Integrity
Integrated Process: Communication and
    Documentation
Content Area: Adult Health/Oncology

References
Black, J., & Hawks, J. (2005). *Medical-surgical nursing: Clinical management for positive outcomes* (7th ed., p. 380). Philadelphia: Saunders.
Potter, P., & Perry, A. (2005). *Fundamentals of nursing* (6th ed., p. 437). St. Louis: Mosby.

1255. A client with an endotracheal tube gets easily frustrated when trying to communicate personal needs to the nurse. The nurse determines that which of the following methods for communication may be the easiest for the client?
1 Use a picture or word board.
2 Have the family interpret needs.
3 Devise a system of hand signals.
4 Use a pad of paper and a pencil.

Level of Cognitive Ability: Analysis
Client Needs: Psychosocial Integrity
Integrated Process: Communication and
    Documentation
Content Area: Adult Health/Respiratory

Answer: 1
Rationale: The client with an endotracheal tube in place cannot speak, so the nurse devises an alternative communication system with the client. The use of a picture or word board is the simplest method of communication, because it requires only pointing at the word or object. A pad of paper and a pencil is an acceptable alternative, but it requires more client effort and time. The use of hand signals may not be a reliable method, because it may not meet all needs, and it is subject to misinterpretation. The family does not need to bear the burden of communicating the client's needs, and they may not understand them either.

Test-Taking Strategy: Note the strategic words "frustrated" and "easiest." Options 3 and 4 are not the "easiest," and they are therefore eliminated first. Because the family may not necessarily know what the client is trying to communicate, option 3 could cause added frustration for the client. Review alternative methods of communication if you had difficulty with this question.

Reference
Black, J., & Hawks, J. (2005). *Medical-surgical nursing: Clinical management for positive outcomes* (7th ed., p. 1893). Philadelphia: Saunders.

1256. The home-care nurse visits a client who is receiving parenteral nutrition, and the client states, "I really miss eating dinner with my family." To reply to the client therapeutically, the nurse says:
1 "What you are feeling is very common."
2 "In a few weeks, you may be allowed to eat."
3 "Tell me more about your family dinners."
4 "You can sit down to dinner even if you do not eat."

Level of Cognitive Ability: Application
Client Needs: Psychosocial Integrity
Integrated Process: Communication and
    Documentation
Content Area: Fundamental Skills

Answer: 3
Rationale: The nurse assists the client with expressing feelings and dealing with the aspects of illness and treatment by clarifying and helping the client to focus on and explore concerns. In option 1, the nurse characterizes and classifies the feelings on the basis of an assumption. Option 2 provides false hope, and option 4 blocks communication by giving advice.

Test-Taking Strategy: Use therapeutic communication techniques. Focus on client feelings first, and then use the process of elimination. This will direct you to option 3. Review therapeutic communication techniques if you had difficulty with this question.

References
Ignatavicius, D., & Workman, M. (2006). *Medical-surgical nursing: Critical thinking for collaborative care* (5th ed., p. 1434). Philadelphia: Saunders.
Potter, P., & Perry, A. (2005). *Fundamentals of nursing* (6th ed., p. 437). St. Louis: Mosby.

1257. A client has been receiving maprotiline (Ludiomil). The nurse notifies the health care provider if which adverse client response to the medication is noted?
1 Increased appetite
2 Increased drowsiness
3 Reported decrease in anxiety
4 Increased sense of well-being

Answer: 2
Rationale: Maprotiline is a tricyclic antidepressant that is used to treat various forms of depression and anxiety. The client is also often in psychotherapy while taking this medication. Expected effects of the medication include an improved sense of well-being, increased appetite and time spent sleeping, and a reduced sense of anxiety. Adverse effects to report to the health care provider include drowsiness, lethargy, and fatigue.

Level of Cognitive Ability: Application
Client Needs: Psychosocial Integrity
Integrated Process: Nursing Process/ Implementation
Content Area: Pharmacology

Test-Taking Strategy: Focus on the subject: an adverse response. Recall that this medication is an antidepressant. It would seem reasonable to expect options 1, 3, and 4 to occur as positive responses to this medication. Review maprotiline if you had difficulty with this question.

Reference
Skidmore-Roth, L. (2005). *Mosby's drug guide for nurses* (6th ed., p. 930). St. Louis: Mosby.

1258. A client who is to undergo thoracentesis is afraid of not being able to tolerate the procedure. The nurse interprets that the client needs honest support and reassurance, which can best be accomplished by which of the following statements?
1 "I'll be right by your side, but the procedure will be totally painless as long as you don't move."
2 "The procedure only takes 1 to 2 minutes, so you might try to get through it by mentally counting up to 120."
3 "The needle hurts when it goes in, and you must remain still. I'll stay with you throughout the entire procedure and help you hold your position."
4 "The needle is a little uncomfortable going in, but this is controlled by rhythmically breathing in and out. I'll be with you to coach your breathing."

Answer: 3
Rationale: The needle insertion for thoracentesis is painful for the client. The nurse tells the client how important it is to remain still during the procedure so that the needle does not injure visceral pleura or lung tissue. The nurse reassures the client during the procedure and helps the client hold the proper position. Options 1, 2, and 4 are inaccurate statements.

Test-Taking Strategy: Use the process of elimination and therapeutic communication techniques. Recalling that the client must remain still during the procedure helps you eliminate option 4 first. Knowing that the procedure may be painful for the client and that it takes longer than 1 to 2 minutes helps you eliminate options 1 and 2. Review thoracentesis if you had difficulty with this question.

Level of Cognitive Ability: Application
Client Needs: Psychosocial Integrity
Integrated Process: Communication and Documentation
Content Area: Adult Health/Respiratory

References
Black, J., & Hawks, J. (2005). *Medical-surgical nursing: Clinical management for positive outcomes* (7th ed., p. 1772). Philadelphia: Saunders.
Lewis, S., Heitkemper, M., Dirksen, S., O'Brien, P., & Bucher, L. (2007). *Medical surgical nursing: Assessment and management of clinical problems* (7th ed., p. 596). St. Louis: Mosby.

1259. A client with chronic respiratory failure is dyspneic. The client becomes anxious, which worsens the feelings of dyspnea. The nurse teaches the client which of the following methods to best interrupt the dyspnea–anxiety–dyspnea cycle?

1 Guided imagery and limiting fluids
2 Relaxation and breathing techniques
3 Biofeedback and coughing techniques
4 Distraction and increased dietary carbohydrates

Level of Cognitive Ability: Application
Client Needs: Psychosocial Integrity
Integrated Process: Teaching and Learning
Content Area: Adult Health/Respiratory

Answer: 2
Rationale: The anxious client with dyspnea should be taught interventions to decrease anxiety, which include relaxation, biofeedback, guided imagery, and distraction. This will stop the escalation of feelings of anxiety and dyspnea. The dyspnea can be further controlled by teaching the client breathing techniques, which include pursed lip and diaphragmatic breathing. Coughing techniques are useful, but breathing techniques are more effective. Limiting fluids will thicken secretions, and increased dietary carbohydrates will increase the production of carbon dioxide by the body.

Test-Taking Strategy: Focus on the subject of relieving anxiety and dyspnea, and note the strategic word "best." Limiting fluids and increasing carbohydrates are contraindicated and therefore eliminated. From the remaining options, recall that breathing techniques are more effective than coughing techniques. This will direct you to option 2. Review the measures used to relieve anxiety and dyspnea in the client with respiratory failure if you had difficulty with this question.

References
Black, J., & Hawks, J. (2005). *Medical-surgical nursing: Clinical management for positive outcomes* (7th ed., p. 1825). Philadelphia: Saunders.
Ignatavicius, D., & Workman, M. (2006). *Medical-surgical nursing: Critical thinking for collaborative care* (5th ed., p. 657). Philadelphia: Saunders.

1260. Immediately after taking a routine evening dose of alprazolam (Xanax), a client says, "I'm not sure I should have taken that stuff." The nurse makes which appropriate statement to the client?

1 "Anxiety is expected with any new experience."
2 "Let's talk about how you feel about Xanax for a while."
3 "You are afraid of the media claims about this medication."
4 "Your depression will fade once the medication begins to work."

Level of Cognitive Ability: Application
Client Needs: Physiological Integrity
Integrated Process: Communication and Documentation
Content Area: Pharmacology

Answer: 2
Rationale: The nurse should focus on determining the reason for the client's concern. The nurse would add anxiety to the client by mentioning media concerns. Alprazolam is used to treat anxiety, not depression. Cliché responses (option 1) do not express concern.

Test-Taking Strategy: Use therapeutic communication techniques. Remembering to address the client's feelings will direct you to option 2. Review these techniques if you had difficulty with this question.

Reference
Lilley, L., Harrington, S., & Snyder J. (2007). *Pharmacology and the nursing process* (5th ed., p. 232). St. Louis: Mosby.

1261. The nurse is caring for a client who has just experienced a pulmonary embolism. The client is restless and very anxious. The nurse uses which approach when communicating with this client?

1 Explaining each treatment in great detail
2 Having the family reinforce the nurse's directions
3 Giving simple, clear directions and explanations
4 Speaking very little to the client until the crisis is over

Level of Cognitive Ability: Application
Client Needs: Psychosocial Integrity
Integrated Process: Communication and Documentation
Content Area: Adult Health/Respiratory

Answer: 3
Rationale: The client who has suffered pulmonary embolism is fearful and apprehensive. The nurse effectively communicates with this client by staying with the client; providing simple, clear, and accurate information; and displaying a calm, efficient manner. Options 1, 2, and 4 will produce more anxiety for the client and the family.

Test-Taking Strategy: Use the process of elimination. Eliminate option 1 because of the words "great detail." Next, eliminate option 4 because of the words "speaking very little." From the remaining options, having the family reinforce the directions may place stress on the family and provide too much sensory input for the client. This will direct you to option 3. Review communication strategies for the client who is restless and anxious if you had difficulty with this question.

Reference
Black, J., & Hawks, J. (2005). *Medical-surgical nursing: Clinical management for positive outcomes* (7th ed., pp. 1832-1833). Philadelphia: Saunders.

1262. A nurse in the emergency department is admitting a client with carbon monoxide poisoning as a result of a suicide attempt. Which of the following services should be initiated first?

1 Psychiatric consult
2 Neurological consult
3 Occupational therapy
4 Pulmonary rehabilitation

Level of Cognitive Ability: Application
Client Needs: Psychosocial Integrity
Integrated Process: Nursing Process/ Implementation
Content Area: Mental Health

Answer: 1
Rationale: The client with carbon monoxide poisoning as a result of a suicide attempt should have a psychiatric consult. The necessity of a neurological consult would depend on the sequelae to the nervous system from the carbon monoxide poisoning, and there are no data in the question that indicate this need. Occupational therapy and pulmonary rehabilitation are not indicated.

Test-Taking Strategy: Focus on the client's diagnosis, and note the strategic word "first." Eliminate occupational therapy first, because there is no indication of the need for that service. The client will need respiratory therapy but not pulmonary rehabilitation, so option 4 is eliminated next. A neurological consult could be beneficial, but only if the client suffers long-term central nervous system damage from this suicide attempt. Review the care of the client who attempted suicide if you had difficulty with this question.

References
Stuart, G., & Laraia, M. (2005). *Principles and practice of psychiatric nursing* (8th ed., pp. 116, 370-371). St. Louis: Mosby.
Varcarolis, E., Carson, V., & Shoemaker, N. (2006). *Foundations of psychiatric mental health nursing* (5th ed., p. 66). Philadelphia: Saunders.

1263. The nurse is caring for a young adult who has been diagnosed with sarcoidosis. The client is angry and tells the nurse that there is no point in learning disease management, because there is no possibility of ever being cured. The nurse formulates which nursing diagnosis for this client?

1 Anxiety
2 Powerlessness
3 Disturbed thought processes
4 Ineffective health maintenance

Level of Cognitive Ability: Analysis
Client Needs: Psychosocial Integrity
Integrated Process: Nursing Process/Analysis
Content Area: Adult Health/Respiratory

Answer: 2
Rationale: The client with Powerlessness expresses feelings of having no control over a situation or outcome. Anxiety is a vague sense of unease. Disturbed thought processes involve the disruption of cognitive abilities or thought. Ineffective health maintenance involves the inability to seek out help that is needed to maintain health.

Test-Taking Strategy: Use the process of elimination, and note the data in the question. Focusing on the subject of anger over a situation in which the client has little control will direct you to option 2. Review the definitions of the listed nursing diagnoses if you had difficulty with this question.

References

Black, J., & Hawks, J. (2005). *Medical-surgical nursing: Clinical management for positive outcomes* (7th ed., pp. 1871-1872). Philadelphia: Saunders.
Stuart, G., & Laraia, M. (2005). *Principles and practice of psychiatric nursing* (8th ed., p. 245). St. Louis: Mosby.

1264. A client who is immobilized in skeletal leg traction complains of being bored and restless. On the basis of these complaints, the nurse formulates which nursing diagnosis for this client?

1 Powerlessness
2 Self-care deficit
3 Impaired physical mobility
4 Deficient diversional activity

Level of Cognitive Ability: Analysis
Client Needs: Psychosocial Integrity
Integrated Process: Nursing Process/Analysis
Content Area: Adult Health/Musculoskeletal

Answer: 4
Rationale: A major defining characteristic of Deficient diversional activity is the expression of boredom by the client. The question also does not identify client feelings of a lack of control (Powerlessness) or an inability to perform activities of daily living (Self-care deficit). The question does not identify difficulties with coordination, range of motion, or muscle strength, which would indicate Impaired physical mobility.

Test-Taking Strategy: Use the process of elimination, and focus on the data in the question. Noting the strategic words "bored and restless" will direct you to option 4. Review the defining characteristics of Deficient diversional activity if you had difficulty with this question.

References

Black, J., & Hawks, J. (2005). *Medical-surgical nursing: Clinical management for positive outcomes* (7th ed., p. 637). Philadelphia: Saunders.
Potter, P., & Perry, A. (2005). *Fundamentals of nursing* (6th ed., pp. 462-463). St. Louis: Mosby.
Stuart, G., & Laraia, M. (2005). *Principles and practice of psychiatric nursing* (8th ed., p. 783). St. Louis: Mosby.

1265. A client who is being mechanically ventilated after experiencing a fat embolus is visibly anxious. The nurse would take which appropriate action?

1 Ask a family member to stay with the client at all times.
2 Ask the physician for an order for succinylcholine (Anectine).
3 Encourage the client to sleep until the arterial blood gas results improve.
4 Provide reassurance to the client, and give small doses of morphine sulfate intravenously, as prescribed.

Answer: 4
Rationale: The nurse always speaks to the client calmly and provides reassurance to the anxious client. Morphine sulfate is often prescribed for pain and anxiety for the client who is receiving mechanical ventilation. It is not beneficial to ask the family to take on the burden of remaining with the client at all times. Succinylcholine is a paralyzing agent, but it has no antianxiety properties. In option 3, the nurse does nothing to reassure or help the client.

Level of Cognitive Ability: Application
Client Needs: Psychosocial Integrity
Integrated Process: Nursing Process/
  Implementation
Content Area: Adult Health/Respiratory

Test-Taking Strategy: Use the process of elimination. Note that the client is anxious. Option 4 is the only option in which the nurse interacts with the client. Also note the words "provide reassurance" in the correct option. Review the measures used to relieve anxiety if you had difficulty with this question.

References

Black, J., & Hawks, J. (2005). *Medical-surgical nursing: Clinical management for positive outcomes* (7th ed., p. 1891). Philadelphia: Saunders.

Lewis, S., Heitkemper, M., Dirksen, S., O'Brien, P., & Bucher, L. (2007). *Medical-surgical nursing: Assessment and management of clinical problems* (7th ed., p. 370). St. Louis: Mosby.

1266. The nurse establishes the goal of diminishing the risk of disturbed thought processes for an older post-stroke client who is confused after being admitted to the hospital with a fractured hip. Which is the priority client information for the nurse to use when planning care to keep the client at the highest level of cognitive functioning?

1 First admission to this hospital
2 Hip fracture causing client upset
3 Expressive aphasia caused by stroke
4 Hearing aid and new battery on hand

Level of Cognitive Ability: Analysis
Client Needs: Psychosocial Integrity
Integrated Process: Nursing Process/Assessment
Content Area: Fundamental Skills

Answer: 4

Rationale: Reduced clarity of the client's environmental awareness can result in confusion in an older client who was not confused before the hospital admission; thus the most important client information for the nurse to consider when planning care is the presence of the hearing aid, because it is most likely to help the client understand and interact properly with the environment. In addition, helping the client hear provides for accurate follow-up client assessment data. Many factors can lead to confusion in an older adult, including unfamiliar settings, acute distress, infection, dehydration, and hypoxia; however, most of these issues are unlikely to be quickly or easily resolved. Residual effects of a stroke can also impair the client's ability to interact with the environment, but this client's aphasia is an input rather than a reception impairment with regard to interaction with the environment.

Test-Taking Strategy: Note the strategic word "priority." This word cues you to select the client data that provide the best information, along with the nurse's goal, for helping to keep the client at the highest level of cognitive functioning. Client distress about an unfamiliar setting (option 1), the fracture (option 2), and the residual effects of a stroke (option 3) can impair a client's cognitive function. Eliminate these options, because they are unlikely to be resolved quickly. The hearing aide enhances client interaction with the environment immediately, and, thus, it is a better piece of information to consider when planning care. Review the factors that place a hospitalized client at risk for disturbed thought processes if you had difficulty with this question.

References

Black, J., & Hawks, J. (2005). *Medical-surgical nursing: Clinical management for positive outcomes* (7th ed., p. 641). Philadelphia: Saunders.

Lewis, S., Heitkemper, M., Dirksen, S., O'Brien, P., & Bucher, L. (2007). *Medical-surgical nursing: Assessment and management of clinical problems* (7th ed., p. 1577). St. Louis: Mosby.

1267. A client is admitted to the nursing unit after a left below-the-knee amputation after a crush injury to the foot and lower leg. The client tells the nurse, "I think I'm going crazy. I can feel my left foot itching." The nurse interprets the client's statement to be:

1 A normal response that indicates the presence of phantom limb pain
2 A normal response that indicates the presence of phantom limb sensation
3 An abnormal response that indicates that the client is in denial about the limb loss
4 An abnormal response that indicates that the client needs more psychological support

Level of Cognitive Ability: Analysis
Client Needs: Psychosocial Integrity
Integrated Process: Nursing Process/Analysis
Content Area: Adult Health/Cardiovascular

Answer: 2
Rationale: Phantom limb sensations are felt in the area of the amputated limb. These can include itching, warmth, and cold. The sensations are caused by intact peripheral nerves in the residual limb area. Whenever possible, clients should be told that they may experience these sensations. The client may also feel painful sensations in the area of the amputated limb (phantom limb pain). The origin of the pain is less well understood, but the client should be prepared for this, too, whenever possible. This is not an abnormal response.

Test-Taking Strategy: Focus on the client's complaint: itching. Recalling that sensation and pain may be felt in the area of the amputated limb eliminates options 3 and 4 first, because these feelings are not abnormal responses. From the remaining options, select option 2, because the client has complained of itching rather than pain. Review the expected findings of a client who had an amputation if you had difficulty with this question.

Reference
Black, J., & Hawks, J. (2005). *Medical-surgical nursing: Clinical management for positive outcomes* (7th ed., p. 450). Philadelphia: Saunders.

1268. A male client who had a spinal fusion with hardware insertion is extremely concerned that the lengthy rehabilitation period will cause financial and work-related problems for him. To address the client's concerns, to which member of the health care team does the nurse refer the client?

1 Social worker
2 Neurosurgeon
3 Physical therapist
4 Clinical nurse specialist

Level of Cognitive Ability: Application
Client Needs: Psychosocial Integrity
Integrated Process: Nursing Process/Planning
Content Area: Fundamental Skills

Answer: 1
Rationale: After spinal surgery, financial and work-related concerns are managed by a social worker whose role is to assist the client with health care–related social issues by making use of community agencies and resources. A physical therapist has the best knowledge of techniques for increasing mobility, endurance, flexibility, and strength. The clinical nurse specialist and the neurosurgeon are specialists who are important in the physical care of the neurosurgical client and who can make the referral to the social worker.

Test-Taking Strategy: Use the process of elimination. Focus on the client's concerns about finances and work, and think about the roles of each member of the health care team identified in the options to direct you to option 1. Review the roles of the listed health care professions if you had difficulty with this question.

References
Ignatavicius, D., & Workman, M. (2006). *Medical-surgical nursing: Critical thinking for collaborative care* (5th ed., p. 120). Philadelphia: Saunders.
Lewis, S., Heitkemper, M., Dirksen, S., O'Brien, P., & Bucher, L. (2007). *Medical-surgical nursing: Assessment and management of clinical problems* (7th ed., p. 91). St. Louis: Mosby.

1269. A client is fearful about having an arm cast removed. Which action by the nurse would be helpful for alleviating the client's fear?
1 Telling the client that the saw makes a frightening noise
2 Stating that the hot cutting blades have rarely caused burns
3 Showing the client the cast cutter and explaining how it works
4 Reassuring the client that no one has had an arm lacerated yet

Level of Cognitive Ability: Application
Client Needs: Psychosocial Integrity
Integrated Process: Nursing Process/
  Implementation
Content Area: Adult Health/Musculoskeletal

Answer: 3
Rationale: Clients may be fearful of having a cast removed because of the cast-cutting blade. The nurse should show the cast cutter to the client before it is used and explain that the client may feel heat, vibration, and pressure. The cast cutter resembles a small electric saw with a circular blade. The nurse should reassure the client that the blade does not cut like a saw but instead cuts the cast by vibrating side to side. Options 1, 2, and 4 are inappropriate and may increase the client's fear.

Test-Taking Strategy: Use the process of elimination, and note the strategic word "helpful." Focusing on the subject of the client's fear will direct you to option 3. Option 3 gives the client the most reassurance, because it best prepares the client for what will occur when the cast is removed. Review the measures used to relieve fear in a client preparing for a procedure if you had difficulty with this question.

References
Ignatavicius, D., & Workman, M. (2006). *Medical-surgical nursing: Critical thinking for collaborative care* (5th ed., p. 1198). Philadelphia: Saunders.
Perry, A., & Potter, P. (2006). *Clinical nursing skills & techniques* (6th ed., pp. 313-316). St. Louis: Mosby.

1270. A client has several fractures of the lower leg and has been placed in an external fixation device. The client is upset about the appearance of the leg, which is very edematous. The nurse formulates which nursing diagnosis for the client?
1 Social isolation
2 Activity intolerance
3 Disturbed body image
4 Risk for impaired physical mobility

Level of Cognitive Ability: Analysis
Client Needs: Psychosocial Integrity
Integrated Process: Nursing Process/Analysis
Content Area: Adult Health/Musculoskeletal

Answer: 3
Rationale: The client is at risk for Disturbed body image related to a change in the structure and function of the affected leg. There are no data in the question to support a diagnosis of (actual) Activity intolerance or Social isolation. The client has actual Impaired mobility (rather than a risk for it) because of the fixation device.

Test-Taking Strategy: Use the process of elimination, and focus on the data in the question. Noting the strategic words "upset about the appearance of the leg" will direct you to option 3. Review the defining characteristics of Disturbed body image if you had difficulty with this question.

Reference
Black, J., & Hawks, J. (2005). *Medical-surgical nursing: Clinical management for positive outcomes* (7th ed., p. 1423). Philadelphia: Saunders.

1271. A client and her husband are being discharged from the hospital after giving birth to a fetal demise. They ask about the possibility of attending a bereavement support group in the community. The nurse is aware that this is an indication of:
1 Anger
2 Denial
3 Normal grieving
4 Prolonged sadness

Answer: 3
Rationale: A perinatal bereavement support group can help the parents work through their pain with the nonjudgmental sharing of feelings. It is a necessary part of normal grieving. The parents' request is not indicative of denial, prolonged sadness, or anger.

Test-Taking Strategy: Use the process of elimination, and focus on the subject of the question. Focus on the parents' request, which will direct you to option 3. Review the normal grieving process if you had difficulty with this question.

Level of Cognitive Ability: Comprehension
Client Needs: Psychosocial Integrity
Integrated Process: Nursing Process/Assessment
Content Area: Maternity/Postpartum

References
Murray, S., & McKinney, E. (2006). *Foundations of maternal-newborn nursing* (4th ed., pp. 24-25, 610-612). Philadelphia: Saunders.
Potter, P., & Perry, A. (2005). *Fundamentals of nursing* (6th ed., p. 437). St. Louis: Mosby.

1272. A school nurse is teaching a class of high school students about the risk of sexually transmitted infections (STIs). What opening statement will best encourage participation within the group?

 1 "Please feel free to share your personal experiences with the group."

 2 "At the end of the class, condoms will be distributed to everyone in class."

 3 "Our goal today is to describe ways to prevent acquiring a sexually transmitted infection."

 4 "The topic today is very personal. For this reason, anything shared with the group will remain confidential."

Level of Cognitive Ability: Application
Client Needs: Psychosocial Integrity
Integrated Process: Communication and Documentation
Content Area: Child Health

Answer: 4
Rationale: Option 4 identifies the rules for confidentiality, which will help to develop trust for sharing sensitive issues with the group. Option 1 provides no protection of confidentiality. Option 2 may be an incentive for those attending to stay, but participation is not required to get the reward. Option 3 does not foster trust, especially among those students who may already have an STI.

Test-Taking Strategy: Focus on the subjects of confidentiality, trust building, and sharing. Option 4 is the only option that addresses the subject of confidentiality. Review the concepts related to group process if you had difficulty with this question.

Reference
Hockenberry, M., Wilson, D., & Winkelstein, M. (2005). *Wong's essentials of pediatric nursing* (7th ed., pp. 106-107, 529). St. Louis: Mosby.

ALTERNATE ITEM FORMATS

1273. An emergency department nurse is caring for a female client who is in the acute phase of rape trauma syndrome. Which nursing interventions apply to the care of the client? Select all that apply.

 ☐ 1 Assess the degree of injury sustained during the rape.

 ☐ 2 Encourage the client to talk about what she did to cause the rape.

 ☐ 3 Obtain the client's written permission for examination and treatment.

 ☐ 4 Inform the client that she needs to press charges if the offender is caught.

 ☐ 5 Leave the client alone so that she will feel more comfortable crying and expressing sorrow.

 ☐ 6 Explain to the client that her responses are normal and that they may continue for weeks after the rape.

Answers: 1, 3, 6
Rationale: Rape trauma syndrome is the acute or immediate phase of psychological disorganization and the long-term process of reorganization that occurs as a result of attempted or actual assault. During the acute phase, which occurs immediately after the assault, emergency assessment and treatment are provided, and forensic evidence is collected. The nurse would always assess the degree of injury sustained during the rape and immediately treat any life-threatening injury. The client should not be left alone at this time and should be provided with calm and supportive interventions. Encouraging the client to talk about the cause of the rape is inappropriate. The nurse needs to encourage the client to talk about any mixed feelings that she may have and remind the client that she is in no way responsible for the rape. The nurse would obtain the client's written permission for examination and treatment. This is necessary, because two types of specimens will be collected. One part of the specimen will be sent to the laboratory for evaluation, and another part will be sent to a forensic laboratory and will be considered evidence in the event that the offender is caught and the client presses charges. The decision to press charges is made by the client, and the nurse needs to support the client in the decision-making process. Sexual assault is the ultimate invasion of privacy and safety. The nurse needs to explain to the client that her emotional responses to the attack are normal and that they may continue for weeks after the rape.

Level of Cognitive Ability: Application
Client Needs: Psychosocial Integrity
Integrated Process: Caring
Content Area: Mental Health

Test-Taking Strategy: Read each intervention carefully. Use the principles of a therapeutic nurse–client relationship and ethical and legal guidelines to select the correct interventions. Review the principles and guidelines for care of the rape victim if you had difficulty with this question.

Reference
Varcarolis, E., Carson, V., & Shoemaker, N. (2006). *Foundations of psychiatric mental health nursing* (5th ed., p. 533). Philadelphia: Saunders.

1274. A client is experiencing acute alcohol withdrawal, and 7.5 mg of diazepam (Valium) intravenously has been prescribed. The medication bottle indicates that there are 5 mg per milliliter. The nurse draws how many milliliters into the syringe to administer the correct dose?

Answer: _____ mL

Level of Cognitive Ability: Application
Client Needs: Psychosocial Integrity
Integrated Process: Nursing Process/
  Implementation
Content Area: Pharmacology

Answer: 1.5
Rationale: Use the following formula for calculating medication dosages:

$$\frac{\text{Desired}}{\text{Available}} \times \text{Volume} = \text{mL per dose}$$

$$\frac{7.5 \text{ mg}}{5 \text{ mg}} \times 1 \text{ mL} = 1.5 \text{ mL}$$

Test-Taking Strategy: Identify what the question is asking. In this case, the question asks for the number of milliliters per dose. Set up the formula knowing that the desired dose is 7.5 mg and that the available dose is 5 mg per 1 mL. Review medication calculations if you had difficulty with this question.

References
Hodgson, B., & Kizior, R. (2008). *Saunders nursing drug handbook 2008* (p. 350). Philadelphia: Saunders.
Kee, J. & Marshall, S. (2004). *Clinical calculations: With applications to general and specialty areas* (4th ed., pp. 80-81, 180). Philadelphia: Saunders.

1275. A male client who is discharged to home is occasionally forgetful about medication, exercise, and diet instructions. He needs daily dressing changes for a small leg ulcer, and he requires assistance with activities of daily living (ADLs) as a result of deconditioning. Which service(s) should the nurse request for this client in the home? Select all that apply.
☐ **1** Dietitian
☐ **2** Home health aide
☐ **3** Physical therapist
☐ **4** Skilled nursing care
☐ **5** Wound care specialist
☐ **6** Occupational therapist

Level of Cognitive Ability: Application
Client Needs: Psychosocial Integrity
Integrated Process: Nursing Process/Planning
Content Area: Fundamental Skills

Answers: 2, 3, 4
Rationale: This client needs help with self-care and disease management, so the nurse requests skilled nursing care to manage the dressing, diet, and medications; a home health aide to assist with ADLs; and a physical therapist to increase endurance, flexibility, and strength. Although the client is forgetful, dietary services are not indicated, because the client's dietary needs are related more to cognitive impairment than to a knowledge deficit. A wound care specialist assesses and evaluates the type of care needed for wound care and healing, but there is no indication that this service is needed. The occupational therapist helps clients to adapt to physical handicaps through new vocational skills and adaptive techniques for ADLs.

Test-Taking Strategy: Use the process of elimination, and focus on the client's needs as identified by the question. Recalling the role of each of these health care team members and focusing on the client's needs will direct you to options 2, 3, and 4. Review the roles of these health care team members if you had difficulty with this question.

Reference

Potter, P., & Perry, A. (2005). *Fundamentals of nursing* (6th ed., p. 36). St. Louis: Mosby.

REFERENCES

Ackley, B., & Ladwig, G. (2006). *Nursing diagnosis handbook: A guide for planning care* (7th ed.). St. Louis: Mosby.

Black, J., & Hawks, J. (2005). *Medical-surgical nursing: Clinical management for positive outcomes* (7th ed.). Philadelphia: Saunders.

Chernecky, C., & Berger, B. (2008). *Laboratory tests and diagnostic procedures* (5th ed.). Philadelphia: Saunders.

Giger, J., & Davidhizar, R. (2004). *Transcultural nursing* (5th ed.). St. Louis: Mosby.

Hockenberry, M., & Wilson, D. (2007). *Nursing care of infants and children* (8th ed.). St. Louis: Mosby.

Hockenberry, M., Wilson, D., & Winkelstein, M. (2005). *Wong's essentials of pediatric nursing* (7th ed.). St. Louis: Mosby.

Hodgson, B., & Kizior, R. (2007). *Saunders nursing drug handbook 2007.* Philadelphia: Saunders.

Hodgson, B., & Kizior, R. (2008). *Saunders nursing drug handbook 2008.* Philadelphia: Saunders.

Huber, D. (2006). *Leadership and nursing care management* (3rd ed.). Philadelphia: Saunders.

Ignatavicius, D., & Workman, M. (2006). *Medical-surgical nursing: Critical thinking for collaborative care* (5th ed.). Philadelphia: Saunders.

Kee, J., & Marshall, S. (2004). *Clinical calculations: With applications to general and specialty areas* (4th ed.). Philadelphia: Saunders.

Lehne, R. (2007). *Pharmacology for nursing care* (6th ed.). Philadelphia: Saunders.

Lewis, S., Heitkemper, M., Dirksen, S., O'Brien, P., & Bucher, L. (2007). *Medical-surgical nursing: Assessment and management of clinical problems* (7th ed.). St. Louis: Mosby.

McKinney, E., James, S., Murray, S., & Ashwill, J. (2005). *Maternal-child nursing* (2nd ed.). St. Louis: Saunders.

Monahan, F., Sands, J., Neighbors, M., Marek, J., & Green, C. (2007). *Phipps' medical-surgical nursing: Health and illness perspectives* (8th ed.). St. Louis: Mosby.

Murray, S., & McKinney, E. (2006). *Foundations of maternal-newborn nursing* (4th ed.). Philadelphia: Saunders.

National Council of State Boards of Nursing (Eds.). (2007). *2007 NCLEX-RN® Detailed Test Plan.* Chicago: Author.

Pagana, K., & Pagana, T. (2005). *Mosby's diagnostic and laboratory test reference* (7th ed.). St. Louis: Mosby.

Perry, A., & Potter, P. (2006). *Clinical nursing skills & techniques* (6th ed.). St. Louis: Mosby.

Potter, P., & Perry, A. (2005). *Fundamentals of nursing* (6th ed.). St. Louis: Mosby.

Skidmore-Roth, L. (2005). *Mosby's drug guide for nurses* (6th ed.). St. Louis: Mosby.

Skidmore-Roth, L. (2007). *2007 Mosby's nursing drug reference* (20th ed.). St. Louis: Mosby.

Skidmore-Roth, L. (2008). *Mosby's nursing drug reference* (21st ed.). St. Louis: Mosby.

Stuart, G., & Laraia, M. (2005). *Principles and practice of psychiatric nursing* (8th ed.). St. Louis: Mosby.

Varcarolis, E., Carson, V., & Shoemaker, N. (2006). *Foundations of psychiatric mental health nursing* (5th ed.). Philadelphia: Saunders.

Wong, D., Hockenberry, M., Perry, S., Lowdermilk, D., & Wilson, D. (2006). *Maternal-child nursing care* (3rd ed.). St. Louis: Mosby.

Integrated Processes

Integrated Processes and the NCLEX-RN® Test Plan

INTEGRATED PROCESSES

In the new test plan implemented in April 2007, the National Council of State Boards of Nursing (NCSBN) identified a test plan framework based on Client Needs. This framework was selected on the basis of the analysis of the findings in a practice analysis study of newly licensed registered nurses in the United States. This study identified the nursing activities performed by entry-level nurses across all settings for all clients. The NCSBN identified four major categories of Client Needs. These categories—Safe and Effective Care Environment, Health Promotion and Maintenance, Psychosocial Integrity, and Physiological Integrity—are described in Chapter 6.

The 2007 NCLEX-RN test plan also identifies four processes that are fundamental to the practice of nursing. These processes are integrated throughout the four major categories of Client Needs. The test plan for NCLEX-RN identifies these components as Integrated Processes, and they are as follows: Caring, Communication and Documentation, Teaching and Learning, and Nursing Process (Box 11-1).

CARING

Caring is the essence of nursing, and it is basic to any helping relationship. Caring is central to every encounter that a nurse may have with a client. Through caring, the nurse humanizes the client. Treating the client with respect and dignity is a true expression of caring. In the technological environment of health care, emphasizing the client's individuality counteracts any potential process of depersonalization. Caring is an Integrated Process of the test plan for NCLEX-RN. This means that this concept is nuclear to all Client Needs components of the test plan.

For the NCLEX-RN, the concept of caring is primary. It is very easy to become involved with looking at a question from a technological viewpoint. However, the concept of caring needs to be addressed when reading a test question and when selecting an option. Always address the client's feelings and provide support. Remember that this examination is all about nursing and that nursing is caring (Box 11-2)!

COMMUNICATION AND DOCUMENTATION

The process of communication occurs as a nurse interacts either verbally or nonverbally with a client. Therapeutic communication techniques are key to an effective nurse-client relationship. Communication-type test questions are integrated throughout the NCLEX-RN test plan, and they may address a client situation in any health care setting.

When answering a question on the NCLEX-RN, the use of therapeutic communication techniques indicates a correct option, and the use of nontherapeutic communication techniques indicates an incorrect option. In additional, some communication-type questions may focus on psychosocial issues or issues related to client anxiety, fears, or concerns. For communication-type questions, always focus on the client's feelings first. If an option reflects the client's feelings, anxiety, or concerns, select that option.

Box 11-1 ▲ INTEGRATED PROCESSES

Caring
Communication and Documentation
Teaching and Learning
Nursing Process

Documentation is a critical component of a nurse's responsibilities. The process of documentation serves many purposes; it provides a comprehensive representation of the client's health status and the care given by all members of the health care team. There are many methods of documentation, but the responsibilities surrounding this practice remain the same.

When answering a question on the NCLEX-RN related to documentation, consider the ethical and legal responsibilities related to documentation and the specific guidelines related to both narrative and computerized documentation systems (Box 11-3).

TEACHING AND LEARNING

Client and family education is a primary nursing responsibility. The NCSBN describes this process as facilitating the acquisition of knowledge, skills, and attitudes that lead to a change in behavior.

The principles related to the teaching and learning process are used when the nurse functions in the role of a teacher. The nurse needs to remember that the assessment of the client's readiness and motivation to learn is the initial step in the teaching and learning process.

When answering a question on the NCLEX-RN related to the teaching and learning process, use the principles related to teaching and learning theory. If a test question addresses client education, remember that client motivation and readiness to learn is the first priority (Box 11-4).

NURSING PROCESS

The steps of the nursing process provide a systematic and organized method of problem solving and providing care to clients. These steps include assessment, analysis, planning, implementation, and evaluation (Box 11-5).

Assessment

Assessment is the first step of the nursing process. It involves a systematic method of collecting data about a client to identify actual and potential client health problems and to establish a database. The database provides the foundation for the remaining steps of the nursing process; therefore, a thorough and adequate database is essential. Data collection begins with the first contact with the client. During all successive contacts, the nurse continues to collect information that is significant and relevant to the needs of that client.

During the assessment process, the nurse collects data about the client from a variety of sources. The client is the primary source of data. Family members and significant others are secondary sources of assessment data, and these sources may supplement or verify the information provided by the client. Data may also be obtained from the client's record through the medical history, laboratory results, and diagnostic reports. Medical records from previous admissions may provide additional information about the client. The nurse may also obtain information through consultation with other health care team members who have had contact with the client.

Box 11-2 ▲ CARING

A woman comes into the emergency department in a severe state of anxiety after a car accident. The priority nursing intervention at this time would be to:
  1 Remain with the client.
  2 Put the client in a quiet room.
  3 Teach the client deep-breathing exercises.
  4 Encourage the client to talk about her feelings and concerns.

Level of Cognitive Ability: Application
Client Needs: Psychosocial Integrity
Integrated Process: Caring
Content Area: Mental Health

Answer: 1
Rationale: If the client is left alone with severe anxiety, she may feel abandoned and become overwhelmed. Placing the client in a quiet room is also indicated, but the nurse must stay with the client. It is not possible to teach the client deep-breathing or relaxation exercises until the anxiety decreases. Encouraging the client to discuss her concerns and feelings would not take place until the anxiety has decreased.

Test-Taking Strategy: Note the strategic words "severe state of anxiety." Because the anxiety state is severe, eliminate options 3 and 4. From the remaining options, consider the word "priority" in the question. This should direct you to option 1. Review the care of the client with severe anxiety if you had difficulty with this question.

Reference
Varcarolis, E., Carson, V., & Shoemaker, N. (2006). *Foundations of psychiatric mental health nursing* (5th ed., p. 216). Philadelphia: Saunders.

Box 11-3 ▲ COMMUNICATION AND DOCUMENTATION

COMMUNICATION

A client with type 2 diabetes mellitus was recently hospitalized for hyperglycemic hyperosmolar nonketotic syndrome (HHNS). Upon discharge from the hospital, the client expresses concerns about the recurrence of HHNS. The nurse makes which statement to the client?
  1 "I'm sure this won't happen again."
  2 "Don't worry. Your family will help you."
  3 "I think you might need to go to the nursing home."
  4 "You have concerns about the treatment of your condition?"

Level of Cognitive Ability: Application
Client Needs: Psychosocial Integrity
Integrated Process: Communication and Documentation
Content Area: Adult Health/Endocrine

Answer: 4
Rationale: The nurse should provide time and listen to the client's concerns. In option 4, the nurse is attempting to clarify the client's feelings. Option 1 and 2 provide inappropriate false hope. Additionally, the nurse should not tell the client to not worry. Option 3 is not an appropriate nursing response, because it disregards the client's concerns and gives advice.

Test-Taking Strategy: Use therapeutic communication techniques. Remembering to always address the client's feelings will direct you to option 4. Review therapeutic communication techniques if you had difficulty with this question.

References
Ignatavicius, D., & Workman, M. (2006). *Medical-surgical nursing: Critical thinking for collaborative care* (5th ed., pp. 1545-1546). Philadelphia: Saunders.
Potter, P., & Perry, A. (2005). *Fundamentals of nursing* (6th ed., p. 437). St. Louis: Mosby.

DOCUMENTATION

A client calls out for help. The nurse hurries into the client's room. The client is lying on the floor. The nurse performs a thorough assessment, assists the client back into the bed, notifies the physician of the incident, and completes an incident report. Which of the following would the nurse document on the incident report?
  1 The client fell out of bed.
  2 The client climbed over the side rails.
  3 The client was found lying on the floor.
  4 The client was restless and got out of bed.

Level of Cognitive Ability: Application
Client Needs: Safe and Effective Care Environment
Integrated Process: Communication and Documentation
Content Area: Fundamental Skills

Answer: 3
Rationale: The incident report should contain the client's name, age, and diagnosis. It should contain a factual description of the incident, any injuries experienced by those involved, and the outcome of the situation. Option 3 is the only option that describes the facts as observed by the nurse. Options 1, 2, and 4 are interpretations of the situation and are not factual data as observed by the nurse.

Test-Taking Strategy: Use general documentation guidelines and principles to answer the question. Remember to focus on factual information when documenting and to avoid including interpretations. This will direct you to option 3. Review the documentation principles related to incident reports if you had difficulty with this question.

Reference
Potter, P., & Perry, A. (2005). *Fundamentals of nursing* (6th ed, pp. 419, 497). St. Louis: Mosby.

Box 11-4 ▲ TEACHING AND LEARNING

A nurse is giving dietary instructions to a client who has been prescribed cyclosporine (Sandimmune). Which of the following food items would the nurse instruct the client to avoid?
  1 Red meats
  2 Orange juice
  3 Grapefruit juice
  4 Green leafy vegetables

Level of Cognitive Ability: Application
Client Needs: Physiological Integrity
Integrated Process: Teaching and Learning
Content Area: Pharmacology

Answer: 3
Rationale: A compound in grapefruit juice inhibits the metabolism of cyclosporine. Thus, drinking grapefruit juice can raise cyclosporine levels by 50% to 100%, greatly increasing the risk of toxicity. The foods in options 1, 2, and 4 are acceptable to consume.

Test-Taking Strategy: Note the strategic word "avoid." Recalling the substances that inhibit the metabolism of cyclosporine, such as grapefruit juice, will direct you to option 3. Review cyclosporine if you had difficulty with this question.

Reference
Hodgson, B., & Kizior, R. (2008). *Saunders nursing drug handbook 2008* (pp. 303-305). Philadelphia: Saunders.

A thorough database is obtained with the use of a health history and a physical assessment. The information collected by the nurse includes both subjective and objective data. Subjective data include the information that the client states. Objective data are the observable, measurable pieces of information about the client, including measurements such as vital signs and laboratory findings as well as information obtained by observing the client. Objective data also include clinical manifestations, such as the signs and symptoms of an illness or disease.

The process of assessment additionally consists of confirming and verifying client data, communicating information obtained through the assessment process, and documenting assessment findings in a thorough and accurate manner.

On the NCLEX-RN, remember that assessment is the first step of the nursing process. When answering these types of questions, focus on the data in the question, and select the option that addresses an assessment action. In addition, use the skills of prioritizing and the ABCs—airway, breathing, and circulation—to answer the question (Box 11-6).

Box 11-5 ▲ STEPS OF THE NURSING PROCESS

Assessment
Analysis
Planning
Implementation
Evaluation

Analysis

Analysis is the second step of the nursing process. During this step, the nurse focuses on the data gathered during the assessment process and identifies actual or potential health care needs, problems, or both. During this process, the nurse summarizes and interprets the assessment data, organizes and validates the data, and determines the need for additional data. Client assessment data are compared with the normal expected findings and behaviors for the client's age, education, and cultural background. The nurse then draws conclusions regarding the client's unique needs and health care risks or problems.

Client health problems are categorized as at risk problems that require prevention or as actual problems that are being managed or that require interventions. The nurse reports the results of the analysis to the appropriate members of the health care team and documents the client's unique health care problems, needs, or both.

On the NCLEX-RN, questions that address the process of analysis are difficult questions, because they require an understanding of the principles of physiological responses as well as an interpretation of the data on the basis of assessment findings. Analysis questions require critical thinking and determining the rationale for therapeutic interventions that may be addressed in the case event. These questions may address the formulation of a nursing diagnosis and the communication and documentation of the results of the process of analysis (Box 11-7).

Box 11-6 ▲ NURSING PROCESS: ASSESSMENT

A nurse is admitting a child with a diagnosis of irritable bowel syndrome to the hospital. Which data would the nurse expect to obtain during the assessment of the child?

  1 Reports of frothy diarrhea
  2 Reports of foul-smelling ribbon stools
  3 Reports of profuse, watery diarrhea and vomiting
  4 Reports of diffuse abdominal pain unrelated to meals or activity

Level of Cognitive Ability: Analysis
Client Needs: Physiological Integrity
Integrated Process: Nursing Process/
  Assessment
Content Area: Child Health

Answer: 4
Rationale: Irritable bowel syndrome causes diffuse abdominal pain unrelated to meals or activity. Alternating constipation and diarrhea with the presence of undigested food and mucus in the stools may also be noted. Option 1 is a clinical manifestation of lactose intolerance. Option 2 is a clinical manifestation of Hirschsprung's disease. Option 3 is a clinical manifestation of celiac disease.

Test-Taking Strategy: Focus on the child's diagnosis. Noting the name of the syndrome will direct you to option 4, because you would expect abdominal pain to occur in clients with this disorder. Review the clinical manifestations associated with irritable bowel syndrome if you had difficulty with this question.

References
Hockenberry, M., & Wilson, D. (2007). *Nursing care of infants and children* (8th ed., p. 1403). St. Louis: Mosby.
McKinney, E., James, S., Murray, S., & Ashwill, J. (2005). *Maternal-child nursing* (2nd ed., p. 1125). St. Louis: Saunders.

Planning

Planning is the third step of the nursing process. This step involves the functions of setting priorities, determining goals of care, planning actions, collaborating with other health care team members, establishing evaluative criteria, and communicating the plan of care.

Setting priorities assists the nurse with organizing and planning care that solves the most urgent problems. Priorities may change as the client's level of wellness changes. Both actual and at risk problems should be considered when establishing priorities. Actual problems are usually more important than at risk problems. However, at risk problems may at times take precedence over actual problems.

After priorities are established, the client and the nurse mutually decide on the expected goals. The selected goals serve as a guide for the selection of nursing interventions and for determining the criteria for evaluation. Before nursing actions are implemented, mechanisms to determine goal achievement and the effectiveness of nursing interventions are established. Unless criteria have been predetermined, it is difficult to know whether the goal has been achieved or if the problem has been resolved.

It is important for the nurse to both identify health or social resources available to the client and to collaborate with other health care team members when planning the delivery of care. The nurse needs to communicate the plan of care, review the plan of care with the client, and document the plan of care thoroughly and accurately.

When answering questions on the NCLEX-RN, remember that this is a nursing examination. In addition, remember that actual problems are usually more important than at risk problems and that physiological needs are usually the priority (Box 11-8).

Box 11-7 ▲ NURSING PROCESS: ANALYSIS

A client is admitted to the cardiac unit and placed on telemetry. A nurse reviews the client's laboratory values and notes that the client's potassium level is 6.3 mEq/L. When analyzing the cardiac rhythm, the nurse would expect to note which electrocardiogram (ECG) finding?

  1 A sinus tachycardia with an extra U wave
  2 A sinus rhythm with a tall, peaked T wave
  3 A sinus rhythm with a depressed ST segment
  4 A sinus tachycardia with a prolonged QT interval

Level of Cognitive Ability: Analysis
Client Needs: Physiological Integrity
Integrated Process: Nursing Process/Analysis
Content Area: Adult Health/Cardiovascular

Answer: 2
Rationale: A potassium level of more than 5.1 mEq/L indicates hyperkalemia, which can be detected on ECG by the presence of a tall, peaked T wave. A U wave and a depressed ST segment are present with hypokalemia. A prolonged QT interval indicates hypocalcemia.

Test-Taking Strategy: In this question, it is necessary to know that the client is experiencing hyperkalemia as evidenced by the potassium level of 6.3 mEq/L. After this has been determined, it is necessary to know the ECG changes that occur with hyperkalemia: a tall, peaked T wave. Review the ECG changes noted in a client with hyperkalemia if you had difficulty with this question.

Reference
Ignatavicius, D., & Workman, M. (2006). *Medical-surgical nursing: Critical thinking for collaborative care* (5th ed., p. 232). Philadelphia: Saunders.

Box 11-8 ▲ NURSING PROCESS: PLANNING

A nurse is caring for a client with dementia who has a nursing diagnosis of Self-Care Deficit, feeding. The nurse plans for which appropriate goal for this client?

  1 Client will be free of hallucinations.
  2 Client will feed self with cueing within 24 hours.
  3 Client will be oriented to place by the time of discharge.
  4 Client will correctly identify objects in his or her room by the time of discharge.

Level of Cognitive Ability: Analysis
Client Needs: Physiological Integrity
Integrated Process: Nursing Process/Analysis
Content Area: Fundamental Skills

Answer: 2
Rationale: Option 2 identifies a goal that is directly related to the client's ability to care for him- or herself. Options 1, 3, and 4 are not related to the nursing diagnosis of Self-Care Deficit.

Test-Taking Strategy: Focus on the nursing diagnosis. Option 2 is the only option that addresses a physiological need. In addition, on the basis of Maslow's Hierarchy of Needs theory, physiological needs take precedence. This will direct you to option 2. Review the goals for a client with a nursing diagnosis of Self-Care Deficit if you had difficulty with this question.

Reference
Ackley, B., & Ladwig, G. (2006). *Nursing diagnosis handbook: A guide to planning care* (7th ed., p. 1025). St. Louis: Mosby.

Implementation

Implementation is the fourth step of the nursing process. It includes initiating and completing nursing actions that are required to accomplish defined goals. This step is the action phase that involves counseling, teaching, organizing and managing client care, providing care to achieve established goals, supervising and coordinating the delivery of client care, and communicating and documenting the nursing interventions and client responses.

During implementation, the nurse uses intellectual skills, interpersonal skills, and technical skills. Intellectual skills involve critical thinking, problem solving, and making judgments. Interpersonal skills involve the ability to communicate, listen, and convey compassion. Technical skills relate to the performance of treatments and procedures and to the use of necessary equipment when providing care to the client.

The nurse independently implements actions that include activities that do not require a physician's order. The nurse also implements actions collaboratively on the basis of the physician's orders. Sound nursing judgment and working with other health care members is incorporated into the process of implementation. The implementation step concludes when the nurse's actions are completed and when these actions, including their effects and the client's response, are communicated and documented.

The NCLEX-RN is an examination about nursing, so focus on the nursing action rather than the medical action, unless the question is asking what prescribed medical action is anticipated (Box 11-9).

Evaluation

Evaluation is the fifth and final step of the nursing process. The process of evaluation identifies the degree to which the nursing diagnoses, plans for care, and interventions have been successful.

Although evaluation is the final step of the nursing process, it is an ongoing and integral component of each step. The process of data collection and assessment is reviewed to determine if sufficient information was obtained and whether the information obtained was specific and appropriate. The nursing diagnoses are evaluated for accuracy and completeness on the basis of the client's specific needs. The plan and expected outcomes are examined to determine whether they are realistic, achievable, measurable, and effective. Interventions are examined to determine their effectiveness for achieving the expected outcomes.

Because evaluation is an ongoing process, it is vital to all steps of the nursing process. It is the continuous process of comparing actual outcomes with the expected outcomes of care, and it provides the means for determining the need to modify the plan of care. Inherent in this step of the nursing process is the communication of evaluation findings and the process of documenting the client's response to treatment, care, and teaching.

Evaluation-type questions on the NCLEX-RN may be written to address a client's response to treatment measures or to determine a client's understanding of the prescribed treatment measures (Box 11-10).

Box 11-9 ▲ NURSING PROCESS: IMPLEMENTATION

A client with heart failure is receiving furosemide (Lasix) and digoxin (Lanoxin) daily. When the nurse enters the room to administer the morning doses, the client complains of anorexia, nausea, and yellow vision. Which of the following should the nurse do first?

1 Contact the physician.
2 Administer the medications.
3 Check the morning serum digoxin level.
4 Check the morning serum potassium level.

Level of Cognitive Ability: Application
Client Needs: Physiological Integrity
Integrated Process: Nursing Process/
  Implementation
Content Area: Adult Health/Cardiovascular

Answer: 3
Rationale: The nurse should check the result of the digoxin level that was drawn, because the client's symptoms are compatible with digoxin toxicity. A low potassium level may contribute to digoxin toxicity, so checking the serum potassium level may give useful additional information, but the digoxin level should be checked first. The medications should be withheld until both levels are known. If the digoxin level is elevated or if the potassium level is not within the normal range, then the physician should be notified. If the morning digoxin level is within the therapeutic range, then the client's complaints are unrelated to the digoxin.

Test-Taking Strategy: Note the strategic word "first." This will assist you with determining that the nurse's action is to further investigate the cause of the client's complaints. Recalling the manifestations of digoxin toxicity and noting the relationship of the name of the medication and option 3 will direct you to the correct option. Review the nursing interventions if digoxin toxicity is suspected if you had difficulty with this question.

References
Hodgson, B., & Kizior, R. (2008). *Saunders nursing drug handbook 2008* (pp. 362-363). Philadelphia: Saunders.
Ignatavicius, D., & Workman, M. (2006). *Medical-surgical nursing: Critical thinking for collaborative care* (5th ed., p. 762). Philadelphia: Saunders.

Box 11-10 ▲ NURSING PROCESS: EVALUATION

A client has been taking nadolol (Corgard) for the past month. Which finding would indicate a therapeutic effect of the medication?
 1 The client is afebrile.
 2 The client has clear breath sounds.
 3 The client reports no episodes of headache.
 4 The client has a blood pressure of 118/72 mm Hg.

Level of Cognitive Ability: Analysis
Client Needs: Physiological Integrity
Integrated Process: Nursing Process/ Evaluation
Content Area: Pharmacology

Answer: 4
Rationale: Nadolol is a β-adrenergic blocking agent that is used to treat hypertension. Therefore, a blood pressure within the normal range would indicate an effective response to the medication. Options 1, 2, and 3 are unrelated to the action of this medication.

Test-Taking Strategy: Focus on the strategic words "therapeutic effect." Remember that an evaluation-type question addresses a client's response to a treatment measure. In addition, prerecalling that medication names that end with *-lol* are β-blocking agents will direct you to option 4. Review the therapeutic effects of nadolol if you had difficulty with this question.

Reference
Hodgson, B., & Kizior, R. (2008). *Saunders nursing drug handbook 2008* (p. 805). Philadelphia: Saunders.

REFERENCES

Ackley, B., & Ladwig, G. (2006). *Nursing diagnosis handbook: A guide to planning care* (7th ed.). St. Louis: Mosby.

Hockenberry, M., & Wilson, D. (2007). *Nursing care of infants and children* (8th ed.). St. Louis: Mosby.

Hodgson, B., & Kizior, R. (2008). *Saunders nursing drug handbook 2008.* Philadelphia: Saunders.

Ignatavicius, D., & Workman, M. (2006). *Medical surgical nursing: Critical thinking for collaborative care* (5th ed.). Philadelphia: Saunders.

McKinney, E., James, S., Murray, S., & Ashwill, J. (2005). *Maternal-child nursing* (2nd ed.). St. Louis: Saunders.

National Council of State Boards of Nursing (Eds.). (2007). *2007 NCLEX-RN® detailed test plan.* Chicago: Author.

National Council of State Boards of Nursing. NCSBN Web Site: www.ncsbn.org. Accessed May 12, 2008.

Potter, P., & Perry, A. (2005). *Fundamentals of nursing* (6th ed.). St. Louis: Mosby.

Stuart, G., & Laraia, M. (2005). *Principles and practice of psychiatric nursing* (8th ed.). St. Louis: Mosby.

Varcarolis, E., Carson, V., & Shoemaker, N. (2006). *Foundations of psychiatric mental health nursing* (5th ed.). Philadelphia: Saunders.

Integrated Processes

CARING

1276. Family members of a Cuban-American client who is terminally ill are visibly upset and crying loudly in the hallways. What is the best intervention for the nurse to implement?

1 Close the doors of the other clients' rooms.
2 Direct the family members to the chapel.
3 Provide a private room for the family and client.
4 Ask the family to quiet down when in the hallways.

Level of Cognitive Ability: Application
Client Needs: Psychosocial Integrity
Integrated Process: Caring
Content Area: Fundamental Skills

Answer: 3

Rationale: In the Cuban-American culture, loud crying and other physical manifestations of grief are acceptable. The nurse provides culturally sensitive care and a caring approach to the client and family by providing a private room for grieving while still fulfilling the duty owed to the other clients. The nurse can direct the family to the chapel upon their request. Closing the doors to other clients' rooms can increase the risk of client injury and annoyance. Asking the grieving family to be considerate can be misinterpreted as being disrespectful to their culture.

Test-Taking Strategy: Focus on the client and the family who are Cuban Americans. Recall the characteristics of this culture, the importance of cultural sensitivity, and the duty owed to all clients, and use the process of elimination. This will direct you to option 3. Review the characteristics of the Cuban-American culture if you had difficulty with this question.

References
Giger, J., & Davidhizar, R. (2004). *Transcultural nursing* (5th ed., p. 623). St. Louis: Mosby.
Lewis, S., Heitkemper, M., Dirksen, S., O'Brien, P., & Bucher, L. (2007). *Medical-surgical nursing: Assessment and management of clinical problems* (7th ed., p. 155). St. Louis: Mosby.

1277. An older female client who has end-stage cancer is admitted to a long-term care facility from her home. Which intervention should the nurse implement to address the client's psychosocial needs?

1 Administer total care for the client.
2 Engage the client in social activities.
3 Allow the client to verbalize feelings.
4 Provide pain medication every 4 hours.

Level of Cognitive Ability: Application
Client Needs: Psychosocial Integrity
Integrated Process: Caring
Content Area: Fundamental Skills

Answer: 3
Rationale: The client is experiencing loss from two life-changing experiences: her poor prognosis and the loss of control over the environment, independence, and privacy that accompanies admission to a long-term care facility. To meet the client's psychosocial needs, the nurse promotes a therapeutic relationship and allows the client to verbalize her feelings. Options 1 and 4 help to manage physical needs. Although total care may be necessary, it does not necessarily facilitate a therapeutic relationship. Providing pain medication is indicated as part of effective pain management; however, this can interfere with therapeutic communication if the client is too sedated. Engaging the client in social activities is unlikely to effectively meet the client's psychosocial needs relating to loss; it is more likely to help diminish loneliness and isolation.

Test-Taking Strategy: Focus on the strategic words "psychosocial needs." Eliminate options 1 and 4 first, because these options deal with physiological needs. From the remaining options, recall that the client's feelings should be addressed first. This will direct you to option 3. Review the care of the client experiencing loss if you had difficulty with this question.

References
Meiner, S., & Leuckenotte, A. (2006). *Gerontologic nursing* (3rd ed, pp. 352-353). St. Louis: Mosby.
Potter, P., & Perry, A. (2005). *Fundamentals of nursing* (6th ed., pp. 573, 605). St. Louis: Mosby.

1278. A male client who has diabetes mellitus requires the amputation of a leg to preserve tissue and his life. The client is very upset and states, "This is the doctor's fault! I did everything that I was told to do!" The nurse responds to the client's statement by:

1 Asking the client to list all previous health care
2 Allowing the client to use this coping mechanism
3 Notifying the agency's risk management department
4 Helping the client to consider alternatives to treatment

Level of Cognitive Ability: Application
Client Needs: Psychosocial Integrity
Integrated Process: Caring
Content Area: Fundamental Skills

Answer: 2
Rationale: Anger is a stage in the grieving process and an expected response to impending loss. Usually a client directs the anger toward him- or herself, God or another spiritual being, or the caregivers; thus far the client's behavior demonstrates effective coping. Analyzing previous health care and alternative treatment options is likely to interfere with effective coping, and it can delay life-saving treatment. Notifying the risk management department is premature, especially since the client has said nothing about legal action.

Test-Taking Strategy: Focus on the data provided in the question, and use the process of elimination to choose a suitable nursing response to the client. Noting that the client is blaming the doctor and knowledge of the stages of grief associated with loss will direct you to option 2. Review the stages of grief and expected client expressions if you had difficulty with this question.

Reference
Black, J., & Hawks, J. (2005). *Medical-surgical nursing: Clinical management for positive outcomes* (7th ed., p. 1524). Philadelphia: Saunders.

1279. The nurse has an established relation-ship with the family of a client whose death is imminent. Which should the nurse provide to help the family deal with this experience?
1 Effective coping mechanisms
2 Requested information and help
3 Spiritual leadership and guidance
4 Individual family member privacy

Level of Cognitive Ability: Application
Client Needs: Psychosocial Integrity
Integrated Process: Caring
Content Area: Fundamental Skills

Answer: 2
Rationale: Maintaining effective and open communication among family members affected by death and grief is important to facili-tate decision making and effective coping. The nurse maintains and enhances communication and preserves the family's sense of self-direction and control by providing information and resources for decision making. However, the nurse cannot provide coping mechanisms for family members, because coping mechanisms directed by the nurse are unlikely to be as effective as the methods that the individuals choose for themselves. In addition, the nurse's role does not include making decisions for the client or family or leading spiritual practices. Isolating individuals is likely to interfere with communication.

Test-Taking Strategy: Recall the concepts related to therapeutic communication and the role of the nurse in grieving and loss, and then use the process of elimination to choose suitable nursing assistance for the family. Review the therapeutic techniques for individuals in crisis if you had difficulty with this question.

Reference
Black, J., & Hawks, J. (2005). *Medical-surgical nursing: Clinical management for positive outcomes* (7th ed., p. 500). Philadelphia: Saunders.

1280. A client is dead on arrival (DOA) to the emergency department, and the family of the client states that they do not want an autopsy. Which statement should the nurse use in response to the family?
1 "I will notify the medical examiner of your request."
2 "Autopsies are mandatory for clients who are DOA."
3 "Federal law requires autopsies for clients who are DOA."
4 "The medical examiner makes the decision about autopsies."

Level of Cognitive Ability: Application
Client Needs: Safe and Effective Care Environment
Integrated Process: Caring
Content Area: Fundamental Skills

Answer: 1
Rationale: The nurse should notify the medical examiner or the coroner when a family wishes to avoid having an autopsy on a deceased family member. Many states require an autopsy in specific circumstances, including sudden death, a suspicious death, and death within 24 hours of admission to the hospital. Autopsy is not a requirement under federal law. Depending on the state, it is not mandatory for every client who is DOA to have an autopsy.

Test-Taking Strategy: Use your knowledge regarding the laws and issues surrounding autopsy and therapeutic communica-tion techniques to answer the question. Eliminate options 2 and 3, because these statements are not accurate. From the remaining options, option 1 is the most therapeutic and caring response to the family. Review the issues and laws surrounding autopsies if you had difficulty with this question.

Reference
Potter, P., & Perry, A. (2005). *Fundamentals of nursing* (6th ed., pp. 412, 589). St. Louis: Mosby.

1281. The nurse prepares an older client who lives alone for discharge to home. The client states, "This is confusing. How am I going to take care of myself?" Which should the nurse implement before discharge to ensure effective health maintenance for the client at home?

1 Request a home health care referral from the provider.
2 Notify a family member that the client needs assistance.
3 Ask the provider to delay discharge for additional teaching.
4 Advise social services to provide follow-up communication.

Level of Cognitive Ability: Application
Client Needs: Safe and Effective Care Environment
Integrated Process: Caring
Content Area: Fundamental Skills

Answer: 1
Rationale: With managed care demanding earlier hospital discharges, clients return home with more problems and more serious problems. To make a successful transition to self-care at home for effective health maintenance, clients potentially require support from a home health agency until they can function independently. Engaging a family member in the client's transition to home does not guarantee effective health maintenance for the client; in addition, there may not be a family member available. The provider may not be able to delay the discharge for client teaching when those services can be provided in the home. Social services cannot assist with postdischarge surveillance of the client's health care, because that is not their area of expertise or responsibility.

Test-Taking Strategy: Focus on the subject of effective health maintenance, and remember the client's concern. Use the process of elimination, and note that option 1 is the only action that will ensure that the client receives the necessary assistance until independence is achieved. Review home-care support services if you had difficulty with this question.

References
Ignatavicius, D., & Workman, M. (2006). *Medical-surgical nursing: Critical thinking for collaborative care* (5th ed., pp. 19-20). Philadelphia: Saunders.
Potter, P., & Perry, A. (2005). *Fundamentals of nursing* (6th ed., pp. 35-36). St. Louis: Mosby.

1282. The nurse is interacting with the family of a client who is unconscious as a result of a head injury. Which approach should the nurse use to help the family cope with this situation?

1 Discourage the family from touching the client.
2 Explain equipment and procedures on an ongoing basis.
3 Encourage the family to not give in to their feelings of grief.
4 Enforce adherence to visiting hours to ensure the client's rest.

Level of Cognitive Ability: Application
Client Needs: Psychosocial Integrity
Integrated Process: Caring
Content Area: Adult Health/Neurological

Answer: 2
Rationale: Families often need assistance to cope with the sudden severe illness of a loved one. The nurse should explain all equipment, treatments, and procedures, and he or she should supplement or reinforce the information given by the physician. The family should be encouraged to touch and speak to the client and to become involved in the client's care in some way if they are comfortable with doing so. The nurse should allow the family to stay with the client whenever possible. The nurse also encourages the family to eat properly and to obtain enough sleep to maintain their strength.

Test-Taking Strategy: Use therapeutic communication techniques to answer this question. Each of the incorrect options puts distance between the family and the client. Review therapeutic techniques that assist the family with dealing with a sudden illness if you had difficulty with this question.

References
Lewis, S., Heitkemper, M., Dirksen, S., O'Brien, P., & Bucher, L. (2007). *Medical-surgical nursing: Assessment and management of clinical problems* (7th ed., pp. 161-162). St. Louis: Mosby.
Potter, P., & Perry, A. (2005). *Fundamentals of nursing* (6th ed., pp. 103, 437). St. Louis: Mosby.

1283. The nurse admits a female client who has right-sided weakness, aphasia, and urinary incontinence. The woman's daughter states, "If this is a stroke, it's the kiss of death." The nurse responds to the family member by saying:

1 "You should not think like that."
2 "You feel your mother is dying?"
3 "These symptoms are reversible."
4 "A stroke is not the kiss of death."

Level of Cognitive Ability: Application
Client Needs: Psychosocial Integrity
Integrated Process: Caring
Content Area: Fundamental Skills

Answer: 2
Rationale: Option 2 allows the daughter to verbalize her feelings, to begin coping, and to adapt to what is happening. By restating, the nurse seeks clarification of the daughter's feelings and offers information that potentially helps ease some of the fears and concerns related to the client's condition and prognosis. Option 1 is a disapproving comment that is likely to interfere with communication. Option 3 is potentially misleading and offers false hope. The nurse could reflect back the statement in option 4 to the daughter to promote communication; as it stands, option 4 is a barrier to communication that puts the daughter's feelings on hold.

Test-Taking Strategy: Use the principles of therapeutic communication and the process of elimination. Option 2 is the only option that addresses the daughter's feelings. Review therapeutic communication techniques if you had difficulty with this question.

References
Ignatavicius, D., & Workman, M. (2006). *Medical-surgical nursing: Critical thinking for collaborative care* (5th ed., p. 1029). Philadelphia: Saunders.
Potter, P., & Perry, A. (2005). *Fundamentals of nursing* (6th ed., p. 437). St. Louis: Mosby.

1284. A female client and her infant have undergone testing for human immunodeficiency virus (HIV), and both clients were found to be positive. The news is devastating, and the mother is crying. The nurse determines that which intervention will meet the client's needs at this time?

1 Examining with the mother how she got HIV
2 Listening quietly while the mother talks and cries
3 Describing the progressive stages and treatments of HIV
4 Calling an HIV counselor and making an appointment for the mother and infant

Level of Cognitive Ability: Application
Client Needs: Psychosocial Integrity
Integrated Process: Caring
Content Area: Fundamental Skills

Answer: 2
Rationale: This client has just received devastating news and needs to have someone present with her as she begins to cope with this issue. The nurse needs to sit and actively listen while the mother talks and cries. Calling an HIV counselor may be helpful, but it is not what the client needs at this time. The other options are not appropriate for this stage of coping with the news that both she and her infant have HIV. Remember to address the client's feelings and to support the client. The nurse should sit, listen, and provide support, because this is the most caring intervention.

Test-Taking Strategy: Use therapeutic communication techniques, and remember to focus on the client's feelings. This will direct you to option 2. Review therapeutic communication techniques if you had difficulty with this question.

Reference
Potter, P., & Perry, A. (2005). *Fundamentals of nursing* (6th ed., pp. 103, 437). St. Louis: Mosby.

1285. The nurse cared for a client who died a few minutes ago. Which statement supports the nurse's belief that the client died with dignity?

1 A new nurse states that it is difficult to give that kind of care to a dying client.

2 The nurse gave increasing doses of pain medication to keep the client well sedated.

3 The provider recognizes that all of the orders were carried out and there were no questions.

4 The family thanks the nurse and states that the client was not in pain and was peaceful at the end.

Level of Cognitive Ability: Analysis
Client Needs: Psychosocial Integrity
Integrated Process: Caring
Content Area: Fundamental Skills

Answer: 4

Rationale: The family response is an external perception, and it is extremely important. Families derive a great deal of comfort from knowing that their loved one received the best care possible. Option 4 provides external validation that the client received comprehensive, quality care. Option 1 focuses on the feelings of a new nurse, who may be expressing his or her own anxiety. Option 2 reflects on only one aspect of the care of a dying client. Option 3 focuses on the provider's orders rather than client care.

Test-Taking Strategy: Use the process of elimination, and focus on the subject of whether the client died with dignity. The only option that addresses this subject is option 4. Review the concepts related to death and dying if you had difficulty with this question.

References
Black, J., & Hawks, J. (2005). *Medical-surgical nursing: Clinical management for positive outcomes* (7th ed., pp. 500-501). Philadelphia: Saunders.
Potter, P., & Perry, A. (2005). *Fundamentals of nursing* (6th ed., p. 576). St. Louis: Mosby.

1286. The family of a client with Parkinson's disease tells the nurse that the client is having difficulty adjusting to the disorder and that they do not know what to do to help. The nurse advises the family that which of the following would be therapeutic for assisting the client with coping with the disease?

1 Plan only a few activities for the client during the day.

2 Assist the client with activities of daily living as much as possible.

3 Cluster activities at the end of the day, when the client is restless and bored.

4 Encourage and praise client efforts to exercise and perform activities of daily living.

Level of Cognitive Ability: Application
Client Needs: Psychosocial Integrity
Integrated Process: Caring
Content Area: Adult Health/Neurological

Answer: 4

Rationale: The client with Parkinson's disease has a tendency to become withdrawn and depressed, which can be limited by encouraging the client to be an active participant in his or her own care. The family should also give the client encouragement and praise for his or her perseverance in these efforts. The family should plan activities intermittently throughout the day to inhibit daytime sleeping and boredom.

Test-Taking Strategy: Use the process of elimination. Eliminate option 3 first, because clustering activities at one time will tire the client. Eliminate option 1 next because of the use of the close-ended word "only." From the remaining options, recalling that the client should be an active participant in his or her own care will direct you to option 4. Review therapeutic techniques for the client with Parkinson's disease to assist with adjustment to the disease if you had difficulty with this question.

Reference
Ignatavicius, D., & Workman, M. (2006). *Medical-surgical nursing: Critical thinking for collaborative care* (5th ed., p. 961). Philadelphia: Saunders.

1287. A community health nurse is caring for a group of homeless people. When planning for the potential needs of this group, what is the most immediate concern?

1 Peer support through structured groups
2 Finding affordable housing for the group
3 Setting up a 24-hour crisis center and hotline
4 Meeting the basic needs to ensure that adequate food, shelter, and clothing are available

Level of Cognitive Ability: Analysis
Client Needs: Physiological Integrity
Integrated Process: Caring
Content Area: Delegating/Prioritizing

Answer: 4

Rationale: The question asks about the immediate concern. The ABCs of community health are always attending to people's basic needs of food, shelter, and clothing. Options 1, 2, and 3 are other activities that may be completed at a later time.

Test-Taking Strategy: Use Maslow's Hierarchy of Needs theory to answer the question. Option 4 addresses basic physiological needs. Although options 1, 2, and 3 are also appropriate actions, option 4 is the immediate concern. Review the needs of the homeless population if you had difficulty with this question.

Reference
Potter, P., & Perry, A. (2005). *Fundamentals of nursing* (6th ed., pp. 51-52, 143). St. Louis: Mosby.

1288. A stillborn baby was delivered a few hours ago. After the birth, the family has remained together, holding and touching the baby. Which statement by the nurse would further assist the family during their initial period of grief?

1 "What did you name your baby?"
2 "You seem upset. Do you need a tranquilizer?"
3 "I feel so bad. I don't understand why this happened either."
4 "You can hold the baby for another 15 minutes, but then I need to take the baby away."

Level of Cognitive Ability: Application
Client Needs: Psychosocial Integrity
Integrated Process: Caring
Content Area: Maternity/Postpartum

Answer: 1

Rationale: Nurses should be able to explore measures that assist the family with creating memories of the infant so that the existence of the child is confirmed and the parents can complete the grieving process. Option 1 identifies this measure and also demonstrates a caring and empathetic response. Option 2 devalues the parents' feelings and is inappropriate. Option 3 is inappropriate and reflects a lack of knowledge on the nurse's part. Option 4 is uncaring.

Test-Taking Strategy: Note the strategic words "further assist the family during their initial period of grief." Use the process of elimination and therapeutic communication techniques. Choose the option that demonstrates a caring and empathetic response by the nurse and that meets the psychosocial needs of the client and family. Review therapeutic communication techniques and the grief process if you had difficulty with this question.

Reference
Murray, S., & McKinney, E. (2006). *Foundations of maternal-newborn nursing* (4th ed., pp. 611-612). Philadelphia: Saunders.

1289. While counseling a prenatal client about her dietary and alcohol consumption habits, the nurse observes that the client has difficulty concentrating and appears agitated. The nurse should proceed with the assessment using which guideline?

1 A nonjudgmental approach may help the nurse to gain maternal trust.

2 Provoking maternal guilt may help the woman recognize her problem and seek support services.

3 A discussion of the possible consequences of drinking alcohol during pregnancy should be avoided.

4 Women respond negatively to a hopeful message of the potential benefits of drinking cessation during pregnancy.

Level of Cognitive Ability: Application
Client Needs: Psychosocial Integrity
Integrated Process: Caring
Content Area: Maternity/Antepartum

Answer: 1
Rationale: The potential effects of alcohol abuse during pregnancy for both the mother and fetus have been well documented. The nurse who expresses genuine concern with suspected abusers may motivate positive behavioral changes during the prenatal period. The maternal behaviors of lack of concentration and agitation are frequently seen among childbearing women who are abusing alcohol. Options 2, 3, and 4 are inappropriate guidelines for the nurse to follow in this situation, and they do not address a caring approach.

Test-Taking Strategy: Use therapeutic communication techniques and the process of elimination. Remember that it is important to display a caring and nonjudgmental attitude. This will direct you to option 1. Review therapeutic communication techniques if you had difficulty with this question.

Reference
Murray, S., & McKinney, E. (2006). *Foundations of maternal-newborn nursing* (4th ed., pp. 24-25, 601). Philadelphia: Saunders.

1290. A nurse is caring for a client who, while drinking, was responsible for an automobile accident that resulted in the death of her only daughter. The nurse observes that the client is withdrawn. What is the nurse's initial action?

1 Let the client have some time alone to grieve over the loss.

2 Tell the client that her daughter's death was a result of alcohol abuse.

3 Inform the physician of the client's depression, and request medication to assist with coping.

4 Communicate with the client in a manner that reflects back to the client that he or she appears upset.

Level of Cognitive Ability: Application
Client Needs: Psychosocial Integrity
Integrated Process: Caring
Content Area: Mental Health

Answer: 4
Rationale: The nurse needs to encourage the client to express her feelings. Reflection statements tend to elicit a deeper awareness of feelings. Additionally, option 4 validates the perception that the client is upset. A well-timed reflection can reveal an emotion that has escaped the client's notice. Options 1 and 3 address interventions before assessing the situation. Option 2 is inappropriate and is a block to communication.

Test-Taking Strategy: Note the strategic word "initial." Use therapeutic communication techniques and the process of elimination. Select the option that encourages the client to express her feelings and talk more. Remember to always address the client's feelings. Review therapeutic communication techniques if you had difficulty with this question.

References
Stuart, G., & Laraia, M. (2005). *Principles and practice of psychiatric nursing* (8th ed., pp. 30-34). St. Louis: Mosby.
Varcarolis, E., Carson, V., & Shoemaker, N. (2006). *Foundations of psychiatric mental health nursing* (5th ed., p. 721). Philadelphia: Saunders.

1291. An emergency department nurse is assigned to care for an older client who has been identified as a victim of physical abuse. When planning care for this client, the nurse's priority is to:
1 Refer the abusing family member for treatment.
2 Comply with the mandatory abuse-reporting laws.
3 Encourage the client to file charges against the abuser.
4 Remove the client from any immediate sources of danger.

Level of Cognitive Ability: Application
Client Needs: Safe and Effective Care Environment
Integrated Process: Caring
Content Area: Mental Health

Answer: 4
Rationale: Whenever the abused client remains in the abusive environment, priority must be placed on ascertaining whether the person is in any immediate danger. If so, emergency action must be taken to remove the person from the abusive situation. Options 1 and 2 may be appropriate interventions, but they are not the priority. Option 3 is not an appropriate intervention at this time, and it may produce increased fear and anxiety in the client.

Test-Taking Strategy: Use the process of elimination, and eliminate option 3 first, knowing that this action may produce increased fear and anxiety in the client. Use Maslow's Hierarchy of Needs theory to select from the remaining options, remembering that, if a physiological need is not present, then safety is the priority. This should direct you to option 4, which is the only option that directly addresses client safety. Review the principles related to caring for the abused client if you had difficulty with this question.

Reference
Varcarolis, E., Carson, V., & Shoemaker, N. (2006). *Foundations of psychiatric mental health nursing* (5th ed., p. 512). Philadelphia: Saunders.

1292. A community health nurse is working with older residents who were involved in a recent flood. Many of the residents are emotionally despondent, and they refused to leave their homes for days. When planning for the rescue and relocation of these older residents, what is the first item that the nurse needs to consider?
1 Contacting the older residents' families
2 Attending to the emotional needs of the older residents
3 Arranging for ambulance transportation for the oldest residents
4 Attending to the nutritional status and basic needs of the older residents

Level of Cognitive Ability: Application
Client Needs: Physiological Integrity
Integrated Process: Caring
Content Area: Delegating/Prioritizing

Answer: 4
Rationale: The question asks about the first thing that the nurse needs to consider. The ABCs of community health are always attending to people's basic needs of food, shelter, and clothing. Options 1, 2, and 3 are other activities that may or may not be needed at a later date.

Test-Taking Strategy: Use Maslow's Hierarchy of Needs theory to answer the question. Option 4 addresses basic physiological needs. Although options 1, 2, and 3 may be appropriate actions at a later time, option 4 is the immediate concern. Review the care of clients experiencing crisis if you had difficulty with this question.

References
Ignatavicius, D., & Workman, M. (2006). *Medical-surgical nursing: Critical thinking for collaborative care* (5th ed., pp. 167-168). Philadelphia: Saunders.
Stuart, G., & Laraia, M. (2005). *Principles and practice of psychiatric nursing* (8th ed., pp. 234-235, 244). St. Louis: Mosby.

1293. A nurse is assisting with planning the care for a suicidal client who has been newly admitted to the mental health unit. To provide a caring, therapeutic environment, which of the following should be included in the nursing care plan?

1 Placing the client in a private room to ensure privacy and confidentiality
2 Establishing a therapeutic relationship and conveying unconditional positive regard
3 Placing the client in charge of a meaningful unit activity, such as the morning chess tournament
4 Maintaining a distance of 10 inches at all times to ensure for the client that control will be provided

Level of Cognitive Ability: Application
Client Needs: Psychosocial Integrity
Integrated Process: Caring
Content Area: Mental Health

Answer: 2

Rationale: The establishment of a therapeutic relationship with the suicidal client increases feelings of acceptance. Although the suicidal behavior and thinking of the client are unacceptable, the use of unconditional positive regard acknowledges the client in a human-to-human context and increases the client's sense of self-worth. The client would not be placed in a private room, because this is an unsafe action that may intensify the client's feelings of worthlessness. Placing the client in charge of the morning chess game is a premature intervention that can overwhelm the client and cause him or her to fail; this can reinforce the client's feelings of worthlessness. Distances of 18 inches or less between two individuals constitutes intimate space. The invasion of this space may be misinterpreted by the client and increase the client's tension and feelings of helplessness.

Test-Taking Strategy: Use the process of elimination. Eliminate option 1, because isolation is not the safe and therapeutic intervention. Option 3 may produce feelings of worthlessness. Eliminate option 4, because a distance of 10 inches is restrictive. Option 2 is the only option that addresses a caring and therapeutic environment. Review the care of the suicidal client if you had difficulty with this question.

Reference
Varcarolis, E., Carson, V., & Shoemaker, N. (2006). *Foundations of psychiatric mental health nursing* (5th ed., p. 480). Philadelphia: Saunders.

1294. Fifteen minutes after a client dies, the nurse asks the family about funeral arrangements, but the family refuses to discuss the issue. Which intervention should the nurse implement?

1 Display acceptance.
2 Provide information.
3 Probe for information.
4 Remain with the family.

Level of Cognitive Ability: Application
Client Needs: Psychosocial Integrity
Integrated Process: Caring
Content Area: Fundamental Skills

Answer: 4

Rationale: The family is exhibiting the first stage of grief: denial. By staying with the family, the nurse demonstrates acceptance of their feelings and allows the family to process the death. Option 1 is a suitable intervention for the acceptance or reorganization and restitution stage. Options 2 and 3 can be suitable when the family is ready to receive information, because probing will help to clarify the information that the family needs and wants.

Test-Taking Strategy: Note the stage of grief that the family is demonstrating, and focus on the subject of the family refusing to discuss the funeral arrangements. The question asks for the response or action by the nurse that is suitable for the family's stage of grief. Recognizing that the family is in denial will direct you to choose option 4. Review the grieving process if you had difficulty with this question.

References
Black, J., & Hawks, J. (2005). *Medical-surgical nursing: Clinical management for positive outcomes* (7th ed., pp. 500-502). Philadelphia: Saunders.
Ignatavicius, D., & Workman, M. (2006). *Medical-surgical nursing: Critical thinking for collaborative care* (5th ed., pp. 113-114). Philadelphia: Saunders.

1295. A female client has incurable cancer with a life expectancy of a few weeks. Which response by the client's husband indicates that he is reacting with a normal and expected coping response?

1 He refuses to visit his wife.
2 He expresses anger with God.
3 He will not allow his wife to die at home.
4 He sends the children to live with a relative.

Level of Cognitive Ability: Application
Client Needs: Psychosocial Integrity
Integrated Process: Caring
Content Area: Fundamental Skills

Answer: 2

Rationale: The expression of anger is a normal response to impending loss, and often the anger is directed internally or at the dying person, God or another spiritual being, or the caregivers. In option 1, the husband is denying his wife's situation and her needs by refusing to visit her. Options 3 and 4 indicate hasty, unilateral decisions made by the husband without considering anyone else's feelings.

Test-Taking Strategy: Note the strategic words "a normal and expected coping response." Recalling the stages of grief associated with loss will direct you to option 2. Review effective coping mechanisms if you had difficulty with this question.

Reference
Black, J., & Hawks, J. (2005). *Medical-surgical nursing: Clinical management for positive outcomes* (7th ed., p. 390). Philadelphia: Saunders.

COMMUNICATION AND DOCUMENTATION

1296. A client says to the nurse, "I'm going to die, and I wish my family would stop hoping for a cure! I get so angry when they carry on like this! After all, I'm the one who's dying." The nurse makes which therapeutic response to the client?

1 "Have you shared your feelings with your family?"
2 "I think we should talk more about your anger with your family."
3 "You're feeling angry that your family continues to hope for you to be cured?"
4 "Well, it sounds like you're being pretty pessimistic. After all, years ago, before antibiotics were discovered, people died of pneumonia."

Level of Cognitive Ability: Application
Client Needs: Psychosocial Integrity
Integrated Process: Communication and Documentation
Content Area: Fundamental Skills

Answer: 3

Rationale: Reflection is the therapeutic communication technique that redirects the client's feelings back to him or her to validate what the client is saying. Option 3 uses the therapeutic technique of reflection. In option 1, the nurse is attempting to assess the client's ability to openly discuss his or her feelings with family members. Although this is an appropriate response to this client, the timing is somewhat premature, and it closes off the facilitation of the client's feelings. In option 2, the nurse attempts to use focusing, but the attempt to discuss central issues seems premature. In option 4, the nurse makes a judgment, which is not therapeutic for the one-to-one relationship.

Test-Taking Strategy: Use therapeutic communication techniques. Remembering to always address the client's feelings will direct you to option 3. Review therapeutic communication techniques if you had difficulty with this question.

Reference
Potter, P., & Perry, A. (2005). *Fundamentals of nursing* (6th ed., p. 437). St. Louis: Mosby.

1297. The husband of a client who has a Sengstaken-Blakemore tube tells the nurse, "I thought having this tube down her nose the first time would convince my wife to quit drinking." The nurse makes which response to the client's husband?

1 "I think you are a good person to stay with your wife."

2 "Alcoholism is a disease that affects the whole family."

3 "Have you discussed this subject at the Al-Anon meetings?"

4 "You sound frustrated with dealing with your wife's drinking problem."

Level of Cognitive Ability: Application
Client Needs: Psychosocial Integrity
Integrated Process: Communication and Documentation
Content Area: Adult Health/Gastrointestinal

Answer: 4
Rationale: In option 4, the nurse uses the therapeutic communication techniques of clarifying and focusing to assist the client (the husband) with expressing his feelings about his wife's chronic illness. Showing approval (option 1), stereotyping (option 2), and changing the subject (option 3) are nontherapeutic techniques that block communication.

Test-Taking Strategy: Use therapeutic communication techniques. Remembering to always address the client's feelings will direct you to option 4. Review therapeutic communication techniques if you had difficulty with this question.

References
Ignatavicius, D., & Workman, M. (2006). *Medical-surgical nursing: Critical thinking for collaborative care* (5th ed., pp. 1378-1379). Philadelphia: Saunders.
Potter, P., & Perry, A. (2005). *Fundamentals of nursing* (6th ed., p. 437). St. Louis: Mosby.

1298. The nurse has an order to institute aneurysm precautions for a client with a cerebral aneurysm. Which item should the nurse document on the plan of care for this client?

1 Limit out-of-bed activities to twice daily.

2 Allow the client to read and watch television.

3 Encourage the client to take his or her own daily bath.

4 Instruct the client to not strain with bowel movements.

Level of Cognitive Ability: Application
Client Needs: Physiological Integrity
Integrated Process: Communication and Documentation
Content Area: Adult Health/Neurological

Answer: 4
Rationale: Aneurysm precautions include placing the client on bedrest in a quiet setting. Lights are kept dim to minimize environmental stimulation. Any activity that increases the blood pressure (BP) or that impedes venous flow from the brain is prohibited, such as pushing, pulling, sneezing, coughing, or straining. The nurse provides all physical care to minimize increases in the BP. For the same reason, visitors, radio, television, and reading materials are prohibited or limited. Stimulants such as caffeine and nicotine are prohibited. The nurse documents that the client is instructed to avoid straining with bowel movements.

Test-Taking Strategy: Recall that the components of aneurysm precautions are to limit the amount of stimulation (in any form) that the client receives and to prevent increased intracranial pressure (ICP). With this in mind, eliminate options 1 and 3 first. From the remaining options, recall that straining can increase ICP, so it is appropriate to tell the client not to do so. Review the components of aneurysm precautions if you had difficulty with this question.

References
Ignatavicius, D., & Workman, M. (2006). *Medical-surgical nursing: Critical thinking for collaborative care* (5th ed., pp. 1053-1064). Philadelphia: Saunders.
Lewis, S., Heitkemper, M., Dirksen, S., O'Brien, P., & Bucher, L. (2007). *Medical-surgical nursing: Assessment and management of clinical problems* (7th ed., p. 898). St. Louis: Mosby.
Monahan, F., Sands, J., Neighbors, M., Marek, J., & Green, C. (2007). *Phipps' medical-surgical nursing: Health and illness perspectives* (8th ed., p. 1441). St. Louis: Mosby.

1299. A client with myasthenia gravis is having difficulty with the motor aspects of speech. The client has difficulty forming words, and the voice has a nasal tone. The nurse should plan to use which communication strategy when working with this client?

1 Encourage the client to speak quickly.
2 Nod continuously while the client is speaking.
3 Repeat what the client has said to verify the message.
4 Engage the client in lengthy discussions to strengthen the voice.

Level of Cognitive Ability: Application
Client Needs: Psychosocial Integrity
Integrated Process: Communication and Documentation
Content Area: Adult Health/Neurological

Answer: 3

Rationale: The client has speech that is nasal in tone because of cranial nerve involvement in the muscles that govern speech. The nurse listens attentively and verbally verifies what the client has said. Other helpful techniques involve asking questions that require a "yes" or "no" response and developing alternative communication methods (e.g., letter board, picture board, pen and paper, flash cards). Encouraging the client to speak quickly is inappropriate and counterproductive. Continuous nodding may be distracting and is unnecessary. Lengthy discussions will tire the client rather than strengthen the voice.

Test-Taking Strategy: Use the process of elimination and the basic principles of communication techniques to answer this question. This will direct you to option 3. Review myasthenia gravis and effective communication strategies if you had difficulty with this question.

Reference
Ignatavicius, D., & Workman, M. (2006). *Medical-surgical nursing: Critical thinking for collaborative care* (5th ed., p. 1016). Philadelphia: Saunders.

1300. The nurse assesses the client's peripheral intravenous (IV) site and notes that it is cool, pale, swollen, and not infusing. The nurse documents in the client's record that which of the following has probably occurred?

1 Phlebitis
2 Infection
3 Infiltration
4 Thrombosis

Level of Cognitive Ability: Application
Client Needs: Physiological Integrity
Integrated Process: Communication and Documentation
Content Area: Fundamental Skills

Answer: 3

Rationale: The pallor, coolness, and swelling of the IV site are the result of IV fluid infusing into the subcutaneous tissue. When the pressure in the tissue exceeds the pressure in the tubing, the infusion stops. An IV site is infiltrated when it becomes dislodged from the vein and is lying in subcutaneous tissue, so the nurse concludes that the IV is infiltrated. The nurse needs to remove the infiltrated catheter and insert a new IV. The remaining options are likely to be accompanied by warmth at the site. Options 1 and 2 also involve the site appearing to be reddened.

Test-Taking Strategy: Use the process of elimination and your knowledge regarding the clinical indicators of the complications associated with IV therapy. Focusing on the data in the question and noting the words "cool," "pale," and "swollen" will direct you to option 3. Review the signs of infiltration if you had difficulty with this question.

References
Ignatavicius, D., & Workman, M. (2006). *Medical-surgical nursing: Critical thinking for collaborative care* (5th ed., p. 259). Philadelphia: Saunders.
Potter, P., & Perry, A. (2005). *Fundamentals of nursing* (6th ed., p. 1189). St. Louis: Mosby.

1301. A nurse is observing a nursing assistant talking to a client who is hearing impaired. The nurse would intervene if which of the following is performed by the nursing assistant during communication with the client?

1 The nursing assistant is speaking in a normal tone.
2 The nursing assistant is speaking clearly to the client.
3 The nursing assistant is facing the client when speaking.
4 The nursing assistant is speaking directly into the impaired ear.

Level of Cognitive Ability: Analysis
Client Needs: Safe and Effective Care Environment
Integrated Process: Communication and Documentation
Content Area: Leadership/Management

Answer: 4
Rationale: When communicating with a hearing-impaired client, the nurse should speak in a normal tone to the client and should not shout. The nurse should talk directly to the client while facing the client, and he or she should speak clearly. If the client does not seem to understand what is being said, the nurse should express the statement differently. Moving closer to the client and toward the better ear may facilitate communication, but the nurse needs to avoid talking directly into the impaired ear.

Test-Taking Strategy: Note the strategic words "the nurse would intervene." These words indicate a negative event query and ask you to select an option that involves an incorrect action by the nursing assistant. Knowledge regarding effective communication techniques for the hearing-impaired client will direct you to option 4. Review therapeutic communication techniques if you had difficulty with this question.

References
Ignatavicius, D., & Workman, M. (2006). *Medical-surgical nursing: Critical thinking for collaborative care* (5th ed., p. 1139). Philadelphia: Saunders.
Lewis, S., Heitkemper, M., Dirksen, S., O'Brien, P., & Bucher, L. (2007). *Medical-surgical nursing: Assessment and management of clinical problems* (7th ed., p. 445). St. Louis: Mosby.

1302. A nurse is assigned to care for a client who has been diagnosed with catatonic stupor. When the nurse enters the client's room, the client is found lying on the bed with the body pulled into a fetal position. The nurse should:

1 Ask the client direct questions to encourage talking.
2 Take the client into the dayroom to be with other clients.
3 Leave the client alone and continue with providing care to other clients.
4 Sit beside the client in silence and occasionally ask open-ended questions.

Level of Cognitive Ability: Application
Client Needs: Psychosocial Integrity
Integrated Process: Communication and Documentation
Content Area: Mental Health

Answer: 4
Rationale: Clients who are withdrawn may be immobile and mute, and they require consistent, repeated approaches. Intervention includes the establishment of interpersonal contact. Communication with withdrawn clients requires much patience from the nurse. The nurse facilitates communication with the client by sitting in silence, asking open-ended questions, and pausing to provide opportunities for the client to respond. The client would not be left alone. Asking direct questions to the client is not therapeutic. It is not appropriate at this time to place the client in a public place, such as a dayroom.

Test-Taking Strategy: Use the process of elimination. Eliminate option 1, because asking direct questions to this client is not therapeutic. Eliminate option 2, because it is not appropriate to place the client in a public space. Eliminate option 3, because you would not leave the client alone. Option 4 is the best action, because it provides client supervision and communication with the client. Review the care of the client with catatonic stupor if you had difficulty with this question.

References
Stuart, G., & Laraia, M. (2005). *Principles and practice of psychiatric nursing* (8th ed., pp. 30-34, 404). St. Louis: Mosby.
Varcarolis, E., Carson, V., & Shoemaker, N. (2006). *Foundations of psychiatric mental health nursing* (5th ed., pp. 414-415). Philadelphia: Saunders.

1303. The nurse develops a plan of care to facilitate effective communication for a client. Which should the nurse include in the plan of care?

1 Direct the client discussions.
2 Focus on the client's message.
3 Reflect facts only to the client.
4 React excitedly when conversing.

Level of Cognitive Ability: Application
Client Needs: Psychosocial Integrity
Integrated Process: Communication and Documentation
Content Area: Fundamental Skills

Answer: 2
Rationale: For effective communication, the nurse uses active listening and assesses for verbal and nonverbal communication to receive the client's intended message, thus creating an environment in which the client feels comfortable expressing his or her feelings. An authoritarian approach is directive and not permissive, and it is unlikely to create an environment for the free exchange of thoughts and ideas. Reacting enthusiastically can be an ineffective strategy for facilitating communication. Reflecting facts only is a barrier to effective communication, because subjective information can also provide a stimulus for effective communication.

Test-Taking Strategy: Use the process of elimination and therapeutic communication techniques. This will direct you to option 2. Review therapeutic communication techniques if you had difficulty with this question.

References
Perry, A., & Potter, P. (2006). *Clinical nursing skills & techniques* (6th ed., pp. 23-24). St. Louis: Mosby.
Potter, P., & Perry, A. (2005). *Fundamentals of nursing* (6th ed., p. 437). St. Louis: Mosby.

1304. The nurse made an error when documenting vital signs on a client's medical record. As part of the proper procedure for correcting an error, the nurse:

1 Documents a late entry
2 Draws a line through the error
3 Covers the error using a marker
4 Conceals the error with correction fluid

Level of Cognitive Ability: Application
Client Needs: Safe and Effective Care Environment
Integrated Process: Communication and Documentation
Content Area: Fundamental Skills

Answer: 2
Rationale: If the nurse makes a documentation error in the client's record, the nurse should follow agency policy to correct the error. This usually includes drawing one line through the error, initialing and dating the line, and then providing the correct information. The nurse avoids concealing the error with a marker or correction fluid, because these actions raise the suspicion of wrongdoing. The nurse uses a later entry to document additional information that was not documented at the time that it occurred.

Test-Taking Strategy: Use the process of elimination and the principles related to documentation. Recalling that the nurse avoids alterations to a client's record will direct you to eliminate options 3 and 4. From the remaining options, focusing on the subject of the question will direct you to eliminate option 1, because the subject relates to errors in the medical record rather than to omitted data. Review the principles related to documentation if you had difficulty with this question.

Reference
Potter, P., & Perry, A. (2005). *Fundamentals of nursing* (6th ed., p. 480). St. Louis: Mosby.

1305. The nurse finds a client lying on the floor. The nurse performs an assessment, assists the client back to bed, and completes an incident report. Which should the nurse document on the incident report?

1 The client fell onto the floor.
2 The client climbed over the side rails.
3 The client was found lying on the floor.
4 The nurse was the only responder to the event.

Level of Cognitive Ability: Application
Client Needs: Safe and Effective Care Environment
Integrated Process: Communication and Documentation
Content Area: Fundamental Skills

Answer: 3
Rationale: The incident report should contain the client's name, age, and diagnosis as well as a factual description of the incident, any injuries experienced by those involved, and the outcome of the situation. Option 3 is the only option that describes the facts as observed by the nurse, and it is thus a suitable response. The nurse did not witness the events that led up to finding the client on the floor; thus he or she cannot comment on how the client got to the floor (options 1 and 2). Option 4 is unsuitable documentation on an incident report, because it implies that other staff members failed to respond to the event.

Test-Taking Strategy: Use general documentation guidelines and principles to answer the question. Remember to focus on factual information when documenting and to avoid including interpretations. This will direct you to option 3. Review the documentation principles related to incident reports if you had difficulty with this question.

Reference
Potter, P., & Perry, A. (2005). *Fundamentals of nursing* (6th ed, pp. 419, 497). St. Louis: Mosby.

1306. A client diagnosed with angina pectoris appears to be very anxious and states, "So, I had a heart attack, right?" The nurse makes which response to the client?

1 "Yes, that is why you are here."
2 "Yes, but there is minimal damage to your heart."
3 "No, and we will see to it that you do not have a heart attack."
4 "No, but the doctor wants to monitor you and control or eliminate your pain."

Level of Cognitive Ability: Application
Client Needs: Psychosocial Integrity
Integrated Process: Communication and Documentation
Content Area: Adult Health/Cardiovascular

Answer: 4
Rationale: Angina pectoris occurs as a result of an inadequate blood supply to the myocardium. The term *myocardial infarction* refers to a heart attack. Option 3 provides false reassurance. Neither the nurse nor the physician can guarantee that a heart attack will not occur.

Test-Taking Strategy: Use therapeutic communication techniques and your knowledge regarding the definition of angina pectoris to eliminate options 1 and 2. From the remaining options, eliminate option 3, because it provides false reassurance. Review the pathophysiology associated with angina pectoris and therapeutic communication techniques if you had difficulty with this question.

Reference
Ignatavicius, D., & Workman, M. (2006). *Medical-surgical nursing: Critical thinking for collaborative care* (5th ed., pp. 840, 845). Philadelphia: Saunders.

1307. A nurse is caring for a client who has been diagnosed with depression and who is silent. Which statement would be appropriate for the nurse to make when caring for the client?
  1 "Do you feel like talking today?"
  2 "You are wearing your new shoes."
  3 "Can you tell me how you slept last night?"
  4 "Can you tell me how you are feeling today?"

Level of Cognitive Ability: Application
Client Needs: Psychosocial Integrity
Integrated Process: Communication and Documentation
Content Area: Mental Health

Answer: 2
Rationale: When a depressed client is mute or silent, the nurse should use the communication technique of making observations. A statement such as "you are wearing your new shoes" is an appropriate statement to make to the client. When the client is not ready to talk, direct questions such as options 1, 3, and 4 can raise the client's anxiety level. Pointing out commonalties in the environment draws the client into and reinforces reality.

Test-Taking Strategy: Use therapeutic communication techniques. Eliminate options 1, 3, and 4 because they are comparable or alike. These options are direct questions that require a response from the client. Review communication techniques for the depressed client if you had difficulty with this question.

Reference
Stuart, G., & Laraia, M. (2005). *Principles and practice of psychiatric nursing* (8th ed., pp. 30-34, 334). St. Louis: Mosby.

1308. A nurse is caring for a client with delirium who states, "Look at the spiders on the wall." How should the nurse respond?
  1 "Would you like me to kill the spiders for you?"
  2 "I can see the spiders on the wall, but they are not going to hurt you."
  3 "I know that you are frightened, but I do not see any spiders on the wall."
  4 "You are having a hallucination; there are no spiders in this room at all."

Level of Cognitive Ability: Application
Client Needs: Psychosocial Integrity
Integrated Process: Communication and Documentation
Content Area: Mental Health

Answer: 3
Rationale: When hallucinations are present, the nurse should reinforce reality with the client. In option 3, the nurse addresses the client's feelings and reinforces reality. Options 1 and 2 do not reinforce reality. Option 4 reinforces reality but does not address the client's feelings

Test-Taking Strategy: Use therapeutic communication techniques. Eliminate options 1 and 2, because they reinforce the client's hallucination. Eliminate option 4, because, although it reinforces reality, it diminishes the importance of the client's feelings. Review therapeutic communication techniques for the client experiencing disturbed thought processes if you had difficulty with this question.

Reference
Stuart, G., & Laraia, M. (2005). *Principles and practice of psychiatric nursing* (8th ed., pp. 30-34, 411). St. Louis: Mosby.

1309. While in the hospital, the female client was diagnosed with coronary heart disease (CHD). Which question by the nurse is likely to elicit the most useful client response for determining her adjustment to the new diagnosis?
  1 "Can anyone help with housework and shopping?"
  2 "How do you feel about making changes to your lifestyle?"
  3 "Do you understand the schedule for your new medications?"
  4 "Did you make a follow-up appointment with your provider?"

Answer: 2
Rationale: Exploring feelings assists with determining the individualized plan of care for the client who is adjusting to a new diagnosis. Option 2 is the best question to ask the client, because it is likely to elicit the most revealing information about the client's feelings about CHD and the requisite lifestyle changes that can help to maintain health and wellness. The remaining options are aspects of posthospital care, but they are unlikely to uncover as much information about the client's adjustment to CHD as option 2, because they are close-ended questions.

Level of Cognitive Ability: Analysis
Client Needs: Health Promotion and
  Maintenance
Integrated Process: Communication and
  Documentation
Content Area: Fundamental Skills

Test-Taking Strategy: Use therapeutic communication techniques. Open-ended questions are needed to explore the client's reactions to or feelings about an identified situation. Close-ended responses generally elicit a "yes" or "no" response exclusively. All of the incorrect options are close-ended responses. Review therapeutic communication techniques if you had difficulty with this question.

References

Ignatavicius, D., & Workman, M. (2006). *Medical-surgical nursing: Critical thinking for collaborative care* (5th ed., p. 862). Philadelphia: Saunders.
Potter, P., & Perry, A. (2005). *Fundamentals of nursing* (6th ed., p. 437). St. Louis: Mosby.

1310. A female client with a long leg cast has been using crutches to ambulate for 1 week. She comes to the clinic with complaints of pain, fatigue, and frustration with crutch walking. She states, "I feel like I have a crippled leg." The nurse makes which response to the client?
  1 "Tell me what is bothersome for you."
  2 "I know how you feel. I had to use crutches before, too."
  3 "Why don't you take a couple of days off of work and rest."
  4 "Just remember, you'll be done with the crutches in another month."

Answer: 1

Rationale: Option 1 demonstrates the therapeutic communication technique of clarification and validation and indicates that the nurse is dealing with the client's problem from the client's perspective. Option 2 devalues the client's feelings and thus blocks communication. Option 3 gives advice and is a communication block. Option 4 provides false reassurances, because the client may not be done with the crutches in another month. Additionally, it does not focus on the present problem.

Test-Taking Strategy: Use therapeutic communication techniques. Option 1 is the only response that encourages communication. Review therapeutic communication techniques if you had difficulty with this question.

Level of Cognitive Ability: Application
Client Needs: Psychosocial Integrity
Integrated Process: Communication and
  Documentation
Content Area: Adult Health/Musculoskeletal

References

Ignatavicius, D., & Workman, M. (2006). *Medical-surgical nursing: Critical thinking for collaborative care* (5th ed., p. 1198). Philadelphia: Saunders.
Potter, P., & Perry, A. (2005). *Fundamentals of nursing* (6th ed., p. 437). St. Louis: Mosby.

1311. An 18-year-old male client is discharged from the hospital after surgery with instructions to use a cane for the next 6 months. What is the best question for the nurse to use to assess the client's feelings about the use of the cane?
  1 "What do you think about ambulating with a cane?"
  2 "Are you worried about what your friends will think?"
  3 "What types of obstacles will interfere with ambulation?"
  4 "Do you have questions about ambulating with a cane?"

Answer: 1

Rationale: The nurse poses an open-ended question to the client to elicit assessment data about his psychosocial status. Option 2 is a close-ended question, because the client can respond with a single word. Options 3 and 4 are also close-ended questions, but they deal with physical issues.

Test-Taking Strategy: Use therapeutic communication techniques. Avoid responses that include communication blocks or that fail to focus on the subject of psychosocial assessment. Remember to address the client's feelings first. Review therapeutic communication techniques if you had difficulty with this question.

Level of Cognitive Ability: Analysis
Client Needs: Psychosocial Integrity
Integrated Process: Communication and
  Documentation
Content Area: Fundamental Skills

References
Ignatavicius, D., & Workman, M. (2006). *Medical-surgical nursing: Critical thinking for collaborative care* (5th ed., p. 123). Philadelphia: Saunders.
Potter, P., & Perry, A. (2005). *Fundamentals of nursing* (6th ed., p. 437). St. Louis: Mosby.

1312. After the surgical repair of a fractured hip, a client who is 85 years old has a poor appetite and refuses to get out of bed. Which statement by the nurse is therapeutic and accurate for this client?
  1 "Physical therapy will strengthen your bones."
  2 "We can give you calcium if you are not walking."
  3 "Turn yourself in bed to keep your bones strong."
  4 "Getting out of bed helps to maintain strong bones."

Level of Cognitive Ability: Application
Client Needs: Physiological Integrity
Integrated Process: Communication and
  Documentation
Content Area: Fundamental Skills

Answer: 4
Rationale: Early ambulation during the postoperative period is very important, because, if a client does not engage in weight-bearing activity, the bones lose calcium and muscles atrophy. In addition, postoperative ambulation helps to decrease the risk of other complications, including atelectasis, pneumonia, constipation, deconditioning, and pressure ulcers. Physical therapy helps to maintain range of motion and to slow bone demineralization, but it does not strengthen bones while the client is on bedrest. Engaging clients in their care can be an effective strategy for implementing the plan of care; however, the nurse remains responsible for ensuring that the plan is implemented, and he or she cannot delegate the responsibility to the client. Calcium supplements in an immobile client can elevate the serum calcium level and potentially lead to kidney stones.

Test-Taking Strategy: Use the process of elimination, the principles of therapeutic communication, and your knowledge regarding the effects of immobility and bone metabolism. Eliminate options 1 and 2, because they are inaccurate. Eliminate option 3, because the nurse is delegating responsibility for the client's care to the client. Review the complications associated with immobility if you had difficulty with this question.

References
Black, J., & Hawks, J. (2005). *Medical-surgical nursing: Clinical management for positive outcomes* (7th ed., pp. 642, 645). Philadelphia: Saunders.
Lewis, S., Heitkemper, M., Dirksen, S., O'Brien, P., & Bucher, L. (2007). *Medical-surgical nursing: Assessment and management of clinical problems* (7th ed., p. 1655). St. Louis: Mosby.

1313. A client has thrombophlebitis of the left leg. Which intervention should the nurse document in the client's plan of care while the client is on bedrest?
  1 Elevating the left leg
  2 Keeping the left leg flat
  3 Engaging in activity as tolerated
  4 Maintaining bathroom privileges

Answer: 1
Rationale: The nurse plans to elevate the affected extremity, because this facilitates venous return by using gravity to improve blood return to the heart, it decreases venous pressure, and it helps to relieve edema and pain. Options 3 and 4 are unsuitable activities for a client on bedrest. Option 2 does not facilitate venous return and thus is not indicated for a client with thrombophlebitis.

Test-Taking Strategy: Use the process of elimination. Focus on the client's diagnosis, and think about how gravity affects venous blood flow and edema. This will direct you to option 1. Review the nursing care for a client with a venous disorder if you had difficulty with this question.

Level of Cognitive Ability: Application
Client Needs: Physiological Integrity
Integrated Process: Communication and
   Documentation
Content Area: Fundamental Skills

References
Black, J., & Hawks, J. (2005). *Medical-surgical nursing: Clinical management for positive outcomes* (7th ed., pp. 1537, 1541). Philadelphia: Saunders.
Monahan, F., Sands, J., Neighbors, M., Marek, J., & Green, C. (2007). *Phipps' medical-surgical nursing: Health and illness perspectives* (8th ed., pp. 888, 1707). St. Louis: Mosby.

1314. A client who is experiencing disordered thinking about food being poisoned is admitted to the mental health unit. The nurse uses which communication technique to encourage the client to eat dinner?

   1 Using open-ended questions and silence
   2 Offering personal opinions about the need to eat
   3 Verbalizing reasons that the client may choose to not eat
   4 Focusing on self-disclosure of the nurse's own food preferences

Level of Cognitive Ability: Application
Client Needs: Physiological Integrity
Integrated Process: Communication and
   Documentation
Content Area: Mental Health

Answer: 1
Rationale: Open-ended questions and silence are strategies that are used to encourage clients to discuss their problem in a descriptive manner. Options 2 and 3 are not helpful to the client, because they do not encourage the client to express his or her feelings. Option 4 is not a client-centered intervention.

Test-Taking Strategy: Use the process of elimination and therapeutic communication techniques. Eliminate options 2 and 3 first, because they do not support client expression of feelings. Eliminate option 4 next, because it is not a client-centered response. Review therapeutic communication techniques if you had difficulty with this question.

Reference
Stuart, G., & Laraia, M. (2005). *Principles and practice of psychiatric nursing* (8th ed., pp. 30-34). St. Louis: Mosby.

1315. A nurse is engaged in preparing a client for electroconvulsive therapy (ECT). After the client signs the informed consent form, a family member states, "I don't know. I don't think that this ECT will be helpful if it makes people's memory worse." The nurse should:

   1 Ask other family members and the client if they think that ECT makes people worse.
   2 Immediately reassure the client and family that ECT will help and that the memory loss is only temporary.
   3 Involve the family member in a dialogue to ascertain how the family member arrived at this conclusion.
   4 Reinforce with the client and the family member that depression causes more memory impairment than ECT.

Level of Cognitive Ability: Application
Client Needs: Psychosocial Integrity
Integrated Process: Communication and
   Documentation
Content Area: Mental Health

Answer: 3
Rationale: In option 3, the nurse is looking for data to assist with clarifying information about the procedure with the family. Option 1 may place family members on the defensive and promote conflict among family members. Option 2 would not acknowledge the family member's statement and concerns. Option 4 addresses content clarification but not the assessment process, and it is not the most therapeutic action.

Test-Taking Strategy: Use therapeutic communication techniques and the nursing process. Remember that assessment is the first step in the nursing process. In option 3, the nurse gathers more data and addresses the family member's thoughts and feelings. Review therapeutic communication techniques if you had difficulty with this question.

Reference
Stuart, G., & Laraia, M. (2005). *Principles and practice of psychiatric nursing* (8th ed., pp. 30-34, 605). St. Louis: Mosby.

TEACHING AND LEARNING

1316. A client with tuberculosis (TB) is preparing for discharge from the hospital, and the nurse provides instructions to the client about home care. Which client statement indicates that further instructions are necessary?

1 "I need to place used tissues in a plastic bag when I am home."
2 "I need to eat foods that are high in iron, protein, and vitamin C."
3 "It is not necessary to maintain respiratory isolation when I am at home."
4 "If I miss a dose of medication because of nausea, I just skip that dose and then resume my regular schedule."

Level of Cognitive Ability: Analysis
Client Needs: Physiological Integrity
Integrated Process: Teaching and Learning
Content Area: Adult Health/Respiratory

Answer: 4
Rationale: Because of the resistant strains of TB, the nurse must emphasize that noncompliance regarding medication could lead to an infection that is difficult to treat and that may cause total drug resistance. Clients may prevent nausea related to the medications by taking the daily dose at bedtime, and antinausea medications may also prevent this symptom. Medication doses should not be skipped. Options 1, 2, and 3 are correct statements.

Test-Taking Strategy: Note the strategic words "further instructions are necessary." These words indicate a negative event query and ask you to select an option that is an incorrect statement. General principles related to medication administration will direct you to option 4. Review medication therapy and its importance for the treatment of TB if you had difficulty with this question.

Reference
Ignatavicius, D., & Workman, M. (2006). *Medical-surgical nursing: Critical thinking for collaborative care* (5th ed., pp. 643-644). Philadelphia: Saunders.

1317. The nurse is planning to teach a client who has been newly diagnosed with tuberculosis (TB) about how to prevent the spread of TB. Which instruction would be the least effective for preventing the spread of TB?

1 Teach the client to sterilize dishes at home.
2 Teach the client to properly dispose of facial tissues.
3 Teach the client to cover the mouth when coughing.
4 Teach the client that close contacts should be tested for TB.

Level of Cognitive Ability: Application
Client Needs: Safe and Effective Care Environment
Integrated Process: Teaching and Learning
Content Area: Adult Health/Respiratory

Answer: 1
Rationale: Options 2, 3, and 4 would assist with breaking the chain of infection. Option 1 is impractical, and no evidence exists that suggests that sterilizing dishes would break the chain of infection with pulmonary TB.

Test-Taking Strategy: Note the strategic words "least effective." These words indicate a negative event query and ask you to select the option that is not helpful for preventing the spread of TB. Recalling the methods of transmission of TB will direct you to option 1. Review the home-care principles related to TB if you had difficulty with this question.

Reference
Ignatavicius, D., & Workman, M. (2006). *Medical-surgical nursing: Critical thinking for collaborative care* (5th ed., p. 644). Philadelphia: Saunders.

1318. A client is receiving intravenous (IV) antibiotic therapy at home for 1 week via a heparin lock (intermittent IV catheter). Which does the nurse include in client teaching for the early detection of complications of IV therapy?
1 Protect the heparin lock continually.
2 Keep the heparin lock clean and dry.
3 Report regional pain, drainage, or edema.
4 Apply pressure to the IV site if it dislodges.

Level of Cognitive Ability: Analysis
Client Needs: Safe and Effective Care Environment
Integrated Process: Teaching and Learning
Content Area: Fundamental Skills

Answer: 3
Rationale: The nurse instructs the client to report clinical indicators of an IV site infection, including pain, drainage, and edema, because the early detection of infection decreases the risk of septicemia, tissue loss, and devastating complications. The remaining options are reasonable aspects of client teaching for IV therapy at home, but they are not surveillance methods.

Test-Taking Strategy: Note the strategic words "early detection of complications," and use the process of elimination to choose a method of surveillance for complications of IV therapy. Eliminate option 1, 2, and 4, because these choices describe aspects of IV care to help prevent complications, but they do not contribute to early detection. Review the principles of IV insertion site care if you had difficulty with this question.

References
Perry, A., & Potter, P. (2006). *Clinical nursing skills & techniques* (6th ed., pp. 910-911). St. Louis: Mosby.
Potter, P., & Perry, A. (2005). *Fundamentals of nursing* (6th ed., p. 1194). St. Louis: Mosby.

1319. The home-care nurse provides instructions to a client with jaundice who is experiencing pruritus. The nurse determines that the client needs additional instructions if the client states the need to:
1 Wear loose cotton clothing.
2 Use tepid water for bathing.
3 Maintain a warm house temperature.
4 Take the prescribed antihistamines to relieve the itch.

Level of Cognitive Ability: Analysis
Client Needs: Health Promotion and Maintenance
Integrated Process: Teaching and Learning
Content Area: Adult Health/Gastrointestinal

Answer: 3
Rationale: Pruritus is caused by the accumulation of bile salts in the skin and results from obstructed biliary excretion. Antihistamines may relieve the itching, as will tepid water and emollient baths. The client should avoid the use of alkaline soap, and he or she should wear loose, soft, cotton clothing. The client is instructed to keep the house temperature cool.

Test-Taking Strategy: Use the process of elimination, and note the strategic words "needs additional instructions." These words indicate a negative event query and ask you to select an option that is an incorrect statement. Recalling that heat causes vasodilation will assist with directing you to option 3. Review the measures that assist with alleviating pruritus if you had difficulty with this question.

Reference
Ignatavicius, D., & Workman, M. (2006). *Medical-surgical nursing: Critical thinking for collaborative care* (5th ed., pp. 1575-1576). Philadelphia: Saunders.

1320. The nurse provides home-care instructions to a client who has been hospitalized for a transurethral resection of the prostate (TURP). Which statement by the client indicates the need for further instructions?

1 "I need to include prune juice in my diet."

2 "I need to avoid strenuous activity for 4 to 6 weeks."

3 "I can lift and push objects up to 30 pounds in weight."

4 "I need to maintain a daily intake of 6 to 8 glasses of water."

Level of Cognitive Ability: Analysis
Client Needs: Health Promotion and Maintenance
Integrated Process: Teaching and Learning
Content Area: Adult Health/Renal

Answer: 3
Rationale: The client needs to be advised to avoid strenuous activity for 4 to 6 weeks and to avoid lifting items that weigh more than 20 pounds. Straining during defecation is avoided to prevent bleeding. Prune juice is a satisfactory bowel stimulant. The client needs to consume a daily intake of at least 6 to 8 glasses of nonalcoholic fluids to minimize clot formation.

Test-Taking Strategy: Note the strategic words "need for further instructions." These words indicate a negative event query and ask you to select an option that is an incorrect statement. Options 2 and 4 can be eliminated first, because they are general postoperative teaching points. Considering the anatomical location of the surgical procedure, it is reasonable to think that constipation needs to be avoided; therefore, eliminate option 1. Also note that lifting items that weigh 30 pounds is excessive. Review TURP discharge teaching points if you had difficulty with this question.

Reference
Ignatavicius, D., & Workman, M. (2006). *Medical-surgical nursing: Critical thinking for collaborative care* (5th ed., p. 1864). Philadelphia: Saunders.

1321. A nurse is providing home-care instructions to a client who will be receiving intravenous (IV) therapy at home. The nurse teaches the client that the important action to prevent an infection at the IV site is to:

1 Protect the insertion site continually.

2 Assess the IV site for redness and edema.

3 Change the IV tubing every 48 to 72 hours.

4 Wash your hands before handling the IV site.

Level of Cognitive Ability: Analysis
Client Needs: Safe and Effective Care Environment
Integrated Process: Teaching and Learning
Content Area: Fundamental Skills

Answer: 4
Rationale: Option 4 emphasizes the need to perform thorough handwashing before handling the IV site or equipment to reduce the risk of introducing potential pathogens that are likely to cause an infection, and it is the only option that does so. Option 1 helps to maintain the IV catheter securely to prevent creating a mode of entry for potential pathogens. Changing the IV fluid and tubing (option 3) helps to reduce the risk of overgrowth of microorganisms from within the system. Option 2 helps with the early detection of infection.

Test-Taking Strategy: Note the strategic word "important," and focus on the subject: preventing infection. Remember that the top priority for infection prevention always includes proper handwashing technique. Review standard precautions and their role in preventing infection if you had difficulty with this question.

References
Ignatavicius, D., & Workman, M. (2006). *Medical-surgical nursing: Critical thinking for collaborative care* (5th ed., pp. 512-513). Philadelphia: Saunders.
Potter, P., & Perry, A. (2005). *Fundamentals of nursing* (6th ed., pp. 789, 1194). St. Louis: Mosby.

1322. A 64-year-old client is being treated for an atrial dysrhythmia with quinidine gluconate and the nurse provides instructions to the client about the medication. Which statement by the client indicates that the client understands the instructions?

1 "If I miss a dose, I should call my doctor."

2 "If I miss a dose, I should take the next prescribed dose as usual."

3 "If I miss a dose, I should take the dose in the evening, if I remember."

4 "If I miss a dose, I take two doses of the medication at the next scheduled time."

Level of Cognitive Ability: Analysis
Client Needs: Health Promotion and Maintenance
Integrated Process: Teaching and Learning
Content Area: Pharmacology

Answer: 2

Rationale: The client should be instructed to not take an extra dose, to take the medication if remembered within 2 hours of the missed dose, or to omit the dose and then resume the normal schedule. Quinidine gluconate needs to be taken exactly as prescribed. There is no need to call the doctor.

Test-Taking Strategy: Use the process of elimination and general principles related to medication administration. Eliminate option 4, because this action is inaccurate and could cause toxic effects. There is no need to call the doctor unless toxic effects occur; therefore, eliminate option 1. From the remaining options, recalling that a missed dose can be taken within 2 hours if remembered will direct you to option 2. Review the basic principles associated with medication administration if you had difficulty with this question.

Reference
Lilley, L., Harrington, S., & Snyder, J. (2007). *Pharmacology and the nursing process* (5th ed., pp. 340-342, 351). St. Louis: Mosby.

1323. In the event of a fire, which is the best recommendation for the nurse to provide to a client to save lives and to prevent burn injuries in the home?

1 Place escape ladders in the bedrooms.

2 Install a whole-house sprinkler system.

3 Keep fresh batteries in smoke detectors.

4 Mount fire extinguishers in several areas.

Level of Cognitive Ability: Application
Client Needs: Safe and Effective Care Environment
Integrated Process: Teaching and Learning
Content Area: Fundamental Skills

Answer: 3

Rationale: The early detection of smoke using a smoke detector and immediate evacuation from the house have significant and positive effects on mortality rates. This is because the smoke alarm activates before the appearance of open flames, which gives people in the house a chance to evacuate without burn injuries. Option 1 helps people in the house to escape from second-story rooms safely, but it does not alert the people to the fire before flames are evident, thus exposing them to the risk of burn injury. Installing a sprinkler system is very expensive (option 2), and this is usually not done in private residences. Fire extinguishers are a good idea to have in the kitchen and other areas for small fires, but they are not designed to extinguish large fires.

Test-Taking Strategy: Use the process of elimination, and look for the safety prevention measure that is simple to implement and that will alert individuals to the need to evacuate a residence. This will direct you to option 3. Review fire safety if you had difficulty with this question.

References
Black, J., & Hawks, J. (2005). *Medical-surgical nursing: Clinical management for positive outcomes* (7th ed., p. 1435). Philadelphia: Saunders.
Potter, P., & Perry, A. (2005). *Fundamentals of nursing* (6th ed., pp. 991-992). St. Louis: Mosby.

1324. A client has had same-day surgery to insert a ventilating tube into the tympanic membrane. The nurse determines that the client understands the discharge instructions if the client states the need to:
1 Use a shower cap if taking a shower.
2 Swim only with the head above water.
3 Avoid taking any medications for pain.
4 Wash the hair quickly, in 2 minutes or less.

Level of Cognitive Ability: Analysis
Client Needs: Health Promotion and Maintenance
Integrated Process: Teaching and Learning
Content Area: Adult Health/Ear

Answer: 1
Rationale: After the insertion of tubes into the tympanic membrane, it is important to avoid getting water in the ears. For this reason, swimming, showering, and washing the hair are avoided after surgery until the time frame designated for each is identified by the surgeon. A shower cap or earplug may be used when showering, if allowed by the physician. The client should take medication as advised for postoperative discomfort.

Test-Taking Strategy: Use the process of elimination, and note the strategic words "understands the discharge instructions." Eliminate option 2 because of the close-ended word "only," and eliminate option 4 because of the word "quickly." From the remaining options, focusing on the anatomical location of the surgery will direct you to option 1. Review client instructions after the insertion of ventilating tubes into the tympanic membrane if you had difficulty with this question.

Reference
Ignatavicius, D., & Workman, M. (2006). *Medical-surgical nursing: Critical thinking for collaborative care* (5th ed., p. 1130). Philadelphia: Saunders.

1325. The nurse has completed diet teaching for a client on a low-sodium diet for the treatment of hypertension. The nurse determines that further teaching is necessary if the client makes which statement?
1 "Frozen foods are lowest in sodium."
2 "This diet will help lower my blood pressure."
3 "This diet is not a replacement for my antihypertensive medications."
4 "The reason I need to lower my salt intake is to reduce fluid retention."

Level of Cognitive Ability: Analysis
Client Needs: Health Promotion and Maintenance
Integrated Process: Teaching and Learning
Content Area: Adult Health/Cardiovascular

Answer: 1
Rationale: A low-sodium diet is used as an adjunct to antihypertensive medications for the treatment of hypertension. Sodium retains fluid, which leads to hypertension as a result of increased fluid volume. Frozen foods use salt as a preservative and should not be encouraged as part of a low-sodium diet; fresh foods are best.

Test-Taking Strategy: Note the strategic words "further teaching is necessary." These words indicate a negative event query and ask you to select an option that is an incorrect statement. Use the process of elimination, and eliminate options 2, 3, and 4, because these are accurate statements related to hypertension. Review the treatment of hypertension and foods high in sodium if you had difficulty with this question.

References
Lewis, S., Heitkemper, M., Dirksen, S., O'Brien, P., & Bucher, L. (2007). *Medical-surgical nursing: Assessment and management of clinical problems* (7th ed., p. 834). St. Louis: Mosby.
Nix, S. (2005). *Williams' basic nutrition & diet therapy* (12th ed., p. 359). St. Louis: Mosby.

1326. A nurse is preparing a plan regarding home-care instructions for the parents of a child with generalized tonic-clonic seizures who is being treated with oral phenytoin (Dilantin). The nurse includes instructions in the plan regarding:

1 Monitoring the child's intake and output daily
2 Providing oral hygiene, especially care of the gums
3 Administering the medication 1 hour before food intake
4 Checking the child's blood pressure before the administration of the medication

Level of Cognitive Ability: Application
Client Needs: Physiological Integrity
Integrated Process: Teaching and Learning
Content Area: Pharmacology

Answer: 2
Rationale: Phenytoin causes gum bleeding and hyperplasia, and, therefore, a soft toothbrush and gum massage should be instituted to diminish this complication and to prevent trauma. Intake, output, and blood pressure are not affected by this medication. Directions for administration of this medication include administering it with food to minimize gastrointestinal upset.

Test-Taking Strategy: Use the process of elimination. Correlate phenytoin with gum bleeding and hyperplasia. In addition, note the word "oral" in the question and in the correct option. Review the side effects and the method of administration of phenytoin if you had difficulty with this question.

Reference
Kee, J., Hayes, E., & McCuistion, L. (2006). *Pharmacology: A nursing process approach* (5th ed., p. 341). Philadelphia: Saunders.

1327. A nurse performs an initial assessment on a pregnant client and determines that the client is at risk for toxoplasmosis. The nurse would teach the client which of the following to prevent exposure to this disease?

1 Eat raw meats.
2 Wash your hands only before meals.
3 Avoid exposure to litter boxes used by cats.
4 Use topical corticosteroid treatments prophylactically.

Level of Cognitive Ability: Application
Client Needs: Safe and Effective Care Environment
Integrated Process: Teaching and Learning
Content Area: Maternity/Antepartum

Answer: 3
Rationale: Infected house cats transmit toxoplasmosis through the feces. Handling litter boxes can transmit the disease to the pregnant client. Meats that are undercooked can harbor microorganisms that can cause infection. Hands should be washed frequently throughout the day. The use of topical corticosteroids will not prevent exposure to the disease.

Test-Taking Strategy: Use the process of elimination. Eliminate option 2 because of the close-ended word "only." Option 1 represents an extreme statement and can also be eliminated. From the remaining options, focusing on the strategic words "prevent exposure" in the question will direct you to option 3. Review the causes of toxoplasmosis if you had difficulty with this question.

Reference
Wong, D., Hockenberry, M., Perry, S., Lowdermilk, D., & Wilson, D. (2006). *Maternal-child nursing care* (3rd ed., pp. 410, 836). St. Louis: Mosby.

1328. A home-care nurse is instructing a mother of a child with cystic fibrosis (CF) about the appropriate dietary measures. The nurse tells the mother that the child needs to consume a:

1 Low-calorie, low-fat diet
2 High-calorie, restricted fat
3 Low-calorie, low-protein diet
4 High-calorie, high-protein diet

Answer: 4
Rationale: Children with CF are managed with a high-calorie, high-protein diet. Pancreatic enzyme replacement therapy and fat-soluble vitamin supplements are administered. Fat restriction is not necessary.

Test-Taking Strategy: Use the process of elimination. Eliminate options 1 and 2 first, because they both indicate the need to restrict fat in the diet. From the remaining options, thinking about the pathophysiology related to CF will direct you to option 4. Review the diet plan for the child with CF if you had difficulty with this question.

Level of Cognitive Ability: Application
Client Needs: Physiological Integrity
Integrated Process: Teaching and Learning
Content Area: Child Health

References

Hockenberry, M., Wilson, D., & Winkelstein, M. (2005). *Wong's essentials of pediatric nursing* (7th ed., p. 827). St. Louis: Mosby.

Wong, D., Hockenberry, M., Perry, S., Lowdermilk, D., & Wilson, D. (2006). *Maternal-child nursing care* (3rd ed., p. 1462). St. Louis: Mosby.

1329. The nurse in the ambulatory care unit is reviewing the surgical instructions with a client who will be admitted for knee replacement surgery. The nurse informs the client that crutches will be needed for ambulation after surgery and that the client will be instructed regarding the use of the crutches:

1 Before surgery
2 On the first postoperative day
3 On the second postoperative day
4 At the time of discharge after surgery

Level of Cognitive Ability: Application
Client Needs: Physiological Integrity
Integrated Process: Teaching and Learning
Content Area: Adult Health/Musculoskeletal

Answer: 1

Rationale: It is best to assess crutch-walking ability and to instruct the client with regard to the use of the crutches before surgery, because this task can be difficult to learn when the client is in pain and not used to the imbalance that may occur after surgery. Options 2, 3, and 4 are not the appropriate times to teach a client about crutch walking.

Test-Taking Strategy: Use the process of elimination. Note that options 2, 3, and 4 are comparable or alike in that they all address the postoperative period. Review preoperative teaching principles if you had difficulty with this question.

References

Black, J., & Hawks, J. (2005). *Medical-surgical nursing: Clinical management for positive outcomes* (7th ed., pp. 596, 2501). Philadelphia: Saunders.

Ignatavicius, D., & Workman, M. (2006). *Medical surgical nursing: Critical thinking for collaborative care* (5th ed., p. 1204). Philadelphia: Saunders.

1330. A client with a short leg plaster cast complains of an intense itching under the cast. The nurse provides instructions to the client regarding relief measures for the itching. Which statement by the client indicates an understanding of the measures used to relieve the itching?

1 "I can use the blunt part of a ruler to scratch the area."
2 "I can trickle small amounts of water down inside the cast."
3 "I need to obtain assistance when placing an object into the cast for the itching."
4 "I can use a hair dryer on the low setting and allow the air to blow into the cast."

Level of Cognitive Ability: Analysis
Client Needs: Safe and Effective Care Environment
Integrated Process: Teaching and Learning
Content Area: Adult Health/Musculoskeletal

Answer: 4

Rationale: Itching is a common complaint of clients with casts. Objects should not be put inside a cast because of the risk of scratching the skin and providing a point of entry for bacteria. A plaster cast can break down when wet. Therefore, the best way to relieve itching is with the forceful injection of air inside the cast.

Test-Taking Strategy: Use the process of elimination, and eliminate options 1 and 3 first, because they both involve the use of an object being placed inside the cast. Recalling that water can soften a plaster cast and cause maceration of the skin will direct you to option 4. Review client teaching regarding cast care if you had difficulty with this question.

References

Perry, A., & Potter, P. (2006). *Clinical nursing skills & techniques* (6th ed., p. 312). St. Louis: Mosby.

Monahan, F., Sands, J., Neighbors, M., Marek, J., & Green, C. (2007). *Phipps' medical-surgical nursing: Health and illness perspectives* (8th ed., p. 1536). St. Louis: Mosby.

1331. Disulfiram (Antabuse) has been prescribed for a client, and the nurse provides instructions to the client about the medication. Which statement by the client indicates the need for further instructions?

1 "I must be careful taking cold medicines."

2 "I will have to check my aftershave lotion."

3 "As long as I don't drink alcohol, I'll be fine."

4 "I will have to be more careful with the ingredients I use for cooking."

Level of Cognitive Ability: Analysis
Client Needs: Physiological Integrity
Integrated Process: Teaching and Learning
Content Area: Pharmacology

Answer: 3

Rationale: Clients who are taking disulfiram must be taught that substances that contain alcohol can trigger an adverse reaction. Sources of hidden alcohol include foods (soups, sauces, vinegars), medicine (cold medicine), mouthwashes, and skin preparations (alcohol rubs, aftershave lotions).

Test-Taking Strategy: Note the strategic words "need for further instructions." These words indicate a negative event query and ask you to select an option that is an incorrect statement. Remember that disulfiram is used for clients who have alcoholism and that any form of alcohol needs to be avoided with this medication. Review disulfiram and the health teaching that is indicated when this medication is prescribed if you had difficulty with this question.

References

Lilley, L., Harrington, S., & Snyder, J. (2007). *Pharmacology and the nursing process* (5th ed., pp. 90-91, 95). St. Louis: Mosby.

McKenry, L., Tressler, E., & Hogan, M. (2006). *Mosby's pharmacology in nursing* (22nd ed., pp. 170, 175). St. Louis: Mosby.

Skidmore-Roth, L. (2007). *2007 Mosby's nursing drug reference* (20th ed., p. 375). St. Louis: Mosby.

1332. The nurse has provided instructions to a client who is receiving external radiation therapy. Which statement by the client indicates a need for further instructions regarding self-care related to the radiation therapy?

1 "I need to eat a high-protein diet."

2 "I need to avoid exposure to sunlight."

3 "I need to wash my skin with a mild soap and pat it dry."

4 "I need to apply pressure on the irritated area to prevent bleeding."

Level of Cognitive Ability: Application
Client Needs: Physiological Integrity
Integrated Process: Teaching and Learning
Content Area: Adult Health/Oncology

Answer: 4

Rationale: The client should avoid pressure on the irritated area and wear loose-fitting clothing. Specific physician instructions would be necessary to obtain if an alteration in skin integrity occurred as a result of the radiation therapy. Options 1, 2, and 3 are accurate measures regarding radiation therapy.

Test-Taking Strategy: Note the strategic words "need for further instructions." These words indicate a negative event query and ask you to select an option that is an incorrect statement. The word "pressure" in option 4 is an indication that this is an inappropriate measure. Review the client teaching points related to skin care and radiation therapy if you had difficulty with this question.

Reference

Ignatavicius, D., & Workman, M. (2006). *Medical-surgical nursing: Critical thinking for collaborative care* (5th ed., p. 491). Philadelphia: Saunders.

1333. The nurse has provided instructions to a client regarding the testicular self-examination (TSE). Which statement by the client indicates that the client needs further instructions regarding TSE?

1 "I know to report any small lumps."

2 "I should examine myself every 2 months."

3 "I should examine myself after I take a warm shower."

4 "I should feel the spermatic cord in the back and going up."

Answer: 2

Rationale: TSE should be performed every month. Small lumps or abnormalities should be reported. The spermatic cord finding is normal. After a warm bath or shower, the scrotum is relaxed, which makes it easier to perform TSE.

Test-Taking Strategy: Use the process of elimination. Remembering that breast self-examination needs to be performed monthly may assist you with recalling that TSE is also performed monthly. Review the procedure for TSE if you had difficulty with this question.

Level of Cognitive Ability: Analysis
Client Needs: Health Promotion and Maintenance
Integrated Process: Teaching and Learning
Content Area: Adult Health/Oncology

Reference
Black, J., & Hawks, J. (2005). *Medical-surgical nursing: Clinical management for positive outcomes* (7th ed., p. 1005). Philadelphia: Saunders.

1334. A client with acquired immunodeficiency syndrome (AIDS) has a nursing diagnosis of fatigue. The nurse teaches the client which strategy to conserve energy after discharge from the hospital?

1 Bathe before eating breakfast.
2 Sit for as many activities as possible.
3 Stand in the shower instead of taking a bath.
4 Group all tasks to be performed early in the morning.

Level of Cognitive Ability: Application
Client Needs: Health Promotion and Maintenance
Integrated Process: Teaching and Learning
Content Area: Adult Health/Immune

Answer: 2

Rationale: The client is taught to conserve energy by sitting for as many activities as possible, including dressing, shaving, preparing food, ironing, and so on. The client should also sit in a shower chair instead of standing while bathing. The client needs to prioritize activities such as eating breakfast before bathing, and he or she should intersperse each major activity with a period of rest.

Test-Taking Strategy: Focus on the subject of conserving energy. Think about the amount of exertion required by the client to perform each of the activities described in the options. Options 3 and 4 are obviously taxing for the client and are thus eliminated first. From the remaining options, recall that bathing may take away energy that could be used for eating and so is not helpful. Review the measures that conserve energy if you had difficulty with this question.

Reference
Black, J., & Hawks, J. (2005). *Medical-surgical nursing: Clinical management for positive outcomes* (7th ed., p. 2395). Philadelphia: Saunders.

1335. The nurse has provided self-care activity instructions to a client after the insertion of an internal cardioverter-defibrillator (ICD). The nurse determines that further instruction is needed if the client makes which statement?

1 "I need to avoid doing anything where there would be rough contact with the ICD insertion site."
2 "I can perform activities such as swimming, driving, or operating heavy equipment as I need to do them."
3 "I should try to avoid doing strenuous things that would make my heart rate go up to or above the rate cutoff on the ICD."
4 "I should keep away from electromagnetic sources such as transformers, large electrical generators, and metal detectors as well as running motors."

Answer: 2

Rationale: Postdischarge instructions typically include avoiding the following: tight clothing or belts over the ICD insertion site; rough contact with the ICD insertion site; electromagnetic fields, such as those surrounding electrical transformers; radio, television, and radar transmitters; metal detectors; and the running motors of cars or boats. Clients must also alert physicians or dentists to the presence of the device, because certain procedures such as diathermy, electrocautery, and magnetic resonance imaging may need to be avoided to prevent device malfunction. Clients should follow the specific advice of a physician regarding activities that are potentially hazardous to the self or others, such as swimming, driving, or operating heavy equipment.

Test-Taking Strategy: Use the process of elimination, and note the strategic words "further instruction is needed." These words indicate a negative event query and ask you to select an option that is an incorrect statement. Options 1 and 4 can be eliminated first, because they are similar to standard postpacemaker insertion instructions. From the remaining options, noting the words "heavy equipment" in option 2 will direct you to this option. Review the client teaching points for ICD if you had difficulty with this question.

Level of Cognitive Ability: Analysis
Client Needs: Safe and Effective Care
  Environment
Integrated Process: Teaching and Learning
Content Area: Adult Health/Cardiovascular

References
Ignatavicius, D., & Workman, M. (2006). *Medical-surgical nursing: Critical thinking for collaborative care* (5th ed., p. 746). Philadelphia: Saunders.
Lewis, S., Heitkemper, M., Dirksen, S., O'Brien, P., & Bucher, L. (2007). *Medical-surgical nursing: Assessment and management of clinical problems* (7th ed., p. 858). St. Louis: Mosby.

1336. A 10-year-old child who is very active socially and who is often away from his parents has been diagnosed with type 1 diabetes mellitus. The nurse prepares to educate the family about the disorder and plans to teach:

1 The child to monitor insulin requirements and administer his own insulin
2 The parents to always be available to monitor the child's insulin requirements
3 The child's schoolteacher to monitor insulin requirements and to administer the child's insulin
4 All of the friends and family involved with the child's activities to monitor the child's insulin requirements

Level of Cognitive Ability: Application
Client Needs: Health Promotion and
  Maintenance
Integrated Process: Teaching and Learning
Content Area: Child Health

Answer: 1
Rationale: Most children 9 years old or older can understand the principles of monitoring their own insulin requirements. They are usually responsible enough to determine the appropriate intervention needed to maintain their health. The schoolteacher should not be expected to take responsibility for health care interventions. Parents, friends, and family cannot always be available.

Test-Taking Strategy: Noting the age of the child will indicate that the child is able to take control and responsibility regarding his health care situation. Eliminate option 4 first because of the close-ended word "all." From the remaining options, note that options 2 and 3 rely on other individuals to care for the child. Review the growth and development of a 10-year-old child if you had difficulty with this question.

Reference
Hockenberry, M., Wilson, D., & Winkelstein, M. (2005). *Wong's essentials of pediatric nursing* (7th ed., p. 1088). St. Louis: Mosby.

1337. The nurse instructs a client with candidiasis (thrush) of the oral cavity about how to care for the disorder. The nurse determines that the client needs additional instructions if the client states the need to:

1 Eat foods that are liquid or pureed.
2 Eliminate spicy foods from the diet.
3 Eliminate citrus juices and hot liquids from the diet.
4 Rinse the mouth 4 times daily with a commercial mouthwash.

Level of Cognitive Ability: Application
Client Needs: Physiological Integrity
Integrated Process: Teaching and Learning
Content Area: Adult Health/Immune

Answer: 4
Rationale: Clients with thrush cannot tolerate commercial mouthwashes, because the high alcohol concentration in these products can cause pain and discomfort of the lesions. A solution of warm water or mouthwash formulas without alcohol are better tolerated and may promote healing. A change in diet to liquid or pureed food often eases the discomfort of eating. The client should avoid spicy foods, citrus juices, and hot liquids.

Test-Taking Strategy: Use the process of elimination, and note the strategic words "needs additional instructions." These words indicate a negative event query and ask you to select an option that is an incorrect statement. In addition, noting the words "commercial mouthwash" in option 4 will direct you to this option. Review the client teaching points related to candidiasis (thrush) if you had difficulty with this question.

References
Ignatavicius, D., & Workman, M. (2006). *Medical-surgical nursing: Critical thinking for collaborative care* (5th ed., p. 1249). Philadelphia: Saunders.
Lewis, S., Heitkemper, M., Dirksen, S., O'Brien, P., & Bucher, L. (2007). *Medical-surgical nursing: Assessment and management of clinical problems* (7th ed., p. 1000). St. Louis: Mosby.

1338. The nurse has given instructions about site care to a hemodialysis client who had an implantation of an arteriovenous (AV) fistula in the right arm. The nurse determines that the client needs further instructions if the client states the need to:

1 Sleep on the right side.
2 Avoid carrying heavy objects with the right arm.
3 Perform range-of-motion exercises routinely on the right arm.
4 Report an increased temperature, redness, or drainage at the site.

Level of Cognitive Ability: Analysis
Client Needs: Health Promotion and Maintenance
Integrated Process: Teaching and Learning
Content Area: Adult Health/Renal

Answer: 1
Rationale: Routine instructions to the client with an AV fistula, graft, or shunt include reporting signs and symptoms of infection, performing routine range-of-motion exercises of the affected extremity, avoiding sleeping with the body weight on the extremity with the access site, and avoiding carrying heavy objects or compressing the extremity that has the access site.

Test-Taking Strategy: Use the process of elimination, and note the strategic words "needs further instructions." These words indicate a negative event query and ask you to select an option that is an incorrect statement. Recalling the importance of maintaining the patency of the AV fistula will direct you to option 1. Review the home-care instructions for a client with an AV fistula if you had difficulty with this question.

Reference
Ignatavicius, D., & Workman, M. (2006). *Medical-surgical nursing: Critical thinking for collaborative care* (5th ed , p. 1754). Philadelphia: Saunders.

1339. A nurse provides instructions to a client about applying nitroglycerin patch (Nitrodisc). The nurse determines that the client is using correct technique when applying the patch if the client:

1 Applies a second patch if chest pain occurs
2 Applies the patch to any nonhairy area of the body
3 Removes the patch when bathing and reapplies it after the bath
4 Applies the patch directly to the skin, then gently rubs the patch to activate the medication

Level of Cognitive Ability: Analysis
Client Needs: Physiological Integrity
Integrated Process: Teaching and Learning
Content Area: Pharmacology

Answer: 2
Rationale: Nitroglycerin ointment is used on a scheduled basis, and it is not prescribed specifically for the occurrence of chest pain. The ointment is not rubbed into the skin; it is reapplied only as directed. It is applied to a nonhairy part of the body.

Test-Taking Strategy: Use the process of elimination, and focus on the subject of using correct technique. Noting the word "nonhairy" in option 2 will direct you to this option. Review these client teaching points if you had difficulty with this question.

References
Kee, J., Hayes, E., & McCuistion, L. (2006). *Pharmacology: A nursing process approach* (5th ed., p. 618). Philadelphia: Saunders.
McKenry, L., Tressier, E., & Hogan, M. (2006). *Mosby's pharmacology in nursing* (22nd ed., pp. 609-610). St. Louis: Mosby.

1340. A nurse is giving medication instructions to a client who is receiving furosemide (Lasix). The nurse determines that further teaching is necessary if the client makes which of the following statements?

1 "I need to change positions slowly."
2 "I need to talk to my physician about the use of alcohol."
3 "I need to be careful to not get overheated in warm weather."
4 "I need to avoid the use of salt substitutes, because they contain potassium."

Answer: 4
Rationale: Furosemide is a potassium-losing diuretic, so there is no need to avoid high-potassium products, such as a salt substitute. Orthostatic hypotension is a risk, and the client must use caution when changing positions and with exposure to warm weather. The client needs to discuss the use of alcohol with the physician.

Level of Cognitive Ability: Analysis
Client Needs: Physiological Integrity
Integrated Process: Teaching and Learning
Content Area: Pharmacology

Test-Taking Strategy: Use the process of elimination, and note the strategic words "further teaching is necessary." These words indicate a negative event query and ask you to select an option that is an incorrect statement. Recalling that furosemide is a potassium-losing diuretic and that diuretic therapy can induce orthostatic hypotension will direct you to option 4. Review furosemide if you had difficulty with this question.

References

Kee, J., Hayes, E., & McCuistion, L. (2006). *Pharmacology: A nursing process approach* (5th ed., pp. 634, 920-921). Philadelphia: Saunders.

McKenry, L., Tressier, E., & Hogan, M. (2006). *Mosby's pharmacology in nursing* (22nd ed., pp. 676-677). St. Louis: Mosby.

1341. A client has been prescribed a clonidine patch (Catapres-TTS), and the nurse has instructed the client regarding the use of the patch. The nurse determines that further instruction is needed if the nurse noted that the client:

1 Intended to change the patch every 7 days
2 Trimmed the patch because one edge was loose
3 Selected a hairless site on the torso for application
4 Planned to leave the patch in place during bathing or showering

Level of Cognitive Ability: Analysis
Client Needs: Physiological Integrity
Integrated Process: Teaching and Learning
Content Area: Pharmacology

Answer: 2

Rationale: The clonidine patch should be applied to a hairless site on the torso or the upper arm. It is changed every 7 days, and it is left in place when bathing or showering. The patch should not be trimmed, because it will alter the medication dose. If it becomes slightly loose, it should be covered with an adhesive overlay from the medication package. If it becomes very loose or falls off, it should be replaced. The patch is discarded by folding it in half with the adhesive sides together.

Test-Taking Strategy: Use the process of elimination, and note the strategic words "further instruction is needed." These words indicate a negative event query and ask you to select an option that is an incorrect statement. Noting the words "trimmed the patch" will direct you to option 2, because this client action would alter the medication dose. Review the clonidine patch if you had difficulty with this question.

References

McKenry, L., Tressier, E., & Hogan, M. (2006). *Mosby's pharmacology in nursing* (22nd ed., pp. 576-579). St. Louis: Mosby.

Skidmore-Roth, L. (2007). *2007 Mosby's nursing drug reference* (20th ed., p. 292). St. Louis: Mosby.

1342. Cholestyramine (Questran) is prescribed, and the nurse provides instructions to the client about the medication. The nurse determines that further instructions are needed if the client makes which statement?

1 "I should take this medication with meals."
2 "I need to mix the medicine with juice or applesauce."
3 "I should call my doctor immediately if it causes constipation."
4 "I should increase my fluid intake while taking this medication."

Answer: 3

Rationale: This medication should not be taken dry, and it can be mixed in water, juice, carbonated beverages, applesauce, or soup. Common side effects include constipation, nausea, indigestion, and flatulence. Increasing fluids will minimize the constipating effects of the medication. Questran must be administered with food to be effective.

Test-Taking Strategy: Use the process of elimination, and note the strategic words "further instructions are needed." These words indicate a negative event query and ask you to select an option that is an incorrect statement. Select option 3 because of the word "immediately" and because normally measures can be taken to prevent constipation rather than immediately calling the physician. Review cholestyramine if you are unfamiliar with it.

Level of Cognitive Ability: Analysis
Client Needs: Physiological Integrity
Integrated Process: Teaching and Learning
Content Area: Pharmacology

References
McKenry, L., Tressier, E., & Hogan, M. (2006). *Mosby's pharmacology in nursing* (22nd ed., pp. 654-656). St. Louis: Mosby.
Skidmore-Roth, L. (2007). *2007 Mosby's nursing drug reference* (20th ed., p. 268). St. Louis: Mosby.

1343. A nurse is preparing written medication instructions for a client who is receiving colestipol hydrochloride (Colestid). The nurse includes instructions about the need for the client to take which of the following to counteract unintended medication effects?

1 Vitamin C
2 Vitamin B12
3 B-complex vitamins
4 Fat-soluble vitamins

Level of Cognitive Ability: Application
Client Needs: Physiological Integrity
Integrated Process: Teaching and Learning
Content Area: Pharmacology

Answer: 4

Rationale: Colestipol, which is a bile-sequestering agent, is used to lower blood cholesterol levels. However, the bile salts (which are rich in cholesterol) interfere with the absorption of the fat-soluble vitamins A, D, E, and K as well as folic acid. With ongoing therapy, the client is at risk for the deficiency of these vitamins and is counseled to take them as supplements.

Test-Taking Strategy: Use the process of elimination. Recalling that bile-sequestering agents interfere with the absorption of fat-soluble vitamins will assist you with eliminating options 1, 2 and 3. Also, select option 4, because it is the umbrella option. Review client teaching points regarding colestipol hydrochloride if you had difficulty with this question.

References
McKenry, L., Tressier, E., & Hogan, M. (2006). *Mosby's pharmacology in nursing* (22nd ed., pp. 642-644). St. Louis: Mosby.
Skidmore-Roth, L. (2007). *2007 Mosby's nursing drug reference* (20th ed., p. 302). St. Louis: Mosby.

NURSING PROCESS

Assessment

1344. A clinic nurse in a well-baby clinic is collecting data regarding the motor development of a 15-month-old child. Which of the following is the highest level of development that the nurse would expect to observe in this child?

1 The child turns a doorknob.
2 The child unzips a large zipper.
3 The child builds a tower of two blocks.
4 The child puts on simple clothes independently.

Level of Cognitive Ability: Analysis
Client Needs: Health Promotion and Maintenance
Integrated Process: Nursing Process/Assessment
Content Area: Child Health

Answer: 3

Rationale: At the age of 15 months, the nurse would expect that the child could build a tower of two blocks. A 24-month-old child would be able to turn a doorknob and unzip a large zipper. At the age of 30 months, the child would be able to put on simple clothes independently.

Test-Taking Strategy: Note the age of the child and the strategic words "highest level of development." Visualize each of the motor skills presented in the options to assist you with selecting the correct option. Review these developmental milestones if you had difficulty with this question.

Reference
Hockenberry, M., Wilson, D., & Winkelstein, M. (2005). *Wong's essentials of pediatric nursing* (7th ed., p. 398). St. Louis: Mosby.

1345. A child with hemophilia is brought into the emergency department after being hit on the neck with a baseball. The nurse immediately assesses the child for:

1 Airway obstruction
2 Factor VIII deficiency
3 Spontaneous hematuria
4 Headache and slurred speech

Level of Cognitive Ability: Analysis
Client Needs: Physiological Integrity
Integrated Process: Nursing Process/Assessment
Content Area: Child Health

Answer: 1
Rationale: Trauma to the neck may cause bleeding into the tissues of the neck, which may compromise the airway. Although hematuria is a symptom of hemophilia, it is not associated with neck injury. Headache and slurred speech are associated with head trauma. Factor VIII deficiency is not a symptom of hemophilia but rather a common form of the disease.

Test-Taking Strategy: Use the ABCs—airway, breathing, and circulation—to answer this question. Remember that airway assessment is always a first priority. This will direct you to option 1. Review the care of the child with hemophilia if you had difficulty with this question.

References
McKinney, E., James, S., Murray, S., & Ashwill, J. (2005). *Maternal-child nursing* (2nd ed., pp. 1316, 1320). St. Louis: Saunders.
Ward, K., & Hagemann, T. (2006). *Mosby's pediatric drug consult* (pp. 651-658). St. Louis: Mosby.

1346. A nurse is caring for a child who has been diagnosed with rubeola (measles). The nurse notes that the physician has documented the presence of Koplik's spots. On the basis of this documentation, which of the following would the nurse expect to note during the assessment of the child?

1 Pinpoint petechiae noted on both legs
2 Whitish vesicles located across the chest
3 Petechiae spots that are reddish and pinpoint on the soft palate
4 Small, blue-white spots with a red base found on the buccal mucosa

Level of Cognitive Ability: Analysis
Client Needs: Physiological Integrity
Integrated Process: Nursing Process/Assessment
Content Area: Child Health

Answer: 4
Rationale: Koplik's spots appear approximately 2 days before the appearance of the rash. These are small, blue-white spots with a red base that are found on the buccal mucosa. The spots last approximately 3 days, after which time they slough off. Options 1, 2, and 3 are incorrect.

Test-Taking Strategy: Use the process of elimination. Eliminate options 1 and 3 first, because they are comparable or alike and address petechiae spots. From the remaining options, recalling that Koplik's spots are located on the buccal mucosa will direct you to option 4. Review the presentation of Koplik's spots if you had difficulty with this question.

Reference
Hockenberry, M., Wilson, D., & Winkelstein, M. (2005). *Wong's essentials of pediatric nursing* (7th ed., pp. 440-441). St. Louis: Mosby.

1347. A child is hospitalized with a diagnosis of nephrotic syndrome. Which assessment finding would the nurse expect to note in the child?
1 Weight loss
2 Constipation
3 Hypotension
4 Abdominal pain

Answer: 4
Rationale: Clinical manifestations associated with nephrotic syndrome include edema, anorexia, fatigue, and abdominal pain from the presence of extra fluid in the peritoneal cavity. Diarrhea caused by the edema of the bowel occurs and may cause the decreased absorption of nutrients. Increased weight and a normal blood pressure are noted.

Test-Taking Strategy: Think about the physiology associated with nephrotic syndrome. Recalling that edema is a clinical manifestation will direct you to option 4. Review the clinical manifestations of nephrotic syndrome if you had difficulty with this question.

Level of Cognitive Ability: Analysis
Client Needs: Physiological Integrity
Integrated Process: Nursing Process/Assessment
Content Area: Child Health

Reference
Hockenberry, M., Wilson, D., & Winkelstein, M. (2005). *Wong's essentials of pediatric nursing* (7th ed., p. 996). St. Louis: Mosby.

1348. A child is admitted to the hospital with a suspected diagnosis of von Willebrand's disease. On assessment of the child, which symptom would most likely be noted?
1 Hematuria
2 Presence of hematomas
3 Presence of hemarthrosis
4 Bleeding from the mucous membranes

Level of Cognitive Ability: Analysis
Client Needs: Physiological Integrity
Integrated Process: Nursing Process/Assessment
Content Area: Child Health

Answer: 4

Rationale: The primary clinical manifestations of von Willebrand's disease are bruising and mucous membrane bleeding from the nose, mouth, and gastrointestinal tract. Prolonged bleeding after trauma and surgery, including tooth extraction, may be the first evidence of abnormal hemostasis in those with mild disease. In females, menorrhagia and profuse postpartum bleeding may occur. Bleeding associated with von Willebrand's disease may be severe and lead to anemia and shock, but, unlike what is seen in clients with hemophilia, deep bleeding into joints and muscles is rare. Options 1, 2, and 3 are characteristic of those signs found in clients with hemophilia.

Test-Taking Strategy: Specific knowledge regarding the clinical manifestations associated with von Willebrand's disease is required to answer this question. Recalling that options 1, 2, and 3 are characteristic of hemophilia will assist you with eliminating these options and direct you to option 4. Review the clinical manifestations of hemophilia if you are unfamiliar with this disorder.

Reference
Hockenberry, M., Wilson, D., & Winkelstein, M. (2005). *Wong's essentials of pediatric nursing* (7th ed., pp. 952-953). St. Louis: Mosby.

1349. A female client with narcolepsy has been prescribed dextroamphetamine (Dexedrine). The client complains to the nurse that she cannot sleep well anymore at night and that she does not want to take the medication any longer. The nurse then asks the client if the medication is taken at which appropriate time?
1 Before a bedtime snack
2 Just before going to sleep
3 Two hours before bedtime
4 At least 6 hours before bedtime

Level of Cognitive Ability: Application
Client Needs: Physiological Integrity
Integrated Process: Nursing Process/Assessment
Content Area: Pharmacology

Answer: 4

Rationale: Dextroamphetamine is a central nervous system (CNS) stimulant that acts by releasing norepinephrine from the nerve endings. The client should take the medication at least 6 hours before going to bed at night to prevent disturbances with sleep. Therefore, options 1, 2, and 3 are incorrect.

Test-Taking Strategy: Use the process of elimination. Recall that this medication causes CNS stimulation and interferes with sleep. Evaluate each of the options in terms of how far removed the scheduled dose is from the client's bedtime. This will direct you to option 4. Review dextroamphetamine if you had difficulty with this question.

Reference
Skidmore-Roth, L. (2008). *Mosby's nursing drug reference* (21st ed., p. 351). St. Louis: Mosby.

1350. A nurse is assessing the level of consciousness of a child with a head injury and documents that the child is obtunded. On the basis of this documentation, which observation did the nurse note?

  1 The child is unable to think clearly and rapidly.

  2 The child is unable to recognize place or person.

  3 The child requires considerable stimulation for arousal.

  4 The child sleeps unless aroused and, when aroused, has limited interaction with the environment.

Level of Cognitive Ability: Analysis
Client Needs: Physiological Integrity
Integrated Process: Nursing Process/Assessment
Content Area: Child Health

Answer: 4

Rationale: If the child is obtunded, the child sleeps unless aroused and, when aroused, has limited interaction with the environment. Option 1 describes confusion. Option 2 describes disorientation. Option 3 describes stupor.

Test-Taking Strategy: Note the strategic word "obtunded." Knowledge regarding the standard terms used to identify level of consciousness will direct you to option 4. Review the assessment of the level of consciousness if you had difficulty with this question.

References

Hockenberry, M., & Wilson, D. (2007). *Nursing care of infants and children* (8th ed., p. 1619). St. Louis: Mosby.

Hockenberry, M., Wilson, D., & Winkelstein, M. (2005). *Wong's essentials of pediatric nursing* (7th ed., p. 1013). St. Louis: Mosby.

1351. The home-care nurse is visiting a client who is in a body cast. The nurse is performing an assessment of the psychosocial adjustment of the client to the cast. During the assessment, the nurse would most appropriately assess:

  1 The need for sensory stimulation

  2 The amount of home-care support available

  3 The ability to perform activities of daily living

  4 The type of transportation available for follow-up care

Level of Cognitive Ability: Analysis
Client Needs: Psychosocial Integrity
Integrated Process: Nursing Process/Assessment
Content Area: Adult Health/Musculoskeletal

Answer: 1

Rationale: A psychosocial assessment of the client who is immobilized would most appropriately include the need for sensory stimulation. This assessment should also include such factors as body image, past and present coping skills, and the coping methods used during the period of immobilization. Although home-care support, the ability to perform activities of daily living, and transportation are components of an assessment, they are not specifically related to psychosocial adjustment.

Test-Taking Strategy: Use the process of elimination, and focus on the strategic words "psychosocial adjustment" and "most appropriately." Option 3 can be eliminated first, because it relates to physiological integrity rather than psychosocial integrity. Eliminate options 2 and 4 next, because they are most closely related to the physical support of, rather than the psychosocial needs of, the client. Review the components of a psychosocial assessment if you had difficulty with this question.

References

Black, J., & Hawks, J. (2005). *Medical-surgical nursing: Clinical management for positive outcomes* (7th ed., p. 645). Philadelphia: Saunders.

Ignatavicius, D., & Workman, M. (2006). *Medical-surgical nursing: Critical thinking for collaborative care* (5th ed., p. 1196). Philadelphia: Saunders.

Lewis, S., Heitkemper, M., Dirksen, S., O'Brien, P., & Bucher, L. (2007). *Medical-surgical nursing: Assessment and management of clinical problems* (7th ed., pp. 1647-1648). St. Louis: Mosby.

1352. The nurse is caring for a client with acquired immunodeficiency syndrome (AIDS). Which finding noted in the client indicates the presence of an opportunistic respiratory infection?

1 Loss of sight
2 Ulcerated perirectal lesions
3 White plaques located on the oral mucosa
4 Fever, exertional dyspnea, and nonproductive cough

Level of Cognitive Ability: Analysis
Client Needs: Physiological Integrity
Integrated Process: Nursing Process/Assessment
Content Area: Adult Health/Immune

Answer: 4
Rationale: Fever, exertional dyspnea, and a nonproductive cough are signs of *Pneumocystis jiroveci* pneumonia, which is a common, life-threatening opportunistic infection that afflicts those with AIDS. Options 1, 2, and 3 are not associated with respiratory infection. Option 1 describes the viral infection herpes zoster (shingles) when it has spread to involve the ophthalmic nerve. Option 2 describes herpes simplex, which can occur in homosexual men. Option 3 describes the fungal infection oral candidiasis *(Candida albicans)*, which is also called *thrush.*

Test-Taking Strategy: Use the process of elimination, and focus on the subject: respiratory infection. Option 4 is the only option that identifies symptoms that are related to the respiratory system. Review the signs of respiratory infection if you had difficulty with this question.

References
Black, J., & Hawks, J. (2005). *Medical-surgical nursing: Clinical management for positive outcomes* (7th ed., p. 2392). Philadelphia: Saunders.
Ignatavicius, D., & Workman, M. (2006). *Medical-surgical nursing: Critical thinking for collaborative care* (5th ed., pp. 432-434). Philadelphia: Saunders.

1353. An adult client seeks treatment in an ambulatory care clinic for complaints of a left earache, nausea, and a full feeling in the left ear. The client has an elevated temperature. The nurse first questions the client about:

1 If hearing is magnified in that ear
2 A history of a recent brain abscess
3 If acetaminophen (Tylenol) relieves the pain
4 A history of a recent upper respiratory infection (URI)

Level of Cognitive Ability: Analysis
Client Needs: Physiological Integrity
Integrated Process: Nursing Process/Assessment
Content Area: Adult Health/Ear

Answer: 4
Rationale: Otitis media in the adult is typically one sided and presents as an acute process with earache, nausea, and possible vomiting, fever, and fullness in the ear. The client may complain of diminished hearing in that ear. The nurse takes a client history first, assessing whether the client has had a recent URI. It is unnecessary to question the client about a brain abscess. The nurse may ask the client if anything relieves the pain, but ear infection pain is usually not relieved until antibiotic therapy is initiated.

Test-Taking Strategy: Use the process of elimination. Recalling the relationship between a URI and otitis media will direct you to option 4. Review otitis media if you had difficulty with this question.

Reference
Black, J., & Hawks, J. (2005). *Medical-surgical nursing: Clinical management for positive outcomes* (7th ed., p. 1984). Philadelphia: Saunders.

1354. The home-care nurse visits an 83-year-old client who is upset about urinary incontinence. Which of the following does the nurse determine is a potential environmental contributor to the client's problem?

1 Nightlights in the hallways
2 Large, unmovable furniture
3 A bathroom at each end of the house
4 The commode seat being at a 15-inch height

Answer: 4
Rationale: A bathroom with a low commode seat is a potential barrier to voiding for an older adult. The low seat is likely to increase the time that it takes for the client to lower the body down onto the seat. This increases the risk of incontinence, because reaching a low level can be very difficult for a client with limited range of motion who is at risk for falls or who needs an assistive device for ambulation. The nurse helps to resolve the client's problem with incontinence by recommending a raised toilet seat that can be attached to a standard commode or toilet. Nightlights, a fixed floor plan as a result of heavy furniture, and conveniently located bathrooms should facilitate voiding.

Level of Cognitive Ability: Analysis
Client Needs: Health Promotion and
  Maintenance
Integrated Process: Nursing Process/Assessment
Content Area: Fundamental Skills

Test-Taking Strategy: Focus on the subject of an environmental barrier to normal voiding, and use the process of elimination. Eliminate option 1, 2, and 3, because they contribute to the client safely reaching the bathroom for voiding. Review the measures that promote normal voiding if you had difficulty with this question.

References

Ignatavicius, D., & Workman, M. (2006). *Medical-surgical nursing: Critical thinking for collaborative care* (5th ed., p. 1695). Philadelphia: Saunders.
Meiner, S., & Leuckenotte, A. (2006). *Gerontologic nursing* (3rd ed., p. 632). St. Louis: Mosby.

1355. The nurse prepares to administer a continuous intravenous (IV) infusion through a peripheral IV to a client who has dehydration. Which is the priority nursing assessment before initiating the IV infusion?
  1 Checking a daily body weight
  2 Checking the serum electrolytes
  3 Checking intake and output records
  4 Asking the client about the dominant side

Level of Cognitive Ability: Analysis
Client Needs: Physiological Integrity
Integrated Process: Nursing Process/Assessment
Content Area: Fundamental Skills

Answer: 1
Rationale: The nurse obtains the client's baseline body weight before beginning the IV infusion, because body weight is a sensitive and specific indicator of fluid volume status when body weights are compared on a daily basis. This means that, as a client receives or accumulates fluid, body weight quickly and proportionately increases and vice versa. The remaining options are reasonable assessments to complete before initiating an IV infusion. Determining the client's dominant side assists in deciding a site for inserting the initial IV catheter, but it provides no information about fluid volume status. Intake, output, and serum electrolytes are potentially affected by more confounding factors, and, thus, they are less specific and sensitive to fluctuations in body fluid.

Test-Taking Strategy: Focus on the client's diagnosis. Review the options to determine the best method for the nurse to use to evaluate fluid status. Body weight is the best option, because it is the most sensitive and specific measurement listed. Review the care of the dehydrated client if you had difficulty with this question.

References

Black, J., & Hawks, J. (2005). *Medical-surgical nursing: Clinical management for positive outcomes* (7th ed., p. 209). Philadelphia: Saunders.
Lewis, S., Heitkemper, M., Dirksen, S., O'Brien, P., & Bucher, L. (2007). *Medical-surgical nursing: Assessment and management of clinical problems* (7th ed., p. 322). St. Louis: Mosby.

1356. A client is scheduled for an arteriogram using a radiopaque dye. The nurse assesses which most critical item before the procedure?
  1 Vital signs
  2 Intake and output
  3 Height and weight
  4 Allergy to iodine or shellfish

Answer: 4
Rationale: Allergy to iodine or seafood is associated with allergy to the radiopaque dye that is used for medical imaging examinations. Informed consent is necessary, because an arteriogram requires the injection of a radiopaque dye into the blood vessel. Although options 1, 2, and 3 are components of the preprocedure assessment, the risks of allergic reaction and possible anaphylaxis are the most critical.

Level of Cognitive Ability: Application
Client Needs: Physiological Integrity
Integrated Process: Nursing Process/Assessment
Content Area: Delegating/Prioritizing

Test-Taking Strategy: Use the process of elimination, and note the strategic words "most critical." Recalling the risk of anaphylaxis related to the dye will direct you to option 4. Review the preprocedure care for angiography if you had difficulty with this question.

References

Chernecky, C., & Berger, B. (2008). *Laboratory tests and diagnostic procedures* (5th ed., p. 167). Philadelphia: Saunders.

Pagana, K., & Pagana, T. (2005). *Mosby's diagnostic and laboratory test reference* (7th ed., p. 127). St. Louis: Mosby.

1357. The nurse is performing a cardiovascular assessment on a client. Which item would the nurse assess to obtain the best information about the client's left-sided heart function?

1 The status of breath sounds
2 The presence of peripheral edema
3 The presence of hepatojugular reflux
4 The presence of jugular vein distention

Level of Cognitive Ability: Application
Client Needs: Physiological Integrity
Integrated Process: Nursing Process/Assessment
Content Area: Adult Health/Cardiovascular

Answer: 1
Rationale: The client with heart failure may present different symptoms depending on whether the right or the left side of the heart is failing. Peripheral edema, hepatojugular reflux, and jugular vein distention are all signs of right-sided heart function. The assessment of breath sounds provides information about left-sided heart function.

Test-Taking Strategy: Use the process of elimination, and focus on the subject: the status of left-sided heart function. Remember "left" and "lungs." Options 2, 3, and 4 reflect right-sided heart failure. Review the signs of right- and left-sided heart failure if you had difficulty with this question.

References

Black, J., & Hawks, J. (2005). *Medical-surgical nursing: Clinical management for positive outcomes* (7th ed., p. 1653). Philadelphia: Saunders.

Ignatavicius, D., & Workman, M. (2006). *Medical-surgical nursing: Critical thinking for collaborative care* (5th ed., pp. 753-754). Philadelphia: Saunders.

1358. The nurse is obtaining a history from a client who was admitted to the hospital with a thrombotic brain attack (stroke). The nurse assesses the client, knowing that, before the stroke occurred, the client most likely experienced:

1 No symptoms at all
2 Throbbing headaches
3 Transient hemiplegia and loss of speech
4 Unexplained episodes of loss of consciousness

Level of Cognitive Ability: Application
Client Needs: Physiological Integrity
Integrated Process: Nursing Process/Assessment
Content Area: Adult Health/Neurological

Answer: 3
Rationale: Cerebral thrombosis does not occur suddenly. During the few hours or days before a thrombotic stroke, the client may experience a transient loss of speech, hemiplegia, or paresthesias on one side of the body. Other signs and symptoms of thrombotic stroke vary, but they may include dizziness, cognitive changes, or seizures. Headache is rare, and a loss of consciousness is not likely to occur.

Test-Taking Strategy: Use the process of elimination. Option 1 is eliminated first, because the client experiencing a stroke will likely experience symptoms. From the remaining options, focus on the type of stroke addressed in the question to direct you to option 3. Review the signs and symptoms of a thrombotic stroke if you had difficulty with this question.

Reference

Black, J., & Hawks, J. (2005). *Medical-surgical nursing: Clinical management for positive outcomes* (7th ed., p. 2111). Philadelphia: Saunders.

1359. A client in a long-term care facility has had a series of gastrointestinal (GI) diagnostic tests, including an upper GI series and endoscopies. Upon return to the long-term care facility, the priority nursing assessment should focus on:
  1 The comfort level
  2 Activity tolerance
  3 The level of consciousness
  4 The hydration and nutrition status

Level of Cognitive Ability: Application
Client Needs: Physiological Integrity
Integrated Process: Nursing Process/Assessment
Content Area: Delegating/Prioritizing

Answer: 4
Rationale: Many of the diagnostic studies to identify GI disorders require that the GI tract be cleaned (usually with laxatives and enemas) before testing. In addition, the client most often takes nothing by mouth before and during the testing period. Because the studies may be done over a period that exceeds 24 hours, the client may become dehydrated and/or malnourished. Although options 1, 2, and 3 may be components of the assessment, option 4 is the priority.

Test-Taking Strategy: Note the strategic words "priority nursing assessment." Use Maslow's Hierarchy of Needs theory to direct you to option 4. Hydration and nutrition are the priorities. Review the care of the client after diagnostic GI tests if you had difficulty with this question.

Reference
Ignatavicius, D., & Workman, M. (2006). *Medical-surgical nursing: Critical thinking for collaborative care* (5th ed., pp. 1242-1243). Philadelphia: Saunders.

1360. A nurse plans to assess a client for the vegetative signs of depression. The nurse assesses for these signs by determining the client's:
  1 Level of self-esteem
  2 Level of suicidal ideation
  3 Appetite, weight, sleep patterns, and psychomotor activity
  4 Ability to think, concentrate, and make rational decisions

Level of Cognitive Ability: Analysis
Client Needs: Physiological Integrity
Integrated Process: Nursing Process/Assessment
Content Area: Mental Health

Answer: 3
Rationale: The vegetative signs of depression are changes in physiological functioning that occur during depression. These include changes in appetite, weight, sleep patterns, and psychomotor activity. Options 1, 2, and 4 represent psychological assessment categories.

Test-Taking Strategy: Focus on the subject of the vegetative signs of depression. Recalling that these are physiological changes will direct you to option 3. Review the assessment of depression if you had difficulty with this question.

Reference
Varcarolis, E., Carson, V., & Shoemaker, N. (2006). *Foundations of psychiatric mental health nursing* (5th ed., pp. 334, 336). Philadelphia: Saunders.

1361. A nurse is caring for a client who has been diagnosed with cirrhosis of the liver and who is receiving 50 mg of oral spironolactone (Aldactone) daily. Which of the following would indicate to the nurse that the client is experiencing a side effect related to the medication?
  1 Dry skin
  2 Excitability
  3 Constipation
  4 Hyperkalemia

Answer: 4
Rationale: Spironolactone is a potassium-sparing diuretic. Side effects include hyperkalemia, dehydration, hyponatremia, and lethargy. Although the concern with most diuretics is hypokalemia, this is a potassium-sparing medication, which means that the concern with the administration of this medication is hyperkalemia. Additional side effects include nausea, vomiting, cramping, diarrhea, headache, ataxia, drowsiness, confusion, and fever.

Test-Taking Strategy: Focus on the name of the medication. Recalling that this is a potassium-sparing medication will direct you to option 4. Review the potassium-sparing diuretics if you had difficulty with this question.

Level of Cognitive Ability: Analysis
Client Needs: Physiological Integrity
Integrated Process: Nursing Process/Assessment
Content Area: Pharmacology

References
Lehne, R. (2007). *Pharmacology for nursing care* (6th ed., p. 443). Philadelphia: Saunders.
Skidmore-Roth, L. (2008). *Mosby's nursing drug reference* (21st ed., pp. 940-941). St. Louis: Mosby.

1362. A nurse is preparing a woman in labor for an amniotomy. The nurse would assess which priority data before the procedure?
1 Fetal heart rate
2 Maternal heart rate
3 Fetal scalp sampling
4 Maternal blood pressure

Level of Cognitive Ability: Application
Client Needs: Physiological Integrity
Integrated Process: Nursing Process/Assessment
Content Area: Maternity/Antepartum

Answer: 1
Rationale: Fetal well-being must be confirmed before and after amniotomy. Fetal heart rate should be checked by Doppler or with the application of the external fetal monitor. Although maternal vital signs may be assessed, fetal heart rate is the priority. A fetal scalp sampling cannot be done when the membranes are intact.

Test-Taking Strategy: Note the strategic word "priority." Eliminate option 3 first, knowing that a fetal scalp sampling cannot be done before an amniotomy. Eliminate options 2 and 4 next, noting that they are comparable or alike and that they address maternal vital signs. Option 1 addresses fetal well-being. Review preprocedure care for amniotomy if you had difficulty with this question.

Reference
Murray, S., & McKinney, E. (2006). *Foundations of maternal-newborn nursing* (4th ed., pp. 281-282, 366). Philadelphia: Saunders.

1363. A nurse is monitoring a client who is receiving an oxytocin (Pitocin) infusion for the induction of labor. The nurse would suspect water intoxication if which of the following were noted?
1 Fatigue
2 Lethargy
3 Sleepiness
4 Tachycardia

Level of Cognitive Ability: Analysis
Client Needs: Physiological Integrity
Integrated Process: Nursing Process/Assessment
Content Area: Maternity/Intrapartum

Answer: 4
Rationale: During an oxytocin infusion, the woman is monitored closely for signs of water intoxication, including tachycardia, cardiac dysrhythmias, shortness of breath, nausea, and vomiting.

Test-Taking Strategy: Focus on the subject of water intoxication. Think about the physiological response that occurs when fluid overload exists to direct you to option 4. In addition, note that options 1, 2, and 3 are comparable or alike and eliminate these options. Review the signs of water intoxication if you had difficulty with this question.

Reference
Murray, S., & McKinney, E. (2006). *Foundations of maternal-newborn nursing* (4th ed., p. 371). Philadelphia: Saunders.

1364. The nurse reviews the record of a client who is receiving external radiation therapy and notes the documentation of a skin finding noted as moist desquamation. The nurse expects to note which of the following on assessment of the client?
1 A rash
2 Dermatitis
3 Reddened skin
4 Weeping of the skin

Answer: 4
Rationale: Moist desquamation occurs when the basal cells of the skin are destroyed. The dermal level is exposed, which results in the leakage of serum. Reddened skin, a rash, and dermatitis may occur with external radiation, but these conditions are not described as moist desquamation.

Level of Cognitive Ability: Analysis
Client Needs: Physiological Integrity
Integrated Process: Nursing Process/Assessment
Content Area: Adult Health/Oncology

Test-Taking Strategy: Use the process of elimination. Options 1, 2, and 3 are eliminated, because they are comparable or alike, and they describe a dry rather than a moist skin alteration. In addition, note the relationship between the word "moist" in the question and the word "weeping" in the correct option. Review the signs associated with moist desquamation if you had difficulty with this question.

References
Black, J., & Hawks, J. (2005). *Medical-surgical nursing: Clinical management for positive outcomes* (7th ed., p. 386). Philadelphia: Saunders.
Gulanick, M., & Myers, J. (2007). *Nursing care plans: Nursing diagnosis and interventions* (6th ed., p. 828). St. Louis: Mosby.
Lewis, S., Heitkemper, M., Dirksen, S., O'Brien, P., & Bucher, L. (2007). *Medical-surgical nursing: Assessment and management of clinical problems* (7th ed., p. 299). St. Louis: Mosby.

1365. A nurse is performing an assessment on a pregnant client with a history of cardiac disease. The nurse checks which body area for venous congestion, knowing that it is most commonly noted in this area?
  1 Vulva
  2 Around the eyes
  3 Fingers of the hands
  4 Around the abdomen

Level of Cognitive Ability: Application
Client Needs: Physiological Integrity
Integrated Process: Nursing Process/Assessment
Content Area: Maternity/Antepartum

Answer: 1
Rationale: Assessment of the cardiovascular system includes observation for venous congestion that can develop into varicosities. Venous congestion is most commonly noted in the legs, the vulva, or the rectum. It would be difficult to assess for edema in the abdominal area of a client who is pregnant. Although edema may be noted in the fingers and around the eyes, edema in these areas would not be directly associated with venous congestion.

Test-Taking Strategy: Focus on the strategic words "venous congestion." From the options provided, the only body area in which venous congestion would be noted is the vulva. Review the physical assessment of the cardiovascular system of a pregnant client if you had difficulty with this question.

Reference
McKinney, E., James, S., Murray, S., & Ashwill, J. (2005). *Maternal-child nursing* (2nd ed., p. 269). St. Louis: Saunders.

1366. A client who has been receiving long-term diuretic therapy is admitted to the hospital with a diagnosis of dehydration. The nurse would assess for which sign or symptom that correlates with this fluid imbalance?
  1 Decreased pulse
  2 Bibasilar crackles
  3 Increased blood pressure
  4 Decreased central venous pressure (CVP)

Answer: 4
Rationale: A client with dehydration has a low CVP. The normal CVP is between 4 and 11 mm H_2O. Other assessment findings with fluid volume deficit are increased pulse and respirations, weight loss, poor skin turgor, dry mucous membranes, decreased urine output, concentrated urine with increased specific gravity, increased hematocrit, and altered level of consciousness. The assessment signs in options 1, 2, and 3 occur with excess fluid volume.

Test-Taking Strategy: Use the process of elimination, and focus on the client's diagnosis. Remember that CVP reflects the pressure under which blood is returned to the right atrium and that pressure (volume) decreases with deficient fluid volume. Review the signs and symptoms of deficient fluid volume if you had difficulty with this question.

Level of Cognitive Ability: Analysis
Client Needs: Physiological Integrity
Integrated Process: Nursing Process/Assessment
Content Area: Fundamental Skills

References
Black, J., & Hawks, J. (2005). *Medical-surgical nursing: Clinical management for positive outcomes* (7th ed., pp. 208-209, 2494). Philadelphia: Saunders.
Ignatavicius, D., & Workman, M. (2006). *Medical-surgical nursing: Critical thinking for collaborative care* (5th ed., p. 212). Philadelphia: Saunders.

1367. A nurse is preparing a plan of care for a child with Reye's syndrome. The nurse identifies nursing interventions and plans to monitor the child for:
1 Signs of hyperglycemia
2 Signs of a bacterial infection
3 The presence of protein in the urine
4 Signs of increased intracranial pressure (ICP)

Level of Cognitive Ability: Application
Client Needs: Physiological Integrity
Integrated Process: Nursing Process/Assessment
Content Area: Child Health

Answer: 4
Rationale: Intracranial pressure, encephalopathy, and hepatic dysfunction are major symptoms of Reye's syndrome. Protein is not present in the urine. Reye's syndrome is related to a history of viral infections, and hypoglycemia is a symptom of this disease.

Test-Taking Strategy: Focus on the diagnosis. Recalling that increased ICP is a major symptom of Reye's syndrome will direct you to option 4. Review the care of the child with Reye's syndrome if you had difficulty with this question.

Reference
Hockenberry, M., Wilson, D., & Winkelstein, M. (2005). *Wong's essentials of pediatric nursing* (7th ed., p. 1045). St. Louis: Mosby.

1368. The clinic nurse reads the chart of a client who was seen by the physician and notes that the physician has documented that the client has stage III Lyme disease. On assessment of the client, which clinical manifestation would the nurse expect to note?
1 Palpitations
2 A cardiac dysrhythmia
3 A generalized skin rash
4 Enlarged and inflamed joints

Level of Cognitive Ability: Analysis
Client Needs: Physiological Integrity
Integrated Process: Nursing Process/Assessment
Content Area: Adult Health/Integumentary

Answer: 4
Rationale: Stage III Lyme disease develops within a month to several months after initial infection. It is characterized by arthritic symptoms such as arthralgia and enlarged or inflamed joints, which can persist for several years after the initial infection. A rash occurs during stage I, and cardiac and neurological dysfunction occur during stage II.

Test-Taking Strategy: Use the process of elimination. Eliminate options 1 and 2 first, because they are both cardiac symptoms. From the remaining options, recalling that a rash occurs during stage I will direct you to option 4. Review the clinical manifestations associated with Lyme disease if you had difficulty with this question.

References
Black, J., & Hawks, J. (2005). *Medical-surgical nursing: Clinical management for positive outcomes* (7th ed., p. 2372). Philadelphia: Saunders.
Ignatavicius, D., & Workman, M. (2006). *Medical-surgical nursing: Critical thinking for collaborative care* (5th ed., p. 418). Philadelphia: Saunders.

1369. A nurse is assigned to care for a child with a basilar skull fracture. The nurse reviews the child's record and notes that the physician has documented the presence of Battle's sign. Which of the following would the nurse expect to note in the child?
1 Bruising behind the ear
2 The presence of epistaxis
3 A bruised periorbital area
4 An edematous periorbital area

Answer: 1
Rationale: The most serious type of skull fracture is a basilar skull fracture. Two classic findings associated with this type of skull fracture are Battle's sign and raccoon eyes. Battle's sign is the presence of bruising or ecchymosis behind the ear caused by a leaking of blood into the mastoid sinuses. Raccoon eyes occur as a result of blood leaking into the frontal sinus and causing an edematous and bruised periorbital area.

Level of Cognitive Ability: Analysis
Client Needs: Physiological Integrity
Integrated Process: Nursing Process/Assessment
Content Area: Child Health

Test-Taking Strategy: Use the process of elimination. Eliminate options 3 and 4 first, because they are comparable or alike. From the remaining options, recalling the description of Battle's sign will direct you to option 1. Review Battle's sign if you had difficulty with this question.

Reference
Wong, D., Hockenberry, M., Perry, S., Lowdermilk, D., & Wilson, D. (2006). *Maternal-child nursing care* (3rd ed., p. 1685). St. Louis: Mosby.

1370. A mother brings her child to the health care clinic. The child has been complaining of severe headaches and has been vomiting. The child has a high fever, and the nurse notes the presence of nuchal rigidity and suspects a possible diagnosis of bacterial meningitis. The nurse continues to assess the child for the presence of Kernig's sign. Which finding would indicate the presence of this sign?
1 Calf pain when the foot is dorsiflexed
2 Pain when the chin is pulled down to the chest
3 The flexion of the hips when the neck is flexed from a lying position
4 The inability of the child to extend the legs fully when lying supine

Level of Cognitive Ability: Analysis
Client Needs: Physiological Integrity
Integrated Process: Nursing Process/Assessment
Content Area: Child Health

Answer: 4
Rationale: Kernig's sign is the inability of the child to extend the legs fully when lying supine. Brudzinski's sign is flexion of the hips when the neck is flexed from a supine position. Both of these signs are frequently present in clients with bacterial meningitis. Nuchal rigidity is also present with bacterial meningitis, and it occurs when pain prevents the child from touching the chin to the chest. Homan's sign is elicited when pain occurs in the calf region when the foot is dorsiflexed; it is present in clients with thrombophlebitis.

Test-Taking Strategy: Use the process of elimination, and focus on the child's diagnosis. Option 1 is eliminated first, because this is an assessment test for the presence of thrombophlebitis rather than meningitis. Eliminate option 2 next, because this option identifies the presence of nuchal rigidity. From the remaining options, it is necessary to be able to distinguish between Kernig's sign and Brudzinski's sign. Review the assessment findings of meningitis if you had difficulty with this question.

References
Hockenberry, M., & Wilson, D. (2007). *Nursing care of infants and children* (8th ed., p. 1645). St. Louis: Mosby.
Hockenberry, M., Wilson, D., & Winkelstein, M. (2005). *Wong's essentials of pediatric nursing* (7th ed., p. 1042). St. Louis: Mosby.

1371. A home-care nurse assesses an older client's functional status and ability to perform activities of daily living (ADLs). The nurse focuses the assessment on:
1 Everyday routines
2 Self-care activities
3 Household management
4 Endurance and flexibility

Level of Cognitive Ability: Comprehension
Client Needs: Health Promotion and Maintenance
Integrated Process: Nursing Process/Assessment
Content Area: Fundamental Skills

Answer: 2
Rationale: To evaluate the client's functional status, the nurse assesses the client's ability to perform self-care or ADLs, including bathing, toileting, ambulating, dressing, and feeding. Everyday routines (option 1), household management (option 3), and physical condition (option 4) are not components of functional status.

Test-Taking Strategy: Use the process of elimination, and focus on the subject of the ability to perform ADLs. Recalling that ADLs refer to self-care needs will direct you to option 2. Review the concepts of ADLs if you had difficulty with this question.

Reference
Potter, P., & Perry, A. (2005). *Fundamentals of nursing* (6th ed., pp. 256, 347). St. Louis: Mosby.

1372. The nurse is assessing a client with Addison's disease for signs of hyperkalemia. The nurse expects to note which of the following if hyperkalemia is present?
1 Polyuria
2 Cardiac dysrhythmias
3 Dry mucous membranes
4 Prolonged bleeding time

Level of Cognitive Ability: Analysis
Client Needs: Physiological Integrity
Integrated Process: Nursing Process/Assessment
Content Area: Adult Health/Endocrine

Answer: 2
Rationale: The inadequate production of aldosterone in clients with Addison's disease causes the inadequate excretion of potassium and results in hyperkalemia. The clinical manifestations of hyperkalemia are the result of altered nerve transmission. The most harmful consequence of hyperkalemia is its effect on cardiac function. Options 1, 3, and 4 are not manifestations that are associated with Addison's disease or hyperkalemia.

Test-Taking Strategy: Use the process of elimination, and focus on the subject of hyperkalemia. Remember that hyperkalemia has a direct effect on cardiac function. This will direct you to option 2. Review the pathophysiology associated with Addison's disease and the effects of hyperkalemia if you had difficulty with this question.

Reference
Black, J., & Hawks, J. (2005). *Medical-surgical nursing: Clinical management for positive outcomes* (7th ed., p. 1220). Philadelphia: Saunders.

1373. A client goes into respiratory distress, and blood for an arterial blood gas (ABG) assessment is drawn from the radial artery. The nurse performs Allen's test before the blood is drawn to determine the adequacy of the:
1 Ulnar circulation
2 Carotid circulation
3 Brachial circulation
4 Femoral circulation

Level of Cognitive Ability: Application
Client Needs: Physiological Integrity
Integrated Process: Nursing Process/Assessment
Content Area: Adult Health/Respiratory

Answer: 1
Rationale: Before radial puncture for obtaining an arterial specimen for ABGs, Allen's test is performed to determine adequate ulnar circulation. Failure to assess collateral circulation could result in severe ischemic injury to the hand if damage to the radial artery occurs with arterial puncture. Allen's test does not determine the adequacy of femoral, brachial, or carotid circulation.

Test-Taking Strategy: Use the process of elimination, and note the strategic words "radial artery" in the question. Using your knowledge of the anatomy of the cardiovascular system, eliminate options 2, 3, and 4. Review the purpose and procedure of Allen's test if you had difficulty with this question.

Reference
Black, J., & Hawks, J. (2005). *Medical-surgical nursing: Clinical management for positive outcomes* (7th ed., pp. 258, 1483). Philadelphia: Saunders.

1374. A pregnant client with diabetes mellitus arrives at the health care clinic for a follow-up visit. What priority assessment should the nurse monitor?
1 Urine for specific gravity
2 For the presence of edema
3 Urine for glucose and ketones
4 Blood pressure, pulse, and respirations

Answer: 3
Rationale: The nurse assesses the pregnant client with diabetes mellitus for glucose and ketones in the urine at each prenatal visit, because the physiological changes of pregnancy can drastically alter insulin requirements. The assessment of blood pressure, pulse, respirations, urine for specific gravity, and the presence of edema are more related to the client with gestational hypertension.

Test-Taking Strategy: Use the process of elimination, and focus on the client's diagnosis. The only option that specifically addresses diabetes mellitus is option 3. Review the prenatal care of the client with diabetes mellitus if you had difficulty with this question.

Level of Cognitive Ability: Application
Client Needs: Physiological Integrity
Integrated Process: Nursing Process/Assessment
Content Area: Maternity/Antepartum

Reference
Murray, S., & McKinney, E. (2006). *Foundations of maternal-newborn nursing* (4th ed., p. 666). Philadelphia: Saunders.

Analysis

1375. A client had arterial blood gases drawn. The results are a pH of 7.34, a partial pressure of carbon dioxide of 37 mm Hg, a partial pressure of oxygen of 79 mm Hg, and a bicarbonate level of 19 mEq/L. The nurse interprets that the client is experiencing:

1 Metabolic acidosis
2 Metabolic alkalosis
3 Respiratory acidosis
4 Respiratory alkalosis

Level of Cognitive Ability: Analysis
Client Needs: Physiological Integrity
Integrated Process: Nursing Process/Analysis
Content Area: Adult Health/Respiratory

Answer: 1

Rationale: Metabolic acidosis occurs when the pH falls to less than 7.35 and the bicarbonate level falls to less than 22 mEq/L. With respiratory acidosis, the pH drops to less than 7.35 and the carbon dioxide level rises to more than 45 mm Hg. With respiratory alkalosis, the pH rises to more than 7.45 and the carbon dioxide level falls to less than 35 mm Hg. With metabolic alkalosis, the pH rises to more than 7.45 and the bicarbonate level rises to more than 26 mEq/L.

Test-Taking Strategy: Use the process of elimination. Knowing that a pH of 7.34 is acidotic assists you with eliminating options 2 and 4 first. From the remaining options, knowing that a metabolic condition exists when the bicarbonate follows the same up or down pattern as the pH helps you to choose option 1 over option 3. Review the analysis of arterial blood gas results if you had difficulty with this question.

References
Ignatavicius, D., & Workman, M. (2006). *Medical-surgical nursing: Critical thinking for collaborative care* (5th ed., p. 282). Philadelphia: Saunders.
Pagana, K., & Pagana, T. (2005). *Mosby's diagnostic and laboratory test reference* (7th ed., p. 119). St. Louis: Mosby.

1376. A client with advanced cirrhosis of the liver is not tolerating protein well, as evidenced by abnormal laboratory values. The nurse anticipates that which of the following medications will be prescribed for the client?

1 Folic acid (Folvite)
2 Lactulose (Chronulac)
3 Thiamine (Vitamin B1)
4 Ethacrynic acid (Edecrin)

Level of Cognitive Ability: Analysis
Client Needs: Physiological Integrity
Integrated Process: Nursing Process/Analysis
Content Area: Pharmacology

Answer: 2

Rationale: The client with cirrhosis has an impaired ability to metabolize protein as a result of liver dysfunction. The administration of lactulose aids in the clearance of ammonia via the gastrointestinal tract. Ethacrynic acid is a diuretic. Folic acid and thiamine are vitamins, which may be used as supplemental therapy to treat clients with liver disease.

Test-Taking Strategy: To answer this question correctly, it is necessary to know that ammonia levels are elevated with advanced liver disease and that lactulose is a standard form of medication therapy for this condition. Review advanced cirrhosis of the liver and the purpose of lactulose if you had difficulty with this question.

Reference
Skidmore-Roth, L. (2008). *Mosby's nursing drug reference* (21st ed., p. 503). St. Louis: Mosby.

1377. A nurse is caring for a child with renal disease and is analyzing the child's laboratory results. The nurse notes a sodium level of 148 mEq/L. On the basis of this finding, which clinical manifestation would the nurse expect to note in the child?
1 Lethargy
2 Diaphoresis
3 Cold, wet skin
4 Dry, sticky mucous membranes

Level of Cognitive Ability: Analysis
Client Needs: Physiological Integrity
Integrated Process: Nursing Process/Analysis
Content Area: Child Health

Answer: 4
Rationale: Hypernatremia occurs when the sodium level is more than 145 mEq/L. Clinical manifestations include intense thirst, oliguria, agitation, restlessness, flushed skin, peripheral and pulmonary edema, dry and sticky mucous membranes, nausea, and vomiting. Options 1, 2, and 3 are not associated with the clinical manifestations of hypernatremia.

Test-Taking Strategy: First, determine that the sodium level is elevated and that the child is experiencing hypernatremia. Eliminate options 2 and 3 next, because they are comparable or alike. From the remaining options, recalling that agitation and restlessness (not lethargy) are associated with hypernatremia will direct you to option 4. Review the normal sodium level and the clinical manifestations associated with an imbalance if you had difficulty with this question.

Reference
Hockenberry, M., Wilson, D., & Winkelstein, M. (2005). *Wong's essentials of pediatric nursing* (7th ed., p. 842). St. Louis: Mosby.

1378. A nurse is caring for an infant who is admitted to the hospital with a diagnosis of hemolytic disease. The nurse reviews the laboratory results, expecting to note which of the following in this infant?
1 Decreased bilirubin count
2 Elevated blood glucose level
3 Decreased red blood cell count
4 Decreased white blood cell count

Level of Cognitive Ability: Analysis
Client Needs: Physiological Integrity
Integrated Process: Nursing Process/Analysis
Content Area: Child Health

Answer: 3
Rationale: The two primary pathophysiologic alterations associated with hemolytic disease are anemia and hyperbilirubinemia. The red blood cell count is decreased, because red blood cell production cannot keep pace with red blood cell destruction. Hyperbilirubinemia results from the red blood cell destruction that accompanies this disorder as well as from the normally decreased ability of the neonate's liver to conjugate and excrete bilirubin efficiently from the body. Hypoglycemia is associated with hypertrophy of the pancreatic islet cells and increased levels of insulin. The white blood cell count is not related to this disorder.

Test-Taking Strategy: Focus on the infant's diagnosis. Noting the word "hemolytic" in the diagnosis will direct you to option 3. Review the clinical manifestations associated with hemolytic disease if you had difficulty with this question.

Reference
Hockenberry, M., Wilson, D., & Winkelstein, M. (2005). *Wong's essentials of pediatric nursing* (7th ed., p. 999). St. Louis: Mosby.

1379. A nurse is performing an assessment of a child who is to receive a measles, mumps, and rubella (MMR) vaccine. The nurse notes that the child is allergic to eggs. Which of the following would the nurse anticipate being prescribed for this child?
1 Eliminating this vaccine from the immunization schedule
2 Administering epinephrine (Adrenalin) before the administration of the MMR
3 Taking a careful history about the allergy and reporting this to the physician before administering the MMR vaccine
4 Administering diphenhydramine (Benadryl) and acetaminophen (Tylenol) before the administering of the MMR vaccine

Level of Cognitive Ability: Analysis
Client Needs: Health Promotion and Maintenance
Integrated Process: Nursing Process/Analysis
Content Area: Child Health

Answer: 3
Rationale: Live measles vaccine is produced by chick embryo cell culture, so the possibility of an anaphylactic hypersensitivity in children with egg allergies should be considered. The nurse should take a thorough history of the allergy to a previous MMR and report this to the physician. If this is the first MMR, the physician should be aware of the egg sensitivity before administering the vaccine.

Test-Taking Strategy: Use the process of elimination. Option 1 can be eliminated first, because a vaccine would not be eliminated from the immunization schedule. Options 2 and 4 can be eliminated next, knowing that the use of medications before a vaccine is not normal procedure. Also note that option 3 addresses the first step of the nursing process, assessment. Review the procedures related to the administration of vaccines if you had difficulty with this question.

References
Hockenberry, M., & Wilson, D. (2007). *Nursing care of infants and children* (8th ed., p. 546). St. Louis: Mosby.
Kee, J., Hayes, E., & McCuistion, L. (2006). *Pharmacology: A nursing process approach.* (5th ed., p. 473). Philadelphia: Saunders.

1380. Intravenous immune globulin (IVIG) therapy is prescribed for a child with idiopathic thrombocytopenic purpura (ITP). The nurse determines that this medication is prescribed for the child to:
1 Increase the number of circulating platelets.
2 Provide immunity to the child against infection.
3 Decrease the production of antiplatelet antibodies.
4 Prevent infection after exposure to communicable diseases.

Level of Cognitive Ability: Analysis
Client Needs: Physiological Integrity
Integrated Process: Nursing Process/Analysis
Content Area: Child Health

Answer: 1
Rationale: IVIG is usually effective to rapidly increase the platelet count. It is thought to act by interfering with the attachment of antibody-coded platelets to receptors on the macrophage cells of the reticuloendothelial system. Corticosteroids may be prescribed to enhance vascular stability and to decrease the production of antiplatelet antibodies. Options 2, 3, and 4 are unrelated to the administration of this medication.

Test-Taking Strategy: Note the relationship between the name of the diagnosis "thrombocytopenic purpura" and the word "platelets" in the correct option. This relationship may assist with directing you to the correct option. Review ITP and the purpose of IVIG if you had difficulty with this question.

References
Gahart, B., & Nazareno, A. (2006). *2006 intravenous medications* (22nd ed., pp. 676, 681). St. Louis: Mosby.
Hockenberry, M., & Wilson, D. (2007). *Nursing care of infants and children* (8th ed., p. 1541). St. Louis: Mosby.

1381. A child was diagnosed with acute post-streptococcal glomerulonephritis and renal insufficiency. Which laboratory result will the nurse expect to note in the child?
1 Negative protein in the urinalysis
2 Negative red blood cells in the urinalysis
3 An elevated white blood cell (WBC) count
4 Elevated blood urea nitrogen (BUN) and creatinine levels

Level of Cognitive Ability: Analysis
Client Needs: Physiological Integrity
Integrated Process: Nursing Process/Analysis
Content Area: Child Health

Answer: 4
Rationale: With poststreptococcal glomerulonephritis, a urinalysis will reveal hematuria with red cell casts. Proteinuria is also present. If renal insufficiency is severe, the BUN and creatinine levels will be elevated. The WBC is usually within normal limits, and mild anemia is common.

Test-Taking Strategy: Use the process of elimination, and focus on the child's diagnosis. Recalling that the BUN and creatinine levels are laboratory studies that relate to the renal system will direct you to option 4. Review the clinical manifestations associated with acute poststreptococcal glomerulonephritis if you had difficulty with this question.

Reference
Wong, D., Hockenberry, M., Perry, S., Lowdermilk, D., & Wilson, D. (2006). *Maternal-child nursing care* (3rd ed., p. 1656). St. Louis: Mosby.

1382. A child is admitted to the hospital with a suspected diagnosis of bacterial endocarditis. The child has been experiencing fever, malaise, anorexia, and a headache, and diagnostic studies are performed on the child. Which of the following studies will primarily confirm the diagnosis?
1 A blood culture
2 A sedimentation rate
3 A white blood cell count
4 An electrocardiogram (ECG)

Level of Cognitive Ability: Analysis
Client Needs: Physiological Integrity
Integrated Process: Nursing Process/Analysis
Content Area: Child Health

Answer: 1
Rationale: The diagnosis of bacterial endocarditis is primarily established on the basis of a positive blood culture of the organisms and the visualization of vegetation on echocardiographic studies. Other laboratory tests that may help to confirm the diagnosis are an elevated sedimentation rate and the C-reactive protein level. An ECG is not usually helpful for the diagnosis of bacterial endocarditis.

Test-Taking Strategy: Note the strategic words "primarily confirm." Use the process of elimination, and recall that bacterial endocarditis is caused by an organism. The only test that will confirm the presence of an organism is the blood culture. Review the diagnostic studies associated with bacterial endocarditis if you had difficulty with this question.

Reference
Wong, D., Hockenberry, M., Perry, S., Lowdermilk, D., & Wilson, D. (2006). *Maternal-child nursing care* (3rd ed., p. 1584). St. Louis: Mosby.

1383. The nurse is caring for a client with an intracranial aneurysm. The nurse interprets that which of the following is related to the dysfunction of cranial nerve III?
1 Mild drowsiness
2 Ptosis of the left eyelid
3 Slight slurring of speech
4 Less frequent spontaneous speech

Answer: 2
Rationale: Ptosis of the eyelid is caused by pressure on and the dysfunction of cranial nerve III. Options 1, 3, and 4 identify early signs of a deteriorating level of consciousness.

Test-Taking Strategy: Note the strategic words "cranial nerve III." Recalling the function of this nerve will direct you to option 2. Review the function of cranial nerve III if you had difficulty with this question.

Level of Cognitive Ability: Analysis
Client Needs: Physiological Integrity
Integrated Process: Nursing Process/Analysis
Content Area: Adult Health/Neurological

References
Ignatavicius, D., & Workman, M. (2006). *Medical-surgical nursing: Critical thinking for collaborative care* (5th ed., p. 931). Philadelphia: Saunders.
Lewis, S., Heitkemper, M., Dirksen, S., O'Brien, P., & Bucher, L. (2007). *Medical-surgical nursing: Assessment and management of clinical problems* (7th ed., pp. 1450, 1457). St. Louis: Mosby.

1384. A client with thrombotic brain attack (stroke) experiences periods of emotional lability. The client alternately laughs and cries and intermittently becomes irritable and demanding. The nurse interprets that this behavior indicates:
  1 That the client is not adapting well to the disability
  2 That the problem is likely to get worse before it gets better
  3 That the client is experiencing the usual sequelae of a stroke
  4 That the client is experiencing the side effects of prescribed anticoagulants

Level of Cognitive Ability: Analysis
Client Needs: Psychosocial Integrity
Integrated Process: Nursing Process/Analysis
Content Area: Adult Health/Neurological

Answer: 3
Rationale: After a brain attack (stroke), the client often experiences periods of emotional lability, which are characterized by sudden bouts of laughing or crying or by irritability, depression, confusion, or being demanding. This is a normal part of the clinical picture of the client with this health problem, although it may be difficult for health care personnel and family members to deal with it. The other options are incorrect.

Test-Taking Strategy: Use the process of elimination. Eliminate option 4 first because anticoagulants do not cause emotional lability. From the remaining options, recalling the emotional changes that accompany a brain attack (stroke) will direct you to option 3. Review the effects of a brain attack (stroke) if you had difficulty with this question.

References
Black, J., & Hawks, J. (2005). *Medical-surgical nursing: Clinical management for positive outcomes* (7th ed., p. 2132). Philadelphia: Saunders.
Ignatavicius, D., & Workman, M. (2006). *Medical-surgical nursing: Critical thinking for collaborative care* (5th ed., p. 1031). Philadelphia: Saunders.

1385. A nonstress test is performed on a client, and the results are documented as "two or more fetal heart rate (FHR) accelerations of 15 beats/min, lasting 15 seconds in association with fetal movement." The nurse interprets these findings as:
  1 Unsatisfactory
  2 A reactive nonstress test
  3 A nonreactive nonstress test
  4 Unclear for accurate interpretation

Level of Cognitive Ability: Analysis
Client Needs: Physiological Integrity
Integrated Process: Nursing Process/Analysis
Content Area: Maternity/Antepartum

Answer: 2
Rationale: A reactive nonstress test (normal/negative) indicates a healthy fetus. It is described as two or more FHR accelerations of at least 15 beats/min and lasting at least 15 seconds from the beginning of the acceleration to the end in association with fetal movement during a 20-minute period. A nonreactive nonstress test (abnormal) is described as no accelerations or accelerations of less than 15 beats/min or lasting less than 15 seconds in duration throughout any fetal movement during the testing period. An unsatisfactory test cannot be interpreted because of the poor quality of the FHR.

Test-Taking Strategy: Focus on the data in the question. Eliminate options 1 and 4 first, because they are comparable or alike. From the remaining options, remembering that a reactive nonstress test is a normal or negative test will assist with directing you to option 2. Review the nonstress test if you had difficulty answering this question.

Reference
Murray, S., & McKinney, E. (2006). *Foundations of maternal-newborn nursing* (4th ed., p. 214). Philadelphia: Saunders.

1386. The nurse is developing a plan of care for a client in Buck's traction regarding measures to prevent complications. The nurse determines that the priority nursing diagnosis to be included in the plan is which of the following?
  1 Potential for infection at pin sites
  2 Impaired physical mobility related to traction
  3 Deficient diversional activity related to bedrest
  4 Bathing/hygiene self-care deficit related to the need for traction

Level of Cognitive Ability: Analysis
Client Needs: Physiological Integrity
Integrated Process: Nursing Process/Analysis
Content Area: Adult Health/Musculoskeletal

Answer: 2
Rationale: The priority nursing diagnosis for the client in Buck's traction is impaired physical mobility. Options 3 and 4 may also be appropriate for the client in traction, but immobility presents the greatest risk for the development of complications. Buck's traction is a skin traction, and there are no pin sites.

Test-Taking Strategy: Use the process of elimination. Eliminate option 1 first, because there are no pin sites with Buck's traction. From the remaining options, focus on the strategic word "priority," recalling that the client experiences immobility when in traction. This will direct you to option 2. Review the care of the client in Buck's traction if you had difficulty with this question.

References
Black, J., & Hawks, J. (2005). *Medical-surgical nursing: Clinical management for positive outcomes* (7th ed., p. 637). Philadelphia: Saunders.
Ignatavicius, D., & Workman, M. (2006). *Medical-surgical nursing: Critical thinking for collaborative care* (5th ed., pp. 1200-1201). Philadelphia: Saunders.

1387. A pregnant client with mitral valve prolapse is receiving anticoagulant therapy during pregnancy. The nurse reviews the client's medical record, expecting to note that which medication is prescribed?
  1 Oral intake of warfarin (Coumadin) 15 mg daily
  2 Intravenous infusion of heparin sodium 5000 units daily
  3 Subcutaneous administration of terbutaline (Brethine) daily
  4 Subcutaneous administration of heparin sodium 5000 units daily

Level of Cognitive Ability: Analysis
Client Needs: Physiological Integrity
Integrated Process: Nursing Process/Analysis
Content Area: Maternity/Antepartum

Answer: 4
Rationale: Pregnant women with mitral valve prolapse are frequently given anticoagulant therapy during pregnancy, because they are at greater risk for thromboembolic disease during the antenatal, intrapartal, and postpartum periods. Warfarin (Coumadin) is contraindicated during pregnancy, because it passes the placental barrier and causes potential fetal malformations and hemorrhagic disorders. Heparin, which does not pass the placental barrier, is a safe anticoagulant therapy during pregnancy, and it would be administered by the subcutaneous route. Terbutaline is a medication that is indicated for preterm labor management.

Test-Taking Strategy: Use the process of elimination and your knowledge regarding the medications that are safe during pregnancy to assist you with answering the question. Eliminate options 1 and 3 first, because warfarin is contraindicated, and terbutaline is indicated, for preterm labor management. From the remaining options, select option 4 because of the word "subcutaneous." Review the treatment measures for the pregnant client with mitral valve prolapse if you had difficulty with this question.

Reference
Murray, S., & McKinney, E. (2006). *Foundations of maternal-newborn nursing* (4th ed., p. 674). Philadelphia: Saunders.

1388. A nurse continues to assess a client who is in the late first stage of labor for progress and fetal well-being. At the last vaginal exam, the client was fully effaced, 8 centimeters dilated, vertex presentation, and station −1. Which observation would indicate that the fetus was in fetal distress?

1 The fetal heart rate slowly drops to 110 beats/min during strong contractions, recovering to 138 beats/min immediately afterward.

2 Fresh meconium is found on the examiner's gloved fingers after a vaginal exam, and the fetal monitor pattern remains essentially unchanged.

3 Fresh, thick meconium is passed with a small gush of liquid, and the fetal monitor shows late decelerations with a variable descending baseline.

4 The vaginal exam continues to reveal some old meconium staining, and the fetal monitor demonstrates a U-shaped pattern of deceleration during contractions, recovering to a baseline of 140 beats/min.

Level of Cognitive Ability: Analysis
Client Needs: Physiological Integrity
Integrated Process: Nursing Process/Analysis
Content Area: Maternity/Intrapartum

Answer: 3

Rationale: Meconium staining alone is not a sign of fetal distress. Meconium passage is a normal physiological function that is frequently noted with a fetus of more than 38 weeks' gestation. Old meconium staining may be the result of a prenatal trauma that is resolved. It is not unusual for the fetal heart rate to drop to less than the 140 to 160 beats/min range in late labor during contractions, and, in a healthy fetus, the fetal heart rate will recover between contractions. Fresh meconium in combination with late decelerations and a variable descending baseline is an ominous signal of fetal distress caused by fetal hypoxia.

Test-Taking Strategy: Use the process of elimination, and note the subject of fetal distress. Eliminate options 1 and 4 first, because they both indicate a recovering fetal heart rate. From the remaining options, eliminate option 2 because of the words "fetal monitor pattern remains essentially unchanged." Review signs of fetal distress if you had difficulty with this question.

References
McKinney, E., James, S., Murray, S., & Ashwill, J. (2005). *Maternal-child nursing* (2nd ed., p. 410). St. Louis: Saunders.
Wong, D., Hockenberry, M., Perry, S., Lowdermilk, D., & Wilson, D. (2006). *Maternal-child nursing care* (3rd ed., pp. 474-475). St. Louis: Mosby.

1389. A nurse is caring for a child with complex partial seizures who is being treated with carbamazepine (Tegretol). The nurse reviews the laboratory report for the results of the drug plasma level and determines that the plasma level is in a therapeutic range if which of the following is noted?

1 1 mcg/mL
2 10 mcg/mL
3 18 mcg/mL
4 20 mcg/mL

Level of Cognitive Ability: Analysis
Client Needs: Physiological Integrity
Integrated Process: Nursing Process/Analysis
Content Area: Pharmacology

Answer: 2

Rationale: When carbamazepine is administered, plasma levels of the medication need to be monitored periodically to check for the child's absorption of the medication. The amount of the medication prescribed is based on the results of this laboratory test. The therapeutic plasma level of carbamazepine is 3 to 14 mcg/mL. Option 1 indicates a low level that possibly necessitates an increased medication dose. Options 3 and 4 identify elevated levels that indicate the need to decrease the medication dose.

Test-Taking Strategy: Use the process of elimination and your knowledge of the therapeutic plasma level of carbamazepine to answer the question. Recalling that the therapeutic plasma level is 3 to 14 mcg/mL will direct you to option 2. Review the therapeutic plasma level of carbamazepine if you had difficulty with this question.

Reference
McKenry, L., Tressier, E., & Hogan, M. (2006). *Mosby's pharmacology in nursing* (22nd ed., p. 369). St. Louis: Mosby.

1390. A nurse performs an assessment on a client with a history of congestive heart failure. The client has been taking diuretics on a long-term basis. The nurse reviews the medication record, knowing that which medication, if prescribed for this client, would place the client at risk for hypokalemia?

1 Bumetanide (Bumex)
2 Triamterene (Dyrenium)
3 Spironolactone (Aldactone)
4 Amiloride and hydrochlorothiazide (Midamor)

Level of Cognitive Ability: Analysis
Client Needs: Physiological Integrity
Integrated Process: Nursing Process/Analysis
Content Area: Pharmacology

Answer: 1
Rationale: Bumetanide (Bumex) is a loop diuretic. The client on this medication would be at risk for hypokalemia. Spironolactone (Aldactone), triamterene (Dyrenium), and amiloride and hydrochlorothiazide (Midamor) are potassium-sparing diuretics.

Test-Taking Strategy: Use the process of elimination and your knowledge of potassium-sparing diuretics. Recalling that bumetanide is a loop diuretic will direct you to option 1. Review loop diuretics if you had difficulty with this question.

Reference
Skidmore-Roth, L. (2008). *Mosby's nursing drug reference* (21st ed., p. 199). St. Louis: Mosby.

1391. The home-care nurse is preparing to visit a client with a diagnosis of Meniere's disease. The nurse reviews the physician orders and expects to note that which of the following dietary measures is prescribed?

1 A low-fiber diet with decreased fluids
2 A low-sodium diet and fluid restriction
3 A low fat diet with a restriction of citrus fruits
4 A low-carbohydrate diet and the elimination of red meats

Level of Cognitive Ability: Analysis
Client Needs: Physiological Integrity
Integrated Process: Nursing Process/Analysis
Content Area: Adult Health/Ear

Answer: 2
Rationale: Dietary changes such as salt and fluid restrictions that reduce the amount of endolymphatic fluid are sometimes prescribed for clients with Meniere's disease. Options 1, 3, and 4 are not prescribed for this disorder.

Test-Taking Strategy: Use the process of elimination, and focus on the client's diagnosis. Recalling that salt and fluid restrictions are sometimes necessary to reduce the amount of endolymphatic fluid will assist with directing you to option 2. Review the pathophysiology and treatment of Meniere's disease if you had difficulty with this question.

Reference
Ignatavicius, D., & Workman, M. (2006). *Medical-surgical nursing: Critical thinking for collaborative care* (5th ed., p. 1132). Philadelphia: Saunders.

1392. A nurse is caring for a client who has been diagnosed with tuberculosis. The client is receiving 600 mg of oral rifampin (Rifadin) daily. Which laboratory finding would indicate to the nurse that the client is experiencing an adverse reaction?

1 A total bilirubin level of 0.5 mg/dL
2 A white blood cell count of 6000/μL
3 A sedimentation rate of 15 mm/hour
4 An alkaline phosphatase level of 25 King-Armstrong units/dL

Answer: 4
Rationale: Adverse reactions or toxic effects of rifampin include hepatotoxicity, hepatitis, blood dyscrasias, Stevens-Johnson syndrome, and antibiotic-related colitis. The nurse monitors for increased liver function, bilirubin, blood urea nitrogen, and uric acid levels, because elevations indicate an adverse reaction. The normal alkaline phosphatase is 4.5 to 13 King-Armstrong units/dL. The normal total bilirubin level is less than 1.5 mg/dL. A normal white blood cell count is 4500 to 11,000/μL. The normal sedimentation rate is 0 to 30 mm/hour.

Level of Cognitive Ability: Analysis
Client Needs: Physiological Integrity
Integrated Process: Nursing Process/Analysis
Content Area: Pharmacology

Test-Taking Strategy: Use the process of elimination. Recalling that the medication is metabolized in the liver will assist you with eliminating options 2 and 3, because these laboratory studies are not directly related to assessing liver function. From the remaining options, a knowledge of normal laboratory values will direct you to option 4. Review oral rifampin and these common laboratory values if you had difficulty with this question.

Reference
McKenry, L., Tressier, E., & Hogan, M. (2006). *Mosby's pharmacology in nursing* (22nd ed., p. 1059). St. Louis: Mosby.

1393. A home-care nurse is assessing a client who is taking prazosin (Minipress). Which statement by the client would support the nursing diagnosis of Noncompliance with medication therapy?

1 "If I feel dizzy, I'll skip my dose for a few days."
2 "I can't see the numbers on the label to know how much salt is in the food."
3 "I don't understand why I have to keep taking the pills when my blood pressure is normal."
4 "If I have a cold, I shouldn't take any over-the-counter remedies without consulting my doctor."

Level of Cognitive Ability: Analysis
Client Needs: Health Promotion and Maintenance
Integrated Process: Nursing Process/Analysis
Content Area: Pharmacology

Answer: 1
Rationale: The side effects of prazosin are dizziness and impotence. The client needs to be instructed to call the physician if these side effects occur. Holding (skipping) medication will cause an abrupt rise in blood pressure. Option 2 indicates a self-care deficit. Option 3 indicates a knowledge deficit. Option 4 indicates client understanding regarding the medication.

Test-Taking Strategy: Focus on the nursing diagnosis of Noncompliance to select the correct option. Noting the strategic words "I'll skip my dose" will direct you to option 1. Review the defining characteristics of Noncompliance if you had difficulty with this question.

References
Kee, J., Hayes, E., & McCuistion, L. (2006). *Pharmacology: A nursing process approach* (5th ed., pp. 650-651). Philadelphia: Saunders.
Skidmore-Roth, L. (2008). *Mosby's nursing drug reference* (21st ed., p. 841). St. Louis: Mosby.

1394. A client manages peptic ulcer disease (PUD) with excessive amounts of oral antacids. The client is at risk for which acid-base imbalance?

1 Metabolic acidosis
2 Metabolic alkalosis
3 Respiratory acidosis
4 Respiratory alkalosis

Answer: 2
Rationale: Oral antacids can be effective treatment for PUD when administered properly, but, when they are taken in excess, they can lead to metabolic alkalosis (a pH of more than 7.45 and a bicarbonate ion [HCO_3] level of more than 26 mEq/L). As effective therapy for PUD, antacids bind with the hydrochloric acid (HCl^-) of gastric secretions and halt the corrosive action of the HCl^-. However, antacids are alkaline substances, and excessive administration can exceed the kidney's ability to clear the excess HCO_3, which leads to the accumulation of HCO_3, an increased pH, and metabolic alkalosis. Metabolic acidosis occurs when the pH is low and the HCO_3 is low, respiratory acidosis occurs when the pH is low and the partial pressure of carbon dioxide (pCO_2) is high, and respiratory alkalosis occurs when the pH is high and the pCO_2 is low.

Level of Cognitive Ability: Analysis
Client Needs: Physiological Integrity
Integrated Process: Nursing Process/Analysis
Content Area: Fundamental Skills

Test-Taking Strategy: Note the strategic word "antacids" and the fact that the question indicates that the problem is not respiratory in nature. With this in mind, eliminate options 3 and 4 first, because they both refer to disorders that involve respiratory components. Knowing that the word "antacids" means "working against acids" helps you to choose the correct option, because an agent that works against an acid will increase the pH. Review the causes of metabolic alkalosis if you had difficulty with this question.

Reference
Ignatavicius, D., & Workman, M. (2006). *Medical-surgical nursing: Critical thinking for collaborative care* (5th ed., p. 289). Philadelphia: Saunders.

1395. A nurse is assessing a 39-year-old Caucasian female client. The client has a blood pressure (BP) of 152/92 mm Hg at rest, a total cholesterol level of 190 mg/dL, and a fasting blood glucose level of 110 mg/dL. The nurse would place priority on which risk factor for coronary heart disease (CHD) in this client?
1 Age
2 Hypertension
3 Hyperlipidemia
4 Glucose intolerance

Level of Cognitive Ability: Analysis
Client Needs: Health Promotion and Maintenance
Integrated Process: Nursing Process/Analysis
Content Area: Delegating/Prioritizing

Answer: 2
Rationale: Hypertension, cigarette smoking, and hyperlipidemia are major risk factors for CHD. Glucose intolerance, obesity, and response to stress are also contributing factors. An age of more than 40 years is a nonmodifiable risk factor. A cholesterol level of 190 mg/dL and a blood glucose level of 110 mg/dL are within the normal range. The nurse places priority on major risk factors that need modification.

Test-Taking Strategy: Focus on the data in the question, and note the strategic word "priority." Note that the only abnormal value is the BP. Review the risk factors associated with CHD if you had difficulty with this question.

References
Ignatavicius, D., & Workman, M. (2006). *Medical-surgical nursing: Critical thinking for collaborative care* (5th ed., pp. 784, 842-843). Philadelphia: Saunders.
Lewis, S., Heitkemper, M., Dirksen, S., O'Brien, P., & Bucher, L. (2007). *Medical surgical nursing: Assessment and management of clinical problems* (7th ed., p. 766). St. Louis: Mosby.

1396. The nurse is caring for a client who has just returned to the nursing unit after an intravenous pyelogram (IVP). The nurse determines that which of the following is the priority for the postprocedure care of this client?
1 Maintaining the client on bedrest
2 Ambulating the client in the hallway
3 Encouraging the increased intake of oral fluids
4 Encouraging the client to try to void frequently

Level of Cognitive Ability: Analysis
Client Needs: Physiological Integrity
Integrated Process: Nursing Process/Analysis
Content Area: Adult Health/Renal

Answer: 3
Rationale: After IVP, the client should take in increased fluids to aid in the clearance of the dye used for the procedure. It is unnecessary to void frequently after the procedure. The client is usually allowed activity as tolerated, without any specific activity guidelines.

Test-Taking Strategy: Use the process of elimination, and note the strategic word "priority." Option 4 has no useful purpose and is eliminated first. From the remaining options, recall that there are no activity guidelines after this procedure. Recalling that fluids are necessary to promote the clearance of the dye from the client's system will direct you to option 3. Review IVP if you had difficulty with this question.

Reference
Chernecky, C., & Berger, B. (2008). *Laboratory tests and diagnostic procedures* (5th ed., p. 682). Philadelphia: Saunders.

1397. The nurse is caring for a client with myasthenia gravis. The client is vomiting and complaining of abdominal cramps and diarrhea. The nurse also notes that the client is hypotensive and experiencing facial muscle twitching. The nurse interprets that these symptoms are compatible with:
1 Myasthenic crisis
2 Cholinergic crisis
3 Systemic infection
4 A reaction to plasmapheresis

Level of Cognitive Ability: Analysis
Client Needs: Physiological Integrity
Integrated Process: Nursing Process/Analysis
Content Area: Adult Health/Neurological

Answer: 2
Rationale: Signs and symptoms of cholinergic crisis include nausea, vomiting, abdominal cramping, diarrhea, blurred vision, pallor, facial muscle twitching, pupillary miosis, and hypotension. It is caused by overmedication with cholinergic (anticholinesterase) medications, and it is treated by withholding medications. Myasthenic crisis is an exacerbation of myasthenic symptoms caused by undermedication with anticholinesterase medications. There are no data in the question to support options 1, 3, and 4.

Test-Taking Strategy: Use the process of elimination. Note the client's diagnosis, and think about the treatment for this disorder. Recalling the effects of cholinergic medications and focusing on the data in the question will direct you to option 2. Review the clinical manifestations associated with cholinergic crisis if you had difficulty with this question.

Reference
Ignatavicius, D., & Workman, M. (2006). *Medical-surgical nursing: Critical thinking for collaborative care* (5th ed., p. 1015). Philadelphia: Saunders.

1398. A nurse is assigned to care for a child with juvenile idiopathic arthritis (JIA). The nurse reviews the plan of care, knowing that which of the following is a priority nursing diagnosis?
1 Acute pain, related to inflammatory process
2 Risk for self-care deficit, related to immobility
3 Disturbed body image, related to activity intolerance
4 Risk for injury, related to impaired physical mobility

Level of Cognitive Ability: Analysis
Client Needs: Physiological Integrity
Integrated Process: Nursing Process/Analysis
Content Area: Delegating/Prioritizing

Answer: 1
Rationale: All of the nursing diagnoses are appropriate for the child with JIA; however, acute pain needs to be managed before other problems can be addressed.

Test-Taking Strategy: Note the strategic word "priority." Use Maslow's Hierarchy of Needs theory, and remember that physiological needs (option 1) receive the highest priority. Option 4 addresses safety and security needs. Option 3 addresses body image. Option 2 identifies a risk for a problem rather than an actual problem. Review the care of a child with JIA if you had difficulty with this question.

Reference
Wong, D., Hockenberry, M., Perry, S., Lowdermilk, D., & Wilson, D. (2006). *Maternal-child nursing care* (3rd ed., p. 1834). St. Louis: Mosby.

1399. A child is admitted to the hospital with a suspected diagnosis of idiopathic thrombocytopenic purpura (ITP), and diagnostic studies are performed. Which of the following diagnostic results are indicative of this disorder?
1 An elevated platelet count
2 Elevated hemoglobin and hematocrit levels
3 A bone marrow examination showing an increased number of megakaryocytes
4 A bone marrow examination indicating an increased number of immature white blood cells

Answer: 3
Rationale: The laboratory manifestations of ITP include the presence of a low platelet count of usually less than 20,000 cells/mm^3. Thrombocytopenia is the only laboratory abnormality expected with ITP. If there has been significant blood loss, there is evidence of anemia in the blood cell count. If a bone marrow examination is performed, the results with ITP show a normal or increased number of megakaryocytes, which are the precursors of platelets. Option 4 indicates the bone marrow result that would be found in a child with leukemia.

Level of Cognitive Ability: Analysis
Client Needs: Physiological Integrity
Integrated Process: Nursing Process/Analysis
Content Area: Child Health

Test-Taking Strategy: Focus on the diagnosis. Recalling that megakaryocytes are the precursors of platelets will assist with directing you to option 3. Review ITP and its associated clinical manifestations if you had difficulty with this question.

Reference

Wong, D., Hockenberry, M., Perry, S., Lowdermilk, D., & Wilson, D. (2006). *Maternal-child nursing care* (3rd ed., p. 1616). St. Louis: Mosby.

1400. An infant is brought to the health care clinic, and the mother tells the nurse that her infant has been vomiting after meals. The mother explains that the vomiting is now becoming more frequent and forceful and that the infant seems to be constipated. During the assessment, the nurse notes visible peristaltic waves moving from left to right across the infant's abdomen. On the basis of this finding, the nurse would suspect which of the following?
1 Colic
2 Intussusception
3 Pyloric stenosis
4 Congenital megacolon

Level of Cognitive Ability: Analysis
Client Needs: Physiological Integrity
Integrated Process: Nursing Process/Analysis
Content Area: Child Health

Answer: 3

Rationale: In pyloric stenosis, the vomitus contains sour, undigested food but no bile, the child is constipated, and visible peristaltic waves move from left to right across the abdomen. A movable, palpable, firm, olive-shaped mass in the right upper quadrant may be noted. Crying during the evening hours, appearing to be in pain, but eating well and gaining weight are clinical manifestations of colic. An infant who suddenly becomes pale, cries out, and draws the legs up to the chest is demonstrating physical signs of intussusception. Ribbon-like stool, bile-stained emesis, the absence of peristalsis, and abdominal distention are symptoms of congenital megacolon (Hirschsprung's disease).

Test-Taking Strategy: Focus on the data provided in the question. Consider each condition presented in the options, and think about the clinical manifestations of each. Recalling the manifestations associated with pyloric stenosis will direct you to option 3. Review the clinical manifestations of pyloric stenosis if you had difficulty with this question.

Reference

Wong, D., Hockenberry, M., Perry, S., Lowdermilk, D., & Wilson, D. (2006). *Maternal-child nursing care* (3rd ed., p. 1533). St. Louis: Mosby.

1401. A nurse is reviewing the laboratory analysis of cerebrospinal fluid (CSF) obtained during a lumbar puncture from a child who is suspected of having bacterial meningitis. Which of the following results would most likely confirm this diagnosis?
1 Clear CSF with low protein and low glucose
2 Cloudy CSF with low protein and low glucose
3 Cloudy CSF with high protein and low glucose
4 Decreased pressure and cloudy CSF with high protein

Answer: 3

Rationale: A diagnosis of meningitis is made by testing CSF obtained by lumbar puncture. In the case of bacterial meningitis, findings usually include increased pressure and cloudy CSF with high protein and low glucose. Options 1, 2, and 4 are incorrect.

Test-Taking Strategy: Use the process of elimination. Eliminate options 1 and 4 first, because clear CSF and decreased pressure are not likely to be found with an infectious process such as meningitis. From the remaining options, recalling that high protein indicates a possible diagnosis of meningitis will direct you to option 3. Review the findings in bacterial meningitis if you had difficulty with this question.

Level of Cognitive Ability: Analysis
Client Needs: Physiological Integrity
Integrated Process: Nursing Process/Analysis
Content Area: Child Health

References
Hockenberry, M., & Wilson, D. (2007). *Nursing care of infants and children* (8th ed., p. 1648). St. Louis: Mosby.
Hockenberry, M., Wilson, D., & Winkelstein, M. (2005). *Wong's essentials of pediatric nursing* (7th ed., pp. 1041-1042). St. Louis: Mosby.

1402. A child is admitted to the pediatric unit with a diagnosis of acute gastroenteritis. The nurse monitors the child for signs of hypovolemic shock as a result of fluid and electrolyte losses that have occurred in the child. Which finding would indicate the presence of compensated shock?

1 Bradycardia
2 Hypotension
3 Profuse diarrhea
4 A capillary refill time of more than 2 seconds

Level of Cognitive Ability: Analysis
Client Needs: Physiological Integrity
Integrated Process: Nursing Process/Analysis
Content Area: Child Health

Answer: 4
Rationale: Shock may be classified as compensated or decompensated. In compensated shock, the child becomes tachycardic in an effort to increase the cardiac output. The blood pressure remains normal. The capillary refill time may be prolonged and more than 2 seconds, and the child may become irritable as a result of increasing hypoxia. The most prevalent cause of hypovolemic shock is fluid and electrolyte losses associated with gastroenteritis. Diarrhea is not a sign of shock; rather, it is a cause of the fluid and electrolyte imbalance.

Test-Taking Strategy: Use the process of elimination, and focus on the strategic words "compensated shock." Recalling that hypotension is a late sign of shock in children will assist you with eliminating option 2. Recalling that tachycardia rather than bradycardia occurs in shock will assist you with eliminating option 1. From the remaining options, focusing on the subject of signs of shock will direct you to option 4. Review the signs of compensated shock in a child if you had difficulty with this question.

References
Hockenberry, M., Wilson, D., & Winkelstein, M. (2005). *Wong's essentials of pediatric nursing* (7th ed., p. 933). St. Louis: Mosby.
Wong, D., Hockenberry, M., Perry, S., Lowdermilk, D., & Wilson, D. (2006). *Maternal-child nursing care* (3rd ed., p. 1595). St. Louis: Mosby.

1403. A mother brings her child to the health care clinic for a routine examination. The mother tells the nurse that the teacher has reported that the child appears to be daydreaming and staring off into space. The teacher tells the mother that this occurs numerous times throughout the day, yet, during the remainder of the day, the child is alert and participates in classroom activities. The nurse documents the findings and suspects that which of the following is occurring with this child?

1 The child probably has school phobia.
2 The child is experiencing absence seizures.
3 The child is showing signs of a behavioral problem.
4 The child has attention-deficit/hyperactivity syndrome and is in need of medication.

Answer: 2
Rationale: Absence seizures are a type of generalized seizure. They consist of a sudden, brief (usually 5 to 10 seconds) arrest of the child's motor activities accompanied by a blank stare and a loss of awareness. The child's posture is maintained at the end of the seizure, and the child returns to activity that was in process as though nothing has happened. A child with attention-deficit/hyperactivity syndrome becomes easily distracted, is fidgety, and has difficulty following directions. School phobia includes physical symptoms that usually occur at home and that may prevent the child from attending school. Behavior problems would be noted by more overt symptoms than the ones described in this question.

Test-Taking Strategy: Use the process of elimination, and focus on the information provided in the question. Note the relationship of the information and option 2. Review absence seizures if you had difficulty with this question.

Level of Cognitive Ability: Analysis
Client Needs: Physiological Integrity
Integrated Process: Nursing Process/Analysis
Content Area: Child Health

Reference

Hockenberry, M., & Wilson, D. (2007). *Wong's nursing care of infants and children* (8th ed., p. 1655). St. Louis: Mosby.

1404. A mother and her 3-week-old infant arrive at the well-baby clinic for a rescreening test for phenylketonuria (PKU). The nurse reviews the results of the serum phenylalanine levels and notes that the level is 1.0 mg/dL. The nurse interprets this level as:

1 Normal
2 Inconclusive
3 Requiring a repeat study
4 Elevated and indicating PKU

Level of Cognitive Ability: Analysis
Client Needs: Physiological Integrity
Integrated Process: Nursing Process/Analysis
Content Area: Maternity/Postpartum

Answer: 1

Rationale: The normal PKU level is less than 2 mg/dL. With early postpartum discharge, screening is often performed when the infant is less than 2 days old because of the concern that the infant will be lost to follow up. Infants should be rescreened by the time that they are 14 days old if the initial screening was done when the infant was 24 to 48 hours old.

Test-Taking Strategy: Use the process of elimination and your knowledge regarding the normal phenylalanine level. Recalling that the normal level is less than 2 mg/dL will direct you to option 1. Review the PKU screening test if you had difficulty with this question.

Reference

Hockenberry, M., Wilson, D., & Winkelstein, M. (2005). *Wong's essentials of pediatric nursing* (7th ed., pp. 742, 864). St. Louis: Mosby.

Planning

1405. The nurse is caring for a client who is receiving parenteral nutrition through a central venous catheter. Which action should the nurse plan to implement to decrease the risk of infection in this client?

1 Track the client's oral temperature.
2 Administer antibiotics intravenously.
3 Evaluate the differential of the leukocytes.
4 Use aseptic technique for dressing changes.

Level of Cognitive Ability: Application
Client Needs: Safe and Effective Care Environment
Integrated Process: Nursing Process/Planning
Content Area: Fundamental Skills

Answer: 4

Rationale: Aseptic technique is vital during dressing changes, because parenteral nutrition is administered through a central venous catheter (CVC). CVCs are large-bore catheters that can serve as a direct-entry point for microorganisms into the heart and circulatory system. Using aseptic technique helps to avoid catheter related infections by preventing the introduction of potential pathogens to the site. Options 1, 2, and 3 are reasonable nursing interventions for a client with a CVC; however, none of these actions prevents infection. Options 1 and 3 are assessment methods, and option 2 is implemented after the confirmation of an existing infection.

Test-Taking Strategy: Focus on the subject of preventing infection. Note the relationship between "infection" in the question and "aseptic" in the correct option. In addition, the only option that will prevent infection is option 4. Review the care of a client receiving parenteral nutrition if you had difficulty with this question.

References

Black, J., & Hawks, J. (2005). *Medical-surgical nursing: Clinical management for positive outcomes* (7th ed., p. 709). Philadelphia: Saunders.

Ignatavicius, D., & Workman, M. (2006). *Medical-surgical nursing: Critical thinking for collaborative care* (5th ed., p. 1431). Philadelphia: Saunders.

1406. The nurse develops a plan of care for a client with a spica cast that covers a lower extremity. Which action should the nurse include in the daily plan of care to promote bowel elimination?
1 Use a bedside commode.
2 Use a low-profile bedpan.
3 Ambulate to the bathroom.
4 Administer an enema daily.

Level of Cognitive Ability: Application
Client Needs: Physiological Integrity
Integrated Process: Nursing Process/Planning
Content Area: Fundamental Skills

Answer: 2
Rationale: A client with a spica cast (body cast) that covers a lower extremity cannot bend at the hips to sit up. A low-profile bedpan or fracture pan is designed for use by clients with body or leg casts and for clients who have difficulty raising the hips to use a standard bedpan; therefore, using a commode or the bathroom is contraindicated. Daily enemas are not a part of routine care.

Test-Taking Strategy: Focus on the words "covers a lower extremity." Use the process of elimination to choose a facet of daily care that promotes elimination for a client who cannot flex the hip. Review the care of the client with a spica cast if you had difficulty with this question.

Reference
Potter, P., & Perry, A. (2005). *Fundamentals of nursing* (6th ed., p. 1395). St. Louis: Mosby.

1407. A nurse is caring for a postpartum client with thromboembolytic disease. When planning care to prevent the complication of pulmonary embolism, the nurse plans specifically to:
1 Enforce bedrest.
2 Monitor the vital signs frequently.
3 Assess the breath sounds frequently.
4 Administer and monitor anticoagulant therapy as prescribed.

Level of Cognitive Ability: Application
Client Needs: Physiological Integrity
Integrated Process: Nursing Process/Planning
Content Area: Maternity/Postpartum

Answer: 4
Rationale: The purposes of anticoagulant therapy for the treatment of thromboembolytic disease are to prevent the formation of a clot and to prevent a clot from moving to another area, thus preventing pulmonary embolism. Although options 1, 2, and 3 may be implemented for a client with thromboembolytic disease, option 4 will specifically assist in the prevention of pulmonary embolism.

Test-Taking Strategy: Focus on the subject of preventing the complication of pulmonary embolism. Note the strategic word "specifically." Recall that anticoagulant therapy is prescribed to treat thromboembolytic disease. In addition, noting the words "as prescribed" in option 4 will direct you to this option. Review the interventions for the client with thromboembolytic disease that will prevent pulmonary embolism if you had difficulty with this question.

Reference
Murray, S., & McKinney, E. (2006). *Foundations of maternal-newborn nursing* (4th ed., pp. 743-744). Philadelphia: Saunders.

1408. After reviewing a client's serum electrolyte levels, the provider prescribes an isotonic intravenous (IV) infusion. Which IV solution should the nurse plan to administer?
1 5% dextrose in water
2 10% dextrose in water
3 3% sodium chloride solution
4 0.45% sodium chloride solution

Answer: 1
Rationale: Five percent dextrose in water is an isotonic solution, which means that the osmolality of this solution matches normal body fluids. Other examples of isotonic fluids include 0.9% sodium chloride solution (normal saline) and lactated Ringer's solution. Ten percent dextrose in water and 3% sodium chloride solution are hypertonic solutions, and 0.45% sodium chloride solution is hypotonic.

Level of Cognitive Ability: Comprehension
Client Needs: Physiological Integrity
Integrated Process: Nursing Process/Planning
Content Area: Fundamental Skills

Test-Taking Strategy: To answer this question accurately, you must be familiar with the tonicity of various IV solutions. Note the strategic word "isotonic," and recall that 5% dextrose in water and 0.9% normal saline are isotonic. Review the tonicity of IV fluids if you had difficulty with this question.

References

Lewis, S., Heitkemper, M., Dirksen, S., O'Brien, P., & Bucher, L. (2007). *Medical-surgical nursing: Assessment and management of clinical problems* (7th ed., p. 340). St. Louis: Mosby.

Potter, P., & Perry, A. (2005). *Fundamentals of nursing* (6th ed., p. 1160). St. Louis: Mosby.

1409. The nurse is admitting a client to the hospital who recently had a bilateral adrenalectomy. Which intervention is essential for the nurse to include in the client's plan of care?
1 Prevent social isolation.
2 Consider occupational therapy.
3 Discuss changes in body image.
4 Avoid stress-producing situations and procedures.

Level of Cognitive Ability: Application
Client Needs: Physiological Integrity
Integrated Process: Nursing Process/Planning
Content Area: Adult Health/Endocrine

Answer: 4
Rationale: Adrenalectomy can lead to adrenal insufficiency. Adrenal hormones are essential to maintaining homeostasis in response to stressors. Options 1, 2, and 3 are not essential interventions specific to this client's problem.

Test-Taking Strategy: Note the strategic word "essential." This indicates the need to prioritize. Remember that, according to Maslow's Hierarchy of Needs theory, physiological needs come first. The stress reaction involves physiological processes. Review the postoperative effects of an adrenalectomy if you had difficulty with this question.

Reference

Black, J., & Hawks, J. (2005). *Medical-surgical nursing: Clinical management for positive outcomes* (7th ed., p. 1227). Philadelphia: Saunders.

1410. A perinatal client is admitted to the obstetric unit during an exacerbation of a heart condition. When planning for the nutritional requirements of the client, the nurse would consult with the dietitian to ensure which of the following?
1 A low-calorie diet to prevent weight gain
2 A diet adequate in fluids and fiber to decrease constipation
3 A diet low in fluids and fiber to decrease blood volume
4 Unlimited sodium intake to increase circulating blood volume

Level of Cognitive Ability: Analysis
Client Needs: Physiological Integrity
Integrated Process: Nursing Process/Planning
Content Area: Maternity/Antepartum

Answer: 2
Rationale: Constipation can cause the client to use Valsalva's maneuver. This maneuver can cause blood to rush to the heart and overload the cardiac system. A low-calorie diet is not recommended during pregnancy. Diets low in fluid and fiber can cause a decrease in blood volume that can deprive the fetus of nutrients. Therefore, adequate fluid intake and high-fiber foods are important. Sodium should be restricted to some degree as prescribed by the physician, because this will cause an overload to the circulating blood volume and contribute to cardiac complications.

Test-Taking Strategy: Use the process of elimination. Think about the physiology of the cardiac system, the maternal and fetal needs, and the factors that increase the workload on the heart to answer the question. Review nursing measures for the pregnant client with cardiac disease if you had difficulty with this question.

Reference

Wong, D., Hockenberry, M., Perry, S., Lowdermilk, D., & Wilson, D. (2006). *Maternal-child nursing care* (3rd ed., pp. 350-351). St. Louis: Mosby.

1411. The nurse is developing a plan of care for a client on bedrest. During the planning, the nurse includes measures to limit the complications of prolonged immobility. The nurse includes which essential item in the plan?

1 Maintain the client in a supine position.
2 Provide a daily fluid intake of 1000 mL.
3 Limit the intake of milk and milk products.
4 Monitor for signs of a low serum calcium level.

Level of Cognitive Ability: Application
Client Needs: Physiological Integrity
Integrated Process: Nursing Process/Planning
Content Area: Adult Health/Musculoskeletal

Answer: 3
Rationale: The formation of renal and urinary calculi is a complication of immobility. Daily fluid intake should be 2000 mL or more per day. The nurse should monitor for signs and symptoms of hypercalcemia, such as nausea, vomiting, polydipsia, polyuria, and lethargy. A supine position increases urinary stasis; therefore, this position should be limited or avoided. Limiting milk and milk products is the best measure to prevent the formation of calcium stones.

Test-Taking Strategy: Focus on the subject of the complications of prolonged immobility. Option 1 should be eliminated immediately, because it refers to maintaining an immobile client in one position. Eliminate option 2 next, noting the amount of fluid in this option. From the remaining options, recalling the effect of the movement of calcium into the blood from the bones will direct you to option 3. Review the complications of immobility if you had difficulty with this question.

Reference
Black, J., & Hawks, J. (2005). *Medical-surgical nursing: Clinical management for positive outcomes* (7th ed., pp. 644-645, 885). Philadelphia: Saunders.

1412. The nurse determines that a Mantoux tuberculin skin test is positive. To most accurately diagnose tuberculosis (TB), the nurse plans to consult with the physician to follow up the skin test with a:

1 Chest x-ray
2 Sputum culture
3 Complete blood cell count
4 Computed tomography scan of the chest

Level of Cognitive Ability: Application
Client Needs: Physiological Integrity
Integrated Process: Nursing Process/Planning
Content Area: Adult Health/Respiratory

Answer: 2
Rationale: Although the findings of the chest X-ray examination are important, it is not possible to make a diagnosis of TB solely on the basis of this examination, because other diseases can mimic the appearance of TB. The demonstration of tubercle bacilli bacteriologically is essential for establishing a diagnosis. The microscopic examination of sputum for acid-fast bacilli is usually the first bacteriologic evidence of the presence of tubercle bacilli. Options 3 and 4 will not diagnose TB.

Test-Taking Strategy: Note the strategic words "most accurately diagnose tuberculosis." Recalling that the presence of tubercle bacilli indicates TB will direct you to option 2. Review the tests used to diagnose TB if you had difficulty with this question.

Reference
Black, J., & Hawks, J. (2005). *Medical-surgical nursing: Clinical management for positive outcomes* (7th ed., p. 1846). Philadelphia: Saunders.

1413. The home-care nurse is preparing a plan of care for a client with Meniere's disease who is experiencing severe vertigo. Which nursing intervention should the nurse include in the plan of care to assist the client with controlling the vertigo?

1 Encourage the client to increase the daily fluid intake.
2 Instruct the client to cut down on cigarette smoking.
3 Encourage the client to avoid sudden head movements.
4 Instruct the client to increase the amount of sodium in the diet.

Answer: 3
Rationale: The nurse instructs the client to make slow head movements to prevent worsening of the vertigo. Dietary changes such as salt and fluid restrictions that reduce the amount of endolymphatic fluid are sometimes prescribed. Clients are advised to stop smoking because of its vasoconstrictive effects.

Level of Cognitive Ability: Application
Client Needs: Physiological Integrity
Integrated Process: Nursing Process/Planning
Content Area: Adult Health/Ear

Test-Taking Strategy: Identify the subject of the question: severe vertigo. Note the relationship between the words "severe vertigo" and the correct option, which recommends the avoidance of sudden head movements. Recalling that salt and fluid restrictions are sometimes prescribed will also assist you with eliminating options 1 and 4. Noting the words "cut down" in option 2 will assist you with eliminating this option. Review the measures that will reduce vertigo in the client with Meniere's disease if you had difficulty with this question.

Reference
Ignatavicius, D., & Workman, M. (2006). *Medical-surgical nursing: Critical thinking for collaborative care* (5th ed., p. 1132). Philadelphia: Saunders.

1414. An 18-year-old woman is admitted to a mental health unit with the diagnosis of anorexia nervosa. The nurse plans care, knowing that health promotion should focus on:

1 Providing a supportive environment
2 Examining intrapsychic conflicts and past issues
3 Emphasizing social interaction with clients who are withdrawn
4 Helping the client identify and examine dysfunctional thoughts and beliefs

Level of Cognitive Ability: Application
Client Needs: Psychosocial Integrity
Integrated Process: Nursing Process/Planning
Content Area: Mental Health

Answer: 4
Rationale: Health promotion focuses on helping clients identify and examine dysfunctional thoughts as well as identifying and examining the values and beliefs that maintain these thoughts. Providing a supportive environment is important, but it is not as primary as option 4 for this client. Emphasizing social interaction is not appropriate at this time. Examining intrapsychic conflicts and past issues is not directly related to the client's problem.

Test-Taking Strategy: Use the process of elimination, and focus on the subject of health promotion. Option 4 is the only option that is specifically client centered. This option also focuses on assessment, which is the first step of the nursing process. Review the care of the client with anorexia nervosa if you had difficulty with this question.

Reference
Varcarolis, E., Carson, V., & Shoemaker, N. (2006). *Foundations of psychiatric mental health nursing* (5th ed., p. 314). Philadelphia: Saunders.

1415. A nurse is preparing discharge plans for a hospitalized client who attempted suicide. The nurse includes which of the following in the plan?

1 Weekly follow-up appointments
2 Contracts and immediately available crisis resources
3 Providing phone numbers for the hospital and physician
4 Encouraging family and friends to be with the client at all times

Level of Cognitive Ability: Application
Client Needs: Psychosocial Integrity
Integrated Process: Nursing Process/Planning
Content Area: Mental Health

Answer: 2
Rationale: Crisis times may occur between appointments. Contracts facilitate clients feeling a responsibility for keeping a promise, which gives the client control. Family and friends cannot always be present. Providing phone numbers will not ensure available and immediate crisis intervention.

Test-Taking Strategy: Focus on the subject: the availability of immediate resources for the client. Eliminate option 4 first, because this is unrealistic. Options 1 and 3 will not necessarily provide immediate resources. In addition, note the word "immediately" in the correct option. Review the discharge plans for the client who attempted suicide if you had difficulty with this question.

Reference
Stuart, G., & Laraia, M. (2005). *Principles and practice of psychiatric nursing* (8th ed., pp. 367, 374). St. Louis: Mosby.

1416. A nurse is developing a plan of care for a newborn infant diagnosed with bilateral club feet. The nurse includes instructions in the plan to tell the parents that:

1 The regimen of manipulation and casting is effective in all cases of bilateral club feet.

2 Genetic testing is wise for future pregnancies, because other children born to this couple may also be affected.

3 If casting is needed, it will begin at birth and continue for 12 weeks, at which time the condition will be reevaluated.

4 Surgery performed immediately after birth has been found to be the most effective for achieving a complete recovery.

Level of Cognitive Ability: Application
Client Needs: Physiological Integrity
Integrated Process: Nursing Process/Planning
Content Area: Child Health

Answer: 3
Rationale: Casting should begin at birth and continue for at least 12 weeks or until maximum correction is achieved. At this time, corrective shoes may provide support to maintain alignment, or surgery can be performed. Surgery is usually delayed until the child is 4 to 12 months old. Options 1 and 4 are inaccurate. Option 2 does not specifically address the subject of the question.

Test-Taking Strategy: Focus on the subject of parental instructions for the child with bilateral club feet. Eliminate option 2, because it does not specifically address the subject of the question, and it relates to the future. Eliminate option 4 because of the word "immediately." From the remaining options, note that option 3 provides accurate information and that option 1 contains the close-ended word "all." Review the treatment plan for bilateral club feet if you had difficulty with this question.

Reference
Wong, D., Hockenberry, M., Perry, S., Lowdermilk, D., & Wilson, D. (2006). *Maternal-child nursing care* (3rd ed., pp. 1820-1821). St. Louis: Mosby.

1417. The nurse is planning to assist with obtaining a set of arterial blood gas measurements for a client. The nurse plans to provide which of the following items to optimally maintain the integrity of the specimen?

1 A syringe that contains a preservative

2 A heparinized syringe and a bag of ice

3 A heparinized syringe and a preservative

4 A syringe that contains a preservative and a bag of ice

Level of Cognitive Ability: Application
Client Needs: Physiological Integrity
Integrated Process: Nursing Process/Planning
Content Area: Adult Health/Respiratory

Answer: 2
Rationale: The arterial blood gas sample is obtained using a heparinized syringe. The sample of blood is placed on ice and sent to the laboratory immediately. A preservative is not used.

Test-Taking Strategy: Specific knowledge regarding this procedure is needed to answer this question. Remember that an arterial blood gas sample is obtained using a heparinized syringe, placed on ice, and sent to the laboratory immediately. Review arterial blood gas measurement if you had difficulty with this question.

References
Pagana, K., & Pagana, T. (2005). *Mosby's diagnostic and laboratory test reference* (7th ed., p. 123). St. Louis: Mosby.
Perry, A., & Potter, P. (2006). *Clinical nursing skills & techniques* (6th ed., p. 1458). St. Louis: Mosby.

1418. A client is experiencing diabetes insipidus as a result of cranial surgery. The nurse who is caring for the client plans to implement which of these anticipated therapies?

1 Fluid restriction

2 Administering diuretics

3 Increased sodium intake

4 Intravenous (IV) replacement of fluid losses

Answer: 4
Rationale: The client with diabetes insipidus excretes large amounts of extremely dilute urine. This usually occurs as a result of decreased synthesis or the release of antidiuretic hormone in clients with conditions such as head injury, surgery near the hypothalamus, or increased intracranial pressure. Corrective measures include allowing ample oral fluid intake, administering IV fluid as needed to replace sensible and insensible losses, and administering vasopressin (Pitressin). Sodium is not administered, because the serum sodium level is usually high, as is the serum osmolality. Diuretics are not administered.

Level of Cognitive Ability: Analysis
Client Needs: Physiological Integrity
Integrated Process: Nursing Process/Planning
Content Area: Adult Health/Neurological

Test-Taking Strategy: Focus on the client's diagnosis, and recall that a large fluid loss is the problem in this client. This will assist you with eliminating options 1 and 2. From the remaining options, recalling that the serum sodium level is already elevated in clients with this disorder or knowing that fluid replacement is the most direct form of therapy for fluid loss will direct you to option 4. Review the treatment for diabetes insipidus if you had difficulty with this question.

Reference
Ignatavicius, D., & Workman, M. (2006). *Medical-surgical nursing: Critical thinking for collaborative care* (5th ed., p. 1467). Philadelphia: Saunders.

1419. A nurse is planning care for a child with an infectious and communicable disease. The nurse determines that the primary goal is that the:
  1 Child will experience mild discomfort.
  2 Public health department will be notified.
  3 Child will not spread the infection to others.
  4 Child will experience only minor complications.

Level of Cognitive Ability: Analysis
Client Needs: Health Promotion and
  Maintenance
Integrated Process: Nursing Process/Planning
Content Area: Child Health

Answer: 3
Rationale: The primary goal is to prevent the spread of the infection to others. The child should experience no complications. Although the health department may need to be notified at some point, it is not the primary goal. It is also important to prevent discomfort as much as possible.

Test-Taking Strategy: Use the process of elimination. Note the strategic words "primary goal." Note the relationship between the words "infectious and communicable disease" in the question and "infection" in the correct option. Review the goals of the care of a child with an infectious and communicable disease if you had difficulty with this question.

Reference
Wong, D., Hockenberry, M., Perry, S., Lowdermilk, D., & Wilson, D. (2006). *Maternal-child nursing care* (3rd ed., p. 1128). St. Louis: Mosby.

1420. A nurse is preparing to care for an infant with pertussis. When planning care, the nurse addresses which critical problem?
  1 Risk for infection
  2 Excess fluid volume
  3 Disturbed sleep pattern
  4 Ineffective airway clearance

Level of Cognitive Ability: Application
Client Needs: Physiological Integrity
Integrated Process: Nursing Process/Planning
Content Area: Child Health

Answer: 4
Rationale: The most important problem relates to adequate air exchange. Because of the copious, thick secretions that occur with pertussis and the small airways of an infant, air exchange is critical. A deficient fluid volume is more likely to occur in this infant because of the thick secretions and vomiting. Sleep patterns may be disturbed because of the coughing, but this is not the critical issue. Infection is an important consideration, but airway is the priority.

Test-Taking Strategy: Use the process of elimination and the ABCs—airway, breathing, and circulation. Airway is always the most critical concern. This should direct you to option 4. Review the care of the infant with pertussis if you had difficulty with this question.

Reference
Wong, D., Hockenberry, M., Perry, S., Lowdermilk, D., & Wilson, D. (2006). *Maternal-child nursing care* (3rd ed., p. 1135). St. Louis: Mosby.

1421. A nurse is planning care for an infant who has pyloric stenosis. To most effectively meet the infant's preoperative needs, the nurse includes which of the following in the plan of care?

1 Administer enemas until returns are clear.
2 Provide the mother privacy to breast-feed every 2 hours.
3 Monitor the intravenous (IV) infusion, intake, output, and weight.
4 Provide small, frequent feedings of glucose, water, and electrolytes.

Level of Cognitive Ability: Application
Client Needs: Physiological Integrity
Integrated Process: Nursing Process/Planning
Content Area: Child Health

Answer: 3
Rationale: Preoperatively, important nursing responsibilities include monitoring the IV infusion, intake, output, and weight and obtaining urine specific gravity measurements. Additionally, weighing the infant's diapers provides information regarding output. Preoperatively, the infant receives nothing by mouth (unless otherwise prescribed by the physician). Enemas until clear would further compromise the fluid volume status.

Test-Taking Strategy: Use the process of elimination, and note the strategic word "preoperative." Eliminate options 2 and 4, because the infant needs to receive nothing by mouth during the preoperative period. Eliminate option 1, because enemas would further compromise the fluid balance status. Review the preoperative care of the infant with pyloric stenosis if you had difficulty with this question.

Reference
Wong, D., Hockenberry, M., Perry, S., Lowdermilk, D., & Wilson, D. (2006). *Maternal-child nursing care* (3rd ed., p. 1534). St. Louis: Mosby.

1422. A client who was a victim of a gunshot incident states, "I feel like I am losing my mind. I keep hearing the gunshots and seeing my friend lying on the ground." The nurse initially plans strategies to formulate a therapeutic relationship that will include:

1 Teaching the client a variety of relaxation techniques
2 Asking the psychiatrist to order appropriate medication
3 Encouraging the client to talk about the incident and feelings related to it
4 Encouraging the client to think about just how lucky he or she is to still be alive

Level of Cognitive Ability: Application
Client Needs: Psychosocial Integrity
Integrated Process: Nursing Process/Planning
Content Area: Mental Health

Answer: 3
Rationale: When developing a therapeutic relationship, it is important to acknowledge and validate the client's feelings. Although teaching the client relaxation techniques may be helpful at some point, it is not related to the subject of the question. Options 2 and 4 are nontherapeutic techniques, and they do not promote a therapeutic relationship.

Test-Taking Strategy: Use therapeutic communication techniques. Eliminate options 2 and 4, because they do not encourage further discussion about the client's feelings. Teaching the client how to relax may be helpful at some point, but not at the beginning of the therapeutic relationship. Remember to address the client's feelings. Review therapeutic communication techniques if you had difficulty with this question.

References
Black, J., & Hawks, J. (2005). *Medical-surgical nursing: Clinical management for positive outcomes* (7th ed., p. 2487). Philadelphia: Saunders.
Stuart, G., & Laraia, M. (2005). *Principles and practice of psychiatric nursing* (8th ed., pp. 30-34). St. Louis: Mosby.

1423. A nurse is caring for a hospitalized child with a diagnosis of rheumatic fever who has developed carditis. The mother asks the nurse to explain the meaning of carditis. The nurse plans to respond, knowing that which of the following most appropriately describes this complication of rheumatic fever?

1 Involuntary movements affecting the legs, arms, and face
2 Inflammation of all parts of the heart, primarily the mitral valve
3 Tender, painful joints, especially in the elbows, knees, ankles, and wrists
4 Red skin lesions that start as flat or slightly raised macules, usually over the trunk, and that spread peripherally

Level of Cognitive Ability: Application
Client Needs: Physiological Integrity
Integrated Process: Nursing Process/Planning
Content Area: Child Health

Answer: 2
Rationale: Carditis is the inflammation of all parts of the heart, primarily the mitral valve, and it is a complication of rheumatic fever. Option 1 describes chorea. Option 3 describes polyarthritis. Option 4 describes erythema marginatum.

Test-Taking Strategy: Use the process of elimination. Note the relationship between the word "carditis" in the question and "heart" in the correct option. Review carditis if you had difficulty with this question.

References
Hockenberry, M., & Wilson, D. (2007). *Nursing care of infants and children* (8th ed., p. 1479). St. Louis: Mosby.
McKinney, E., James, S., Murray, S., & Ashwill, J. (2005). *Maternal-child nursing* (2nd ed., p. 1287). St. Louis: Saunders.

1424. A nurse receives a telephone call from the emergency department and is told that a 7-month-old infant with febrile seizures will be admitted to the pediatric unit. When planning care for the admission of the infant, the nurse would anticipate the need for which of the following?

1 Restraints at the bedside
2 A code cart at the bedside
3 Suction equipment at the bedside
4 A padded tongue blade taped to the head of the bed

Level of Cognitive Ability: Application
Client Needs: Physiological Integrity
Integrated Process: Nursing Process/Planning
Content Area: Child Health

Answer: 3
Rationale: During a seizure, the infant should be placed in a side-lying position, but he or she should not be restrained. Suctioning may be required during a seizure to remove secretions that obstruct the airway. It is not necessary to place a code cart at the bedside, but a cart should be readily available on the nursing unit. A padded tongue blade should never be used; in fact, nothing should be placed in the mouth during a seizure.

Test-Taking Strategy: Use the process of elimination and the ABCs—airway, breathing, and circulation—to answer the question. Option 3 is the only option that specifically relates to the airway. Review nursing interventions for an infant with seizures if you had difficulty with this question.

References
Hockenberry, M., Wilson, D., & Winkelstein, M. (2005). *Wong's essentials of pediatric nursing* (7th ed., pp. 1052-1053). St. Louis: Mosby.
McKinney, E., James, S., Murray, S., & Ashwill, J. (2005). *Maternal-child nursing* (2nd ed., p. 1520). St. Louis: Saunders.

1425. A 10-month-old infant is hospitalized for respiratory syncytial virus (RSV). The nurse develops a plan of care for the infant. On the basis of the developmental stage of the infant, the nurse includes which of the following in the plan of care?

1 Restrain the infant with a total body restraint to prevent any tubes from being dislodged.
2 Wash hands, wear a mask when caring for the infant, and keep the infant as quiet as possible.
3 Provide a consistent routine, and touch, rock, and cuddle the infant throughout the hospitalization.
4 Follow the home feeding schedule, and allow the infant to be held only when the parents visit.

Level of Cognitive Ability: Application
Client Needs: Physiological Integrity
Integrated Process: Nursing Process/Planning
Content Area: Child Health

Answer: 3
Rationale: A 10-month-old infant is in the trust versus mistrust stage of psychosocial development, according to Erik Erikson, and the sensorimotor period of cognitive development, according to Jean Piaget. RSV is not airborne (a mask is not required), and it is usually transmitted by the hands. Touching and holding the infant only when the parents visit will not provide adequate stimulation and interpersonal contact for the infant. Total body restraint is unnecessary and an incorrect action. Hospitalization may have an adverse effect. A consistent routine accompanied by touching, rocking, and cuddling will help the child develop trust and provide sensory stimulation.

Test-Taking Strategy: Note the age and diagnosis of the infant. Focusing on the strategic words "developmental stage of the infant" will direct you to option 3. Review the psychosocial needs of an infant if you had difficulty with this question.

References
Hockenberry, M., Wilson, D., & Winkelstein, M. (2005). *Wong's essentials of pediatric nursing* (7th ed., p. 805). St. Louis: Mosby.
McKinney, E., James, S., Murray, S., & Ashwill, J. (2005). *Maternal-child nursing* (2nd ed., p. 1215). St. Louis: Saunders.

1426. A pediatric nurse receives a telephone call from the admission office and is informed that a child with a diagnosis of Reye's syndrome is being admitted to the hospital. The nurse develops a plan of care for the child and includes which critical nursing action in the plan?

1 Monitoring for hearing loss
2 Monitoring intake and output (I&O)
3 Repositioning the child every 2 hours
4 Providing a quiet environment with low, dimmed lighting

Level of Cognitive Ability: Application
Client Needs: Physiological Integrity
Integrated Process: Nursing Process/Planning
Content Area: Child Health

Answer: 4
Rationale: Cerebral edema is a progressive part of the disease process of Reye's syndrome. A major component of care for a child with Reye's syndrome is maintaining effective cerebral perfusion and controlling intracranial pressure. Decreasing stimuli in the environment would decrease the stress on the cerebral tissue as well as neuron responses. Hearing loss does not occur in clients with this disorder. Although monitoring I&O may be a component of the plan, it is not the critical nursing action. Changing the body position every 2 hours would not affect the cerebral edema and intracranial pressure directly. The child should be in a head-elevated position to decrease the progression of cerebral edema and to promote the drainage of cerebrospinal fluid.

Test-Taking Strategy: Note the strategic word "critical." Recalling that increased intracranial pressure is a concern for clients with Reye's syndrome will direct you to option 4. Review the plan of care for the child with Reye's syndrome if you had difficulty with this question.

References
Hockenberry, M., & Wilson, D. (2007). *Nursing care of infants and children* (8th ed., p. 1651). St. Louis: Mosby.
McKinney, E., James, S., Murray, S., & Ashwill, J. (2005). *Maternal-child nursing* (2nd ed., p. 1528). St. Louis: Saunders.

1427. A nursing student is preparing to conduct a clinical conference regarding cerebral palsy. Which characteristic related to this disorder will the student plan to include in the discussion?

1 Cerebral palsy is an infectious disease of the central nervous system.
2 Cerebral palsy is an inflammation of the brain as a result of a viral illness.
3 Cerebral palsy is a congenital condition that results in moderate to severe retardation.
4 Cerebral palsy is a chronic disability characterized by difficulty with controlling the muscles.

Level of Cognitive Ability: Application
Client Needs: Physiological Integrity
Integrated Process: Nursing Process/Planning
Content Area: Child Health

Answer: 4
Rationale: Cerebral palsy is a chronic disability that is characterized by difficulty with controlling the muscles because of an abnormality in the extrapyramidal or pyramidal motor system. Meningitis is an infectious process of the central nervous system. Encephalitis is an inflammation of the brain that occurs as a result of viral illness or central nervous system infections. Down syndrome is an example of a congenital condition that results in moderate to severe retardation.

Test-Taking Strategy: Use the process of elimination. Eliminate options 1 and 2 first, because they are comparable or alike. From the remaining options, note the relationship between "palsy" in the question and "muscles" in the correct option. Review the characteristics associated with cerebral palsy if you had difficulty with this question.

Reference
Wong, D., Hockenberry, M., Perry, S., Lowdermilk, D., & Wilson, D. (2006). *Maternal-child nursing care* (3rd ed., p. 1842). St. Louis: Mosby.

1428. A nursing student is asked to conduct a clinical conference about autism. The student plans to include in the discussion that the primary characteristic associated with autism is:

1 Normal social play
2 Lack of social interaction and awareness
3 The consistent imitation of others' actions
4 Normal verbal but abnormal nonverbal communication

Level of Cognitive Ability: Application
Client Needs: Psychosocial Integrity
Integrated Process: Nursing Process/Planning
Content Area: Child Health

Answer: 2
Rationale: Autism is a severe developmental disorder that begins in infancy or toddlerhood. A primary characteristic is a lack of social interaction and awareness. Social behaviors in children with autism include a lack of or abnormal imitations of others' actions and a lack of or abnormal social play. Additional characteristics include a lack of or impaired verbal communication and marked abnormal nonverbal communication.

Test-Taking Strategy: Use the process of elimination. Eliminate options 1 and 4 first, because they address normal behaviors. From the remaining options, recalling that the autistic child lacks social interaction and awareness will direct you to option 2. Review the characteristics associated with autism if you had difficulty with this question.

Reference
Hockenberry, M., Wilson, D., & Winkelstein, M. (2005). *Wong's essentials of pediatric nursing* (7th ed., p. 618). St. Louis: Mosby.

1429. A charge nurse reviews the plan of care formulated by a new nursing graduate for a child returning from the operating room after a tonsillectomy. The charge nurse assists the new nursing graduate with changing the plan if which incorrect intervention is documented?

1 Suction whenever necessary.
2 Offer clear, cool liquids when awake.
3 Monitor for bleeding from the surgical site.
4 Eliminate milk or milk products from the diet.

Answer: 1
Rationale: After tonsillectomy, suction equipment should be available, but suctioning is not performed unless there is an airway obstruction. Clear, cool liquids are encouraged. Milk and milk products are avoided initially because they coat the throat; this causes the child to clear the throat, thereby increasing the risk of bleeding. Option 3 is an important intervention after any type of surgery.

Level of Cognitive Ability: Application
Client Needs: Physiological Integrity
Integrated Process: Nursing Process/Planning
Content Area: Leadership/Management

Test-Taking Strategy: Use the process of elimination, and note the strategic words "incorrect intervention." Eliminate option 3 first, because this is an expected general nursing procedure. From the remaining options, thinking about the anatomical location of the surgery will direct you to option 1. Suctioning after tonsillectomy will disrupt the integrity of the surgical site and can cause bleeding. Review postoperative care for tonsillectomy if you had difficulty with this question.

References
Hockenberry, M., Wilson, D., & Winkelstein, M. (2005). *Wong's essentials of pediatric nursing* (7th ed., pp. 796-797). St. Louis: Mosby.
McKinney, E., James, S., Murray, S., & Ashwill, J. (2005). *Maternal-child nursing* (2nd ed., p. 1202). St. Louis: Saunders.

1430. A nurse is preparing a plan of care for a child being admitted to the hospital with a diagnosis of congestive heart failure (CHF). The nurse avoids including which of the following in the plan?
1 Elevating the head of the bed
2 Providing oxygen during stressful periods
3 Limiting the time that the child is allowed to bottle-feed
4 Waking the child for feedings to ensure adequate nutrition

Level of Cognitive Ability: Application
Client Needs: Physiological Integrity
Integrated Process: Nursing Process/Planning
Content Area: Child Health

Answer: 4
Rationale: Measures that will decrease the workload on the heart include limiting the time that the child is allowed to bottle- or breast-feed, elevating the head of the bed, allowing for uninterrupted rest periods, and providing oxygen during stressful periods.

Test-Taking Strategy: Note the strategic word "avoids." Review each option carefully, and recall that the goal for a child with CHF is to decrease the workload on the heart. Option 4 is the only option that will not ensure this goal. Review the measures associated with caring for the child with CHF if you had difficulty with this question.

Reference
Hockenberry, M., Wilson, D., & Winkelstein, M. (2005). *Wong's essentials of pediatric nursing* (7th ed., pp. 908, 910). St. Louis: Mosby.

1431. A nurse is preparing a plan of care for a child with leukemia who is scheduled to receive chemotherapy. Which intervention will the nurse include in the plan of care?
1 Monitor rectal temperatures every 4 hours.
2 Monitor the mouth and anus each shift for signs of breakdown.
3 Encourage the child to consume fresh fruits and vegetables to maintain nutritional status.
4 Provide meticulous mouth care several times daily using an alcohol-based mouthwash and a toothbrush.

Answer: 2
Rationale: When the child is receiving chemotherapy, the nurse should avoid taking rectal temperatures. Oral temperatures are also avoided if mouth ulcers are present. Axillary temperatures should be taken to prevent alterations in skin integrity. Meticulous mouth care should be performed, but the nurse should avoid alcohol-based mouthwashes and should use a soft-bristled toothbrush. The nurse should assess the mouth and anus each shift for ulcers, erythema, or breakdown. Bland, nonirritating foods and liquids should be provided to the child. Fresh fruits and vegetables need to be avoided, because they can harbor organisms. Chemotherapy can cause neutropenia, and the child should be maintained on a low-bacteria diet if the white blood cell count is low.

Test-Taking Strategy: Use the process of elimination, and read each option carefully. Thinking about the side effects that can occur with chemotherapy will direct you to option 2. Review the care of the child receiving chemotherapy if you had difficulty with this question.

Level of Cognitive Ability: Application
Client Needs: Physiological Integrity
Integrated Process: Nursing Process/Planning
Content Area: Child Health

References
Hockenberry, M., & Wilson, D. (2007). *Nursing care of infants and children* (8th ed., p. 1543). St. Louis: Mosby.
Hockenberry, M., Wilson, D., & Winkelstein, M. (2005). *Wong's essentials of pediatric nursing* (7th ed., pp. 960-961). St. Louis: Mosby.

1432. The nurse is assisting with preparing to admit a client from the postanesthesia care unit who has had microvascular decompression of the trigeminal nerve. The nurse asks the nursing assistant to make sure that which of the following equipment is at the bedside when the client arrives?
1 Flashlight and pulse oximeter
2 Blood pressure cuff and cardiac monitor
3 Cardiac monitor and suction equipment
4 Padded bed rails and suction equipment

Level of Cognitive Ability: Application
Client Needs: Physiological Integrity
Integrated Process: Nursing Process/Planning
Content Area: Adult Health/Neurological

Answer: 1
Rationale: The postoperative care of the client having microvascular decompression of the trigeminal nerve is the same as for the client undergoing craniotomy. This client requires hourly neurological assessment as well as monitoring of the cardiovascular and respiratory statuses. Cardiac monitoring and padded bed rails are not indicated unless there is a special need based on a client history of cardiac disease or seizures, respectively. Suctioning is performed cautiously and only when necessary after craniotomy to avoid increasing the intracranial pressure.

Test-Taking Strategy: Use the process of elimination, and focus on the data in the question. The client is not necessarily at risk for seizures postoperatively, so option 4 is eliminated first. Eliminate options 2 and 3 next, because no data in the question indicate that the client had a history of a cardiac problem. In addition, knowing that the procedure is performed via craniotomy enables you to recall that suctioning is done cautiously and only when necessary and also that neurological assessment is needed, so a flashlight would be required to perform a neurological assessment. Review the care of the client after microvascular decompression of the trigeminal nerve if you had difficulty with this question.

References
Ignatavicius, D., & Workman, M. (2006). *Medical-surgical nursing: Critical thinking for collaborative care* (5th ed., p. 1024). Philadelphia: Saunders.
Lewis, S., Heitkemper, M., Dirksen, S., O'Brien, P., & Bucher, L. (2007). *Medical-surgical nursing: Assessment and management of clinical problems* (7th ed., p. 1582). St. Louis: Mosby.

1433. The nurse is receiving a client from the emergency department who has a diagnosis of Guillain-Barré syndrome. The client's chief complaint is an ascending paralysis that has reached the level of the waist. The nurse plans to have which items available for emergency use?
1 Nebulizer and pulse oximeter
2 Blood pressure cuff and flashlight
3 Flashlight and incentive spirometer
4 Cardiac monitor and intubation tray

Answer: 4
Rationale: The client with Guillain-Barré syndrome is at risk for respiratory failure as a result of ascending paralysis. An intubation tray should be available for emergency use. Another complication of this syndrome is cardiac dysrhythmias, which necessitates the need for cardiac monitoring. Although some of the items in options 1, 2, and 3 may be kept at the bedside (e.g., pulse oximeter blood pressure cuff, flashlight, pulse oximeter), they are not necessarily needed for emergency use in this situation.

Test-Taking Strategy: Note the strategic words "emergency use." These tell you that the correct answer will be an option that contains equipment that is not routinely used to provide care. With this in mind, eliminate options 2 and 3 first, because a flashlight is needed for routine neurological assessment. From the remaining options, recalling the complications of this syndrome will direct you to option 4. Review the nursing care measures for the client with Guillain-Barré syndrome if you had difficulty with this question.

Level of Cognitive Ability: Application
Client Needs: Physiological Integrity
Integrated Process: Nursing Process/Planning
Content Area: Adult Health/Neurological

References
Black, J., & Hawks, J. (2005). *Medical-surgical nursing: Clinical management for positive outcomes* (7th ed., p. 2182). Philadelphia: Saunders.
Ignatavicius, D., & Workman, M. (2006). *Medical-surgical nursing: Critical thinking for collaborative care* (5th ed., p. 1009). Philadelphia: Saunders.

1434. A nurse in the newborn nursery receives a telephone call and is informed that a newborn infant whose mother is Rh negative will be admitted to the nursery. When planning care for the infant's arrival, the nurse takes which important action?

1 Obtains the newborn infant's blood type and direct Coombs' results from the laboratory
2 Obtains the necessary equipment from the blood bank needed for an exchange transfusion
3 Calls the maintenance department and asks for a phototherapy unit to be brought to the nursery
4 Obtains a vial of vitamin K from the pharmacy and prepares to administer an injection to prevent isoimmunization

Level of Cognitive Ability: Application
Client Needs: Physiological Integrity
Integrated Process: Nursing Process/Planning
Content Area: Maternity/Postpartum

Answer: 1

Rationale: To further plan for the newborn infant's care, the infant's blood type and direct Coombs' results must be known. Umbilical cord blood is taken at the time of delivery to determine blood type, Rh factor, and antibody titer (direct Coombs' test) of the newborn infant. The nurse should obtain these results from the laboratory. Options 2 and 3 are inappropriate at this time, and additional data are needed to determine whether these actions are needed. Option 4 is incorrect, because vitamin K is given to prevent hemorrhagic disease of the newborn infant.

Test-Taking Strategy: Use the process of elimination, and focus on the subject of the mother being RH negative. Note the relationship between the subject of the question and option 1. In addition, note that option 1 is the only option that addresses assessment. Review Rh incompatibilities if you had difficulty with this question.

References
McKinney, E., James, S., Murray, S., & Ashwill, J. (2005). *Maternal-child nursing* (2nd ed., pp. 642-643). St. Louis: Saunders.
Wong, D., Hockenberry, M., Perry, S., Lowdermilk, D., & Wilson, D. (2006). *Maternal-child nursing care* (3rd ed., pp. 853-854). St. Louis: Mosby.

1435. The nurse is planning to instruct a client with chronic vertigo about safety measures to prevent the exacerbation of symptoms or injury. The nurse plans to teach the client that it is important to:

1 Turn the head slowly when spoken to.
2 Remove throw rugs and clutter in the home.
3 Drive at times when the client does not feel dizzy.
4 Go to the bedroom and lie down when vertigo is experienced.

Level of Cognitive Ability: Application
Client Needs: Safe and Effective Care Environment
Integrated Process: Nursing Process/Planning
Content Area: Adult Health/Ear

Answer: 2

Rationale: The client should maintain the home in a state that is free of clutter and that has throw rugs removed, because the effort of trying to regain balance after slipping could trigger the onset of vertigo. The client with chronic vertigo should avoid driving and using public transportation, because the sudden movements involved in each could precipitate an attack. To further prevent vertigo attacks, the client should change positions slowly, and he or she should turn the entire body rather than just the head when spoken to. If vertigo does occur, the client should immediately sit down or grasp the nearest piece of furniture.

Test-Taking Strategy: Use the process of elimination, and focus on the subject of safety. Eliminate options 3 and 4 first, because they put the client at greatest risk of injury as a result of vertigo. Choose option 2 over option 1, because it is the safer intervention of the remaining options. Review the safety measures for the client with vertigo if you had difficulty with this question.

References
Black, J., & Hawks, J. (2005). *Medical-surgical nursing: Clinical management for positive outcomes* (7th ed., p. 1991). Philadelphia: Saunders.
Ignatavicius, D., & Workman, M. (2006). *Medical-surgical nursing: Critical thinking for collaborative care* (5th ed., p. 1132). Philadelphia: Saunders.

1436. A male client who initially denied abusing alcohol is being discharged from the mental health unit. The client now states that he will "get some help" to live a healthier lifestyle. The nurse should provide the client with information concerning which of the following support groups?

1 Al-Anon
2 Fresh Start
3 Families Anonymous
4 Alcoholics Anonymous

Level of Cognitive Ability: Application
Client Needs: Health Promotion and Maintenance
Integrated Process: Nursing Process/Planning
Content Area: Mental Health

Answer: 4
Rationale: Alcoholics Anonymous is a major self-help organization for the treatment of alcoholism. Option 1 is a group for families of alcoholics. Option 2 is for nicotine addicts. Option 3 is for the parents of children who abuse substances.

Test-Taking Strategy: Use the process of elimination. Note the relationship between "abusing alcohol" in the question and "Alcoholics" in the correct option. Review the purposes of specific support groups if you had difficulty with this question.

References
Black, J., & Hawks, J. (2005). *Medical-surgical nursing: Clinical management for positive outcomes* (7th ed., p. 24). Philadelphia: Saunders.
Varcarolis, E., Carson, V., & Shoemaker, N. (2006). *Foundations of psychiatric mental health nursing* (5th ed., p. 566). Philadelphia: Saunders.

1437. A client with a brain attack (stroke) is prepared for discharge from the hospital. The physician has prescribed range-of-motion (ROM) exercises for the client's right side. When planning for the client's care, the home-care nurse:

1 Implements ROM exercises to the point of pain for the client
2 Considers the use of active, passive, or active-assisted exercises in the home
3 Encourages the client to be dependent on the home-care nurse to complete the exercise program
4 Develops a schedule that involves ROM exercises every 2 hours while awake, even if the client is fatigued

Level of Cognitive Ability: Application
Client Needs: Physiological Integrity
Integrated Process: Nursing Process/Planning
Content Area: Adult Health/Neurological

Answer: 2
Rationale: The home-care nurse must consider all forms of ROM for the client. Even if the client has right hemiplegia, the client can assist with some of his or her own rehabilitative care. In addition, the goal of home-care nursing is for the client to assume as much self-care and independence as possible. The nurse needs to teach so that the client becomes self-reliant. Options 1 and 4 are incorrect from a physiological standpoint.

Test-Taking Strategy: Use the process of elimination. Options 1 and 4 can be eliminated first, because these actions may be harmful to the client. From the remaining options, recall that dependency is not in the best interest of a client's sense of health promotion, which will help you to eliminate option 3. In addition, note that option 2 is the umbrella option. Review basic knowledge related to ROM exercises if you had difficulty with this question.

Reference
Black, J., & Hawks, J. (2005). *Medical-surgical nursing: Clinical management for positive outcomes* (7th ed., p. 2123). Philadelphia: Saunders.

Implementation

1438. A nurse in the postpartum unit checks the temperature of a client who delivered a healthy newborn infant 4 hours ago. The mother's temperature is 100.8°F. The nurse provides oral hydration to the mother and encourages fluids. Four hours later, the nurse rechecks the temperature and notes that it is still 100.8°F. Which nursing action is appropriate?
1 Notify the physician.
2 Document the temperature.
3 Increase the intravenous fluids.
4 Continue hydration and recheck the temperature 4 hours later.

Level of Cognitive Ability: Application
Client Needs: Physiological Integrity
Integrated Process: Nursing Process/ Implementation
Content Area: Maternity/Postpartum

Answer: 1
Rationale: A temperature of more than 100.4°F at two consecutive readings is considered febrile, and the physician should be notified. Options 2, 3, and 4 are inappropriate actions at this time.

Test-Taking Strategy: Use the process of elimination. Option 3 can be eliminated first, because this action requires a physician order. From the remaining options, noting that the temperature has remained unchanged after a nursing intervention should provide you with a clue that further intervention is necessary and direct you to option 1. Review the normal and abnormal findings of the postpartum period if you had difficulty with this question.

Reference
Murray, S., & McKinney, E. (2006). *Foundations of maternal-newborn nursing* (4th ed., p. 409). Philadelphia: Saunders.

1439. A nurse is checking the fundus of a postpartum woman and notes that the uterus is soft and spongy. Which nursing action is appropriate initially?
1 Notify the physician.
2 Encourage the mother to ambulate.
3 Massage the fundus gently until it is firm.
4 Document fundal position, consistency, and height.

Level of Cognitive Ability: Application
Client Needs: Physiological Integrity
Integrated Process: Nursing Process/ Implementation
Content Area: Maternity/Postpartum

Answer: 3
Rationale: If the fundus is boggy (soft), it should be massaged gently until it is firm and observed for increased bleeding or clots. Option 2 is an inappropriate action at this time. The nurse should document the fundal position, consistency, and height; the need to perform fundal massage; and the client's response to the intervention. The physician will need to be notified if uterine massage is not helpful.

Test-Taking Strategy: Note the strategic words "appropriate initially." Note the relationship of the data in the question ("soft and spongy") and the data in the correct option ("massage the fundus gently until it is firm"). Review the nursing interventions related to uterine atony if you had difficulty with this question.

Reference
Murray, S., & McKinney, E. (2006). *Foundations of maternal-newborn nursing* (4th ed., p. 409). Philadelphia: Saunders.

1440. A primipara is being evaluated in the clinic during her second trimester of pregnancy. The nurse checks the fetal heart rate (FHR) and notes that it is 190 beats/min. The appropriate nursing action would be to:
1 Document the finding.
2 Consult with the physician.
3 Tell the client that the FHR is normal.
4 Recheck the FHR with the client in the standing position.

Answer: 2
Rationale: The FHR should be between 110 and 160 beats/min throughout pregnancy. In this situation, the FHR is elevated from the normal range, and the nurse should consult with the physician. The FHR would be documented, but option 2 is the appropriate action. The nurse would not tell the client that the FHR is normal, because this is not true information. Option 4 is an inappropriate action.

Level of Cognitive Ability: Application
Client Needs: Physiological Integrity
Integrated Process: Nursing Process/
  Implementation
Content Area: Maternity/Antepartum

Test-Taking Strategy: Focus on the data in the question. Recalling that the normal FHR is between 110 and 160 beats/min will direct you to option 2. Review the normal FHR if you had difficulty with this question.

Reference
Murray, S., & McKinney, E. (2006). *Foundations of maternal-newborn nursing* (4th ed., pp. 127, 311). Philadelphia: Saunders.

1441. A female client tells the clinic nurse that her skin is very dry and irritated. Which product would the nurse suggest that the client apply to the dry skin?
  1 Myoflex
  2 Aspercreme
  3 Glycerin emollient
  4 Acetic acid solution

Level of Cognitive Ability: Application
Client Needs: Health Promotion and
  Maintenance
Integrated Process: Nursing Process/
  Implementation
Content Area: Pharmacology

Answer: 3
Rationale: Glycerin is an emollient that is used for dry, cracked, and irritated skin. Aspercreme and Myoflex are used to treat muscular aches. Acetic acid solution is used for irrigating, cleansing, and packing wounds infected with *Pseudomonas aeruginosa*.

Test-Taking Strategy: Use the process of elimination. Noting the strategic words "skin is very dry and irritated" will direct you to option 3. Review the listed products if you had difficulty with this question.

References
Lilley, L., Harrington, S., & Snyder, J. (2007). *Pharmacology and the nursing process* (5th ed., pp. 868-869). St. Louis: Mosby.
McKenry, L., Tressler, E., & Hogan, M. (2006). *Mosby's pharmacology in nursing* (22nd ed., p. 1124). St. Louis: Mosby.

1442. A client with a history of hypertension has been prescribed triamterene (Dyrenium). The nurse provides information to the client about the medication and tells the client to avoid consuming which of the following fruits?
  1 Pears
  2 Apples
  3 Bananas
  4 Cranberries

Level of Cognitive Ability: Application
Client Needs: Health Promotion and
  Maintenance
Integrated Process: Nursing Process/
  Implementation
Content Area: Adult Health/Cardiovascular

Answer: 3
Rationale: Triamterene is a potassium-sparing diuretic, and the client should avoid foods that are high in potassium. Fruits that are naturally higher in potassium include avocados, bananas, fresh oranges, mangoes, nectarines, papayas, and dried prunes.

Test-Taking Strategy: Recall that triamterene is a potassium-sparing diuretic, and then identify the high-potassium food. Review triamterene and food items that are high in potassium if you had difficulty with this question.

References
Kee, J., Hayes, E., & McCuistion, L. (2006). *Pharmacology: A nursing process approach* (5th ed., p. 638). Philadelphia: Saunders.
Skidmore-Roth, L. (2007). *Mosby's drug guide for nurses* (7th ed., pp. 938-939). St. Louis: Mosby.

1443. A client in the late, active, first stage of labor has just reported a gush of vaginal fluid. The nurse observes a fetal monitor pattern of variable decelerations during contractions followed by a brief acceleration. After that, there is a return to baseline until the next contraction, when the pattern is repeated. On the basis of this data, the nurse prepares to initially:
1 Take the client's vital signs.
2 Perform a Leopold's maneuver.
3 Perform a manual sterile vaginal exam.
4 Test the vaginal fluid with a nitrazine strip.

Level of Cognitive Ability: Application
Client Needs: Health Promotion and Maintenance
Integrated Process: Nursing Process/Implementation
Content Area: Maternity/Intrapartum

Answer: 3
Rationale: Variable deceleration with brief acceleration after a gush of amniotic fluid is a common clinical manifestation of cord compression caused by occult or frank prolapse of the umbilical cord. A manual vaginal exam can detect the presence of the cord in the vagina, which confirms the problem. On the basis of the data in the question, options 1, 2, and 4 are not initial actions.

Test-Taking Strategy: Use the process of elimination, and note the word "initially." Focusing on the data in the question and determining the significance of the data will direct you to option 3. Review the signs of cord compression if you had difficulty with this question.

References
McKinney, E., James, S., Murray, S., & Ashwill, J. (2005). *Maternal-child nursing* (2nd ed., p. 406). St. Louis: Saunders.
Wong, D., Hockenberry, M., Perry, S., Lowdermilk, D., & Wilson, D. (2006). *Maternal-child nursing care* (3rd ed., p. 479). St. Louis: Mosby.

1444. The nurse prepares to administer an enteral feeding to a client through a nasogastric tube (NGT). Which is the priority intervention for the nurse to complete before administering the feeding?
1 Determining tube placement
2 Auscultating the bowel sounds
3 Measuring the intake and output
4 Establishing the client's baseline weight

Level of Cognitive Ability: Analysis
Client Needs: Physiological Integrity
Integrated Process: Nursing Process/Implementation
Content Area: Fundamental Skills

Answer: 1
Rationale: The nurse avoids injecting any substance into a client's NGT before verifying tube placement, because NGTs can migrate out of the stomach. If the NGT is not in the correct location, subsequent injections or feedings through the tube can lead to serious complications such as aspiration. Options 2, 3, and 4 are not priorities before administering an enteral feeding.

Test-Taking Strategy: Note the strategic word "priority." Use the ABCs—airway, breathing, and circulation—and the nursing process to answer the question. Option 1 relates to assessment and to the risk of aspiration. Review the nursing interventions when initiating a tube feeding if you had difficulty with this question.

References
Lewis, S., Heitkemper, M., Dirksen, S., O'Brien, P., & Bucher, L. (2007). *Medical-surgical nursing: Assessment and management of clinical problems* (7th ed., p. 962). St. Louis: Mosby.
Perry, A., & Potter, P. (2006). *Clinical nursing skills & techniques* (6th ed., pp. 1015, 1021). St. Louis: Mosby.

1445. The nurse teaches a client with a rib fracture to cough and deep breathe. The client resists directions by the nurse because of the pain. The nurse appropriately:
1 Continues to give the client gentle encouragement to do so
2 Requests that the physician perform a nerve block to deaden the pain
3 Premedicates the client and assists the client with splinting the area during these exercises
4 Explains in detail the potential complications that may result from not coughing and deep breathing

Level of Cognitive Ability: Application
Client Needs: Physiological Integrity
Integrated Process: Nursing Process/
Implementation
Content Area: Adult Health/Respiratory

Answer: 3
Rationale: Shallow respirations that occur with rib fracture predispose the client to developing atelectasis and pneumonia. It is essential that the client perform coughing and deep breathing exercises to prevent these complications. The nurse accomplishes this most effectively by premedicating the client with pain medication and assisting the client with splinting during the exercises. Options 2 and 4 are inappropriate. Option 2 is an extreme measure, and the nurse would not explain in detail potential complications as identified in option 4. Because the client is resisting directions, "gentle encouragement" may not be adequate.

Test-Taking Strategy: Use the process of elimination. Options 2 and 4 are likely to be the most extreme or unrealistic options, respectively, and they should be eliminated first. From the remaining options, premedication and assistance are more likely than continued gentle encouragement to be effective. Review the care of the client with a rib fracture if you had difficulty with this question.

References
Black, J., & Hawks, J. (2005). *Medical-surgical nursing: Clinical management for positive outcomes* (7th ed., p. 1901). Philadelphia: Saunders.
Lewis, S., Heitkemper, M., Dirksen, S., O'Brien, P., & Bucher, L. (2007). *Medical-surgical nursing: Assessment and management of clinical problems* (7th ed., pp. 587-588). St. Louis: Mosby.

1446. A client who has episodes of bronchospasm and a history of tachydysrhythmias is admitted to the hospital. The nurse reviews the physician's orders and contacts the physician to verify which medication, if it has been prescribed?
1 Albuterol (Proventil)
2 Metaproterenol (Alupent)
3 Epinephrine (Primatene Mist)
4 Salmeterol/fluticasone (Advair)

Level of Cognitive Ability: Analysis
Client Needs: Safe and Effective Care Environment
Integrated Process: Nursing Process/
Implementation
Content Area: Pharmacology

Answer: 3
Rationale: A client with a history of tachydysrhythmias should not be given bronchodilators that contain catecholamines, such as epinephrine and isoproterenol hydrochloride (Isuprel). Other sympathomimetics that are noncatecholamines should be used instead. These include metaproterenol, albuterol, and salmeterol.

Test-Taking Strategy: Focus on the client's diagnosis of tachydysrhythmias, and use the process of elimination. Recalling that epinephrine is a catecholamine will direct you to option 3. Review the effects of epinephrine if you had difficulty with this question.

Reference
Skidmore-Roth, L. (2007). *2007 Mosby's nursing drug reference* (20th ed., p. 1086). St. Louis: Mosby.

1447. A client with obsessive-compulsive rituals often misses the unit's morning activities because of a bed-making ritual. Which nursing action would be therapeutic?

1 Verbalize tactful, mild disapproval of the behavior.
2 Discuss the ridiculousness of the behavior with the client.
3 Help the client to make the bed so that the task can be finished quicker.
4 Offer reflective feedback, such as "I see that you have made your bed several times."

Level of Cognitive Ability: Application
Client Needs: Psychosocial Integrity
Integrated Process: Nursing Process/
  Implementation
Content Area: Mental Health

Answer: 4
Rationale: Verbalizing disapproval would increase the client's anxiety and reinforce the need to perform the ritual. Helping with the ritual is nontherapeutic and also reinforces the behavior. The client is usually aware of the irrationality (ridiculousness) of the behavior. Reflective feedback acknowledges the client's behavior.

Test-Taking Strategy: Use the process of elimination. Recalling that the purpose of the ritual is to relieve anxiety would assist you with eliminating options 1 and 2, because these actions would increase the client's anxiety. Eliminate option 3, because there is no therapeutic value in participating in the ritual. Review the appropriate interventions for the client with compulsive behavior if you had difficulty with this question.

References
Stuart, G., & Laraia, M. (2005). *Principles and practice of psychiatric nursing* (8th ed., p. 273). St. Louis: Mosby.
Varcarolis, E., Carson, V., & Shoemaker, N. (2006). *Foundations of psychiatric mental health nursing* (5th ed., pp. 234-235). Philadelphia: Saunders.

1448. An older client who has undergone internal fixation after fracturing a left hip has developed a reddened left heel. The nurse obtains which of the following as a priority item to manage this problem?

1 Trapeze
2 Sheepskin
3 Bed cradle
4 Draw sheet

Level of Cognitive Ability: Application
Client Needs: Physiological Integrity
Integrated Process: Nursing Process/
  Implementation
Content Area: Adult Health/Musculoskeletal

Answer: 2
Rationale: The reddened heel results from the pressure of the foot against the mattress. The nurse obtains a sheepskin, heel protectors, or an alternating pressure mattress. The bed cradle will keep the linens off of the client's lower extremities but will not assist with the management of a reddened heel. A draw sheet and trapeze are of general use for this client, but they are not specific for dealing with the reddened heel.

Test-Taking Strategy: Note the subject of the question: a reddened left heel. Eliminate option 3 first, because it is unnecessary and not helpful. Eliminate options 1 and 4 next, because, although they are generally helpful for the client's mobility, they are not related to the subject of the question. Option 2 addresses the problem stated in the question. Review the measures that prevent skin breakdown in the immobile client if you had difficulty with this question.

References
Black, J., & Hawks, J. (2005). *Medical-surgical nursing: Clinical management for positive outcomes* (7th ed., pp. 1406, 1410-1411). Philadelphia: Saunders.
Ignatavicius, D., & Workman, M. (2006). *Medical-surgical nursing: Critical thinking for collaborative care* (5th ed., p. 991). Philadelphia: Saunders.

1449. A nurse is caring for an infant after pyloromyotomy performed to treat hypertrophic pyloric stenosis. The nurse places the infant in which position after surgery?
1 Flat on the operative side
2 Flat on the unoperative side
3 Prone with the head of the bed elevated
4 Supine with the head of the bed elevated

Level of Cognitive Ability: Application
Client Needs: Physiological Integrity
Integrated Process: Nursing Process/
    Implementation
Content Area: Child Health

Answer: 3
Rationale: After pyloromyotomy, the head of the bed is elevated, and the infant is placed prone to reduce the risk of aspiration. Options 1, 2, and 4 are incorrect positions after this type of surgery.

Test-Taking Strategy: Consider the anatomical location of the surgical procedure and the risks associated with the procedure to answer the question. Visualize each of the positions identified in the options. Keeping in mind that aspiration is a major concern will direct you to option 3. Review the nursing care measures after pyloromyotomy if you had difficulty with this question.

References
Hockenberry, M., Wilson, D., & Winkelstein, M. (2005). *Wong's essentials of pediatric nursing* (7th ed., p. 881). St. Louis: Mosby.
Wong, D., Hockenberry, M., Perry, S., Lowdermilk, D., & Wilson, D. (2006). *Maternal-child nursing care* (3rd ed., p. 1534). St. Louis: Mosby.

1450. A mother of a child with mumps calls the health care clinic to tell the nurse that the child has been lethargic and vomiting. The nurse tells the mother:
1 To continue to monitor the child
2 To bring the child to the clinic to be seen by the physician
3 That lethargy and vomiting are normal manifestations of mumps
4 That, as long as there is no fever, there is nothing to be concerned about

Level of Cognitive Ability: Application
Client Needs: Physiological Integrity
Integrated Process: Nursing Process/
    Implementation
Content Area: Child Health

Answer: 2
Rationale: Mumps generally affects the salivary glands, but it can also affect multiple organs. The most common complication is septic meningitis, with the virus being identified in the cerebrospinal fluid. Common signs include nuchal rigidity, lethargy, and vomiting. The child should be seen by the physician.

Test-Taking Strategy: Focus on the signs and symptoms presented in the question. Recalling that meningitis is a complication of mumps will direct you to option 2. Review the complications of mumps and the associated clinical manifestations if you had difficulty with this question.

References
Hockenberry, M., Wilson, D., & Winkelstein, M. (2005). *Wong's essentials of pediatric nursing* (7th ed., pp. 440-441). St. Louis: Mosby.
McKinney, E., James, S., Murray, S., & Ashwill, J. (2005). *Maternal-child nursing* (2nd ed., pp. 1026-1027). St. Louis: Saunders.

1451. A nurse is reviewing the physician's orders for a child who was admitted to the hospital with vaso-occlusive pain crisis from sickle cell anemia. Which of the following physician orders would the nurse question?
1 Bedrest
2 Intravenous fluids
3 Supplemental oxygen
4 Meperidine hydrochloride (Demerol) for pain

Answer: 4
Rationale: Meperidine hydrochloride is contraindicated for ongoing pain management because of the increased risk of seizures associated with the use of the medication. The management of vaso-occlusive pain generally includes the use of strong opioid analgesics such as morphine sulfate or hydromorphone (Dilaudid). These medications are usually most effective when given as a continuous infusion or at regular intervals around the clock. Options 1, 2, and 3 are appropriate prescriptions for treating vaso-occlusive pain crisis.

Level of Cognitive Ability: Application
Client Needs: Safe and Effective Care
  Environment
Integrated Process: Nursing Process/
  Implementation
Content Area: Child Health

Test-Taking Strategy: Use the process of elimination. Note the strategic words "orders would the nurse question." Recalling that oxygen, fluids, and bedrest are components of care will direct you to option 4. In addition, remember that meperidine hydrochloride is associated with an increased risk of seizures. Review the care of the child with sickle cell crisis if you had difficulty with this question.

Reference
Hockenberry, M., Wilson, D., & Winkelstein, M. (2005). *Wong's essentials of pediatric nursing* (7th ed., pp. 945-946). St. Louis: Mosby.

1452. A nurse is caring for an infant with laryngomalacia (congenital laryngeal stridor). Which position would the nurse place the infant in to decrease the incidence of stridor?
  1 Prone
  2 Supine
  3 Supine with the neck flexed
  4 Prone with the neck hyperextended

Level of Cognitive Ability: Application
Client Needs: Physiological Integrity
Integrated Process: Nursing Process/
  Implementation
Content Area: Child Health

Answer: 4
Rationale: The prone position with the neck hyperextended improves the child's breathing. Options 1, 2, and 3 are not appropriate positions.

Test-Taking Strategy: Use the process of elimination, and note the strategic words "decrease the incidence of stridor." Visualize each of the positions identified in the options to assist with directing you to option 4. Review the care of the infant with laryngomalacia if you had difficulty with this question.

References
Hockenberry, M., Wilson, D., & Winkelstein, M. (2005). *Wong's essentials of pediatric nursing* (7th ed., p. 802). St. Louis: Mosby.
McKinney, E., James, S., Murray, S., & Ashwill, J. (2005). *Maternal-child nursing* (2nd ed., p. 1203). St. Louis: Saunders.

1453. A nurse in the newborn nursery prepares to admit a newborn infant with spina bifida, meningomyelocele type. Which nursing action is most important for the care for this infant?
  1 Monitoring the temperature
  2 Monitoring the blood pressure
  3 Monitoring the specific gravity of the urine
  4 Inspecting the anterior fontanel for bulging

Answer: 4
Rationale: Intracranial pressure is a complication that is associated with spina bifida. A sign of intracranial pressure in the newborn infant with spina bifida is a bulging anterior fontanel. The newborn infant is at risk for infection before the surgical procedure and the closure of the gibbus, and monitoring the temperature is an important intervention; however, assessing the anterior fontanel for bulging is most important. A normal saline dressing is placed over the affected site to maintain the moisture of the gibbus and its contents. This prevents tearing or breakdown of skin integrity at the site. Blood pressure is difficult to assess during the newborn period, and it is not the best indicator of infection or a potential complication. Urine concentration is not well developed during the newborn stage of development.

Test-Taking Strategy: Use the process of elimination, and focus on the strategic words "most important." Eliminate options 2 and 3 first, because blood pressure and specific gravity are common assessments, but they are not as reliable indications of changes in the status of a newborn as they would be for an older child. From the remaining options, focusing on the strategic words will direct you to option 4. Review the care of the infant with spina bifida if you had difficulty with this question.

Level of Cognitive Ability: Application
Client Needs: Physiological Integrity
Integrated Process: Nursing Process/
Implementation
Content Area: Maternity/Postpartum

References
McKinney, E., James, S., Murray, S., & Ashwill, J. (2005). *Maternal-child nursing* (2nd ed., p. 1502). St. Louis: Saunders.
Murray, S., & McKinney, E. (2006). *Foundations of maternal-newborn nursing* (4th ed., p. 826). Philadelphia: Saunders.

1454. During the assessment of a child, a nurse notes that the child's genitals are swollen. The nurse suspects that the child is being sexually abused. Which action by the nurse is of primary importance?

1 Document the child's physical findings.
2 Refer the family to appropriate support groups.
3 Report the case in which the abuse is suspected.
4 Assist the family with identifying resources and support systems.

Level of Cognitive Ability: Application
Client Needs: Psychosocial Integrity
Integrated Process: Nursing Process/
Implementation
Content Area: Child Health

Answer: 3
Rationale: The primary legal responsibility of the nurse when child abuse is suspected is to report the case. All 50 states require health care professionals to report all cases of suspected abuse. Although documenting the assessment findings, assisting the family, and referring the family to appropriate resources and support groups is important, the primary legal responsibility is to report the case.

Test-Taking Strategy: Use the process of elimination. In addition to the many implications associated with child abuse, recall that abuse is a crime. Keeping this in mind will direct you to option 3. Review the responsibilities of the nurse when child abuse is suspected if you had difficulty with this question.

Reference
Wong, D., Hockenberry, M., Perry, S., Lowdermilk, D., & Wilson, D. (2006). *Maternal-child nursing care* (3rd ed., pp. 1144-1145). St. Louis: Mosby.

1455. A nurse is planning care for an infant with a diagnosis of encephalocele located in the occipital area. Which item would the nurse use to assist with positioning the child to avoid pressure on the encephalocele?

1 Sandbags
2 Sheepskin
3 Feather pillows
4 Foam half donut

Level of Cognitive Ability: Application
Client Needs: Physiological Integrity
Integrated Process: Nursing Process/
Implementation
Content Area: Child Health

Answer: 4
Rationale: The infant is positioned to avoid pressure on the lesion. If the encephalocele is in the occipital area, a foam half donut may be useful for positioning to prevent this pressure. A sheepskin, a feather pillow, or a sandbag will not protect the encephalocele from pressure.

Test-Taking Strategy: Note the strategic word "occipital," and use the process of elimination. Note that options 1, 2, and 3 are comparable or alike in that they would require the head to remain flat and therefore would not protect the lesion. Review the nursing care associated with a child with an encephalocele if you had difficulty with this question.

References
Hockenberry, M., Wilson, D., & Winkelstein, M. (2005). *Wong's essentials of pediatric nursing* (7th ed., p. 1200). St. Louis: Mosby.
Wong, D., Hockenberry, M., Perry, S., Lowdermilk, D., & Wilson, D. (2006). *Maternal-child nursing care* (3rd ed., p. 1853). St. Louis: Mosby.

1456. A nurse is caring for a child with a head injury. During the review of the record, the nurse notes that the physician has documented decorticate posturing. During the assessment of the child, the nurse notes the extension of the upper extremities and the internal rotation of the upper arms and wrists. The nurse also notes that the lower extremities are extended, with some internal rotation noted at the knees and feet. On the basis of these findings, which of the following is the appropriate nursing action?

1 Notify the physician.
2 Document the findings.
3 Attempt to flex the child's lower extremities.
4 Continue to monitor the child for any posturing.

Level of Cognitive Ability: Application
Client Needs: Physiological Integrity
Integrated Process: Nursing Process/ Implementation
Content Area: Child Health

Answer: 1
Rationale: Decorticate posturing refers to the flexion of the upper extremities and the extension of the lower extremities. Plantar flexion of the feet may also be observed. Decerebrate posturing involves the extension of the upper extremities with the internal rotation of the upper arms and wrists. The lower extremities will extend with some internal rotation noted at the knees and feet. The progression from decorticate to decerebrate posturing usually indicates deteriorating neurological function and warrants physician notification.

Test-Taking Strategy: Focus on the data in the question, and use your knowledge regarding the assessment findings associated with decerebrate and decorticate positioning. Recalling that progression from decorticate to decerebrate posturing usually indicates deteriorating neurological function will direct you to option 1. Review posturing if you had difficulty with this question.

Reference
Hockenberry, M., Wilson, D., & Winkelstein, M. (2005). *Wong's essentials of pediatric nursing* (7th ed., pp. 1015-1016). St. Louis: Mosby.

1457. A child with a diagnosis of hepatitis B is being cared for at home. The mother of the child calls the health care clinic and tells the nurse that the jaundice seems to be worsening. The nurse makes which response to the mother?

1 "The hepatitis may be spreading."
2 "It is necessary to isolate the child from the others."
3 "The jaundice may appear to get worse before it resolves."
4 "You need to bring the child to the health care clinic to see the physician."

Level of Cognitive Ability: Application
Client Needs: Physiological Integrity
Integrated Process: Nursing Process/ Implementation
Content Area: Child Health

Answer: 3
Rationale: The parents should be instructed that jaundice may appear to get worse before it resolves. The parents of a child with hepatitis should also be taught the danger signs that could indicate a worsening of the child's condition, specifically changes in neurological status, bleeding, and fluid retention. The statements in options 1, 2, and 4 are incorrect.

Test-Taking Strategy: Use your knowledge regarding the physiology associated with hepatitis to answer this question. Remember that jaundice worsens before it resolves. This will direct you to the correct option. Review the instructions for the parents of a child with hepatitis if you had difficulty with this question.

References
McKinney, E., James, S., Murray, S., & Ashwill, J. (2005). *Maternal-child nursing* (2nd ed., p. 1149). St. Louis: Saunders.
Wong, D., Hockenberry, M., Perry, S., Lowdermilk, D., & Wilson, D. (2006). *Maternal-child nursing care* (3rd ed., p. 1522). St. Louis: Mosby.

1458. A nurse is preparing to suction a tracheotomy on an infant. The nurse prepares the equipment for the procedure and turns the suction to which setting?
1 60 mm Hg
2 90 mm Hg
3 110 mm Hg
4 120 mm Hg

Level of Cognitive Ability: Application
Client Needs: Physiological Integrity
Integrated Process: Nursing Process/
   Implementation
Content Area: Child Health

Answer: 2
Rationale: The suctioning procedure for pediatric clients varies from that used for adults. Suctioning in infants and children requires the use of a smaller suction catheter and lower suction settings as compared with those used for adults. Suction settings for a neonate are 60 to 80 mm Hg; for an infant, they are 80 to 100 mm Hg; and, for larger children, they are 100 to 120 mm Hg.

Test-Taking Strategy: Use the process of elimination, and note the strategic word "infant." Recalling the procedure that is used for an adult will assist with directing you to option 2. Review the suctioning procedure of a tracheotomy on an infant if you had difficulty with this question.

References
Hockenberry, M., Wilson, D., & Winkelstein, M. (2005). *Wong's essentials of pediatric nursing* (7th ed., p. 774). St. Louis: Mosby.
McKinney, E., James, S., Murray, S., & Ashwill, J. (2005). *Maternal-child nursing* (2nd ed., p. 963). St. Louis: Saunders.

1459. The nurse is caring for a client who begins to experience seizure activity while in bed. The nurse implements which action to prevent aspiration?
1 Raises the head of the bed
2 Loosens restrictive clothing
3 Removes the pillow and raises the padded side rails
4 Positions the client on the side if possible, with the head flexed forward

Level of Cognitive Ability: Application
Client Needs: Physiological Integrity
Integrated Process: Nursing Process/
   Implementation
Content Area: Adult Health/Neurological

Answer: 4
Rationale: Positioning the client on one side with the head flexed forward allows the tongue to fall forward and facilitates the drainage of secretions, which could help prevent aspiration. The nurse would also remove restrictive clothing and the pillow and raise the padded side rails, if present, but these actions would not decrease the risk of aspiration. Rather, they are general safety measures to use during seizure activity. The nurse would not raise the head of the client's bed.

Test-Taking Strategy: Note the strategic words "prevent aspiration." Eliminate option 3 first, because it is unrelated to the subject of the question. Visualize the effect that each of the remaining options would have on airway and aspiration to direct you to option 4. Review the care of the client with seizures to prevent aspiration if you had difficulty with this question.

References
Black, J., & Hawks, J. (2005). *Medical-surgical nursing: Clinical management for positive outcomes* (7th ed., p. 2077). Philadelphia: Saunders.
Lewis, S., Heitkemper, M., Dirksen, S., O'Brien, P., & Bucher, L. (2007). *Medical-surgical nursing: Assessment and management of clinical problems* (7th ed., p. 1540). St. Louis: Mosby.

1460. A client with a brain attack (stroke) has episodes of coughing while swallowing liquids. The client has developed a temperature of 101°F, an oxygen saturation of 91% (down from 98% previously), slight confusion, and noticeable dyspnea. The nurse would take which appropriate action?

1 Notify the physician.
2 Encourage the client to cough and deep breathe.
3 Administer an acetaminophen (Tylenol) suppository.
4 Administer a bronchodilator ordered on an as-needed basis.

Level of Cognitive Ability: Application
Client Needs: Physiological Integrity
Integrated Process: Nursing Process/ Implementation
Content Area: Adult Health/Neurological

Answer: 1
Rationale: The client is exhibiting clinical signs and symptoms of aspiration, which include fever, dyspnea, decreased arterial oxygen levels, and confusion. Other symptoms that occur with this complication are difficulty with managing saliva or coughing or choking while eating. Because the client has developed a complication that requires medical intervention, the most appropriate action is to contact the physician.

Test-Taking Strategy: Focusing on the data in the question will indicate that aspiration has most likely occurred. Eliminate options 2, 3, and 4, because these actions will not assist with alleviating this life-threatening condition. Review the findings of the client who is aspirating and the appropriate nursing interventions if you had difficulty with this question.

Reference
Black, J., & Hawks, J. (2005). *Medical-surgical nursing: Clinical management for positive outcomes* (7th ed., pp. 2124-2125). Philadelphia: Saunders.

1461. The nurse is providing care to a client after a bone biopsy. Which action should the nurse take as part of aftercare for this procedure?

1 Monitor the vital signs once per day.
2 Keep the area in a dependent position.
3 Administer intramuscular opioid analgesics.
4 Monitor the site for swelling, bleeding, or hematoma formation.

Level of Cognitive Ability: Application
Client Needs: Physiological Integrity
Integrated Process: Nursing Process/ Implementation
Content Area: Adult Health/Musculoskeletal

Answer: 4
Rationale: Nursing care after bone biopsy includes monitoring the site for swelling, bleeding, or hematoma formation. The biopsy site is elevated for 24 hours to reduce edema. The vital signs are monitored every 4 hours for 24 hours. The client usually requires mild analgesics; more severe pain usually indicates that complications are arising.

Test-Taking Strategy: Begin to answer this question by recalling that, after this procedure, the client must have periodic assessments. With this in mind, eliminate option 1, because the time frame is too infrequent. Knowing that the procedure is done under local anesthesia helps you to eliminate option 3 next. From the remaining options, recall the principles related to circulation and positioning to direct you to option 4. Review the care of a client after bone biopsy if you had difficulty with this question.

References
Black, J., & Hawks, J. (2005). *Medical-surgical nursing: Clinical management for positive outcomes* (7th ed., p. 577). Philadelphia: Saunders.
Chernecky, C., & Berger, B. (2008). *Laboratory tests and diagnostic procedures* (5th ed., p. 243). Philadelphia: Saunders.

1462. A nurse is caring for a client who is going to have an arthrogram involving the use of a contrast medium. Which action by the nurse is the highest priority?

1 Determining the presence of client allergies
2 Asking if the client has any last-minute questions
3 Telling the client to try to void before leaving the unit
4 Emphasizing to the client the importance of remaining still during the procedure

Level of Cognitive Ability: Application
Client Needs: Physiological Integrity
Integrated Process: Nursing Process/
    Implementation
Content Area: Delegating/Prioritizing

Answer: 1
Rationale: Because of the risk of allergy to contrast medium, the nurse places the highest priority on assessing whether the client has an allergy to iodine or shellfish. The nurse also reinforces information about the test and reminds the client about the need to remain still during the procedure. It is helpful to have the client void before the procedure for comfort.

Test-Taking Strategy: Use the process of elimination, and note the strategic words "contrast medium" and "highest priority." Recalling the risk associated with the administration of contrast medium will direct you to option 1. Review the preprocedure care for an arthrogram if you had difficulty with this question.

Reference
Pagana, K., & Pagana, T. (2005). *Mosby's diagnostic and laboratory test reference* (7th ed., p. 137). St. Louis: Mosby.

1463. The nurse responds to a call bell and finds a client lying on the floor after a fall. The nurse suspects that the client's arm may be broken. The nurse takes which immediate action?

1 Immobilizes the arm
2 Takes a set of vital signs
3 Calls the radiology department
4 Tells the client that there is no permanent damage

Level of Cognitive Ability: Application
Client Needs: Physiological Integrity
Integrated Process: Nursing Process/
    Implementation
Content Area: Adult Health/Musculoskeletal

Answer: 1
Rationale: When a fracture is suspected, it is imperative that the area be splinted before the client is moved. Emergency help should be called for if the client is external to a hospital, and a physician is called if the client is hospitalized. The nurse should remain with the client and provide realistic reassurance. The client would not be told that there is no permanent damage. Vital signs would be taken, but this is not the immediate action. The physician rather than the nurse prescribes an x-ray examination.

Test-Taking Strategy: Use the process of elimination, and note the strategic word "immediate." Eliminate option 3, because the physician will order radiology films. Option 4 is eliminated next, because the nurse does not make statements to the client that could provide false reassurance. From the remaining options, noting that a fracture is suspected will direct you to option 1. Review the care of the client with a suspected extremity fracture if you had difficulty with this question.

Reference
Black, J., & Hawks, J. (2005). *Medical-surgical nursing: Clinical management for positive outcomes* (7th ed., p. 2501). Philadelphia: Saunders.

1464. A nurse is caring for a 14-year-old child who is hospitalized and placed in Crutchfield traction. The child is having difficulty adjusting to the length of the hospital confinement. Which nursing action would be appropriate to meet the child's needs?
  1 Allow the child to play loud music in the hospital room.
  2 Allow the child to have his or her hair dyed if the parent agrees.
  3 Let the child wear his or her own clothing when friends visit.
  4 Allow the child to keep the shades closed and the room darkened at all times.

Level of Cognitive Ability: Application
Client Needs: Psychosocial Integrity
Integrated Process: Nursing Process/ Implementation
Content Area: Child Health

Answer: 3
Rationale: An adolescent needs to identify with peers and has a strong need to belong to a group. The child should be allowed to wear his or her own clothes to feel a sense of belonging to the group. The adolescent likes to dress like the group and to wear similar hairstyles. Loud music may disturb others in the hospital. Because Crutchfield traction involves the use of skeletal pins, hair dye is not appropriate. The child's request for a darkened room is indicative of a possible problem with depression that may require further evaluation and intervention.

Test-Taking Strategy: Use the process of elimination, and focus on the subjects of Crutchfield traction and a 14-year-old child. Knowledge of Crutchfield traction and its limitations as well as of growth and development concepts will direct you to option 3. Review growth and development and the care of the child in traction if you had difficulty with this question.

References
Hockenberry, M., & Wilson, D. (2007). *Nursing care of infants and children* (8th ed., pp. 826, 1074). St. Louis: Mosby.
Potter, P., & Perry, A. (2005). *Fundamentals of nursing* (6th ed., pp. 208-209). St. Louis: Mosby.

1465. A nurse receives a telephone call from the emergency department and is told that a client in leg traction will be admitted to the nursing unit. The nurse prepares for the arrival of the client and asks the nursing assistant to obtain which item that will be essential for helping the client move in bed while in leg traction?
  1 A foot board
  2 Extra pillows
  3 A bed trapeze
  4 An electric bed

Level of Cognitive Ability: Application
Client Needs: Physiological Integrity
Integrated Process: Nursing Process/ Implementation
Content Area: Leadership/Management

Answer: 3
Rationale: A trapeze is essential to allow the client to lift straight up while being moved so that the amount of pull exerted on the limb in traction is not altered. A foot board and extra pillows do not facilitate moving. Either an electric bed or a manual bed can be used for traction, but this does not specifically assist the client with moving in bed.

Test-Taking Strategy: Note the strategic words "essential" and "move in bed." Attempt to visualize the items identified in the options, and focus on the subject of helping the client to move in bed. Using the process of elimination will direct you to option 3. Review the care of the client in traction if you had difficulty with this question.

References
Monahan, F., Sands, J., Marek, J., Neighbors, M., & Green, C. (2007). *Phipps' medical-surgical nursing: Health and illness perspectives* (8th ed., p. 1535). St. Louis: Mosby.
Potter, P., & Perry, A. (2005). *Fundamentals of nursing* (6th ed., pp. 1455-1456). St. Louis: Mosby.

1466. A pregnant client is receiving rehabilitative services for alcohol abuse. The nurse would provide supportive care by:

1 Minimizing communication with supportive family members
2 Encouraging the client to stop counseling after the infant is born
3 Avoiding the discussion of the alcohol problem and recovery with the client
4 Encouraging the client to participate in care and identifying supportive strategies that are helpful

Level of Cognitive Ability: Application
Client Needs: Health Promotion and Maintenance
Integrated Process: Nursing Process/ Implementation
Content Area: Maternity/Antepartum

Answer: 4
Rationale: The nurse provides supportive care by encouraging the client to participate in care. The nurse should not avoid discussing the client's problem with the client, and communication with family members is important. Counseling needs to continue after the infant is born.

Test-Taking Strategy: Use the process of elimination, and note the strategic words "supportive care." Option 4 provides the client with an active role in care. Options 1, 2, and 3 create barriers for long-term success in dealing with the problem. Review the measures that provide supportive nursing care for the pregnant client who abuses alcohol if you had difficulty with this question.

References
Murray, S., & McKinney, E. (2006). *Foundations of maternal-newborn nursing* (4th ed., p. 147). Philadelphia: Saunders.
Wong, D., Hockenberry, M., Perry, S., Lowdermilk, D., & Wilson, D. (2006). *Maternal-child nursing care* (3rd ed., p. 367). St. Louis: Mosby.

1467. A client in the second trimester of pregnancy is being assessed at the health care clinic. The nurse performing the assessment notes that the fetal heart rate is 100 beats/min. Which nursing action would be appropriate?

1 Notify the physician.
2 Document the findings.
3 Inform the mother that the assessment is normal and that everything is fine.
4 Instruct the mother to return to the clinic in 1 week for the reevaluation of the fetal heart rate.

Level of Cognitive Ability: Application
Client Needs: Physiological Integrity
Integrated Process: Nursing Process/ Implementation
Content Area: Maternity/Antepartum

Answer: 1
Rationale: The fetal heart rate should be between 110 and 160 beats/ min during pregnancy. A fetal heart rate of 100 beats/min would require that the physician be notified and that the client be further evaluated. Although the nurse would document the findings, the most appropriate nursing action is to notify the physician. Options 3 and 4 are inaccurate nursing actions.

Test-Taking Strategy: Use the process of elimination. Options 3 and 4 are comparable or alike as well as inaccurate, and they can be eliminated first. From the remaining options, recalling that the range for the fetal heart rate is between 110 and 160 beats/ min will direct you to option 1. Review the normal findings of the pregnant client if you had difficulty with this question.

References
Murray, S., & McKinney, E. (2006). *Foundations of maternal-newborn nursing* (4th ed., p. 317). Philadelphia: Saunders.
Wong, D., Hockenberry, M., Perry, S., Lowdermilk, D., & Wilson, D. (2006). *Maternal-child nursing care* (3rd ed., p. 471). St. Louis: Mosby.

1468. A client is admitted to the hospital with a diagnosis of a leaking cerebral aneurysm and is scheduled for surgery. The nurse implements which of the following during the preoperative period?

1 Places the client on strict bedrest
2 Allows the client to ambulate to the bathroom
3 Obtains a bedside commode for the client's use
4 Encourages the client to be up at least twice per day

Answer: 1
Rationale: The client is placed on aneurysm precautions, and the client's activity is kept to a minimum to prevent Valsalva's maneuver. Clients often hold their breath and strain while pulling up to get out of bed. This exertion may cause a rise in blood pressure, which increases bleeding. Clients who have bleeding aneurysms in any vessel will have activity curtailed. Therefore, options 2, 3, and 4 are incorrect actions.

Level of Cognitive Ability: Application
Client Needs: Physiological Integrity
Integrated Process: Nursing Process/
   Implementation
Content Area: Adult Health/Neurological

Test-Taking Strategy: Use the process of elimination, and focus on the client's diagnosis and the strategic words "preoperative period." Eliminate options 2, 3, and 4, because they are comparable or alike in that they all involve out-of-bed activity. Review aneurysm precautions if you had difficulty with this question.

Reference
Ignatavicius, D., & Workman, M. (2006). *Medical-surgical nursing: Critical thinking for collaborative care* (5th ed., pp. 1058, 1060, 1064). Philadelphia: Saunders.

1469. A provider calls the nurse to obtain the daily laboratory results of a client who is receiving parenteral nutrition. Which is the most important laboratory result for the nurse to present to the provider?
   1 White blood cell count
   2 Serum electrolyte levels
   3 Arterial blood gas levels
   4 Hemoglobin and hematocrit levels

Level of Cognitive Ability: Analysis
Client Needs: Physiological Integrity
Integrated Process: Nursing Process/
   Implementation
Content Area: Fundamental Skills

Answer: 2
Rationale: Parenteral nutrition solutions contain amino acids and dextrose in solution with electrolytes, trace elements, and other agents added. The provider uses the electrolyte values (including sodium, potassium, chloride) and the glucose level to determine the effectiveness of the solution, to make changes to the solution as necessary, and to decrease the client's risk of a fluid and electrolyte imbalance. It is important to monitor the serum glucose, because parenteral nutrition is usually composed of 10% or more dextrose in water. Options 1, 3, and 4 can be suitable tests for a client who is receiving parenteral nutrition, but these results cover a narrower range of information than serum electrolytes.

Test-Taking Strategy: Note the strategic words "most important," and use the process of elimination to choose the laboratory test that provides better information than the other options. Eliminate options 1, 3, and 4 first, because the results of these tests provide less information than serum electrolytes. Review the composition of parenteral nutrition if you had difficulty with this question.

References
Black, J., & Hawks, J. (2005). *Medical-surgical nursing: Clinical management for positive outcomes* (7th ed., p. 706). Philadelphia: Saunders.
Lewis, S., Heitkemper, M., Dirksen, S., O'Brien, P., & Bucher, L. (2007). *Medical-surgical nursing: Assessment and management of clinical problems* (7th ed., p. 965). St. Louis: Mosby.

Evaluation

1470. The nurse is evaluating the effects of care for the client with nephrotic syndrome. The nurse determines that the client showed the least amount of improvement if which of the following information was obtained serially over 2 days of care?
   1 Serum albumin 1.9 g/dL, up to 2.0 g/dL
   2 Initial weight 208 pounds, down to 203 pounds
   3 Blood pressure 160/90 mm Hg, down to 130/78 mm Hg
   4 Daily intake and output record of 2100 mL intake and 1900 mL output and 2000 mL intake and 2900 mL output

Answer: 1
Rationale: The goal of therapy in nephrotic syndrome is to heal the leaking glomerular membrane. This would then control edema by stopping the loss of protein in the urine. Fluid balance and albumin levels are monitored to determine the effectiveness of therapy. Option 2 represents a loss of fluid that slightly exceeds 2 L and that represents a significant improvement. Option 3 shows improvement, because both systolic and diastolic blood pressures are lower. Option 4 represents a total fluid loss of 700 mL over the 2 days, which is also helpful. The least amount of improvement is in the serum albumin level, because the normal albumin level is 3.5 to 5.0 g/dL.

Level of Cognitive Ability: Analysis
Client Needs: Physiological Integrity
Integrated Process: Nursing Process/Evaluation
Content Area: Adult Health/Renal

Test-Taking Strategy: Use the process of elimination, and note the strategic words "least amount of improvement." Option 2 illustrates the greatest improvement and is eliminated first. Option 4 is also a significant improvement and is eliminated next. From the remaining options, noting that the blood pressure has decreased significantly will direct you to option 1. Review the care of the client with nephrotic syndrome if you had difficulty with this question.

Reference
Ignatavicius, D., & Workman, M. (2006). *Medical-surgical nursing: Critical thinking for collaborative care* (5th ed., p. 1719). Philadelphia: Saunders.

1471. A client is being discharged to home after the application of a plaster leg cast. The nurse determines that the client understands the proper care of the cast if the client states the need to:
1 Avoid getting the cast wet.
2 Use the fingertips to lift and move the leg.
3 Cover the casted leg with warm blankets.
4 Use a padded coat hanger end to scratch under the cast.

Level of Cognitive Ability: Analysis
Client Needs: Physiological Integrity
Integrated Process: Nursing Process/Evaluation
Content Area: Adult Health/Musculoskeletal

Answer: 1
Rationale: A plaster cast must remain dry to keep its strength. The cast should be handled using the palms of the hands rather than the fingertips until it is fully dry. Air should circulate freely around the cast to help it dry. Additionally, the cast also gives off heat as it dries. The client should never scratch under the cast. A cool hair dryer may be used to relieve an itch.

Test-Taking Strategy: Use the process of elimination, and note the strategic word "plaster." Option 4 is dangerous to skin integrity and is eliminated first. Knowing that a wet cast can be dented with the fingertips causing pressure underneath helps you to eliminate option 2. Recalling that the cast needs to dry eliminates option 3. Remember that plaster casts, when they have dried after application, should not become wet. Review the home-care instructions for a client with a plaster cast if you had difficulty with this question.

References
Black, J., & Hawks, J. (2005). *Medical-surgical nursing: Clinical management for positive outcomes* (7th ed., p. 631). Philadelphia: Saunders.
Ignatavicius, D., & Workman, M. (2006). *Medical-surgical nursing: Critical thinking for collaborative care* (5th ed., p. 1198). Philadelphia: Saunders.

1472. A client is being discharged to home while recovering from acute renal failure (ARF). The client indicates an understanding of the therapeutic dietary regimen if the client states the need to eat foods that are lower in:
1 Fats
2 Vitamins
3 Potassium
4 Carbohydrates

Answer: 3
Rationale: Most of the excretion of potassium and the control of potassium balance are normal functions of the kidneys. In the client with renal failure, potassium intake must be restricted as much as possible (30 to 50 mEq/day). The primary mechanism of potassium removal during ARF is dialysis. Options 1, 2, and 4 are not normally restricted in the client with ARF unless a secondary health problem warrants the need to do so.

Test-Taking Strategy: Noting the diagnosis of the client will assist you with answering this question. Recalling that potassium balance and excretion are controlled by the kidney will direct you to option 3. Review the therapeutic diet for the client with ARF if you had difficulty with this question.

Level of Cognitive Ability: Analysis
Client Needs: Physiological Integrity
Integrated Process: Nursing Process/Evaluation
Content Area: Adult Health/Renal

Reference
Black, J., & Hawks, J. (2005). *Medical-surgical nursing: Clinical management for positive outcomes* (7th ed., p. 946). Philadelphia: Saunders.

1473. The nurse teaches the client with a history of anxiety and command hallucinations to harm the self or others appropriate management techniques. The nurse determines that the client understands these techniques when the client says:
1 "I can go to group and talk about my feelings."
2 "I can call my counselor so that I can talk about my feelings and not hurt anyone."
3 "If I get enough sleep and eat well, I won't be as likely to get anxious and hear things."
4 "If I always take my prescribed medication as I'm supposed too, I won't be as anxious."

Level of Cognitive Ability: Analysis
Client Needs: Psychosocial Integrity
Integrated Process: Nursing Process/Evaluation
Content Area: Mental Health

Answer: 2
Rationale: There may be an increased risk for impulsive or aggressive behavior if a client is receiving command hallucinations to harm the self or others. The client should be asked if he or she has intentions to hurt himself or herself or others. Talking about auditory hallucinations can interfere with the subvocal muscular activity that is associated with a hallucination. Options 1, 3, and 4 are general interventions, but they are not specific to anxiety and hallucinations.

Test-Taking Strategy: Use the process of elimination, and focus on the subject of anxiety and hallucinations. Options 1, 3, and 4 are all interventions that a client can do to aid wellness. Option 2 is specific to the subject and indicates self-responsible commitment and control over the client's own behavior. Review the interventions for anxiety and hallucinations if you had difficulty with this question.

Reference
Varcarolis, E., Carson, V., & Shoemaker, N. (2006). *Foundations of psychiatric mental health nursing* (5th ed., pp. 217, 403). Philadelphia: Saunders.

1474. A perinatal client has been instructed about the prevention of genital tract infections. Which statement by the client indicates an understanding of these preventive measures?
1 "I can douche anytime I want."
2 "I can wear my tight-fitting jeans."
3 "I should avoid the use of condoms."
4 "I should wear underwear with a cotton panel liner."

Level of Cognitive Ability: Comprehension
Client Needs: Health Promotion and Maintenance
Integrated Process: Nursing Process/Evaluation
Content Area: Maternity/Antepartum

Answer: 4
Rationale: Condoms should be used to minimize the spread of genital tract infections. Wearing tight clothes irritates the genital area and does not allow for air circulation. Douching is to be avoided. Wearing items with a cotton panel liner allows for air movement in and around the genital area.

Test-Taking Strategy: Use the process of elimination, and note the strategic words "indicates an understanding." Options 1, 2, and 3 are all incorrect statements regarding client self-care. Review the prevention measures associated with genital tract infections if you had difficulty with this question.

Reference
Murray, S., & McKinney, E. (2006). *Foundations of maternal-newborn nursing* (4th ed., p. 914). Philadelphia: Saunders.

1475. A nurse has given a client information about the use of sublingual nitroglycerin tablets. The client has an order for as-needed use if chest pain occurs. The nurse determines that the client understands how to self-administer the medication if the client stated the need to:

1 Keep the nitroglycerin in a shirt pocket close to the body.

2 Avoid using the medication until chest pain actually begins and intensifies.

3 Take acetylsalicylic acid (aspirin) to treat a headache that occurs with the early use of nitroglycerin.

4 Discard unused nitroglycerin tablets 3 to 6 months after the bottle is opened, and obtain a new prescription.

Level of Cognitive Ability: Analysis
Client Needs: Physiological Integrity
Integrated Process: Nursing Process/Evaluation
Content Area: Pharmacology

Answer: 4

Rationale: Nitroglycerin may be self-administered sublingually 5 to 10 minutes before an activity that triggers chest pain. Tablets should be discarded 3 to 6 months after opening the bottle (per expiration date), and a new bottle of pills should be obtained from the pharmacy. Nitroglycerin is unstable and is affected by heat and cold, so it should not be kept close to the body (warmth) in a shirt pocket; rather, it should be kept in a jacket pocket or a purse. Headache often occurs with early use and diminishes in time. Acetaminophen (Tylenol) may be used to treat headache.

Test-Taking Strategy: Use the process of elimination, and note the strategic words "understands how to self-administer the medication." Recalling that nitroglycerin loses its potency in 3 to 6 months will direct you to option 4. Review the client teaching points related to nitroglycerin if you had difficulty with this question.

References

Ignatavicius, D., & Workman, M. (2006). *Medical-surgical nursing: Critical thinking for collaborative care* (5th ed., p. 848). Philadelphia: Saunders.
Lewis, S., Heitkemper, M., Dirksen, S., O'Brien, P., & Bucher, L. (2007). *Medical-surgical nursing: Assessment and management of clinical problems* (7th ed., p. 798). St. Louis: Mosby.

1476. A client has had a laryngectomy for throat cancer and has started oral intake. The nurse determines that the client has tolerated the first stage of dietary advancement if the client takes which of the following types of diet without aspirating or choking?

1 Bland

2 Full liquids

3 Clear liquids

4 Semisolid foods

Level of Cognitive Ability: Analysis
Client Needs: Physiological Integrity
Integrated Process: Nursing Process/Evaluation
Content Area: Adult Health/Oncology

Answer: 4

Rationale: Oral intake after laryngectomy is started with semisolid foods. When the client can manage this type of food, liquids may be introduced. Thin liquids are not given until the risk of aspiration is negligible. A bland diet is not appropriate. The client may not be able to tolerate the texture of some of the solid foods that would be included in a bland diet.

Test-Taking Strategy: Use the process of elimination. Eliminate options 2 and 3 first, and recall that a client with swallowing difficulty will not be able to manage liquids. From the remaining options, recall that a bland diet provides no control over the consistency or texture of the food. Review the dietary measures for a client after laryngectomy if you had difficulty with this question.

References

Black, J., & Hawks, J. (2005). *Medical-surgical nursing: Clinical management for positive outcomes* (7th ed., p. 1791). Philadelphia: Saunders.
Ignatavicius, D., & Workman, M. (2006). *Medical-surgical nursing: Critical thinking for collaborative care* (5th ed., pp. 576-580). Philadelphia: Saunders.

1477. An older male client who is a victim of elder abuse and his family have been attending counseling sessions for the past month. Which statement, if made by the abusive family member, would indicate that he or she has learned more positive coping skills?

1 "I will be more careful to make sure that my father's needs are 100% met."
2 "I am so sorry and embarrassed that the abusive event occurred. It won't happen again."
3 "I feel better equipped to care for my father now that I know where to turn if I need assistance."
4 "Now that my father is going to move into my home with me, I will have to stop drinking alcohol."

Level of Cognitive Ability: Analysis
Client Needs: Psychosocial Integrity
Integrated Process: Nursing Process/Evaluation
Content Area: Mental Health

Answer: 3
Rationale: Elder abuse is sometimes caused by family members who are being expected to care for their aging parents. This care can cause the family to become overextended, frustrated, or financially depleted. Knowing where to turn in the community for assistance with caring for an aging family member can bring much-needed relief. Using these alternatives is a positive coping skill for many families. Options 1, 2, and 4 are statements of good faith or promises, which may or may not be kept in the future.

Test-Taking Strategy: Focus on the subject of positive coping skills, and use the process of elimination. Option 3 is the only option that identifies a means of coping with the issues and that outlines a definitive plan for how to handle the pressure associated with the father's care. Review the concepts related to elder abuse if you had difficulty with this question.

Reference
Varcarolis, E., Carson, V., & Shoemaker, N. (2006). *Foundations of psychiatric mental health nursing* (5th ed., pp. 521-523). Philadelphia: Saunders.

1478. A nurse is caring for a term infant who is 24 hours old who had a confirmed episode of hypoglycemia when 1 hour old. Which observation by the nurse would indicate the need for further evaluation?

1 Weight loss of 4 ounces and dry, peeling skin
2 Blood glucose level of 40 mg/dL before the last feeding
3 Breast-feeding for 20 minutes or more, with strong sucking
4 High-pitched cry, drinking 10 to 15 mL of formula per feeding

Level of Cognitive Ability: Analysis
Client Needs: Physiological Integrity
Integrated Process: Nursing Process/Evaluation
Content Area: Maternity/Postpartum

Answer: 4
Rationale: At 24 hours old, a term infant should be able to consume at least 1 ounce of formula per feeding. A high-pitched cry is indicative of neurological involvement. Blood glucose levels are acceptable at 40 mg/dL during the first few days of life. Weight loss over the first few days of life and dry, peeling skin are normal findings for term infants. Breast-feeding for 20 minutes with a strong suck is an excellent finding. Hypoglycemia causes central nervous system symptoms (high-pitched cry), and it is also exhibited by a lack of strength for eating enough for growth.

Test-Taking Strategy: Use the process of elimination, and note the strategic words "need for further evaluation." Eliminate options 1, 2, and 3, because these are normal findings. The words "high-pitched cry" should direct you to option 4. Review normal newborn findings and the indications of hypoglycemia if you had difficulty with this question.

Reference
Wong, D., Hockenberry, M., Perry, S., Lowdermilk, D., & Wilson, D. (2006). *Maternal-child nursing care* (3rd ed., p. 740). St. Louis: Mosby.

1479. A home-care nurse visits a child with a diagnosis of celiac disease. Which finding best indicates that a gluten-free diet is being maintained and has been effective?
  1 The child is free of diarrhea.
  2 The child is free of bloody stools.
  3 The child tolerates dietary wheat and rye.
  4 A balanced fluid and electrolyte status is noted on the laboratory results.

Level of Cognitive Ability: Analysis
Client Needs: Physiological Integrity
Integrated Process: Nursing Process/Evaluation
Content Area: Child Health

Answer: 1
Rationale: Watery diarrhea is a frequent clinical manifestation of celiac disease. The absence of diarrhea indicates effective treatment. Bloody stools are not associated with this disease. The grains of wheat and rye contain gluten and are not allowed. A balance of fluids and electrolytes does not necessarily demonstrate the improved status of celiac disease.

Test-Taking Strategy: Focus on the subject: a lack of signs and symptoms related to celiac disease. Recalling that watery diarrhea is a manifestation of celiac disease will direct you to option 1. Review the manifestations of celiac disease if you had difficulty with this question.

References
Hockenberry, M., Wilson, D., & Winkelstein, M. (2005). *Wong's essentials of pediatric nursing* (7th ed., p. 886). St. Louis: Mosby.
McKinney, E., James, S., Murray, S., & Ashwill, J. (2005). *Maternal-child nursing* (2nd ed., p. 1147). St. Louis: Saunders.

1480. A nurse is assisting with caring for a woman in labor who is receiving oxytocin (Pitocin) by intravenous infusion. The nurse monitors the client, knowing that which of the following indicates an adequate contraction pattern?
  1 One contraction per minute, with resultant cervical dilation
  2 Four contractions every 5 minutes, with resultant cervical dilation
  3 One contraction every 10 minutes, without resultant cervical dilation
  4 Three to five contractions in a 10-minute period, with resultant cervical dilation

Level of Cognitive Ability: Analysis
Client Needs: Physiological Integrity
Integrated Process: Nursing Process/Evaluation
Content Area: Maternity/Intrapartum

Answer: 4
Rationale: The preferred oxytocin dosage is the minimal amount necessary to maintain an adequate contraction pattern characterized by three to five contractions in a 10-minute period, with resultant cervical dilation. If contractions are more frequent than every 2 minutes, contraction quality may be decreased.

Test-Taking Strategy: Use the process of elimination. Focusing on the subject of an adequate contraction pattern will assist you with eliminating option 3. Eliminate options 1 and 2 next, because they are comparable or alike. Review the expected effects of oxytocin if you had difficulty with this question.

References
Gahart, B., & Nazareno, A. (2006). *2006 intravenous medications* (22nd ed., pp. 925-926). St. Louis: Mosby.
Wong, D., Hockenberry, M., Perry, S., Lowdermilk, D., & Wilson, D. (2006). *Maternal-child nursing care* (3rd ed., p. 568). St. Louis: Mosby.

1481. A home-care nurse is assigned to visit a preschooler who has a diagnosis of scarlet fever and is on bedrest. What data obtained by the nurse would indicate that the child is coping with the illness and bedrest?
  1 The child insists that his mother stay in the room.
  2 The child is coloring and drawing pictures in a notebook.
  3 The mother keeps providing new activities for the child to do.
  4 The child sucks his thumb whenever he does not get what he asked for.

Answer: 2
Rationale: According to Jean Piaget, for the preschooler, play is the best way for children to understand and adjust to life's experiences. They are able to use pencils and crayons, and they can draw stick figures and other rudimentary things. A child with scarlet fever needs quiet play, and drawing will provide that. Options 1, 3, and 4 do not address positive coping mechanisms.

Level of Cognitive Ability: Analysis
Client Needs: Health Promotion and
    Maintenance
Integrated Process: Nursing Process/Evaluation
Content Area: Child Health

Test-Taking Strategy: Think about the developmental level of a preschooler. Note the subject: an analysis of data by the nurse to determine if the child is coping with the disease and bedrest. Option 2 is a positive coping mechanism for preschoolers. Options 1, 3, and 4 do not address positive coping mechanisms. Review the expected developmental level of a preschooler and the effects of bedrest on a child if you had difficulty with this question.

Reference
Hockenberry, M., Wilson, D., & Winkelstein, M. (2005). *Wong's essentials of pediatric nursing* (7th ed., pp. 88-89, 444-445). St. Louis: Mosby.

1482. A client has just taken a dose of trimetho-benzamide (Tigan). The nurse determines that the medication has been effective if the client states relief of:
  1 Heartburn
  2 Constipation
  3 Abdominal pain
  4 Nausea and vomiting

Level of Cognitive Ability: Analysis
Client Needs: Physiological Integrity
Integrated Process: Nursing Process/Evaluation
Content Area: Pharmacology

Answer: 4
Rationale: Trimethobenzamide (Tigan) is an antiemetic agent that is used for the treatment of nausea and vomiting. The medication is not used to treat heartburn, constipation, or abdominal pain.

Test-Taking Strategy: Use the process of elimination. Recalling that trimethobenzamide is an antiemetic will direct you to option 4. Review the action of trimethobenzamide if you had difficulty with this question.

Reference
Skidmore-Roth, L. (2008). *Mosby's nursing drug reference* (21st ed., p. 1034). St. Louis: Mosby.

1483. A nurse is providing instructions to the mother of a child with a diagnosis of strabismus of the left eye, and the nurse reviews the procedure for patching the child. The nurse determines that the mother understands the procedure if the mother makes which statement?
  1 "I will place the patch on both eyes."
  2 "I will place the patch on the left eye."
  3 "I will place the patch on the right eye."
  4 "I will alternate the patch from the right eye to the left eye every hour."

Level of Cognitive Ability: Analysis
Client Needs: Physiological Integrity
Integrated Process: Nursing Process/Evaluation
Content Area: Child Health

Answer: 3
Rationale: Patching may be used for the treatment of strabismus to strengthen the weak eye. With this treatment, the good eye is patched; this encourages the child to use the weaker eye. The treatment is most successful when it is performed during the preschool years. The schedule for patching is individualized and prescribed by the ophthalmologist.

Test-Taking Strategy: Use the process of elimination. Remembering that this condition involves a lazy eye will direct you to the correct option. It makes sense to patch the unaffected eye to strengthen the muscles in the affected eye. Review the procedure for patching if you had difficulty with this question.

References
Hockenberry, M., Wilson, D., & Winkelstein, M. (2005). *Wong's essentials of pediatric nursing* (7th ed., p. 611). St. Louis: Mosby.
McKinney, E., James, S., Murray, S., & Ashwill, J. (2005). *Maternal-child nursing* (2nd ed., pp. 1585-1586). St. Louis: Saunders.

1484. A nurse is assessing a client with gestational hypertension who was admitted to the hospital 48 hours ago. Which of the following data obtained would indicate that the condition has not yet resolved?
1 Urinary output is increased
2 Presence of trace urinary protein
3 Client complaints of blurred vision
4 Blood pressure reading at prenatal baseline

Level of Cognitive Ability: Analysis
Client Needs: Physiological Integrity
Integrated Process: Nursing Process/Evaluation
Content Area: Maternity/Antepartum

Answer: 3
Rationale: Client complaints of headache or blurred vision indicate a worsening of the condition and warrant immediate further evaluation. Options 1, 2, and 4 are all signs that the gestational hypertension is being resolved.

Test-Taking Strategy: Note the strategic words "has not yet resolved." These words indicate a negative event query and ask you to select the option that identifies a symptom of gestational hypertension. Options 1 and 4 can be eliminated first, because they are normal findings. From the remaining options, note that option 2 contains the word "trace" and is the most normal finding of these two options. Review the clinical manifestations associated with gestational hypertension if you had difficulty with this question.

References
McKinney, E., James, S., Murray, S., & Ashwill, J. (2005). *Maternal-child nursing* (2nd ed., p. 632). St. Louis: Saunders
Wong, D., Hockenberry, M., Perry, S., Lowdermilk, D., & Wilson, D. (2006). *Maternal-child nursing care* (3rd ed., p. 376). St. Louis: Mosby.

1485. A client has begun medication therapy with betaxolol (Kerlone). The nurse determines that the client is experiencing the intended effect of therapy if which of the following is noted?
1 Edema present at 3+
2 Weight loss of 5 pounds
3 Pulse rate increased from 58 to 74 beats/minute
4 Blood pressure decreased from 142/94 mm Hg to 128/82 mm Hg

Level of Cognitive Ability: Analysis
Client Needs: Physiological Integrity
Integrated Process: Nursing Process/Evaluation
Content Area: Pharmacology

Answer: 4
Rationale: Betaxolol is a β-adrenergic blocking agent used to lower blood pressure, relieve angina, or eliminate dysrhythmias. Side effects include bradycardia and symptoms of congestive heart failure, such as weight gain and increased edema.

Test-Taking Strategy: Note that the question asks for the "intended effect" of the medication. Remember that β-adrenergic blocking agent medication names end with the suffix *-lol*. Recalling the action of the medication will direct you to option 4. Review the intended effects of betaxolol if you had difficulty with this question.

Reference
Skidmore-Roth, L. (2008). *Mosby's nursing drug reference* (21st ed., p. 1034). St. Louis: Mosby.

1486. A nurse has taught a client who is taking a xanthine bronchodilator about beverages to avoid. The nurse determines that the client understands the information if the client chooses which of the following beverages from the dietary menu?
1 Cola
2 Coffee
3 Chocolate milk
4 Cranberry juice

Answer: 4
Rationale: Cola, coffee, and chocolate contain xanthine and should be avoided by the client who is taking a xanthine bronchodilator. This could lead to an increased incidence of cardiovascular and central nervous system side effects that can occur with the use of these types of bronchodilators.

Test-Taking Strategy: Use the process of elimination. Note that options 1, 2, and 3 are comparable or alike in that they all contain some form of stimulant. Review the dietary measures for the client taking a xanthine bronchodilator if you had difficulty with this question.

Level of Cognitive Ability: Analysis
Client Needs: Physiological Integrity
Integrated Process: Nursing Process/Evaluation
Content Area: Pharmacology

References
Kee, J., Hayes, E., & McCuistion, L. (2006). *Pharmacology: A nursing process approach.* (5th ed., p. 593). Philadelphia: Saunders.
McKenry, L., Tressier, E., & Hogan, M. (2006). *Mosby's pharmacology in nursing* (22nd ed., p. 724). St. Louis: Mosby.

1487. A client is started on tolbutamide (Orinase) once daily. The nurse observes for which of the following intended effect of this medication?

1 Weight loss
2 Resolution of infection
3 Decreased blood glucose
4 Decreased blood pressure

Level of Cognitive Ability: Analysis
Client Needs: Physiological Integrity
Integrated Process: Nursing Process/Evaluation
Content Area: Pharmacology

Answer: 3

Rationale: Tolbutamide is an oral hypoglycemic agent that is taken in the morning. It is not used to decrease blood pressure, enhance weight loss, or treat infection.

Test-Taking Strategy: Note the strategic words "intended effect." Recalling that this medication is an oral hypoglycemic will direct you to option 3. Review the action of tolbutamide if you had difficulty with this question.

References
Kee, J., Hayes, E., & McCuistion, L. (2006). *Pharmacology: A nursing process approach* (5th ed., p. 784). Philadelphia: Saunders.
McKenry, L., Tressier, E., & Hogan, M. (2006). *Mosby's pharmacology in nursing* (22nd ed., pp. 880, 1218). St. Louis: Mosby.

1488. A client who regularly takes nonsteroidal antiinflammatory drugs (NSAIDs) has been taking misoprostol (Cytotec). The nurse would monitor the client to see if the client experienced the relief of which of the following symptoms?

1 Diarrhea
2 Bleeding
3 Infection
4 Epigastric pain

Level of Cognitive Ability: Analysis
Client Needs: Physiological Integrity
Integrated Process: Nursing Process/Evaluation
Content Area: Pharmacology

Answer: 4

Rationale: The client who regularly takes NSAIDs is prone to gastric mucosal injury, which gives the client epigastric pain as a symptom. Misoprostol is administered to prevent this occurrence. Diarrhea can be a side effect of the medication, but it is not an intended effect. Bleeding and infection are unrelated to the question.

Test-Taking Strategy: Note the strategic words "NSAIDs" and "relief." This tells you that the medication is being given to treat or prevent the occurrence of a specific symptom. Recalling that NSAIDs can cause gastric mucosal injury will direct you to option 4. Review the action and indications for the use of misoprostol if you had difficulty with this question.

Reference
McKenry, L., Tressier, E., & Hogan, M. (2006). *Mosby's pharmacology in nursing* (22nd ed., pp. 769-770). St. Louis: Mosby.

1489. A client has received a dose of an as-needed medication called loperamide (Imodium). The nurse evaluates the client after administration to see if the client has relief of:

1 Diarrhea
2 Tarry stools
3 Constipation
4 Abdominal pain

Answer: 1

Rationale: Loperamide is an antidiarrheal agent, and it is commonly administered after loose stools. It is used for the management of acute diarrhea and also for chronic diarrhea, such as with inflammatory bowel disease. It can also be used to reduce the volume of drainage from an ileostomy.

Test-Taking Strategy: Use the process of elimination. Recalling that this medication is an antidiarrheal agent will direct you to option 1. Review the purpose of loperamide if you had difficulty with this question.

Level of Cognitive Ability: Analysis
Client Needs: Physiological Integrity
Integrated Process: Nursing Process/Evaluation
Content Area: Pharmacology

Reference
McKenry, L., Tressier, E., & Hogan, M. (2006). *Mosby's pharmacology in nursing* (22nd ed., p. 223). St. Louis: Mosby.

1490. A nurse has reinforced discharge instructions to the parent of a child who has undergone heart surgery. Which statement by the parent would indicate the need for further instruction?

1 "My child can return to school for full days 2 weeks after discharge."
2 "I should allow my child to play inside but omit outside play at this time."
3 "I should have my child avoid crowds and people for 1 week after discharge."
4 "I should call the physician if my child develops faster or harder breathing than normal."

Level of Cognitive Ability: Analysis
Client Needs: Safe and Effective Care Environment
Integrated Process: Nursing Process/Evaluation
Content Area: Child Health

Answer: 1
Rationale: The child may return to school the third week after hospital discharge, but he or she should go to school for half days for the first week. Outside play should be omitted for several weeks, with inside play allowed as tolerated. The child should avoid crowds of people for 1 week after discharge, including crowds at day care centers and churches. If any difficulty with breathing occurs, the parent should notify the physician.

Test-Taking Strategy: Note the strategic words "indicate the need for further instruction." These words indicate a negative event query and ask you to select an option that is an incorrect statement. Recalling the principles related to the prevention of infection and the complications of surgery will direct you to option 1. Review the home-care instructions for a child after heart surgery if you had difficulty with this question.

Reference
McKinney, E., James, S., Murray, S., & Ashwill, J. (2005). *Maternal-child nursing* (2nd ed., p. 1283). St. Louis: Saunders.

1491. A client has been given a prescription for a course of azithromycin (Zithromax). The nurse determines that the medication is having the intended effect if which of the following is noted?

1 Pain is relieved.
2 Blood pressure is lowered.
3 Joint discomfort is reduced.
4 Signs and symptoms of infection are relieved.

Level of Cognitive Ability: Analysis
Client Needs: Physiological Integrity
Integrated Process: Nursing Process/Evaluation
Content Area: Pharmacology

Answer: 4
Rationale: Azithromycin is a macrolide antibiotic that is used to treat infection. It is not ordered for the treatment of pain, joint discomfort, or blood pressure.

Test-Taking Strategy: Use the process of elimination. Eliminate options 1 and 3 first, because they are comparable or alike. From the remaining options, recalling the action of this medication will direct you to option 4. Review the action and purpose of azithromycin if you had difficulty with this question.

References
Lehne, R. (2007). *Pharmacology for nursing care* (6th ed., p. 986). Philadelphia: Saunders.
McKenry, L., Tressier, E., & Hogan, M. (2006). *Mosby's pharmacology in nursing* (22nd ed., p. 1030). St. Louis: Mosby.

1492. A nurse is assigned to care for a client with acquired immunodeficiency syndrome who is receiving amphotericin B (Fungizone) for a fungal respiratory infection. Which of the following would indicate an adverse reaction to the medication?

1 Hypokalemia
2 Hyperkalemia
3 Hypocalcemia
4 Hypercalcemia

Level of Cognitive Ability: Analysis
Client Needs: Physiological Integrity
Integrated Process: Nursing Process/Evaluation
Content Area: Pharmacology

Answer: 1
Rationale: Clients receiving amphotericin B may develop hypokalemia, which can be severe and lead to extreme muscle weakness and electrocardiogram changes. Distal renal tubular acidosis commonly occurs, and this contributes to the development of hypokalemia. High potassium levels do not occur. The medication does not cause calcium levels to fluctuate.

Test-Taking Strategy: Note that amphotericin B is an antifungal. Recalling that hypokalemia is an adverse reaction to this medication will direct you to option 1. Review amphotericin B if you had difficulty with this question.

Reference
McKenry, L., Tressier, E., & Hogan, M. (2006). *Mosby's pharmacology in nursing* (22nd ed., p. 1015). St. Louis: Mosby.

1493. A client is seen in the health care clinic, and a diagnosis of conjunctivitis is made. The nurse provides instructions to the client regarding the care of the disorder while at home. Which statement by the client indicates the need for further instruction?

1 "I can use an ophthalmic analgesic ointment at night if I have eye discomfort."
2 "I do not need to be concerned about spreading this infection to others in my family."
3 "I should apply warm compresses before instilling antibiotic drops if purulent discharge is present in my eye."
4 "I should perform a saline eye irrigation before instilling the antibiotic drops into my eye if purulent discharge is present."

Level of Cognitive Ability: Analysis
Client Needs: Safe and Effective Care Environment
Integrated Process: Nursing Process/Evaluation
Content Area: Adult Health/Eye

Answer: 2
Rationale: Conjunctivitis is highly contagious. Antibiotic drops are usually administered four times a day. Ophthalmic analgesic ointment or drops may be instilled, especially at bedtime, because discomfort becomes more noticeable when the eyelids are closed. When purulent discharge is present, saline eye irrigations or applications of warm compresses to the eye may be necessary before instilling the medication.

Test-Taking Strategy: Use the process of elimination, and note the strategic words "need for further instruction." Knowing that this disorder is considered highly contagious will direct you to option 2. Review the management of the client with conjunctivitis if you had difficulty with this question.

References
Black, J., & Hawks, J. (2005). *Medical-surgical nursing: Clinical management for positive outcomes* (7th ed., p. 1963). Philadelphia: Saunders.
Ignatavicius, D., & Workman, M. (2006). *Medical-surgical nursing: Critical thinking for collaborative care* (5th ed., p. 1090). Philadelphia: Saunders.

1494. A nurse reviews the nursing care plan of a hospitalized child who is immobilized as a result of skeletal traction. The nurse notes a nursing diagnosis of Delayed Growth and Development related to immobilization and hospitalization. Which evaluative statement indicates a positive outcome for the child?

1 The fracture heals without complications.
2 The caregivers verbalize safe and effective home care.
3 The child maintains normal joint and muscle integrity.
4 The child displays age-appropriate developmental behaviors.

Level of Cognitive Ability: Analysis
Client Needs: Health Promotion and Maintenance
Integrated Process: Nursing Process/Evaluation
Content Area: Child Health

Answer: 4
Rationale: Regression and inappropriate developmental behaviors may be displayed in response to immobilization and hospitalization. With individualized care planning, a positive outcome of age-appropriate behavior can be achieved. Options 1, 2, and 3 are appropriate evaluative statements for an immobilized child, but they do not directly address the nursing diagnosis of Delayed Growth and Development.

Test-Taking Strategy: Focus on the subject: a nursing diagnosis of Delayed Growth and Development. Recalling that Delayed Growth and Development involves an individual not performing age-appropriate tasks will direct you to option 4. All options are evaluative statements, but only option 4 addresses this nursing diagnosis. Review the defining characteristics and appropriate outcomes for Delayed Growth and Development if you had difficulty with this question.

Reference
Hockenberry, M., Wilson, D., & Winkelstein, M. (2005). *Wong's essentials of pediatric nursing* (7th ed., pp. 1150-1151). St. Louis: Mosby.

1495. A nurse has been encouraging the intake of oral fluids for a client in labor to improve hydration. Which of the following indicates a successful outcome of this action?

1 Ketones in the urine
2 A urine specific gravity of 1.020
3 A blood pressure of 150/90 mm Hg
4 The continued leaking of amniotic fluid during labor

Level of Cognitive Ability: Analysis
Client Needs: Physiological Integrity
Integrated Process: Nursing Process/Evaluation
Content Area: Maternity/Intrapartum

Answer: 2
Rationale: Urine specific gravity measures the concentration of the urine. During the first stage of labor, the renal system has a tendency to concentrate urine. Labor and birth require hydration and caloric intake to replenish energy expenditure and to promote efficient uterine function. An elevated blood pressure and ketones in the urine are not expected outcomes related to labor and hydration. After the membranes have ruptured, it is expected that amniotic fluid may continue to leak.

Test-Taking Strategy: Use the process of elimination, and focus on the subject of a successful outcome related to oral intake. Recalling the relationship of oral intake to urine concentration will direct you to option 2. Review the importance of hydration for the woman in labor if you had difficulty with this question.

References
McKinney, E., James, S., Murray, S., & Ashwill, J. (2005). *Maternal-child nursing* (2nd ed., p. 1160). St. Louis: Saunders.
Murray, S., & McKinney, E. (2006). *Foundations of maternal-newborn nursing* (4th ed., pp. 182, 714). Philadelphia: Saunders.

1496. A postpartum client has a nursing diagnosis of Risk for Infection. A goal has been developed that states: "The client will remain free of infection during her hospital stay." Which assessment data would support that the goal has been met?
1 Loss of appetite
2 Absence of fever
3 Presence of chills
4 Abdominal tenderness

Level of Cognitive Ability: Analysis
Client Needs: Physiological Integrity
Integrated Process: Nursing Process/Evaluation
Content Area: Maternity/Postpartum

Answer: 2
Rationale: Fever is the first indication of an infection. Chills, abdominal tenderness, and loss of appetite can indicate the presence of an infection. Therefore, the absence of a fever indicates that an infection is not present.

Test-Taking Strategy: Use the process of elimination, and note the strategic words "that the goal has been met." The question is asking for a means of evaluating the effectiveness of a goal that relates to infection. Options 1, 3, and 4 indicate possible signs of infection and that the goal has not been met. Review the signs of postpartum infection if you had difficulty with this question.

Reference
Wong, D., Hockenberry, M., Perry, S., Lowdermilk, D., & Wilson, D. (2006). *Maternal-child nursing care* (3rd ed., p. 668). St. Louis: Mosby.

1497. The nurse is monitoring the nutritional status of a client who is receiving enteral nutrition. Which does the nurse monitor as the best clinical indicator of the client's nutritional status?
1 Daily weight
2 Calorie count
3 Skinfold measurement
4 Serum prealbumin level

Level of Cognitive Ability: Analysis
Client Needs: Physiological Integrity
Integrated Process: Nursing Process/Evaluation
Content Area: Fundamental Skills

Answer: 4
Rationale: A serum prealbumin level is the most important parameter for determining the effectiveness of a client's nutritional management and nutritional status. Because prealbumin is a major plasma protein with a short half-life, it is sensitive to changes in protein synthesis and catabolism, and it is thus the best clinical indicator of nutritional status. It is a better nutritional index than a daily weight, because body weight can be skewed quickly by changes in total body fluid. It is also a better index than anthropomorphic measurements, because nutritional status is not necessarily related to skinfold thickness. The calorie count reports the total calories provided to the client without data regarding the client's use of the calories and nutrients.

Test-Taking Strategy: Note the strategic word "best." This tells you that the correct option is a better indicator of nutritional status than the remaining options. Review the methods of monitoring nutritional status if you had difficulty with this question.

Reference
Lewis, S., Heitkemper, M., Dirksen, S., O'Brien, P., & Bucher, L. (2007). *Medical-surgical nursing: Assessment and management of clinical problems* (7th ed., p. 963). St. Louis: Mosby.

1498. An adult client with hyperkalemia receives sodium polystyrene sulfonate (Kayexalate). Which serum potassium level is a clinical indicator of effective therapy?
1 4.9 mEq/L
2 5.4 mEq/L
3 5.8 mEq/L
4 6.2 mEq/L

Answer: 1
Rationale: The normal serum potassium level for an adult is 3.5 to 5.1 mEq/L. Option 1 is the only option that reflects a value within this range. Options 2, 3, and 4 identify hyperkalemic levels.

Level of Cognitive Ability: Analysis
Client Needs: Physiological Integrity
Integrated Process: Nursing Process/Evaluation
Content Area: Fundamental Skills

Test-Taking Strategy: Note the strategic word "hyperkalemia," and use the process of elimination. Without knowing the mechanism of action of sodium polystyrene sulfonate, compare each value with normal serum potassium levels. Note that only one value is within normal limits and that effective therapy is very likely to achieve normal results. Review the expected effects of this medication and the normal potassium level if you had difficulty with this question.

References

Hodgson, B., & Kizior, R. (2007). *Saunders nursing drug handbook 2007* (pp. 1065-1066). Philadelphia: Saunders.

Pagana, K., & Pagana, T. (2005). *Mosby's diagnostic and laboratory test reference* (7th ed., p. 733). St. Louis: Mosby.

1499. The nurse assesses a client after abdominal surgery who has a nasogastric tube (NG) in place that is connected to suction. Which observation by the nurse indicates most reliably that the tube is functioning properly?

1 The suction gauge reads low intermittent suction.
2 The client indicates that pain is a 3 on a scale of 1 to 10.
3 The distal end of the NG tube is pinned to the client's gown.
4 The client denies nausea and has 250 mL of fluid in the suction collection container.

Level of Cognitive Ability: Analysis
Client Needs: Physiological Integrity
Integrated Process: Nursing Process/Evaluation
Content Area: Adult Health/Gastrointestinal

Answer: 4

Rationale: An NG tube connected to suction is used postoperatively to decompress and rest the bowel. The gastrointestinal tract lacks peristaltic activity as a result of manipulation during surgery. Although the nurse makes pertinent observations of the tube to ensure that it is secure and properly connected to suction, the client is assessed for the effect. The client should not experience symptoms of ileus (nausea and vomiting) if the tube is functioning properly. A pain indicator of 3 is an expected finding in a postoperative client.

Test-Taking Strategy: Focus on the subject of the tube functioning properly. Recalling the purpose of an NG tube in a postoperative client will direct you to option 4. Review the care of the client with an NG tube if you had difficulty with this question.

References

Ignatavicius, D., & Workman, M. (2006). *Medical-surgical nursing: Critical thinking for collaborative care* (5th ed., p. 345). Philadelphia: Saunders.

Potter, P., & Perry, A. (2005). *Fundamentals of nursing* (6th ed., p. 1408). St. Louis: Mosby.

1500. The nurse is caring for a client who has returned from the postanesthesia care unit after prostatectomy. The client has a three-way Foley catheter with an infusion of continuous bladder irrigation (CBI). The nurse determines that the flow rate is adequate if the color of the urinary drainage is:

1 Dark cherry
2 Clear as water
3 Pale yellow or slightly pink
4 Concentrated yellow with small clots

Answer: 3

Rationale: The infusion of bladder irrigant is not at a preset rate; rather, it is increased or decreased to maintain urine that is a clear, pale yellow color or that has just a slight pink tinge. The infusion rate should be increased if the drainage is cherry colored or if clots are seen. Alternatively, the rate can be slowed down slightly if the returns are as clear as water.

Test-Taking Strategy: Note the subject of the question: an adequate flow rate. With this in mind, eliminate option 4, because clots are not expected. Next, eliminate options 1 and 2 as reflecting inadequate or excessive irrigation flow, respectively. Review the care of the client with CBI if you had difficulty with this question.

Level of Cognitive Ability: Analysis
Client Needs: Physiological Integrity
Integrated Process: Nursing Process/Evaluation
Content Area: Adult Health/Renal

Reference
Ignatavicius, D., & Workman, M. (2006). *Medical-surgical nursing: Critical thinking for collaborative care* (5th ed., pp. 1862-1863). Philadelphia: Saunders.

1501. The nurse who is caring for a client with Graves' disease notes a nursing diagnosis of "Imbalanced Nutrition: less than body requirements related to the effects of the hypercatabolic state" in the care plan. Which of the following indicates a successful outcome for this diagnosis?

1 The client verbalizes the need to avoid snacking between meals.
2 The client discusses the relationship between mealtime and the blood glucose level.
3 The client maintains the normal weight or gradually gains weight if it is below normal.
4 The client demonstrates knowledge regarding the need to consume a diet that is high in fat and low in protein.

Level of Cognitive Ability: Analysis
Client Needs: Physiological Integrity
Integrated Process: Nursing Process/Evaluation
Content Area: Adult Health/Endocrine

Answer: 3

Rationale: Graves' disease causes a state of chronic nutritional and caloric deficiency caused by the metabolic effects of excessive T3 and T4. Clinical manifestations are weight loss and increased appetite. Therefore, it is a nutritional goal that the client will not lose additional weight and that he or she will gradually return to the ideal body weight, if necessary. To accomplish this, the client must be encouraged to eat frequent high-calorie, high-protein, and high-carbohydrate meals and snacks.

Test-Taking Strategy: Use the process of elimination, and focus on the strategic words "hypercatabolic state." Options 1 and 4 would not be beneficial for a client in a hypercatabolic state. Option 2 can be eliminated, because discussing the fluctuation in the blood glucose level will not be helpful for a client who is hypermetabolic. Review imbalanced nutrition and Graves' disease if you had difficulty with this question.

Reference
Black, J., & Hawks, J. (2005). *Medical-surgical nursing: Clinical management for positive outcomes* (7th ed., p. 1196). Philadelphia: Saunders.

1502. A nurse in the physician's office is reviewing the results of a client's phenytoin (Dilantin) level that was drawn that morning. The nurse determines that the client had a therapeutic drug level if the client's result was:

1 3 mcg/mL
2 8 mcg/mL
3 15 mcg/mL
4 24 mcg/mL

Level of Cognitive Ability: Analysis
Client Needs: Physiological Integrity
Integrated Process: Nursing Process/Evaluation
Content Area: Pharmacology

Answer: 3

Rationale: The therapeutic range for serum phenytoin levels is 10 to 20 mcg/mL in clients with normal serum albumin levels and renal function. A level below this range indicates that the client is not receiving sufficient medication and is at risk for seizure activity. In this case, the medication dose should be adjusted upward. A level above the therapeutic range indicates that the client is entering the toxic range and is at risk for toxic side effects of the medication. In this case, the dose should be adjusted downward.

Test-Taking Strategy: Recalling that the therapeutic drug serum level for phenytoin is 10 to 20 mcg/mL will direct you to option 3. Review phenytoin if you had difficulty with this question.

Reference
Skidmore-Roth, L. (2008). *Mosby's nursing drug reference* (21st ed., p. 817). St. Louis: Mosby.

1503. A nurse instructs a parent regarding the appropriate actions to take when the toddler has a temper tantrum. Which statement by the parent indicates a successful outcome of the teaching?

1 "I will ignore the tantrums as long as there is no physical danger."
2 "I will give frequent reminders that only bad children have tantrums."
3 "I will send my child to a room alone for 10 minutes after every tantrum."
4 "I will reward my child with candy at the end of each day without a tantrum."

Level of Cognitive Ability: Analysis
Client Needs: Health Promotion and Maintenance
Integrated Process: Nursing Process/Evaluation
Content Area: Child Health

Answer: 1
Rationale: Ignoring a negative attention-seeking behavior is considered the best way to extinguish it, provided that the child is safe from injury. Option 2 is untrue and negative. Option 3 gives attention to the tantrum and also exceeds the recommended time of 1 minute per year of age for a time-out. Providing candy for rewards is unhealthy and unlikely to be effective at the end of the day.

Test-Taking Strategy: Use the process of elimination. Recalling that ignoring a tantrum is the best way to extinguish it will direct you to option 1. Review the interventions for the child who has temper tantrums if you had difficulty with this question.

Reference
Wong, D., Hockenberry, M., Perry, S., Lowdermilk, D., & Wilson, D. (2006). *Maternal-child nursing care* (3rd ed., p. 1097). St. Louis: Mosby.

1504. A nurse is caring for a client who is in seclusion. The nurse determines that the seclusion is no longer necessary when the client says:

1 "I am in control of myself now."
2 "I need to use the restroom right away."
3 "I'd like to go back to my room and be alone for a while."
4 "I can't breathe in here. It feels like the walls are closing in on me."

Level of Cognitive Ability: Analysis
Client Needs: Psychosocial Integrity
Integrated Process: Nursing Process/Evaluation
Content Area: Mental Health

Answer: 1
Rationale: Option 1 indicates that the client may be safely removed from seclusion. The client in seclusion must be assessed at regular intervals (usually every 15 to 30 minutes) for physical needs, safety, and comfort. Option 2 indicates a physical need that could be met with a urinal, a bedpan, or a commode; it does not indicate that the client has calmed down enough to leave the seclusion room. Option 3 could be an attempt to manipulate the nurse; it gives no indication that the client will control himself or herself when alone in the room. Option 4 could be handled by supportive communication or an as-needed medication, if indicated; it does not necessitate discontinuing seclusion.

Test-Taking Strategy: Focus on the subject of the question: removing a client from seclusion. Recalling the purpose and the use of seclusion will direct you to option 1. Review seclusion procedures if you had difficulty with this question.

References
Stuart, G., & Laraia, M. (2005). *Principles and practice of psychiatric nursing* (8th ed., p. 646). St. Louis: Mosby.
Varcarolis, E., Carson, V., & Shoemaker, N. (2006). *Foundations of psychiatric mental health nursing* (5th ed., pp. 496-497). Philadelphia: Saunders.

1505. The nurse has developed a plan of care for a client who is in traction and documents a nursing diagnosis of Bathing/Hygiene Self-Care Deficit. The nurse evaluates the plan of care and determines that which observation indicates a successful outcome?

1 The client refuses care.

2 The client allows the family to assist in the care.

3 The client assists in self-care as much as possible.

4 The client allows the nurse to complete the care on a daily basis.

Level of Cognitive Ability: Analysis
Client Needs: Physiological Integrity
Integrated Process: Nursing Process/Evaluation
Content Area: Adult Health/Musculoskeletal

Answer: 3
Rationale: A successful outcome for the nursing diagnosis of Bathing/Hygiene Self-Care Deficit is for the client to do as much of the self-care as possible. The nurse should promote independence in the client and allow the client to perform as much self-care as is optimal considering the client's condition. The nurse would determine that the outcome is unsuccessful if the client refused care or allows others to perform the care.

Test-Taking Strategy: Focus on the strategic words "successful outcome." Option 1 can be eliminated first, because the client is refusing care. Note that options 2 and 4 are comparable or alike in that they indicate relying on others to perform care. Review successful outcomes related to the nursing diagnosis of Bathing/Hygiene Self-Care Deficit if you had difficulty with this question.

References
Black, J., & Hawks, J. (2005). *Medical-surgical nursing: Clinical management for positive outcomes* (7th ed., p. 643). Philadelphia: Saunders.
Ignatavicius, D., & Workman, M. (2006). *Medical-surgical nursing: Critical thinking for collaborative care* (5th ed., pp. 127, 1196). Philadelphia: Saunders.

ALTERNATE ITEM FORMATS

1506. The provider's prescription reads "Tobramycin sulfate (Nebcin) 7.5 mg intramuscularly twice daily." The medication label reads "10 mg/mL." How much tobramycin sulfate should the nurse administer for one dose?

Answer: _____ mL

Level of Cognitive Ability: Application
Client Needs: Physiological Integrity
Integrated Process: Nursing Process/ Implementation
Content Area: Fundamental Skills

Answer: 0.75
Rationale: Use the following formula to calculate the medication dose:

$$\frac{\text{Desired}}{\text{Available}} \times \text{Volume} = \text{mL per dose}$$

$$\frac{7.5 \text{ mg}}{10 \text{ mg}} \times 1 \text{ mL} = 0.75 \text{ mL}$$

Test-Taking Strategy: Identify what the question is asking. In this case, the question asks for the mL per dose. Use the formula to determine the correct dosage, and use a calculator to verify your answer. Review the formula for calculating a medication dose if you had difficulty with this question.

Reference
Kee, J., & Marshall, S. (2004). *Clinical calculations: With applications to general and specialty areas* (4th ed., p. 80). Philadelphia: Saunders.

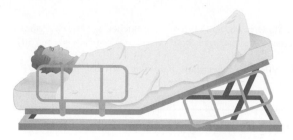

From Black, J., & Hawks, J. (2005). *Medical-surgical nursing: Clinical management for positive outcomes* (7th ed.). Philadelphia: Saunders.

1507. The nurse is asked to assist another health care team member with providing care for a client. On entering the client's room, the nurse notes that the client is placed in this position. (Refer to figure).

The nurse interprets that the client is most likely being treated for:

1 Shock

2 A head injury

3 Respiratory insufficiency

4 Increased intracranial pressure

Level of Cognitive Ability: Analysis
Client Needs: Physiological Integrity
Integrated Process: Nursing Process/Analysis
Content Area: Adult Health/Cardiovascular

Answer: 1
Rationale: A client in shock is placed in a modified Trendelenburg's position that includes elevating the legs, leaving the trunk flat, and elevating the head and shoulders slightly. This position promotes increased venous return from the lower extremities without compressing the abdominal organs against the diaphragm. Options 2, 3, and 4 identify conditions in which the head of the client's bed would be elevated.

Test-Taking Strategy: Focus on the position identified in the question. Eliminate options 2 and 4 first, because they are comparable or alike, and they both relate to a neurological condition. From the remaining options, eliminate option 3, recalling that the head of the bed is elevated for respiratory conditions. Review the care of the client with shock if you had difficulty with this question.

Reference
Black, J., & Hawks, J. (2005). *Medical-surgical nursing: Clinical management for positive outcomes* (7th ed., p. 2461). Philadelphia: Saunders.

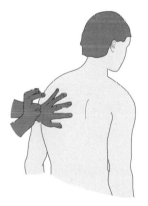

From Potter, P., & Perry, A. (2005). *Fundamentals of nursing* (6th ed.). St. Louis: Mosby.

1508. The clinic nurse is performing a complete physical assessment on a client. During the respiratory assessment, the nurse is using which physical assessment technique?

1 Palpation

2 Inspection

3 Percussion

4 Auscultation

Answer: 3
Rationale: To perform percussion, the nurse places the middle finger of the nondominant hand against the body's surface. The tip of the middle finger of the dominant hand strikes the top of the middle finger of the nondominant hand. Auscultation involves listening to the sounds produced by the body. Palpation is performed using the sense of touch. Inspection is the process of observation.

Test-Taking Strategy: Use the process of elimination. Recalling the definition of each technique listed in the options will direct you to option 3. Remember that inspection is observing, palpation uses the sense of touch, and ausculating is listening. Review physical assessment techniques if you had difficulty with this question.

Level of Cognitive Ability: Application
Client Needs: Health Promotion and
    Maintenance
Integrated Process: Nursing Process/Assessment
Content Area: Adult Health/Respiratory

References
Lewis, S., Heitkemper, M., Dirksen, S., O'Brien, P., & Bucher, L. (2007). *Medical-surgical nursing: Assessment and management of clinical problems* (7th ed., p. 750). St. Louis: Mosby.
Potter, P., & Perry, A. (2005). *Fundamentals of nursing* (6th ed., pp. 676-677). St. Louis: Mosby.

1509. The nurse assesses a client upon arrival in the postanesthesia care unit after a colectomy. List the initial assessment actions in order of priority from the first action performed to the last action performed.

  ___ Checks for airway patency
  ___ Checks abdominal dressing
  ___ Measures the respiratory rate
  ___ Evaluates heart rate and rhythm
  ___ Documents postoperative findings
  ___ Asks the client about any concerns

Level of Cognitive Ability: Application
Client Needs: Physiological Integrity
Integrated Process: Nursing Process/Assessment
Content Area: Fundamental Skills

Answer: 1, 4, 2, 3, 6, 5
Rationale: Postoperative assessment begins with the evaluation of the client's ABCs—airway, breathing, and circulation; thus, the nurse assesses airway patency first to ensure adequate oxygenation to the body organs and tissues. Next, the rate and quality of the client's respirations are determined, and breath sounds are auscultated throughout all lung fields to ensure adequate ventilation. The client's heart rate and rhythm are determined, and the client's blood pressure is checked after the respiratory assessment and according to the hierarchy of the ABCs. After the ABCs are complete, the nurse assesses the neurological status and the remaining organ systems and performs other assessments, including dressings, drains, tubes, and pain as part of a comprehensive assessment. Finally, the nurse asks the client about any concerns and then documents the assessment findings.

Test-Taking Strategy: Note the words "order of priority." Use the ABCs—airway, breathing, and circulation—to assist with determining the correct order of action. In addition, Maslow's Hierarchy of Needs theory can be used to determine that physiological needs come first. Review the initial care of the postoperative client if you had difficulty with this question.

References
Lewis, S., Heitkemper, M., Dirksen, S., O'Brien, P., & Bucher, L. (2007). *Medical-surgical nursing: Assessment and management of clinical problems* (7th ed., pp. 377-378). St. Louis: Mosby.
Potter, P., & Perry, A. (2005). *Fundamentals of nursing* (6th ed., pp. 1628-1630). St. Louis: Mosby.

1510. A nurse is providing home-care instructions to the spouse of a client who is confused and who will be cared for at home. Select all instructions that the nurse provides to the spouse:

☐ 1 Turn the lights off at dusk.

☐ 2 Maintain a predictable routine.

☐ 3 Use simple, clear communication.

☐ 4 Limit the number of choices given to the client.

☐ 5 Encourage frequent visits from family and friends.

☐ 6 Display a calendar and a clock in the client's room.

Level of Cognitive Ability: Application
Client Needs: Psychosocial Integrity
Integrated Process: Teaching and Learning
Content Area: Mental Health

Answer: 2, 3, 4, 6
Rationale: The caregiver of a confused client is taught measures and techniques that will keep the client oriented and calm. Sensory overload or tasks and activities that are overwhelming for the client will cause disorientation and additional confusion. Therefore, any measures or activities that will increase sensory overload are avoided. Some helpful techniques include displaying a calendar and a clock around the house and in the client's room; maintaining a predictable routine; limiting the number of visitors who come to see the client; limiting the number of choices given to the client; using simple, clear communication; and turning the lights on at dusk to avoid the sundown syndrome of increased confusion and combative behavior.

Test-Taking Strategy: Focus on the subject: measures that will keep the client oriented and calm. Think about each listed intervention, and remember that measures or activities that will increase sensory overload or that are overwhelming for the client are to be avoided. This principle will assist you with selecting the correct measures. Review the care of the confused client if you had difficulty with this question.

Reference
Stuart, G., & Laraia, M. (2005). *Principles and practice of psychiatric nursing* (8th ed., pp. 465-467). St. Louis: Mosby.

REFERENCES

Black, J., & Hawks, J. (2005). *Medical-surgical nursing: Clinical management for positive outcomes* (7th ed.). Philadelphia: Saunders.

Chernecky, C., & Berger, B. (2008). *Laboratory tests and diagnostic procedures* (5th ed.). Philadelphia: Saunders.

Gahart, B., & Nazareno, A. (2006). *2006 intravenous medications* (22nd ed.). St. Louis: Mosby.

Giger, J., & Davidhizar, R. (2004). *Transcultural nursing* (5th ed.). St. Louis: Mosby.

Gulanick, M., & Myers, J. (2007). *Nursing care plans: Nursing diagnosis and interventions* (6th ed.). St. Louis: Mosby.

Hockenberry, M., & Wilson, D. (2007). *Nursing care of infants and children* (8th ed.). St. Louis: Mosby.

Hockenberry, M., Wilson, D., & Winkelstein, M. (2005). *Wong's essentials of pediatric nursing* (7th ed.). St. Louis: Mosby.

Hodgson, B., & Kizior, R. (2007). *Saunders nursing drug handbook 2007*. Philadelphia: Saunders.

Ignatavicius, D., & Workman, M. (2006). *Medical-surgical nursing: Critical thinking for collaborative care* (5th ed.). Philadelphia: Saunders.

Kee, J., Hayes, E., & McCuistion, L. (2006). *Pharmacology: A nursing process approach* (5th ed.). Philadelphia: Saunders.

Kee, J., & Marshall, S. (2004). *Clinical calculations: With applications to general and specialty areas* (5th ed.). Philadelphia: Saunders.

Lehne, R. (2007). *Pharmacology for nursing care* (6th ed.). Philadelphia: Saunders.

Lewis, S., Heitkemper, M., Dirksen, S., O'Brien, P., & Bucher, L. (2007). *Medical-surgical nursing: Assessment and management of clinical problems* (7th ed.). St. Louis: Mosby.

Lilley, L., Harrington, S., & Snyder, J. (2007). *Pharmacology and the nursing process* (5th ed.). St. Louis: Mosby.

Meiner, S., & Leuckenotte, A. (2006). *Gerontologic nursing* (3rd ed.). St. Louis: Mosby.

McKenry, L., Tessier, E., & Hogan, M. (2006). *Mosby's pharmacology in nursing* (22nd ed.). St. Louis: Mosby.

McKinney, E., James, S., Murray, S., & Ashwill, J. (2005). *Maternal-child nursing* (2nd ed.). St. Louis: Saunders.

Monahan, F., Sands, J., Marek, J., Neighbors, M., & Green, C. (2007). *Phipps' medical-surgical nursing: Health and illness perspectives* (8th ed.). St. Louis: Mosby.

Murray, S., & McKinney, E. (2006). *Foundations of maternal-newborn nursing* (4th ed.). Philadelphia: Saunders.

National Council of State Boards of Nursing (Eds.). (2007). *2007 NCLEX-RN® detailed test plan*. Chicago: Author.

Nix, S. (2005). *Williams' basic nutrition & diet therapy* (12th ed.). St. Louis: Mosby.

Pagana, K., & Pagana, T. (2005). *Mosby's diagnostic and laboratory test reference* (7th ed.). St. Louis: Mosby.

Perry, A., & Potter, P. (2006). *Clinical nursing skills & techniques* (6th ed.). St. Louis: Mosby.

Potter, P., & Perry, A. (2005). *Fundamentals of nursing* (6th ed.). St. Louis: Mosby.

Skidmore-Roth, L. (2007). *2007 Mosby's nursing drug reference* (20th ed.). St. Louis: Mosby.

Skidmore-Roth, L. (2008). *Mosby's nursing drug reference* (21st ed.). St. Louis: Mosby.

Stuart, G., & Laraia, M. (2005). *Principles and practice of psychiatric nursing* (8th ed.). St. Louis: Mosby.

Varcarolis, E., Carson, V., & Shoemaker, N. (2006). *Foundations of psychiatric mental health nursing* (5th ed.). Philadelphia: Saunders.

Wong, D., Hockenberry, M., Perry, S., Lowdermilk, D., & Wilson, D. (2006). *Maternal-child nursing care* (3rd ed.). St. Louis: Mosby.

Comprehensive Test

1511. The nurse monitors a client who is receiving a blood transfusion when the client complains of diaphoresis, warmth, and a backache. After stopping the blood transfusion, which intervention should the nurse implement?

1 Hang D$_5$W.
2 Discontinue the IV catheter.
3 Convert the IV to a heparin lock.
4 Hang 0.9% sodium chloride solution.

Level of Cognitive Ability: Application
Client Needs: Physiological Integrity
Integrated Process: Nursing Process/
   Implementation
Content Area: Fundamental Skills

Answer: 4
Rationale: The nurse recognizes that the client is most likely experiencing a transfusion reaction. The nurse stops the transfusion and prevents the infusion of any additional blood; then, the nurse hangs a bag of normal saline solution. This maintains IV access and helps maintain the client's intravascular volume. The nurse avoids hanging D$_5$W because any remaining blood in the IV catheter is likely to coagulate in the presence of dextrose and occlude the IV line. To preserve the IV access, the nurse avoids discontinuing the IV site. The nurse avoids converting the IV site to a heparin lock because the client is likely to receive additional IV fluids as a result of the reactions.

Test-Taking Strategy: Use the process of elimination and knowledge regarding blood transfusions and transfusion reactions to answer the question. Recalling that normal saline is compatible with blood will direct you to option 4. Review interventions if a transfusion reaction occurs if you had difficulty with this question.

References
Black, J., & Hawks, J. (2005). *Medical-surgical nursing: Clinical management for positive outcomes* (7th ed., p. 2284). Philadelphia: Saunders.
Ignatavicius, D., & Workman, M. (2006). *Medical-surgical nursing: Critical thinking for collaborative care* (5th ed., p. 913). Philadelphia: Saunders.

1512. A nurse assesses a client admitted to the hospital with rib fractures in order to identify the risk for potential complications. The nurse notes that the client has a history of emphysema. Following the assessment, the nurse ensures that which of the following interventions is documented in the plan of care? Select all that apply.

☐ 1 Collect sputum specimens at hour of sleep.
☐ 2 Maintain the client in a position of comfort.
☐ 3 Offer medication to suppress cough as needed.
☐ 4 Administer small, frequent meals with plenty of fluids.
☐ 5 Have the client cough and breathe deeply 20 minutes after pain medication is given.
☐ 6 Administer 4 to 6 liters of oxygen when the client's pulse oximetry drops below 90%.

Answer: 2, 4, 5
Rationale: If sputum specimen collection is prescribed, the specimen should be collected early in the morning upon the client's awakening. Productive cough is more likely to occur after the client has slept. Clients with emphysema are not given cough suppressants because expectoration of sputum is essential to airway clearance. Giving the client with emphysema a high flow of oxygen (option 6) would halt the hypoxic drive and cause apnea. Options 2, 4, and 5 are appropriate interventions.

Test-Taking Strategy: Focus on the data in the question and note that the client has emphysema. Recalling the pathophysiology associated with emphysema will assist in determining the correct options. Review the complications that can occur in the client with emphysema if you had difficulty with this question.

Level of Cognitive Ability: Application
Client Needs: Physiological Integrity
Integrated Process: Nursing Process/Planning
Content Area: Adult Health/Respiratory

References
Ignatavicius, D., & Workman, M. (2006). *Medical-surgical nursing: Critical thinking for collaborative care* (5th ed., p. 913). Philadelphia: Saunders.
Lewis, S., Heitkemper, M., Dirksen, S., O'Brien, P., & Bucher, L. (2007). *Medical-surgical nursing: Assessment and management of clinical problems* (7th ed., p. 638). St. Louis: Mosby.

1513. A client has been given a prescription to begin using nitroglycerin transdermal patches in the management of coronary artery disease. The nurse instructs the client about this medication administration system and tells the client to:

1 Apply a new system every 7 days.
2 Wait 1 day to apply a new system if it becomes dislodged.
3 Place the system in the area of a skin fold to promote better adherence.
4 Apply the system in the morning and leave it in place for 12 to 16 hours as directed.

Level of Cognitive Ability: Application
Client Needs: Physiological Integrity
Integrated Process: Teaching and Learning
Content Area: Pharmacology

Answer: 4
Rationale: Nitroglycerin is a coronary vasodilator used in the management of coronary artery disease. The client is generally advised to apply a new system each morning and leave it in place for 12 to 16 hours as per physician directions. This prevents the client from developing tolerance (as happens with 24-hour use). The client should avoid placing the system in skin folds or excoriated areas. The client can apply a new system if it becomes dislodged because the dose is released continuously in small amounts through the skin.

Test-Taking Strategy: Specific information related to this type of medication administration system is needed to answer this question. Recalling that tolerance can occur with this medication will direct you to option 4. Review the procedures related to transdermal medication systems if you had difficulty with this question.

Reference
Mosby. (2007). *Mosby's nursing drug reference* (20th ed., p. 729). St. Louis: Mosby.

1514. A 9-year-old child is newly diagnosed with type 1 diabetes mellitus. The nurse is planning for home care with the child and his family and determines that an age-appropriate activity for this child for health maintenance is:

1 Independently self-administering insulin
2 Administering insulin drawn up by an adult
3 Making independent decisions with regard to sliding-scale coverage of insulin
4 Having an adult assist in the self-administration of insulin and glucose monitoring

Level of Cognitive Ability: Analysis
Client Needs: Health Promotion and Maintenance
Integrated Process: Nursing Process/Planning
Content Area: Child Health

Answer: 1
Rationale: School-age children have the cognitive and motor skills to independently administer insulin with adult supervision. Developmentally, they do not yet have the maturity to make situational decisions without adult validation. Options 2 and 4 suppress the maximum level of independence appropriate to the level of this child.

Test-Taking Strategy: Use the process of elimination. Focusing on the age of the child will assist in eliminating options 2 and 4. From the remaining options, recalling that in this age group decision making is a cognitive skill that develops later than motor skills will direct you to option 1. Review growth and development of the 9-year-old if you had difficulty with this question.

References
Hockenberry, M., & Wilson, D. (2007). *Nursing care of infants and children* (8th ed., p. 1088). St. Louis: Mosby.
McKinney, E., James, S., Murray, S., & Ashwill, J. (2005). *Maternal-child nursing* (2nd ed., pp. 1472-1474). St. Louis: Saunders.

1515. A nurse is reviewing a plan of care formulated by a nursing student who is working in the health care clinic and is preparing to instruct a pregnant client to perform Kegel exercises. The nurse asks the student to explain the purpose of the Kegel exercises. Which response by the student indicates an understanding of the purpose of these types of exercises?

1 "The exercises will help reduce backache."
2 "The exercises will help prevent ankle edema."
3 "The exercises will help prevent urinary tract infections."
4 "The exercises will help strengthen the pelvic floor in preparation for delivery."

Level of Cognitive Ability: Analysis
Client Needs: Health Promotion and Maintenance
Integrated Process: Nursing Process/Planning
Content Area: Maternity/Antepartum

Answer: 4
Rationale: Kegel exercises assist to strengthen the pelvic floor (pubococcygeal muscle). Pelvic tilt exercises help reduce backaches. Instructing a client to drink 8 ounces of fluids six times a day helps prevent urinary tract infections. Leg elevation assists in preventing ankle edema.

Test-Taking Strategy: Focus on the subject—Kegel exercises. Remember that Kegel exercises will help strengthen the pelvic floor muscles. Review the purpose of Kegel exercises if you had difficulty with this question.

Reference
Wong, D., Hockenberry, M., Perry, S., Lowdermilk, D., & Wilson, D. (2006). *Maternal-child nursing care.* (3rd ed., pp. 277, 614-615). St. Louis: Mosby.

1516. The provider's prescription reads as follows: piperacillin sodium (Pipracil) 650 mg intravenously every 6 hours. The medication label reads as follows: reconstitute with 4.8 mL of bacteriostatic water to yield piperacillin sodium 2 grams in 5 mL. How much piperacillin sodium should the nurse withdraw from the vial for one dose? (Round answer to the tenth position.)

Answer: _____mL

Level of Cognitive Ability: Application
Client Needs: Physiological Integrity
Integrated Process: Nursing Process/Implementation
Content Area: Fundamental Skills

Answer: 1.6
Rationale: Convert 2 g to mg and then use the formula for calculating medication doses. In the metric system, to convert larger to smaller, multiply by 1000 or move the decimal three places to the right. Therefore, 2 g = 2000 mg.

Formula:

$$\frac{\text{Desired}}{\text{Available}} \times \text{mL} = \text{mL per dose}$$

$$\frac{650 \text{ mg}}{2000 \text{ mg}} \times 5 \text{ mL} = 1.625 \text{ mL}$$

Test-Taking Strategy: Identify the strategic components of the question and what the question is asking. In this case, the question asks for the milliliters per dose. Convert grams to milligrams first. Next, use the formula to determine the correct dose, knowing that 2000 mg = 5.0 mL. Finally, round the answer to the tenth position. Review medication calculation formulas if you had difficulty with this question.

Reference
Kee, J., & Marshall, S. (2004). *Clinical calculations: With applications to general and specialty areas* (5th ed., p. 80). Philadelphia: Saunders.

1517. A child with sickle cell disease is admitted to the hospital for treatment of vasoocclusive pain crisis. A nursing student is assigned to care for the child, and the nurse reviews the plan of care with the student. Which intervention, if included in the plan of care, indicates a need for further research by the student?

1 Increased fluid intake
2 Oxygen administration
3 IV fluids for rehydration
4 Meperidine hydrochloride (Demerol) for pain management

Level of Cognitive Ability: Analysis
Client Needs: Physiological Integrity
Integrated Process: Teaching and Learning
Content Area: Child Health

Answer: 4
Rationale: Management of the severe pain that occurs with vasoocclusive crisis includes the use of strong opioid analgesics, such as morphine sulfate and hydromorphone hydrochloride (Dilaudid). Meperidine hydrochloride is contraindicated because of its side effects and increased risk of seizures. Oxygen is administered to increase tissue perfusion. Fluids are necessary to promote hydration.

Test-Taking Strategy: Note the strategic words "need for further research." These words indicate a negative event query and the need to select the incorrect intervention. Eliminate options 1 and 3 first, knowing that hydration is necessary, and because these options are comparable or alike. From the remaining options, use the ABCs—airway, breathing, and circulation—to eliminate option 2. Review care of the client with sickle cell disease if you had difficulty with this question.

Reference
Hockenberry, M., Wilson, D., & Winkelstein, M. (2005). *Wong's essentials of pediatric nursing* (7th ed., p. 946). St. Louis: Mosby.

1518. A newborn infant receives the first dose of hepatitis B vaccine within 12 hours of birth. The nurse instructs the mother regarding the immunization schedule for this vaccine and tells the mother that the second vaccine is administered at:

1 8 months of age and then 1 year after the initial dose
2 3 years of age and then during the adolescent years
3 6 months of age and then 8 months after the initial dose
4 1 to 2 months of age and then 6 months after the initial dose

Level of Cognitive Ability: Application
Client Needs: Health Promotion and Maintenance
Integrated Process: Teaching and Learning
Content Area: Child Health

Answer: 4
Rationale: The vaccination schedule for an infant whose mother tests negative for hepatitis B consists of a series of three immunizations given at 0 months (birth), 1 to 2 months of age, and then 6 months after the initial dose. An infant whose mother tests positive receives hepatitis B immune globulin along with the first dose of the hepatitis vaccine within 12 hours of birth.

Test-Taking Strategy: Knowledge regarding the immunization schedule for hepatitis B vaccine is required to answer this question. Remember that the vaccination schedule consists of a series of three immunizations given at 0 months (birth), 1 to 2 months of age, and then 6 months after the initial dose. Review this schedule if you are unfamiliar with it.

Reference
Hockenberry, M. & Wilson, D. (2007). *Nursing care of infants and children* (8th ed., p. 335). St. Louis: Mosby.

1519. The nurse assesses the client with a diagnosis of thyroid storm. Which classic signs and symptoms associated with thyroid storm indicate the priority need for immediate nursing intervention?

1 Polyuria, nausea, and severe headaches
2 Hypotension, translucent skin, and obesity
3 Fever, tachycardia, and systolic hypertension
4 Profuse diaphoresis, flushing, and constipation

Level of Cognitive Ability: Analysis
Client Needs: Physiological Integrity
Integrated Process: Nursing Process/Assessment
Content Area: Adult Health/Endocrine

Answer: 3
Rationale: The excessive amounts of thyroid hormone cause a rapid increase in the metabolic rate, thereby causing the classic signs and symptoms of thyroid storm such as fever, tachycardia, and hypertension. When these signs present themselves, the nurse must take quick action to prevent deterioration of the client's health because death can ensue. Priority interventions include maintaining a patent airway and stabilizing the hemodynamic status. Options 1, 2, and 4 do not indicate the need for immediate nursing intervention.

Test-Taking Strategy: Note the words "the priority need for immediate nursing intervention" and use the process of elimination. Tachycardia, hypertension, and a fever indicate hemodynamic instability and take precedence over the signs and symptoms identified in options 1, 2, and 4. Additionally, option 3 is the only option that identifies all the signs and symptoms of thyroid storm. Review thyroid storm if you had difficulty with this question.

References
Black, J., & Hawks, J. (2005). *Medical-surgical nursing: Clinical management for positive outcomes* (7th ed., p. 1202). Philadelphia: Saunders.
Ignatavicius, D., & Workman, M. (2006). *Medical-surgical nursing: Critical thinking for collaborative care* (5th ed., pp. 1487-1488). Philadelphia: Saunders.

1520. A client is hospitalized for ingesting an overdose of acetaminophen (Tylenol). The nurse prepares to administer which specific antidote for this medication overdose?

1 Protamine sulfate
2 Acetylcysteine (Mucomyst)
3 Vitamin K (AquaMephyton)
4 Naloxone hydrochloride (Narcan)

Level of Cognitive Ability: Analysis
Client Needs: Physiological Integrity
Integrated Process: Nursing Process/Planning
Content Area: Pharmacology

Answer: 2
Rationale: Acetylcysteine restores sulfhydryl groups that are depleted by acetaminophen metabolism. Protamine sulfate is the antidote for heparin. Vitamin K is the antidote for warfarin sodium (Coumadin). Naloxone hydrochloride reverses respiratory depression.

Test-Taking Strategy: Use the process of elimination. Recalling the specific antidotes for both heparin and warfarin sodium will assist in eliminating options 1 and 3. Next, recalling that naloxone hydrochloride reverses respiratory depression will assist in eliminating option 4. Review these antidotes if you had difficulty with this question.

Reference
Hodgson, B., & Kizior, R. (2007). *Saunders nursing drug handbook 2007* (p. 13). Philadelphia: Saunders.

1521. A nurse is caring for a client at risk for suicide. Which client behavior is most indicative that the client may be contemplating suicide?

 1 The client shares that he is finally happy.
 2 The client sits and cries for long periods of time.
 3 The client reports a variety of sleep pattern disturbances.
 4 The client prefers to spend long periods of time alone.

Level of Cognitive Ability: Analysis
Client Needs: Physiological Integrity
Integrated Process: Nursing Process/Analysis
Content Area: Mental Health

Answer: 1

Rationale: If a client displays a suicidal ideation and is able to share a plan, the client should be taken very seriously and suicide precautions should be implemented. Option 1 shows a contentment that is often a sign that a sucide plan has been created. Options 2, 3 and 4 are indicative of depression but are not as definitive as option 1 in regard to suicide.

Test-Taking Strategy: Note the strategic words "most indicative" and focus on the subject—suicide. Recalling that a cardinal sign of suicidal ideation is the formulation of a suicidal plan will direct you to option 1. Review assessment of the client at risk for suicide if you had difficulty with this question.

Reference
Varcarolis, E., Carson, V, & Shoemaker, N. (2006) *Foundations of psychiatric mental health nursing* (5th ed., pp. 477-478). Philadelphia: Saunders.

1522. A nurse is reviewing the record of a client who was admitted to the hospital for diagnostic studies following a fainting spell. The nurse notes that the client is receiving olanzapine (Zyprexa). Which disorder or condition would the nurse suspect in the client?

 1 History of schizophrenia
 2 History of diabetes mellitus
 3 History of diabetes insipidus
 4 History of coronary artery disease

Level of Cognitive Ability: Analysis
Client Needs: Physiological Integrity
Integrated Process: Nursing Process/Analysis
Content Area: Pharmacology

Answer: 1

Rationale: Zyprexa is an antipsychotic medication used in the management of manifestations associated with psychotic disorders. It is the first-line treatment for schizophrenia targeting both the positive and the negative symptoms. Options 2, 3, and 4 are not indicated uses for this medication.

Test-Taking Strategy: Focus on the name of the medication. Recalling that this medication is an antipsychotic will direct you to option 1. Review this content if you are unfamiliar with the action and use of this medication.

Reference
Lehne, R. (2007) *Pharmacology for nursing care* (6th ed., p. 322) Philadelphia: Saunders.

1523. A client is admitted to the hospital for a thyroidectomy. While preparing the client for surgery, the nurse assesses the client for psychosocial problems that may cause preoperative anxiety, knowing that a realistic source of anxiety is fear of:

 1 Sexual dysfunction and infertility
 2 Imposed dietary restrictions after discharge
 3 Developing gynecomastia and hirsutism postoperatively
 4 Changes in body image secondary to the location of the incision

Answer: 4

Rationale: Because the incision is in the neck area, the client may be fearful of having a large scar postoperatively. Sexual dysfunction and infertility could possibly occur if the entire thyroid gland was removed and if the client was not placed on thyroid replacement medications. The client will not have specific dietary restrictions after discharge. Having all or part of the thyroid gland removed will not cause the client to experience gynecomastia or hirsutism.

Test-Taking Strategy: Use the process of elimination, focusing on the surgical procedure. Recalling the location of the thyroid gland will direct you to option 4. Review the psychosocial concerns of the client following thyroidectomy if you had difficulty with this question.

Level of Cognitive Ability: Analysis
Client Needs: Psychosocial Integrity
Integrated Process: Nursing Process/Assessment
Content Area: Adult Health/Endocrine

References
Black, J., & Hawks, J. (2005). *Medical-surgical nursing: Clinical management for positive outcomes* (7th ed., p. 1202). Philadelphia: Saunders.
Ignatavicius, D., & Workman, M. (2006). *Medical-surgical nursing: Critical thinking for collaborative care* (5th ed., p. 1496). Philadelphia: Saunders.
Lewis, S., Heitkemper, M., Dirksen, S., O'Brien, P., & Bucher, L. (2007). *Medical-surgical nursing: Assessment and management of clinical problems* (7th ed., p. 1304). St. Louis: Mosby.

1524. A provider prescribes intralipids intravenously for a client. Before initiating the intralipids, which should the nurse assess that is related to the infusion?
1 Allergies
2 Vital signs
3 History of seizures
4 Serum glucose level

Level of Cognitive Ability: Application
Client Needs: Physiological Integrity
Integrated Process: Nursing Process/Assessment
Content Area: Fundamental Skills

Answer: 1
Rationale: Before administering any medication, the nurse assesses for allergies to all of the agent's components. Fat emulsions such as intralipids contain an emulsifying agent made from egg yolks, so clients who are hypersensitive to eggs are at risk for developing hypersensitivity reactions. Options 2, 3, and 4 are unrelated to administering fat emulsion.

Test-Taking Strategy: Note the strategic words "Before initiating" and "related to the infusion." This will direct you to option 1. Review the content related to the administration of this solution if you had difficulty with this question.

Reference
Gahart, B., & Nazareno, A. (2006). *2006 Intravenous medications* (22nd ed., p. 540). St. Louis: Mosby.

1525. A client is admitted to the hospital with a myocardial infarction and is not experiencing chest pain at this time. The nurse reviews the ECG rhythm strip and notes that the PR intervals are 0.16 seconds. The nurse determines that this measurement indicates:
1 A normal finding
2 An abnormal finding
3 First-degree A-V block
4 An impending reinfarction

Level of Cognitive Ability: Analysis
Client Needs: Physiological Integrity
Integrated Process: Nursing Process/Analysis
Content Area: Adult Health/Cardiovascular

Answer: 1
Rationale: The PR interval represents the time it takes for the cardiac impulse to spread from the atria to the ventricles. The PR interval range is 0.12 to 0.2 seconds. Therefore, the finding is normal.

Test-Taking Strategy: Use the process of elimination and knowledge regarding ECG readings. Eliminate options 2, 3, and 4 because they are comparable or alike and all indicate an abnormal finding. Review basic ECG findings if you had difficulty with this question.

Reference
Black, J., & Hawks, J. (2005). *Medical-surgical nursing: Clinical management for positive outcomes* (7th ed., p. 1584). Philadelphia: Saunders.

1526. A nurse administers 30 units of NPH insulin at 7:00 AM to a client with a blood glucose level of 200 mg/dL. The nurse monitors the client for a hypoglycemic reaction, knowing that NPH insulin peaks in approximately how many hours following administration?
1 2 hours
2 3 to 4 hours
3 6 to 14 hours
4 16 to 24 hours

Answer: 3
Rationale: NPH is an intermediate-acting insulin with an onset of action in 60 to 120 minutes, a peak time in 6 to 14 hours, and a duration time of 16 to 24 hours.

Test-Taking Strategy: Knowledge of the onset, peak, and duration of NPH insulin is required. Recalling that NPH is an intermediate-acting insulin will direct you to option 3. Review the various types of insulin if you had difficulty with this question.

Level of Cognitive Ability: Application
Client Needs: Physiological Integrity
Integrated Process: Nursing Process/Assessment
Content Area: Pharmacology

Reference
Lehne, R. (2007). *Pharmacology for nursing care* (6th ed., pp. 652-653). Philadelphia: Saunders.

1527. A client with a psychotic disorder is being treated with haloperidol (Haldol). The nurse monitors the client for which of the following that indicates the presence of an adverse effect of this medication?

1 Nausea
2 Hypotension
3 Blurred vision
4 Excessive salivation

Level of Cognitive Ability: Application
Client Needs: Physiological Integrity
Integrated Process: Nursing Process/Assessment
Content Area: Pharmacology

Answer: 4
Rationale: Adverse effects of this medication include extrapyramidal symptoms such as marked drowsiness and lethargy, excessive salivation, a fixed stare, akathisia, acute dystonias, and tardive dyskinesia. Hypotension, nausea, and blurred vision are occasional side effects.

Test-Taking Strategy: Focus on the subject—an adverse effect. Use the process of elimination and select option 4 because of the word "excessive" in this option. Review the adverse effects of this medication if you had difficulty with this question.

Reference
Hodgson, B., & Kizior, R. (2007). *Saunders nursing drug handbook 2007* (p. 569). Philadelphia: Saunders.

1528. A home care nurse visits an older client with acute gouty arthritis. Indomethacin (Indocin) has been prescribed for the client, and the nurse teaches the client about the medication. Which statement by the client indicates that further teaching is necessary?

1 "I'll rest if I am having pain."
2 "I need to call the doctor if I notice a rash."
3 " I can take a pill whenever I need to for pain."
4 "I'll watch for any swollen feet or fingers or any stomach distress."

Level of Cognitive Ability: Analysis
Client Needs: Physiological Integrity
Integrated Process: Teaching and Learning
Content Area: Pharmacology

Answer: 3
Rationale: Indomethacin (Indocin) may be prescribed to treat gouty arthritis. It may alleviate pain but is administered on a scheduled time frame, not on an as-needed schedule. When pain occurs, the client will usually limit movement and rest. A rash should be reported because it could indicate hypersensitivity to the medication. The client should be instructed to monitor for swelling and gastric distress, which can be caused by the medication.

Test-Taking Strategy: Note the strategic words "further teaching is necessary." These words indicate a negative event query and the need to select the incorrect client statement. Recalling the action and purpose of indomethacin will direct you to option 3. Review this medication if you had difficulty with this question.

References
Hodgson, B., & Kizior, R. (2007). *Saunders nursing drug handbook 2007* (p. 617). Philadelphia: Saunders.
Lehne, R. (2007). *Pharmacology for nursing care* (6th ed., p. 818). Philadelphia: Saunders.

1529. A nurse is providing information to a community group about violence in the family. Which statement by a group member would indicate a need to provide additional information?

1 "Abusers use fear and intimidation."
2 "Abusers usually have poor self-esteem."
3 "Abusers are often jealous or self-centered."
4 "Abuse occurs more in low-income families."

Level of Cognitive Ability: Analysis
Client Needs: Psychosocial Integrity
Integrated Process: Teaching and Learning
Content Area: Mental Health

Answer: 4
Rationale: Personal characteristics of abusers include low self-esteem, immaturity, dependence, insecurity, and jealousy. Abusers will often use fear and intimidation to the point where their victims will do anything just to avoid further abuse. The statement that abuse occurs more in low-income families is inaccurate.

Test-Taking Strategy: Note the strategic words "need to provide additional information." These words indicate a negative event query and the need to select the incorrect statement. Use knowledge regarding the characteristics related to family violence to direct you to option 4. Review the characteristics of an abuser and family violence if you had difficulty with this question.

References
Stuart, G., & Laraia, M. (2005). *Principles and practice of psychiatric nursing* (8th ed., p. 805). St. Louis: Mosby.
Varcarolis, E., Carson, V., & Shoemaker, N. (2006) *Foundations of psychiatric mental health nursing* (5th ed., pp. 514-515, 519). Philadelphia: Saunders.

1530. Which of the following measures should the nurse plan to implement to prevent ventilator-associated pneumonia (VAP) in the client who is intubated and on mechanical ventilation?

1 Practice meticulous hand hygiene.
2 Maintain head of the bed elevation at 10 degrees.
3 Perform suctioning of oral cavity secretions every 4 hours.
4 Have the respiratory therapist change the ventilator circuit tubing every 4 hours.

Level of Cognitive Ability: Application
Client Needs: Physiological Integrity
Integrated Process: Nursing Process/Planning
Content Area: Adult Health/Respiratory

Answer: 1
Rationale: Because normal upper airway defenses are bypassed, clients who are intubated with mechanical ventilation are at risk for VAP. Prevention includes effective hand washing before and after suctioning, when touching ventilator equipment, and when in contact with respiratory secretions. The client will need oral suctioning more frequently than every 4 hours and at least 30-degree head of the bed elevation. It is not necessary to change the ventilator circuit tubing every 4 hours. The more frequently the circuit is broken, the greater the risk for pathogen entry.

Test-Taking Strategy: Use the process of elimination. Eliminate options 2 and 3 first because to prevent aspiration of colonized secretions from the oral cavity the client will need more frequent oral suctioning and at least 30 degrees head of the bed elevation. From the remaining options, eliminate option 4 because the more frequently the circuit is broken, the greater the risk for pathogen entry. Review measures to prevent VAP in the client who is intubated and on mechanical ventilation if you had difficulty with this question.

References
Ignatavicius, D., & Workman, M. (2006). *Medical-surgical nursing: Critical thinking for collaborative care* (5th ed., pp. 667-668). Philadelphia: Saunders.
Lewis, S., Heitkemper, M., Dirksen, S., O'Brien, P., & Bucher, L. (2007). *Medical-surgical nursing: Assessment and management of clinical problems* (7th ed., pp. 1764-1765). St. Louis: Mosby.

1531. A registered nurse asks a nursing student about suicide and suicide intentions. The registered nurse determines that the student understands the concepts associated with this topic if the student makes which statement?

  1 "Only the psychotic individual commits suicide."

  2 "Suicidal attempts are attention-seeking behaviors."

  3 "Suicide runs in the family, so there is nothing that health care personnel can do about it."

  4 "Many individuals who commit suicide have talked about their suicidal intentions to others."

Level of Cognitive Ability: Analysis
Client Needs: Psychosocial Integrity
Integrated Process: Teaching and Learning
Content Area: Mental Health

Answer: 4

Rationale: Most people who do commit suicide have given definite clues or warnings about their intentions. Suicide is not an inherited condition. A suicide attempt is not an attention-seeking behavior, and each act should be taken very seriously. The individual who is suicidal is not necessarily psychotic. Options 1, 2, and 3 are considered myths regarding suicide.

Test-Taking Strategy: Use the process of elimination. Eliminate option 1 because of the word "only." Eliminate option 2 because of the statement "attention-seeking behaviors." Eliminate option 3 because of the statement "there is nothing that health care personnel can do about it." Review concepts related to suicide if you had difficulty with this question.

Reference
Stuart, G., & Laraia, M. (2005). *Principles and practice of psychiatric nursing* (8th ed., p. 367). St. Louis: Mosby.

1532. A client wanders in and out of other clients' rooms, taking their possessions while singing to herself and then giggling for no apparent reason. The nurse reacts therapeutically by taking which action?

  1 Putting arms around the client, saying "You're okay. You just need a hug."

  2 Saying "I can see you are very anxious today. Let's go and play the piano."

  3 Taking the client to the seclusion room until she cooperates with unit rules.

  4 Taking the client to the lounge and saying "Sit here and try to behave yourself."

Level of Cognitive Ability: Application
Client Needs: Psychosocial Integrity
Integrated Process: Nursing Process/ Implementation
Content Area: Mental Health

Answer: 2

Rationale: The use of a defense mechanism allows a person to avoid the painful experience of anxiety or to transform it into a more tolerable symptom, such as regression. Regression allows the threatened client to move backward developmentally to a stage in which more security is felt. The recognition of regression is a signal that the client feels anxious. Option 2 will help the client feel less anxious. Option 1 does not address the client's anxiety. Options 3 and 4 are restrictive and degrading.

Test-Taking Strategy: Use the process of elimination. Recall that because anxiety consumes energy, it should be redirected into a healthier task. This will direct you to the correct option. Review defense mechanisms if you had difficulty with this question.

Reference
Stuart, G., & Laraia, M. (2005). *Principles and practice of psychiatric nursing* (8th ed., p. 280). St. Louis: Mosby.

1533. A nurse is caring for a human immuno-deficiency virus (HIV)-positive pregnant client. To help prevent the transmission of HIV from the woman to her fetus during the intrapartum period, the nurse plans to initiate measures to avoid:
1 Cesarean birth
2 Epidural anesthesia
3 External fetal monitoring
4 Direct (internal) fetal heart rate monitoring

Level of Cognitive Ability: Application
Client Needs: Safe and Effective Care Environment
Integrated Process: Nursing Process/ Implementation
Content Area: Maternity/Intrapartum

Answer: 4
Rationale: Health care professionals must use caution during the intrapartal period to reduce the risk of the transmission of HIV to the fetus. Any procedure that exposes blood or body fluids from the mother to the fetus should be avoided. Direct (internal) fetal monitoring is a procedure that may expose the fetus to maternal blood or body fluids and therefore should be avoided. Options 1, 2, and 3 are not invasive measures that place the fetus at risk in the intrapartum period.

Test-Taking Strategy: Note the strategic word "avoid." This word indicates a negative event query and the need to select the incorrect intervention. All of the options address procedures that may take place during the intrapartum period, but only option 4 is invasive with regard to the fetus. Recalling that transmission of HIV occurs primarily by the exchange of body fluids will direct you to option 4. Review this content area if you had difficulty with this question.

Reference
Murray, S., & McKinney, E. (2006). *Foundations of maternal-newborn nursing* (4th ed., p. 689). Philadelphia: Saunders.

1534. During electroconvulsive therapy (ECT), the client receives oxygen by mask via positive pressure ventilation. The nurse assisting with this procedure knows that positive pressure ventilation is necessary because:
1 Grand mal seizure activity depresses respirations.
2 Anesthesia is routinely administered during the ECT procedure.
3 Muscle relaxants given to prevent injury depress respirations.
4 Decreased oxygen to the brain increases confusion and disorientation.

Level of Cognitive Ability: Analysis
Client Needs: Physiological Integrity
Integrated Process: Nursing Process/Analysis
Content Area: Mental Health

Answer: 3
Rationale: A short-acting skeletal muscle relaxant such as succinylcholine (Anectine) is administered during this procedure to prevent injuries during the seizure. The client receives positive pressure ventilation until the muscle relaxant is metabolized, usually within 2 to 3 minutes. Options 1, 2, and 4 do not address the subject of the question and the specific reason for positive pressure ventilation.

Test-Taking Strategy: Use the process of elimination and focus on the subject. Recalling that a muscle relaxant is administered will direct you to option 3. Review this content if you are unfamiliar with the procedure for ECT.

Reference
Stuart, G., & Laraia, M. (2005). *Principles and practice of psychiatric nursing* (8th ed., pp. 606-607). St. Louis: Mosby.

1535. A client is in a coma of unknown cause, and the physician has written several orders for the client including the need for intubation. Which procedure should the nurse withhold until the client was properly intubated?
1 Gastric feeding
2 Urethral catheterization
3 Fingerstick for blood glucose level
4 Venipuncture for complete blood cell (CBC) count

Level of Cognitive Ability: Application
Client Needs: Physiological Integrity
Integrated Process: Nursing Process/ Implementation
Content Area: Adult Health/Neurological

Answer: 1
Rationale: Intubation should always precede gastric feeding to prevent pulmonary aspiration. All other options identify procedures that can be initiated before intubation of the client.

Test-Taking Strategy: Use the process of elimination and the ABCs—airway, breathing, and circulation. Recalling that the comatose client is at risk for aspiration will direct you to option 1. Review care of the comatose client if you had difficulty with this question.

References
Black, J., & Hawks, J. (2005). *Medical-surgical nursing: Clinical management for positive outcomes* (7th ed., pp. 2058, 2060). Philadelphia: Saunders.
Lewis, S., Heitkemper, M., Dirksen, S., O'Brien, P., & Bucher, L. (2007). *Medical-surgical nursing: Assessment and management of clinical problems* (7th ed., p. 1755). St. Louis: Mosby.

1536. A manic client is placed in a seclusion room after an outburst of violent behavior that included a physical assault on another client. As the client is secluded, the nurse should:
1 Remain silent because verbal interaction would be too stimulating.
2 Tell the client that he will be allowed to rejoin the others when he can behave.
3 Ask the client if he understands why the use of therapeutic seclusion is necessary.
4 Inform the client that he is being secluded for the purpose of helping regain control of self.

Level of Cognitive Ability: Application
Client Needs: Psychosocial Integrity
Integrated Process: Nursing Process/ Implementation
Content Area: Mental Health

Answer: 4.
Rationale: The client is removed to a nonstimulating environment as a result of behavior. Options 1, 2, and 3 are nontherapeutic. In addition, option 2 implies punishment. It is best to directly inform the client of the purpose of the seclusion.

Test-Taking Strategy: Use the process of elimination. Look for the option that presents reality most clearly to the client. Option 4 is the only option that provides a clear and direct purpose of the seclusion. Review care of the client requiring seclusion if you had difficulty with this question.

Reference
Stuart, G., & Laraia, M. (2005). *Principles and practice of psychiatric nursing* (8th ed., pp. 644, 646). St. Louis: Mosby.

1537. A nurse is providing instructions to a client regarding quinapril hydrochloride (Accupril). The nurse tells the client to:
1 Take the medication with food only.
2 Expect a therapeutic effect immediately.
3 Discontinue the medication if nausea occurs.
4 Rise slowly from a lying to a sitting position.

Answer: 4
Rationale: Accupril is an angiotensin-converting enzyme (ACE) inhibitor. It is used in the treatment of hypertension. The client should be instructed to rise slowly from a lying to sitting position and to permit the legs to dangle from the bed momentarily before standing to reduce the hypotensive effect. The medication does not need to be taken with meals. It may be given without regard to food. If nausea occurs, the client should be instructed to take a non-cola carbonated beverage and salted crackers or dry toast. A full therapeutic effect may be noted in 1 to 2 weeks.

Level of Cognitive Ability: Application
Client Needs: Physiological Integrity
Integrated Process: Teaching and Learning
Content Area: Pharmacology

Test-Taking Strategy: Use the process of elimination. Eliminate option 1 because of the close-ended word "only." From the remaining options, focus on the medication classification. Recalling that medication names that end with the letters "pril" indicate that the medication is an ACE inhibitor and that ACE inhibitors are used in the treatment of hypertension will direct you to option 4. Review the action of this medication and the associated client teaching points if you had difficulty with this question.

Reference

Hodgson, B., & Kizior, R. (2007). *Saunders nursing drug handbook 2007* (p. 996). Philadelphia: Saunders.

1538. A nurse is providing emergency treatment for a client in ventricular tachycardia and is preparing to defibrillate the client. Which nursing action provides for the safest environment during a defibrillation attempt?

  1 Ensuring that no lubricant is on the paddles
  2 Placing the charged paddles one at a time on the client's chest
  3 Holding the client's upper torso stable while the defibrillation is performed
  4 Performing a visual and verbal check that all assisting personnel are clear of the client and the client's bed

Level of Cognitive Ability: Application
Client Needs: Safe and Effective Care Environment
Integrated Process: Nursing Process/ Implementation
Content Area: Adult Health/Cardiovascular

Answer: 4
Rationale: Safety during defibrillation is essential for preventing injury to the client and to the personnel assisting with the procedure. The person performing the defibrillation ensures that all personnel are standing clear of the bed by a verbal and visual check of "all clear." For the shock to be effective, some type of conductive medium (e.g., lubricant, gel) must be placed between the paddles and the skin. Both paddles are placed on the client's chest.

Test-Taking Strategy: Use the process of elimination, focusing on the subject—safest environment. Option 4 involves a verbal and visual check of "all clear" providing for the safety of all involved. Review the procedure for defibrillation if you had difficulty with this question.

References

Black, J., & Hawks, J. (2005). *Medical-surgical nursing: Clinical management for positive outcomes* (7th ed., pp. 1685, 1689). Philadelphia: Saunders.
Lewis, S., Heitkemper, M., Dirksen, S., O'Brien, P., & Bucher, L. (2007). *Medical-surgical nursing: Assessment and management of clinical problems* (7th ed., p. 857). St. Louis: Mosby.

1539. A client is admitted to the emergency department with complaints of severe, radiating chest pain. The client is extremely restless, frightened, and dyspneic. Immediate admission orders include oxygen by nasal cannula at 4 liters per minute, troponin, creatinine phosphokinase and isoenzymes blood levels, a chest x-ray, and a 12-lead ECG. Which action should the nurse take first?

  1 Obtain the 12-lead ECG.
  2 Draw the blood specimens.
  3 Apply the oxygen to the client.
  4 Call radiology to order the chest x-ray study.

Answer: 3
Rationale: The first action would be to apply the oxygen because the client can be experiencing myocardial ischemia. The ECG can provide evidence of cardiac damage and the location of myocardial ischemia. However, oxygen is the priority to prevent further cardiac damage. Drawing the blood specimens would be done after oxygen administration and just before or after the ECG, depending on the situation. Although the chest x-ray can show cardiac enlargement, having the chest x-ray would not influence immediate treatment.

Test-Taking Strategy: Note the strategic word "first." Remember that the immediate goal of therapy is to prevent myocardial ischemia. The only option that will achieve that goal is option 3. Also, use the ABCs—airway, breathing, and circulation—to direct you to option 3. Review care of the client with a myocardial infarction if you had difficulty with this question.

Level of Cognitive Ability: Application
Client Needs: Physiological Integrity
Integrated Process: Nursing Process/
  Implementation
Content Area: Adult Health/Cardiovascular

References
Black, J., & Hawks, J. (2005). *Medical-surgical nursing: Clinical management for positive outcomes* (7th ed., p. 1721). Philadelphia: Saunders.
Lewis, S., Heitkemper, M., Dirksen, S., O'Brien, P., & Bucher, L. (2007). *Medical-surgical nursing: Assessment and management of clinical problems* (7th ed., p. 806). St. Louis: Mosby.

1540. Chemical cardioversion is prescribed for the client with atrial fibrillation. The nurse who is assisting in preparing the client would expect that which medication specific for chemical cardioversion will be needed?
  1 Nitroglycerin
  2 Nifedipine (Procardia)
  3 Lidocaine (Xylocaine)
  4 Amiodarone (Cordarone)

Level of Cognitive Ability: Analysis
Client Needs: Physiological Integrity
Integrated Process: Nursing Process/Analysis
Content Area: Adult Health/Cardiovascular

Answer: 4
Rationale: Amiodarone is an antidysrhythmic that is useful in restoring normal sinus rhythm for the client experiencing atrial fibrillation. Both nitroglycerin and nifedipine are vasodilators. Lidocaine is used for control of ventricular dysrhythmias.

Test-Taking Strategy: Note the strategic words "chemical cardioversion." Recalling the action of these medications and that amiodarone is an antidysrhythmic for both atrial and ventricular dysrhythmias will direct you to option 4. Review this content if you are unfamiliar with these medications or with preprocedure care.

References
Black, J., & Hawks, J. (2005). *Medical-surgical nursing: Clinical management for positive outcomes* (7th ed., p. 1679). Philadelphia: Saunders.
Hodgson, B., & Kizior, R. (2007). *Saunders nursing drug handbook 2007* (pp. 997-998). Philadelphia: Saunders.

1541. A registered nurse is observing a nursing student auscultate the breath sounds of a client. The registered nurse intervenes if the nursing student performs which incorrect action?
  1 Uses the bell of the stethoscope
  2 Asks the client to sit straight up
  3 Places the stethoscope directly on the client's skin
  4 Has the client breathe slowly and deeply through the mouth

Level of Cognitive Ability: Analysis
Client Needs: Health Promotion and
  Maintenance
Integrated Process: Nursing Process/Assessment
Content Area: Leadership/Management

Answer: 1
Rationale: The bell of the stethoscope is not used to auscultate breath sounds. The client ideally should sit up and breathe slowly and deeply through the mouth. The diaphragm of the stethoscope, which is warmed before use, is placed directly on the client's skin, not over a gown or clothing.

Test-Taking Strategy: Note the strategic words "intervenes" and "incorrect." These words indicate a negative event query and the need to select the incorrect action by the nursing student. Visualizing each action and the procedure for auscultating breath sounds will direct you to option 1. Review auscultation as a basic physical assessment technique if you had difficulty with this question.

References
Huber, D. (2006). *Leadership and nursing care management* (3rd ed., p. 75). Philadelphia: Saunders.
Lewis, S., Heitkemper, M., Dirksen, S., O'Brien, P., & Bucher, L. (2007). *Medical-surgical nursing: Assessment and management of clinical problems* (7th ed., pp. 522-523). St. Louis: Mosby.

1542. The home care nurse cares for an obese adult client. The client has a sprained right ankle, has not exercised for more than 1 week, and has missed the last two physical therapy appointments. The client says, "I attend therapy for my ankle and I do my exercises three times a day." Which response should the nurse use with the client?

1 "Show me the exercises that you perform in physical therapy."
2 "You will never heal if you skip the physical therapy sessions."
3 "Your progress sounds fine. Is more physical therapy scheduled?"
4 "I see that you missed the last two physical therapy appointments."

Level of Cognitive Ability: Application
Client Needs: Psychosocial Integrity
Integrated Process: Communication and Documentation
Content Area: Fundamental Skills

Answer: 4
Rationale: In option 4, the nurse employs the therapeutic communication technique of confrontation. Because the client is employing avoidance, the nurse presents the facts according to the medical record to assess the client's perspective without accusing, threatening, or humiliating the client about the missed physical therapy. By confronting, the nurse assists the client with problem solving. Option 1 is potentially helpful when the client is complying with therapy. In option 2, the nurse provides an opinion and this statement admonishes the client for the behavior. In option 3, the nurse is nontherapeutic in giving approval and is mirroring the client's avoidance and passivity by not dealing directly with the problem of missed appointments.

Test-Taking Strategy: Use therapeutic communication techniques and the process of elimination. Option 4 is the only option that promotes problem solving by additional client assessment. Review therapeutic communication techniques if you had difficulty with this question.

Reference
Potter, P., & Perry, A. (2005) *Fundamentals of nursing* (6th ed., p. 437). St. Louis: Mosby.

1543. A client with unstable ventricular tachycardia (VT) loses consciousness and becomes pulseless after an initial treatment with a dose of lidocaine (Xylocaine) intravenously. The nurse caring for the client would immediately obtain which of the following needed items?

1 A pacemaker
2 A defibrillator
3 A second dose of lidocaine
4 An electrocardiogram machine

Level of Cognitive Ability: Application
Client Needs: Physiological Integrity
Integrated Process: Nursing Process/ Implementation
Content Area: Adult Health/Cardiovascular

Answer: 2
Rationale: For the client with VT who becomes pulseless, the physician or qualified advanced cardiac life support personnel immediately defibrillates the client. In the absence of this equipment, cardiopulmonary resuscitation is initiated immediately. Options 1, 3, and 4 are not items that are needed immediately in this situation.

Test-Taking Strategy: Use the process of elimination, noting the strategic word "immediately" and that the client is in VT. Options 3 and 4 should be eliminated first, because option 3 was unsuccessful and option 4 is of no use. From the remaining options, focusing on the subject will direct you to option 2. Review the immediate measures for VT if you had difficulty with this question.

References
Gahart, B., & Nazareno, A. (2006). *2006 Intravenous medications* (22nd ed., p. 758). St. Louis: Mosby.
Ignatavicius, D., & Workman, M. (2006). *Medical-surgical nursing: Critical thinking for collaborative care* (5th ed., pp. 729, 731). Philadelphia: Saunders.

1544. The nurse has done preoperative teaching with a client scheduled for percutaneous insertion of an inferior vena cava (IVC) filter. The nurse determines that the client needs further clarification if the client stated that the procedure:

1 Is done under general anesthesia
2 Is rarely associated with complications
3 Eliminates the need for anticoagulant therapy
4 May cause congestion when clots get trapped at the filter

Level of Cognitive Ability: Analysis
Client Needs: Physiological Integrity
Integrated Process: Teaching and Learning
Content Area: Adult Health/Cardiovascular

Answer: 1
Rationale: Complications after insertion of an IVC filter are rare. When they do occur, they include air embolism, improper placement, and filter migration. The percutaneous approach uses local anesthesia. There is usually no need for anticoagulant therapy after surgery. Venous congestion can occur from accumulation of thrombi on the filter, but the process usually occurs gradually.

Test-Taking Strategy: Note the strategic words "needs further clarification." These words indicate a negative event query and the need to select the incorrect client statement. Noting the words "percutaneous insertion" in the question should direct you to option 1. General anesthesia is not used in this procedure. Review this procedure if you had difficulty with this question.

References
Ignatavicius, D., & Workman, M. (2006). *Medical-surgical nursing: Critical thinking for collaborative care* (5th ed., p. 815). Philadelphia: Saunders.
Lewis, S., Heitkemper, M., Dirksen, S., O'Brien, P., & Bucher, L. (2007). *Medical-surgical nursing: Assessment and management of clinical problems* (7th ed., p. 915). St. Louis: Mosby.

1545. A client with a head injury and a feeding tube continuously tries to remove the tube. The nurse contacts the physician who prescribes the use of restraints. After checking the agency's policy and procedure regarding the use of restraints, the nurse uses which method in restraining the client?

1 Vest restraint
2 Waist restraint
3 Wrist restraints
4 Mitten restraints

Level of Cognitive Ability: Application
Client Needs: Physiological Integrity
Integrated Process: Nursing Process/ Implementation
Content Area: Adult Health/Neurological

Answer: 4
Rationale: Mitten restraints are useful for this client because the client cannot pull against them, creating resistance that could lead to increased intracranial pressure (ICP). Wrist restraints cause resistance. Vest and waist restraints prevent the client from getting up or falling out of bed but do nothing to limit hand movement.

Test-Taking Strategy: Use the process of elimination and focus on the subject—a restraint that safely limits hand movement for this client. Eliminate options 1 and 2 because they do not address this subject. From the remaining options, thinking about the concern of ICP in a client with a head injury will direct you to option 4. Review care of the client with a head injury if you had difficulty with this question.

References
Ignatavicius, D., & Workman, M. (2006). *Medical-surgical nursing: Critical thinking for collaborative care* (5th ed., p. 1053). Philadelphia: Saunders.
Potter, P., & Perry, A. (2005) *Fundamentals of nursing* (6th ed., p. 986). St. Louis: Mosby.

1546. A nurse has oriented a new employee to basic procedures for continuous electro-cardiogram (ECG) monitoring. The nurse would intervene if the new employee did which of the following while initiating cardiac monitoring on a client?

1 Clipped small areas of hair under the area planned for electrode placement
2 Stated the need to change the electrodes and inspect the skin every 24 hours
3 Stated the need to use hypoallergenic electrodes for clients who are sensitive
4 Cleansed the skin with Betadine (povidone-iodine) before applying the electrodes

Level of Cognitive Ability: Application
Client Needs: Safe and Effective Care Environment
Integrated Process: Teaching and Learning
Content Area: Leadership/Management

Answer: 4
Rationale: The skin is cleansed with soap and water (not Betadine), denatured with alcohol, and allowed to air-dry before electrodes are applied. The other three options are correct.

Test-Taking Strategy: Note the strategic word "intervene." This word indicates a negative event query and the need to select the incorrect action. Eliminate options 2 and 3 because they are correct procedure. From the remaining options, remember that Betadine is used to cleanse the skin usually before some type of invasive procedure that breaks the skin barrier. ECG monitoring does not break the skin. Review the procedure for initiating cardiac monitoring if you had difficulty with this question.

References
Black, J., & Hawks, J. (2005). *Medical-surgical nursing: Clinical management for positive outcomes* (7th ed., p. 1583). Philadelphia: Saunders.
Potter, P., & Perry, A. (2005) *Fundamentals of nursing* (6th ed., p. 1513). St. Louis: Mosby.

1547. A client has been defibrillated three times using an automatic external defibrillator (AED). The nurse observes that the attempts to convert the ventricular fibrillation (VF) were unsuccessful. Based on an evaluation of the situation, the nurse determines that which action would be best?

1 Terminating the resuscitation effort
2 Preparing for the administration of sodium bicarbonate intravenously
3 Performing cardiopulmonary resuscitation (CPR) for 5 minutes, then defibrillating three more times at 400 joules
4 Performing cardiopulmonary resuscitation (CPR) for 1 minute, then defibrillating up to three more times at 360 joules

Level of Cognitive Ability: Analysis
Client Needs: Physiological Integrity
Integrated Process: Nursing Process/Analysis
Content Area: Adult Health/Cardiovascular

Answer: 4
Rationale: After three unsuccessful defibrillation attempts, CPR should be done for 1 minute, followed by three more shocks, each delivered at 360 joules. There is no information in the question to indicate that life support should be terminated. Sodium bicarbonate may be prescribed but is not the best action. Giving CPR for 5 minutes may not help oxygenation to the brain and myocardium and is not the best action. It would be best to administer CPR for 1 minute and then resume attempts to convert the rhythm to a viable one.

Test-Taking Strategy: Use the process of elimination and knowledge regarding the treatment for VF. There is no information in the question to indicate that life support should be terminated, so option 1 is eliminated first. From the remaining options, focusing on the strategic word "best" and recalling the treatment for VF will direct you to option 4. Review the treatment for VF if you had difficulty with this question.

Reference
Ignatavicius, D., & Workman, M. (2006). *Medical-surgical nursing: Critical thinking for collaborative care* (5th ed., p. 742). Philadelphia: Saunders.

1548. The nurse is inserting an oropharyngeal airway into an assigned client. The nurse plans to use which correct insertion procedure?

1 Flex the client's neck
2 Leave any dentures in place
3 Suction the client's mouth once per shift
4 Insert the airway with the tip pointed upward

Answer: 4
Rationale: Before insertion of an oropharyngeal airway, any dentures or partial plates should be removed from the client's mouth. An airway should be selected that is an appropriate size. The client should be positioned supine, with the neck hyperextended if possible. The airway is inserted with the tip pointed upward and is then rotated downward once the flange has reached the client's teeth. Following insertion, the client's mouth is suctioned every hour or as necessary. The airway is removed for inspection of the mouth every 2 to 4 hours.

Level of Cognitive Ability: Application
Client Needs: Physiological Integrity
Integrated Process: Nursing Process/Planning
Content Area: Adult Health/Respiratory

Test-Taking Strategy: Note the strategic words "correct insertion procedure." Eliminate option 3 because this is not part of the insertion procedure. Next eliminate option 1, because the neck is hyperextended (unless contraindicated) to open the airway. From the remaining options, recall that dentures should be removed because they are a potential source of airway obstruction. Review this procedure if you had difficulty with this question.

Reference
Perry, A., & Potter, P. (2006) *Clinical nursing skills & techniques* (6th ed., pp. 881-882). St. Louis: Mosby.

1549. The home care nurse visits a client who started wandering around at 10:00 PM each evening and got out of the house for the first time last night. The family asks for help. Which response should the nurse make to the family?
   1 "What prevented her from leaving the house in the past?"
   2 "You cannot handle this alone because she could get hurt."
   3 "I think you need to consider a nursing home immediately."
   4 "This is a common problem known as sundowner's syndrome."

Level of Cognitive Ability: Application
Client Needs: Psychosocial Integrity
Integrated Process: Nursing Process/
   Implementation
Content Area: Fundamental Skills

Answer: 1
Rationale: The nurse responds to the family by assessing the situation and collecting additional data regarding the change in the client's behavior. The best response focuses on the family's problem so the nurse can help develop potential strategies. Option 2 is giving advice. Option 3 is histrionic, invalidates the family's attempt to manage the client's care, and potentially causes resentment. Option 4 provides the nurse's conclusion based on an incomplete assessment; other factors may be causing confusion.

Test-Taking Strategy: Use therapeutic communication techniques and the steps of the nursing process because the nurse needs more information before planning care; thus, determining that the correct option must be assessment directs you to option 1. Review therapeutic communication techniques and interventions for caregivers if you had difficulty with this question.

Reference
Potter, P., & Perry, A. (2005) *Fundamentals of nursing* (6th ed., pp. 19, 609-610). St. Louis: Mosby.

1550. The home care nurse visits an older adult female client who asks the nurse to buy some groceries for her because she is not feeling well today. Which statement should the nurse use in response?
   1 "I am not allowed to buy groceries for clients."
   2 "Let's discuss how we can solve this problem."
   3 "Do you have any support systems for shopping?"
   4 "Nurses are professionals and do not run errands."

Level of Cognitive Ability: Application
Client Needs: Psychosocial Integrity
Integrated Process: Communication and
   Documentation
Content Area: Fundamental Skills

Answer: 2
Rationale: The nurse's duty is to help the client; but, in helping the client, the nurse's first action is to finish the assessment and then find immediate and long-term solutions to the problem. In option 1, the nurse uses a passive approach and hides behind policies and rules, even though this can be true. In option 3, the nurse asks a closed-ended question, which is unlikely to further nurse-client communication. Option 4 is inappropriate and indicates that the nurse thinks more of status than of helping the client.

Test-Taking Strategy: Use the process of elimination and therapeutic communication techniques. Option 2 is the only option that addresses the client's problem and provides the means to problem solve. Review therapeutic communication techniques if you had difficulty with this question.

Reference
Potter, P., & Perry, A. (2005) *Fundamentals of nursing* (6th ed., p. 437). St. Louis: Mosby.

1551. A nurse is caring for a client who is being treated with an intravenous (IV) bolus of lidocaine hydrochloride (Xylocaine). The nurse understands the actions and the effects of the medication and plans to monitor which of the following?

1 Urinary pH
2 Radial pulse
3 Temperature
4 Respiratory status and blood pressure

Level of Cognitive Ability: Application
Client Needs: Physiological Integrity
Integrated Process: Nursing Process/ Implementation
Content Area: Pharmacology

Answer: 4
Rationale: The nurse is responsible for monitoring the client's respiratory status and blood pressure while the client is being treated with an IV bolus of lidocaine hydrochloride. The urinary pH and temperature are not related to this medication. It is best to monitor the apical pulse in this client.

Test-Taking Strategy: Use the ABCs—airway, breathing, and circulation—to answer the question. This should direct you to option 4. Review nursing responsibilities when a client receives lidocaine hydrochloride if you had difficulty with this question.

References
Gahart, B., & Nazareno, A. (2006). *2006 Intravenous medications* (22nd ed., p. 761). St. Louis: Mosby.
Mosby. (2007). *Mosby's nursing drug reference* (20th ed., p. 606). St. Louis: Mosby.

1552. A client has an order for seizure precautions, and a nursing student develops a plan of care for the client. The registered nurse reviews the plan of care with the student and will instruct the student to remove which of the following interventions?

1 Keep all the lights on in the room at night.
2 Assist the client to ambulate in the hallway.
3 Monitor the client closely while the client is showering.
4 Push the lock-out button on the electric bed to keep the bed in the lowest position.

Level of Cognitive Ability: Application
Client Needs: Safe and Effective Care Environment
Integrated Process: Teaching and Learning
Content Area: Leadership/Management

Answer: 1
Rationale: A quiet, restful environment is provided as part of seizure precautions. This includes undisturbed times for sleep, while using a nightlight for safety. The client should be accompanied during activities such as bathing and walking, so that assistance is readily available and injury is minimized if a seizure begins. The bed is maintained in low position for safety.

Test-Taking Strategy: Note the strategic words "instruct the student to remove." These words indicate a negative event query and the need to select the incorrect intervention. Focus on the subject, seizure precautions. Noting the word "all" in option 1 and thinking about the importance of a quiet, restful environment will direct you to this option. Review care of the client on seizure precautions if you had difficulty with this question.

Reference
Ignatavicius, D., & Workman, M. (2006). *Medical-surgical nursing: Critical thinking for collaborative care* (5th ed., pp. 953-954). Philadelphia: Saunders.

1553. A nurse is caring for a child who sustained a head injury from a fall. The nurse avoids which of the following in the care of this child?

1 Forcing fluids
2 Performing neurological assessments
3 Keeping the child in a sitting-up position
4 Keeping the child awake as much as possible

Answer: 1
Rationale: A child with a head injury is at risk for increased intracranial pressure (ICP). Neurological assessments need to be performed to monitor for increased ICP. Sitting up will decrease fluid retention in cerebral tissue and promote drainage. Keeping the child awake will assist in accurate evaluation of any cerebral edema that is present and will detect early coma. Forcing fluids may cause fluid overload and increased ICP. Additionally, the nurse would not "force" the client to do something.

Level of Cognitive Ability: Application
Client Needs: Physiological Integrity
Integrated Process: Nursing Process/
   Implementation
Content Area: Child Health

Test-Taking Strategy: Note the strategic word "avoids." Use the process of elimination and knowledge regarding increased ICP. Eliminate options 2, 3, and 4 because they are correct in terms of monitoring for and preventing increased ICP. Additionally, noting the word "forcing" in option 1 will direct you to this option. Review measures to prevent increased ICP if you had difficulty with this question.

References

Hockenberry, M., & Wilson, D. (2007). *Nursing care of infants and children* (8th ed., p. 1020). St. Louis: Mosby.
McKinney, E., James, S., Murray, S., & Ashwill, J. (2005). *Maternal-child nursing* (2nd ed., p. 1500). St. Louis: Saunders.

1554. A nurse has conducted a stress-management seminar for clients in an ambulatory care setting. Which statement by a client would indicate that further instruction is needed?
1 "Biofeedback might be nice, but I don't like the idea of having to use equipment."
2 "Using confrontation with coworkers should solve my problems at work quickly."
3 "I can use those guided imagery techniques I've learned anywhere and anytime."
4 "The progressive muscle relaxation technique should ease my tension headaches."

Level of Cognitive Ability: Analysis
Client Needs: Psychosocial Integrity
Integrated Process: Teaching and Learning
Content Area: Mental Health

Answer: 2
Rationale: Biofeedback, progressive muscle relaxation, meditation, and guided imagery are techniques that the nurse can teach the client to reduce the physical impact of stress on the body and promote a feeling of self-control for the client. Biofeedback entails electronic equipment, whereas the others require no adjuncts, such as tapes, once the technique is learned. Confrontation is a communication technique, not a stress-management technique. It may also exacerbate stress, at least in the short term, rather than alleviate it.

Test-Taking Strategy: Note the strategic words "further instruction is needed." These words indicate a negative event query and the need to select the incorrect statement. Recalling the methods of stress management techniques guides you to option 2, which is a communication technique rather than a stress-management technique. Review stress-management techniques if you had difficulty with this question.

References

Stuart, G., & Laraia, M. (2005). *Principles and practice of psychiatric nursing* (8th ed., pp. 292-293). St. Louis: Mosby.
Varcarolis, E., Carson, V., & Shoemaker, N. (2006) *Foundations of psychiatric mental health nursing* (5th ed., pp. 724-725). Philadelphia: Saunders.

1555. The nurse is caring for a client with a peptic ulcer. In assessing the client for gastrointestinal perforation, the nurse monitors for:
1 Slow, strong pulses
2 Increase in bowel sounds
3 Positive guaiac stool tests
4 Sudden, severe abdominal pain

Answer: 4
Rationale: Sudden, severe abdominal pain is the most indicative sign of perforation. When perforation of an ulcer occurs, the nurse may be unable to hear bowel sounds at all. When perforation occurs, the pulse will more likely be weak and rapid. Positive guaiac stool results indicate the presence of bleeding but are not necessarily indicative of perforation.

Test-Taking Strategy: Use the process of elimination, focusing on the subject—the signs of perforation. Correlate perforation with sudden, severe abdominal pain. Remember that the nurse may be unable to hear bowel sounds and that the pulse will most likely be weak and rapid. Positive guaiac stool results are not specific to perforation. Review the signs of perforation if you had difficulty with this question.

Level of Cognitive Ability: Application
Client Needs: Physiological Integrity
Integrated Process: Nursing Process/Assessment
Content Area: Adult Health/Gastrointestinal

References
Ignatavicius, D., & Workman, M. (2006). *Medical-surgical nursing: Critical thinking for collaborative care* (5th ed., pp. 1289, 1294, 1296). Philadelphia: Saunders.
Lewis, S., Heitkemper, M., Dirksen, S., O'Brien, P., & Bucher, L. (2007). *Medical-surgical nursing: Assessment and management of clinical problems* (7th ed., p. 1532). St. Louis: Mosby.

1556. Human albumin (Albuminar) administered intravenously is prescribed for a client with burns of the anterior chest and both legs. The nurse reviews the client's medical record to identify the presence of any existing conditions that would be a contraindication in the use of human albumin. The nurse contacts the physician before administering the human albumin if which of the following is noted in the client's record?
1 Diabetes mellitus
2 Multiple myeloma
3 Renal insufficiency
4 Lymphocytic leukemia

Level of Cognitive Ability: Application
Client Needs: Safe and Effective Care Environment
Integrated Process: Nursing Process/ Implementation
Content Area: Pharmacology

Answer: 3
Rationale: Human albumin (Albuminar) is classified as a blood derivative and is contraindicated in severe anemia, cardiac failure, history of allergic reaction, renal insufficiency, and when no albumin deficiency is present. It is used with caution in clients with low cardiac reserve, pulmonary disease, or hepatic or renal failure.

Test-Taking Strategy: Use the process of elimination and focus on the subject—a contraindication. Eliminate options 2 and 4 first because they are comparable or alike in that they are oncological disorders. From the remaining options, recalling that albumin restores intravascular volume will assist in directing you to option 3. Review this blood derivative if you had difficulty with this question.

References
Gahart, B., & Nazareno, A. (2006). *2006 Intravenous medications* (22nd ed., p. 22). St. Louis: Mosby.
Mosby. (2007). *Mosby's nursing drug reference* (20th ed., p. 88). St. Louis: Mosby.

1557. A male newborn is in the neonatal intensive care unit for respiratory distress syndrome (RDS) and surfactant replacement therapy has been given. The nurse evaluates the infant 1 hour after the surfactant therapy and determines that the infant's condition has improved somewhat. Which of the following, if observed by the nurse, indicates improvement?
1 Unequal breath sounds
2 Increased work of breathing
3 Decreased need for supplemental oxygen
4 Increased level of carbon dioxide (CO_2) in the blood gas analysis

Level of Cognitive Ability: Analysis
Client Needs: Physiological Integrity
Integrated Process: Nursing Process/Evaluation
Content Area: Child Health

Answer: 3
Rationale: A decreased need for supplemental oxygen indicates an improvement in the infant's ability to use oxygen. The increased work of breathing indicates air hunger and the need for further support. Unequal breath sounds may indicate atelectasis or blocked airways. Increased levels of CO_2 would indicate increasing respiratory acidosis and not improvement of oxygenation.

Test-Taking Strategy: Use the process of elimination, focusing on the strategic word "improvement." Noting the word "increased" in options 2 and 4 will assist in eliminating these options. From the remaining options, recall that "unequal" does not indicate improvement. Review the expected effects of surfactant therapy if you had difficulty with this question.

Reference
Wong, D., Hockenberry, M., Perry, S., Lowdermilk, D. & Wilson, D. (2006). *Maternal-child nursing care.* (3rd ed., p. 814). St. Louis: Mosby.

1558. The nurse is evaluating the effectiveness of antimicrobial therapy for a client with infective endocarditis. The nurse determines that which finding documented in the client's health record is the least reliable indicator of effectiveness?
1 Clear breath sounds
2 Systolic heart murmur
3 Temperature of 98.8° F
4 Negative blood cultures

Level of Cognitive Ability: Analysis
Client Needs: Physiological Integrity
Integrated Process: Nursing Process/Evaluation
Content Area: Adult Health/Cardiovascular

Answer: 2
Rationale: A systolic heart murmur, once present, will not resolve spontaneously and is therefore the least reliable indicator. Negative blood cultures and normothermia indicate resolution of infection. Clear breath sounds are a normal finding, and in this instance could mean resolution of heart failure, if that was accompanying the endocarditis.

Test-Taking Strategy: Note the strategic words "least reliable indicator." The question is worded to look for the finding that will not respond to antimicrobial therapy and that is an abnormal finding. The only option that meets these criteria is option 2, which does not resolve once it has developed. Review care of the client with infective endocarditis if you had difficulty with this question.

References
Ignatavicius, D., & Workman, M. (2006). *Medical-surgical nursing: Critical thinking for collaborative care* (5th ed., p. 768). Philadelphia: Saunders.
Lewis, S., Heitkemper, M., Dirksen, S., O'Brien, P., & Bucher, L. (2007). *Medical-surgical nursing: Assessment and management of clinical problems* (7th ed., p. 867). St. Louis: Mosby.

1559. The nurse is caring for a client with continuous electrocardiogram (ECG) monitoring. The nurse notes that the ECG complexes are very small and hard to evaluate. The nurse checks which setting on the ECG monitor console?
1 Power button
2 Low rate alarm
3 High rate alarm
4 Amplitude or "gain"

Level of Cognitive Ability: Application
Client Needs: Physiological Integrity
Integrated Process: Nursing Process/ Implementation
Content Area: Adult Health/Cardiovascular

Answer: 4
Rationale: The power button turns the machine on and off. The low and high alarm settings indicate the heart rate limits beyond which an alarm will sound. The amplitude, commonly called "gain," regulates the size of the complex and can be adjusted up and down to some degree.

Test-Taking Strategy: Focus on the subject—the complexes are small and hard to evaluate. Eliminate options 2 and 3 first because they are comparable or alike. From the remaining options, noting the relation of the subject to the word "amplitude" (meaning size or strength) in option 4 will direct you to this option. Review the procedure for the use of an ECG monitor if you had difficulty with this question.

References
Black, J., & Hawks, J. (2005). *Medical-surgical nursing: Clinical management for positive outcomes* (7th ed., p. 1586). Philadelphia: Saunders.
Ignatavicius, D., & Workman, M. (2006). *Medical-surgical nursing: Critical thinking for collaborative care* (5th ed., p. 711). Philadelphia: Saunders.

1560. The nurse is monitoring a client who has received antidysrhythmic therapy for the treatment of premature ventricular contractions (PVCs). The nurse would determine this therapy as being less than optimal if the client's PVCs continued to:
1 Occur in pairs
2 Be unifocal in appearance
3 Be fewer than six per minute
4 Fall after the end of the T wave

Answer: 1
Rationale: PVCs are considered dangerous when they are frequent (more than six per minute), occur in pairs or couplets, are multifocal (multiform), or fall on the T wave.

Level of Cognitive Ability: Analysis
Client Needs: Physiological Integrity
Integrated Process: Nursing Process/Evaluation
Content Area: Adult Health/Cardiovascular

Test-Taking Strategy: Note the strategic words "less than optimal." These words indicate a negative event query and the need to select the option that identifies ineffective treatment. Knowledge regarding the occurrence of PVCs and the situations in which they may be dangerous to the client will direct you to option 1. Review this basic information if you had difficulty with this question.

Reference

Black, J., & Hawks, J. (2005). *Medical-surgical nursing: Clinical management for positive outcomes* (7th ed., p. 1682). Philadelphia: Saunders.

1561. The nurse is reviewing the client's arterial blood gas results. Which finding would indicate that the client had respiratory acidosis?

1 pH 7.5, Pco_2 30
2 pH 7.3, Pco_2 50
3 pH 7.3, Pco_2 19
4 pH 7.5, Pco_2 30

Level of Cognitive Ability: Analysis
Client Needs: Physiological Integrity
Integrated Process: Nursing Process/Analysis
Content Area: Adult Health/Respiratory

Answer: 2

Rationale: In respiratory acidosis, the pH is decreased and an opposite effect is seen in the Pco_2 (pH decreased, Pco_2 elevated). Option 1 indicates respiratory alkalosis; option 3 indicates possible metabolic acidosis; and option 4 indicates possible metabolic alkalosis.

Test-Taking Strategy: Use the process of elimination. Recalling that the pH is decreased in acidosis will assist in eliminating options 1 and 4. Next, remember that in respiratory acidosis the Pco_2 has an opposite effect from the pH. This will direct you to option 2. Review these basic interpretations if you had difficulty with this question.

References

Black, J., & Hawks, J. (2005). *Medical-surgical nursing: Clinical management for positive outcomes* (7th ed., p. 254). Philadelphia: Saunders.
Ignatavicius, D., & Workman, M. (2006). *Medical-surgical nursing: Critical thinking for collaborative care* (5th ed., p. 283). Philadelphia: Saunders.

1562. The nurse is assigned to care for a client with a chest tube attached to closed chest drainage. The nurse determines that the client's lung has completely expanded if:

1 Pleuritic chest pain has resolved
2 The oxygen saturation is greater than 92%
3 Fluctuations in the water-seal chamber ceased
4 Suction in the chest drainage system is no longer needed

Answer: 3

Rationale: When the lung has completely expanded, there is no longer air or fluid in the pleural space to be drained into the water-seal chamber. Thus, an indication that a chest tube is ready for removal is when fluctuations in the water-seal chamber cease and drainage of fluid into the collection bottle/chamber ceases. Adequate oxygen saturation does not imply that the lung has fully reexpanded. Although air is known to be an irritant to pleural tissue, cessation of pleuritic pain does not indicate that the lung is expanded. The chest tube acts as an irritant and therefore contributes to pain. Use or nonuse of suction in the chest drainage system is not necessarily governed by the degree of lung expansion. Suction is indicated when gravity is not sufficient to drain air and pleural fluid or if the client has a poor respiratory effort and cough. Suction increases the speed at which air and fluid is removed from the pleural space.

Level of Cognitive Ability: Analysis
Client Needs: Physiological Integrity
Integrated Process: Nursing Process/Evaluation
Content Area: Adult Health/Respiratory

Test-Taking Strategy: Note the strategic words "completely expanded." Eliminate options 1 and 2 because they are not directly related to a chest tube drainage system. From the remaining options, recalling the functioning of chest tubes will direct you to option 3. Review chest tube drainage systems if you had difficulty with this question.

Reference

Black, J., & Hawks, J. (2005). *Medical-surgical nursing: Clinical management for positive outcomes* (7th ed., p. 1866). Philadelphia: Saunders.

1563. A nurse is caring for a child with leukemia and notes that the platelet count is 20,000/mm³. Based on this finding, the nurse plans to delete which of the following from the plan of care?
  1 Monitor stools for blood.
  2 Clean oral cavity with soft swabs.
  3 Provide appropriate play activities.
  4 Administer acetaminophen (Tylenol) suppositories for fever.

Level of Cognitive Ability: Application
Client Needs: Physiological Integrity
Integrated Process: Nursing Process/Planning
Content Area: Child Health

Answer: 4
Rationale: A platelet count of 20,000/mm³ places the child at risk for bleeding. Options 1, 2, and 3 are accurate interventions. The use of suppositories is avoided because of the risk of rectal bleeding.

Test-Taking Strategy: Note the strategic word "deletes." This word indicates a negative event query and the need to select the intervention that is contraindicated. Noting the subject of the question—bleeding—and recalling the interventions related to bleeding precautions will direct you to option 4. Review interventions for the child at risk for bleeding if you had difficulty with this question.

References

Hockenberry, M., Wilson, D., & Winkelstein, M. (2005). *Wong's essentials of pediatric nursing* (7th ed., p. 960). St. Louis: Mosby.
McKinney, E., James, S., Murray, S., & Ashwill, J. (2005). *Maternal-child nursing* (2nd ed., p. 1340). St. Louis: Saunders.

1564. It has been 12 hours since the client's delivery of a newborn. The nurse assesses the client for the process of involution and documents that it is progressing normally when palpation of the client's fundus is noted at which level?
  1 At the umbilicus
  2 One fingerbreadth below the umbilicus
  3 Two fingerbreadths above the umbilicus
  4 Two fingerbreadths below the umbilicus

Answer: 1
Rationale: The term "involution" is used to describe the rapid reduction in size and the return of the uterus to a normal condition similar to its pregnant state. Immediately following the delivery of the placenta, the uterus contracts to the size of a large grapefruit. The fundus is situated in the midline between the symphysis pubis and the umbilicus. Within 6 to 12 hours after birth, the fundus of the uterus rises to the level of the umbilicus. The top of the fundus remains at the level of the umbilicus for about a day and then descends into the pelvis approximately one fingerbreadth on each succeeding day.

Test-Taking Strategy: Note the strategic words "it has been 12 hours." Attempt to visualize the process of assessment of involution and the expected finding at this time to answer the question. Remember that within 6 to 12 hours after birth, the fundus of the uterus rises to the level of the umbilicus, remaining at this level for about a day, and then descends into the pelvis approximately one fingerbreadth on each succeeding day. Review this process if you had difficulty with this question.

Level of Cognitive Ability: Application
Client Needs: Health Promotion and Maintenance
Integrated Process: Nursing Process/Assessment
Content Area: Maternity/Postpartum

Reference
Murray, S., & McKinney, E. (2006). *Foundations of maternal-newborn nursing* (4th ed., p. 394). Philadelphia: Saunders.

1565. The nurse evaluates the arterial blood gas (ABG) results of a client who is receiving supplemental oxygen. Which finding would indicate that the oxygen level was adequate?

    1 A Po_2 of 80 mm Hg
    2 A Po_2 of 60 mm Hg
    3 A Po_2 of 50 mm Hg
    4 A Po_2 of 45 mm Hg

Level of Cognitive Ability: Comprehension
Client Needs: Physiological Integrity
Integrated Process: Nursing Process/Evaluation
Content Area: Adult Health/Respiratory

Answer: 1
Rationale: The normal Po_2 level is 80 to 100 mm Hg. Options 2, 3, and 4 are low values and do not indicate adequate oxygen levels.

Test-Taking Strategy: Focus on the subject—oxygen level was adequate. Use the process of elimination and select the option that identifies the highest oxygen level. This will direct you to option 1. Review interpretation of the results of ABGs if you had difficulty with this question.

Reference
Black, J., & Hawks, J. (2005). *Medical-surgical nursing: Clinical management for positive outcomes* (7th ed., pp. 252-253, 1764). Philadelphia: Saunders.

1566. A client has been taking lisinopril (Prinivil) for 3 months. The client complains to the nurse of a persistent dry cough that began about 1 month ago. The nurse interprets that this is most likely:

    1 Caused by neutropenia as a result of therapy
    2 Caused by a concurrent upper respiratory infection
    3 An expected, though bothersome, side effect of therapy
    4 An indication that the client will show signs of heart failure

Level of Cognitive Ability: Analysis
Client Needs: Physiological Integrity
Integrated Process: Nursing Process/Analysis
Content Area: Pharmacology

Answer: 3
Rationale: A frequent side effect of therapy with any of the angiotensin-converting enzyme (ACE) inhibitors, such as lisinopril, is the appearance of a persistent, dry cough. The cough generally does not improve while the client is taking the medication. Clients are advised to notify the physician if the cough becomes very troublesome to them. The other options are incorrect.

Test-Taking Strategy: Use the process of elimination. Eliminate options 1 and 2 first because they are comparable or alike and focus on infection. From the remaining options, it is necessary to know the frequent side effects of this medication to direct you to option 3. Review the side effects of ACE inhibitor therapy if you had difficulty with this question.

Reference
Mosby. (2007). *Mosby's nursing drug reference* (20th ed., p. 613). St. Louis: Mosby.

1567. The nurse is developing a plan of care for a client with acquired immunodeficiency syndrome (AIDS). The nurse documents which appropriate goal in the plan of care?

    1 The client has no increased platelet aggregation.
    2 The client has a urinary output of 50 mL per hour.
    3 The client does not experience respiratory distress.
    4 The client has no evidence of dissecting aortic aneurysm.

Answer: 3
Rationale: A common, life-threatening opportunistic infection that attacks clients with AIDS is *Pneumocystis jiroveci* pneumonia. Its symptoms include fever, exertional dyspnea, and nonproductive cough. The absence of respiratory distress is one of the goals that the nurse sets as a priority. Options 1, 2, and 4 are not specifically related to the subject of the question.

Level of Cognitive Ability: Application
Client Needs: Physiological Integrity
Integrated Process: Nursing Process/
    Implementation
Content Area: Adult Health/Respiratory

Test-Taking Strategy: Note the subject of the question. Option 3 is the only option that is directly related to the client's diagnosis. In addition, use the ABCs—airway, breathing, and circulation—to answer the question. Review care of the client with AIDS if you had difficulty with this question.

Reference
Ignatavicius, D., & Workman, M. (2006). *Medical-surgical nursing: Critical thinking for collaborative care* (5th ed., p. 433). Philadelphia: Saunders.

1568. A client with active tuberculosis (TB) is to be admitted to a medical-surgical unit. When planning a bed assignment, the nurse:
  1 Places the client in a private, well-ventilated room
  2 Assigns the client to a double room because intravenous antibiotics will be administered
  3 Assigns the client to a double room and places a "strict handwashing" sign outside the door
  4 Plans to transfer the client to the intensive care unit

Level of Cognitive Ability: Application
Client Needs: Safe and Effective Care
    Environment
Integrated Process: Nursing Process/Planning
Content Area: Leadership/Management

Answer: 1
Rationale: According to category-specific (respiratory) isolation precautions, a client with TB requires a private room. The room needs to be well-ventilated and should have at least six exchanges of fresh air per hour and should be ventilated to the outside if possible. Therefore, option 1 is the only correct option.

Test-Taking Strategy: Note that the question states "active tuberculosis." Eliminate options 2 and 3 because they are comparable or alike in that they involve assignment to a double room. From the remaining options, recalling the need for respiratory isolation precautions will direct you to option 1. Review care of the client with active tuberculosis if you had difficulty with this question.

Reference
Ignatavicius, D., & Workman, M. (2006). *Medical-surgical nursing: Critical thinking for collaborative care* (5th ed., p. 644). Philadelphia: Saunders.

1569. A client develops an irregular heart rate. Which statement by the client indicates to the nurse that the client is ready for learning?
  1 "I feel weak with an irregular pulse."
  2 "What is it like to have a pacemaker?"
  3 "All my medications will be changed now."
  4 "How can this heart rate problem affect me?"

Answer: 4
Rationale: Learning depends on two things: physical and emotional readiness to learn. Without one or the other, teaching can occur, but learning may not take place. A good time to teach is when the client indicates an interest in learning, is motivated, and is physically capable of concentrating on learning. Option 4 addresses the client's readiness because the client is directly asking about the disorder. Option 1 indicates that the client is potentially incapable of learning at this time. The client indicates wanting to learning about pacemakers in option 2; however, the client has formed a hasty conclusion because the need for a pacemaker has not been determined. In option 3, by assuming that the medications will change, the client is emotionally unprepared for learning because the statement is based on incomplete data.

Test-Taking Strategy: Use the process of elimination. Note that option 4 directly addresses the client's diagnosis. Review teaching-learning principles if you had difficulty with this question.

Level of Cognitive Ability: Comprehension
Client Needs: Psychosocial Integrity
Integrated Process: Teaching and Learning
Content Area: Fundamental Skills

References
Ignatavicius, D., & Workman, M. (2006). *Medical-surgical nursing: Critical thinking for collaborative care* (5th ed., pp. 8, 680). Philadelphia: Saunders.
Lewis, S., Heitkemper, M., Dirksen, S., O'Brien, P., & Bucher, L. (2007). *Medical-surgical nursing: Assessment and management of clinical problems* (7th ed., pp. 54-55). St. Louis: Mosby.

1570. A provider prescribes intralipids for a client who is receiving parenteral nutrition (PN). The nurse explains to the client that the fat emulsion is administered:
1 To provide essential fatty acids
2 As a supplement to fluid intake
3 To decrease the risk of phlebitis
4 During the night in place of parenteral nutrition

Level of Cognitive Ability: Application
Client Needs: Physiological Integrity
Integrated Process: Teaching and Learning
Content Area: Fundamental Skills

Answer: 1
Rationale: Intralipids are a brand of intravenous fat emulsion administered to clients who are at risk for developing an essential fatty acid deficiency, such as clients receiving PN. Fat emulsions help to meet caloric and nutritional needs that cannot be met by glucose administration alone. Fat emulsions are not administered to increase the amount of body fluids (option 2) and they do not decrease the incidence of phlebitis (option 3). Fat emulsions neither replace PN nor do they require infusion during the night (option 4).

Test-Taking Strategy: Focus on the subject—intravenous fat emulsion—and use the principles about intralipids to choose the correct option. Remember that fat emulsion is administered to prevent fatty acid deficiency. Review the purpose of administering fat emulsion during PN therapy if you had difficulty with this question.

References
Black, J., & Hawks, J. (2005). *Medical-surgical nursing: Clinical management for positive outcomes* (7th ed., p. 706). Philadelphia: Saunders.
Gahart, B., & Nazareno, A. (2006). *2006 Intravenous medications* (22nd ed., p. 540). St. Louis: Mosby.

1571. A client with valvular heart disease is at risk for developing congestive heart failure. The nurse assesses which of the following closely when monitoring for congestive heart failure?
1 Heart rate
2 Breath sounds
3 Blood pressure
4 Activity tolerance

Level of Cognitive Ability: Analysis
Client Needs: Physiological Integrity
Integrated Process: Nursing Process/Assessment
Content Area: Delegating/Prioritizing

Answer: 2
Rationale: Breath sounds are the best way to assess for the onset of congestive heart failure. The presence of crackles or an increase in crackles is an indicator of fluid in the lungs caused by congestive heart failure. Options 1, 3, and 4 are components of the assessment but are less reliable indicators of congestive heart failure.

Test-Taking Strategy: Use the process of elimination, thinking about the pathophysiology that occurs with congestive heart failure. Use of the ABCs—airway, breathing, and circulation—will direct you to option 2. Review assessment of congestive heart failure if you had difficulty with this question.

References
Black, J., & Hawks, J. (2005). *Medical-surgical nursing: Clinical management for positive outcomes* (7th ed., p. 1653, 1655). Philadelphia: Saunders.
Ignatavicius, D., & Workman, M. (2006). Medical-surgical nursing: Critical thinking for collaborative care (5th ed., pp. 750, 764-765). Philadelphia: Saunders.

1572. The nurse is caring for a client receiving fludrocortisone acetate (Florinef) for the treatment of Addison's disease. The nurse monitors the client for improvement, knowing that the anticipated therapeutic effect of this medication is to:

1 Promote electrolyte balance.
2 Stimulate thyroid production.
3 Stimulate the immune response.
4 Stimulate thyrotropin production.

Level of Cognitive Ability: Analysis
Client Needs: Physiological Integrity
Integrated Process: Nursing Process/Evaluation
Content Area: Adult Health/Endocrine

Answer: 1
Rationale: Florinef is a long-acting oral medication with mineralocorticoid and moderate glucocorticoid activity that is used for long-term management of Addison's disease. Mineralocorticoids act on the renal distal tubules to enhance the reabsorption of sodium and chloride ions and the excretion of potassium and hydrogen ions. The client can rapidly develop hypotension and fluid and electrolyte imbalance if the medication is discontinued abruptly. The medication does not affect the immune response or thyroid or thyrotropin production.

Test-Taking Strategy: Remember that Addison's disease produces deficiencies of glucocorticoids, mineralocorticoids, and androgens. Eliminate options 2 and 4 first because they are comparable or alike. From the remaining options, recalling that Addison's disease is not related to the immune system will direct you to option 1. Review the action of this medication if you had difficulty with this question.

References
Black, J., & Hawks, J. (2005). *Medical-surgical nursing: Clinical management for positive outcomes* (7th ed., p. 1219). Philadelphia: Saunders.
Hodgson, B., & Kizior, R. (2007). *Saunders nursing drug handbook 2007* (p. 488). Philadelphia: Saunders.
Ignatavicius, D., & Workman, M. (2006). *Medical-surgical nursing: Critical thinking for collaborative care* (5th ed., p. 1473). Philadelphia: Saunders.

1573. The nurse is assessing the leg pain of a client who has just undergone right femoral-popliteal artery bypass grafting. Which question would be most useful in determining whether the client is experiencing graft occlusion?

1 "Can you describe what the pain feels like?"
2 "Can you rate the pain on a scale of 1 to 10?"
3 "Did you get any relief from the last dose of pain medication?"
4 "Can you compare this pain to the pain you felt before surgery?"

Level of Cognitive Ability: Application
Client Needs: Physiological Integrity
Integrated Process: Nursing Process/Assessment
Content Area: Adult Health/Cardiovascular

Answer: 4
Rationale: The most frequent indication that a graft is occluding is the return of pain that is similar to that experienced preoperatively. Standard pain assessment techniques also include the items described in options 1, 2, and 3, but these will not help differentiate current pain from preoperative pain.

Test-Taking Strategy: Focus on the subject—the assessment question that will help differentiate expected postoperative pain from pain that indicates graft occlusion. Eliminate options 1, 2, and 3 because they are comparable or alike and are standard pain assessment questions. Review care of the client following this type of surgery if you had difficulty with this question.

Reference
Black, J., & Hawks, J. (2005). *Medical-surgical nursing: Clinical management for positive outcomes* (7th ed., pp. 1518-1519). Philadelphia: Saunders.

1574. A client has implemented dietary and other lifestyle changes to manage hypertension. The nurse determines that the client has been most successful if the client has a follow-up blood pressure reading of:

1 156/89 mm Hg
2 128/84 mm Hg
3 164/90 mm Hg
4 140/94 mm Hg

Level of Cognitive Ability: Comprehension
Client Needs: Physiological Integrity
Integrated Process: Nursing Process/Evaluation
Content Area: Adult Health/Cardiovascular

Answer: 2
Rationale: Normal blood pressure readings are less than 120/80 mm Hg. A blood pressure reading between 120/80 mm Hg and 139/89 mm Hg is considered to be a prehypertensive state. From the readings provided in the options, option 2 identifies the most successful outcome, although the reading indicates a prehypertensive state.

Test-Taking Strategy: Note the strategic words "most successful." Option 2 identifies a reading that is closest to normal even though it identifies a prehypertensive state. Review the definitions of prehypertension and hypertension if you had difficulty with this question.

References
Black, J., & Hawks, J. (2005). *Medical-surgical nursing: Clinical management for positive outcomes* (7th ed., p. 1497). Philadelphia: Saunders.
Monahan, F., Sands, J., Marek, J., Neighbors, M., & Green, C. (2007). *Medical-surgical nursing: Health and illness perspectives* (8th ed., p. 859). St. Louis: Mosby.

1575. A client is scheduled to have surgery. The nurse should place highest priority on determining whether the surgeon wants which of the following medications held in the preoperative period?

1 Furosemide (Lasix)
2 Famotidine (Pepcid)
3 Warfarin (Coumadin)
4 Multivitamin with minerals

Level of Cognitive Ability: Analysis
Client Needs: Physiological Integrity
Integrated Process: Nursing Process/Analysis
Content Area: Adult Health/Cardiovascular

Answer: 3
Rationale: The nurse is careful to question the surgeon about whether warfarin should be administered in the preoperative period. This medication is often withheld for a period of time preoperatively to minimize the risk of hemorrhage during surgery. The other medications may also be withheld if specifically ordered, but usually they are discontinued as part of an NPO (nothing by mouth) after midnight order.

Test-Taking Strategy: Note the strategic words "highest priority." Recalling that warfarin is an anticoagulant and that when a client is taking an anticoagulant a risk for bleeding exists will direct you to option 3. Review anticoagulant medication therapy and preoperative nursing care if you had difficulty with this question.

References
Black, J., & Hawks, J. (2005). *Medical-surgical nursing: Clinical management for positive outcomes* (7th ed., pp. 1832-1833). Philadelphia: Saunders.
Lewis, S., Heitkemper, M., Dirksen, S., O'Brien, P., & Bucher, L. (2007). *Medical-surgical nursing: Assessment and management of clinical problems* (7th ed., pp. 915-916). St. Louis: Mosby.

1576. A client's medical record states a history of intermittent claudication. In collecting data about this symptom, the nurse would ask the client about which symptom?

1 Leg pain that is sharp and occurs with exercise
2 Chest pain that is dull and feels like heartburn
3 Chest pain that is sudden and occurs with exertion
4 Leg pain that is achy and gets worse as the day progresses

Answer: 1
Rationale: Intermittent claudication is a symptom characterized by a sudden onset of leg pain that occurs with exercise and is relieved by rest. It is the classic symptom of peripheral arterial insufficiency. Venous insufficiency is characterized by an achy type of leg pain that intensifies as the day progresses. Chest pain can occur for a variety of reasons, including indigestion (option 2) or angina pectoris (option 3).

Level of Cognitive Ability: Application
Client Needs: Physiological Integrity
Integrated Process: Nursing Process/Assessment
Content Area: Adult Health/Cardiovascular

Test-Taking Strategy: Use the process of elimination. Focusing on the strategic word "intermittent" in the question will direct you to option 1. Review this content area if you had difficulty with this question or if you are unfamiliar with the term "intermittent claudication."

Reference

Black, J., & Hawks, J. (2005). *Medical-surgical nursing: Clinical management for positive outcomes* (7th ed., p. 1476). Philadelphia: Saunders.

1577. A client has just been diagnosed with right leg deep vein thrombosis (DVT). The nurse immediately implements which intervention?

1 Ice packs to the right leg
2 Elevation of the right leg
3 Hourly calf measurements
4 Vigorous range of motion to the right leg

Level of Cognitive Ability: Application
Client Needs: Physiological Integrity
Integrated Process: Nursing Process/ Implementation
Content Area: Adult Health/Cardiovascular

Answer: 2

Rationale: Treatment for DVT may require bedrest, leg elevation, and application of warm moist heat to the affected leg. The client may have calf measurements ordered once per shift or once per day, but they would not be obtained hourly. Option 1 is incorrect because heat may be prescribed, not cold. Option 4 is dangerous to the client, because vigorous activity after clot formation can cause pulmonary embolus.

Test-Taking Strategy: Focus on the client's diagnosis and use knowledge of the treatment for DVT as well as concepts related to gravity and the applications of heat and cold to answer the question. Review the interventions for this disorder if you had difficulty with this question.

Reference

Black, J., & Hawks, J. (2005). *Medical-surgical nursing: Clinical management for positive outcomes* (7th ed., pp. 1540-1541). Philadelphia: Saunders

---

1578. A client is scheduled to have a serum digoxin (Lanoxin) level obtained. The nurse should plan to have the blood sample drawn:

1 Just before a dose is given
2 One hour after a dose is given
3 Just after a dose has been given
4 One-half hour after a dose is given

Level of Cognitive Ability: Application
Client Needs: Physiological Integrity
Integrated Process: Nursing Process/Planning
Content Area: Adult Health/Cardiovascular

Answer: 1

Rationale: The purpose of a serum digoxin (Lanoxin) level is to record the serum concentration of the medication to ensure that it is in the therapeutic range. Serum digoxin levels are most often drawn before a dose, although they may be drawn 6 to 8 hours after a dose was administered. Drawing the medication before a dose ensures that the level is not falsely elevated.

Test-Taking Strategy: Eliminate options 2, 3, and 4 because they are comparable or alike. Each of these options requires the blood sample to be drawn within a relatively short period after the client has been given the medication. Review this laboratory test if you had difficulty with this question.

References

Ignatavicius, D., & Workman, M. (2006). *Medical-surgical nursing: Critical thinking for collaborative care* (5th ed., p. 762). Philadelphia: Saunders.

Kee, J., Hayes, E., & McCuistion, L. (2006). *Pharmacology: A nursing process approach.* (5th ed., p. 610). Philadelphia: Saunders.

1579. The nurse assesses the environmental safety of a client receiving home oxygen therapy. Which observation does the nurse use to plan additional client teaching?
1 Oxygen used 30 feet from a gas stove
2 Oxygen tank stored in the tank holder
3 "No smoking" sign posted at the front door
4 Oxygen concentrator propped against a wall

Level of Cognitive Ability: Analysis
Client Needs: Safe and Effective Care Environment
Integrated Process: Nursing Process/Assessment
Content Area: Fundamental Skills

Answer: 4
Rationale: The oxygen concentrator should be free and clear of walls or other enclosed spaces to allow adequate air circulation around the unit; otherwise the unit can overheat and increase the risk of fire. Clients should avoid using oxygen within 10 feet or more of open flames because oxygen fuels a fire (option 1). Oxygen tanks are secured in a holder to stabilize and protect the tank (option 2), and a "no smoking" sign should be in plain view to alert visitors about the risk (option 3).

Test-Taking Strategy: Note the strategic words "the client needs instructions." These words indicate a negative event query and the need to select the incorrect client action. Recalling the principles of safe oxygen use will direct you to option 4. Review these safety principles if you had difficulty with this question.

References
Lewis, S., Heitkemper, M., Dirksen, S., O'Brien, P., & Bucher, L. (2007). *Medical-surgical nursing: Assessment and management of clinical problems* (7th ed., p. 644). St. Louis: Mosby.
Potter, P., & Perry, A. (2005) *Fundamentals of nursing* (6th ed., p. 1122). St. Louis: Mosby.

1580. The nurse has finished suctioning the tracheostomy of a client. The nurse determines the effectiveness of the procedure by monitoring which item?
1 Breath sounds
2 Capillary refill
3 Respiratory rate
4 Oxygen saturation level

Level of Cognitive Ability: Analysis
Client Needs: Physiological Integrity
Integrated Process: Nursing Process/Evaluation
Content Area: Adult Health/Respiratory

Answer: 1
Rationale: After suctioning a client either with or without an artificial airway, the breath sounds are auscultated to determine the extent to which the airways have been cleared of respiratory secretions. The other assessment items are not as precise as breath sounds for this purpose.

Test-Taking Strategy: Use the process of elimination, focusing on the subject—evaluating the effectiveness of suctioning. Recalling that the purpose of suctioning is to clear the airways of secretions will direct you to option 1. Review the procedure for suctioning if you had difficulty with this question.

Reference
Potter, P., & Perry, A. (2005) *Fundamentals of nursing* (6th ed., pp. 1101, 1108-1109). St. Louis: Mosby.

1581. A nurse has given a client directions for proper use of aluminum hydroxide tablets (Alu-Caps). The client indicates an understanding of the medication if which statement is made?
1 "I should take the tablet at the same time as an antacid."
2 "I should take each dose with a laxative to prevent constipation."
3 "I should swallow the tablet whole with a full glass of water."
4 "I should chew the tablet thoroughly and then drink 4 ounces of water."

Answer: 4
Rationale: Aluminum hydroxide tablets should be chewed thoroughly before swallowing. This prevents them from entering the small intestine undissolved. They should not be swallowed whole. Antacids should be taken at least 2 hours apart from other medications to prevent interactive effects. Constipation is a side effect of the use of aluminum products, but the client should not take a laxative with each dose. This promotes laxative abuse. The client should first try other means to prevent constipation.

Level of Cognitive Ability: Analysis
Client Needs: Physiological Integrity
Integrated Process: Nursing Process/Evaluation
Content Area: Pharmacology

Test-Taking Strategy: Use the process of elimination. Eliminate option 2 first because it does not promote healthy bowel function. Next, eliminate option 1 using general knowledge of antacid interactive effects. From the remaining options, use principles of digestion and medication use to direct you to option 4. Review client teaching points related to the use of this medication if you had difficulty with this question.

References
Kee, J., Hayes, E., & McCuistion, L. (2006). *Pharmacology: A nursing process approach.* (5th ed., p. 712). Philadelphia: Saunders.
Lehne, R. (2007). *Pharmacology for nursing care* (6th ed., p. 901). Philadelphia: Saunders.

1582. The nurse is checking a client's disposable closed chest drainage system at the beginning of the shift and notes continuous bubbling in the water-seal chamber. The nurse interprets that:
1 The system is intact.
2 A pneumothorax is resolving.
3 The suction to the system is shut off.
4 There is an air leak somewhere in the system.

Level of Cognitive Ability: Analysis
Client Needs: Physiological Integrity
Integrated Process: Nursing Process/Evaluation
Content Area: Adult Health/Respiratory

Answer: 4
Rationale: Continuous bubbling in the water-seal chamber through both inspiration and expiration indicates that air is leaking into the system. A resolving pneumothorax would show intermittent bubbling in the water-seal chamber with respiration. Shutting the suction off to the system stops bubbling in the suction control chamber, but does not affect the water-seal chamber.

Test-Taking Strategy: Use the process of elimination and focus on the subject—continuous bubbling in the water-seal chamber. The words "continuous bubbling" should provide you with the clue that an air leak is present. Review the concepts associated with a chest tube drainage system if you had difficulty with this question.

Reference
Black, J., & Hawks, J. (2005). *Medical-surgical nursing: Clinical management for positive outcomes* (7th ed., p. 1863). Philadelphia: Saunders.

1583. A client is suspected of having pulmonary tuberculosis. The nurse assesses the client for which signs and symptoms of tuberculosis?
1 High fever and chest pain
2 Increased appetite, dyspnea, and chills
3 Weight gain, insomnia, and night sweats
4 Low-grade fever, fatigue, and productive cough

Level of Cognitive Ability: Application
Client Needs: Physiological Integrity
Integrated Process: Nursing Process/Assessment
Content Area: Adult Health/Respiratory

Answer: 4
Rationale: The client with pulmonary tuberculosis generally has a productive or nonproductive cough, anorexia and weight loss, fatigue, low-grade fever, chills and night sweats, dyspnea, hemoptysis, and chest pain. Breath sounds may reveal crackles.

Test-Taking Strategy: Use the process of elimination. Remember that when an option has more than one part, all of the parts of that option must be correct if the entire option is to be correct. Eliminate options 2 and 3 first because the client will not have an increased appetite or weight gain. From the remaining options, it is necessary to know that the fever will be low grade. Review findings related to tuberculosis if you had difficulty with this question.

Reference
Black, J., & Hawks, J. (2005). *Medical-surgical nursing: Clinical management for positive outcomes* (7th ed., pp. 1845-1846). Philadelphia: Saunders.

1584. A nurse is preparing to implement emergency care measures for the client who has just experienced pulmonary embolism. The nurse implements which of the following physician orders first?
1 Apply oxygen.
2 Administer morphine sulfate.
3 Start an intravenous (IV) line.
4 Obtain an electrocardiogram (ECG).

Level of Cognitive Ability: Application
Client Needs: Physiological Integrity
Integrated Process: Nursing Process/
  Implementation
Content Area: Delegating/Prioritizing

Answer: 1
Rationale: The client needs immediate oxygen because of hypoxemia, which is most often accompanied by respiratory distress and cyanosis. The client should have an IV line for the administration of emergency medications such as morphine sulfate. An ECG is useful in determining the presence of possible right ventricular hypertrophy. All of the interventions listed are appropriate, but the client needs the oxygen first.

Test-Taking Strategy: Note the strategic word "first." Use the process of elimination and the ABCs—airway, breathing, and circulation. This will direct you to option 1. Review care of the client with pulmonary embolism if you had difficulty with this question.

Reference
Ignatavicius, D., & Workman, M. (2006). *Medical-surgical nursing: Critical thinking for collaborative care* (5th ed., p. 652). Philadelphia: Saunders.

1585. A client is scheduled for bronchoscopy, and the registered nurse reviews the plan of care written by a nursing student. The registered nurse discusses revision of the plan with the nursing student if which incorrect intervention was documented?
1 Removing any dentures
2 Removing contact lenses
3 Letting the client eat or drink
4 Obtaining a signed informed consent

Level of Cognitive Ability: Application
Client Needs: Physiological Integrity
Integrated Process: Nursing Process/
  Implementation
Content Area: Leadership/Management

Answer: 3
Rationale: The client is not allowed to eat or drink for usually 6 to 8 hours (or as specified by the physician) before the procedure. The client must sign an informed consent, because the procedure is invasive. If the client has any contact lenses, dentures, or other prostheses, they are removed before sedation is administered to the client.

Test-Taking Strategy: Note the strategic words "incorrect intervention." These words indicate a negative event query and the need to select the incorrect intervention. Recalling that for many invasive procedures the client must be on nothing by mouth status (NPO) will direct you to option 3. Review care of the client undergoing bronchoscopy if you had difficulty with this question.

References
Chernecky, C., & Berger, B. (2008). *Laboratory tests and diagnostic procedures* (5th ed., p. 263). Philadelphia: Saunders.
Pagana, K., & Pagana, T. (2005). *Mosby's diagnostic and laboratory test reference* (7th ed., p. 207). St. Louis: Mosby.

1586. A client who has no history of immunosuppressive disease and is at low risk for tuberculosis has a Mantoux test. The results indicate an area of induration that is 8 mm in size. The nurse interprets that the client:
1 Has active tuberculosis
2 Has a negative response
3 Has a history of tuberculosis
4 Has been exposed to tuberculosis

Answer: 2
Rationale: Induration of 15 mm or more is considered positive for clients in low-risk groups. More than 5 mm of induration is considered a positive result for clients with known or suspected human immunodeficiency virus infection, intravenous drug users, people in close contact with a known case of tuberculosis, and the client with a chest x-ray study suggestive of previous tuberculosis. More than 10 mm of induration is considered positive in all other high-risk groups.

Level of Cognitive Ability: Analysis
Client Needs: Physiological Integrity
Integrated Process: Nursing Process/Analysis
Content Area: Adult Health/Respiratory

Test-Taking Strategy: Use the process of elimination and note the strategic words "at low risk." Noting that the area of induration measures 8 mm will direct you to option 2. Review the normal parameters for this test if you had difficulty with this question.

Reference
Black, J., & Hawks, J. (2005). *Medical-surgical nursing: Clinical management for positive outcomes* (7th ed., p. 1846). Philadelphia: Saunders.

1587. A client has an order to have a set of arterial blood gases (ABGs) drawn, and the intended site is the radial artery. The nurse ensures that which of the following is positive before the ABGs are drawn?
1 Allen test
2 Homans' sign
3 Babinski reflex
4 Brudzinski's sign

Level of Cognitive Ability: Analysis
Client Needs: Physiological Integrity
Integrated Process: Nursing Process/Analysis
Content Area: Adult Health/Respiratory

Answer: 1
Rationale: The Allen test is performed before drawing ABGs. Each of the radial and ulnar arteries is occluded in turn and then released. Observation is made in the distal circulation. If the results are positive, then the client has adequate circulation, and that site may be used. Homans' sign tests for deep vein thrombosis with dorsiflexion of the foot. The Babinski reflex is checked by stroking upward on the sole of the foot. Brudzinski's sign tests for nuchal rigidity by bending the head down toward the chest.

Test-Taking Strategy: Note the strategic words "radial artery." Recalling the purpose of each test listed in the options will direct you to option 1. Review these tests if you had difficulty with this question.

Reference
Pagana, K., & Pagana, T. (2005). *Mosby's diagnostic and laboratory test reference* (7th ed., p. 122). St. Louis: Mosby.

1588. A client has been taking benzonatate (Tessalon) as ordered. The nurse tells the client that this medication should do which of the following?
1 Increase comfort level.
2 Decrease anxiety level.
3 Calm the persistent cough.
4 Take away nausea and vomiting.

Level of Cognitive Ability: Application
Client Needs: Physiological Integrity
Integrated Process: Teaching and Learning
Content Area: Pharmacology

Answer: 3
Rationale: Benzonatate is a locally acting antitussive. Its effectiveness is measured by the degree to which it decreases the intensity and frequency of cough, without eliminating the cough reflex. Options 1, 2, and 4 are not intended effects of this medication.

Test-Taking Strategy: Use the process of elimination and focus on the medication classification. Recalling that benzonatate is a locally acting antitussive will direct you to option 3. Review this content if you had difficulty with this question or if you are unfamiliar with this medication.

References
Kee, J., Hayes, E., & McCuistion, L. (2006). *Pharmacology: A nursing process approach.* (5th ed., p. 584). Philadelphia: Saunders.
Mosby. (2007). *Mosby's nursing drug reference* (20th ed., p. 174). St. Louis: Mosby.

1589. The nurse is assessing a client with a suspected rib fracture. The nurse observes for which typical symptoms?
  1 Pain on expiration, deep rapid respirations
  2 Pain on inspiration, deep rapid respirations
  3 Pain on expiration, shallow guarded respirations
  4 Pain on inspiration, shallow guarded respirations

Level of Cognitive Ability: Application
Client Needs: Physiological Integrity
Integrated Process: Nursing Process/Assessment
Content Area: Adult Health/Respiratory

Answer: 4
Rationale: The client with fractured ribs typically has pain over the fracture site with inspiration and to palpation. Respirations are shallow, and guarding of the area is often noted. Bruising may or may not be present.

Test-Taking Strategy: Focus on the client's diagnosis. Think about the movement of the chest wall on inspiration and expiration. Remember that pain will occur on inspiration and respirations will be shallow. Review the signs related to a rib fracture if you had difficulty with this question.

Reference
Ignatavicius, D., & Workman, M. (2006). *Medical-surgical nursing: Critical thinking for collaborative care* (5th ed., p. 670). Philadelphia: Saunders.

1590. A client with a flail chest caused by four fractured rib segments is experiencing severe pain when trying to breathe. The nurse observes the client for which characteristics of a flail chest?
  1 Cyanosis and slow respirations
  2 Slight tachypnea with shallow breaths
  3 Pallor and paradoxical chest movement
  4 Severe dyspnea and paradoxical chest movement

Level of Cognitive Ability: Analysis
Client Needs: Physiological Integrity
Integrated Process: Nursing Process/Assessment
Content Area: Adult Health/Respiratory

Answer: 4
Rationale: The client with flail chest is in obvious respiratory distress. The client has severe dyspnea and cyanosis accompanied by paradoxical chest movement. Respirations are shallow, rapid, and grunting in nature.

Test-Taking Strategy: Use the process of elimination. Remember that for an option to be correct, all of the parts of that option must also be correct. With this in mind, eliminate options 2 and 3 because of the words "slight" and "pallor." Choose between the remaining options, knowing that this client would be tachypneic, rather than having slow respirations. Review the clinical manifestations associated with flail chest if you had difficulty with this question.

Reference
Ignatavicius, D., & Workman, M. (2006). *Medical-surgical nursing: Critical thinking for collaborative care* (5th ed., p. 670). Philadelphia: Saunders.

1591. The nurse is assigned to care for a client with pneumonia. The nurse reviews the nursing care plan and notes documentation of a nursing diagnosis of Activity intolerance. The nurse implements which of the following in the client's care?
  1 Encourages deep, rapid breathing during activity
  2 Provides stimulation in the environment to maintain client alertness
  3 Observes vital signs and oxygen saturation periodically during activity
  4 Schedules activities before giving respiratory medications or treatments

Answer: 3
Rationale: The nurse monitors vital signs, including oxygen saturation, before, during, and after activity to gauge client response. Activities should be planned after giving the client respiratory medications or treatments to increase activity tolerance. The client should use pursed-lip and diaphragmatic breathing to lower oxygen consumption during activity. Finally, the environment should be conducive to rest, because the client is easily fatigued.

Test-Taking Strategy: Focus on the subject—activity intolerance—and note the client's diagnosis. Use the ABCs—airway, breathing, and circulation—to direct you to option 3. Review the interventions for a client with pneumonia and Activity intolerance if you had difficulty with this question.

Level of Cognitive Ability: Application
Client Needs: Physiological Integrity
Integrated Process: Nursing Process/
  Implementation
Content Area: Adult Health/Respiratory

References
Black, J., & Hawks, J. (2005). *Medical-surgical nursing: Clinical management for positive outcomes* (7th ed., p. 1843). Philadelphia: Saunders.
Lewis, S., Heitkemper, M., Dirksen, S., O'Brien, P., & Bucher, L. (2007). *Medical-surgical nursing: Assessment and management of clinical problems* (7th ed., pp. 565, 569). St. Louis: Mosby.

1592. A nurse is assisting in admitting a newborn infant to the nursery and notes that the physician has documented that the newborn has gastroschisis. The nurse plans care, knowing that in this condition the viscera are:

1 Inside the abdominal cavity and under the skin
2 Inside the abdominal cavity and under the dermis
3 Outside the abdominal cavity and not covered with a sac
4 Outside the abdominal cavity but inside a translucent sac covered with peritoneum and amniotic membrane

Level of Cognitive Ability: Application
Client Needs: Physiological Integrity
Integrated Process: Nursing Process/Planning
Content Area: Maternity/Postpartum

Answer: 3
Rationale: Gastroschisis is an abdominal wall defect in which the viscera are outside the abdominal cavity and not covered with a sac. Embryonal weakness in the abdominal wall causes herniation of the gut on one side of the umbilical cord during early development. Options 1 and 2 describe an umbilical hernia. Option 4 describes an omphalocele.

Test-Taking Strategy: Use the process of elimination. Eliminate options 1 and 2 first because they are comparable or alike. From the remaining options, recalling the definition of gastroschisis will direct you to option 3. Review this disorder if you are unfamiliar with it.

Reference
Wong, D., Hockenberry, M., Perry, S., Lowdermilk, D., & Wilson, D. (2006). *Maternal-child nursing care.* (3rd ed., p. 859). St. Louis: Mosby.

1593. A nurse is performing an assessment on a 6-month-old infant suspected of having hydrocephalus. Which finding is associated with this diagnosis?

1 A bulging anterior fontanel
2 An elevated apical heart rate
3 The presence of protein in the urine
4 A drop in blood pressure from baseline

Level of Cognitive Ability: Analysis
Client Needs: Physiological Integrity
Integrated Process: Nursing Process/Assessment
Content Area: Child Health

Answer: 1
Rationale: A bulging anterior fontanel indicates an increase in cerebrospinal fluid collection in the cerebral ventricle, which occurs in hydrocephalus. Proteinuria, an elevated apical heart rate, and a drop in blood pressure are not specifically related to increasing cerebrospinal fluid in the brain tissue.

Test-Taking Strategy: Use the principles associated with excessive fluid buildup in the cranial cavity to answer this question. Remember that fluid accumulation in the cranial cavity will exert pressure on the soft brain tissue. This will cause the anterior fontanel to expand. Additionally, correlate the word "hydrocephalus" in the question with "anterior fontanel" in option 1. Review the findings associated with hydrocephalus if you had difficulty with this question.

Reference
Hockenberry, M., Wilson, D., & Winkelstein, M. (2005). *Wong's essentials of pediatric nursing* (7th ed., pp. 1019, 1057, 1059). St. Louis: Mosby.

1594. A 10-day postpartum breast-feeding client telephones the postpartum unit complaining of a reddened, painful breast and elevated temperature. Based on assessment of the client's complaints, the nurse tells the client to:
  1 "Breast-feed only with the unaffected breast."
  2 "Notify your physician because you may need medication."
  3 "Stop breast-feeding because you probably have an infection."
  4 "Continue breast-feeding because this is a normal response in breast-feeding mothers."

Level of Cognitive Ability: Application
Client Needs: Physiological Integrity
Integrated Process: Nursing Process/ Implementation
Content Area: Maternity/Postpartum

Answer: 2
Rationale: Based on the signs and symptoms presented by the client (particularly the elevated temperature), the physician needs to be notified because an antibiotic that is tolerated by the infant as well as the mother may be prescribed. The mother should continue to nurse on both breasts, but should start the infant on the unaffected breast while the affected breast lets down.

Test-Taking Strategy: Focus on the data in the question and note that the client has an elevated temperature. Option 4 can be eliminated first because the client's complaints are not normal. Eliminate option 3 because it does not encourage the continuation of breast-feeding or notification of the physician. Option 1 also does not encourage continuation of normal breast-feeding and could possibly lead to engorgement, creating more discomfort and pain for the mother. Review postpartum complications if you had difficulty with this question.

Reference
Murray, S., & McKinney, E. (2006). *Foundations of maternal-newborn nursing* (4th ed., pp. 749-751). Philadelphia: Saunders.

1595. The nurse notes that the physician has written an order for prednisone (Deltasone) for a client. The nurse contacts the physician about revision of the client's medication plan if which medication is noted on the client's medication record?
  1 Oxycodone (Oxycontin)
  2 Propoxyphene (Darvon)
  3 Acetaminophen (Tylenol)
  4 Acetylsalicylic acid (aspirin)

Level of Cognitive Ability: Application
Client Needs: Safe and Effective Care Environment
Integrated Process: Nursing Process/ Implementation
Content Area: Pharmacology

Answer: 4
Rationale: Prednisone is irritating to the gastrointestinal (GI) tract, which could be worsened by the use of other products that have the same side effect. Therefore, products such as aspirin and nonsteroidal anti-inflammatory drugs are not used during corticosteroid therapy.

Test-Taking Strategy: Use the process of elimination and think about the side effects of prednisone. Recalling that aspirin is irritating to the GI tract will assist in answering the question. Review the side effects of prednisone if you had difficulty with this question.

Reference
Lehne, R. (2007). *Pharmacology for nursing care* (6th ed., p. 836). Philadelphia: Saunders.

1596. The nurse talks to students at a high school about sexually transmitted infections (STIs). Which effective methods of preventing STIs does the nurse include in the discussion? Select all that apply.

☐ **1** Some birth control pills prevent STIs.

☐ **2** STIs do not transmit through oral sex.

☐ **3** Diaphragms are a barrier against STIs.

☐ **4** Abstinence prevents transmission of STIs.

☐ **5** Multiple sex partners increases risk of STIs.

☐ **6** Proper condom use provides STI protection.

Level of Cognitive Ability: Application
Client Needs: Safe and Effective Care Environment
Integrated Process: Teaching and Learning
Content Area: Fundamental Skills

Answer: 4, 5, 6

Rationale: Effective measures to avoid STIs include abstinence, using condoms, and avoiding multiple partners and the nurse should provide this factual information to the high school students. The nurse also includes information about ineffective methods of preventing STIs, including oral sex, birth control pills, and diaphragms.

Test-Taking Strategy: Focus on the subject—preventing STIs—not pregnancy. This focus will eliminate options 1, 2, and 3. Review the methods of protection against STIs if you had difficulty with this question.

Reference
Lewis, S., Heitkemper, M., Dirksen, S., O'Brien, P., & Bucher, L. (2007). *Medical-surgical nursing: Assessment and management of clinical problems* (7th ed., pp. 1377). St. Louis: Mosby.

1597. The home care nurse is caring for a client who has just been discharged from the hospital after implantation of a permanent pacemaker. A priority nursing action to maintain a safe environment for the client would be to assess the client's home for the presence of:

1 Hair dryers

2 Electric blankets

3 Electric toothbrushes

4 Electrical items that have strong electric currents or magnetic fields

Level of Cognitive Ability: Application
Client Needs: Safe and Effective Care Environment
Integrated Process: Nursing Process/Assessment
Content Area: Adult Health/Cardiovascular

Answer: 4

Rationale: A pacemaker is shielded from interference from most electrical devices. Radios, televisions, electric blankets, toasters, microwave ovens, heating pads, and hair dryers are considered to be safe. Devices to be forewarned about include those with a strong electric current or magnetic field, such as antitheft devices in stores, metal detectors used in airports, and radiation therapy (if applicable and which might require relocation of the pacemaker).

Test-Taking Strategy: Use the process of elimination. Note that option 4 uses the word "strong" and is the umbrella option addressing items with strong electric currents or magnetic fields. Review home care measures for the client with a pacemaker if you had difficulty with this question.

References
Ignatavicius, D., & Workman, M. (2006). *Medical-surgical nursing: Critical thinking for collaborative care* (5th ed., p. 745). Philadelphia: Saunders.
Monahan, F., Sands, J., Neighbors, M., Marek, J., & Green, C. (2007). *Phipps' medical-surgical nursing: Health and illness perspectives* (8th ed., p. 794). St. Louis: Mosby.

1598. A client with low back pain asks the nurse which type of exercise will best strengthen the lower back muscles. The nurse tells the client to participate in which beneficial exercise?

1 Tennis
2 Diving
3 Canoeing
4 Swimming

Level of Cognitive Ability: Application
Client Needs: Health Promotion and Maintenance
Integrated Process: Nursing Process/ Implementation
Content Area: Adult Health/Musculoskeletal

Answer: 4
Rationale: Walking and swimming are very beneficial in strengthening back muscles for the client with low back pain. The other options involve twisting and pulling of the back muscles, which is not helpful to the client experiencing back pain.

Test-Taking Strategy: Recalling that low back pain is aggravated by any activity that twists or turns the spine, evaluate each of the options according to this guideline. This will enable you to eliminate options 1, 2, and 3. Review home care measures for the client with low back pain if you had difficulty with this question.

Reference
Ignatavicius, D., & Workman, M. (2006). *Medical-surgical nursing: Critical thinking for collaborative care* (5th ed., p. 978). Philadelphia: Saunders.

1599. A nurse is caring for a child with a diagnosis of Kawasaki disease, and the mother of the child asks the nurse about the disorder. The nurse bases the response to the mother on which description of this disorder?

1 It is an acquired cell-mediated immunodeficiency disorder.
2 It is a chronic multisystem autoimmune disease characterized by the inflammation of connective tissue.
3 It is an inflammatory autoimmune disease that affects the connective tissue of the heart, joints, and subcutaneous tissues.
4 It is also called mucocutaneous lymph node syndrome and is a febrile generalized vasculitis of unknown etiology.

Level of Cognitive Ability: Application
Client Needs: Physiological Integrity
Integrated Process: Nursing Process/ Implementation
Content Area: Child Health

Answer: 4
Rationale: Kawasaki disease, also called *mucocutaneous lymph node syndrome,* is a febrile generalized vasculitis of unknown etiology. Option 1 describes human immunodeficiency virus infection. Option 3 describes rheumatic fever. Option 2 describes systemic lupus erythematosus.

Test-Taking Strategy: Knowledge regarding the description of Kawasaki disease is required to answer this question. Remember Kawasaki disease is a febrile generalized vasculitis of unknown etiology. Review this content if you are unfamiliar with this disorder.

Reference
Wong, D., Hockenberry, M., Perry, S., Lowdermilk, D., & Wilson, D. (2006). *Maternal-child nursing care.* (3rd ed., pp. 1593-1594). St. Louis: Mosby.

1600. A nurse is preparing to teach the parents of a child with anemia about the dietary sources of iron that are easy for the body to absorb. Which food item would the nurse include in the teaching plan?

1 Fruits
2 Poultry
3 Apricots
4 Vegetables

Answer: 2
Rationale: Dietary sources of iron that are easy for the body to absorb include meat, poultry, and fish. Vegetables, fruits, cereals, and breads are also dietary sources of iron, but they are harder for the body to absorb.

Level of Cognitive Ability: Application
Client Needs: Health Promotion and
 Maintenance
Integrated Process: Teaching and Learning
Content Area: Child Health

References
McKinney, E., James, S., Murray, S., & Ashwill, J. (2005). *Maternal-child nursing* (2nd ed., pp.1304-1306). St. Louis: Saunders.
Nix, S. (2005) *Williams' basic nutrition & diet therapy* (12th ed., pp. 142-143). St. Louis: Mosby.

1601. A nurse is caring for a child with a patent ductus arteriosus. The nurse reviews the child's assessment data, knowing that which of the following is characteristic of this disorder?
 1 It produces abnormalities in the atrial septum.
 2 It involves an opening between the two atria.
 3 It involves an opening between the two ventricles.
 4 It involves an artery that connects the aorta and the pulmonary artery during fetal life.

Level of Cognitive Ability: Comprehension
Client Needs: Physiological Integrity
Integrated Process: Nursing Process/Assessment
Content Area: Child Health

Answer: 4
Rationale: Patent ductus arteriosus is described as an artery that connects the aorta and the pulmonary artery during fetal life. It generally closes spontaneously within a few hours to several days after birth. It allows abnormal blood flow from the high-pressure aorta to the low-pressure pulmonary artery, resulting in a left-to-right shunt. Options 1, 2, and 3 are not characteristics of this cardiac defect.

Reference
Hockenberry, M., Wilson, D., & Winkelstein, M. (2005). *Wong's essentials of pediatric nursing* (7th ed., p. 898). St. Louis: Mosby.

1602. The nurse is caring for a client who has returned to the physician's office for follow-up after a parathyroidectomy with autotransplantation of some parathyroid tissue into the forearm. The client has been taking oral calcium and vitamin D supplements since discharge 2 weeks ago. Which statement by the client indicates an understanding of the medical management following this type of surgical procedure?
 1 "Do you think I'll always have to take these pills?"
 2 "The thought of taking these pills for the rest of my life makes me shudder!"
 3 "I can't wait for the transplant to start working. I'm tired of taking all these pills!"
 4 "Well, I guess the transplant isn't working because my calcium levels are still low."

Answer: 3
Rationale: The purpose of autotransplantation of some parathyroid tissue is to regain function of the parathyroid gland. Autotransplantation of parathyroid tissue takes some time to mature. Oral calcium and vitamin D supplements must be taken to prevent hypoparathyroidism until the transplant matures and becomes an active endocrine gland.

Level of Cognitive Ability: Analysis
Client Needs: Physiological Integrity
Integrated Process: Nursing Process/Evaluation
Content Area: Adult Health/Endocrine

References
Black, J., & Hawks, J. (2005). *Medical-surgical nursing: Clinical management for positive outcomes* (7th ed., p. 2284). Philadelphia: Saunders.
Ignatavicius, D., & Workman, M. (2006). *Medical-surgical nursing: Critical thinking for collaborative care* (5th ed., p. 1487). Philadelphia: Saunders.

1603. Desmopressin (DDAVP) is prescribed via intranasal route for a child with von Willebrand's disease, and the nurse instructs the parents regarding the administration of this medication. Which statement by the parents indicates a need for further instructions?

1 "We need to refrigerate the DDAVP."
2 "We do not need to reduce our child's fluid intake."
3 "Nausea and abdominal cramps can occur as a side effect of the medication."
4 "Headache and drowsiness may be a sign of water intoxication that can occur with the medication."

Level of Cognitive Ability: Analysis
Client Needs: Physiological Integrity
Integrated Process: Teaching and Learning
Content Area: Child Health

Answer: 2
Rationale: Parents should be instructed to reduce fluid intake during initial treatment, since the treatment will prevent continued fluid loss and the result will be fluid buildup. The medication should be refrigerated, but freezing should be avoided. Side effects of the medication include facial flushing, nasal congestion, increased blood pressure, nausea, abdominal cramps, decreased urination, and vulval pain. Signs and symptoms of water intoxication include headache, drowsiness and confusion, weight gain, seizures, and coma.

Test-Taking Strategy: Note the strategic words "need for further instructions." These words indicate a negative event query and the need to select the incorrect client statement. Noting the word "reduce" in option 2 will direct you to this option. Review the action, use, and side effects of this medication if you had difficulty with this question.

References
Hockenberry, M., & Wilson, D. (2007). *Nursing care of infants and children* (8th ed., p. 1540). St. Louis: Mosby.
Lehne, R. (2007). *Pharmacology for nursing care* (6th ed., p. 694). Philadelphia: Saunders.

1604. A child is brought to the emergency department after being bitten in the arm by a neighborhood dog. The nurse performs a focused assessment, cleanses the wound as prescribed, and continues to perform a thorough assessment on the child. Which of the following is the priority question for the nurse to ask the mother of the child?

1 "How old is the dog?"
2 "Did the dog have rabies?"
3 "Are the child's immunizations up-to-date?"
4 "Did the dog have all of its recommended shots?"

Level of Cognitive Ability: Application
Client Needs: Health Promotion and Maintenance
Integrated Process: Nursing Process/Assessment
Content Area: Child Health

Answer: 3
Rationale: When a bite occurs, the injury site of the bite should be cleansed carefully and the child should be given tetanus prophylaxis if immunizations are not up-to-date. Option 3 is the priority consideration. Options 1, 2, and 4 identify information that may have to be obtained, but are not the priority questions. Additionally, the mother may not have the answers to these questions.

Test-Taking Strategy: Use the process of elimination and note the strategic word "priority." Option 3 is the only option that focuses on the needs of the child. Review this content if you are unfamiliar with the assessment and care of a child who receives a dog bite.

Reference
Hockenberry, M., Wilson, D., & Winkelstein, M. (2005). *Wong's essentials of pediatric nursing* (7th ed., p. 1120). St. Louis: Mosby.

1605. A nurse is providing instructions to the mother of a child who had a myringotomy with insertion of tympanostomy tubes. The nurse tells the mother that if the tubes fall out:

1 "Bring the child to the emergency room immediately."

2 "It is not an emergency, but it is best to call the health care clinic."

3 "It is important to replace them immediately so that the surgical opening does not close."

4 "Clean the tubes with half-strength hydrogen peroxide for 30 minutes and then replace them into the child's ears."

Level of Cognitive Ability: Application
Client Needs: Physiological Integrity
Integrated Process: Teaching and Learning
Content Area: Child Health

Answer: 2

Rationale: The mother should be assured that if the tympanostomy tubes fall out, it is not an emergency, but it is best if the physician or health care clinic is notified. The size and appearance of the tympanostomy tubes should be described to the mother following surgery so that she will be familiar with their appearance. Options 1, 3, and 4 are incorrect.

Test-Taking Strategy: Use the process of elimination. Option 1 is eliminated first because it will cause concern in the mother. Next eliminate options 3 and 4 because they are comparable or alike and relate to replacing the tubes. Review home care instructions following this procedure if you had difficulty with this question.

Reference
McKinney, E., James, S., Murray, S., & Ashwill, J. (2005). *Maternal-child nursing* (2nd ed., p. 1199). St. Louis: Saunders.

1606. The mother of a child calls the health care clinic and tells a nurse that the child has developed a bloody nose. The nurse instructs the mother to do which of the following?

1 Pinch the nostrils for 5 minutes and then recheck for bleeding.

2 Maintain the child in a sitting position with the head tilted backward.

3 Lay the child down with a pillow tucked under the neck and stay with the child to keep the child calm.

4 Have the child sit with the head tilted forward and hold pressure on the soft part of the nose for a period of 10 minutes.

Level of Cognitive Ability: Application
Client Needs: Physiological Integrity
Integrated Process: Nursing Process/ Implementation
Content Area: Child Health

Answer: 4

Rationale: The child should be positioned erect, sitting with head tilted forward to avoid blood dripping posteriorly to the pharynx. The soft part of the nose should be tightly pinched against the center wall for 10 minutes, and the mother should be instructed that this pinch should be timed by a clock, not estimated. The mother should be told not to release pressure for 10 minutes. The child is encouraged to remain calm and quiet and to breathe through the mouth.

Test-Taking Strategy: Use the process of elimination, focusing on the subject—controlling a bloody nose. Visualize the positions presented in the options to direct you to option 4. Review the interventions used when epistaxis occurs if you had difficulty with question.

Reference
Hockenberry, M., Wilson, D., & Winkelstein, M. (2005). *Wong's essentials of pediatric nursing* (7th ed., p. 957). St. Louis: Mosby.

1607. A nurse is assessing a child admitted to the hospital with a diagnosis of rheumatic fever. The nurse asks the child's mother which significant question during the assessment?

1 "Has your child had difficulty urinating?"

2 "Has your child been exposed to anyone with chickenpox?"

3 "Has any family member had a sore throat within the past few weeks?"

4 "Has any family member had a gastrointestinal disorder in the past few weeks?"

Level of Cognitive Ability: Application
Client Needs: Physiological Integrity
Integrated Process: Nursing Process/Assessment
Content Area: Child Health

Answer: 3
Rationale: Rheumatic fever characteristically presents 2 to 6 weeks following an untreated or partially treated group A beta-hemolytic streptococcal infection of the respiratory tract. Initially, the nurse determines whether any family member has had a sore throat or unexplained fever within the past few weeks. Options 1, 2, and 4 are unrelated to the assessment findings of rheumatic fever.

Test-Taking Strategy: Note the strategic word "significant." Recalling that rheumatic fever characteristically presents 2 to 6 weeks following a streptococcal infection of the respiratory tract will direct you to the correct option. Review this content if you are unfamiliar with the etiology and the pathophysiology associated with this disorder.

Reference
Hockenberry, M., Wilson, D., & Winkelstein, M. (2005). *Wong's essentials of pediatric nursing* (7th ed., p. 923). St. Louis: Mosby.

1608. The parents of a child with mumps express concern that their child will develop orchitis as a result of having mumps and ask the nurse about the signs of this complication. The nurse tells the parents that which of the following is a sign of this complication?

1 Fever

2 Facial swelling

3 Swollen glands

4 Difficulty urinating

Level of Cognitive Ability: Application
Client Needs: Physiological Integrity
Integrated Process: Teaching and Learning
Content Area: Child Health

Answer: 1
Rationale: Unilateral orchitis occurs more frequently than bilateral orchitis. About 1 week after the appearance of parotitis, there is an abrupt onset of testicular pain, tenderness, fever, chills, headache, and vomiting. The affected testicle becomes red, swollen, and tender. Atrophy, resulting in sterility, occurs only in a small number of cases. Difficulty urinating is not a sign of this complication. Swollen glands and facial swelling normally occur in mumps.

Test-Taking Strategy: Use the process of elimination. Eliminate options 2 and 3 first because they are comparable or alike. From the remaining options, focus on the word "orchitis." Recalling that "itis" indicates inflammation will direct you to option 1. Review the characteristics of orchitis if you had difficulty with this question.

Reference
Hockenberry, M., Wilson, D., & Winkelstein, M. (2005). *Wong's essentials of pediatric nursing* (7th ed., pp. 440-441). St. Louis: Mosby.

1609. A maternity nurse is teaching a pregnant client about the physiological effects and hormone changes that occur in pregnancy. The client asks the nurse about the purpose of estrogen. The nurse bases the response on which of the following?

1 It maintains the uterine lining for implantation.

2 It stimulates metabolism of glucose and converts the glucose to fat.

3 It prevents the involution of the corpus luteum and maintains the production of progesterone until the placenta is formed.

4 It stimulates uterine development to provide an environment for the fetus and stimulates the breasts to prepare for lactation.

Level of Cognitive Ability: Application
Client Needs: Physiological Integrity
Integrated Process: Teaching and Learning
Content Area: Maternity/Antepartum

Answer: 4

Rationale: Estrogen stimulates uterine development to provide an environment for the fetus and stimulates the breasts to prepare for lactation. Progesterone maintains the uterine lining for implantation and relaxes all smooth muscle. Human placental lactogen stimulates the metabolism of glucose and converts the glucose to fat. Human chorionic gonadotropin prevents involution of the corpus luteum and maintains the production of progesterone until the placenta is formed.

Test-Taking Strategy: Knowledge regarding the functions of various hormones related to pregnancy is required to answer this question. Remember that estrogen stimulates uterine development to provide an environment for the fetus and stimulates the breasts to prepare for lactation. Review this content if you had difficulty with this question or are unfamiliar with these hormones.

References

McKinney, E., James, S., Murray, S., & Ashwill, J. (2005). *Maternal-child nursing* (2nd ed., p. 258). St. Louis: Saunders.

Murray, S., & McKinney, E., (2006). *Foundations of maternal-newborn nursing* (4th ed., p.120). Philadelphia: Saunders.

1610. The nurse has explained the reason that the physician has chosen laser surgery to treat a client's cervical cancer. Which statement by the client indicates an understanding of the explanation?

1 "I want to be asleep during my procedure."

2 "I have too much cancer to be removed with surgery."

3 "The doctor is able to see all the edges of my cancer clearly."

4 "I am young and the laser prevents cancer tissue from regrowing."

Level of Cognitive Ability: Analysis
Client Needs: Physiological Integrity
Integrated Process:Nursing Process/Evaluation
Content Area: Adult Health/Oncology

Answer: 3

Rationale: Laser therapy is performed in an outpatient setting and is used when all boundaries of the lesion are visible. Option 1 is not the reason for performing laser surgery. Laser surgery is painless, and the client would not receive general anesthesia. Laser therapy does not prevent regrowth.

Test-Taking Strategy: Use the process of elimination and focus on the subject—laser surgery. Thinking about the procedure involved in laser surgery will direct you to option 3. Review this type of treatment for cervical cancer if you had difficulty with this question.

References

Black, J., & Hawks, J. (2005). *Medical-surgical nursing: Clinical management for positive outcomes* (7th ed., p. 1075-1076). Philadelphia: Saunders.

Ignatavicius, D., & Workman, M. (2006). *Medical-surgical nursing: Critical thinking for collaborative care* (5th ed., pp. 1846-1847). Philadelphia: Saunders.

1611. A physician orders 1000 mL of ½-normal saline to infuse over 8 hours. The drop factor is 15 drops (gtt) per 1 mL. The nurse sets the flow rate at how many drops per minute? (Round to the nearest whole number.)

Answer: _____ gtt/minute

Answer: 31

Rationale: Use the IV flow rate formula.

Formula:

$$\frac{\text{Total volume} \times \text{gtt factor}}{\text{Time in minutes}} = \text{gtt/minute}$$

$$\frac{1000 \text{ mL} \times 15 \text{ gtt}}{480 \text{ minutes}} = 31.2 \text{ or } 31 \text{ gtt/minute}$$

Level of Cognitive Ability: Application
Client Needs: Physiological Integrity
Integrated Process: Nursing Process/
    Implementation
Content Area: Fundamental Skills

Test-Taking Strategy: Use the formula for calculating IV flow rates when answering the question. Use a calculator to verify the answer and remember to round to the nearest whole number. Review IV infusion rates if you had difficulty with this question.

Reference

Kee, J., & Marshall, S. (2004). *Clinical Calculations: With applications to general and specialty areas* (4th ed., p. 202). Philadelphia: Saunders.

1612. The nurse is monitoring the function of a client's chest tube. The chest tube is attached to a chest drainage system. The nurse notes that the fluid in the water-seal chamber is below the 2-cm mark. The nurse determines that:
  1 There is a leak in the system.
  2 Suction should be added to the system.
  3 This is caused by client pneumothorax.
  4 Water should be added to the chamber.

Level of Cognitive Ability: Analysis
Client Needs: Physiological Integrity
Integrated Process: Nursing Process/Analysis
Content Area: Adult Health/Respiratory

Answer: 4
Rationale: The water-seal chamber should be filled to the 2-cm mark to provide an adequate water seal between the external environment and the client's pleural cavity. The water seal prevents air from reentering the pleural cavity. Because evaporation of water can occur, the nurse should remedy this problem by adding water until the level is again at the 2-cm mark. The other interpretations are incorrect.

Test-Taking Strategy: Focus on the subject—the water-seal chamber is below the 2-cm mark. Recalling that the chamber needs to be filled to the 2-cm mark will direct you to option 4. Review the principles associated with care of chest tubes if you had difficulty with this question.

References

Black, J., & Hawks, J. (2005). *Medical-surgical nursing: Clinical management for positive outcomes* (7th ed., pp. 1862-1863). Philadelphia: Saunders.
Lewis, S., Heitkemper, M., Dirksen, S., O'Brien, P., & Bucher, L. (2007). *Medical-surgical nursing: Assessment and management of clinical problems* (7th ed., pp. 589, 591). St. Louis: Mosby.

1613. A client has decided to use transcutaneous electrical nerve stimulation (TENS) as prescribed by the physician for the relief of chronic pain, and the nurse has provided instructions to the client regarding the TENS unit. Which statement by the client would indicate a need for further instructions regarding this pain relief measure?
  1 "I understand that this will help relieve the pain."
  2 "This unit will eliminate the need for taking so many pain medications."
  3 "I am not real happy that I have to stay in the hospital for this treatment."
  4 "I am not sure that I am going to like those electrodes attached to my skin."

Level of Cognitive Ability: Analysis
Client Needs: Physiological Integrity
Integrated Process: Teaching and Learning
Content Area: Pharmacology

Answer: 3
Rationale: The TENS unit is a portable unit, and the client controls the system for relieving pain and reducing the need for analgesics. It is attached to the skin of the body by electrodes. It is not necessary for the client to remain in the hospital for this treatment.

Test-Taking Strategy: Note the words "need for further instructions." These words indicate a negative event query and the need to select the incorrect client statement. Options 1 and 2 can be eliminated first because they are comparable or alike. From the remaining options, select option 3, because it would not be a very cost-effective pain management technique if the client required hospitalization. Review the principles related to the TENS unit if you had difficulty with this question.

References

Black, J., & Hawks, J. (2005). *Medical-surgical nursing: Clinical management for positive outcomes* (7th ed., pp. 476-477). Philadelphia: Saunders.
Ignatavicius, D., & Workman, M. (2006). *Medical-surgical nursing: Critical thinking for collaborative care* (5th ed., pp. 84, 385). Philadelphia: Saunders.

1614. A client with chronic renal failure has a protein restriction in the diet. The nurse should include in a teaching plan to avoid which of the following sources of incomplete protein in the diet?

1 Fish
2 Eggs
3 Milk
4 Nuts

Level of Cognitive Ability: Application
Client Needs: Health Promotion and Maintenance
Integrated Process: Teaching and Learning
Content Area: Adult Health/Renal

Answer: 4

Rationale: The client whose diet has a protein restriction should be careful to ensure that the proteins eaten are complete proteins with the highest biological value. Foods such as meat, fish, milk, and eggs are complete proteins, which are optimal for the client with chronic renal failure.

Test-Taking Strategy: Focus on the subject—protein composition of various foods. Eliminate options 2 and 3 first because they are comparable or alike and are dairy products. From the remaining options, note the strategic words "avoid" and "incomplete protein" to direct you to option 4. Review foods that are complete and incomplete proteins if you had difficulty with this question.

References

Lewis, S., Heitkemper, M., Dirksen, S., O'Brien, P., & Bucher, L. (2007). *Medical-surgical nursing: Assessment and management of clinical problems* (7th ed., pp. 1211-1212). St. Louis: Mosby.

Nix, S. (2005) Williams, *Basic nutrition & diet therapy* (12th ed., pp. 46-47). St. Louis: Mosby.

1615. A newborn infant is diagnosed with imperforate anus. The nurse plans care, knowing that which of the following appropriately describes a characteristic of this disorder?

1 The presence of fecal incontinence
2 Incomplete development of the anus
3 The infrequent and difficult passage of dry stools
4 Invagination of a section of the intestine into the distal bowel

Level of Cognitive Ability: Application
Client Needs: Physiological Integrity
Integrated Process: Nursing Process/Planning
Content Area: Maternity/Postpartum

Answer: 2

Rationale: Imperforate anus (anal atresia, anal agenesis) is the incomplete development or absence of the anus in its normal position in the perineum. Option 1 describes encopresis. Encopresis generally affects preschool and school-age children. Option 3 describes constipation. Constipation can affect any child at any time, although it peaks at age 2 to 3 years. Option 4 describes intussusception.

Test-Taking Strategy: Use the process of elimination. Noting the relationship between the disorder "imperforate anus" and "incomplete development of the anus" in option 2 should direct you to this option. Review this disorder if you had difficulty with this question.

References

Hockenberry, M. & Wilson, D. (2007). *Nursing care of infants and children* (8th ed., pp. 474-475). St. Louis: Mosby.

McKinney, E., James, S., Murray, S., & Ashwill, J. (2005). *Maternal-child nursing* (2nd ed., p. 1116). St. Louis: Saunders.

1616. A nurse is providing bottle-feeding instructions to the mother of a newborn infant. The nurse provides instructions regarding the amount of formula to be given, knowing that the stomach capacity for a newborn infant is approximately:

1 5 to 10 mL
2 10 to 20 mL
3 30 to 90 mL
4 75 to 100 mL

Answer: 2

Rationale: The stomach capacity of a newborn infant is approximately 10 to 20 mL. It is 30 to 90 mL for a 1-week-old infant, and 75 to 100 mL for a 2- to 3-week-old infant.

Test-Taking Strategy: Use the process of elimination. Note the strategic words "newborn infant." This should assist in eliminating options 3 and 4. From the remaining options, visualize the amounts in options 1 and 2. Noting that 5 mL is a very small amount should assist in directing you to option 2. Review these pediatric differences if you had difficulty with this question.

Level of Cognitive Ability: Application
Client Needs: Health Promotion and Maintenance
Integrated Process: Teaching and Learning
Content Area: Maternity/Postpartum

References
Murray, S., & McKinney, E. (2006). *Foundations of maternal-newborn nursing* (4th ed., p. 459). Philadelphia: Saunders.
Wong, D., Hockenberry, M., Perry, S., Lowdermilk, D. & Wilson, D. (2006). *Maternal-child nursing care.* (3rd ed., p. 696). St. Louis: Mosby.

1617. A mother who is breast-feeding her newborn infant is experiencing nipple soreness, and the nurse provides instructions regarding measures to relieve the soreness. Which statement by the mother indicates an understanding of the instructions?

  1 "I need to avoid rotating breast-feeding positions so that the nipple will toughen."
  2 "I need to stop nursing during the period of nipple soreness to allow the nipples to heal."
  3 "I need to nurse less frequently and substitute a bottle feeding until the nipples become less sore."
  4 "I need to position my infant with her ear, shoulder, and hip in straight alignment and place her stomach against me."

Level of Cognitive Ability: Analysis
Client Needs: Health Promotion and Maintenance
Integrated Process: Nursing Process/Evaluation
Content Area: Maternity/Postpartum

Answer: 4
Rationale: Comfort measures for nipple soreness include positioning the infant with the ear, shoulder, and hip in straight alignment and with the infant's stomach against the mother's. Additional measures include rotating breast-feeding positions; breaking suction with the little finger; nursing frequently; beginning feeding on the less sore nipple; not allowing the infant to chew on the nipple or to sleep holding the nipple in the mouth; and applying tea bags soaked in warm water to the nipple. Options 1, 2, and 3 are incorrect.

Test-Taking Strategy: Use the process of elimination, focusing on the strategic words "indicates an understanding." Visualize each of the options in terms of how they may or may not lessen the nipple soreness to direct you to option 4. Review these measures if you had difficulty answering the question.

Reference
Murray, S., & McKinney, E. (2006). *Foundations of maternal-newborn nursing* (4th ed., p. 553). Philadelphia: Saunders.

1618. A client with acute myocardial infarction receives therapy with alteplase recombinant, or tissue plasminogen activator (t-PA). Which finding indicates to the nurse that the client is experiencing a possible complication?

  1 Epistaxis
  2 Vomiting
  3 ECG changes
  4 Absent pedal pulses

Level of Cognitive Ability: Analysis
Client Needs: Physiological Integrity
Integrated Process: Nursing Process/Analysis
Content Area: Pharmacology

Answer: 1
Rationale: Bleeding is a major side effect of t-PA therapy. The bleeding can be superficial or internal and can be spontaneous. Options 2, 3, and 4 are not side or adverse effects of t-PA therapy.

Test-Taking Strategy: Use the process of elimination. Recalling that this medication is a thrombolytic and that epistaxis is a bloody nose will direct you to option 1. Review the side and adverse effects of t-PA if you had difficulty with this question.

Reference
Mosby. (2007). *Mosby's nursing drug reference* (20th ed., p. 102). St. Louis: Mosby.

1619. A nurse is performing an assessment on a mother who just delivered a healthy newborn infant. The nurse checks the uterine fundus, expecting to note that the fundus is positioned:
1 To the right of the abdomen
2 At the level of the umbilicus
3 Above the level of the umbilicus
4 One fingerbreadth above the symphysis pubis

Level of Cognitive Ability: Analysis
Client Needs: Physiological Integrity
Integrated Process: Nursing Process/Assessment
Content Area: Maternity/Postpartum

Answer: 2
Rationale: Immediately after delivery, the uterine fundus should be at the level of the umbilicus or one to three fingerbreadths below it and in the midline of the abdomen. If the fundus is above the umbilicus, this may indicate that blood clots in the uterus need to be expelled by fundal massage. A fundus that is not located in the midline may indicate a full bladder.

Test-Taking Strategy: Use the process of elimination, noting the strategic words "just delivered." Use knowledge regarding normal anatomy and visualize each description in the options to direct you to option 2. Review normal post-delivery findings if you had difficulty with this question.

Reference
Murray, S., & McKinney, E. (2006). *Foundations of maternal-newborn nursing* (4th ed., p. 410). Philadelphia: Saunders.

1620. A nurse obtains the vital signs on a mother who delivered a healthy newborn infant 2 hours ago and notes that the mother's temperature is 102° F. The appropriate nursing action would be to:
1 Notify the physician.
2 Remove the blanket from the client's bed.
3 Document the finding and recheck the temperature in 4 hours.
4 Administer acetaminophen (Tylenol) and recheck the temperature in 4 hours.

Level of Cognitive Ability: Application
Client Needs: Physiological Integrity
Integrated Process: Nursing Process/ Implementation
Content Area: Maternity/Postpartum

Answer: 1
Rationale: Vital signs return to normal within the first hour postpartum if no complications arise. If the temperature is greater than 2° F above normal, this may indicate infection, and the physician should be notified. Options 2, 3, and 4 are inaccurate nursing interventions for a temperature of 102° F 2 hours following delivery.

Test-Taking Strategy: Note that the mother delivered 2 hours ago. Use the process of elimination and think about the normal postpartum findings. It is most appropriate in this situation to report the findings because a temperature of 102° F can indicate infection. Review normal vital signs following delivery and the appropriate nursing interventions if the vital signs are not within the normal range.

References
McKinney, E., James, S., Murray, S., & Ashwill, J. (2005). *Maternal-child nursing* (2nd ed., p. 477). St. Louis: Saunders.
Murray, S., & McKinney, E. (2006). *Foundations of maternal-newborn nursing* (4th ed., p. 409). Philadelphia: Saunders.

1621. A nurse in the postpartum unit is caring for a mother following vaginal delivery of a healthy newborn infant. The client received epidural anesthesia for the delivery. One-half hour after admission to the postpartum unit, the nurse checks the client and suspects the presence of a vaginal hematoma. Which finding would be the best indicator of the presence of this type of hematoma?
1 Changes in vital signs
2 Signs of vaginal bruising
3 Client complaints of a tearing sensation
4 Client complaints of intense vaginal pressure

Answer: 1
Rationale: Changes in vital signs indicate hypovolemia in the anesthetized postpartum woman with a vaginal hematoma. Because the client received anesthesia, she would not feel pain or pressure. Vaginal bruising may be present, but this may be a result of the delivery process and additionally is not the best indicator of the presence of a hematoma.

Test-Taking Strategy: Focus on the data presented in the question. Noting that the client received an epidural anesthetic will assist in eliminating options 3 and 4. From the remaining options, recalling the pathophysiology associated with the development of a hematoma and use of the ABCs—airway, breathing, and circulation—will direct you to option 1. Review the signs of a vaginal hematoma if you had difficulty with this question.

Level of Cognitive Ability: Analysis
Client Needs: Physiological Integrity
Integrated Process: Nursing Process/Assessment
Content Area: Maternity/Postpartum

References
McKinney, E., James, S., Murray, S., & Ashwill, J. (2005). *Maternal-child nursing* (2nd ed., p. 705). St. Louis: Saunders.
Murray, S., & McKinney, E. (2006). *Foundations of maternal-newborn nursing* (4th ed., p. 737). Philadelphia: Saunders.

1622. A client with acute renal failure has an elevated blood urea nitrogen (BUN). The client is experiencing difficulty remembering information due to uremia. The nurse avoids which of the following when communicating with this client?

1 Giving simple, clear directions
2 Including the family in discussions related to care
3 Giving thorough, lengthy explanations of procedures
4 Explaining treatments using understandable language

Level of Cognitive Ability: Application
Client Needs: Psychosocial Integrity
Integrated Process: Communication and Documentation
Content Area: Adult Health/Renal

Answer: 3
Rationale: The client with acute renal failure may have difficulty remembering information and instructions because of anxiety and the increased level of the BUN. The nurse should avoid giving lengthy explanations about procedures because this information may not be remembered by the client and could increase client anxiety. Communications should be clear, simple, and understandable. The family should be included whenever possible.

Test-Taking Strategy: Use the process of elimination and note the strategic word "avoids." Use knowledge of the basic principles of effective communication to eliminate each of the incorrect options. Review basic communication techniques if you had difficulty with this question.

References
Black, J., & Hawks, J. (2005). *Medical-surgical nursing: Clinical management for positive outcomes* (7th ed., pp. 941, 948). Philadelphia: Saunders.
Lewis, S., Heitkemper, M., Dirksen, S., O'Brien, P., & Bucher, L. (2007). *Medical-surgical nursing: Assessment and management of clinical problems* (7th ed., p. 1256). St. Louis: Mosby.
Potter, P., & Perry, A. (2005) *Fundamentals of nursing* (6th ed., p. 437). St. Louis: Mosby.

1623. A nurse in the newborn nursery receives a telephone call from the delivery room and is told that a post-term small for gestational age (SGA) newborn will be admitted to the nursery. The nurse develops a plan of care for the newborn and documents that the priority nursing action is to monitor:

1 Urinary output
2 Blood glucose levels
3 Total bilirubin levels
4 Hemoglobin and hematocrit

Level of Cognitive Ability: Application
Client Needs: Physiological Integrity
Integrated Process: Nursing Process/Planning
Content Area: Maternity/Postpartum

Answer: 2
Rationale: The most common metabolic complication in the SGA newborn is hypoglycemia, which can produce central nervous system abnormalities and mental retardation if not corrected immediately. Urinary output, although important, is not the highest priority action because the post-term SGA newborn is typically dehydrated from placental dysfunction. Hemoglobin and hematocrit levels are monitored because the post-term SGA newborn exhibits polycythemia, although this also does not require immediate attention. The polycythemia contributes to increased bilirubin levels, usually beginning on the second day after delivery.

Test-Taking Strategy: Note the strategic words "priority nursing action." Recalling that the most common metabolic complication in the SGA newborn is hypoglycemia will direct you to option 2. Review the SGA newborn content if you had difficulty with this question.

Reference
Murray, S., & McKinney, E. (2006). *Foundations of maternal-newborn nursing* (4th ed., p. 793). Philadelphia: Saunders.

1624. A nurse in the postpartum unit reviews a client's record and notes that a new mother was administered methylergonovine (Methergine) intramuscularly following delivery. The nurse understands that this medication was administered to:

1 Decrease uterine contractions.
2 Prevent postpartum hemorrhage.
3 Maintain a normal blood pressure.
4 Reduce the amount of lochia drainage.

Level of Cognitive Ability: Analysis
Client's Needs: Physiological Integrity
Integrated Process: Nursing Process/Analysis
Content Area: Pharmacology

Answer: 2
Rationale: Methylergonovine, an oxytocic, is an agent used to prevent or control postpartum hemorrhage by contracting the uterus. The first dose is usually administered intramuscularly, and then if it needs to be continued, it is given by mouth. It increases the strength and frequency of contractions and may elevate blood pressure. There is no relationship between the action of this medication and lochial drainage.

Test-Taking Strategy: Use the process of elimination, focus on the medication name, and note the client is postpartum. Recalling that this medication is an oxytocic agent will direct you to option 2. Review its action and use if you are unfamiliar with this medication.

Reference
Mosby. (2007). *Mosby's nursing drug reference* (20th ed., p. 661). St. Louis: Mosby.

1625. A nurse in the newborn nursery receives a telephone call and is informed that a newborn infant with Apgar scores of 1 and 4 will be brought to the nursery. The nurse quickly prepares for the arrival of the newborn and determines that the priority intervention is to:

1 Connect the resuscitation bag to the oxygen
2 Turn on the apnea and cardiorespiratory monitor
3 Prepare for the insertion of an intravenous (IV) line with D_5W
4 Set up the radiant warmer control temperature at 36.5° C (97.6° F)

Level of Cognitive Ability: Application
Client Needs: Physiological Integrity
Integrated Process: Nursing Process/ Implementation
Content Area: Delegating/Prioritizing

Answer: 1
Rationale: The priority action for a newborn infant with low Apgar scores is airway, which would involve preparing respiratory resuscitation equipment. Options 2, 3, and 4 are also important, although they are of lower priority. Setting up an IV with D_5W would provide circulatory support. The radiant warmer will provide an external heat source, which is necessary to prevent further respiratory distress. The newborn infant's cardiopulmonary status would be monitored by a cardiorespiratory monitoring device.

Test-Taking Strategy: Note the strategic words "priority intervention." This question asks you to prioritize care planning based on information about a newborn infant's condition. Use the ABCs—airway, breathing, and circulation—to direct you to option 1. Although options 2, 3, and 4 are a component of the plan of care, option 1 is the priority. Review care of the newborn infant with a low Apgar score if you had difficulty with this question.

Reference
Murray, S., & McKinney, E. (2006). *Foundations of maternal-newborn nursing* (4th ed., p. 298). Philadelphia: Saunders.

1626. A nurse is caring for a client in labor who has butorphanol tartrate (Stadol) prescribed for the relief of labor pain. During the administration of the medication, the nurse would ensure that which priority item was readily available?

1 Naloxone (Narcan)
2 Meperidine hydrochloride (Demerol)
3 An intravenous form of an antiemetic
4 An intravenous solution of normal saline

Answer: 1
Rationale: Butorphanol tartrate is an opioid analgesic that provides systemic pain relief during labor. The nurse would ensure that naloxone and resuscitation equipment are readily available to treat respiratory depression, should it occur. Although an antiemetic may be prescribed for vomiting, antiemetics may enhance the respiratory depressant effects of the butorphanol tartrate. Although an IV access is desirable, the administration of normal saline is unrelated to the administration of this medication. Meperidine hydrochloride is also an opioid analgesic that may be used for pain relief, but it also causes respiratory depression.

Level of Cognitive Ability: Application
Client Needs: Physiological Integrity
Integrated Process: Nursing Process/Planning
Content Area: Maternity/Intrapartum

Test-Taking Strategy: Use the process of elimination, focusing on the strategic words "readily available" in the question. Recalling that butorphanol tartrate causes respiratory depression will direct you to option 1. Review this medication and its use during labor if you had difficulty with this question.

Reference
Murray, S., & McKinney, E. (2006). *Foundations of maternal-newborn nursing* (4th ed., p. 348). Philadelphia: Saunders.

1627. Methylergonovine (Methergine) is prescribed for a woman who has just delivered a healthy newborn infant. The priority assessment before administering the medication is to check the client's:
1 Lochia
2 Uterine tone
3 Blood pressure
4 Deep tendon reflexes

Level of Cognitive Ability: Application
Client Needs: Physiological Integrity
Integrated Process: Nursing Process/Assessment
Content Area: Maternity/Postpartum

Answer: 3
Rationale: Methergine, an oxytocic, is an agent used to prevent or control postpartum hemorrhage by contracting the uterus. The immediate dose is administered intramuscularly, and then if still needed, it is administered orally. It causes constant uterine contractions and may elevate the blood pressure. A priority assessment before administration of methylergonovine is blood pressure. Methylergonovine is to be administered cautiously in the presence of hypertension, and the physician should be notified if hypertension is present. Options 1 and 2 are general components of care in the postpartum period. Option 4 is most specifically related to the administration of magnesium sulfate.

Test-Taking Strategy: Use the process of elimination. Options 1 and 2 can be eliminated first because lochia and uterine tone are comparable or alike and are general assessments related to the postpartum period. Next, note the strategic word "priority" and use the ABCs—airway, breathing, and circulation—to direct you to option 3. Blood pressure is a method of assessing circulation. Additionally, option 4 can be eliminated because it most specifically relates to the administration of magnesium sulfate. Review the nursing responsibilities related to the administration of methylergonovine if you had difficulty with this question.

Reference
Murray, S., & McKinney, E. (2006). *Foundations of maternal-newborn nursing* (4th ed., p. 411). Philadelphia: Saunders.

1628. A nurse provides instructions to a client who is taking allopurinol (Zyloprim) for the treatment of gout. Which statement by the client indicates an understanding of the medication?
1 "I should put ice on my lips if they swell."
2 "I need to take the medication 2 hours after I eat."
3 "I need to drink at least eight glasses of fluid every day."
4 "I can use an antihistamine lotion if I get a rash that is itchy."

Answer: 3
Rationale: Clients taking allopurinol are encouraged to drink 3000 mL of fluid a day. Allopurinol is to be given with or immediately following meals or milk. If the client develops a rash, irritation of the eyes, or swelling of the lips or mouth, he or she should contact the physician because this may indicate hypersensitivity.

Level of Cognitive Ability: Analysis
Client Needs: Physiological Integrity
Integrated Process: Nursing Process/Evaluation
Content Area: Pharmacology

Test-Taking Strategy: Use the process of elimination, noting the strategic words "indicates an understanding." Options 1 and 4 can be eliminated first because they indicate a hypersensitivity, which is not a normal expected response. From the remaining options, recalling that the medication should be taken with food or milk will direct you to option 3. Review client instructions related to allopurinol if you had difficulty with this question.

Reference
Mosby. (2007). *Mosby's nursing drug reference* (20th ed., p. 98). St. Louis: Mosby.

1629. A rubella vaccine is administered to a client who delivered a healthy newborn infant 2 days ago. The nurse provides instructions to the client regarding the potential risks associated with this vaccination. Which statement by the client indicates an understanding of the medication?

1 "I need to stay out of the sunlight for 3 days."
2 "The injection site may itch, but I can scratch it if I need to."
3 "I need to avoid sexual intercourse for 2 to 3 months after the vaccination."
4 "I need to prevent becoming pregnant for 2 to 3 months after the vaccination."

Level of Cognitive Ability: Analysis
Client Needs: Health Promotion and Maintenance
Integrated Process: Nursing Process/Evaluation
Content Area: Maternity/Postpartum

Answer: 4
Rationale: Rubella vaccine is a live attenuated virus that evokes an antibody response and provides immunity for approximately 15 years. Because rubella is a live vaccine, it will act as the virus and is potentially teratogenic in the organogenesis phase of fetal development. The client needs to be informed about the potential effects this vaccine may have and the need to avoid becoming pregnant for a period of 2 to 3 months afterward. Abstinence from sexual intercourse is not necessary, unless another form of effective contraception is not being used. The vaccine may cause local or systemic reactions, but all are mild and short-lived. Sunlight has no effect on the person who is vaccinated.

Test-Taking Strategy: Use the process of elimination, recalling the effect of live vaccines on pregnancy and fetal development. Remembering that viruses can cross the placental barrier will direct you to option 4. Review the potential risks associated with the administration of this vaccine if you had difficulty with this question.

Reference
Murray, S., & McKinney, E. (2006). *Foundations of maternal-newborn nursing* (4th ed., p. 684). Philadelphia: Saunders.

1630. The school nurse is planning to give a class on testicular self-examination (TSE) at a local high school. The nurse plans to include which instruction on a written handout to be given to the students?

1 Perform the self-examination every other month
2 Perform the self-examination after a cold shower
3 Expect the self-examination to be slightly painful
4 Roll the testicle between the thumb and forefinger

Answer: 4
Rationale: TSE is a self-screening examination for testicular cancer, which predominantly affects men in their late teens and twenties. The self-examination is performed once a month, as is breast self-examination. As an aid to remember to do it, the examination should be done on the same day each month. The scrotum is held in one hand and the testicle is rolled between the thumb and forefinger of the other hand. The self-examination should not be painful. It is easiest to do either during or after a warm shower (or bath) when the scrotum is relaxed.

Level of Cognitive Ability: Application
Client Needs: Health Promotion and
   Maintenance
Integrated Process: Teaching and Learning
Content Area: Adult Health/Oncology

Test-Taking Strategy: Focus on the subject—self-examination—and read each option carefully. Knowledge of physical examination techniques will direct you to option 4. Review this content if you are unfamiliar with the procedure for TSE.

References
Black, J., & Hawks, J. (2005). *Medical-surgical nursing: Clinical management for positive outcomes* (7th ed., p. 1005). Philadelphia: Saunders.
Lewis, S., Heitkemper, M., Dirksen, S., O'Brien, P., & Bucher, L. (2007). *Medical-surgical nursing: Assessment and management of clinical problems* (7th ed., pp. 1432-1433). St. Louis: Mosby.

1631. A 32-year-old female client has a history of fibrocystic disorder of the breasts. The nurse determines that the client understands the nature of the disorder if the client states that symptoms are more likely to occur:

   1 After menses
   2 Before menses
   3 In the spring months
   4 In the winter months

Level of Cognitive Ability: Analysis
Client Needs: Physiological Integrity
Integrated Process: Nursing Process/Evaluation
Content Area: Adult Health/Oncology

Answer: 2
Rationale: The client with fibrocystic breast disorder experiences worsening of symptoms (breast lumps, painful breasts, and possible nipple discharge) before the onset of menses. This is associated with cyclical hormone changes. Clients should understand that this is part of the clinical picture of this disorder. Options 1, 3, and 4 are incorrect.

Test-Taking Strategy: Note the strategic words "more likely." This implies that there is a predictable variation in symptoms. Focus on the disorder and use knowledge of the effects of the various hormonal changes that occur in the body to direct you to option 2. Review the cyclical hormonal changes that occur in the female and the characteristics of fibrocystic disorder of the breasts if you had difficulty with this question.

References
Black, J., & Hawks, J. (2005). *Medical-surgical nursing: Clinical management for positive outcomes* (7th ed., p. 1120). Philadelphia: Saunders.
Ignatavicius, D., & Workman, M. (2006). *Medical-surgical nursing: Critical thinking for collaborative care* (5th ed., p. 1794). Philadelphia: Saunders.
Lewis, S., Heitkemper, M., Dirksen, S., O'Brien, P., & Bucher, L. (2007). *Medical-surgical nursing: Assessment and management of clinical problems* (7th ed., p. 1347). St. Louis: Mosby.

1632. A client has received a dose of dimenhydrinate (Dramamine). The nurse determines that the medication is effective if the client obtains relief of:

   1 Chills
   2 Headache
   3 Ringing in the ears
   4 Nausea and vomiting

Level of Cognitive Ability: Analysis
Client Needs: Physiological Integrity
Integrated Process: Nursing Process/Evaluation
Content Area: Pharmacology

Answer: 4
Rationale: Dimenhydrinate is used to treat and prevent the symptoms of dizziness, vertigo, and nausea and vomiting that accompany motion sickness. The other options are incorrect.

Test-Taking Strategy: Focus on the subject—medication effectiveness. Recalling that this medication is used to treat motion sickness will direct you to option 4. Review its action and uses if this medication is unfamiliar to you.

Reference
Mosby. (2007). *Mosby's nursing drug reference* (20th ed., p. 98). St. Louis: Mosby.

1633 A client is preparing for discharge 10 days after a radical vulvectomy. The nurse determines that the client has the best understanding of the measures to prevent complications if the client plans to do which of the following after discharge?

1 Walk
2 Drive a car
3 Do housework
4 Sit in a chair all day

Level of Cognitive Ability: Analysis
Client Needs: Physiological Integrity
Integrated Process: Nursing Process/Evaluation
Content Area: Adult Health/Oncology

Answer: 1
Rationale: The client should resume activity slowly, and walking is a beneficial activity. The client should know to rest when fatigue occurs. Activities to be avoided include driving, heavy housework, wearing tight clothing, crossing the legs, and prolonged standing or sitting. Sexual activity is usually prohibited for 4 to 6 weeks after surgery.

Test-Taking Strategy: Note the strategic words "to prevent complications." With this in mind, evaluate each of the options in terms of the stress or harm it could cause to the perineal area. This will direct you to option 1. Review teaching points for the client following radical vulvectomy if you had difficulty with this question.

References
Black, J., & Hawks, J. (2005). *Medical-surgical nursing: Clinical management for positive outcomes* (7th ed., pp. 1086-1087). Philadelphia: Saunders.
Lewis, S., Heitkemper, M., Dirksen, S., O'Brien, P., & Bucher, L. (2007). *Medical-surgical nursing: Assessment and management of clinical problems* (7th ed., p. 1406). St. Louis: Mosby.

1634. The nurse is caring for the client with silicosis who has massive pulmonary fibrosis. The nurse monitors the client for emotional reactions related to the chronic respiratory disease. Which emotional reaction if expressed by the client indicates a need for immediate intervention?

1 Anxiety
2 Depression
3 Suicidal ideation
4 Ineffective coping

Level of Cognitive Ability: Analysis
Client Needs: Psychosocial Integrity
Integrated Process: Nursing Process/Analysis
Content Area: Adult Health/Respiratory

Answer: 3
Rationale: Common emotional reactions to a disease such as massive pulmonary fibrosis may be the same as for chronic airflow limitation and include anxiety, ineffective coping, and depression. Suicidal ideation is not a normal emotional reaction with this condition. If it is expressed, it warrants immediate intervention.

Test-Taking Strategy: Use the process of elimination. Noting the strategic words "need for immediate intervention" will direct you to option 3. Review the common emotional reactions that occur in chronic diseases and nursing interventions if suicidal ideation is expressed by the client if you had difficulty with this question.

Reference
Ignatavicius, D., & Workman, M. (2006). *Medical-surgical nursing: Critical thinking for collaborative care* (5th ed., p. 659). Philadelphia: Saunders.

1635. At the beginning of the work shift, the nurse is checking a client who has returned from the post-anesthesia care unit following transurethral resection of the prostate (TURP). The client has bladder irrigation running via a three-way Foley catheter. The nurse should notify the physician if which color of urine is noted in the urinary drainage bag?

1 Pale pink
2 Bright red
3 Dark pink
4 Tea-colored

Answer: 2
Rationale: Bright red bleeding should be reported, because it could indicate complications related to active bleeding. If the bladder irrigation is infusing at a sufficient rate, the urinary drainage will be pale pink. A dark pink color (sometimes referred to as punch-colored) indicates that the speed of the irrigation should be increased. Tea-colored urine is not seen after TURP, but may be noted in the client with renal failure or other renal disorders.

Level of Cognitive Ability: Application
Client Needs: Physiological Integrity
Integrated Process: Nursing Process/
    Implementation
Content Area: Adult Health/Renal

Test-Taking Strategy: Use the process of elimination, recalling that hemorrhage is a complication following any surgical procedure. Remember also that the purpose of bladder irrigation is to flush out blood and clots that could otherwise accumulate in the bladder following surgery. With this in mind, select option 2 because bright red drainage would indicate a potential complication such as bleeding. Review care of the client following TURP if you had difficulty with this question.

Reference
Ignatavicius, D., & Workman, M. (2006). *Medical-surgical nursing: Critical thinking for collaborative care* (5th ed., p. 1863). Philadelphia: Saunders.

1636. Phenelzine sulfate (Nardil) is being administered to a client with depression. The client suddenly complains of a severe occipital headache radiating frontally, and neck stiffness and soreness, and is vomiting. On further assessment, the client exhibits signs of hypertensive crisis. Which medication would the nurse prepare anticipating that it will be prescribed as the antidote for hypertensive crisis?

1 Vitamin K
2 Phentolamine
3 Protamine sulfate
4 Calcium gluconate

Level of Cognitive Ability: Analysis
Client Needs: Physiological Integrity
Integrated Process: Nursing Process/Planning
Content Area: Pharmacology

Answer: 2
Rationale: The manifestations of hypertensive crisis include hypertension, occipital headache radiating frontally, neck stiffness and soreness, nausea, vomiting, sweating, fever and chills, clammy skin, dilated pupils, and palpitations. Tachycardia, bradycardia, and constricting chest pain may also be present. The antidote for hypertensive crisis is phentolamine and a dosage by intravenous injection is administered. Protamine sulfate is the antidote for heparin, and vitamin K is the antidote for warfarin (Coumadin) overdose. Calcium gluconate is used for magnesium overdose.

Test-Taking Strategy: Knowledge regarding the antidotes for various medications and disorders is required to answer this question. Remember that the antidote for hypertensive crisis is phentolamine. Review this content if you are unfamiliar with the antidotes associated with the use of certain medications and conditions.

References
Hodgson, B., & Kizior, R. (2007). *Saunders nursing drug handbook 2007* (p. 921). Philadelphia: Saunders.
Varcarolis, E., Carson, V, & Shoemaker, N. (2006) *Foundations of psychiatric mental health nursing* (5th ed., p. 350). Philadelphia: Saunders.

1637. The nurse is caring for a 25-year-old single client who will undergo bilateral orchiectomy for testicular cancer. The nurse should make it a priority to explore which potential psychological concern with this client?

1 Postoperative pain
2 Postoperative swelling
3 Loss of reproductive ability
4 Length of recuperative period

Answer: 3
Rationale: Although the client will need factual information about the postoperative period and recuperation, the nurse would place priority on addressing loss of reproductive ability as a psychological concern. The radical effects of this surgery in the reproductive area make it likely that the client may have some difficulty in adjustment to this consequence of surgery.

Test-Taking Strategy: Use the process of elimination, focusing on the client's diagnosis and surgical procedure. Eliminate options 1, 2, and 4 because they are general concerns of any surgical procedure. Option 3 is specific to a bilateral orchiectomy. Review the psychosocial issues related to an orchiectomy if you had difficulty with this question.

Level of Cognitive Ability: Application
Client Needs: Psychosocial Integrity
Integrated Process: Caring
Content Area: Adult Health/Oncology

Reference
Ignatavicius, D., & Workman, M. (2006). *Medical-surgical nursing: Critical thinking for collaborative care* (5th ed., pp. 1874-1875). Philadelphia: Saunders.

1638. The nurse is assisting in participating in a prostate screening clinic for men. The nurse questions each client about which sign of prostatism?
1 Absence of postvoid dribbling
2 Ability to stop voiding quickly
3 Excessive force in urinary stream
4 Hesitancy when initiating urinary stream

Level of Cognitive Ability: Application
Client Needs: Health Promotion and Maintenance
Integrated Process: Nursing Process/Assessment
Content Area: Adult Health/Renal

Answer: 4
Rationale: Signs of prostatism that may be reported to the nurse are reduced force and size of urinary stream, intermittent stream, hesitancy in beginning the flow of urine, inability to stop urinating quickly, a sensation of incomplete bladder emptying after voiding, and an increase in episodes of nocturia. These symptoms are the result of pressure of the enlarging prostate on the client's urethra.

Test-Taking Strategy: Use the process of elimination. Eliminate options 1, 2, and 3 because they are comparable or alike and indicate no difficulty with proper emptying of the bladder. Review the signs of prostatism if you had difficulty with this question.

References
Black, J., & Hawks, J. (2005). *Medical-surgical nursing: Clinical management for positive outcomes* (7th ed., p. 1016). Philadelphia: Saunders.
Ignatavicius, D., & Workman, M. (2006). *Medical-surgical nursing: Critical thinking for collaborative care* (5th ed., p. 1879). Philadelphia: Saunders.

1639. A male client being seen in the ambulatory care clinic has a history of being treated for syphilis infection. The nurse interprets that the client has been reinfected if which characteristic is noted in a penile lesion?
1 Papular areas and erythema
2 Cauliflower-like appearance
3 Induration and absence of pain
4 Multiple vesicles, with some that have ruptured

Level of Cognitive Ability: Analysis
Client Needs: Physiological Integrity
Integrated Process: Nursing Process/Assessment
Content Area: Adult Health/Integumentary

Answer: 3
Rationale: The characteristic lesion of syphilis is painless and indurated. The lesion is referred to as a *chancre*. Scabies is characterized by erythematous, papular eruptions. Genital warts are characterized by cauliflower-like growths, or growths that are soft and fleshy. Genital herpes is accompanied by the presence of one or more vesicles that then rupture and heal.

Test-Taking Strategy: To answer this question accurately, it is necessary to be familiar with the characteristics of skin lesions of the various sexually transmitted diseases. Remember that the characteristic lesion of syphilis is painless and indurated. Review the appearance of lesions associated with syphilis if you had difficulty with this question.

References
Black, J., & Hawks, J. (2005). *Medical-surgical nursing: Clinical management for positive outcomes* (7th ed., p. 1133). Philadelphia: Saunders.
Monahan, F., Sands, J., Marek, J., Neighbors, M., & Green, C. (2007). *Phipp's Medical-surgical nursing: Health and illness perspectives* (8th ed., pp. 1790-1791). St. Louis: Mosby.

1640. An adult client has been admitted to the hospital with a 3-day history of uncontrolled vomiting and diarrhea. The nurse assesses for which of the following in this client?
1 Excitability
2 Bradycardia
3 Hypertension
4 Tenting of the skin

Level of Cognitive Ability: Analysis
Client Needs: Physiological Integrity
Integrated Process: Nursing Process/Assessment
Content Area: Adult Health/Gastrointestinal

Answer: 4
Rationale: The client described in the question will most likely be dehydrated. The nurse assesses this client for weight loss, lethargy or headache, sunken eyes, poor skin turgor (such as tenting), flat neck and peripheral veins, tachycardia, and low blood pressure.

Test-Taking Strategy: Use the process of elimination, focusing on the data in the question. Recalling that a client who has a 3-day episode of uncontrolled vomiting and diarrhea is at risk for dehydration will direct you to option 4. Review the signs of dehydration if you had difficulty with this question.

References
Black, J., & Hawks, J. (2005). *Medical-surgical nursing: Clinical management for positive outcomes* (7th ed., pp. 208-209). Philadelphia: Saunders.
Lewis, S., Heitkemper, M., Dirksen, S., O'Brien, P., & Bucher, L. (2007). *Medical-surgical nursing: Assessment and management of clinical problems* (7th ed., p. 323). St. Louis: Mosby.

1641. An adult client with renal insufficiency has been placed on a fluid restriction of 1200 mL per day. The nurse discusses the fluid restriction with the dietitian and then plans to allow the client to have how many milliliters of fluid from 7:00 AM to 3:00 PM?
1 400
2 600
3 800
4 1000

Level of Cognitive Ability: Application
Client Needs: Physiological Integrity
Integrated Process: Nursing Process/Planning
Content Area: Adult Health/Renal

Answer: 2
Rationale: When a client is on a fluid restriction, the nurse informs the dietary department and discusses the allotment of fluid per shift with the dietitian. When calculating how to distribute a fluid restriction, the nurse usually allows half of the daily allotment (600 mL) during the day shift, when the client eats two meals and takes most medications. Another two-fifths (480 mL) is allotted to the evening shift, with the balance (120 mL) allowed during the nighttime.

Test-Taking Strategy: To answer this question accurately, you must be familiar with fluid restriction and the general principles related to fluid distribution over a 24-hour period. Review these principles and calculation of fluid distribution in the client with renal insufficiency if you had difficulty with this question.

Reference
Lewis, S., Heitkemper, M., Dirksen, S., O'Brien, P., & Bucher, L. (2007). *Medical-surgical nursing: Assessment and management of clinical problems* (7th ed., p. 1212). St. Louis: Mosby.

1642. A client with chronic renal failure has learned about managing diet and fluid restriction between dialysis treatments. The nurse determines that the client is compliant with the therapeutic regimen if the client gains no more than how much weight between hemodialysis treatments?
1 2 to 4 kg
2 5 to 6 kg
3 0.5 to 1 kg
4 1 to 1.5 kg

Answer: 4
Rationale: A limit of 1 to 1.5 kg of weight gain between dialysis treatments helps prevent hypotension that tends to occur during dialysis with the removal of larger fluid loads. The nurse determines that the client is compliant with fluid restriction if this weight gain is not exceeded.

Level of Cognitive Ability: Analysis
Client Needs: Physiological Integrity
Integrated Process: Nursing Process/Evaluation
Content Area: Adult Health/Renal

Test-Taking Strategy: It may be helpful in answering this question to recall that 1 L of fluid weighs approximately 1 kg. Recalling that there are approximately 6 L of blood circulating in the body will assist in eliminating options 1 and 2 as being amounts that are too large. Correspondingly, option 3 is eliminated because the amount is too small, representing only 500 to 1000 mL of fluid. Review teaching points for the client with chronic renal failure if you had difficulty with this question.

References

Black, J., & Hawks, J. (2005). *Medical-surgical nursing: Clinical management for positive outcomes* (7th ed., pp. 926-964). Philadelphia: Saunders.

Ignatavicius, D., & Workman, M. (2006). *Medical-surgical nursing: Critical thinking for collaborative care* (5th ed., p. 1736). Philadelphia: Saunders.

Lewis, S., Heitkemper, M., Dirksen, S., O'Brien, P., & Bucher, L. (2007). *Medical-surgical nursing: Assessment and management of clinical problems* (7th ed., p. 1212). St. Louis: Mosby.

1643. A client was admitted to the surgical unit following right total knee replacement performed 2 hours earlier. Which observation by the nurse indicates the need to contact the surgeon?
1 Pale pink and warm right foot
2 Pain relieved by an opioid analgesic
3 Ability to flex and extend the right foot
4 Hemovac wound suction drainage of 175 mL per hour

Level of Cognitive Ability: Analysis
Client Needs: Physiological Integrity
Integrated Process: Nursing Process/Assessment
Content Area: Adult Health/Musculoskeletal

Answer: 4

Rationale: Following total knee replacement, the neurovascular status of the affected leg is assessed, and findings should be within normal limits. The client should have intact capillary refill and adequate color, temperature, sensation, and motion to the limb. Incisional pain should be relieved by opioid analgesic administration. The knee incision may have a wound suction drain in place. Output from the drain is generally less than 300 mL per shift. Drainage of 175 mL per hour is excessive and should be reported.

Test-Taking Strategy: Note the strategic words "need to contact the surgeon." Options 1 and 3 represent normal neurovascular status and are eliminated first. Knowing that surgery causes the client pain, which is then relieved by analgesics, will assist in eliminating option 2. This leaves option 4 as the correct option given the wording of this question. Review expected findings following a total knee replacement if you had difficulty with this question.

References

Black, J., & Hawks, J. (2005). *Medical-surgical nursing: Clinical management for positive outcomes* (7th ed., pp. 595-596). Philadelphia: Saunders.

Lewis, S., Heitkemper, M., Dirksen, S., O'Brien, P., & Bucher, L. (2007). *Medical-surgical nursing: Assessment and management of clinical problems* (7th ed., p. 591). St. Louis: Mosby.

1644. A client is being discharged from the hospital following removal of chest tubes that were inserted following thoracic surgery. The nurse provides home care instructions to the client and determines the need for further instructions if the client states:

1 "I need to avoid heavy lifting for the first 4 to 6 weeks."
2 "I need to take my temperature to detect a possible infection."
3 "I need to report any difficulty with breathing to the physician."
4 "I need to remove the chest tube site dressing as soon as I get home."

Level of Cognitive Ability: Analysis
Client Needs: Health Promotion and Maintenance
Integrated Process: Teaching and Learning
Content Area: Adult Health/Respiratory

Answer: 4
Rationale: Upon removal of a chest tube, a dressing is placed over the chest tube site. This is maintained in place until the physician says it may be removed. The client is taught to monitor and report any respiratory difficulty or increased temperature. The client should avoid heavy lifting for the first 4 to 6 weeks after discharge to facilitate continued wound healing.

Test-Taking Strategy: Use the process of elimination, noting the strategic words "need for further instructions." These words indicate a negative event query and the need to select the incorrect client statement. Recalling that signs of infection and respiratory difficulty should be monitored and reported helps eliminate options 2 and 3 first. From the remaining options, recalling that either heavy lifting should be avoided postoperatively or that removal of the chest tube site dressing disturbs the occlusive seal to the site will direct you to option 4. Review teaching points following removal of a chest tube if you had difficulty with this question.

References
Black, J., & Hawks, J. (2005). *Medical-surgical nursing: Clinical management for positive outcomes* (7th ed., p. 955). Philadelphia: Saunders.
Lewis, S., Heitkemper, M., Dirksen, S., O'Brien, P., & Bucher, L. (2007). *Medical-surgical nursing: Assessment and management of clinical problems* (7th ed., p. 592). St. Louis: Mosby.

1645. The nurse is administering epoetin alfa (Epogen) to a client with chronic renal failure. The nurse monitors the client for which adverse effect of this therapy?

1 Anemia
2 Hypertension
3 Iron intoxication
4 Bleeding tendencies

Level of Cognitive Ability: Analysis
Client Needs: Physiological Integrity
Integrated Process: Nursing Process/Assessment
Content Area: Adult Health/Renal

Answer: 2
Rationale: The client taking epoetin alfa is at risk of hypertension and seizure activity as the most serious adverse effects of therapy. This medication is used to treat anemia. The medication does not cause iron intoxication. Bleeding tendencies is not an adverse effect of this medication.

Test-Taking Strategy: Knowledge regarding the adverse effects of this medication is needed to answer this question. Remember that the client taking epoetin alfa is at risk of hypertension and seizure activity as the most serious adverse effects of therapy. Review this medication if you had difficulty with this question.

References
Black, J., & Hawks, J. (2005). *Medical-surgical nursing: Clinical management for positive outcomes* (7th ed., p. 955). Philadelphia: Saunders.
Hodgson, B., & Kizior, R. (2007). *Saunders nursing drug handbook 2007* (p. 424). Philadelphia: Saunders.

1646. A client is taking lansoprazole (Prevacid) for the chronic management of Zollinger-Ellison syndrome. The nurse determines that the client best understands this disorder and the medication regimen if the client states to take which of the following products for pain?
1 Naprosyn (Aleve)
2 Ibuprofen (Motrin)
3 Acetaminophen (Tylenol)
4 Acetylsalicylic acid (aspirin)

Level of Cognitive Ability: Analysis
Client Needs: Physiological Integrity
Integrated Process: Nursing Process/Evaluation
Content Area: Pharmacology

Answer: 3
Rationale: Zollinger-Ellison syndrome is a hypersecretory condition of the stomach. The client should not take medications that irritate to the stomach lining. Irritants would include aspirin and nonsteroidal anti-inflammatory medications (naprosyn and ibuprofen). The client should take acetaminophen for pain relief.

Test-Taking Strategy: Use the process of elimination. Eliminate options 1 and 2 first because they are both nonsteroidal anti-inflammatory medications. From the remaining options, select acetaminophen over aspirin because it is least irritating to the stomach. Review these medications if you had difficulty with this question.

References
Lehne, R. (2007). *Pharmacology for nursing care* (6th ed., p. 898). Philadelphia: Saunders.
Mosby. (2007). *Mosby's nursing drug reference* (20th ed., p. 590). St. Louis: Mosby.

1647. The client scheduled for a transurethral prostatectomy (TURP) has listened to the surgeon's explanation of the surgery. The client later asks the nurse to explain again how the prostate is going to be removed. The nurse tells the client that the prostate will be removed through:
1 The urethra
2 A lower abdominal incision
3 An upper abdominal incision
4 An incision made in the perineal area

Level of Cognitive Ability: Application
Client Needs: Physiological Integrity
Integrated Process: Nursing Process/ Implementation
Content Area: Adult Health/Renal

Answer: 1
Rationale: A TURP is done through the urethra. An instrument called a resectoscope is used to remove the tissue using high-frequency current. An incision between the scrotum and anus is made when a perineal prostatectomy is performed. A lower abdominal incision is used for suprapubic or retropubic prostatectomy. An upper abdominal incision is not used

Test-Taking Strategy: Use the process of elimination. Note the relationship between the name of the procedure "transurethral" in the question and the word "urethra" in the correct option. Review this procedure if you had difficulty with this question.

References
Black, J., & Hawks, J. (2005). *Medical-surgical nursing: Clinical management for positive outcomes* (7th ed., p. 1020). Philadelphia: Saunders.
Ignatavicius, D., & Workman, M. (2006). *Medical-surgical nursing: Critical thinking for collaborative care* (5th ed., p. 1861). Philadelphia: Saunders.

1648. The nurse tells a client who is scheduled for a bone marrow biopsy that the specimen can be withdrawn from the:
1 Ribs
2 Femur
3 Scapula
4 Sternum

Level of Cognitive Ability: Application
Client Needs: Physiological Integrity
Integrated Process: Nursing Process/ Implementation
Content Area: Fundamental Skills

Answer: 4
Rationale: The most common sites for bone marrow aspiration in the adult are the iliac crest and the sternum. These areas are rich in bone marrow and are easily accessible for testing. The femur, scapula, and ribs are not sites for bone marrow aspiration.

Test-Taking Strategy: Focus on the subject—a bone marrow aspiration. Recalling the anatomy and physiology related to the bones and bone marrow will direct you to option 4. Review the procedure for a bone marrow aspiration if you had difficulty with this question.

Reference
Lewis, S., Heitkemper, M., Dirksen, S., O'Brien, P., & Bucher, L. (2007). *Medical-surgical nursing: Assessment and management of clinical problems* (7th ed., p. 681). St. Louis: Mosby.

1649. A client is taking amiloride (Midamor) 10 mg orally daily for the treatment of hypertension. The nurse gives the client which instruction regarding its use?
1 Take the medication in the morning with breakfast.
2 Withhold the medication if the blood pressure is high.
3 Eat foods with extra sodium while taking this medication.
4 Take the medication 2 hours after lunch on an empty stomach.

Level of Cognitive Ability: Application
Client Needs: Health Promotion and Maintenance
Integrated Process: Teaching and Learning
Content Area: Pharmacology

Answer: 1
Rationale: Amiloride is a potassium-sparing diuretic used to treat edema or hypertension. A daily dose should be taken in the morning to avoid nocturia. The dose should be taken with food to increase bioavailability. Sodium should be restricted if used as an antihypertensive. Increased blood pressure is not a reason to hold the medication, and it may be an indication for its use.

Test-Taking Strategy: Use the process of elimination. Noting the client's diagnosis and recalling that this medication is a potassium-sparing diuretic will direct you to option 1. Review client teaching points related to this medication if you had difficulty with this question.

Reference
Skidmore-Roth, L. (2008). *Mosby's nursing drug reference* (21st ed., p. 112). St. Louis: Mosby.

1650. The nurse is preparing a poster for a booth at a health fair to promote primary prevention of cervical cancer. The nurse includes which recommendation on the poster?
1 Use a commercial douche on a daily basis.
2 Perform monthly breast self-examination (BSE).
3 Seek treatment promptly for infections of the cervix.
4 Use oral contraceptives as a preferred method of birth control.

Level of Cognitive Ability: Application
Client Needs: Health Promotion and Maintenance
Integrated Process: Teaching and Learning
Content Area: Adult Health/Oncology

Answer: 3
Rationale: Early treatment of cervical infection can help prevent chronic cervicitis, which can lead to dysplasia of the cervix. Cervical dysplasia is an early cell change that is considered to be premalignant. Oral contraceptives and douches do not decrease the risk for this type of cancer. BSE is useful for early detection of breast cancer, but is unrelated to cervical cancer.

Test-Taking Strategy: Note the strategic words "primary prevention" and "cervical cancer." Eliminate option 2 because it is unrelated to cervical cancer. From the remaining options, recalling the risk factors associated with this type of cancer will direct you to option 3. Review the risk factors associated with cervical cancer if you had difficulty with this question.

References
Black, J., & Hawks, J. (2005). *Medical-surgical nursing: Clinical management for positive outcomes* (7th ed., pp. 355, 1072). Philadelphia: Saunders.
Lewis, S., Heitkemper, M., Dirksen, S., O'Brien, P., & Bucher, L. (2007). *Medical-surgical nursing: Assessment and management of clinical problems* (7th ed., pp. 1400-1401). St. Louis: Mosby.

1651. The nurse administers diphenhydramine (Benadryl) before a blood transfusion to:
1 Prevent urticaria.
2 Avoid fever and chills.
3 Enhance clotting factors.
4 Expand the blood volume.

Answer: 1
Rationale: The clinical indicators of urticaria are a rash accompanied by pruritus. Urticaria is a manifestation of a transfusion reaction when it occurs during a blood transfusion and is preventable by premedicating the client with an antihistamine, such as diphenhydramine. Options 2, 3, and 4 are incorrect. Clients can also be premedicated with acetaminophen (Tylenol) to help prevent fever and chills.

Level of Cognitive Ability: Analysis
Client Needs: Physiological Integrity
Integrated Process: Nursing Process/Analysis
Content Area: Fundamental Skills

Test-Taking Strategy: Use the process of elimination, focusing on the subject—the purpose of the diphenhydramine. Eliminate options 3 and 4 first because enhancing the blood's clotting factors is undesirable, usually, and the volume of the transfusion expands the client's blood volume. Recalling the classification of diphenhydramine will direct you to option 1. Review the purpose of diphenhydramine if you had difficulty with this question.

References

Black, J., & Hawks, J. (2005). *Medical-surgical nursing: Clinical management for positive outcomes* (7th ed., p. 2320). Philadelphia: Saunders.

Lewis, S., Heitkemper, M., Dirksen, S., O'Brien, P., & Bucher, L. (2007). *Medical-surgical nursing: Assessment and management of clinical problems* (7th ed., p. 733). St. Louis: Mosby.

1652. A client is admitted to the hospital with a diagnosis of infiltrating ductal carcinoma of the breast. The nurse assesses the client for which expected manifestation?

1 Bilateral palpable masses
2 Pain in the breast and edema
3 A fixed, irregularly shaped mass
4 A round-shaped mass that is moveable

Level of Cognitive Ability: Application
Client Needs: Physiological Integrity
Integrated Process: Nursing Process/Assessment
Content Area: Adult Health/Oncology

Answer: 3

Rationale: Infiltrating ductal carcinoma of the breast usually presents as a fixed, irregularly shaped mass. The mass is usually single and unilateral, and is painless, nontender, and hard to the touch.

Test-Taking Strategy: Using principles of anatomy and knowledge regarding the characteristics of a cancerous lesion will assist in eliminating options 1 and 4 first. Choose option 3 over option 2, recalling that pain is generally a late sign of a disorder and that involvement of the ducts makes it more likely that the mass does not move (fixed). Review the characteristics of breast cancer if you had difficulty with this question.

References

Black, J., & Hawks, J. (2005). *Medical-surgical nursing: Clinical management for positive outcomes* (7th ed., p. 1099). Philadelphia: Saunders.

Monahan, F., Sands, J., Marek, J., Neighbors, M., & Green, C. (2007). *Phipps' medical-surgical nursing: Health and illness perspectives* (8th ed., p. 1755). St. Louis: Mosby.

1653. A mother of a 9-year-old child newly diagnosed with diabetes mellitus is very concerned about the child going to school and participating in social events. The nurse develops a plan of care and formulates which goal?

1 The child's normal growth and development will be maintained.
2 The child will use effective coping mechanisms to manage anxiety.
3 The child and family will discuss all aspects of the illness and its treatments.
4 The child and family will integrate diabetes care into patterns of daily living.

Answer: 4

Rationale: In order to effectively manage social events in the child's life, the family and the child need to integrate the care and management of diabetes into their daily living. The other options are goals for the family, but they do not deal with social issues.

Test-Taking Strategy: Use the process of elimination and focus on the subject—social events. Noting the relationship of this subject and the words "into patterns of daily living" will direct you to option 4. Review goals of care for a child with diabetes mellitus if you had difficulty with this question.

Level of Cognitive Ability: Application
Client Needs: Psychosocial Integrity
Integrated Process: Nursing Process/Planning
Content Area: Child Health

Reference
Hockenberry, M., Wilson, D., & Winkelstein, M. (2005). *Wong's essentials of pediatric nursing* (7th ed., pp. 1088-1089). St. Louis: Mosby.

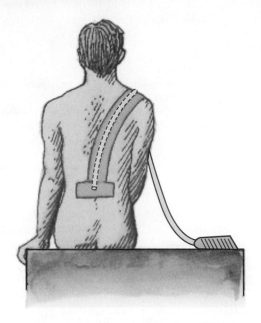

From Perry, A., & Potter, P. (2006). *Clinical nursing skills & techniques* (6th ed.). St. Louis: Mosby.(Courtesy Astra Zeneca Pharmaceuticals, Wilmington, DE.)

1654. A nurse performs an assessment on a client with cancer and notes that the client is receiving pain medication via this type of catheter (see figure). The nurse documents that the client has a(n):
   1. Epidural catheter
   2. Hickman catheter
   3. Central venous catheter (CVC)
   4. Patient-controlled analgesia (PCA) pump

Level of Cognitive Ability: Analysis
Client Needs: Physiological Integrity
Integrated Process: Nursing Process/Assessment
Content Area: Adult Health/Oncology

Answer: 1
Rationale: An epidural catheter is placed in the epidural space. The epidural space lies between the dura mater and the vertebral column. When an opioid is injected into the epidural space, it binds to opiate receptors located on the dorsal horn of the spinal cord and blocks the transmission of pain impulses to the cerebral cortex of the brain. Because the opioid does not cross the blood-brain barrier, pain relief results from drug levels in the spinal cord rather than in the plasma, with little central or systemic distribution of the medication. A Hickman catheter is a vascular access device that is surgically inserted, tunneled through the subcutaneous tissue, and is used to manage long-term intravenous therapy. A CVC is inserted into a large vein (typically the internal or external jugular or the superior vena cava) that leads to the right atrium of the heart. A PCA pump is the device that allows the client to self-administer pain medication.

Test-Taking Strategy: Use the process of elimination and knowledge of anatomy to answer the question. Noting the location of the catheter site will direct you to option 1. Review the placement and use of an epidural catheter if you had difficulty with this question.

References
Ignatavicius, D., & Workman, M. (2006). *Medical-surgical nursing: Critical thinking for collaborative care* (5th ed., pp. 1053-1054). Philadelphia: Saunders.
Perry, A., & Potter, P. (2006) *Clinical nursing skills & techniques* (6th ed., p. 145). St. Louis: Mosby.

1655. A client has had a left mastectomy with axillary lymph node dissection. The nurse determines that the client understands postoperative restrictions and arm care if the client states to:

1 Use gloves when working in the garden.
2 Use a straight razor to shave under the arms.
3 Carry a handbag and heavy objects on the left arm.
4 Allow blood pressures to be taken only on the left arm.

Level of Cognitive Ability: Analysis
Client Needs: Health Promotion and Maintenance
Integrated Process: Nursing Process/Evaluation
Content Area: Adult Health/Oncology

Answer: 1
Rationale: The client is at risk for edema and infection as a result of lymph node dissection. The client should avoid activities that increase edema, such as carrying heavy objects or having blood pressures taken on the affected arm. The client should also use a variety of techniques to avoid trauma to the affected arm. Examples include using an electric razor to shave under the arm, gloves when working in the garden, and pot holders when cooking to prevent burns.

Test-Taking Strategy: Note the surgical procedure and focus on the subject—postoperative restrictions and arm care. Keeping this subject in mind, read each option, noting the potential risk related to edema or trauma. This will direct you to option 1. Review teaching points for the client following mastectomy if you had difficulty with this question.

References
Black, J., & Hawks, J. (2005). *Medical-surgical nursing: Clinical management for positive outcomes* (7th ed., p. 1108). Philadelphia: Saunders.
Monahan, F., Sands, J., Marek, J., Neighbors, M., & Green, C. (2007). *Phipps' medical-surgical nursing: Health and illness perspectives* (8th ed., p. 1771). St. Louis: Mosby.

1656. The nurse is teaching a client about the modifiable risk factors that can reduce the risk for colorectal cancer. The nurse places highest priority on discussing which risk factor with this client?

1 Age older than 30 years
2 High-fat and low-fiber diet
3 Distant relative with colorectal cancer
4 Personal history of ulcerative colitis or gastrointestinal (GI) polyps

Level of Cognitive Ability: Application
Client Needs: Health Promotion and Maintenance
Integrated Process: Teaching and Learning
Content Area: Adult Health/Gastrointestinal

Answer: 2
Rationale: Common risk factors for colorectal cancer that cannot be changed include age older than 40, first-degree relative with colorectal cancer, and history of bowel problems such as ulcerative colitis or familial polyposis. Clients should be aware of modifiable risk factors as part of general health maintenance and primary disease prevention. Modifiable risk factors are those that can be reduced and include a high-fat and low-fiber diet.

Test-Taking Strategy: Focus on the subject—modifiable risk factors related to colorectal cancer. Note the strategic words "reduce the risk" and "highest priority." Recalling that modifiable risk factors are those that can be changed will direct you to option 2. Review modifiable and nonmodifiable risk factors related to colorectal cancer if you had difficulty with this question.

References
Black, J., & Hawks, J. (2005). *Medical-surgical nursing: Clinical management for positive outcomes* (7th ed., pp. 830-831). Philadelphia: Saunders.
Monahan, F., Sands, J., Marek, J., Neighbors, M., & Green, C. (2007). *Phipps' medical-surgical nursing: Health and illness perspectives* (8th ed., p. 1272). St. Louis: Mosby.

1657. A client with gastroesophageal reflux disease (GERD) complains of chest discomfort that feels like heartburn, especially following each meal. After teaching the client to take antacids as prescribed, the nurse suggests that the client lie in which position during sleep?

1 Flat
2 Supine with the head of the bed flat
3 On the stomach with the head of the bed flat
4 With the head of the bed elevated 8 to 12 inches

Level of Cognitive Ability: Application
Client Needs: Physiological Integrity
Integrated Process: Teaching and Learning
Content Area: Adult Health/Gastrointestinal

Answer: 4

Rationale: The discomfort of reflux is aggravated by positions that allow the reflux of gastrointestinal contents. The client is instructed to remain upright for 1 to 2 hours after a meal and to sleep with the head of the bed elevated to approximately 30 degrees (usually on 8 to 12 inch blocks). Lying flat will increase the episodes of reflux, resulting in chest discomfort.

Test-Taking Strategy: Use the process of elimination and think about the physiology associated with this disorder. Eliminate options 1, 2, and 3 because they are comparable or alike and all indicate flat positions. Review measures that will reduce discomfort in the client with GERD if you had difficulty with this question.

References

Ignatavicius, D., & Workman, M. (2006). *Medical-surgical nursing: Critical thinking for collaborative care* (5th ed., p. 1264). Philadelphia: Saunders.

Lewis, S., Heitkemper, M., Dirksen, S., O'Brien, P., & Bucher, L. (2007). *Medical-surgical nursing: Assessment and management of clinical problems* (7th ed., p. 1007). St. Louis: Mosby.

1658. The nurse instructs a female client about collecting a midstream urine sample for culture and sensitivity. Which does the nurse include in client teaching?

1 Bathe before collecting the specimen.
2 Cleanse the perineum from front to back.
3 Label specimen with the provider's name.
4 Collect urine at the beginning of urination.

Level of Cognitive Ability: Application
Client Needs: Physiological Integrity
Integrated Process: Teaching and Learning
Content Area: Fundamental Skills

Answer: 2

Rationale: To prepare properly for collection of a sterile urine specimen, the client cleanses the perineum from front to back using antiseptic swabs. The client should begin the flow of urine and collect the sample after starting the flow of urine and, then, send the specimen to the laboratory as soon as possible. Bathing before a midstream urine collection is unnecessary; however, proper specimen handling is critically important because improper specimen handling can yield inaccurate test results. The specimen should be labeled with the client's name, date, time, and medical record number in addition to the provider's name.

Test-Taking Strategy: Use the process of elimination and recall the principles related to obtaining a midstream urine specimen. Noting the name of the type of sample, "midstream," will assist in eliminating option 4. From the remaining options, use basic principles related to hygiene to assist in directing you to option 2. Review this procedure if you had difficulty with this question.

Reference

Lewis, S., Heitkemper, M., Dirksen, S., O'Brien, P., & Bucher, L. (2007). *Medical-surgical nursing: Assessment and management of clinical problems* (7th ed., p. 1146). St. Louis: Mosby.

1659. The nurse is preparing to care for a client who has undergone esophagogastroduodenoscopy (EGD). After checking the vital signs, what should be the nurse's next priority?

1 Monitor for sharp epigastric pain.
2 Give warm gargles for sore throat.
3 Check for a return of the gag reflex.
4 Monitor for complaints of heartburn.

Level of Cognitive Ability: Application
Client Needs: Physiological Integrity
Integrated Process: Nursing Process/
   Implementation
Content Area: Adult Health/Gastrointestinal

Answer: 3
Rationale: The nurse places highest priority on assessing for the return of the gag reflex, which is part of maintaining the client's airway. The nurse would monitor the client for sharp pain (may indicate a potential complication) and heartburn. The client would also receive warm gargles, but this cannot be done until the gag reflex has returned.

Test-Taking Strategy: Note the strategic word "next." Use the ABCs—airway, breathing, and circulation—to direct you to option 3. Review postprocedure care following an EGD if you had difficulty with question.

References
Ignatavicius, D., & Workman, M. (2006). *Medical-surgical nursing: Critical thinking for collaborative care* (5th ed., p. 1244). Philadelphia: Saunders.
Pagana, K., & Pagana, T. (2005). *Mosby's diagnostic and laboratory test reference*, (7th ed., p. 413). St. Louis: Mosby.

1660. Methylphenidate (Ritalin) is prescribed for a child with a diagnosis of attention deficit hyperactivity disorder (ADHD). The nurse providing information to the mother regarding the administration of the medication instructs the mother to administer the medication:

1 Before dinner and at bedtime
2 At the noontime and evening meals
3 In the morning after breakfast and at bedtime
4 Before breakfast and before the noontime meal

Level of Cognitive Ability: Application
Client Needs: Physiological Integrity
Integrated Process: Teaching and Learning
Content Area: Pharmacology

Answer: 4
Rationale: Methylphenidate is a central nervous stimulant and should be taken before breakfast and before the noontime meal. It should not be taken in the afternoon or evening because the stimulating effect causes insomnia. Options 1, 2, and 3 are incorrect.

Test-Taking Strategy: Use the process of elimination. Noting the name of the medication and the disorder and recalling that this medication is a central nervous system stimulant will direct you to option 4. Review the client teaching points related to the administration of this medication if you had difficulty with this question.

Reference
Mosby. (2007). *Mosby's nursing drug reference* (20th ed., p. 662). St. Louis: Mosby.

1661. A client has been scheduled for a barium swallow (esophagography) the next day. The nurse determines that the client understands preprocedure instructions if the client states to do which of the following before the test?

1 Take all oral medications as scheduled.
2 Eat a regular breakfast on the day of the test.
3 Monitor own bowel movement pattern for constipation.
4 Remove metal objects and jewelry, especially from the neck and chest area.

Answer: 4
Rationale: A barium swallow, or esophagography, is a radiograph that uses a substance called barium for contrast to highlight abnormalities in the gastrointestinal (GI) tract. The client is told to remove metal objects such as medals and jewelry before the test, so they will not interfere with radiographic visualization of the field. The client should fast for a minimum of 8 hours before the test, depending on physician instructions. Some oral medications are withheld before the test, and the client should follow the physician's instructions regarding medication administration. It is important after the procedure to monitor for constipation, which can occur as a result of the presence of barium in the GI tract.

Level of Cognitive Ability: Analysis
Client Needs: Physiological Integrity
Integrated Process: Nursing Process/Evaluation
Content Area: Adult Health/Gastrointestinal

Test-Taking Strategy: Note the strategic words "barium swallow" and "before the test." This tells you that the correct option is an item that the client needs to comply with before the test is done. Eliminate option 3 first, because it is a part of aftercare. Knowing that the procedure is a type of radiographic study that involves barium and that the client needs to remain NPO will assist in eliminating options 1 and 2. Review preprocedure care for a barium swallow if you had difficulty with this question.

References

Chernecky, C., & Berger, B. (2008). *Laboratory tests and diagnostic procedures* (5th ed., p. 186). St. Louis: Saunders.
Ignatavicius, D., & Workman, M. (2006). *Medical-surgical nursing: Critical thinking for collaborative care* (5th ed., p. 1244). Philadelphia: Saunders.

1662. A physician prescribes a chemotherapeutic medication dose that the nurse believes is too high. The nurse calls the physician, but the physician has left the office for the weekend. The nurse appropriately:

1 Reschedules the client's chemotherapy until the following week
2 Telephones the answering service and confers with the on-call physician
3 Withholds giving the medication until the physician's partner makes rounds the following day
4 Checks with the pharmacist, who agrees the dose is too high, and then reduces the dose accordingly

Level of Cognitive Ability: Application
Client Needs: Safe and Effective Care Environment
Integrated Process: Nursing Process/ Implementation
Content Area: Leadership/Management

Answer: 2
Rationale: If the nurse believes a physician's order to be in error, the nurse must clarify the dosage with the client's physician or the physician's substitute before administering the medication. Checking with the pharmacist can assist the nurse in determining whether the dose ordered is incorrect, but the nurse or pharmacist cannot alter the dose without a revised prescription from a licensed health care provider with prescriptive authority. Withholding the medication until the following day is incorrect. Chemotherapy agents must be administered in the proper combinations or sequence in order to be effective. Rescheduling the client's chemotherapy is also incorrect. Chemotherapy must be administered on a specific schedule for maximum effect with minimum adverse effects. Additionally, only a prescriber can withhold or reschedule chemotherapy.

Test-Taking Strategy: Use the process of elimination and knowledge of the legal responsibilities of the nurse in regard to a physician's orders and medication administration. Remember that a nurse cannot alter, withhold, or reschedule a medication dose. Review the legal implications regarding medication administration if you had difficulty with this question.

References

Huber, D. (2006). *Leadership and nursing care management* (3rd ed., pp. 52-54, 858). Philadelphia: Saunders.
Potter, P., & Perry, A. (2005) *Fundamentals of nursing* (6th ed., pp. 419, 842-843). St. Louis: Mosby.

1663. A nurse working in a long-term care setting attended a workshop on creating a restraint-free environment for the residents. Several co-workers firmly believe that their current methods are satisfactory. The nurse can be effective in facilitating change by:

1 Pointing out to co-workers the various mistakes that they are presently making in adhering to outdated restraint procedures

2 Informing the nursing supervisor that current restraint policies must be changed and requesting that all staff be required to comply

3 Writing a new restraint policy over the weekend and distributing it to co-workers for immediate implementation on Monday morning

4 Asking co-workers' to help gather data comparing the facility's restraint procedures and outcomes with those of others using revised procedures

Level of Cognitive Ability: Application
Client Needs: Safe and Effective Care Environment
Integrated Process: Nursing Process/ Implementation
Content Area: Leadership/Management

Answer: 4
Rationale: To be an effective change agent, the nurse must work collaboratively with others to solve common problems. The nurse who works collaboratively with others to facilitate change has a much greater chance of success than one who unilaterally demands or implements change. By enlisting the assistance of others, there is a greater chance that they will support proposed changes in procedures. A punitive atmosphere is not effective in promoting change because it discourages people from taking risks. To focus on errors (perceived or real) serves only to alienate others and is not effective in promoting change.

Test-Taking Strategy: Use the process of elimination, remembering that to facilitate change, collaboration between the nurse and co-workers is important. Additionally, options 1, 2, and 3 focus on unilateral actions by the nurse. Review the change process if you had difficulty with this question.

References
Huber, D. (2006). Leadership and nursing care management (3rd ed., pp. 812-814). Philadelphia: Saunders.
Potter, P., & Perry, A. (2005) *Fundamentals of nursing* (6th ed., p. 385). St. Louis: Mosby.

1664. A client being discharged from the hospital with a diagnosis of gastric ulcer has an order for sucralfate (Carafate) 1 gram by mouth four times daily. The nurse determines that the client understands proper use of the medication if the client states to take it:

1 With meals and at bedtime
2 Every 6 hours around the clock
3 One hour after meals and at bedtime
4 One hour before meals and at bedtime

Level of Cognitive Ability: Analysis
Client Needs: Physiological Integrity
Integrated Process: Nursing Process/Evaluation
Content Area: Pharmacology

Answer: 4
Rationale: Sucralfate (Carafate) is an antiulcer medication. The medication should be scheduled for administration 1 hour before meals and at bedtime. This timing will allow the medication to form a protective coating over the ulcer before it becomes irritated by food intake, gastric acid production, and mechanical movement. The other options are incorrect.

Test-Taking Strategy: Use the process of elimination. Recalling the action of this medication, to form a protective coating, will direct you to option 4. Review client teaching points regarding this medication if you had difficulty with this question.

Reference
Mosby. (2007). *Mosby's nursing drug reference* (20th ed., p. 929). St. Louis: Mosby.

1665. The nurse is assisting a physician with abdominal paracentesis. The nurse assists the client into what position for this procedure?

1 Prone
2 Supine
3 Sitting on the edge of the bed
4 Low Fowler's on the right side

Level of Cognitive Ability: Application
Client Needs: Physiological Integrity
Integrated Process: Nursing Process/ Implementation
Content Area: Adult Health/Gastrointestinal

Answer: 3
Rationale: For abdominal paracentesis, the nurse should position the client in either a semi-Fowler's position an upright position on the edge of the bed with the feet resting on a stool and the back well supported. This position allows the intestine to float posteriorly and helps prevent laceration during catheter insertion. Options 1, 2, and 4 are incorrect positions.

Test-Taking Strategy: Focus on the name and the purpose of the procedure. Eliminate options 1 and 2 because they are comparable or alike. From the remaining options, visualize this procedure and its associated complications to answer the question. Review the procedure for abdominal paracentesis if you had difficulty with this question.

References
Black, J., & Hawks, J. (2005). *Medical-surgical nursing: Clinical management for positive outcomes* (7th ed., p. 1188). Philadelphia: Saunders.
Lewis, S., Heitkemper, M., Dirksen, S., O'Brien, P., & Bucher, L. (2007). *Medical-surgical nursing: Assessment and management of clinical problems* (7th ed., p. 1111). St. Louis: Mosby.

1666. A client was admitted to the hospital with a diagnosis of frequent symptomatic premature ventricular contractions (PVCs). After sitting up in a chair for a few minutes, the client complains of feeling lightheaded. On auscultation of the heartbeat, the nurse should anticipate which of the following findings?

1 A regular apical pulse
2 An irregular apical pulse
3 A very slow regular apical pulse
4 A very rapid regular apical pulse

Level of Cognitive Ability: Analysis
Client Needs: Physiological Integrity
Integrated Process: Nursing Process/Assessment
Content Area: Adult Health/Cardiovascular

Answer: 2
Rationale: The most accurate means of assessing pulse rhythm is by auscultation of the apical pulse. When a client has PVCs, the rate is irregular and if the radial pulse is taken, a true picture of what is occurring is not obtained. A very rapid regular apical pulse indicates tachycardia. A very slow regular apical pulse indicates bradycardia.

Test-Taking Strategy: Use the process of elimination, focusing on the subject—PVCs. Eliminate options 1, 3, and 4 because they are comparable or alike and indicate a regular pulse. Review the manifestations associated with PVCs if you had difficulty with this question.

References
Black, J., & Hawks, J. (2005). *Medical-surgical nursing: Clinical management for positive outcomes* (7th ed., p. 1682). Philadelphia: Saunders.
Potter, P., & Perry, A. (2005) *Fundamentals of nursing* (6th ed., pp. 642, 725). St. Louis: Mosby.

1667. A client with a history of duodenal ulcer is taking calcium carbonate chewable tablets. The nurse monitors the client for relief of which symptom?

1 Flatus
2 Heartburn
3 Rectal pain
4 Muscle twitching

Answer: 2
Rationale: Calcium carbonate is used as an antacid for the relief of heartburn and indigestion. It can also be used as a calcium supplement or to bind phosphorus in the gastrointestinal tract in clients with renal failure. Options 1, 3, and 4 are unrelated to this medication.

Test-Taking Strategy: Use the process of elimination. Focusing on the client's diagnosis will direct you to option 2. Review the action of this medication if you had difficulty with this question.

Level of Cognitive Ability: Analysis
Client Needs: Physiological Integrity
Integrated Process: Nursing Process/Evaluation
Content Area: Pharmacology

Reference
Mosby. (2007). *Mosby's nursing drug reference* (20th ed., p. 210). St. Louis: Mosby.

1668. A child with Hirschsprung's disease is scheduled for surgery, and a temporary colostomy is performed on the child. Postoperatively, the nurse provides instructions to the parents about colostomy care at home. Which statement by the parents indicates their understanding of the instructions?

1 "We will give antidiarrheal medications."

2 "We will report signs of skin breakdown."

3 "We will give saline water enemas if my child doesn't pass stool."

4 "We will apply a heat lamp to any moist red tissue around the stoma."

Level of Cognitive Ability: Analysis
Client Needs: Physiological Integrity
Integrated Process: Nursing Process/Evaluation
Content Area: Child Health

Answer: 2

Rationale: The parents are instructed to report signs of skin breakdown or stomal complications, such as ribbon-like stools, or failure to pass flatus or stools to the physician or the nurse. Moist, red granulation tissue may grow around an ostomy site and does not require special treatment. Options 1 and 3 are incorrect actions and are contraindicated.

Test-Taking Strategy: Use the process of elimination, noting the strategic words "indicates their understanding of the instructions." Focusing on the subject—colostomy care—and careful reading of each option will direct you to option 2. Review parent teaching and colostomy care if you had difficulty with this question.

References
Hockenberry, M., Wilson, D., & Winkelstein, M. (2005). *Wong's essentials of pediatric nursing* (7th ed., p. 855). St. Louis: Mosby.
McKinney, E., James, S., Murray, S., & Ashwill, J. (2005). *Maternal-child nursing* (2nd ed., p. 1144). St. Louis: Saunders.

1669. A client with Bell's palsy is distressed about the change in facial appearance. The nurse tells the client about which characteristic of Bell's palsy to help the client cope with the disorder?

1 It is similar to stroke, but all symptoms will go away eventually.

2 It usually resolves when treated with vasodilator medications.

3 It is not caused by stroke, and many clients recover in 3 to 5 weeks.

4 The symptoms will completely go away once the tumor is removed.

Level of Cognitive Ability: Application
Client Needs: Psychosocial Integrity
Integrated Process: Caring
Content Area: Adult Health/Neurological

Answer: 3

Rationale: Clients with Bell's palsy should be reassured that they have not experienced a stroke and that symptoms often disappear spontaneously in approximately 3 to 5 weeks. The client is given supportive treatment for symptoms. It is not usually caused by a tumor, and the treatment does not involve administering vasodilators.

Test-Taking Strategy: Focus on the subject—helping the client cope with the disorder. Recalling that Bell's palsy is not a stroke and is not caused by a tumor or vasoconstriction will eliminate options 1, 2, and 4. Review the characteristics associated with Bell's palsy if you had difficulty with this question.

References
Black, J., & Hawks, J. (2005). *Medical-surgical nursing: Clinical management for positive outcomes* (7th ed., p. 2154). Philadelphia: Saunders.
Lewis, S., Heitkemper, M., Dirksen, S., O'Brien, P., & Bucher, L. (2007). *Medical-surgical nursing: Assessment and management of clinical problems* (7th ed., p. 1585). St. Louis: Mosby.

1670. A client has been given a prescription for propantheline (Pro-Banthine) as adjunctive treatment for peptic ulcer disease. The nurse tells the client to take this medication:
1 With meals
2 With antacids
3 Just after meals
4 30 minutes before meals

Level of Cognitive Ability: Application
Client Needs: Physiological Integrity
Integrated Process: Teaching and Learning
Content Area: Pharmacology

Answer: 4
Rationale: Propantheline is an antimuscarinic anticholinergic medication that decreases gastrointestinal secretions. It should be administered 30 minutes before meals. The other options are incorrect.

Test-Taking Strategy: Use the process of elimination. Option 2 can be eliminated first because most medications cannot be administered with antacids because of interactive effects. Eliminate options 1 and 3 next because they are comparable or alike and indicate administering the medication with food. Review this medication if you had difficulty with this question.

References
Mosby. (2007). *Mosby's nursing drug reference* (20th ed., p. 844). St. Louis: Mosby.
Skidmore-Roth, L. (2008). *Mosby's nursing drug reference* (21st ed., p. 860). St. Louis: Mosby.

1671. The nurse obtains a fingerstick glucose of 400 mg/dL for a client who receives parenteral nutrition (PN). Which follow-up intervention should the nurse implement?
1 Discontinue the current PN infusion.
2 Decrease the infusion rate of the PN.
3 Replace PN with 5% dextrose solution.
4 Confer with provider for glucose control.

Level of Cognitive Ability: Application
Client Needs: Physiological Integrity
Integrated Process: Nursing Process/ Implementation
Content Area: Fundamental Skills

Answer: 4
Rationale: Hyperglycemia is a complication associated with the administration of PN because the base solution of PN is 10% to 20% glucose in water. This client's capillary glucose is very high, and the hyperglycemia increases the risk of intravascular injury and hyperosmolar crisis. The nurse would not discontinue the infusion, decrease the rate, or replace the solution without a physician's order. Additionally, these actions would not resolve the problem.

Test-Taking Strategy: Use the process of elimination. Eliminate options 1, 2, and 3 because they are counterproductive to the client's nutritional needs. Additionally, recalling the normal glucose level will direct you to option 4. Review this content if you are unfamiliar with the care of the client receiving PN.

References
Black, J., & Hawks, J. (2005). *Medical-surgical nursing: Clinical management for positive outcomes* (7th ed., p. 708). Philadelphia: Saunders.
Ignatavicius, D., & Workman, M. (2006). *Medical-surgical nursing: Critical thinking for collaborative care* (5th ed., p. 1433). Philadelphia: Saunders.
Perry, A., & Potter, P. (2006) *Clinical nursing skills & techniques* (6th ed., p. 1050). St. Louis: Mosby.

1672. Carbamazepine (Tegretol) is prescribed for a client in the management of generalized tonic-clonic seizures. The nurse is providing instructions to the client regarding the side effects of the medication and tells the client to inform the physician if which of the following occurs?
1 Nausea
2 Dizziness
3 Sore throat
4 Drowsiness

Answer: 3
Rationale: Drowsiness, dizziness, nausea, and vomiting are frequent side effects associated with the medication. Adverse reactions include blood dyscrasias. If the client develops a fever, sore throat, mouth ulcerations, unusual bleeding or bruising, or joint pain, this may be indicative of a blood dyscrasia, and the physician should be notified.

Level of Cognitive Ability: Application
Client Needs: Physiological Integrity
Integrated Process: Teaching and Learning
Content Area: Pharmacology

Test-Taking Strategy: Note the strategic words "tells the client to inform the physician." Recalling that blood dyscrasias can occur with the use of carbamazepine will direct you to option 3. Remember that a sore throat is a sign of infection. Review this content if you are unfamiliar with the adverse effects of carbamazepine.

Reference
Skidmore-Roth, L. (2005). *Mosby's drug guide for nurses* (6th ed., p. 137). St. Louis: Mosby.

1673. A medication nurse is supervising a newly hired nurse who is administering pyridostigmine (Mestinon) orally to a client with myasthenia gravis. Which observation by the medication nurse indicates safe practice by the newly hired nurse before administering this medication?

1 Asking the client to take sips of water
2 Asking the client to lie down on her right side
3 Asking the client to look up at the ceiling for 30 seconds
4 Instructing the client to void before taking the medication

Level of Cognitive Ability: Analysis
Client Needs: Safe and Effective Care Environment
Integrated Process: Nursing Process/Evaluation
Content Area: Leadership/Management

Answer: 1

Rationale: Myasthenia gravis can affect the client's ability to swallow. The primary assessment is to determine the client's ability to swallow. Options 2 and 3 are not appropriate. In this situation, there is no reason for the client to lie down to swallow medication or to look up at the ceiling. Additionally, lying down could place the client at risk for aspiration. There is no specific reason for the client to void before taking medication.

Test-Taking Strategy: Note the diagnosis of the client and that the question addresses an oral medication. Recalling that myasthenia gravis can affect the client's ability to swallow will direct you to option 1. Review nursing care of the client with myasthenia gravis if you had difficulty with this question.

References
Ignatavicius, D., & Workman, M. (2006). *Medical-surgical nursing: Critical thinking for collaborative care* (5th ed., p. 1013). Philadelphia: Saunders.
Lewis, S., Heitkemper, M., Dirksen, S., O'Brien, P., & Bucher, L. (2007). *Medical-surgical nursing: Assessment and management of clinical problems* (7th ed., p. 1556). St. Louis: Mosby.

1674. The home care nurse visits a client with chronic obstructive pulmonary disease (COPD) who is on home oxygen at 2 L per minute. The client's respiratory rate is 22 breaths per minute, and the client is complaining of increased dyspnea. The nurse would initially:

1 Determine the need to increase the oxygen.
2 Call emergency services to come to the home.
3 Reassure the client that there is no need to worry.
4 Collect more information about the client's respiratory status.

Answer: 4

Rationale: Completing the assessment and collecting additional information regarding the client's respiratory status is the initial nursing action. The oxygen is not increased without validation of the need for further oxygen and the approval of the physician, especially because clients with COPD can retain carbon dioxide. Calling emergency services is a premature action. Reassuring the client is appropriate, but it is inappropriate to tell the client not to worry.

Test-Taking Strategy: Use the steps of the nursing process. Remember that assessment is the first step. Also, use the ABCs—airway, breathing, and circulation—to direct you to option 4. Review care of the client with COPD if you had difficulty with this question.

Level of Cognitive Ability: Application
Client Needs: Physiological Integrity
Integrated Process: Nursing Process/
  Implementation
Content Area: Adult Health/Respiratory

References
Black, J., & Hawks, J. (2005). *Medical-surgical nursing: Clinical management for positive outcomes* (7th ed., p. 1829). Philadelphia: Saunders.
Ignatavicius, D., & Workman, M. (2006). *Medical-surgical nursing: Critical thinking for collaborative care* (5th ed., p. 601). Philadelphia: Saunders.

1675. A new breast-feeding mother is seen in the clinic with complaints of breast discomfort. The nurse determines that the mother is experiencing breast engorgement and provides the mother with instructions regarding care for the condition. Which statement by the mother indicates an understanding of the measures that will provide comfort for the engorgement?

1 "I will breast-feed using only one breast."
2 "I will apply cold compresses to my breasts."
3 "I will avoid the use of a bra while my breasts are engorged."
4 "I will massage my breasts before feeding to stimulate letdown."

Level of Cognitive Ability: Analysis
Client Needs: Health Promotion and
  Maintenance
Integrated Process: Nursing Process/Evaluation
Content Area: Maternity/Postpartum

Answer: 4
Rationale: Comfort measures for breast engorgement include massaging the breasts before feeding to stimulate letdown; wearing a supportive well-fitting bra at all times; taking a warm shower or applying warm compresses just before feeding; and alternating the breasts during feeding. Options 1, 2, and 3 are incorrect measures.

Test-Taking Strategy: Use the process of elimination, noting the strategic words "indicates an understanding." Visualize each of the descriptions in the options to assist in directing you to option 4. Review the measures to alleviate breast engorgement if you had difficulty with this question.

Reference
Murray, S., & McKinney, E. (2006). *Foundations of maternal-newborn nursing* (4th ed., pp. 555-557). Philadelphia: Saunders.

1676. The nurse fails to recognize that a client's vital signs have deteriorated over the past 4 hours following surgery. Later, the client requires emergency surgery. Which legal consequence does the nurse potentially face due to a failure to act?

1 Tort
2 Statutory law
3 Common law
4 Misdemeanor

Level of Cognitive Ability: Comprehension
Client Needs: Physiological Integrity
Integrated Process: Nursing Process/
  Implementation
Content Area: Fundamental Skills

Answer: 1
Rationale: The nurse's inaction is consistent with a tort offense because a tort is a wrongful act intentionally or unintentionally committed against a person or the person's property. Option 3 describes case law that has evolved over time via precedents. Option 4 is an offense under criminal law. Option 2 describes laws that are enacted by state, federal, or local governments.

Test-Taking Strategy: Focus on the data in the question. Use knowledge regarding the definitions of the items identified in the options to answer this question. Review the definitions related to these items if you had difficulty with this question.

References
Huber, D. (2006). *Leadership and nursing care management* (3rd ed., pp. 735-736). Philadelphia: Saunders.
Potter, P., & Perry, A. (2005) *Fundamentals of nursing* (6th ed., pp. 413-414). St. Louis: Mosby.

1677. A postmastectomy client has been found to have an estrogen-receptor positive tumor. The nurse interprets after reading this information in the pathology report that the client will most likely have which common follow-up treatment prescribed?
1 Removal of the ovaries
2 Administration of estrogen
3 Administration of progesterone
4 Administration of tamoxifen (Nolvadex)

Level of Cognitive Ability: Analysis
Client Needs: Physiological Integrity
Integrated Process: Nursing Process/Analysis
Content Area: Adult Health/Oncology

Answer: 4
Rationale: A common treatment for women with estrogen-receptor positive breast tumors is follow-up treatment with tamoxifen. This medication is classified as an antineoplastic agent and competes with estrogen for binding sites in the breast and other tissues. The medication may be administered for years following surgery. Options 1, 2, and 3 are incorrect.

Test-Taking Strategy: Note the strategic words "estrogen-receptor positive" and "common follow-up treatment." These strategic words will assist in eliminating option 2. From the remaining options, it is necessary to know the action of the tamoxifen. Review the action and use of this medication if you had difficulty with this question.

References
Black, J., & Hawks, J. (2005). *Medical-surgical nursing: Clinical management for positive outcomes* (7th ed., pp. 1096-1097). Philadelphia: Saunders.
Hodgson, B., & Kizior, R. (2007). *Saunders nursing drug handbook 2007* (pp. 1095-1096). Philadelphia: Saunders.

1678. A nurse reviews the client's health care record and notes that the client is taking donepezil hydrochloride (Aricept). Understanding the purpose of this medication, the nurse suspects this client has:
1 Dementia
2 Seizure disorder
3 History of schizophrenia
4 Obsessive-compulsive disorder

Level of Cognitive Ability: Analysis
Client Needs: Physiological Integrity
Integrated Process: Nursing Process/Analysis
Content Area: Pharmacology

Answer: 1
Rationale: Donepezil hydrochloride is a cholinergic agent that is used in the treatment of mild to moderate dementia of the Alzheimer's type. It enhances cholinergic functions by increasing the concentration of acetylcholine. It slows the progression of Alzheimer's disease. Options 2, 3, and 4 are incorrect.

Test-Taking Strategy: Specific knowledge regarding the use of donepezil hydrochloride is required to answer this question. Remember this medication is used in the treatment of mild to moderate dementia of the Alzheimer's type. Review its action and use if you are unfamiliar with this medication.

Reference
Mosby. (2007). *Mosby's nursing drug reference* (20th ed., p. 381). St. Louis: Mosby.

1679. A registered nurse (RN) is supervising a licensed practical nurse (LPN) providing care to a client with end-stage heart failure. The client is withdrawn, reluctant to talk, and shows little interest in participating in hygienic care or activities. Which statement by the LPN to the client indicates that the LPN needs instructions in the use of therapeutic communication skills?
1 "You are very quiet today."
2 "What are your feelings right now?"
3 "Why don't you feel like getting up?"
4 "Tell me more about your difficulty with sleeping at night."

Answer: 3
Rationale: When a "why" question is made to the client, an explanation for feelings and behaviors is requested, and the client may not know the reason. Requesting an explanation is a nontherapeutic communication technique. In option 1, the LPN is using the therapeutic communication technique of acknowledging the client's behavior. In option 2, the LPN is encouraging identification of emotions or feelings. In option 4, the LPN is using the therapeutic communication technique of exploring, which is asking the client to describe something in more detail or to discuss it more fully.

Level of Cognitive Ability: Analysis
Client Needs: Psychosocial Integrity
Integrated Process: Teaching and Learning
Content Area: Leadership/Management

Test-Taking Strategy: Note the strategic words "needs instructions in the use of therapeutic communication skills." These words indicate a negative event query and the need to select the incorrect statement by the LPN. Use the process of elimination, seeking the option that is a block to communication. The word "why" in option 3 should guide you to this option. Review therapeutic communication techniques if you had difficulty with this question.

References
Ignatavicius, D., & Workman, M. (2006). *Medical-surgical nursing: Critical thinking for collaborative care* (5th ed., p. 756). Philadelphia: Saunders.
Potter, P., & Perry, A. (2005). *Fundamentals of nursing* (6th ed., p. 437). St. Louis: Mosby.

1680. A nurse is administering a dose of ondansetron hydrochloride (Zofran) to a client for nausea and vomiting. The nurse tells the client to report which frequent side effect of this medication?
1 Dizziness
2 Blurred vision
3 A warm feeling
4 Urinary frequency

Level of Cognitive Ability: Application
Client Needs: Physiological Integrity
Integrated Process: Teaching and Learning
Content Area: Pharmacology

Answer: 1
Rationale: Ondansetron hydrochloride is a selective receptor antagonist used as an antinausea and antiemetic. Frequent side effects include anxiety, drowsiness, dizziness, headache, fatigue, constipation, diarrhea, urinary retention, and hypoxia. Occasional side effects include abdominal pain, diminished saliva secretion, fever, feeling of cold, paresthesia, and weakness. Rare side effects include hypersensitivity reaction and blurred vision.

Test-Taking Strategy: Focus on the subject—a frequent side effect. Noting that the medication is used to treat nausea and vomiting and that this medication is a selective receptor antagonist will direct you to option 1. Review this content if you had difficulty with this question and are unfamiliar with the side effects associated with the use of this medication.

Reference
Mosby. (2007). *Mosby's nursing drug reference* (20th ed., p. 748). St. Louis: Mosby.

1681. The nurse is reviewing a urinalysis report for a client with acute renal failure and notes that the results are highly positive for proteinuria. The nurse interprets that this client has which type of renal failure?
1 Prerenal failure
2 Postrenal failure
3 Intrinsic renal failure
4 Atypical renal failure

Level of Cognitive Ability: Analysis
Client Needs: Physiological Integrity
Integrated Process: Nursing Process/Analysis
Content Area: Adult Health/Renal

Answer: 3
Rationale: With intrinsic renal failure, there is a fixed specific gravity and the urine tests positive for proteinuria. In prerenal failure, the specific gravity is high, and there is very little or no proteinuria. In postrenal failure, there is a fixed specific gravity and little or no proteinuria. There is no such classification as atypical renal failure.

Test-Taking Strategy: Specific knowledge regarding the types of renal failure is required to answer this question. Remember with intrinsic renal failure, there is a fixed specific gravity and the urine tests positive for proteinuria. Review the manifestations associated with the classifications of renal failure if you had difficulty with this question.

Reference
Ignatavicius, D., & Workman, M. (2006). *Medical-surgical nursing: Critical thinking for collaborative care* (5th ed., pp. 1732, 1734-1735). Philadelphia: Saunders.

1682. A client has undergone a vaginal hysterectomy. The nurse writes on the client's
nursing care plan that which of the following is to be avoided?
  1 Using pneumatic compression boots
  2 Assisting with range of motion leg
  exercises
  3 Removing antiembolism stockings
  twice daily
  4 Elevating the knees with the knee gatch
  on the bed

Level of Cognitive Ability: Application
Client Needs: Physiological Integrity
Integrated Process: Nursing Process/Planning
Content Area: Adult Health/Oncology

Answer: 4
Rationale: The client is at risk for deep vein thrombosis or thrombophlebitis after this surgery, as for any other major surgery. For
this reason, the nurse implements measures that will prevent this
complication. Pneumatic compression boots, range of motion
exercises, and antiembolism stockings are all helpful. The nurse
should avoid elevating the knees using the knee gatch in the bed,
which inhibits venous return, and places the client more at risk for
deep vein thrombosis or thrombophlebitis.

Test-Taking Strategy: Note the strategic word "avoided." This
word indicates a negative event query and the need to select
the incorrect nursing action. Use basic nursing knowledge of
postoperative care to direct you to option 4. Review care of the
client following hysterectomy if you had difficulty with this
question.

References

Ignatavicius, D., & Workman, M. (2006). *Medical-surgical nursing: Critical thinking for collaborative care* (5th ed., pp. 812-813, 1840). Philadelphia: Saunders.
Monahan, F., Sands, J., Neighbors, M., Marek, J. & Green, C. (2007). Phipps' medical-surgical nursing: Health and illness perspectives (8th ed., pp. 1704-1705). St. Louis: Mosby.

1683. Sertraline (Zoloft) is prescribed for a
client in the treatment of depression.
Before administering the medication,
the nurse reviews the client's record and
consults with the physician if which of
the following were noted?
  1 A history of diabetes mellitus
  2 Use of phenelzine sulfate (Nardil)
  3 A history of myocardial infarction
  4 A history of irritable bowel syndrome

Level of Cognitive Ability: Application
Client Needs: Safe and Effective Care
  Environment
Integrated Process: Nursing Process/
  Implementation
Content Area: Pharmacology

Answer: 2
Rationale: Sertraline is a serotonin reuptake inhibitor. Serious
potentially fatal reactions may occur if sertraline is administered
concurrently with a monoamine oxidase inhibitor (MAOI).
Phenelzine sulfate is an MAOI. MAOIs should be stopped at least
14 days before sertraline therapy. Sertraline should also be stopped
at least 14 days before MAOI therapy. Options 1, 3, and 4 are not
concerns with the administration of this medication.

Test-Taking Strategy: Knowledge regarding the interactions and
contraindications associated with the use of sertraline is required
to answer this question. Remember that serious potentially
fatal reactions may occur if sertraline is administered concurrently with an MAOI. Review this content if you are unfamiliar
with the medication interactions and contraindications.

Reference

Mosby. (2007). *Mosby's nursing drug reference* (20th ed., p. 907). St. Louis: Mosby.

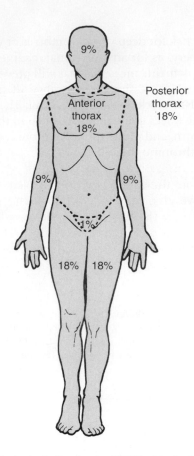

9%

Anterior
thorax
18%

Posterior
thorax
18%

9%   9%

1%

18%   18%

From Black, J., & Hawks, J., (2005). *Medical-surgical nursing: Clinical management for positive outcomes* (7th ed., p. 1443). Philadelphia: Saunders.

1684. An adult client is admitted to the emergency department following a burn injury. The burn initially affected the client's upper half of the anterior torso, and there were circumferential burns to the lower half of both of the arms. The client's clothes caught on fire, and the client ran causing subsequent burn injuries to the entire face (anterior half of the head), and the upper half of the posterior torso. Using the rule of nines, the extent of the burn injury would be what percent?

Answer: _____%

Level of Cognitive Ability: Analysis
Client Needs: Physiological Integrity
Integrated Process: Nursing Process/Assessment
Content Area: Adult Health/Integumentary

Answer: 31.5

Rationale: According to the rule of nines, with the initial burn, the upper half of the anterior torso equals 9% and the lower half of both arms equals 9%. The subsequent burn included the anterior half of head equaling 4.5% and the upper half of posterior torso equaling 9%. This totals 31.5%.

Test-Taking Strategy: Use the rule of nines to answer this question. Remember that the entire head equals 9%, each entire arm equals 9% (both arms 18%), anterior or posterior torso each equals 18% (36% for entire torso), each entire leg equals 18% (both legs equals 36%), perineum equals 1%. Remember: 9 (head), 18 (arms), 36 (torso), 36 (legs), 1 (perineum) equaling 100. If you had difficulty with this question, learn the rule of nines.

References
Black, J., & Hawks, J., (2005). *Medical-surgical nursing: Clinical management for positive outcomes* (7th ed., p. 1443). Philadelphia: Saunders.
Ignatavicius, D., & Workman, M. (2006). *Medical-surgical nursing: Critical thinking for collaborative care* (5th ed., p. 1630). Philadelphia: Saunders.

1685. The clinic nurse provides home care instructions to an adult client diagnosed with influenza. Which instructions should the nurse provide to the client? Select all that apply.

☐ **1** Practice frequent handwashing.

☐ **2** Remain at home until feeling better.

☐ **3** Return in 1 week for an influenza vaccine.

☐ **4** Take acetaminophen (Tylenol) for myalgia.

☐ **5** Cover the nose and mouth when sneezing and coughing.

☐ **6** Completely isolate self in a room from other family members and use a separate bathroom until feeling better.

Level of Cognitive Ability: Application
Client Needs: Safe and Effective Care Environment
Integrated Process: Teaching and Learning
Content Area: Adult Health/Respiratory

Answer: 1, 2, 4, 5
Rationale: Influenza (commonly known as the flu) refers to an acute viral infection of the respiratory tract. It is a communicable disease spread by droplet infection, and measures are instituted to prevent its spread. The client is instructed to practice frequent handwashing, remain at home, and cover the nose and mouth when sneezing and coughing. Supportive measures to relieve fever and myalgia such as the use of acetaminophen are also encouraged. It is unrealistic to completely isolate oneself in a room from other family members, and there is no useful reason to use a separate bathroom because the infection is spread through droplets. Influenza immunization is administered before the start of the "flu" season, not after developing the infection.

Test-Taking Strategy: Focus on the client's diagnosis—influenza. Recalling that this infection is spread by droplets will assist you in selecting the correct instructions. Also remember that the influenza immunization is administered before the start of the "flu" season, not after developing the infection. Review home care measures for treating influenza if you had difficulty with this question.

References
Black, J., & Hawks, J. (2005). *Medical-surgical nursing: Clinical management for positive outcomes* (7th ed., pp. 1838-1839). Philadelphia: Saunders.
Ignatavicius, D., & Workman, M. (2006). *Medical-surgical nursing: Critical thinking for collaborative care* (5th ed., p. 633). Philadelphia: Saunders.

1686. A client who has a positive sputum culture for *Mycobacterium tuberculosis* is receiving streptomycin as part of the treatment. The nurse determines that the client is experiencing toxic effects of the medication if which laboratory result(s) is abnormal?

1 Vision testing

2 Hepatic enzymes

3 Hemoglobin and hematocrit

4 Blood urea nitrogen (BUN) and creatinine

Level of Cognitive Ability: Analysis
Client Needs: Physiological Integrity
Integrated Process: Nursing Process/Analysis
Content Area: Adult Health/Respiratory

Answer: 4
Rationale: BUN and creatinine are measured during therapy with streptomycin because the medication is nephrotoxic. Vision testing is done during treatment with ethambutol (Myambutol). The client taking isoniazid (INH) for tuberculosis is at risk for hepatotoxicity. Hemoglobin and hematocrit are not specifically related to tuberculosis.

Test-Taking Strategy: To answer this question accurately, you must be familiar with the various medications that are used to treat tuberculosis and their associated adverse or toxic effects. Remember that streptomycin is nephrotoxic. Review the adverse effects of streptomycin if you had difficulty with this question.

Reference
Mosby. (2007). *Mosby's nursing drug reference* (20th ed., p. 926). St. Louis: Mosby.

1687. The nurse is planning care for a client with a chest tube attached to a chest drainage system. The nurse avoids which action as part of routine chest tube care?
1 Adding water to the suction chamber as it evaporates
2 Keeping the collection chamber below the client's waist
3 Clamping the chest tube when the client gets out of bed
4 Taping the connection between the chest tube and the drainage system

Level of Cognitive Ability: Application
Client Needs: Physiological Integrity
Integrated Process: Nursing Process/ Implementation
Content Area: Adult Health/Respiratory

Answer: 3
Rationale: To avoid causing tension pneumothorax, the nurse avoids clamping the chest tube for any reason unless specifically ordered. In most instances, clamping of the chest tube is contraindicated by agency policy. Water is added to the suction control chamber as needed to maintain the full suction level ordered. The nurse keeps the drainage collection system below the level of the client's waist to prevent fluid or air from reentering the pleural space. Connections between the chest tube and system are taped to prevent accidental disconnection.

Test-Taking Strategy: Note the strategic word "avoids." This word indicates a negative event query and the need to select the incorrect nursing action. Recalling that clamping chest tubes is contraindicated unless specifically ordered will direct you to option 3. Review care of the client with a chest tube if you had difficulty with this question.

References

Black, J., & Hawks, J. (2005). *Medical-surgical nursing: Clinical management for positive outcomes* (7th ed., pp. 1864-1865). Philadelphia: Saunders.

Lewis, S., Heitkemper, M., Dirksen, S., O'Brien, P., & Bucher, L. (2007). *Medical-surgical nursing: Assessment and management of clinical problems* (7th ed., p. 588). St. Louis: Mosby.

Potter, P., & Perry, A. (2005) *Fundamentals of nursing* (6th ed., pp. 862-863). St. Louis: Mosby.

1688. Ibuprofen (Motrin) 400 mg orally four times daily has been prescribed for an older client with a diagnosis of rheumatoid arthritis. The client asks the nurse about the amount of medication prescribed. The nurse responds based on the understanding that this prescribed dosage is:
1 The normal adult dose
2 Lower than the normal adult dose
3 Higher than the normal adult dose
4 An unusual dosage for this diagnosis

Level of Cognitive Ability: Analysis
Client Needs: Physiological Integrity
Integrated Process: Nursing Process/ Implementation
Content Area: Pharmacology

Answer: 1
Rationale: For acute or chronic rheumatoid arthritis or osteoarthritis, the normal oral adult dose for an older client is 200 to 800 mg three to four times a day. Therefore, options 2, 3, and 4 are incorrect.

Test-Taking Strategy: Knowledge of the normal dosage for ibuprofen is required to answer this question. Remember that the normal oral adult dose for an older client is 200 to 800 mg three to four times a day. Review the normal dosage for this medication if you had difficulty with this question.

Reference

Mosby. (2007). *Mosby's nursing drug reference* (20th ed., p. 540). St. Louis: Mosby.

1689. A nurse is monitoring a client with multiple sclerosis who is receiving baclofen (Lioresal). Which assessment finding would indicate a therapeutic response from the medication?

1 Decreased nausea
2 Decreased muscle spasms
3 Increased muscle tone and strength
4 Increased range of motion of all extremities

Level of Cognitive Ability: Analysis
Client Needs: Physiological Integrity
Integrated Process: Nursing Process/Evaluation
Content Area: Pharmacology

Answer: 2
Rationale: Baclofen is a skeletal muscle relaxant and acts at the spinal cord level to decrease the frequency and amplitude of muscle spasms in clients with spinal cord injuries or diseases, or multiple sclerosis. Options 1, 3, and 4 are unrelated to the effects of this medication.

Test-Taking Strategy: Focus on the client's diagnosis and the subject—a therapeutic response. Recalling that this medication is a skeletal muscle relaxant will direct you to option 2. Review the action of this medication if you had difficulty with this question.

Reference
Mosby. (2007). *Mosby's nursing drug reference* (20th ed., p. 168). St. Louis: Mosby.

1690. An intravenous dose of lorazepam (Ativan) is prescribed for a client. Which of the following facts from the client's history would indicate the need to consult with the physician before administering the medication?

1 History of glaucoma
2 History of hypothyroidism
3 History of diabetes mellitus
4 History of coronary artery disease

Level of Cognitive Ability: Analysis
Client Needs: Safe and Effective Care Environment
Integrated Process: Nursing Process/ Implementation
Content Area: Pharmacology

Answer: 1
Rationale: Lorazepam is contraindicated if hypersensitivity or cross-sensitivity with other benzodiazepines exist. It is also contraindicated in clients who are comatose, with preexisting central nervous system (CNS) depression, with uncontrolled severe pain, and those with narrow-angle glaucoma. It is also not prescribed for clients who are pregnant or breast-feeding.

Test-Taking Strategy: Knowledge regarding the contraindications associated with the use of lorazepam is required to answer this question. Remember that lorazepam is contraindicated in the client with glaucoma. Review this content if you are unfamiliar with these contraindications.

Reference
Mosby. (2007). *Mosby's nursing drug reference* (20th ed., p. 621). St. Louis: Mosby.

1691. The nurse caring for a client immediately following transurethral resection of the prostate (TURP) notices that the client has suddenly become confused and disoriented. The nurse determines that this may be a result of which potential complication of this surgical procedure?

1 Hyponatremia
2 Hypernatremia
3 Hypochloremia
4 Hyperchloremia

Answer: 1
Rationale: The client who suddenly becomes disoriented and confused following TURP could be experiencing early signs of hyponatremia. This may occur because the flushing solution used during the operative procedure is hypotonic. If enough solution is absorbed through the prostate veins during surgery, the client experiences increased circulating volume and dilutional hyponatremia. The nurse needs to report these symptoms.

Test-Taking Strategy: Note the strategic words "potential complication." Specific knowledge about the complications of this procedure will direct you to option 1. Also noting that options 1 and 2 are opposite findings may indicate that one of these options is the correct one. Review the complications related to TURP if you had difficulty with this question.

Level of Cognitive Ability: Analysis
Client Needs: Physiological Integrity
Integrated Process: Nursing Process/Analysis
Content Area: Adult Health/Renal

References
Black, J., & Hawks, J. (2005). *Medical-surgical nursing: Clinical management for positive outcomes* (7th ed., p. 1020). Philadelphia: Saunders.
Ignatavicius, D., & Workman, M. (2006). *Medical-surgical nursing: Critical thinking for collaborative care* (5th ed., pp. 233-234, 1861). Philadelphia: Saunders.

1692. A client hospitalized with a diagnosis of schizophrenia is prescribed risperidone (Risperdal) for the treatment of this disorder. Which laboratory study would the nurse anticipate to be prescribed before the initiation of this medication therapy?
1 Platelet count
2 Blood clotting tests
3 Liver function studies
4 Complete blood count

Level of Cognitive Ability: Analysis
Client Needs: Physiological Integrity
Integrated Process: Nursing Process/Analysis
Content Area: Pharmacology

Answer: 3
Rationale: Risperidone is an antipsychotic medication that suppresses behavioral response in psychosis. Baseline assessment includes renal and liver function tests, and these studies should be done before the initiation of treatment. This medication is used with caution in clients with renal or hepatic impairment, clients with underlying cardiovascular disorders, and in older or debilitated clients. Options 1, 2, and 4 are unrelated to the administration of this medication.

Test-Taking Strategy: Use the process of elimination. Recalling that baseline liver and renal function studies should be done before therapy and that this medication is used cautiously in clients with renal or hepatic impairment will direct you to option 3. Review this content if you are unfamiliar with the contraindications associated with the use of this medication.

Reference
Mosby. (2007). *Mosby's nursing drug reference* (20th ed., p. 885). St. Louis: Mosby.

1693. A nurse has been working with an obese man and is evaluating a weight-reduction plan designed for the client. Which statement by the client indicates the need for additional teaching?
1 "It is so difficult to find food exchanges that taste good and fill me up."
2 "This diet doesn't let me go out for lunch with my friends at work anymore."
3 "I wish my mother could have seen me lose the 60 pounds in the last 9 months."
4 "My wife was kidding me the other night about my being a whole new husband."

Answer: 2
Rationale: Both options 3 and 4 are responses indicating a positive perception of self, that another person has recognized these changes, and that the client wishes to have been able to share these changes with his mother. In the absence of other data, option 1 is a normal response to the changes in eating habits. Option 2 indicates that the client may be having difficulty in making appropriate dietary choices when going out for lunch or that he may perceive his coworkers are uncomfortable with his need to eat differently. A sense of not fitting in can leave the obese individual isolated and therefore make it more difficult for him to maintain his diet at work.

Test-Taking Strategy: Use the process of elimination, noting the strategic words "need for additional teaching." These words indicate a negative event query and the need to select the option that indicates client difficulty with the diet regimen and the need for teaching. Read each option carefully and determine whether it is a positive indicator or a negative one. This will assist in eliminating options 3 and 4 first. Option 1 is a common response by persons who have had to make dietary changes. Option 2 clearly states that the client perceives a definite barrier in pursuing his accustomed lifestyle. Review dietary principles related to weight reduction if you had difficulty with this question.

Level of Cognitive Ability: Analysis
Client Needs: Health Promotion and
Maintenance
Integrated Process: Teaching and Learning
Content Area: Fundamental Skills

References
Ignatavicius, D., & Workman, M. (2006). *Medical-surgical nursing: Critical thinking
for collaborative care* (5th ed., pp. 42-43). Philadelphia: Saunders.
Lewis, S., Heitkemper, M., Dirksen, S., O'Brien, P., & Bucher, L. (2007). *Medical-
surgical nursing: Assessment and management of clinical problems* (7th ed., p. 981).
St. Louis: Mosby.
Potter, P., & Perry, A. (2005). *Fundamentals of nursing* (6th ed., pp. 437, 1279). St.
Louis: Mosby.

1694. A client is complaining of skin irritation
from the edges of a cast that was applied
the previous day, and the nurse notes
that the skin edges are pink and irritated.
The nurse plans to do which of the
following as a corrective action?
1 Petal the edges of the cast with tape.
2 Massage the skin at the rim of the
cast.
3 Shake a small amount of powder
under the cast rim.
4 Use a hair dryer set on a cool high setting to soothe the irritation.

Level of Cognitive Ability: Application
Client Needs: Physiological Integrity
Integrated Process: Nursing Process/Planning
Content Area: Adult Health/Musculoskeletal

Answer: 1
Rationale: The nurse should petal the edges of the cast with tape
to minimize skin irritation. Massaging the skin will not help the
problem. Powder should not be shaken under the cast, because it
could clump, become moist, and cause skin breakdown. A hair
dryer is used on a cool low setting if a nonplaster cast becomes
wet or if the client's skin itches under a cast.

Test-Taking Strategy: Focus on the subject and note the cause of
the client's skin irritation. Because the question tells you that
the cast edges are the cause, you can eliminate options 2, 3, and
4. Review the principles of cast care if you had difficulty with
this question.

Reference
Ignatavicius, D., & Workman, M. (2006). *Medical-surgical nursing: Critical thinking
for collaborative care* (5th ed., p. 1198). Philadelphia: Saunders.

1695. The nurse who has just begun the work
shift is preparing to do tracheostomy
care on a client. The nurse should obtain
which tracheostomy care items from the
supply area?
1 Suction kit and tracheostomy dressing
2 Bottle of sterile saline and a tracheostomy care kit
3 Bottles of sterile saline and water, and
a tracheostomy dressing
4 Tracheostomy care kit, sterile saline
and water, and a suction kit

Level of Cognitive Ability: Application
Client Needs: Physiological Integrity
Integrated Process: Nursing Process/
Implementation
Content Area: Adult Health/Respiratory

Answer: 4
Rationale: Equipment needed to perform tracheostomy care
includes a tracheostomy care kit, sterile water and saline solutions
for cleansing and rinsing, and a suction kit for client suctioning.
As part of tracheostomy care, the client's airway should be
suctioned before cleansing the tracheostomy. New sterile solutions are obtained once per 24 hours, which is often done at the
beginning of the workday. A tracheostomy care kit contains the
needed supplies for cleaning the tracheostomy and for changing
the dressing and holder (tapes).

Test-Taking Strategy: Use the process of elimination. Remember
when an option contains more than one part, all parts of the
option must be complete and correct. Recalling that the key
items needed are the tracheostomy kit and suction kit will
direct you to option 4. Review the procedure for tracheostomy
care if you had difficulty with this question.

References
Ignatavicius, D., & Workman, M. (2006). *Medical-surgical nursing: Critical thinking
for collaborative care* (5th ed., pp. 558-559). Philadelphia: Saunders.
Lewis, S., Heitkemper, M., Dirksen, S., O'Brien, P., & Bucher, L. (2007). *Medical-
surgical nursing: Assessment and management of clinical problems* (7th ed., p. 546).
St. Louis: Mosby.
Potter, P., & Perry, A. (2005). *Fundamentals of nursing* (6th ed., pp. 1113-1114).
St. Louis: Mosby.

1696. A nurse is observing a nursing assistant care for an older client who had a hip pinned following a fracture 4 days ago. To prevent client injury, the nurse intervenes in the care if the nursing assistant:

1 Leaves the side rails down
2 Ensures that the nightlight is working
3 Answers the nurse call signal promptly
4 Places the nurse call signal within reach

Level of Cognitive Ability: Application
Client Needs: Safe and Effective Care Environment
Integrated Process: Nursing Process/ Implementation
Content Area: Leadership/Management

Answer: 1
Rationale: Safe nursing actions intended to prevent injury to the client include keeping the side rails up, bed in low position, and providing a call bell that is within the client's reach. Responding promptly to the client's use of the call bell minimizes the chance that the client will try to get up alone, which could result in a fall. Nightlights are built into the lighting systems of most facilities, and these bulbs should be routinely checked to see that they are functional.

Test-Taking Strategy: Use the process of elimination, noting the strategic word "intervenes." This word indicates a negative event query and the need to select the incorrect action by the nursing assistant. Because options 3 and 4 are standard safety measures, they are eliminated first. Use of a nightlight would help prevent falls, which is also helpful, and can be eliminated next. Review basic safety measures if you had difficulty with this question.

References
Ignatavicius, D., & Workman, M. (2006). *Medical-surgical nursing: Critical thinking for collaborative care* (5th ed., p. 44). Philadelphia: Saunders.
Lewis, S., Heitkemper, M., Dirksen, S., O'Brien, P., & Bucher, L. (2007). *Medical-surgical nursing: Assessment and management of clinical problems* (7th ed., pp. 80, 1654). St. Louis: Mosby.
Potter, P., & Perry, A. (2005). *Fundamentals of nursing* (6th ed., p. 990). St. Louis: Mosby.

1697. A client with chronic renal failure has received dietary counseling about potassium restriction in the diet. The nurse determines that the client has learned the information correctly if the client states to do which of the following for preparation of vegetables?

1 Eat only fresh vegetables.
2 Boil them and discard the water.
3 Use salt substitute on them liberally.
4 Buy frozen vegetables whenever possible.

Level of Cognitive Ability: Analysis
Client Needs: Health Promotion and Maintenance
Integrated Process: Nursing Process/Evaluation
Content Area: Adult Health/Renal

Answer: 2
Rationale: The potassium content of vegetables can be reduced by boiling them and discarding the cooking water. Options 1 and 4 are incorrect. Clients with renal failure should avoid the use of salt substitutes altogether, because they tend to be high in potassium content.

Test-Taking Strategy: Use the process of elimination, recalling which foods are high in potassium and how to reduce their potassium content. Options 3 and 4 can be eliminated first using basic principles of nutrition. Eliminate option 1 next, noting the word "only" in this option. Review client teaching points related to potassium restrictions if you had difficulty with this question.

Reference
Grodner, M., Long, S., & DeYoung, S. (2004). *Foundations and clinical applications of nutrition: A nursing approach.* (3rd ed., p. 609). St. Louis: Mosby.

1698. A client with chronic renal failure has started receiving epoetin alfa (Epogen). The nurse reminds the client about the importance of taking which prescribed medication to enhance the effects of this therapy?

1 Ferrous gluconate
2 Aluminum carbonate
3 Aluminum hydroxide gel
4 Calcium carbonate (Tums)

Level of Cognitive Ability: Application
Client Needs: Physiological Integrity
Integrated Process: Nursing Process/ Implementation
Content Area: Adult Health/Renal

Answer: 1
Rationale: In order to form healthy red blood cells, which is the purpose of epoetin alfa, the body needs adequate stores of iron, folic acid, and vitamin B$_{12}$. The client should take these supplements regularly to enhance the hematocrit-raising benefit of this medication. The other options are incorrect.

Test-Taking Strategy: Use the process of elimination. Recall that this medication is used to stimulate red blood cell formation and that adequate body stores of vitamins and iron are needed to achieve this effect. Also, note that options 2, 3, and 4 are comparable or alike in that they are antacids. Review client teaching points regarding this medication if you had difficulty with this question.

Reference
Mosby. (2007). *Mosby's nursing drug reference* (20th ed., p. 418). St. Louis: Mosby.

1699. A home care nurse is providing instructions to a client who is taking zolpidem (Ambien) for insomnia. To produce a maximal effect of the medication, the nurse tells the client to take the medication:

1 With milk or an antacid
2 At bedtime with a snack
3 Following the evening meal
4 With a full glass of water on an empty stomach

Level of Cognitive Ability: Application
Client Needs: Physiological Integrity
Integrated Process: Teaching and Learning
Content Area: Pharmacology

Answer: 4
Rationale: The client should be instructed to take the medication at bedtime and to swallow the medication whole with a full glass of water. For faster onset of sleep, the client should be instructed not to administer the medication with milk or food, or immediately after a meal. Antacids should be avoided with the administration of the medication because of interactive effects.

Test-Taking Strategy: Use the process of elimination and note the strategic words "maximal effect" in the question. For maximal effectiveness of medications, medications should be taken on an empty stomach with water only. Also note that options 1, 2, and 3 are comparable or alike and indicate taking the medication with food or another substance. Review the principles related to the administration of zolpidem if you had difficulty with this question.

References
Lehne, R. (2007). *Pharmacology for nursing care* (6th ed., p. 368). Philadelphia: Saunders.
Skidmore-Roth, L. (2005). *Mosby's nursing drug guide for nurses* (6th ed., p. 918). St. Louis: Mosby.

1700. A registered nurse is discussing treatment for a client who is hospitalized with acute systemic lupus erythematosus (SLE) with a nursing student assigned to the client. The registered nurse realizes that the nursing student needs to research information about the disease if the student states that which of the following is a clinical manifestation of SLE?

1 Fever
2 Bradycardia
3 Butterfly rash on the face
4 Muscular aches and pains

Answer: 2
Rationale: Manifestations of acute SLE may include fever, musculoskeletal aches and pains, butterfly rash on the face, pleural effusion, basilar pneumonia, generalized lymphadenopathy, pericarditis, tachycardia, hepatosplenomegaly, nephritis, delirium, convulsions, psychosis, and coma.

Test-Taking Strategy: Note the strategic words "needs to research information." These words indicate a negative event query and the need to select the incorrect clinical manifestation. Think about the pathophysiology associated with this disorder to direct you to option 2. Review its clinical manifestations if you are unfamiliar with this disorder.

Level of Cognitive Ability: Analysis
Client Needs: Physiological Integrity
Integrated Process: Teaching and Learning
Content Area: Leadership/Management

References
Black, J., & Hawks, J. (2005). *Medical-surgical nursing: Clinical management for positive outcomes* (7th ed., p. 2354). Philadelphia: Saunders.
Ignatavicius, D., & Workman, M. (2006). *Medical-surgical nursing: Critical thinking for collaborative care* (5th ed., pp. 410-411). Philadelphia: Saunders.

1701. The nurse cares for a client who is pale and complains of fatigue, weakness, and dizziness. Which serum laboratory test result is the nurse's priority for planning care?
1 Hematocrit 43%
2 Sodium 130 mEq/L
3 Potassium 4.8 mEq/L
4 Hemoglobin of 7 g/dL

Level of Cognitive Ability: Analysis
Client Needs: Physiological Integrity
Integrated Process: Nursing Process/Analysis
Content Area: Fundamental Skills

Answer: 4
Rationale: The client's hemoglobin level and sodium level are low; however, the nurse uses the hemoglobin results to plan care because the client's clinical indicators are consistent with anemia. The client is pale because the serum hemoglobin is low; thus the client's tissues are perfused with blood that has a low oxygen-carrying capacity. The client is weak and dizzy because the blood does not carry enough oxygen to meet tissue oxygen demands. While a client who is hyponatremic can also feel weak and dizzy, a hyponatremic client is unlikely to be pale. The hematocrit and the potassium levels are within normal limits.

Test-Taking Strategy: Note that the client has several clinical indicators for anemia. Recalling the normal hemoglobin level will direct you to option 4. Review the normal hemoglobin level and the signs of anemia if you had difficulty with this question.

References
Black, J., & Hawks, J. (2005). *Medical-surgical nursing: Clinical management for positive outcomes* (7th ed., p. 2273). Philadelphia: Saunders.
Pagana, K., & Pagana, T. (2005). *Mosby's diagnostic and laboratory test reference* (7th ed., p. 514). St. Louis: Mosby.

1702. A nurse in the newborn nursery is performing vital signs on the newborn infant. Which finding would indicate a normal respiratory rate?
1 28 breaths per minute
2 50 breaths per minute
3 70 breaths per minute
4 80 breaths per minute

Level of Cognitive Ability: Comprehension
Client Needs: Physiological Integrity
Integrated Process: Nursing Process/Assessment
Content Area: Maternity/Postpartum

Answer: 2
Rationale: The normal respiratory rate for a newborn infant is 30 to 60 breaths per minute. Therefore options 1, 3, and 4 are incorrect.

Test-Taking Strategy: Knowledge of the normal respiratory rate for a newborn infant is required to answer this question. Remember that the normal respiratory rate is 30 to 60 breaths per minute. Review this content if you are unfamiliar with the normal ranges for newborn vital signs.

Reference
Murray, S., & McKinney, E. (2006). *Foundations of maternal-newborn nursing* (4th ed., pp. 469-470). Philadelphia: Saunders.

1703. The nurse is assessing a client with a diagnosis of polycythemia vera. Which clinical manifestation would the nurse expect to note in this client?

1 Pallor
2 Hypertension
3 A low hematocrit level
4 Pale mucous membranes

Level of Cognitive Ability: Analysis
Client Needs: Physiological Integrity
Integrated Process: Nursing Process/Assessment
Content Area: Adult Health/Cardiovascular

Answer: 2
Rationale: Manifestations of polycythemia vera include a ruddy complexion, dusky red mucosa, hypertension, dizziness, headache, and a sense of fullness in the head. Signs of congestive heart failure may also be present. The hematocrit level is usually greater than 54% in men and 49% in women.

Test-Taking Strategy: Focus on the client's diagnosis. Recalling that polycythemia vera is a myeloproliferative disease that causes increased blood viscosity and blood volume will direct you to option 2. Review this content if you are unfamiliar with the clinical manifestations associated with this disorder.

References

Black, J., & Hawks, J. (2005). *Medical-surgical nursing: Clinical management for positive outcomes* (7th ed., pp. 2299-2230). Philadelphia: Saunders.
Lewis, S., Heitkemper, M., Dirksen, S., O'Brien, P., & Bucher, L. (2007). *Medical-surgical nursing: Assessment and management of clinical problems* (7th ed., p. 701). St. Louis: Mosby.

1704. When reviewing the laboratory results of a client with leukemia who is receiving chemotherapy, the registered nurse notes that the neutrophil count is less than 500/mm³. The registered nurse informs the nursing student caring for the client about the results and asks the student to identify the appropriate precautions that need to be instituted. Which intervention identified by the student indicates a need for teaching?

1 Restricting visitors with colds or respiratory infections
2 Removing all live plants, flowers, and stuffed animals in the client's room
3 Placing the client on a low-bacteria diet that excludes raw foods and vegetables
4 Padding the side rails and removing all hazardous and sharp objects from the environment

Level of Cognitive Ability: Analysis
Client Needs: Physiological Integrity
Integrated Process: Teaching and Learning
Content Area: Leadership/Management

Answer: 4
Rationale: When the neutrophil count is less than 500/mm³, visitors should be screened for the presence of infection, and any visitors or staff with colds or respiratory infections should not be allowed in the client's room. All live plants, flowers, and stuffed animals are removed from the client's room. The client is placed on a low-bacteria diet that excludes raw fruits and vegetables. Padding the side rails and removing all hazardous and sharp objects from the environment would be instituted if the client is at risk for bleeding. This client is at risk for infection.

Test-Taking Strategy: Note the strategic words "indicates a need for teaching." These words indicate a negative event query and the need to select the incorrect intervention. Recalling that a low neutrophil count places the client at risk for infection will direct you to option 4. Review this content if you are unfamiliar with the normal neutrophil count and the nursing interventions necessary when the count is low.

Reference

Black, J., & Hawks, J. (2005). *Medical-surgical nursing: Clinical management for positive outcomes* (7th ed., pp. 382, 2408). Philadelphia: Saunders.

1705. The nurse is delivering care to a client who was diagnosed with toxic shock syndrome (TSS). The nurse monitors the client for which complication of this syndrome?

1 Pulmonary embolism
2 Vitamin K deficiency
3 Factor VIII deficiency
4 Disseminated intravascular coagulopathy (DIC)

Level of Cognitive Ability: Analysis
Client Needs: Physiological Integrity
Integrated Process: Nursing Process/Assessment
Content Area: Adult Health/Cardiovascular

Answer: 4
Rationale: TSS is caused by infection and is often associated with tampon use. DIC is a complication of TSS. The nurse monitors the client for signs of this complication, and notifies the physician promptly if signs and symptoms are noted. Options 1, 2, and 3 are not complications of TSS.

Test-Taking Strategy: Familiarity with TSS and knowledge that DIC is a complication is needed to answer this question. Remember DIC is a complication of TSS. Review the complications of TTS if you had difficulty with this question.

Reference
Black, J., & Hawks, J. (2005). *Medical-surgical nursing: Clinical management for positive outcomes* (7th ed., p. 1082). Philadelphia: Saunders.

1706. The nurse is caring for a client with an acute head injury. The nurse carefully assesses which neurological sign as the most sensitive indicator of neurological status?

1 Vital signs
2 Motor function
3 Sensory function
4 Level of consciousness

Level of Cognitive Ability: Application
Client Needs: Physiological Integrity
Integrated Process: Nursing Process/Assessment
Content Area: Adult Health/Neurological

Answer: 4
Rationale: The level of consciousness is the most sensitive indicator of neurological status. An alteration in the level of consciousness occurs before any other changes in neurologic signs or vital signs. Vital sign changes occur late.

Test-Taking Strategy: Noting the subject—neurological status—and the strategic words "most sensitive indicator" will direct you to option 4. Remember that the level of consciousness is the most sensitive indicator of neurological status. Review neurological assessment if you had difficulty with this question.

Reference
Black, J., & Hawks, J. (2005). *Medical-surgical nursing: Clinical management for positive outcomes* (7th ed., pp. 2017, 2024). Philadelphia: Saunders.

1707. A client is admitted to the hospital with Cushing's syndrome. The nurse reviews the results of the client's laboratory studies for which manifestation of this disorder?

1 Hypokalemia
2 Hyperglycemia
3 Decreased plasma cortisol levels
4 Low white blood cell (WBC) count

Level of Cognitive Ability: Analysis
Client Needs: Physiological Integrity
Integrated Process: Nursing Process/Assessment
Content Area: Adult Health/Endocrine

Answer: 2
Rationale: The client with adrenocorticosteroid excess experiences hyperkalemia, hyperglycemia, elevated WBC count, and elevated plasma cortisol and adrenocorticotropic hormone (ACTH) levels. These abnormalities are caused by the effects of excess glucocorticoids and mineralocorticoids on the body.

Test-Taking Strategy: Recalling that an adrenocorticosteroid excess occurs in Cushing's syndrome will direct you to option 2. Also note that options 1, 3, and 4 identify decreased or low levels. Review the manifestations associated with Cushing's syndrome if you had difficulty with this question.

References
Black, J., & Hawks, J. (2005). *Medical-surgical nursing: Clinical management for positive outcomes* (7th ed., p. 1164). Philadelphia: Saunders.
Ignatavicius, D., & Workman, M. (2006). *Medical-surgical nursing: Critical thinking for collaborative care* (5th ed., pp. 1474-1475). Philadelphia: Saunders.

1708. The nurse is going to suction an adult client with a tracheostomy who has copious amounts of secretions. The nurse does which of the following to accomplish this procedure safely and effectively?
 1 Hyperoxygenates the client after the procedure only
 2 Sets the wall suction pressure range between 80 to 120 mm Hg
 3 Applies continuous suction in the airway for up to 20 seconds
 4 Occludes the Y-port of the catheter while advancing it into the tracheostomy

Level of Cognitive Ability: Application
Client Needs: Physiological Integrity
Integrated Process: Nursing Process/ Implementation
Content Area: Adult Health/Respiratory

Answer: 2
Rationale: The safe wall suction range for an adult is 80 to 120 mm Hg making option 2 the action that is consistent with safe and effective practice. The nurse should hyperoxygenate the client both before and after suctioning. The nurse should advance the catheter into the tracheostomy without occluding the Y-port to minimize mucosal trauma and aspiration of the client's oxygen. The nurse should use intermittent suction in the airway (not constant) for up to 10 to 15 seconds.

Test-Taking Strategy: Use the process of elimination. Eliminate option 1 because of the close-ended word "only." From the remaining options, visualize the procedure to direct you to option 2. Review the procedure for suctioning if you had difficulty with this question.

References

Lewis, S., Heitkemper, M., Dirksen, S., O'Brien, P., & Bucher, L. (2007). *Medical-surgical nursing: Assessment and management of clinical problems* (7th ed., p. 571). St. Louis: Mosby.
Potter, P., & Perry, A. (2005). *Fundamentals of nursing* (6th ed., p. 1102). St. Louis: Mosby.

1709. A client experiences postoperative blood loss. Which does the nurse assess to determine that the client is anemic?
 1 Fatigue
 2 Dyspnea
 3 Bradycardia
 4 Muscle cramps

Level of Cognitive Ability: Application
Client Needs: Physiological Integrity
Integrated Process: Nursing Process/Assessment
Content Area: Fundamental Skills

Answer: 1
Rationale: The client with anemia is likely to complain of fatigue caused by deficient hemoglobin leading to a decreased oxygen-carrying capacity of the blood and ability to meet tissue oxygen demands. The respiratory rate can increase to improve oxygenation, but dyspnea (option 2) related to anemia is uncommon. The client is more likely to have tachycardia than bradycardia (option 3), because the heart beats faster to deliver the same amount of oxygen to tissues in compensation for less oxygen in the blood. Muscle cramps, option 4, are an unrelated finding.

Test-Taking Strategy: Use the process of elimination, focusing on the subject—the symptoms associated with anemia. Recalling that anemia causes a reduction in the oxygen-carrying capacity to the tissues will direct you to option 1. Review the manifestations associated with anemia if you had difficulty with this question.

References

Black, J., & Hawks, J. (2005). *Medical-surgical nursing: Clinical management for positive outcomes* (7th ed., pp. 2273, 2275). Philadelphia: Saunders.
Lewis, S., Heitkemper, M., Dirksen, S., O'Brien, P., & Bucher, L. (2007). *Medical-surgical nursing: Assessment and management of clinical problems* (7th ed., p. 687). St. Louis: Mosby.

1710. A nurse employed in a rehabilitation center is planning the client assignments for the day. Which client would the nurse assign to the nursing assistant?

1 A client on strict bedrest for whom a 24-hour urine specimen is being collected

2 A client scheduled for transfer to the hospital for coronary artery bypass surgery

3 A client scheduled for transfer to the hospital for an invasive diagnostic procedure

4 A client who is going through rehabilitation after undergoing a below-the-knee amputation (BKA)

Level of Cognitive Ability: Application
Client Needs: Safe and Effective Care Environment
Integrated Process: Nursing Process/Planning
Content Area: Delegating/Prioritizing

Answer: 1
Rationale: The nurse must assign tasks based on the guidelines of nursing practice acts and the job description of the employing agency. A client who had a BKA, a client scheduled to be transferred to the hospital for coronary artery bypass surgery, and a client scheduled for an invasive diagnostic procedure will require strategies to meet both physiological and psychosocial needs. The nursing assistant has been trained to care for a client on bedrest and to maintain 24-hour urine collections. The nurse would provide instructions to the nursing assistant regarding the tasks, but the tasks required for this client are within the role description of a nursing assistant.

Test-Taking Strategy: Note that the question asks for the assignment to be delegated to the nursing assistant. When asked questions related to delegation, thinking about the role description of the employee and the client needs will direct you to option 1. Review the responsibilities related to delegation and the job description of the nursing assistant if you had difficulty with this question.

References
Huber, D. (2006). Leadership and nursing care management (3rd ed., pp. 546-548). Philadelphia: Saunders.
Potter, P., & Perry, A. (2005). *Fundamentals of nursing* (6th ed., pp. 378-380). St. Louis: Mosby.

1711. The nurse is in the room with a client when a seizure begins. The client's entire body becomes rigid, and the muscles in all four extremities alternate between relaxation and contraction. Following the seizure, the nurse documents that the client has experienced a(n):

1 Partial seizure
2 Absence seizure
3 Tonic-clonic seizure
4 Complex partial seizure

Level of Cognitive Ability: Analysis
Client Needs: Physiological Integrity
Integrated Process: Communication and Documentation
Content Area: Adult Health/Neurological

Answer: 3
Rationale: Tonic-clonic seizures are characterized by body rigidity (tonic phase) followed by rhythmic jerky contraction and relaxation of all body muscles, especially those of the extremities (clonic phase). Absence seizures are characterized by a sudden lapse of consciousness for approximately 2 to 10 seconds and a blank facial expression. There are two types of complex partial seizures: complex partial seizures with automatisms and partial seizures evolving into generalized seizures. Complex partial seizures with automatisms include purposeless repetitive activities such as lip smacking, chewing, or patting the body. Partial seizures evolving into a generalized seizure begin locally and then spread through the body.

Test-Taking Strategy: Use the process of elimination. Eliminate options 1 and 4 first because they are comparable or alike. From the remaining options, focus on the characteristics of the seizure in the question and recall that these characteristics do not occur in an absence seizure. This will direct you to option 3. Review the characteristics of the various types of seizures if you had difficulty with this question.

References
Black, J., & Hawks, J. (2005). *Medical-surgical nursing: Clinical management for positive outcomes* (7th ed., pp. 2075-2076). Philadelphia: Saunders.
Lewis, S., Heitkemper, M., Dirksen, S., O'Brien, P., & Bucher, L. (2007). *Medical-surgical nursing: Assessment and management of clinical problems* (7th ed., p. 1534). St. Louis: Mosby.

1712. The nurse is reviewing the nursing care plan for a client with a right brain attack (stroke) who has left-sided deficits. The nurse notes a nursing diagnosis of Unilateral neglect. The nurse would tell a family member who is assisting the client that it would be least helpful to do which of the following?

  1 Place bedside articles on the left side.
  2 Approach the client from the right side.
  3 Teach the client to scan the environment.
  4 Move the commode and chair to the left side.

Level of Cognitive Ability: Application
Client Needs: Safe and Effective Care
  Environment
Integrated Process: Nursing Process/
  Implementation
Content Area: Adult Health/Neurological

Answer: 2
Rationale: Unilateral neglect is an unawareness of the paralyzed side of the body, which increases the client's risk for injury. The nurse's role is to refocus the client's attention to the affected side. Personal care items, belongings, a bedside chair, and a commode are all placed on the affected side. The client is taught to scan the environment to become aware of that half of the body and is approached on that side by family and caregivers as well.

Test-Taking Strategy: Use the process of elimination, noting the strategic words "left-sided deficits" and "unilateral neglect." Eliminate options 1 and 4 first because they are comparable or alike. For the remaining options, note the strategic words "least helpful." These words indicate a negative event query and the need to select the incorrect intervention. This will direct you to option 2. Review care of the client with unilateral neglect if you had difficulty with this question.

References
Black, J., & Hawks, J. (2005). *Medical-surgical nursing: Clinical management for positive outcomes* (7th ed., pp. 2115, 2131). Philadelphia: Saunders.
Monahan, F., Sands, J., Marek, J., Neighbors, M., & Green, C. (2007). *Phipps' medical-surgical nursing: Health and illness perspectives* (8th ed., p. 1427). St. Louis: Mosby.

1713. The nurse is evaluating the status of a client with myasthenia gravis. The nurse interprets that the client's medication regimen may not be optimal if the client continues to experience fatigue that occurs:

  1 Before meals and at the end of the day
  2 Early in the morning and late in the day
  3 Early in the morning and before lunch
  4 Following exertion and at the end of the day

Level of Cognitive Ability: Analysis
Client Needs: Physiological Integrity
Integrated Process: Nursing Process/Evaluation
Content Area: Adult Health/Neurological

Answer: 4
Rationale: The client with myasthenia gravis has weakness after periods of exertion and near the end of the day. Medication therapy should assist in alleviating the weakness. The medication regimen may not be optimal if the client continues to experience fatigue. The nurse also works with the client to space out activities to conserve energy and regain muscle strength by resting between activities. The client is also instructed to take medication as prescribed.

Test-Taking Strategy: Note the strategic words "may not be optimal if the client continues to experience fatigue." Also remember that when an option has two parts, both parts of the option must be correct in order for the option to be the correct answer. Remember that clients with any form of chronic condition characterized by fatigue experience the greatest amount of fatigue after exertion and at the end of the day. With this concept in mind, eliminate options 1, 2, and 3. Review care of the client with myasthenia gravis if you had difficulty with this question.

References
Ignatavicius, D., & Workman, M. (2006). *Medical-surgical nursing: Critical thinking for collaborative care* (5th ed., p. 1016). Philadelphia: Saunders.
Monahan, F., Sands, J., Neighbors, M., Marek, J. & Green, C. (2007). *Phipps' Medical-surgical nursing: Health and illness perspectives* (8th ed., pp. 1453-1454). St. Louis: Mosby.

1714. Which should the nurse use to administer an injection of iron to a client?
1 Deltoid muscle using an air lock
2 Subcutaneous tissue of the abdomen
3 Gluteal muscle using Z-track technique
4 Anterolateral thigh with 5/8-inch needle

Level of Cognitive Ability: Application
Client Needs: Physiological Integrity
Integrated Process: Nursing Process/
   Implementation
Content Area: Fundamental Skills

Answer: 3
Rationale: The correct technique for administering parenteral iron is deep in the gluteal muscle using Z-track technique to minimize the possibility of staining or irritating the tissues. Administering iron subcutaneously; or with a short needle (options 2 and 4) and using an air lock (option 1) are contraindicated due to iron's irritating nature.

Test-Taking Strategy: Use principles of medication administration by the parenteral route to focus on the subject, an iron injection. Eliminate options 2 and 4 because they both indicate administering the medication subcutaneously. From the remaining options, recall that iron irritates the tissues to direct you to option 3. Review the procedure for administering iron if you had difficulty with this question.

References
Ignatavicius, D., & Workman, M. (2006). *Medical-surgical nursing: Critical thinking for collaborative care* (5th ed., p. 894). Philadelphia: Saunders.
Kee, J., Hayes, E., & McCuistion, L. (2006). *Pharmacology: A nursing process approach* (5th ed., p. 232). Philadelphia: Saunders.

1715. A client is diagnosed with pernicious anemia. The nurse reviews the client's health history for disorders involving which organ responsible for vitamin B_{12} absorption?
1 Liver
2 Ileum
3 Hepatobiliary
4 Gastrointestinal

Level of Cognitive Ability: Comprehension
Client Needs: Physiological Integrity
Integrated Process: Nursing Process/Assessment
Content Area: Fundamental Skills

Answer: 2
Rationale: Pernicious anemia can occur in a client who has a disease involving the ileum, where vitamin B_{12} is absorbed. The nurse checks the client's history for small bowel disorders to detect this risk factor. The liver is not related to impaired B_{12} absorption, usually. Hepatobiliary refers to the liver and gall bladder, and the gastrointestinal refers to the organ system that includes the stomach, liver, gallbladder, and ileum.

Test-Taking Strategy: Focus on the subject—vitamin B_{12} absorption. Recalling that vitamin B_{12} is absorbed in the small intestine will direct you to option 2. Review the physiology associated with the gastrointestinal tract if you had difficulty with this question.

References
Black, J., & Hawks, J. (2005). *Medical-surgical nursing: Clinical management for positive outcomes* (7th ed., pp. 2289-2290). Philadelphia: Saunders.
Lewis, S., Heitkemper, M., Dirksen, S., O'Brien, P., & Bucher, L. (2007). *Medical-surgical nursing: Assessment and management of clinical problems* (7th ed., p. 691). St. Louis: Mosby.

1716. A client had a positive Papanicolaou smear and underwent cryosurgery with laser therapy. The nurse should provide the client with which piece of information before letting the client go home?

1 Sitz baths are soothing to the irritated tissues.
2 Vaginal discharge should be clear and watery.
3 Pain can be relieved with opioid analgesics.
4 There should be absolutely no odor or vaginal discharge.

Level of Cognitive Ability: Application
Client Needs: Physiological Integrity
Integrated Process: Nursing Process/ Implementation
Content Area: Adult Health/Oncology

Answer: 2
Rationale: Cryosurgery is a procedure that involves freezing cervical tissues. Vaginal discharge should be clear and watery following the procedure. The client will then begin to slough off dead cell debris, which may be odorous. This resolves within approximately 8 weeks. Tub and sitz baths are avoided while the area is healing, which takes about 10 weeks. There is mild pain following the procedure, and opioid analgesics would not be required.

Test-Taking Strategy: Specific knowledge about the purpose and effects of this procedure is needed to answer the question. Eliminate option 4 because of the close-ended words "absolutely no." Noting the word "clear" in option 2 will direct you to this option. Review this surgical procedure and the client teaching points if you had difficulty with this question.

References
Black, J., & Hawks, J. (2005). *Medical-surgical nursing: Clinical management for positive outcomes* (7th ed., p. 1076). Philadelphia: Saunders.
Monahan, F., Sands, J., Marek, J., Neighbors, M., & Green, C. (2007). *Phipps' medical-surgical nursing: Health and illness perspectives* (8th ed., pp. 1686-1687). St. Louis: Mosby.

1717. The nurse is planning to do preoperative teaching with a client scheduled for a transurethral resection of the prostate (TURP). The nurse plans to include in the discussion that the most frequent cause of postoperative pain will be:

1 Bladder spasms
2 Bleeding within the bladder
3 Tension on the Foley catheter
4 The lower abdominal incision

Level of Cognitive Ability: Application
Client Needs: Physiological Integrity
Integrated Process: Teaching and Learning
Content Area: Adult Health/Renal

Answer: 1
Rationale: Bladder spasms can occur after this surgery because of postoperative bladder distention or irritation from the balloon on the indwelling urinary catheter. The nurse administers antispasmodic medications, such as belladonna and opium, to treat this type of pain. There is no incision with a TURP (option 4). Options 2 and 3 are not frequent causes of pain. Some surgeons purposefully apply tension to the catheter for a few hours postoperatively to control bleeding.

Test-Taking Strategy: Use the process of elimination, focusing on the surgical procedure. Eliminate option 4, knowing that there is no incision with this procedure. Eliminate options 2 and 3 because they are unrelated to the cause of pain. Review the causes of pain following this type of surgery if you had difficulty with this question.

References
Gulanick, M., & Myers, J. (2007). *Nursing care plans: Nursing diagnosis and interventions* (6th ed., p. 983). St. Louis: Mosby.
Monahan, F., Sands, J., Neighbors, M., Marek, J., & Green, C. (2007). *Phipps' medical-surgical nursing: Health and illness perspectives* (8th ed., p. 1731). St. Louis: Mosby.

1718. A client with gastroesophageal reflux disease (GERD) has just received a breakfast tray. The nurse setting up the tray for the client notices that which of the following foods is the only one that will increase the lower esophageal sphincter (LES) pressure and thus lessen the client's symptoms?

1 Coffee
2 Nonfat milk
3 Fresh scrambled eggs
4 Whole wheat toast with butter

Level of Cognitive Ability: Analysis
Client Needs: Physiological Integrity
Integrated Process: Nursing Process/Analysis
Content Area: Adult Health/Gastrointestinal

Answer: 2
Rationale: Foods that increase the LES pressure will decrease reflux and lessen the symptoms of GERD. The food substance that will increase the LES pressure is nonfat milk. The other substances listed decrease the LES pressure, thus increasing reflux symptoms. Aggravating substances include chocolate, coffee, fatty foods, and alcohol and should be avoided in the diet of a client with GERD.

Test-Taking Strategy: Use the process of elimination and recall the effect of various food substances on LES pressure and GERD. Also, noting the word "nonfat" in option 2 will assist in directing you to this option. Review this content if you are unfamiliar with the LES pressure and the foods that will increase this pressure.

References
Black, J., & Hawks, J. (2005). *Medical-surgical nursing: Clinical management for positive outcomes* (7th ed., pp. 731-733). Philadelphia: Saunders.
Grodner, M., Long, S., & DeYoung, S. (2004). *Foundations and clinical applications of nutrition: A nursing approach.* (3rd ed., p. 505). St. Louis: Mosby.

1719. A nurse is reviewing the serum laboratory test results for a client with sickle cell anemia. Which parameter does the nurse anticipate will be elevated?

1 Sodium
2 Hemoglobin-S
3 Hemoglobin A_{1c}
4 Prothrombin time

Level of Cognitive Ability: Comprehension
Client Needs: Physiological Integrity
Integrated Process: Nursing Process/Assessment
Content Area: Fundamental Skills

Answer: 2
Rationale: Sickle cell anemia is a severe anemia that affects African Americans, predominantly, and is characterized by sickled hemoglobin, or Hgb-S. The client must have two abnormal genes yielding hemoglobin-S to have sickle cell anemia. A client could have sickle cell trait by carrying one hemoglobin-A gene and one hemoglobin-S gene; then, the client has a less severe form of sickle cell anemia. Options 1, 3, and 4 are unrelated to sickle cell anemia.

Test-Taking Strategy: To answer this question, you must know the pathophysiology of sickle cell anemia and how it is reflected in common laboratory studies. Remember that the client with sickle cell anemia must have two abnormal genes yielding hemoglobin-S to have sickle cell anemia. If needed, review the pathophysiology of sickle cell anemia.

References
Ignatavicius, D., & Workman, M. (2006). *Medical-surgical nursing: Critical thinking for collaborative care* (5th ed., p. 888). Philadelphia: Saunders.
Monahan, F., Sands, J., Marek, J., & Neighbors, M. (2003). *Phipps' medical-surgical nursing: Health and illness perspectives* (7th ed., p. 820). St. Louis: Mosby.

1720. Which test result does the nurse examine to determine the compatibility of blood from two different donors?

1 Rh factor
2 ABO typing
3 Direct Coombs'
4 Indirect Coombs'

Answer: 4
Rationale: The indirect Coombs' test detects circulating antibodies against red blood cells (RBCs) and is the screening component of a prescription to "type and screen" a client's blood. This test is used in addition to the ABO typing, which is normally done to determine blood type. The Rh factor is determined at the same time as the ABO type. The direct Coombs' test is used to detect idiopathic hemolytic anemia by detecting the presence of autoantibodies against the client's RBCs.

Level of Cognitive Ability: Comprehension
Client Needs: Physiological Integrity
Integrated Process: Nursing Process/
  Implementation
Content Area: Fundamental Skills

Test-Taking Strategy: Use the process of elimination. Eliminate options 1 and 2 because they are part of blood typing. From the remaining options, it is necessary to know the difference between the two tests. Remember that the indirect Coombs' test is the screening component of a prescription to "type and screen" a client's blood. Review the purpose of the direct and indirect Coombs' test if you had difficulty with this question.

References

Chernecky, C., & Berger, B. (2008). *Laboratory tests and diagnostic procedures* (5th ed., pp. 381-382). Philadelphia: Saunders.
Ignatavicius, D., & Workman, M. (2006). *Medical-surgical nursing: Critical thinking for collaborative care* (5th ed., p. 883). Philadelphia: Saunders.

1721. A client is being discharged to home after undergoing a transurethral resection of the prostate (TURP). The nurse teaches the client to expect which variation in normal urine color for several days following the procedure?

1 Dark red
2 Pink-tinged
3 Clear yellow
4 Cloudy amber

Level of Cognitive Ability: Application
Client Needs: Physiological Integrity
Integrated Process: Teaching and Learning
Content Area: Adult Health/Renal

Answer: 2

Rationale: The client should expect that the urine will be pink-tinged for several days following this procedure. Dark red urine may be present initially, especially with inadequate bladder irrigation, and if it occurs, it must be corrected. Options 3 and 4 are incorrect because urine of these colors is not generally expected for several days following surgery.

Test-Taking Strategy: Note the subject—a client being discharged to home after a resection of the prostate. Eliminate options 3 and 4 first because they are comparable or alike. From the remaining options, focus on the subject to direct you to option 2. Review assessment of the urine for the client who has had this type of surgery if you had difficulty with this question.

References

Black, J., & Hawks, J. (2005) *Medical-surgical nursing: Clinical management for positive outcomes* (7th ed., p. 1024). Philadelphia: Saunders.
Ignatavicius, D., & Workman, M. (2006). *Medical-surgical nursing: Critical thinking for collaborative care* (5th ed., p. 1863). Philadelphia: Saunders.

1722. A client is admitted to the hospital in sickle cell crisis. The nurse monitors the client for which clinical indicator of the disorder?

1 Pain
2 Diarrhea
3 Bradycardia
4 Blurred vision

Answer: 1

Rationale: Sickle cell crisis usually causes severe pain in the bones and joints along with joint swelling. The pain develops as a result of microvascular occlusion from abnormal sickled hemoglobin that occurs with hypoxia. Therapy includes pain management with opioid analgesics, supplemental oxygen, and intravenous fluids. The remaining options are not associated with sickle cell crisis.

Test-Taking Strategy: Note the client's diagnosis. Recalling that the primary treatment of sickle cell crisis focuses on administering fluids and opioid analgesics directs you to option 1. Review the manifestations associated with sickle cell crisis if you had difficulty with this question.

Level of Cognitive Ability: Application
Client Needs: Physiological Integrity
Integrated Process: Nursing Process/Assessment
Content Area: Fundamental Skills

References
Black, J., & Hawks, J. (2005). *Medical-surgical nursing: Clinical management for positive outcomes* (7th ed., pp. 2295-2298). Philadelphia: Saunders.
Lewis, S., Heitkemper, M., Dirksen, S., O'Brien, P., & Bucher, L. (2007). *Medical-surgical nursing: Assessment and management of clinical problems* (7th ed., p. 696). St. Louis: Mosby.

1723. Quinidine gluconate is prescribed for a client. The nurse reviews the client's medical record, knowing that which of the following is a contraindication in the use of this medication?
1 Asthma
2 Infection
3 Muscle weakness
4 Complete atrioventricular (A-V) block

Level of Cognitive Ability: Analysis
Client Needs: Physiological Integrity
Integrated Process: Nursing Process/Analysis
Content Area: Pharmacology

Answer: 4
Rationale: Quinidine gluconate is an antidysrhythmic medication used as prophylactic therapy to maintain normal sinus rhythm after conversion of atrial fibrillation and/or atrial flutter. It is contraindicated in complete A-V block, intraventricular conduction defects, abnormal impulses and rhythms caused by escape mechanisms, and in myasthenia gravis. It is used with caution in clients with preexisting asthma, muscle weakness, infection with fever, and hepatic or renal insufficiency.

Test-Taking Strategy: Note the strategic word "contraindication." Recalling that this medication is an antidysrhythmic medication and has a direct cardiac effect will direct you to option 4. Review this content if you are unfamiliar with this medication and its contraindications.

Reference
Mosby. (2007). *Mosby's nursing drug reference* (20th ed., pp. 862-863). St. Louis: Mosby.

1724. A client with a ruptured intracranial aneurysm has surgery delayed and is still maintained on bedrest with subarachnoid precautions in place. The nurse should question an order for which of the following medications if prescribed for this client?
1 Nimodipine (Nimotop)
2 Heparin sodium (Heparin)
3 Docusate sodium (Colace)
4 Aminocaproic acid (Amicar)

Level of Cognitive Ability: Application
Client Needs: Safe and Effective Care Environment
Integrated Process: Nursing Process/ Implementation
Content Area: Adult Health/Neurological

Answer: 2
Rationale: The nurse should question an order for heparin sodium, which is an anticoagulant. This medication could place the client at risk for rebleeding. Nimodipine is a calcium-channel blocking agent that is useful in the management of vasospasm associated with cerebral hemorrhage. Docusate sodium is a stool softener, which helps prevent straining. Straining would raise intracranial pressure. Aminocaproic acid is an antifibrinolytic agent that prevents clot breakdown or dissolution. It may be prescribed after ruptured intracranial aneurysm and subarachnoid hemorrhage if surgery is delayed or contraindicated.

Test-Taking Strategy: Use the process of elimination. Noting the strategic word "ruptured" in the question suggests that hemorrhage is occurring. It makes sense, knowing the action of heparin sodium, that this medication would be contraindicated. Review care of the client with a ruptured intracranial aneurysm if you had difficulty with this question.

References
Black, J., & Hawks, J. (2005). *Medical-surgical nursing: Clinical management for positive outcomes* (7th ed., p. 2095). Philadelphia: Saunders.
Ignatavicius, D., & Workman, M. (2006). *Medical-surgical nursing: Critical thinking for collaborative care* (5th ed., p. 298). Philadelphia: Saunders.

1725. A client who has a history of chronic ulcerative colitis is diagnosed with anemia. The nurse interprets that which factor is most likely responsible for the anemia?

1 Blood loss
2 Intestinal hookworm
3 Intestinal malabsorption
4 Decreased intake of dietary iron

Level of Cognitive Ability: Analysis
Client Needs: Physiological Integrity
Integrated Process: Nursing Process/Analysis
Content Area: Adult Health/Gastrointestinal

Answer: 1
Rationale: The client with chronic ulcerative colitis is most likely anemic as a result of chronic blood loss in small amounts that occurs with exacerbations of the disease. These clients often have bloody stools and are at increased risk for anemia. There is no information in the question to support options 2 or 4. In ulcerative colitis, the large intestine is involved, not the small intestine where vitamin B_{12} and folic acid are absorbed (option 3).

Test-Taking Strategy: Note the subject—the cause of the anemia. Focusing on the client's diagnosis and recalling the pathophysiology that occurs in this disorder will direct you to option 1. Review the manifestations in ulcerative colitis if you had difficulty with this question.

References
Lewis, S., Heitkemper, M., Dirksen, S., O'Brien, P., & Bucher, L. (2007). *Medical-surgical nursing: Assessment and management of clinical problems* (7th ed., p. 1052). St. Louis: Mosby.
Monahan, F., Sands, J., Marek, J., Neighbors, M., & Green, C. (2007). *Phipps' medical-surgical nursing: Health and illness perspectives* (8th ed., pp. 1250, 1252). St. Louis: Mosby.

1726. A physician has prescribed nimodipine (Nimotop) for a client with subarachnoid hemorrhage. The nurse administering the first dose explains to the client that this medication is a:

1 β-Adrenergic blocker used to decrease blood pressure
2 Vasodilator that has an affinity for cerebral blood vessels
3 Calcium-channel blocker used to decrease the blood pressure
4 Calcium-channel blocker used to decrease cerebral blood vessel spasm

Level of Cognitive Ability: Application
Client Needs: Physiological Integrity
Integrated Process: Nursing Process/ Implementation
Content Area: Adult Health/Neurological

Answer: 4
Rationale: Nimodipine is a calcium-channel blocking agent that has an affinity for cerebral blood vessels. It is used to prevent or control vasospasm in cerebral blood vessels, thereby reducing the chance for further cerebral injury. Options 1, 2, and 3 are incorrect.

Test-Taking Strategy: Use the process of elimination. Recalling that nimodipine is a calcium-channel blocking agent (ends with the suffix "-pine") helps you eliminate options 1 and 2. Recalling that calcium-channel blockers decrease vasospasm helps you select option 4 from the remaining options. Review the action of this medication if you had difficulty with this question.

Reference
Skidmore-Roth, L. (2007). *Mosby's drug guide for nurses* (7th ed., p. 677). St. Louis: Mosby.

1727. A client has been given a prescription to begin using nitroglycerin transdermal patches. The nurse instructs the client about this medication administration system and tells the client to expect which of the following side effects:

1 Sweating
2 Headache
3 Dry mouth
4 Constipation

Answer: 2
Rationale: Nitroglycerin is a coronary vasodilator used in the management of coronary artery disease. A common side effect of this medication is an intense headache. Clients should be instructed about this side effect and that acetaminophen (Tylenol) can be helpful in alleviating discomfort. Options 1, 3, and 4 are not associated with the use of this medication.

Level of Cognitive Ability: Application
Client Needs: Physiological Integrity
Integrated Process: Teaching and Learning
Content Area: Pharmacology

Test-Taking Strategy: Focus on the name of the medication and recall its action. Recalling that it is a vasodilator will direct you to option 2. Review the side effects of this medication if you had difficulty with this question.

Reference
Mosby. (2007). *Mosby's nursing drug reference* (20th ed., p. 729). St. Louis: Mosby.

1728. A nurse is visiting a client who has been started on therapy with topical clotrimazole (Lotrimin AF). The nurse tells the client that this medication will alleviate:
1 Pain
2 Rash
3 Fever
4 Sneezing

Level of Cognitive Ability: Application
Client Needs: Physiological Integrity
Integrated Process: Teaching and Learning
Content Area: Pharmacology

Answer: 2
Rationale: Clotrimazole is a topical antifungal used in the treatment of cutaneous fungal infections and will alleviate an associated rash. The nurse teaches the client that it is used for this purpose. It is not used for sneezing, fever, or pain.

Test-Taking Strategy: Focus on the name of the medication. Recalling that this medication is an antifungal and noting the word "topical" in the question will direct you to option 2. Review the purpose of this anti-infective if you had difficulty with this question.

Reference
Mosby. (2007). *Mosby's nursing drug reference* (20th ed., p. 1089). St. Louis: Mosby.

1729. A nurse is providing care to the client who has received medication therapy with tissue plasminogen activator (t-PA, Activase). As part of standard nursing care for this client, the nurse plans to have which item available for use?
1 Flashlight
2 Pulse oximeter
3 Suction equipment
4 Occult blood test strips

Level of Cognitive Ability: Application
Client Needs: Physiological Integrity
Integrated Process: Nursing Process/Planning
Content Area: Pharmacology

Answer: 4
Rationale: Tissue plasminogen activator is a thrombolytic medication that is used to dissolve thrombi or emboli caused by thrombus. A frequent and potentially adverse effect of therapy is bleeding. The nurse monitors for signs of bleeding in clients receiving this therapy. Equipment needed by the nurse would include occult blood test strips to monitor for occult blood in the urine, stool, or nasogastric drainage. Pulse oximeter and suction equipment would be needed if the client had evidence of respiratory problems. A flashlight may be used for pupil assessment as part of the neurological exam in the client who is neurologically impaired.

Test-Taking Strategy: Focus on the name of the medication. Recalling that this medication is a thrombolytic and that bleeding is an adverse effect of this therapy will direct you to option 4. Review this medication and its adverse effects if you had difficulty with this question.

References
Kee, J., Hayes, E., & McCuistion, L. (2006). *Pharmacology: A nursing process approach.* (5th ed., p. 671). Philadelphia: Saunders.
Skidmore-Roth, L. (2005). *Mosby's drug guide for nurses* (6th ed., p. 31). St. Louis: Mosby.

1730. A client newly diagnosed with angina pectoris has taken two sublingual nitroglycerin tablets for chest pain. The chest pain is relieved, but the client complains of a headache. The nurse interprets that this symptom most likely represents:

1 An early sign of medication tolerance
2 An allergic reaction to the nitroglycerin
3 An expected side effect of the medication
4 A warning that the medication should not be used again

Level of Cognitive Ability: Analysis
Client Needs: Physiological Integrity
Integrated Process: Nursing Process/Analysis
Content Area: Pharmacology

Answer: 3
Rationale: Headache is a frequent side effect of nitroglycerin, because of the vasodilating action of the medication. It usually diminishes in frequency as the client becomes accustomed to the medication and is effectively treated with acetaminophen (Tylenol). The other options are incorrect.

Test-Taking Strategy: Use the process of elimination. Eliminate options 1 and 4 because they are comparable or alike and imply that the medication can no longer be used by the client. From the remaining options, recalling that the medication vasodilates will direct you to option 3. Review the effect of this medication if you had difficulty with this question.

Reference
Mosby. (2007). *Mosby's nursing drug reference* (20th ed., p. 729). St. Louis: Mosby.

1731. A nurse is caring for a client with atrial fibrillation. The physician has prescribed verapamil (Calan) 5 mg intravenously (IV). The nurse ensures that which most essential item is present when administering this medication?

1 Oxygen
2 Pulse oximeter
3 Cardiac monitor
4 Noninvasive blood pressure monitor

Level of Cognitive Ability: Application
Client Needs: Physiological Integrity
Integrated Process: Nursing Process/Planning
Content Area: Pharmacology

Answer: 3
Rationale: Verapamil is a calcium-channel blocking agent that may be used to treat rapid-rate supraventricular tachydysrhythmias, such as atrial flutter and atrial fibrillation. The client must be placed on a cardiac monitor to evaluate the effectiveness of the medication. A noninvasive blood pressure monitor is also helpful but is not as essential as the cardiac monitor. Pulse oximeter and oxygen are related to respiratory care, and although they should be available, they are not directly related to the use of this medication.

Test-Taking Strategy: Note the strategic words "most essential." Eliminate options 1 and 2 first because there is no information about respiratory difficulty in the case situation. From the remaining options, noting the client's diagnosis will direct you to option 3. Review nursing interventions related to the administration of this medication if you had difficulty with this question.

Reference
Gahart, B., & Nazareno, A. (2006). *2006 Intravenous medications* (22nd ed., p. 1227). St. Louis: Mosby.

1732. A client is taking albuterol sulfate (Ventolin Diskus) by inhalation but cannot cough up secretions. The nurse teaches the client to do which of the following to best help clear the bronchial secretions?

1 Get more exercise each day.
2 Use a dehumidifier in the home.
3 Administer an extra dose before bedtime.
4 Increase the amount of fluids consumed every day.

Answer: 4
Rationale: The client should take in increased fluids (2000 to 3000 mL/day unless contraindicated) to make secretions less viscous. This may help the client to expectorate secretions. This is standard advice given to clients receiving any of the adrenergic bronchodilators, such as albuterol, unless the client has another health problem that could be worsened by increased fluid intake. A dehumidifier will dry secretions. The client would not be advised to take additional medication. Additional exercise will not effectively clear bronchial secretions.

Level of Cognitive Ability: Application
Client Needs: Physiological Integrity
Integrated Process: Teaching and Learning
Content Area: Pharmacology

Test-Taking Strategy: Focus on the subject—clearing bronchial secretions. Use general guidelines related to administering medication to eliminate option 3. Next eliminate option 2, recalling that a dehumidifier will dry secretions. From the remaining options, recalling basic respiratory principles will direct you to option 4. Review client teaching points related to this medication if you had difficulty with this question.

References
Hodgson, B., & Kizior, R. (2007). *Saunders nursing drug handbook 2007* (pp. 27-28). Philadelphia: Saunders.
Lewis, S., Heitkemper, M., Dirksen, S., O'Brien, P., & Bucher, L. (2007). *Medical-surgical nursing: Assessment and management of clinical problems* (7th ed., p. 625). St. Louis: Mosby.

1733. A nurse reviews the serum laboratory results for a client taking chlorothiazide (Diuril). The nurse specifically monitors for which of the following most frequent medication side effects on a regular basis?
1 Hypokalemia
2 Hypocalcemia
3 Hypernatremia
4 Hyperphosphatemia

Level of Cognitive Ability: Application
Client Needs: Physiological Integrity
Integrated Process: Nursing Process/Assessment
Content Area: Pharmacology

Answer: 1
Rationale: The client taking a potassium-wasting diuretic such as chlorothiazide (Diuril) needs to be monitored for decreased potassium levels. Other fluid and electrolyte imbalances that occur with the use of this medication include hyponatremia, hypercalcemia, hypomagnesemia, and hypophosphatemia.

Test-Taking Strategy: Focus on the name of the medication and recall that this medication is a potassium-wasting diuretic. Remember that hypokalemia is a concern when a client is taking a potassium-wasting diuretic. Review the side effects of this medication if you had difficulty with this medication.

Reference
Mosby. (2007). *Mosby's nursing drug reference* (20th ed., p. 259). St. Louis: Mosby.

1734. A nurse has administered a dose of diazepam (Valium) to the client. The nurse would take which most important action before leaving the client's room?
1 Draw the shades closed.
2 Give the client a bedpan.
3 Put up the side rails on the bed.
4 Turn the volume on the television set down.

Level of Cognitive Ability: Application
Client Needs: Safe and Effective Care Environment
Integrated Process: Nursing Process/ Implementation
Content Area: Fundamental Skills

Answer: 3
Rationale: Diazepam is a sedative/hypnotic with anticonvulsant and skeletal muscle relaxant properties. The nurse should institute safety measures before leaving the client's room to ensure that the client does not injure self. The most frequent side effects of this medication are dizziness, drowsiness, and lethargy. For this reason, the nurse puts the side rails up on the bed before leaving the room to prevent falls. Options 1, 2, and 4 may be helpful measures that provide a comfortable, restful environment. However, option 3 provides for the client's safety needs.

Test-Taking Strategy: Note the strategic words "most important" and "before leaving the client's room." Recalling that diazepam is a sedative/hypnotic and that safety is a major concern will direct you to option 3. Review care of the client receiving this medication if you had difficulty with this question.

Reference
Mosby. (2007). *Mosby's nursing drug reference* (20th ed., p. 352). St. Louis: Mosby.

1735. A nurse provides home care instructions to a client who is taking lithium carbonate (Eskalith). Which statement by the client indicates a need for further instructions?

1 "I need to take the lithium with meals."
2 "My blood levels must be monitored very closely."
3 "I need to decrease my salt and fluid intake while taking the lithium."
4 "I need to withhold the medication if I have excessive diarrhea, vomiting, or diaphoresis."

Level of Cognitive Ability: Analysis
Client Needs: Physiological Integrity
Integrated Process: Teaching and Learning
Content Area: Pharmacology

Answer: 3
Rationale: Because therapeutic and toxic dosage ranges are so close, lithium blood levels must be monitored very closely, more frequently at first, then once every several months after that. The client should be instructed to withhold the medication if excessive diarrhea, vomiting, or diaphoresis occurs, and to inform the physician if any of these problems occur. Lithium is irritating to the gastric mucosa; therefore, lithium should be taken with meals. A normal diet and normal salt and fluid intake (1500 to 3000 mL per day) should be maintained because lithium decreases sodium reabsorption by the renal tubules, which could cause sodium depletion. A low-sodium intake causes a relative increase in lithium retention and could lead to toxicity.

Test-Taking Strategy: Note the strategic words "need for further instructions." These words indicate a negative event query and the need to select the incorrect client statement. Remember that, generally, it is important that clients be taught to maintain an adequate fluid intake. This principle will direct you to option 3. Review the client teaching points related to the administration of this medication if you had difficulty with this question.

Reference
Mosby. (2007). *Mosby's nursing drug reference* (20th ed., p. 615). St. Louis: Mosby.

1736. A client is brought to the emergency department following a severe burn caused by a fire at home. The burns are extensive, covering greater than 25% of the total body surface area (TBSA). The nurse reviews the laboratory results drawn on the client and would most likely expect to note which of the following?

1 Hematocrit 65%
2 Albumin 4.0 g/dL
3 Sodium 140 mEq/L
4 White blood cell (WBC) count 6000 cells/mm³

Level of Cognitive Ability: Analysis
Client Needs: Physiological Integrity
Integrated Process: Nursing Process/Analysis
Content Area: Adult Health/Integumentary

Answer: 1
Rationale: Extensive burns covering greater than 25% of the TBSA result in generalized body edema in both burned and nonburned tissues and a decrease in circulating intravascular blood volume. Hematocrit levels elevate in the first 24 hours after injury (the emergent phase) as a result of hemoconcentration from the loss of intravascular fluid. The normal hematocrit is 40% to 54% in the male and 38% to 47% in the female. The normal albumin is 3.4 to 5 g/dL. The normal sodium level is 135 to 145 mEq/L. The normal WBC count is 5000 to 10,000 cells/mm³.

Test-Taking Strategy: Use the process of elimination and knowledge regarding physiological alterations and fluid and electrolyte balance during the first 24 hours after injury of a burn client. Note that the only abnormal laboratory value is option 1, the hematocrit. Review normal laboratory values and the immediate postinjury period of burns if you had difficulty with this question.

References
Chernecky, C., & Berger, B. (2008). *Laboratory tests and diagnostic procedures* (5th ed., pp. 615-617). Philadelphia: Saunders.
Monahan, F., Sands, J., Marek, J., Neighbors, M., & Green, C. (2007). *Phipps' medical-surgical nursing: Health and illness perspectives* (8th ed., p. 1926). St. Louis: Mosby.

1737. A nurse is caring for a client with Parkinson's disease who is taking benztropine mesylate (Cogentin) daily. The nurse assesses the client for side effects of this medication and specifically monitors:

1 Pupil response
2 Prothrombin time
3 Skin temperature
4 Intake and output

Level of Cognitive Ability: Application
Client Needs: Physiological Integrity
Integrated Process: Nursing Process/Assessment
Content Area: Pharmacology

Answer: 4
Rationale: Urinary retention is a side effect of benztropine mesylate. The nurse needs to observe for dysuria, distended abdomen, voiding in small amounts, and overflow incontinence. Options 1, 2, and 3 are not side effects of this medication.

Test-Taking Strategy: Focus on the name of the medication. Remember that urinary retention is a concern with this medication. Review this medication and its side effects if you had difficulty with this question.

Reference
Mosby. (2007). *Mosby's nursing drug reference* (20th ed., p. 175). St. Louis: Mosby.

1738. A client has received electroconvulsive therapy (ECT). In the posttreatment area and upon the client's awakening, the nurse will perform which intervention first?

1 Assist the client from the stretcher to a wheelchair
2 Orient the client and monitor the client's vital signs
3 Offer the client frequent reassurance and repeat orientation statements
4 Check for a gag reflex and then encourage the client to eat breakfast and resume activity

Level of Cognitive Ability: Application
Client Needs: Physiological Integrity
Integrated Process: Nursing Process/ Implementation
Content Area: Delegating/Prioritizing

Answer: 2
Rationale: The nurse would first monitor vital signs, orient the client, and review with the client that he or she just received an ECT treatment. The posttreatment area should include accessibility to the anesthesia staff, oxygen, suction, pulse oximeter, vital sign monitoring, and emergency equipment. The nursing interventions outlined in options 1, 3, and 4 will follow accordingly.

Test-Taking Strategy: Use the process of elimination and note the strategic word "first." Use the ABCs—airway, breathing, and circulation—remembering that vital signs are a method of assessing the ABCs. Review care of the client following ECT if you had difficulty with this question.

Reference
Stuart, G., & Laraia, M. (2005). *Principles and practice of psychiatric nursing* (8th ed., p. 607). St. Louis: Mosby.

1739. A client with acquired immunodeficiency syndrome who has cytomegalovirus retinitis is receiving ganciclovir (Cytovene). The nurse plans to do which of the following while the client is taking this medication?

1 Monitor blood glucose levels for elevation.
2 Administer the medication on an empty stomach only.
3 Apply pressure to venipuncture sites for at least 2 minutes.
4 Provide the client with a soft toothbrush and an electric razor.

Answer: 4
Rationale: Ganciclovir causes neutropenia and thrombocytopenia as the most frequent side effects. For this reason, the nurse monitors the client for signs and symptoms of bleeding and implements the same precautions that are used for a client receiving anticoagulant therapy. These include providing a soft toothbrush and electric razor to minimize the risk of trauma that could result in bleeding. Venipuncture sites should be held for approximately 10 minutes. The medication does not have to be taken on an empty stomach. The medication may cause hypoglycemia, but not hyperglycemia.

Level of Cognitive Ability: Application
Client Needs: Safe and Effective Care
  Environment
Integrated Process: Nursing Process/Planning
Content Area: Pharmacology

Test-Taking Strategy: Use the process of elimination. Eliminate option 2 first because of the close-ended word "only." Next eliminate option 3 because of the words "2 minutes." From the remaining options, recalling that ganciclovir causes thrombocytopenia will direct you to option 4. Review the side effects of this medication if you had difficulty with this question.

Reference

Hodgson, B., & Kizior, R. (2007). *Saunders nursing drug handbook 2007* (p. 531). Philadelphia: Saunders.

1740. A client is to be discharged from the hospital on quinidine to control ventricular ectopy, and the nurse provides medication instructions to the client. Which statement by the client would indicate the need for further instructions?
   1 "The best time to schedule this medication is with my meals."
   2 "I need to take this medication regularly, even if my heart feels strong."
   3 "I should avoid alcohol, caffeine, and cigarettes while on this medication."
   4 "If I get diarrhea, nausea, or vomiting, I need to stop the medication immediately and then call my doctor."

Level of Cognitive Ability: Analysis
Client Needs: Physiological Integrity
Integrated Process: Teaching and Learning
Content Area: Pharmacology

Answer: 4
Rationale: Diarrhea, nausea, vomiting, loss of appetite, and dizziness are all common side effects of quinidine. If these should occur, the physician or nurse should be notified, but the medication should never be stopped by the client. A rapid decrease in the medication level of an antidysrhythmic could precipitate dysrhythmia. Options 1, 2, and 3 are accurate client statements.

Test-Taking Strategy: Note the strategic words "need for further instructions." These words indicate a negative event query and the need to select the incorrect client statement. Noting that quinidine is used to control ventricular ectopy and recalling that the client should not stop taking a medication without first consulting the physician will direct you to option 4. Review client teaching points related to this medication if you had difficulty with this question.

Reference

Hodgson, B., & Kizior, R. (2007). *Saunders nursing drug handbook 2007* (p. 998). Philadelphia: Saunders.

1741. A client having a mild panic attack has the following arterial blood gas (ABG) results: pH 7.49, P_{CO_2} 31 mm Hg, Pa_{O_2} 97 mm Hg, HCO_3 22 mEq/L. The nurse reviews the results and determines that the client has which acid-base disturbance?
   1 Metabolic acidosis
   2 Metabolic alkalosis
   3 Respiratory acidosis
   4 Respiratory alkalosis

Answer: 4
Rationale: Acidosis is defined as a pH of less than 7.35, whereas alkalosis is defined as a pH of greater than 7.45. Respiratory alkalosis is present when the P_{CO_2} is less than 35, whereas respiratory acidosis is present when the P_{CO_2} is greater than 45. Metabolic acidosis is present when the HCO_3 is less than 22 mEq/L, whereas metabolic alkalosis is present when the H_{CO_3} is greater than 26 mEq/L. This client's ABGs are consistent with respiratory alkalosis.

Test-Taking Strategy: Note the strategic words "panic attack." This may help you anticipate that the client is having an increased respiratory rate, which makes the client prone to respiratory alkalosis. Otherwise, use the steps for interpreting blood gas results to answer the question. Review these steps if you had difficulty with this question.

Level of Cognitive Ability: Analysis
Client Needs: Physiological Integrity
Integrated Process: Nursing Process/Analysis
Content Area: Adult Health/Respiratory

References
Ignatavicius, D., & Workman, M. (2006). *Medical-surgical nursing: Critical thinking for collaborative care* (5th ed., p. 290). Philadelphia: Saunders.
Monahan, F., Sands, J., Marek, J., Neighbors, M., & Green, C. (2007). *Phipps' medical-surgical nursing: Health and illness perspectives* (8th ed., pp. 393-394). St. Louis: Mosby.

1742. Vasopressin (Pitressin) is prescribed for a client with diabetes insipidus, and the client asks the nurse about the purpose of the medication. The nurse responds, knowing that the action of the medication is to:
1 Decrease peristalsis.
2 Produce vasodilation.
3 Decrease urinary output.
4 Inhibit smooth muscle contraction.

Level of Cognitive Ability: Application
Client Needs: Physiological Integrity
Integrated Process: Teaching and Learning
Content Area: Pharmacology

Answer: 3
Rationale: Vasopressin is a vasopressor and an antidiuretic. It directly stimulates contraction of smooth muscle, causes vasoconstriction, stimulates peristalsis, and increases reabsorption of water by the renal tubules, resulting in decreased urinary output.

Test-Taking Strategy: Use the process of elimination. Eliminate options 1 and 4 first because they are comparable or alike. From the remaining options, recalling the pathophysiology associated with diabetes insipidus will direct you to option 3. Review the actions of this medication if you had difficulty with this question.

Reference
Mosby. (2007). *Mosby's nursing drug reference* (20th ed., p. 1031). St. Louis: Mosby.

1743. The client has diabetes mellitus that has been well controlled with glyburide (DiaBeta), but recently, the client's fasting blood glucose has been reported to be 180 to 200 mg/dL. Which of the following medications, if noted in the client's record, may be contributing to the elevated blood glucose level?
1 Ranitidine (Zantac)
2 Cimetidine (Tagamet)
3 Prednisone (Deltasone)
4 Ciprofloxacin hydrochloride (Cipro)

Level of Cognitive Ability: Analysis
Client Needs: Physiological integrity
Integrated Process: Nursing Process/Analysis
Content Area: Pharmacology

Answer: 3
Rationale: Corticosteroids, thiazide diuretics, and lithium may decrease the effect of glyburide, causing hyperglycemia. Options 1, 2, and 4 may increase the effect of glyburide, leading to hypoglycemia.

Test-Taking Strategy: Knowledge regarding the medications that have an adverse effect if taken concurrently with glyburide is required to answer this question. Remember that corticosteroids can cause hyperglycemia. Review this content if you are unfamiliar with these medications.

References
Mosby. (2007). *Mosby's nursing drug reference* (20th ed., pp. 509-510, 828-829). St. Louis: Mosby.
Skidmore-Roth, L. (2005). *Mosby's drug guide for nurses* (6th ed., p. 714). St. Louis: Mosby.

1744. Buspirone hydrochloride (BuSpar) is prescribed for a client with an anxiety disorder. The nurse instructs the client regarding the medication and tells the client that:
1 The medication is addicting.
2 Dizziness and nervousness may occur.
3 Tolerance can occur with the medication.
4 The medication can produce a sedating effect.

Level of Cognitive Ability: Application
Client Needs: Physiological Integrity
Integrated Process: Teaching and Learning
Content Area: Pharmacology

Answer: 2
Rationale: Buspirone hydrochloride is used in the management of anxiety disorders. The advantages of this medication is that it is not sedating, tolerance does not develop, and it is not addicting. The medication has a more favorable side effect profile than do the benzodiazepines. Dizziness, nausea, headaches, nervousness, lightheadedness, and excitement, which generally are not major problems, are side effects of the medication.

Test-Taking Strategy: Knowledge regarding the side effects and the advantages of buspirone hydrochloride is required to answer this question. Remember that dizziness and nervousness may occur with this medication. Review its characteristics if you are unfamiliar with this medication and its use.

Reference
Mosby. (2007). *Mosby's nursing drug reference* (20th ed., p. 202). St. Louis: Mosby.

1745. Neuroleptic malignant syndrome is suspected in a client who is taking chlorpromazine (Thorazine). Which medication would the nurse prepare in anticipation of being prescribed to treat this adverse reaction related to the use of chlorpromazine?
1 Protamine sulfate
2 Bromocriptine (Parlodel)
3 Phytonadione (Vitamin K)
4 Enalapril maleate (Vasotec)

Level of Cognitive Ability: Analysis
Client Needs: Physiological Integrity
Integrated Process: Nursing Process/Planning
Content Area: Pharmacology

Answer: 2
Rationale: Bromocriptine is an antiparkinson prolactin inhibitor used in the treatment of neuroleptic malignant syndrome. Vitamin K is the antidote for warfarin (Coumadin) overdose. Protamine sulfate is the antidote for heparin overdose. Enalapril maleate is an angiotensin-converting enzyme inhibitor and an antihypertensive that is used in the treatment of hypertension.

Test-Taking Strategy: Use the process of elimination. Recalling that option 3 is the antidote for warfarin overdose and option 1 is the antidote for heparin will assist in eliminating these options. From the remaining options, focus on the medication classifications and eliminate option 4 because it is an antihypertensive. Review neuroleptic malignant syndrome if you had difficulty with this question.

Reference
Lehne, R. (2007). *Pharmacology for nursing care* (6th ed., p. 193). Philadelphia: Saunders.

1746. A client with a fractured leg has learned how to use crutches to assist in ambulation. The nurse determines that the client misunderstood the information if the client states to:
1 Keep spare crutch tips available.
2 Keep crutch tips dry so they don't slip.
3 Inspect the crutch tips for wear from time to time.
4 Keep the set of crutches found in the basement of the home as a spare pair.

Answer: 4
Rationale: The client should use only crutches measured for the client. Crutches belonging to another person should not be used unless they have been adjusted to fit the client. Spare tips and crutches fitted to the client should be available if needed. Crutch tips should remain dry. Water could cause slipping by decreasing the surface friction of the rubber tip on the floor. If crutch tips get wet, the client should dry them with a cloth or paper towel. The tips should be regularly inspected for wear.

Level of Cognitive Ability: Analysis
Client Needs: Safe and Effective Care
  Environment
Integrated Process: Teaching and Learning
Content Area: Adult Health/Musculoskeletal

Test-Taking Strategy: Note the strategic words "misunderstood the information." These words indicate a negative event query and the need to select the incorrect client statement. Option 2 relates to safety and is eliminated first. Eliminate options 1 and 3 next because they are comparable or alike. Review client teaching points related to the use of crutches if you had difficulty with this question.

References

Black, J., & Hawks, J. (2005). *Medical-surgical nursing: Clinical management for positive outcomes* (7th ed., p. 2501). Philadelphia: Saunders.
Ignatavicius, D., & Workman, M. (2006). *Medical-surgical nursing: Critical thinking for collaborative care* (5th ed., p. 1204). Philadelphia: Saunders.

1747. Disulfiram (Antabuse) is prescribed for a client who is seen in the psychiatric health care clinic. The nurse is collecting data from the client and is providing instructions regarding the use of this medication. Which data is important for the nurse to obtain before beginning the administration of this medication?

1 When the last full meal was consumed
2 If the client has a history of diabetes insipidus
3 When the last alcoholic drink was consumed
4 If the client has a history of hyperthyroidism

Level of Cognitive Ability: Analysis
Client Needs: Physiological integrity
Integrated Process: Nursing Process/Assessment
Content Area: Pharmacology

Answer: 3
Rationale: Disulfiram may be used as an adjunct treatment for selected clients with chronic alcoholism who want to remain in a state of enforced sobriety. Clients must abstain from alcohol intake for at least 12 hours before the initial dose of the medication is administered. Therefore, it is important for the nurse to determine when the last alcoholic drink was consumed. The medication is used with caution in clients with diabetes mellitus, hypothyroidism, epilepsy, cerebral damage, nephritis, and hepatic disease. It is also contraindicated in severe heart disease, psychosis, or hypersensitivity related to the medication.

Test-Taking Strategy: Use the process of elimination. Recalling that this medication is used as an adjunct treatment for chronic alcoholism will direct you to option 3. Review this medication if you are unfamiliar with it.

References

McKenry, L., Tressier, E., & Hogan, M. (2006). *Mosby's pharmacology in nursing* (22nd ed., pp. 167-168). St. Louis: Mosby.
Mosby. (2007). *Mosby's nursing drug reference* (20th ed., p. 375). St. Louis: Mosby.

1748. A client with nephrotic syndrome states to the nurse: "Why should I even bother trying to control my diet and the edema? It doesn't really matter what I do, if I can never get rid of this kidney problem anyway!" Based on the client's statement, the nurse addresses which potential client problem?

1 Anxiety
2 Powerlessness
3 Ineffective coping
4 Disturbed body image

Answer: 2
Rationale: Powerlessness is a problem when the client believes that personal actions will not affect an outcome in any significant way. Anxiety occurs when the client has a feeling of unease with a vague or undefined source. Ineffective coping indicates that the client has impaired adaptive abilities or behaviors in meeting the demands or roles expected from the individual. Disturbed body image occurs when the way the client perceives body image is altered.

Test-Taking Strategy: Use the process of elimination, focusing on the data in the question. Note the words "It doesn't really matter what I do…" This implies that the client has a sense of no control of the situation. This will direct you to option 2. Review the defining characteristics of powerlessness if you had difficulty with this question.

Level of Cognitive Ability: Analysis
Client Needs: Psychosocial Integrity
Integrated Process: Nursing Process/Analysis
Content Area: Adult Health/Renal

References
Gulanick, M., & Myers, J. (2007). *Nursing care plans: Nursing diagnosis and interventions* (6th ed., pp. 15, 21, 51, 153). St. Louis: Mosby.
Monahan, F., Sands, J., Neighbors, M., Marek, J., & Green, C. (2007). *Phipps' medical-surgical nursing: Health and illness perspectives* (8th ed., p. 972). St. Louis: Mosby.

1749. Fluoxetine hydrochloride (Prozac) daily is prescribed for a client, and the nurse provides instructions to the client regarding the administration of the medication. Which statement by the client indicates an understanding regarding the administration of the medication?
1 "I should take the medication with food only."
2 "It is best to take the medication in the morning."
3 "I should take the medication at bedtime with a snack."
4 "I should take the medication at noontime with an antacid."

Level of Cognitive Ability: Analysis
Client Needs: Physiological Integrity
Integrated Process: Nursing Process/Evaluation
Content Area: Pharmacology

Answer: 2
Rationale: A daily dose of fluoxetine hydrochloride should be taken in the morning. If the medication is prescribed more than once daily, then the client is instructed to take the last dose of the day before 4:00 PM to avoid insomnia.

Test-Taking Strategy: Use the process of elimination. Eliminate option 1 because of the close-ended word "only." Next eliminate option 4, recalling that generally medications should not be administered with an antacid. From the remaining options, recalling that the medication can cause insomnia will direct you to option 2. Review this content if you are unfamiliar with the use of this medication and the client teaching points.

References
Mosby. (2007). *Mosby's nursing drug reference* (20th ed., p. 471). St. Louis: Mosby.
Skidmore-Roth, L. (2005). *Mosby's drug guide for nurses* (6th ed., p. 367). St. Louis: Mosby.

1750. A nursing student is assigned to care for a client with a diagnosis of Tourette syndrome who is receiving haloperidol decanoate (Haldol deconate). The registered nurse asks the student to describe the action of the medication. The student responds correctly by stating that this medication:
1 Is a serotonin reuptake blocker
2 Inhibits the breakdown of released acetylcholine
3 Blocks the uptake of norepinephrine and serotonin
4 Blocks the binding of dopamine to the post-synaptic dopamine receptors in the brain

Level of Cognitive Ability: Comprehension
Client Needs: Physiological Integrity
Integrated Process: Teaching and Learning
Content Area: Pharmacology

Answer: 4
Rationale: Haloperidol decanoate is a long-acting antipsychotic and acts by blocking the binding of dopamine to the post synaptic dopamine receptors in the brain. Imipramine hydrochloride (Tofranil) blocks the reuptake of norepinephrine and serotonin. Donepezil hydrochloride (Aricept) inhibits the breakdown of released acetylcholine. Fluoxetine hydrochloride (Prozac) is a potent serotonin reuptake blocker.

Test-Taking Strategy: Knowledge regarding the action of haloperidol deconate is required to answer this question. Remember this medication blocks the binding of dopamine. Review its action and use if you are unfamiliar with this medication.

Reference
Mosby. (2007). *Mosby's nursing drug reference* (20th ed., p. 516). St. Louis: Mosby.

1751. A nurse is teaching a client how to mix regular insulin and NPH insulin in the same syringe. The nurse tells the client to first:

1 Draw up the NPH insulin into the syringe first.
2 Keep both bottles in the refrigerator at all times.
3 Take all of the air out of the insulin bottles before mixing.
4 Rotate the NPH insulin bottle in the hands before mixing.

Level of Cognitive Ability: Application
Client Needs: Physiological Integrity
Integrated Process: Teaching and Learning
Content Area: Pharmacology

Answer: 4
Rationale: The NPH insulin bottle needs to be rotated for at least one minute between both hands. This resuspends the insulin. The nurse should not shake the bottles. Shaking causes foaming and bubbles to form, which may trap particles of insulin and alter the dosage. Insulin may be maintained at room temperature. Additional bottles of insulin for future use should be stored in the refrigerator. Regular insulin is drawn up before NPH insulin. Air does not need to be removed from the insulin bottles.

Test-Taking Strategy: Use the process of elimination. Visualizing the procedure for preparing the insulin will direct you to option 4. Review this procedure if you had difficulty with this question.

Reference
Lehne, R. (2007). *Pharmacology for nursing care* (6th ed., p. 669). Philadelphia: Saunders.

1752. A client has undergone mastectomy. The nurse determines that the client is having the most difficulty adjusting to the loss of the breast if which behavior is observed?

1 Performs arm exercises
2 Refuses to look at the dressing
3 Reads the postoperative care booklet
4 Requests pain medication when needed

Level of Cognitive Ability: Analysis
Client Needs: Psychosocial Integrity
Integrated Process: Nursing Process/Evaluation
Content Area: Adult Health/Oncology

Answer: 2
Rationale: The client demonstrates the most difficult adjustment to the loss if she refuses to look at the dressing. This indicates that the client is not ready or willing to begin to acknowledge and cope with the surgery. Performing arm exercises is an action-oriented behavior on the part of the client and is considered a positive sign of adjustment. Reading the postoperative care booklet indicates an interest in self-care and is a positive sign indicating beginning adjustment. Asking for pain medication is an action-oriented option that is helpful, although there is no direct connection to adjustment to the loss of the breast.

Test-Taking Strategy: Note the strategic words "most difficulty adjusting" and focus on the subject. Note that options 1, 3, and 4 are comparable or alike and indicate a positive client action. Review psychosocial responses related to loss if you had difficulty with this question.

References
Gulanick, M., & Myers, J. (2007). *Nursing care plans: Nursing diagnosis and interventions* (6th ed., p. 1006). St. Louis: Mosby.
Lewis, S., Heitkemper, M., Dirksen, S., O'Brien, P., & Bucher, L. (2007). *Medical-surgical nursing: Assessment and management of clinical problems* (7th ed., p. 1357). St. Louis: Mosby.

1753. A client has been taking lansoprazole (Prevacid) for 4 weeks. The nurse monitors the client for relief of which of the following symptoms?

1 Diarrhea
2 Flatulence
3 Heartburn
4 Constipation

Answer: 3
Rationale: Lansoprazole is a gastric pump inhibitor and is classified as an antiulcer agent. The intended effect of the medication is relief of pain from gastric irritation, often referred to as heartburn by clients. The medication does not improve the other symptoms listed.

Level of Cognitive Ability: Analysis
Client Needs: Physiological Integrity
Integrated Process: Nursing Process/Evaluation
Content Area: Pharmacology

Reference
Mosby. (2007). *Mosby's nursing drug reference* (20th ed., p. 590). St. Louis: Mosby.

1754. The nurse is preparing a client who had a total knee replacement with a metal prosthesis for discharge to home and provides the client with discharge instructions. Which statement by the client indicates a need for further instructions?
  1 "I can expect that changes in the shape of the knee will occur."
  2 "I need to tell any future caregivers about the metal prosthesis."
  3 "I need to report bleeding gums or tarry stools to the physician."
  4 "I need to report fever, redness, or increased pain to the physician."

Level of Cognitive Ability: Analysis
Client Needs: Health Promotion and Maintenance
Integrated Process: Teaching and Learning
Content Area: Adult Health/Musculoskeletal

Answer: 1
Rationale: After total knee replacement, the client should be taught to report any changes in the shape of the knee. This is not an expected event during recuperation from surgery. The client must notify caregivers of the metal implant, because the client will need antibiotic prophylaxis for invasive procedures, and because the client will be ineligible for magnetic resonance imaging as a diagnostic procedure. With a metal prosthesis, the client must be on anticoagulant therapy and should report adverse effects of this therapy, such as evidence of bleeding from a variety of sources. Fever, redness, or increased pain may indicate infection.

Test-Taking Strategy: Note the strategic words "metal prosthesis" and "need for further instructions." These words indicate a negative event query and the need to select the incorrect client statement. Recalling that the client will be on prophylactic anticoagulant therapy will assist in eliminating option 3. Eliminate options 2 and 4 next because these are standard postoperative guidelines. Review client teaching points following total knee replacement if you had difficulty with this question.

References
Ignatavicius, D., & Workman, M. (2006). *Medical-surgical nursing: Critical thinking for collaborative care* (5th ed., p. 390). Philadelphia: Saunders.
Monahan, F., Sands, J., Marek, J., Neighbors, M., & Green, C. (2007). *Phipps' medical-surgical nursing: Health and illness perspectives* (8th ed., p. 1630). St. Louis: Mosby.

1755. A nurse administers a dose of scopolamine to a preoperative client. The nurse monitors the client for which common side effect of the medication?
  1 Dry mouth
  2 Diaphoresis
  3 Excessive urination
  4 Pupillary constriction

Level of Cognitive Ability: Application
Client Needs: Physiological Integrity
Integrated Process: Nursing Process/Assessment
Content Area: Pharmacology

Answer: 1
Rationale: Scopolamine is an anticholinergic medication that causes the frequent side effects of dry mouth, urinary retention, decreased sweating, and dilation of the pupils. Each of the incorrect options is the opposite of a side effect of this medication.

Test-Taking Strategy: Focus on the name of the medication. Recalling that this medication is an anticholinergic will direct you to option 1. Review the side effects of anticholinergics if you had difficulty with this question.

Reference
Mosby. (2007). *Mosby's nursing drug reference* (20th ed., p. 901). St. Louis: Mosby.

1756. A nurse is providing medication instructions to a client who is taking imipramine (Tofranil) daily. Which statement by the client indicates a need for further instructions?

  1 "I need to avoid alcohol while taking the medication."
  2 "I need to take the medication in the morning before breakfast."
  3 "The effects of the medication may not be noticed for at least 2 weeks."
  4 "If I miss a dose, I need to take it as soon as possible unless it is almost time for the next dose."

Level of Cognitive Ability: Analysis
Client Needs: Physiological Integrity
Integrated Process: Teaching and Learning
Content Area: Pharmacology

Answer: 2
Rationale: The client should be instructed to take the medication (a single dose) at bedtime and not in the morning because it causes fatigue and drowsiness. The client is instructed to take the medication exactly as directed, and if a dose is missed to take it as soon as possible unless it is almost time for the next dose. The client is told that medication effects may not be noticed for at least 2 weeks, and to avoid alcohol or other central nervous system depressants during therapy.

Test-Taking Strategy: Note the strategic words "need for further instructions." These words indicate a negative event query and the need to select the incorrect client statement. General principles related to medication administration will eliminate options 1 and 4. From the remaining options, recalling that this medication is an antidepressant will eliminate option 3. Review these client teaching points if you are unfamiliar with this medication.

References
Mosby. (2007). *Mosby's nursing drug reference* (20th ed., p. 550). St. Louis: Mosby.
Skidmore-Roth, L. (2008). *Mosby's nursing drug reference* (21st ed., p. 556). St. Louis: Mosby.

1757. The nurse is preparing to assess a client who was admitted to the hospital with a diagnosis of trigeminal neuralgia (tic douloureux). On review of the client's record, the nurse would expect to note that the client experiences:

  1 Bilateral pain in the sixth cranial nerve
  2 Unilateral pain in the sixth cranial nerve
  3 Abrupt onset of pain in the fifth cranial nerve
  4 Chronic, intermittent pain in the seventh cranial nerve

Level of Cognitive Ability: Analysis
Client Needs: Physiological Integrity
Integrated Process: Nursing Process/Assessment
Content Area: Adult Health /Neurological

Answer: 3
Rationale: Trigeminal neuralgia is a chronic syndrome characterized by an abrupt onset of pain. It involves one or more divisions of the trigeminal nerve (cranial nerve V). Options 1, 2, and 4 are incorrect.

Test-Taking Strategy: Focus on the client's diagnosis. Recalling that trigeminal neuralgia affects the fifth cranial nerve will assist in eliminating options 1, 2, and 4. Review the pathophysiology associated with trigeminal neuralgia if you had difficulty with this question.

References
Black, J., & Hawks, J. (2005). *Medical-surgical nursing: Clinical management for positive outcomes* (7th ed., pp. 2153-2154). Philadelphia: Saunders.
Lewis, S., Heitkemper, M., Dirksen, S., O'Brien, P., & Bucher, L. (2007). *Medical-surgical nursing: Assessment and management of clinical problems* (7th ed., p. 1581). St. Louis: Mosby.

1758. A client is taking docusate (Colace). The nurse tells the client to monitor for which of the following to ensure that the medication has the intended effect?

  1 Abdominal pain
  2 Decreased heartburn
  3 Decrease in fatty stools
  4 Regular bowel movements

Answer: 4
Rationale: Docusate is a stool softener that promotes absorption of water into the stool, producing a softer consistency of stool. The intended effect is relief or prevention of constipation. The medication does not relieve abdominal pain, relieve heartburn, or decrease the amount of fat in the stools.

Level of Cognitive Ability: Application
Client Needs: Physiological Integrity
Integrated Process: Teaching and Learning
Content Area: Pharmacology

Test-Taking Strategy: Focus on the name of the medication. Recalling that this medication is a stool softener will direct you to option 4. Review the action of this medication if you had difficulty with this question.

References

Mosby. (2007). *Mosby's nursing drug reference* (20th ed., pp. 378-379). St. Louis: Mosby.
Skidmore-Roth, L. (2008). *Mosby's nursing drug reference* (21st ed., p. 381). St. Louis: Mosby.

1759. A client's laboratory test results reveal a decreased serum transferrin and total iron-binding capacity (TIBC). Which disorder is the most likely cause of the client's anemia?
1 Infection
2 Malnutrition
3 Iron deficiency
4 Sickle cell disease

Level of Cognitive Ability: Comprehension
Client Needs: Physiological Integrity
Integrated Process: Nursing Process/Evaluation
Content Area: Fundamental Skills

Answer: 2
Rationale: Malnutrition can cause reductions in the serum transferrin and the TIBC. Infection is an unrelated option. Sickle cell anemia is diagnosed by determining that the client has hemoglobin S. Iron-deficiency anemia is usually characterized by decreased iron-binding capacity but increased transferrin levels. Additionally, in clinical practice, the hemoglobin level is routinely used to detect iron-deficiency anemia.

Test-Taking Strategy: Focus on the laboratory tests identified in the question. Use these data and knowledge regarding the findings in malnutrition to direct you to option 2. Review the findings in malnutrition if you had difficulty with this question.

References

Chernecky, C., & Berger, B. (2008). *Laboratory tests and diagnostic procedures* (5th ed., pp. 686-687). Philadelphia: Saunders.
Ignatavicius, D., & Workman, M. (2006). *Medical-surgical nursing: Critical thinking for collaborative care* (5th ed., p. 1428). Philadelphia: Saunders.

1760 Which type of anemia is diagnosed with a Schilling test?
1 Aplastic
2 Pernicious
3 Megaloblastic
4 Iron deficiency

Level of Cognitive Ability: Comprehension
Client Needs: Physiological Integrity
Integrated Process: Nursing Process/Assessment
Content Area: Fundamental Skills

Answer: 2
Rationale: The Schilling test is used to determine the cause of vitamin B_{12} deficiency, a potential precursor to pernicious anemia. This test involves the use of a small oral dose of radioactive B_{12} and a large nonradioactive intramuscular dose. A 24-hour urine specimen is then collected to measure the amount of radioactivity in the urine and, thus, radioactive B_{12}. This test is not helpful in diagnosing megaloblastic, iron deficiency, or aplastic anemia.

Test-Taking Strategy: Specific knowledge regarding the Schilling test and its purpose is needed to answer this question. Remember that the Schilling test is used to determine the cause of vitamin B_{12} deficiency. Review this test and the diagnostic tests associated with pernicious anemia if you had difficulty with this question.

References

Chernecky, C., & Berger, B. (2008). *Laboratory tests and diagnostic procedures* (5th ed., p. 995). Philadelphia: Saunders.
Ignatavicius, D., & Workman, M. (2006). *Medical-surgical nursing: Critical thinking for collaborative care* (5th ed., p. 1335). Philadelphia: Saunders.

1761. A physician has written an order for a client with diabetic gastroparesis to receive metoclopramide (Reglan) four times a day. The nurse schedules this medication to be given at which of the following times?

1 With each meal and at bedtime
2 30 minutes before meals and at bedtime
3 One hour after each meal and at bedtime
4 Every 6 hours spaced evenly around the clock

Level of Cognitive Ability: Application
Client Needs: Physiological Integrity
Integrated Process: Nursing Process/ Implementation
Content Area: Pharmacology

Answer: 2
Rationale: Metoclopramide stimulates the motility of the upper gastrointestinal tract and is used to treat gastroparesis (nausea, vomiting, and persistent fullness after meals). The client should be taught to take this medication 30 minutes before meals and at bedtime. The before-meals administration allows the medication time to begin working before the client consumes food that requires digestion. The other options are incorrect.

Test-Taking Strategy: Focus on the client's diagnosis. Noting that the medication is used to treat gastroparesis will direct you to option 2. Remember that it must be taken before meals to enhance digestion. Review the procedure for the administration of this medication if you had difficulty with this question.

Reference
Skidmore-Roth, L. (2008). *Mosby's nursing drug reference* (21st ed., p. 674). St. Louis: Mosby.

1762. The nurse is caring for a client who has just had a mastectomy. The nurse assists the client in doing which of the following exercises during the first 24 hours following surgery?

1 Hand wall climbing
2 Pendulum arm swings
3 Elbow flexion and extension
4 Shoulder abduction and external rotation

Level of Cognitive Ability: Application
Client Needs: Physiological Integrity
Integrated Process: Nursing Process/ Implementation
Content Area: Adult Health/Oncology

Answer: 3
Rationale: During the first 24 hours following surgery, the client is assisted to move the fingers and hands, and to flex and extend the elbow. The client may also use the arm for self-care provided that she does not raise the arm above shoulder level or abduct the shoulder. The exercises identified in options 1, 2, and 4 are done once surgical drains are removed and wound healing is well established.

Test-Taking Strategy: Note the strategic words "during the first 24 hours" and use the process of elimination. Remember that options that are comparable or alike are not likely to be correct. In this situation, each of the incorrect options involves movement of the shoulder joint. Review appropriate exercises for the client following mastectomy if you had difficulty with this question.

References
Black, J., & Hawks, J. (2005). *Medical-surgical nursing: Clinical management for positive outcomes* (7th ed., p. 1109). Philadelphia: Saunders.
Lewis, S., Heitkemper, M., Dirksen, S., O'Brien, P., & Bucher, L. (2007). *Medical-surgical nursing: Assessment and management of clinical problems* (7th ed., p. 1358). St. Louis: Mosby.

1763. The nurse teaches a client about an upcoming endoscopic retrograde cholangiopancreatography (ERCP) procedure. The nurse determines that the client requires additional information if the client states that:

1 An anesthetic throat spray will be used.
2 A signed informed consent is necessary.
3 Medication will be given orally for sedation.
4 It is important to lie still during the procedure.

Level of Cognitive Ability: Application
Client Needs: Physiological Integrity
Integrated Process: Teaching and Learning
Content Area: Adult Health/Gastrointestinal

Answer: 3
Rationale: The client needs to lie still for ERCP, which takes about an hour to perform. The client also has to sign an informed consent form. Intravenous sedation (not oral) is given to relax the client, and an anesthetic throat spray is used to help keep the client from gagging as the endoscope is passed.

Test-Taking Strategy: Note the strategic words "requires additional information" in the question. Recalling that this procedure is endoscopic and noting the word "orally" in option 3 will direct you to this option. Review preprocedure care for an ERCP if you had difficulty with this question.

Reference
Chernecky, C., & Berger, B. (2008). *Laboratory tests and diagnostic procedures* (5th ed., p. 474). Philadelphia: Saunders.

1764. A client has an order to take magnesium citrate to prevent constipation following upper and lower gastrointestinal (GI) barium studies. The nurse tells the client that this medication is best taken:

1 With fruit juice only
2 At room temperature
3 With a tepid glass of water
4 Chilled with a full glass of water

Level of Cognitive Ability: Application
Client Needs: Physiological Integrity
Integrated Process: Nursing Process/
  Implementation
Content Area: Pharmacology

Answer: 4
Rationale: Magnesium citrate is available as an oral solution. It is commonly used as a laxative following certain studies of the GI tract. It should be served chilled and taken with a full glass of water. It should not be allowed to stand for prolonged periods. Allowing the medication to stand would reduce the carbonation and make the solution even less palatable. Options 1, 2, and 3 are incorrect.

Test-Taking Strategy: Use the process of elimination. Eliminate option 1 first because of the close-ended word "only." Next eliminate options 2 and 3 because they identify similar temperatures. Review the procedure for administering this medication if you had difficulty with this question.

References
Mosby. (2007). *Mosby's nursing drug reference* (20th ed., p.630). St. Louis: Mosby.
Skidmore-Roth, L. (2008). *Mosby's nursing drug reference* (21st ed., p. 636). St. Louis: Mosby.

1765. A client has begun medication therapy with pancrelipase (Pancrease). The nurse teaches the client that this medication should:

1 Relieve heartburn
2 Eliminate abdominal pain
3 Help regulate blood glucose
4 Decrease the amount of fat in the stools

Answer: 4
Rationale: Pancrelipase is a pancreatic enzyme used in clients with pancreatitis as a digestive aid. The medication should reduce the amount of fatty stools (steatorrhea). Another intended effect could be improved nutritional status. It is not used to treat abdominal pain or heartburn. It does not regulate blood glucose; this is a function of insulin, a hormone produced in the beta cells of the pancreas.

Test-Taking Strategy: Focus on the name of the medication, which gives an indication of the possible uses of this medication. Also use knowledge of the physiology of the pancreas and recall that the suffix "-ase" in the medication name indicates an enzyme. This will assist in directing you to option 4. Review the action of this medication if you had difficulty with this question.

Level of Cognitive Ability: Application
Client Needs: Physiological Integrity
Integrated Process: Teaching and Learning
Content Area: Pharmacology

Reference
Mosby. (2007). *Mosby's nursing drug reference* (20th ed., p. 768). St. Louis: Mosby.

1766. The nurse is performing tracheostomy care and has replaced the tracheostomy tube holder (tracheostomy ties). The nurse ensures that the holder is not too tight by checking to see if:

1 The client nods that he or she feels comfortable
2 Two fingers can be slid comfortably under the holder
3 Four fingers can be slid comfortably under the holder
4 The tracheostomy does not move more than ½ inch when the client is coughing

Level of Cognitive Ability: Analysis
Client Needs: Physiological Integrity
Integrated Process: Nursing Process/Evaluation
Content Area: Adult Health/Respiratory

Answer: 2
Rationale: There should be enough room for two fingers to slide comfortably under the tracheostomy holder. This ensures that the holder is tight enough to prevent tracheostomy dislocation, while preventing excessive constriction around the neck. The other options are incorrect.

Test-Taking Strategy: Use the process of elimination, focusing on the subject—that the tracheostomy holder is not too tight. Visualize each of the descriptions in the options to direct you to option 2. Review the essentials of this fundamental nursing procedure if you had difficulty with this question.

Reference
Ignatavicius, D., & Workman, M. (2006). *Medical-surgical nursing: Critical thinking for collaborative care* (5th ed., p. 558). Philadelphia: Saunders.

1767. A nurse has assisted the physician in placing a central (subclavian) catheter. Following the procedure, the nurse takes which priority action?

1 Ensures that a chest radiograph is done
2 Obtains a temperature reading to monitor for infection
3 Labels the dressing with the date and time of catheter insertion
4 Monitors the blood pressure (BP) to check for fluid volume overload

Level of Cognitive Ability: Application
Clinical Needs: Physiological Integrity
Integrated Process: Nursing Process/ Implementation
Content Area: Delegating/Prioritizing

Answer: 1
Rationale: A major risk associated with central catheter insertion is the possibility of a pneumothorax developing from an accidental puncture of the lung. Obtaining a chest radiograph and checking the results is the best method to determine if this complication has occurred and to verify catheter tip placement before initiating intravenous (IV) therapy. While a client may develop an infection at the central catheter site, a temperature elevation would not likely occur immediately after placement. While BP assessment is always important in checking a client's status after an invasive procedure, fluid volume overload is not a concern until IV fluids are started. Labeling the dressing site is important, but it is not a priority action in this situation.

Test-Taking Strategy: Use the process of elimination. Noting the strategic words "following the procedure" will assist in eliminating options 2 and 4. Next, noting the words "priority action" will direct you to option 1 from the remaining options. Review postprocedure care following central catheter insertion if you had difficulty with this question.

Reference
Ignatavicius, D., & Workman, M. (2006). *Medical-surgical nursing: Critical thinking for collaborative care* (5th ed., p. 255). Philadelphia: Saunders.

1768. A client is complaining of gas pains following surgery and requests medication. The nurse reviews the medication order sheet to see if which medication is ordered for the relief of gas pains?

1 Droperidol (Inapsine)
2 Simethicone (Mylicon)
3 Acetaminophen (Tylenol)
4 Magnesium hydroxide (MOM)

Level of Cognitive Ability: Analysis
Client Needs: Physiological Integrity
Integrated Process: Nursing Process/Analysis
Content Area: Pharmacology

Answer: 2

Rationale: Simethicone is an antiflatulent used in the relief of pain caused by excessive gas in the gastrointestinal tract. Acetaminophen is a non-opioid analgesic. Magnesium hydroxide is an antacid and laxative. Droperidol is used to treat postoperative nausea and vomiting.

Test-Taking Strategy: Focus on the strategic words "gas pains." Recalling the classifications of each of the medications listed in the options will direct you to option 2. Review the action and purpose of each of the medications listed if you had difficulty with this question.

References
Mosby. (2007). *Mosby's nursing drug reference* (20th ed., p. 910). St. Louis: Mosby.
Skidmore-Roth, L. (2008). *Mosby's nursing drug reference* (21st ed., p. 929). St. Louis: Mosby.

1769. A home care nurse notes that an older client is taking cimetidine (Tagamet). On assessment of the client, the nurse checks for which side effect of this medication?

1 Fatigue
2 Confusion
3 Constipation
4 Blurred vision

Level of Cognitive Ability: Analysis
Client Needs: Physiological Integrity
Integrated Process: Nursing Process/Assessment
Content Area: Pharmacology

Answer: 2

Rationale: Cimetidine is a gastric acid secretion inhibitor. Older clients are especially susceptible to the central nervous system side effects of cimetidine. The most frequent of these is confusion. Less common central nervous system side effects include headache, dizziness, drowsiness, agitation, and hallucinations. Options 1, 3, and 4 are not associated with the use of this medication.

Test-Taking Strategy: Focus on the medication. Recalling that cimetidine causes central nervous system side effects will direct you to option 2. Review the side effects of this medication if you had difficulty with this question.

Reference
Mosby. (2007). *Mosby's nursing drug reference* (20th ed., p. 273). St. Louis: Mosby.

1770. A client is admitted to the hospital after sustaining a fall from a roof. The client has multiple lacerations and a right leg fracture, which has been treated with a plaster cast. The nurse positions the client's leg in which manner to promote optimal circulation?

1 Flat or a level position
2 Flat for 3 hours and elevated for 1 hour
3 Elevated for 3 hours, and then flat for 1 hour
4 Elevated on pillows continuously for 24 to 48 hours

Level of Cognitive Ability: Application
Client Needs: Physiological Integrity
Integrated Process: Nursing Process/Implementation
Content Area: Adult Health/Musculoskeletal

Answer: 4

Rationale: A casted extremity is elevated continuously for the first 24 to 48 hours to minimize swelling and to promote venous drainage. The other options are not part of standard positioning of the newly casted extremity.

Test-Taking Strategy: Focus on the subject—to promote optimal circulation. Recalling that edema occurs after a fracture and can be increased by casting and using the principles of gravity will direct you to option 4. Review appropriate positioning following casting of an extremity if you had difficulty with this question.

References
Ignatavicius, D., & Workman, M. (2006). *Medical-surgical nursing: Critical thinking for collaborative care* (5th ed., p. 1198). Philadelphia: Saunders.
Monahan, F., Sands, J., Neighbors, M., Marek, J. & Green, C. (2007). *Phipps' medical-surgical nursing: Health and illness perspectives* (8th ed., p. 1536). St. Louis: Mosby.

1771. A physical assessment is performed on a suicidal client upon admission to the inpatient unit. The nurse understands its importance because it provides information regarding:
1 The presence of abnormalities
2 Evidence of physical self-harm
3 Both subjective and objective baseline data
4 Existing medical problems and complaints

Level of Cognitive Ability: Analysis
Client Needs: Physiological Integrity
Integrated Process: Nursing Process/Assessment
Content Area: Mental Health

Answer: 2
Rationale: The physical assessment of a suicidal client should be thorough and should focus on the evidence of self-harm or the client's formulation of a plan for the suicide attempt. Although all of the options are correct, option 2 is most appropriate in the context of the suicidal client. Clients with a history of self-harm are greater suicide risks.

Test-Taking Strategy: Use the process of elimination and focus on the client's diagnosis. Remember that assessing for physical evidence of harm is an important component of the assessment process of a suicidal client. Review the characteristics of the client at risk for suicide if you had difficulty with this question.

Reference
Stuart, G., & Laraia, M. (2005). *Principles and practice of psychiatric nursing* (8th ed., p. 367). St. Louis: Mosby.

1772. A client being mechanically ventilated after experiencing a fat embolus is visibly anxious. The nurse takes which appropriate action?
1 Remains with the client and provides reassurance
2 Asks a family member to stay with the client at all times
3 Asks the physician to obtain an order for an antianxiety medication
4 Encourages the client to sleep until arterial blood gas results improve

Level of Cognitive Ability: Application
Client Needs: Psychosocial Integrity
Integrated Process: Caring
Content Area: Adult Health/Respiratory

Answer: 1
Rationale: The nurse always speaks to the client calmly and provides reassurance to the anxious client. Family members are also stressed due to the severity of the situation. Therefore, it is not beneficial to ask the family to take on the burden of remaining with the client at all times. Encouraging the client to sleep will not assist in relieving the client's anxiety. Antianxiety medications are used only if necessary and if other interventions fail to relieve the client's anxiety.

Test-Taking Strategy: Note the strategic words "appropriate action." Use the process of elimination, remembering that it is most important to address the client's feelings. Review care of the client who is anxious if you had difficulty with this question.

References
Black, J., & Hawks, J. (2005). *Medical-surgical nursing: Clinical management for positive outcomes* (7th ed., pp. 1890-1891). Philadelphia: Saunders.
Monahan, F., Sands, J., Marek, J., Neighbors, M., & Green, C. (2007). *Phipps' medical-surgical nursing: Health and illness perspectives* (8th ed., p. 201). St. Louis: Mosby.

1773. A nurse is caring for a client who is receiving colchicine. The nurse understands that the client is responding favorably to the medication if there is a decrease in
1 Headaches
2 Joint inflammation
3 Blood glucose level
4 Serum triglyceride level

Answer: 2
Rationale: Colchicine is classified as an antigout agent. It interferes with the ability of the white blood cells to initiate and maintain an inflammatory response to monosodium urate crystals. The client should report a decrease in pain and inflammation in affected joints, as well as a decrease in the number of gout attacks. The other options are not related to the use of this medication.

Test-Taking Strategy: Focus on the name of the medication. Recalling that this medication is used in the treatment of gout will direct you to option 2. Review the action of this medication if you had difficulty with this question.

Level of Cognitive Ability: Analysis
Client Needs: Physiological Integrity
Integrated Process: Nursing Process/Evaluation
Content Area: Pharmacology

References
Mosby. (2007). *Mosby's nursing drug reference* (20th ed., p. 300). St. Louis: Mosby.
Skidmore-Roth, L. (2008). *Mosby's nursing drug reference* (21st ed., pp. 300-301). St. Louis: Mosby.

1774. A client has an order to begin short-term therapy with enoxaparin (Lovenox). The nurse explains to the client that this medication is being ordered to:
1 Dissolve urinary calculi
2 Relieve migraine headaches
3 Stop progression of multiple sclerosis
4 Reduce the risk of deep vein thrombosis

Level of Cognitive Ability: Application
Client Needs: Physiological Integrity
Integrated Process: Teaching and Learning
Content Area: Pharmacology

Answer: 4
Rationale: Enoxaparin is an anticoagulant that is administered to prevent deep vein thrombosis and thromboembolism in selected clients at risk. It is not used to treat urinary calculi, migraine headaches, or multiple sclerosis.

Test-Taking Strategy: Focus on the name of the medication. Recalling that this medication is an anticoagulant will direct you to option 4. Review the action of this medication if you had difficulty with this question.

References
Mosby. (2007). *Mosby's nursing drug reference* (20th ed., p. 408). St. Louis: Mosby.
Skidmore-Roth, L. (2008). *Mosby's nursing drug reference* (21st ed., pp. 410-411). St. Louis: Mosby.

1775. A client takes aluminum hydroxide (Amphojel) tablets as needed for heartburn. The nurse teaches the client that the most common side effect of this medication is:
1 Dizziness
2 Excitability
3 Muscle pain
4 Constipation

Level of Cognitive Ability: Application
Client Needs: Physiological Integrity
Integrated Process: Teaching and Learning
Content Area: Pharmacology

Answer: 4
Rationale: Because of the antacid's aluminum base, aluminum hydroxide causes constipation as a side effect. The other side effect is hypophosphatemia, which is noted by monitoring serum laboratory studies. The other options are not side effects of this medication.

Test-Taking Strategy: Focus on the medication name and recall that this medication is an antacid. Recalling that aluminum based antacids cause constipation will direct you to option 4. Review the side effects associated with this medication if you had difficulty with this question.

References
McKenry, L., Tressier, E. & Hogan, M. (2006). *Mosby's pharmacology in nursing* (22nd ed., p. 749). St. Louis: Mosby.
Mosby. (2007). *Mosby's nursing drug reference* (20th ed., p. 104). St. Louis: Mosby.

1776. The nurse is caring for a young adult client diagnosed with sarcoidosis. The client is angry and tells the nurse that there is no point in learning disease management, because there is no possibility of ever being cured. Based on the client's statement, the nurse determines that the client is experiencing which potential problem?
1 Anxiety
2 Powerlessness
3 Disturbed thought processes
4 Ineffective health maintenance

Answer: 2
Rationale: The client with powerlessness expresses feelings of having no control over a situation or outcome. Ineffective health maintenance involves the inability to seek out help that is needed to maintain health. Anxiety is a vague sense of unease or dread. Disturbed thought processes involves disruption in cognitive abilities or thought.

Test-Taking Strategy: Focus on the data in the question. Use the process of elimination, noting the strategic words "no point in learning disease management." This will direct you to option 2. Review the defining characteristics of powerlessness if you had difficulty with this question.

Level of Cognitive Ability: Analysis
Client Needs: Psychosocial Integrity
Integrated Process: Nursing Process/Analysis
Content Area: Adult Health/Respiratory

References
Ackley, B., & Ladwig, G. (2008). *Nursing diagnosis handbook: An evidence-based guide to planning care* (8th ed., pp. 139, 412, 650, 834). St. Louis: Mosby.
Monahan, F., Sands, J., Marek, J., Neighbors, M., & Green, C. (2007). *Phipps' medical-surgical nursing: Health and illness perspectives* (8th ed., pp. 642-643). St. Louis: Mosby.

1777. A nurse is providing instructions to the spouse of a client who is taking tacrine (Cognex) for the management of moderate dementia associated with Alzheimer's disease. The nurse tells the spouse:

1 If a dose is missed, double up on the next dose.
2 Do not administer the medication with food.
3 If a change in the color of the stools occurs, notify the physician.
4 If flu-like symptoms occur, it is necessary to notify the physician immediately.

Level of Cognitive Ability: Application
Client Needs: Physiological Integrity
Integrated Process: Teaching and Learning
Content Area: Pharmacology

Answer: 3

Rationale: Tacrine may be administered between meals on an empty stomach, and if gastrointestinal upset occurs, it may be administered with meals. Flu-like symptoms without fever is a frequent side effect that may occur with the use of the medication. The client or spouse should never be instructed to double the dose of any medication if it was missed, and the client and caregiver are instructed to notify the physician if nausea, vomiting, diarrhea, rash, jaundice, or changes in the color of the stool occur. This may be indicative of the potential occurrence of hepatitis.

Test-Taking Strategy: Use the process of elimination. Eliminate option 4 because of the word "immediately." Flu-like symptoms should not be a concern requiring immediate physician notification. Next eliminate option 1 because of the words "double up on the next dose." From the remaining options, recalling that an adverse effect associated with the use of the medication is hepatitis will direct you to option 3. Review this medication if you are unfamiliar with its use and potential adverse effects.

References
Lehne, R. (2007). *Pharmacology for nursing care* (6th ed., p. 201). Philadelphia: Saunders.
Mosby. (2007). *Mosby's nursing drug reference* (20th ed., p. 940). St. Louis: Mosby.

1778. An older client has been using cansonthrol (cascara sagrada) on a long-term basis to treat constipation. The nurse determines that which laboratory finding is a result of the side effects of this medication?

1 Sodium 135 mEq/L
2 Sodium 145 mEq/L
3 Potassium 3.1 mEq/L
4 Potassium 5.0 mEq/L

Level of Cognitive Ability: Analysis
Client Needs: Physiological Integrity
Integrated Process: Nursing Process/Analysis
Content Area: Pharmacology

Answer: 3

Rationale: Hypokalemia can result from long-term use of casanthrol (cascara sagrada), which is a laxative. The medication stimulates peristalsis and alters fluid and electrolyte transport, thus helping fluid to accumulate in the colon. The normal range for potassium is 3.5 to 5.1 mEq/L. The normal range for sodium is 135 to 145 mEq/L. Options 1, 2, and 4 are normal values.

Test-Taking Strategy: Use the process of elimination and knowledge regarding the normal laboratory values for sodium and potassium. The only abnormal value is option 3. Review the effects of this medication if you had difficulty with this question.

References
Mosby. (2007). *Mosby's nursing drug reference* (20th ed., p. 231). St. Louis: Mosby.
Skidmore-Roth, L. (2008). *Mosby's nursing drug reference* (21st ed., p. 213). St. Louis: Mosby.

1779. A client has been started on cyclobenza-prine (Flexeril) for the management of muscle spasms. The nurse teaches the client to observe for which most frequent side effect?
1 Fatigue
2 Irritability
3 Excitability
4 Drowsiness

Level of Cognitive Ability: Application
Client Needs: Physiological Integrity
Integrated Process: Teaching and Learning
Content Area: Pharmacology

Answer: 4
Rationale: The most frequent side effects of cyclobenzaprine are drowsiness, dizziness, and dry mouth. This medication is a centrally acting skeletal muscle relaxant used in the management of muscle spasms that accompany a variety of conditions. Fatigue, nervousness, and confusion are rare side effects of the medication.

Test-Taking Strategy: Note the strategic words "most frequent." Eliminate options 2 and 3 first because they are comparable or alike. Recalling that this medication is a centrally acting skeletal muscle relaxant will direct you to option 4 from the remaining options. Review this medication if you had difficulty with this question.

References
Mosby. (2007). *Mosby's nursing drug reference* (20th ed., p. 310). St. Louis: Mosby.
Skidmore-Roth, L. (2008). *Mosby's nursing drug reference* (21st ed., p. 313). St. Louis: Mosby.

1780. The nurse is caring for a client following shoulder arthroplasty for rheumatoid arthritis and is checking the client for brachial plexus compromise. To assess the status of the median nerve, which of the following would the nurse perform?
1 Have the client spread all of the fingers wide and resist pressure.
2 Monitor for flexion of the biceps by having the client raise the forearm.
3 Have the client move the thumb toward the palm and back to the neutral position.
4 Have the client grasp the nurse's hand while noting the client's strength of the first and second fingers.

Level of Cognitive Ability: Application
Client Needs: Health Promotion and Maintenance
Integrated Process: Nursing Process/Assessment
Content Area: Adult Health/Musculoskeletal

Answer: 4
Rationale: To assess the median nerve status, the client should be instructed to grasp the nurse's hand. The nurse should note the strength of the client's first and second fingers. A weak grip may indicate compromise of the median nerve. Asking the client to spread all fingers wide and resisting pressure is assessing the ulnar nerve status. Monitoring for flexion of the biceps by raising the forearm is assessing for cutaneous nerve status. Asking the client to move the thumb toward the palm and back to neutral position is assessing the radial nerve status.

Test-Taking Strategy: Focus on the subject—assessment of the median nerve. Recalling the location and function of the median nerve will direct you to option 4. Review this assessment technique if you are unfamiliar with this procedure.

Reference
Black, J., & Hawks, J. (2005). *Medical-surgical nursing: Clinical management for positive outcomes* (7th ed., pp. 2010, 2351). Philadelphia: Saunders.

1781. A nurse is preparing to administer heparin sodium (Liquaemin) 5000 units subcutaneously. Which of the following indicates the accurate procedure for administering the medication?
1 Injecting the medication via an infusion device
2 Injecting the medication 1 inch from the umbilicus
3 Massaging the injection site following administration
4 Avoiding aspiration prior to administration of the medication

Level of Cognitive Ability: Application
Client Needs: Physiological Integrity
Integrated Process: Nursing Process/ Implementation
Content Area: Pharmacology

Answer: 4
Rationale: Heparin administered by the subcutaneous route does not require an infusion device. The injection site is above the iliac crest or in the abdominal fat layer. It is injected at least 2 inches from the umbilicus. After administration, the needle is withdrawn, pressure is applied to the injection site, and the site is not massaged. Injection sites are rotated. Aspiration prior to administration should be avoided.

Test-Taking Strategy: Use the process of elimination, focusing on the subject—accurate procedure. Visualize the procedure as you read each option. Recalling the action and effects of heparin will direct you to option 4. Review this procedure if you had difficulty with this question.

References
Mosby. (2007). *Mosby's nursing drug reference* (20th ed., p. 520). St. Louis: Mosby.
Skidmore-Roth, L. (2008). *Mosby's nursing drug reference* (21st ed., p. 527). St. Louis: Mosby.

1782. Which does the nurse assess for in a client who has pernicious anemia?
1 Constipation
2 Shortness of breath
3 Dusky lips and gums
4 Smooth, sore, red tongue

Level of Cognitive Ability: Application
Client Needs: Physiological Integrity
Integrated Process: Nursing Process/Assessment
Content Area: Fundamental Skills

Answer: 4
Rationale: Classic clinical indicators of pernicious anemia include weakness, mild diarrhea, and a smooth, sore red tongue. The client may also have neurological findings, such as paresthesias, confusion, and difficulty with balance. Pernicious anemia does not affect tissue oxygenation, so the mucous membranes do not become dusky, and the client does not exhibit shortness of breath (options 2 and 3). Constipation is an uncommon finding with pernicious anemia.

Test-Taking Strategy: To answer this question, you must be familiar with the clinical indicators of pernicious anemia. Remember that the classic clinical indicators of pernicious anemia include weakness, mild diarrhea, and a smooth, sore red tongue. Review the assessment data related to this disorder if you had difficulty with the question.

References
Ignatavicius, D., & Workman, M. (2006). *Medical-surgical nursing: Critical thinking for collaborative care* (5th ed., p. 895). Philadelphia: Saunders.
Monahan, F., Sands, J., Marek, J., Neighbors, M., & Green, C. (2007). *Phipps' medical-surgical nursing: Health and illness perspectives* (8th ed., p. 921). St. Louis: Mosby.

1783. Benztropine mesylate (Cogentin) is prescribed for a client with a diagnosis of Parkinson's disease. The clinic nurse is providing instructions to the client regarding the medication and tells the client to:

1 Sit in the sun for 30 minutes daily.
2 Avoid driving if drowsiness or dizziness occurs.
3 Expect difficulty swallowing while taking this medication.
4 Expect episodes of vomiting and constipation while taking this medication.

Level of Cognitive Ability: Application
Client Needs: Safe and Effective Care Environment
Integrated Process: Teaching and Learning
Content Area: Pharmacology

Answer: 2

Rationale: The client taking benztropine mesylate should be instructed to avoid driving or operating hazardous equipment if drowsy or dizzy. The client's tolerance to heat may be reduced because of the diminished ability to sweat, and the client should be instructed to plan rest periods in cool places during the day. The client should be instructed to stop taking the medication if difficulty swallowing or speaking or vomiting occurs. The client should also inform the physician if central nervous system effects occur. The client is instructed to monitor urinary output and to watch for signs of constipation.

Test-Taking Strategy: Use the process of elimination. General principles related to safety and medications will direct you to option 2. Review client teaching points related to this medication if you had difficulty with this question.

References

Mosby. (2007). *Mosby's nursing drug reference* (20th ed., p. 175). St. Louis: Mosby
Skidmore-Roth, L. (2008). *Mosby's nursing drug reference* (21st ed., p178). St. Louis: Mosby.

1784. A nurse is preparing to do preoperative teaching with a client scheduled for radical neck dissection. The nurse initially focuses on:

1 Client's usual coping behaviors
2 Client's dependable support systems
3 Postoperative communication techniques
4 Information already supplied by the surgeon

Level of Cognitive Ability: Application
Client Needs: Psychosocial Integrity
Integrated Process: Teaching and Learning
Content Area: Fundamental Skills

Answer: 4

Rationale: The first step in client education is establishing what the client already knows. This allows the nurse to correct any misinformation or misunderstandings, to determine the starting point for teaching, and to plan and implement the education at the client's level. Although options 1, 2, and 3 can be a component of the plan, the first step in client education is establishing what the client already knows.

Test Taking Strategy: Note the strategic word "initially." It is likely that all of the options listed will be included in the teaching plan, but you need to determine what the nurse would focus on initially. Remember, in the teaching and learning process, client motivation and readiness to learn along with what the client already knows are initial assessment items. Review the teaching and learning process if you had difficulty with this question.

References

Ignatavicius, D., & Workman, M. (2006). *Medical-surgical nursing: Critical thinking for collaborative care* (5th ed., pp. 304, 574). Philadelphia: Saunders.
Potter, P., & Perry, A. (2005). *Fundamentals of nursing* (6th ed., pp. 451-454). St. Louis: Mosby.

1785. A client with refractory myasthenia gravis is told by the physician that plasmapheresis therapy is indicated. After the physician leaves the room, the client asks the nurse to repeat the physician's reason for ordering this treatment. The nurse tells the client that this therapy will most likely improve which of the client's symptoms?

  1 Double vision
  2 Difficulty breathing
  3 Urinary incontinence
  4 Pins and needles sensation in the legs

Level of Cognitive Ability: Application
Client Needs: Physiological Integrity
Integrated Process: Nursing Process/
  Implementation
Content Area: Adult Health/Neurological

Answer: 2
Rationale: Plasmapheresis is a process that separates the plasma from the blood elements, so that plasma proteins that contain antibodies can be removed. It is used as an adjunct therapy in myasthenia gravis and may give temporary relief to clients with actual or impending respiratory failure. Usually three to five treatments are required. This therapy is not indicated for the reasons listed in options 1, 3, and 4.

Test-Taking Strategy: Note the strategic word "refractory." This tells you that the client with myasthenia gravis has severe disease, which is not adequately controlled with medication and other measures. Recalling the purpose of plasmapheresis and knowledge of the complications of this disease will direct you to option 2. Review the purpose of this procedure if you had difficulty with this question.

References
Black, J., & Hawks, J. (2005). *Medical-surgical nursing: Clinical management for positive outcomes* (7th ed., p. 2184). Philadelphia: Saunders.
Monahan, F., Sands, J., Marek, J., Neighbors, M., & Green, C. (2007). *Phipps' medical-surgical nursing: Health and illness perspectives* (8th ed., p. 1454). St. Louis: Mosby.

1786. A client is admitted to the hospital in myasthenic crisis. The nurse questions the family about the occurrence of which precipitating factor for this event?

  1 Getting more sleep than usual
  2 Not taking prescribed medication
  3 A decrease in food intake recently
  4 Taking excess prescribed medication

Level of Cognitive Ability: Analysis
Client Needs: Physiological Integrity
Integrated Process: Nursing Process/Assessment
Content Area: Adult Health/Neurological

Answer: 2
Rationale: Myasthenic crisis is often caused by undermedication and responds to the administration of cholinergic medications such as neostigmine (Prostigmin) and pyridostigmine (Mestinon). Cholinergic crisis (the opposite problem) is caused by excess medication and responds to withholding of medications. Change in diet and increased sleep are not precipitating factors. However, overexertion and overeating could possibly trigger myasthenic crisis.

Test-Taking Strategy: Focus on the subject—myasthenic crisis. Recalling that myasthenia gravis is treated with medication will direct you to option 2. Review the causes of myasthenia gravis if you had difficulty with this question.

References
Black, J., & Hawks, J. (2005). *Medical-surgical nursing: Clinical management for positive outcomes* (7th ed., p. 2183). Philadelphia: Saunders.
Monahan, F., Sands, J., Marek, J., Neighbors, M., & Green, C. (2007). *Phipps' medical-surgical nursing: Health and illness perspectives* (8th ed., p. 1454). St. Louis: Mosby.

1787. A client with trigeminal neuralgia asks the nurse what can be done to minimize the episodes of pain. The nurse's response is based on an understanding that the symptoms can be triggered by which of the following?

1 Infection or stress
2 Hypoglycemia and fatigue
3 Sensations of pressure or extreme temperature
4 Excessive watering of the eyes or nasal stuffiness

Level of Cognitive Ability: Analysis
Client Needs: Physiological Integrity
Integrated Process: Nursing Process/ Implementation
Content Area: Adult Health/Neurological

Answer: 3
Rationale: The paroxysms of pain that accompany this neuralgia are triggered by stimulation of the terminal branches of the trigeminal nerve. Symptoms can be triggered by pressure from washing the face, brushing the teeth, shaving, eating and drinking and yawning. Symptoms can also be triggered by thermal stimuli such as a draft of cold air. The items listed in the other options do not trigger the spasm.

Test-Taking Strategy: Recall the pathophysiology of this disorder and that precipitating factors such as pressure or thermal stimuli trigger the spasm. This will direct you to option 3. Review this cranial nerve disorder if you had difficulty with this question.

References
Black, J., & Hawks, J. (2005). *Medical-surgical nursing: Clinical management for positive outcomes* (7th ed., pp. 2153-2154). Philadelphia: Saunders.
Monahan, F., Sands, J., Marek, J., Neighbors, M., & Green, C. (2007). *Phipps' medical-surgical nursing: Health and illness perspectives* (8th ed., p. 1484). St. Louis: Mosby.

1788. A client has been diagnosed with Bell's palsy. The nurse assesses the client to determine if which signs and symptoms are present?

1 Eye paralysis and ptosis of the eyelid
2 Speech difficulties and one-sided facial droop
3 Fixed pupil and an elevated eyelid on one side
4 Twitching of one side of the face and ruddy cheeks

Level of Cognitive Ability: Analysis
Client Needs: Physiological Integrity
Integrated Process: Nursing Process/Assessment
Content Area: Adult Health/Neurological

Answer: 2
Rationale: Bell's palsy is a one sided facial paralysis resulting from compression of the facial nerve (CN VII). There is facial droop from paralysis of the facial muscles, increased lacrimation, painful sensations in the eye, face, or behind the ear, and chewing difficulties. The other items listed are not associated with this disorder.

Test-Taking Strategy: Use the process of elimination. Remember that palsy is a type of paralysis. This will assist in eliminating option 4. Recalling that Bell's palsy results from dysfunction of the facial nerve (CN VII), not the nerves that govern eye movements (CN III, IV, VI), will help to eliminate options 1 and 3. Review the characteristics associated with Bell's palsy if you had difficulty with this question.

References
Black, J., & Hawks, J. (2005). *Medical-surgical nursing: Clinical management for positive outcomes* (7th ed., p. 2154). Philadelphia: Saunders.
Lewis, S., Heitkemper, M., Dirksen, S., O'Brien, P., & Bucher, L. (2007). *Medical-surgical nursing: Assessment and management of clinical problems* (7th ed., p. 1584). St. Louis: Mosby.

1789. A female client arrives at the emergency department and states she was just raped. In preparing a plan of care, the priority intervention is:

1 Providing instructions for medical follow-up
2 Obtaining appropriate counseling for the victim
3 Providing anticipatory guidance for police investigations, medical questions, and court proceedings
4 Exploring safety concerns by obtaining permission to notify significant others who can provide shelter

Level of Cognitive Ability: Analysis
Client Needs: Safe and Effective Care Environment
Integrated Process: Nursing Process/Planning
Content Area: Mental Health

Answer: 4
Rationale: After the provision of medical treatment, the nurse's next priority would be obtaining support and planning for safety. Options 2 and 3 seek to meet the emotional needs related to the rape and emotional readiness for the process of discovery and legal action. Option 1 is concerned with ensuring that the victim understands the importance of and commits to the need for medical follow-up. From the options provided, this is not a priority intervention.

Test-Taking Strategy: Use Maslow's Hierarchy of Needs theory and note the strategic words "priority intervention." Remember that physiological needs are the priority, followed by safety needs. Therefore, select option 4 because it addresses the safety needs. Review care of the rape victim if you had difficulty with this question.

Reference
Stuart, G., & Laraia, M. (2005). *Principles and practice of psychiatric nursing* (8th ed., p. 235). St. Louis: Mosby.

1790. A client has provider instructions to take ibuprofen (Advil) 0.4 g for mild pain. The medication bottle contains ibuprofen (Advil) 200-mg tablets. How many tablets will the nurse instruct the client to take for each dose?

Answer: _____ tablets

Level of Cognitive Ability: Application
Client Needs: Physiological Integrity
Integrated Process: Nursing Process/ Implementation
Content Area: Fundamental Skills

Answer: 2
Rationale: Convert 0.4 g to mg. In the metric system, to convert larger to smaller, multiply by 1000 or move the decimal three places to the right. Then follow the medication calculation formula.

0.4 g = 400 mg

$$\frac{Desired}{Available} \times Quantity = Tablets\ per\ dose$$

$$\frac{400\ mg}{200\ mg} \times 1\ tablet = 2\ tablets$$

Test-Taking Strategy: Use the formula for the calculation of a medication dose. Remember to convert grams to milligrams. Make sure that the calculated dose makes sense, and recheck your answer using a calculator. Review conversions and calculations if you had difficulty with this question.

Reference
Kee, J., & Marshall, S. (2004). *Clinical calculations: With applications to general and specialty areas* (4th ed., p. 80). Philadelphia: Saunders.

1791. The nurse is admitting a client to the hospital who has a diagnosis of Guillain-Barré syndrome. During history-taking, the nurse asks the family member if the client has recently experienced which of the following?
1 Meningitis
2 Seizures or head trauma
3 A back injury or spinal cord trauma
4 A respiratory or gastrointestinal (GI) infection

Answer: 4
Rationale: Guillain-Barré syndrome is a clinical syndrome of unknown origin that involves cranial and peripheral nerves. Many clients report a history of respiratory or GI infection in the 1 to 4 weeks before the onset of neurological deficits. Occasionally, it has been triggered by vaccination or surgery. The other options are not associated with an incidence of this syndrome.

Level of Cognitive Ability: Analysis
Client Needs: Physiological Integrity
Integrated Process: Nursing Process/Assessment
Content Area: Adult Health/Neurological

Test-Taking Strategy: Use the process of elimination. Eliminate options 1, 2, and 3 because they are comparable or alike and relate to neurological problems. Review the etiology associated with Guillain-Barré syndrome if you had difficulty with this question.

References

Black, J., & Hawks, J. (2005). *Medical-surgical nursing: Clinical management for positive outcomes* (7th ed., p. 2182). Philadelphia: Saunders.
Lewis, S., Heitkemper, M., Dirksen, S., O'Brien, P., & Bucher, L. (2007). *Medical-surgical nursing: Assessment and management of clinical problems* (7th ed., pp. 1585-1586). St. Louis: Mosby.

1792. A client is using diphenhydramine (Benadryl) 1% as a topical agent for allergic dermatosis. The nurse evaluates that the medication is having the intended effect if the client reported relief of what complaint?

1 Pain
2 Urticaria
3 Headache
4 Skin redness

Answer: 2
Rationale: Diphenhydramine is an antihistamine medication that has many uses. When used as a topical agent on the skin, it reduces the symptoms of allergic reaction, such as itching or urticaria. It does not act to relieve headache, skin redness, or pain.

Test-Taking Strategy: Note the strategic words "intended effect." Recalling that diphenhydramine is an antihistamine medication will assist in directing you to option 2. Review the action of this medication if you had difficulty with this question.

Level of Cognitive Ability: Analysis
Client Needs: Physiological Integrity
Integrated Process: Nursing Process/Evaluation
Content Area: Pharmacology

References

Mosby. (2007). *Mosby's nursing drug reference* (20th ed., p. 368). St. Louis: Mosby.
Skidmore-Roth, L. (2008). *Mosby's nursing drug reference* (21st ed., p. 373). St. Louis: Mosby.

1793. A client is being treated in the emergency room for a fractured tibia. The skin is not broken, but the nurse can see on the x-ray viewer that the bone is completely fractured across the shaft and has small splintered pieces around it. The nurse interprets that this client's fracture is a:

1 Simple fracture
2 Greenstick fracture
3 Compound fracture
4 Comminuted fracture

Answer: 4
Rationale: A comminuted fracture is a complete fracture across the shaft of a bone, with splintering of the bone into fragments. A simple fracture is a fracture of the bone across its entire shaft with some possible displacement but without breaking the skin. A greenstick fracture is an incomplete fracture, which occurs through part of the cross section of a bone. One side of the bone is fractured, and the other side is bent. A compound fracture, also called an open fracture, is one in which the skin or mucous membrane has been broken, and the wound extends to the depth of the fractured bone.

Test-Taking Strategy: Use the process of elimination, focusing on the strategic words "small splintered pieces." Remember that a comminuted fracture is broken into minute (small) pieces so this will direct you to option 4. Review the characteristics of the types of fractures if you had difficulty with this question.

Level of Cognitive Ability: Analysis
Client Needs: Physiological Integrity
Integrated Process: Nursing Process/Analysis
Content Area: Adult Health/Musculoskeletal

References

Black, J., & Hawks, J. (2005). *Medical-surgical nursing: Clinical management for positive outcomes* (7th ed., p. 624). Philadelphia: Saunders.
Lewis, S., Heitkemper, M., Dirksen, S., O'Brien, P., & Bucher, L. (2007). *Medical-surgical nursing: Assessment and management of clinical problems* (7th ed., p. 1636). St. Louis: Mosby.

1794. The nurse in the emergency department is providing care to a client with a leg fracture. The nurse ensures that which essential item is done first before the fracture is reduced in the casting room?
1 Obtaining an anesthesia consent
2 Administering an opioid analgesic
3 Notifying the operating room staff
4 Obtaining an informed consent for treatment

Level of Cognitive Ability: Application
Client Needs: Safe and Effective Care Environment
Integrated Process: Nursing Process/ Implementation
Content Area: Adult Health/Musculoskeletal

Answer: 4
Rationale: Before a fracture is reduced, an informed consent for treatment is needed. The nurse would reinforce explanations according to the client's needs and ability to understand. Administration of anesthesia would only be done in the operating room for open reduction of fractures. Closed reductions may be done in the emergency department without anesthesia. An analgesic would be administered as prescribed, because the procedure is painful, but the informed consent form needs to be obtained before administering the medication.

Test-Taking Strategy: Note the strategic words "essential" and "first." Note that the question specifically states that the procedure is going to be done in the cast room. This will assist in eliminating options 1 and 3. Recalling that an informed consent form must be obtained before administering sedating medication will direct you to option 4 from the remaining options. Review the procedure related to a closed reduction if you had difficulty with this question.

References
Black, J., & Hawks, J. (2005). *Medical-surgical nursing: Clinical management for positive outcomes* (7th ed., p. 2501). Philadelphia: Saunders.
Ignatavicius, D., & Workman, M. (2006). *Medical-surgical nursing: Critical thinking for collaborative care* (5th ed., pp. 857, 1192, 1197). Philadelphia: Saunders.

1795. The nurse is monitoring a client with a fracture to the left arm. Which sign observed by the nurse is consistent with impaired venous return in the area?
1 Increasing edema
2 Weakened distal pulse
3 Pallor or blotchy cyanosis
4 Continued pain despite medication

Level of Cognitive Ability: Analysis
Client Needs: Physiological Integrity
Integrated Process: Nursing Process/Analysis
Content Area: Adult Health/Musculoskeletal

Answer: 1
Rationale: Impaired venous return is characterized by increasing edema. In the client with a fracture, this is most often prevented by elevating the limb. The other options identify signs of arterial damage, which can occur if the artery is contused, thrombosed, lacerated, or becomes spastic.

Test-Taking Strategy: Note the strategic words "impaired venous return." Use principles of blood flow to answer the question. Each of the incorrect options identifies difficulty with circulation to the extremity and is an arterial sign. The correct option identifies a sign that is consistent with impaired venous return. Review the signs noted in impaired venous return if you had difficulty with this question.

References
Black, J., & Hawks, J. (2005). *Medical-surgical nursing: Clinical management for positive outcomes* (7th ed., pp. 1535-1536). Philadelphia: Saunders.
Ignatavicius, D., & Workman, M. (2006). *Medical-surgical nursing: Critical thinking for collaborative care* (5th ed., p. 1197). Philadelphia: Saunders.

1796. The nurse receives in transfer from the postanesthesia care unit a client who has had skeletal traction applied in the operating room. The nurse takes immediate action to correct which problem noted with the traction setup?

1 Knots are secured tightly
2 Ropes are free of frays or shredding
3 Weights are resting against the foot of the bed
4 Ropes are centered in the wheel grooves of the pulleys

Level of Cognitive Ability: Application
Client Needs: Physiological Integrity
Integrated Process: Nursing Process/ Implementation
Content Area: Adult Health/Musculoskeletal

Answer: 3
Rationale: The traction setup is checked to ensure that the ropes are in the grooves of the pulleys, ropes are not frayed, knots are tied securely, and weights are hanging freely from the ropes. Problems with any of these can interfere with maintenance of proper traction. If any problems are noted, they should be fixed immediately.

Test-Taking Strategy: Use the process of elimination, noting the strategic words "takes immediate action to correct." Recalling that weights exert the pulling force needed in a traction setup will direct you to option 3. Review the principles of setting up traction if you had difficulty with this question.

References
Black, J., & Hawks, J. (2005). *Medical-surgical nursing: Clinical management for positive outcomes* (7th ed., p. 627). Philadelphia: Saunders.
Ignatavicius, D., & Workman, M. (2006). *Medical-surgical nursing: Critical thinking for collaborative care* (5th ed., p. 1201). Philadelphia: Saunders.

1797. A nurse is monitoring for the presence of pitting edema in the prenatal client. The nurse presses the fingertips of the middle and index fingers against the shin and holds pressure for 2 to 3 seconds. The nurse notes that the indentation is approximately 1-inch deep. The nurse documents that the client has which level of pitting edema?

1 +1
2 +2
3 +3
4 +4

Level of Cognitive Ability: Application
Client Needs: Health Promotion and Maintenance
Integrated Process: Nursing Process/Assessment
Content Area: Maternity/Antepartum

Answer: 4
Rationale: When evaluating the presence of pitting edema, the nurse presses the fingertips of the index and middle fingers against the shin and holds pressure for 2 to 3 seconds. An indentation approximately 1-inch deep would be indicative of +4 edema. A slight indentation would indicate +1 edema. An indentation approximately ¼-inch deep indicates +2 edema. An indentation approximately ½-inch deep indicates +3 edema.

Test-Taking Strategy: Focus on the words "indentation is approximately 1-inch deep." Knowledge regarding this technique and the interpretation of the findings will assist in directing you to option 4. Review this content if you are unfamiliar with this technique.

Reference
Murray, S., & McKinney, E. (2006). *Foundations of maternal-newborn nursing* (4th ed., p. 120). Philadelphia: Saunders.

1798. A client has just been diagnosed with acute renal failure. The laboratory calls the nurse to report a serum potassium level of 6.1 mEq/L on the client. The nurse takes which immediate action?

1 Calls the physician
2 Checks the sodium level
3 Encourages an extra 500 mL of fluid intake
4 Teaches the client about foods low in potassium

Answer: 1
Rationale: The client with hyperkalemia is at risk of developing cardiac dysrhythmias and resultant cardiac arrest. Because of this, the physician must be notified at once so that the client may receive definitive treatment. Fluid intake would not be increased because it would contribute to fluid overload and wouldn't effectively lower the serum potassium level. Dietary teaching may be necessary at some point, but this action is not the priority. The nurse might also check the result of a serum sodium level, but this is not a priority action of the nurse.

Level of Cognitive Ability: Application
Client Needs: Physiological Integrity
Integrated Process: Nursing Process/
  Implementation
Content Area: Adult Health/Renal

Test-Taking Strategy: Use the process of elimination, noting the strategic word "immediate." Recalling the normal potassium level and noting that the level identified in the question is elevated will direct you to option 1. Review the normal potassium level if you had difficulty with this question.

References
Chernecky, C., & Berger, B. (2008). *Laboratory tests and diagnostic procedures* (5th ed., pp. 891-893). St. Louis: Saunders.
Ignatavicius, D., & Workman, M. (2006). *Medical-surgical nursing: Critical thinking for collaborative care* (5th ed., pp. 231-232). Philadelphia: Saunders.

1799. A nurse in the postpartum unit is developing a nursing care plan for a client following cesarean delivery. The nurse documents which intervention in the plan of care that will assist in preventing thrombophlebitis?
1 Frequent ambulation
2 Wearing support stockings
3 Applying warm moist packs to the legs
4 Remaining on bedrest with the legs elevated

Level of Cognitive Ability: Application
Client Needs: Physiological Integrity
Integrated Process: Nursing Process/Planning
Content Area: Maternity/Postpartum

Answer: 1
Rationale: Stasis is believed to be a major predisposing factor in the development of thrombophlebitis. Because cesarean delivery is a risk factor for the development of thrombophlebitis, the mother should ambulate early and frequently to promote circulation and prevent stasis. Bedrest is discouraged. Warm moist packs will not prevent thrombophlebitis. Support stockings may be a helpful measure in treating thrombophlebitis.

Test-Taking Strategy: Focus on the subject of the question—to prevent thrombophlebitis. Also, use basic principles related to nursing care and the prevention of complications following any type of abdominal surgery to direct you to option 1. Remember that thrombophlebitis results from the stasis of blood. Review content related to the prevention of thrombophlebitis in the postoperative period if you had difficulty with this question.

Reference
Murray, S., & McKinney, E. (2006). *Foundations of maternal-newborn nursing* (4th ed., p. 415). Philadelphia: Saunders.

1800. A client with glomerulonephritis is at risk of developing acute renal failure. The nurse monitors the client for which sign of this complication?
1 Bradycardia
2 Hypertension
3 Decreased cardiac output
4 Decreased central venous pressure

Answer: 2
Rationale: Acute renal failure caused by glomerulonephritis is classified as intrinsic or intrarenal failure. This form of acute renal failure is commonly manifested by hypertension, tachycardia, oliguria, lethargy, edema, and other signs of fluid overload. Acute renal failure from prerenal causes is characterized by decreased blood pressure or a recent history of the same, tachycardia, and decreased cardiac output and central venous pressure. Bradycardia is not part of the clinical picture for renal failure.

Level of Cognitive Ability: Analysis
Client Needs: Physiological Integrity
Integrated Process: Nursing Process/Assessment
Content Area: Adult Health/Renal

Test-Taking Strategy: Use the process of elimination, focusing on the client's diagnosis. Eliminate option 1 first because bradycardia will not occur. Remember that renal failure is accompanied by fluid overload. This will help you eliminate option 4 next. From the remaining options, recall that hypertension accompanies acute renal failure resulting from intrarenal causes, whereas decreased cardiac output accompanies acute renal failure resulting from prerenal causes. Review the manifestations associated with acute renal failure if you had difficulty with this question.

References
Ignatavicius, D., & Workman, M. (2006). *Medical-surgical nursing: Critical thinking for collaborative care* (5th ed., pp. 1718, 1729, 1732). Philadelphia: Saunders.
Monahan, F., Sands, J., Marek, J., Neighbors, M., & Green, C. (2007). *Phipps' medical-surgical nursing: Health and illness perspectives* (8th ed., p. 968). St. Louis: Mosby.

1801. A client has been prescribed metoprolol (Lopressor) for hypertension. The nurse monitors client compliance carefully because of which common side effect of the medication?
  1 Impotence
  2 Mood swings
  3 Increased appetite
  4 Complete atrioventricular (A-V) block

Level of Cognitive Ability: Analysis
Client Needs: Physiological Integrity
Integrated Process: Nursing Process/Assessment
Content Area: Pharmacology

Answer: 1
Rationale: A common side effect of β-adrenergic blocking agents, such as metoprolol, is impotence. Other common side effects include fatigue and weakness. Central nervous system side effects occur rarely and include mental status changes, nervousness, depression, and insomnia. Increased appetite, complete A-V block, and mood swings are not reported side effects.

Test-Taking Strategy: Focus on the medication name and recall that medication names that end with the letters "-lol" are β-adrenergic blocking agents. Next, focus on the subject—monitoring compliance—and the strategic words "common side effect." Remember that a common side effect of β-adrenergic blocking agents is impotence. This will direct you to option 1. Review the expected side effects of this group of medications if you had difficulty with this question.

Reference
Mosby. (2007). *Mosby's nursing drug reference* (20th ed., p. 669). St. Louis: Mosby.

1802. The nurse is caring for a client with cancer of the lung who is receiving chemotherapy. The nurse reviews the laboratory results and notes that the platelet count is 18,000/mm³. Based on this laboratory result, which of the following would the nurse implement?
  1 Contact precautions
  2 Bleeding precautions
  3 Respiratory precautions
  4 Neutropenic precautions

Answer: 2
Rationale: When the platelet count is less than 20,000/ mm³, the client is at risk for bleeding, and the nurse would institute bleeding precautions. Contact precautions is initiated in a client who has drainage from wounds that may be infectious. Respiratory precautions are instituted for a client with a respiratory infection that is transmitted by the airborne route. Neutropenic precautions would be instituted for a client with a low neutrophil count.

Test-Taking Strategy: Use the process of elimination. Recalling that when the platelet count is low, the client is at risk for bleeding will direct you to option 2. Review the normal platelet count and the nursing interventions necessary when the platelet count is low if you had difficulty with this question.

Level of Cognitive Ability: Application
Client Needs: Physiological Integrity
Integrated Process: Nursing Process/
   Implementation
Content Area: Adult Health/Oncology

References
Ignatavicius, D., & Workman, M. (2006). *Medical-surgical nursing: Critical thinking for collaborative care* (5th ed., pp. 496, 906). Philadelphia: Saunders.
Lewis, S., Heitkemper, M., Dirksen, S., O'Brien, P., & Bucher, L. (2007). *Medical-surgical nursing: Assessment and management of clinical problems* (7th ed., pp. 678-679). St. Louis: Mosby.

1803. A client with a leaking intracranial aneurysm has been placed on aneurysm precautions. A visiting family member wants to take the client to the unit lounge for "just a few minutes." The nurse would use which of the following concepts when explaining why the client must remain in the room?

   1 Clients with aneurysms need isolation to cope with photosensitivity.

   2 A quiet environment promotes more rapid healing of the aneurysm.

   3 Reduced environmental stimuli is needed to prevent aneurysm rupture.

   4 The client has disturbed thought processes and needs reduced stimulation.

Level of Cognitive Ability: Application
Client Needs: Physiological Integrity
Integrated Process: Nursing Process/
   Implementation
Content Area: Adult Health/Neurological

Answer: 3
Rationale: Subarachnoid precautions (or aneurysm precautions) are intended to minimize environmental stimuli, which could increase intracranial pressure and trigger bleeding or rupture of the aneurysm. The client does not need isolation to "cope" with photosensitivity (although photosensitivity may be a problem). The aneurysm will not heal more rapidly with reduced stimuli, and no data indicates that the client has disturbed thought processes.

Test-Taking Strategy: Focus on the subject—the purpose of aneurysm precautions. Recalling that the concern in this client is rupture will direct you to option 3. Review this content if you are unfamiliar with aneurysm precautions and their purpose.

References
Gulanick, M., & Myers, J. (2007). *Nursing care plans: Nursing diagnosis and interventions* (6th ed., p. 559). St. Louis: Mosby.
Monahan, F., Sands, J., Neighbors, M., Marek, J. & Green, C. (2007). *Phipps' medical-surgical nursing: Health and illness perspectives* (8th ed., p. 1441). St. Louis: Mosby.

1804. A client has been taking metoclopramide (Reglan) on a long-term basis. A home care nurse calls the physician immediately if which side effect is noted in this client?

   1 Excitability

   2 Anxiety or irritability

   3 Uncontrolled rhythmic movements of the face or limbs

   4 Dry mouth not minimized by the use of sugar-free hard candy

Level of Cognitive Ability: Application
Client Needs: Physiological Integrity
Integrated Process: Nursing Process/
   Implementation
Content Area: Pharmacology

Answer: 3
Rationale: If the client experiences tardive dyskinesia (rhythmic movements of the face or limbs), the nurse should withhold the medication and call the physician. These side effects may be irreversible. Excitability is not a side effect of this medication. Anxiety, irritability, and dry mouth are milder side effects that are not harmful to the client.

Test-Taking Strategy: Note the strategic words "calls the physician immediately." Select the option that identifies the most serious effect. This will direct you to option 3. Review the side effects of this medication and the signs of tardive dyskinesia if you had difficulty with this question.

Reference
McKenry, L., Tressier, E., & Hogan, M. (2006). *Mosby's pharmacology in nursing* (22nd ed., p. 762). St. Louis: Mosby.

1805. A nurse caring for a client taking clozapine (Clozaril) for the treatment of a schizophrenic disorder, reviews the laboratory studies that have been prescribed for the client. Which laboratory study is the priority to monitor for an adverse effect associated with the use of this medication?

1 Platelet count
2 Cholesterol level
3 Blood urea nitrogen
4 White blood cell count

Level of Cognitive Ability: Analysis
Client Needs: Physiological Integrity
Integrated Process: Nursing Process/Assessment
Content Area: Pharmacology

Answer: 4
Rationale: Hematological reactions can occur in the client taking clozapine and include agranulocytosis and mild leukopenia. The white blood cell count should be assessed before initiating treatment and should be monitored closely during the use of this medication. The client should also be monitored for signs indicating agranulocytosis, which may include sore throat, malaise, and fever. Options 1, 2, and 3 are unrelated to the use of this medication.

Test-Taking Strategy: Recalling that clozapine causes agranulocytosis will direct you to option 4. If you are unfamiliar with the adverse effects of this medication and the laboratory studies that need to be monitored, review this information.

Reference
Mosby. (2007). *Mosby's nursing drug reference* (20th ed., p. 297). St. Louis: Mosby.

1806. A postoperative client has been placed on a clear liquid diet. Which item(s) is(are) the client allowed to consume? Select all that apply.

☐ 1 Tea
☐ 2 Broth
☐ 3 Gelatin
☐ 4 Pudding
☐ 5 Vegetable juice
☐ 6 Pureed vegetables

Level of Cognitive Ability: Application
Client Needs: Physiological Integrity
Integrated Process: Nursing Process/
  Implementation
Content Area: Fundamental Skills

Answer: 1, 2, 3
Rationale: A clear liquid diet consists of foods that are relatively transparent to light, and are clear and liquid at room and body temperature. These foods include such items as water, bouillon, clear broth, carbonated beverages, gelatin, hard candy, lemonade, popsicles, and either regular or decaffeinated coffee or tea. The incorrect food items are items that are allowed on a full liquid diet.

Test-Taking Strategy: Focus on the subject—a clear liquid diet. Recalling that a clear liquid diet consists of foods that are relatively transparent to light, and are clear and liquid at room and body temperature will assist in determining the correct food items. Review foods that are on a clear liquid diet if you had difficulty with this question.

Reference
Grodner, M., Long, S., & DeYoung, S. (2004). *Foundations and clinical applications of nutrition: A nursing approach* (3rd ed., pp. 415-416). St. Louis: Mosby.

1807. A 30-week gestation client is admitted to the maternity unit in preterm labor. Betamethasone is prescribed to be administered and the client asks the nurse about the purpose of the medication. The nurse tells the client that this medication will:

1 Promote fetal lung maturity.
2 Delay delivery for at least 48 hours.
3 Stop the premature uterine contractions.
4 Prevent premature closure of the ductus arteriosus.

Answer: 1
Rationale: Betamethasone, a corticosteroid, is administered to increase the surfactant level and increase fetal lung maturity, reducing the incidence of respiratory distress syndrome in the newborn infant. Surfactant production does not become stable until after 32 weeks' gestation. If adequate amounts of surfactant are not present in the lungs, respiratory distress and death are possible consequences. Delivery needs to be delayed for at least 48 hours after the administration of betamethasone in order to allow time for the lungs to mature. Options 2, 3, and 4 are incorrect.

Level of Cognitive Ability: Application
Client Needs: Physiological Integrity
Integrated Process: Nursing Process/
    Implementation
Content Area: Maternity/Intrapartum

Test-Taking Strategy: Use the process of elimination. Eliminate options 2 and 3 first because they are comparable or alike and both relate to stopping labor. Recalling that respiratory distress syndrome caused by immature lungs is a major concern of prematurity will direct you to option 1 from the remaining options. Review the purpose of this medication if you had difficulty with this question.

Reference
Murray, S., & McKinney, E. (2006). *Foundations of maternal-newborn nursing* (4th ed., p. 718). Philadelphia: Saunders.

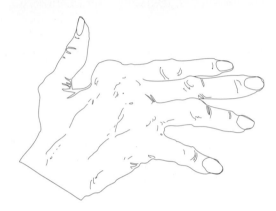

From Black, J., & Hawks, J., (2005). *Medical-surgical nursing: Clinical management for positive outcomes* (7th ed.). Philadelphia: Saunders.

1808. A nurse is performing a physical assessment on a client with rheumatoid arthritis. The nurse assesses the client's hands and notes these characteristic deformities. The nurse identifies this deformity as:
1 Ulnar drift
2 Rheumatoid nodules
3 Swan neck deformity
4 Boutonniere deformity

Level of Cognitive Ability: Analysis
Client Needs: Physiological Integrity
Integrated Process: Nursing Process/Assessment
Content Area: Adult Health/Immune

Answer: 1
Rationale: All of the conditions that are identified in the options can occur in rheumatoid arthritis. Ulnar drift occurs when synovitis stretches and damages the tendons and eventually the tendons become shortened and fixed. This damage causes subluxation (drift) of the joints.

Test-Taking Strategy: Use the process of elimination. Note the relationship between the characteristics in the client's hands and option 1, ulnar drift. Review the deformities that occur in patients with rheumatoid arthritis if you had difficulty with this question.

References
Black, J., & Hawks, J., (2005). *Medical-surgical nursing: Clinical management for positive outcomes* (7th ed., p. 2335). Philadelphia: Saunders.
Ignatavicius, D., & Workman, M. (2006). *Medical-surgical nursing: Critical thinking for collaborative care* (5th ed., p. 395). Philadelphia: Saunders.

1809. A client with a Sengstaken-Blakemore tube in place is admitted to the nursing unit from the emergency department. The nurse plans care knowing that the purpose of this tube is to:
1 Control ascites.
2 Control bleeding from gastritis.
3 Apply pressure to esophageal varices.
4 Remove ammonia-forming bacteria from the gastrointestinal tract.

Level of Cognitive Ability: Application
Client Needs: Physiological Integrity
Integrated Process: Nursing Process/Planning
Content Area: Adult Health/Gastrointestinal

Answer: 3
Rationale: A Sengstaken-Blakemore tube is inserted in clients with cirrhosis who have ruptured esophageal varices. It has esophageal and gastric balloons. The esophageal balloon exerts pressure on the ruptured esophageal varices and stops the bleeding. The gastric balloon holds the tube in correct position and prevents migration of the esophageal balloon. Options 1, 2, and 4 are not the purpose of this tube.

Test-Taking Strategy: Focus on the subject—the purpose of a Sengstaken-Blakemore tube. Recalling the relationship between this tube and ruptured esophageal varices will direct you to option 3. Review the concepts related to this type of tube if you are unfamiliar with them.

References
Ignatavicius, D., & Workman, M. (2006). *Medical-surgical nursing: Critical thinking for collaborative care* (5th ed., pp. 1378-1379). Philadelphia: Saunders.
Lewis, S., Heitkemper, M., Dirksen, S., O'Brien, P., & Bucher, L. (2007). *Medical-surgical nursing: Assessment and management of clinical problems* (7th ed., p. 1108). St. Louis: Mosby.

1810. A nurse is preparing to perform a Mantoux skin test. Which interventions apply in relation to this test? Select all that apply.
☐ 1 Explain the procedure to the client.
☐ 2 Obtain a 3-mL syringe with a ½-inch needle for the injection.
☐ 3 Mark the test area to locate it for reading 48 to 72 hours after injection.
☐ 4 Bunch up the skin and insert the needle with the needle bevel facing downward.
☐ 5 Ask the client about a previous history of a positive purified protein derivative reaction.
☐ 6 Cleanse the injection site on the lower dorsal surface of the forearm with alcohol and allow to dry.

Level of Cognitive Ability: Application
Client Needs: Physiological Integrity
Integrated Process: Nursing Process/Implementation
Content Area: Pharmacology

Answer: 1, 3, 5, 6
Rationale: The nurse would always explain the procedure to the client and then assess the client for a previous history of a positive purified protein derivative reaction. The test should not be administered if the client has such a history. The nurse would use a tuberculin syringe (not a 3-mL syringe) with a ½-inch 26- or 27 gauge needle. The injection site on the lower dorsal surface of the forearm is cleansed with alcohol and allowed to dry. The skin is stretched taut and 0.1 mL of solution containing 0.5 tuberculin units of PPD is injected. The injection is made just under the surface of the skin with the needle bevel facing upward to provide a discrete elevation of the skin (a wheal) 6 to 10 mm in diameter. The test area is marked to locate it for reading and the test area is read 48 to 72 hours after injection.

Test-Taking Strategy: Visualize this procedure and remember that procedures are always explained to the client. Recalling that a Mantoux skin test is a tuberculin test will assist in determining that a tuberculin syringe, not a 3-mL syringe is used for the injection. Also recall that this injection is administered intradermally and that the needle bevel needs to face upward to provide a wheal. Review the procedure for administering a Mantoux test if you had difficulty with this question.

Reference
Chernecky, C., & Berger, B. (2008). *Laboratory tests and diagnostic procedures* (5th ed., pp. 758-759). Philadelphia: Saunders.

REFERENCES

Ackley, B., & Ladwig, G. (2008). *Nursing diagnosis handbook: An evidence-based guide to planning care* (8th ed.). St. Louis: Mosby.

Black, J., & Hawks, J. (2005). *Medical-surgical nursing: Clinical management for positive outcomes* (7th ed.). Philadelphia: Saunders.

Chernecky, C., & Berger, B. (2008). *Laboratory tests and diagnostic procedures* (5th ed.). Philadelphia: Saunders.

Gahart, B., & Nazareno, A. (2006). *2006 Intravenous medications* (22nd ed.). St. Louis: Mosby.

Grodner, M., Long, S., & DeYoung, S. (2004). *Foundations and clinical applications of nutrition: A nursing approach* (3rd ed.). St. Louis: Mosby.

Gulanick, M., & Myers, J. (2007). *Nursing care plans: Nursing diagnosis and interventions* (6th ed.). St. Louis: Mosby.

Hockenberry, M., Wilson, D., & Winkelstein, M. (2005). *Wong's essentials of pediatric nursing* (7th ed.). St. Louis: Mosby.

Hockenberry, M., & Wilson, D. (2007). *Nursing care of infants and children* (8th ed.). St. Louis: Mosby.

Hodgson, B., & Kizior, R. (2007). *Saunders nursing drug handbook 2007.* Philadelphia: Saunders.

Huber, D. (2006). *Leadership and nursing care management* (3rd ed.). Philadelphia: Saunders.

Ignatavicius, D., & Workman, M. (2006). *Medical-surgical nursing: Critical thinking for collaborative care* (5th ed.). Philadelphia: Saunders.

Jarvis, C. (2004). *Physical examination and health assessment* (4th ed.). Philadelphia: Saunders.

Kee, J., Hayes, E., & McCuistion, L. (2006). *Pharmacology: A nursing process approach.* (5th ed.). Philadelphia: Saunders.

Kee, J., & Marshall, S. (2004). *Clinical calculations: With applications to general and specialty areas* (5th ed.). Philadelphia: Saunders

Lehne, R. (2007). *Pharmacology for nursing care* (6th ed.). St. Louis: Saunders.

Lewis, S., Heitkemper, M., Dirksen, S., O'Brien, P., & Bucher, L. (2007). *Medical-surgical nursing: Assessment and management of clinical problems* (7th ed.). St. Louis: Mosby.

McKenry, L., Tressier, E., & Hogan, M. (2006). *Mosby's pharmacology in nursing* (22nd ed.). St. Louis: Mosby.

McKinney, E., James, S., Murray, S., & Ashwill, J. (2005). *Maternal-child nursing* (2nd ed.). St. Louis: Saunders.

Monahan, F., Sands, J., Marek, J., Neighbors, M., & Green, C. (2007). *Phipps' medical-surgical nursing: Health and illness perspectives* (8th ed.). St. Louis: Mosby.

Mosby. (2007). *Mosby's nursing drug reference* (20th ed.). St. Louis: Mosby.

Murray, S., & McKinney, E. (2006). *Foundations of maternal-newborn nursing* (4th ed.). Philadelphia: Saunders.

National Council of State Boards of Nursing (Eds.). (2007). *2007 NCLEX-RN® Detailed Test Plan.* Chicago: Author.

Nix, S. (2005). *Williams' basic nutrition & diet therapy* (12th ed.). St. Louis: Mosby.

Pagana, K., & Pagana, T. (2005). *Mosby's diagnostic and laboratory test reference* (7th ed.). St. Louis: Mosby.

Perry, A., & Potter, P. (2006). *Clinical nursing skills & techniques* (6th ed.). St. Louis: Mosby.

Potter, P., & Perry, A. (2005). *Fundamentals of nursing* (6th ed.). St. Louis: Mosby.

Skidmore-Roth, L. (2008). *Mosby's nursing drug reference* (21st ed.). St. Louis: Mosby.

Skidmore-Roth, L. (2005). *Mosby's nursing drug guide for nurses* (6th ed.). St. Louis: Mosby.

Stuart, G., & Laraia, M. (2005). *Principles and practice of psychiatric nursing* (8th ed.). St. Louis: Mosby.

Varcarolis, E., Carson, V., & Shoemaker, N. (2006) *Foundations of psychiatric mental health nursing* (5th ed.). Philadelphia: Saunders.

Wong, D., Hockenberry, M., Perry, S., Lowdermilk, D., & Wilson, D. (2006). *Maternal-child nursing care.* (3rd ed.). St. Louis: Mosby.